Ferri's
Color Atlas and Text of
CLINICAL MEDICINE

Fred F. Ferri, M.D., F.A.C.P.
Clinical Professor
Alpert Medical School at Brown University
Providence, Rhode Island

SAUNDERS
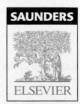
ELSEVIER

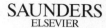

SAUNDERS
ELSEVIER

1600 John F. Kennedy Blvd.
Ste 1800
Philadelphia, PA 19103-2899

FERRI'S COLOR ATLAS AND TEXT OF CLINICAL MEDICINE   ISBN: 978-1-4160-4919-7
Copyright © 2009 by Saunders, an imprint of Elsevier Inc.

Notice

Library of Congress Cataloging-in-Publication Data

Ferri, Fred. F.
    Ferri's color atlas and text of clinical medicine / Fred F. Ferri. -- 1st ed.
        p. ; cm.
    ISBN 978-1-4160-4919-7
    1. Clinical medicine--Handbooks, manuals, etc. 2. Clinical medicine--Atlases. I.
Title. II. Title: Color atlas and text of clinical medicine.
    [DNLM: 1. Clinical Medicine--Atlases. 2. Clinical Medicine--Handbooks. WB 17 F388f
2009]
    RC55.F466 2009
    616--dc22   2008034698

Acquisitions Editor: Druanne Martin
Developmental Editor: Liliana Kim
Publishing Services Manager: Frank Polizzano
Senior Project Manager: Peter Faber
Design Direction: Karen O'Keefe - Owens
Marketing Manager: William Veltre

Printed in China

Last digit is the print number: 9 8 7 6 5 4 3 2 1

Ferri's

Color Atlas and Text of CLINICAL MEDICINE

Diseases/Disorders	ICD-9 CM
Congenital granular epulis	523.8
Congenital melanocytic nevus	M8720/0
Congestive heart failure	428.0
Conjunctivitis	372.30
Contact dermatitis	692
Contraception	V25.09
Corneal ulceration (Keratitis)	370.0
Cor pulmonale	415.0
Cowpox	999.0
Cranial epidural abscess	324.0
Craniopharyngioma	237.0
Creutzfeldt-Jacob disease	046.1
Crohn's colitis	555.9
Cryptococcosis	117.5
Cryptosporidiosis	007.4
Cubital tunnel syndrome	354.2
Cushing's syndrome	255.0
Cutaneous adverse reactions to drugs	693.0
Cutaneous candidiasis	112.3
Cutaneous larva migrans (creeping eruption)	126.9
Cutaneous horn	702.8
Cylindroma	M8200/0
Cysticercosis	123.1
Cystic fibrosis	277.0
Dandy-Walker malformation	742.3
Darier's disease	757.39
Decubitus ulcers	707
Deep vein thrombosis	451.1
Delayed puberty	259.0
Dementia	294.8
Dementia with Lewy bodies	331.82
Denture-associated fibrous hyperplasia	523.8
De Quervain's tenosynovitis	727.04
Dermatitis herpetiformis	694.0
Dermoid cyst	M9084/0
Diabetes insipidus	253.5
Diabetes mellitus type 1	250.1
Diabetes mellitus type 2	250.0
Dilated (congestive) cardiomyopathy	425.4
Discoid eczema (nummular eczema)	692.9
Diphteria	032.9
Disseminated intravascular coagulation (DIC)	286.6
Diverticular disease	526.10
Diverticulitis	562.11
Down syndrome	758.0
Drug-induced hyperpigmentation	709.00
Dupuytren's contracture	728.6
Drug-induced nail discolororation	703.8
Dysplastic nevus syndrome (familial atypical multiple mole melanoma syndrome)	M8720/3
Dystonia	333.6
Ebstein's anomaly	746.2
Eccrine hydrocystoma	M8404/0
Echinococcosis	122.9
Eccrine poroma	M8402/0
Ectopic pregnancy	633
Ectropion	974.10
Ehlers-Danlos syndrome	756.83
Electrical injury	994.8

Diseases/Disorders	ICD-9 CM
Empyema	510.9
Encephalitis	049.9
Endometrial cancer	182
Endometriosis	617.9
Enterobiasis (Pinworms)	127.4
Entropion	374.00
Ephelides (freckles)	709.09
Epicondylitis medial	726.31
Epicondylitis lateral	726.32
Epidermal inclusion cyst	706.2
Epidermal nevus	M8760/0
Epidermoid cyst	706.2
Epidermolysis bullosa acquisita (dermolytic pemphigoid)	757.39
Epididymitis	604.90
Epiglottitis	464.30
Epistaxis	784.7
Epithelial Inclusion Cysts	706.2
Erythema annulare centrifugum	695.0
Erythema infectiosum (fifth disease)	057.0
Erythema multiforme	695.1
Erythrasma	039.0
Esophageal carcinoma	150.8
Esophageal Rings and webs	750.3
Esophageal spasm	530.5
Esophageal varices	456.1
Exanthematous (morbilliform, maculopapular) reactions	782.1
Extradural empyema	324.9
Familial polyposis syndrome	211.3
Felty's syndrome	714.1
Femoral hernia	553.00
Fibrocystic breast	610.1
Fibroepithelial polyp (achrochordon, skin tag)	701.9
Fibromyalgia	729.0
Folliculitis	704.8
Fibroma	M8810/0
Filariasis	125.9
Fistula	569.81
Focal epithelial hyperplasia (Heck's disease)	528.79
Fractures	829.0
Freckles	709.09
Friedreich's ataxia	334.0
Frostbite	991.3
Furuncle (boil)	680.9
Ganglion	727.43
Gardner's syndrome	211.3
Gastric carcinoma	451
Gastritis	535.5
Gastrinoma (Zollinger-Ellison syndrome)	251.5
Gastroesophageal reflux	530.81
Generalized gingival hyperplasia	523.8
Giardiasis	007.1
Gingival nodules	782.2
Glaucoma, chronic open angle	365.1
Glaucoma, primary closed angle	365.2
Giant cell arteritis (temporal arteritis)	446.5
Glomus tumor	M8711/0
Giant cell tumor of tendon sheath	M8003/1

Diseases/Disorders	ICD-9 CM
Glomerulonephritis	583.9
Glucagonoma	M81.52/0
Goodpasture syndrome	446.2
Gout	274.9
Granuloma annulare	695.89
Granuloma inguinale (donovanosis)	099.2
Granulomatous arthritis	716.9
Grover's disease (transient acantholytic dermatosis)	709.9
Guillain-Barre	357.0
Gynecomastia	611.1
Hairy cell leukemia	202.4
Hairy leukoplakia	702.8
Halo nevus	M8723/0
Hammer toes	735.4
Hand eczema (dyshidrotic eczema, pompholyx)	705.81
Hand-foot-mouth disease	074.0
HELPP syndrome	642.50
Hemochromatosis	275.0
Hemolytic-uremic syndrome	283.11
Hemorrhoids	455.6
Henoch-Schonlein purpura	287.0
Hemophilia A	286.0
Hemophilia B	286.1
Hepatic abscess	572.0
Hepatitis A	070.1
Hepatitis B	070.3
Hepatitis C	070.51
Hepatitis D	070.51
Hepatocellular carcinoma	155.0
Hepatorenal syndrome	572.4
Herpangina	074.0
Herpes genital	054.10
Herpes labialis	054.9
Herpes zoster	053.9
Hiatal hernia	750.6
Hirsutism	704.1
Histiocytosis X	277.8
Histoplasmosis	115.90
Hodgkin's lymphoma	201.9
Hookworm	126.35
Hordoleum external	373.11
Hordoleum internal	373.12
Horner's syndrome	337.9
Human Granulocytic Ehrlichiosis (HGE)	082-8
Human Immunodeficiency Virus	044.9
Hydatidiform mole	630
Hydradenitis suppurativa	705.83
Hydrocele	603.9
Hydronephrosis	591
Hyperaldosteronism	255.1
Hypercoagulable state	289.8
Hyperlipidemia	272.4
Hypertension	401.1
Hypertrophic osteoarthropathy	731.2
Hyperparathyroidism	252.0
Hyperthyroidism	242.9
Hypertrophic cardiomyopathy	425.1
Hypoaldosteronism	255.4
Hypocalcemia	275.41
Hypoglycemia	251.2
Hypogonadism	253.4
Hypopituitarism	253.2

Continued on the back endsheet

Expert | CONSULT
Online + Print

Online access activation instructions

This Expert Consult title comes with access to the complete contents online. **Activate your access today** by following these simple instructions:

1. Gently scratch off the surface of the sticker below, using the edge of a coin, to reveal your **activation code.**

2. Visit **www.expertconsultbook.com** and click on the **"Register"** button.

3. **Enter your activation code** along with the other information requested...and begin enjoying your access.

It's that easy! For technical assistance, email **online.help@elsevier.com** or **call 800-401-9962** (inside the US) or **+1-314-995-3200** (outside the US).

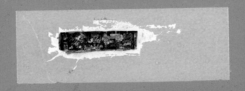

Preface

The goal of this book is to be a comprehensive, current, and clinically relevant medical resource. The idea of this work began while contemplating the enormity of material one needs to master in clinical medicine. Although there are several textbooks available on clinical medicine and a vast number of established atlases dealing primarily with dermatological disorders, there are no established books that combine the information contained within a traditional textbook with the visual imagery of a color atlas. This book aims to provide such a combination.

Visuals are the critical language of medical education. The old adage of "A picture is worth a thousand words" is certainly true in medicine. Recognition of disorders from illustrations remains crucial to early diagnosis and treatment, both of which are usually essential to improve prognosis. In creating this book, care was taken to include the classic examples of common medical disorders in detail. Rare disorders were also included because they are often discussed for purposes of differential diagnosis and because they are frequently referenced in the medical literature and on medical board exams. As such, this book endeavors to provide the student and the newly qualified doctor with a guide to the diagnosis of common clinical disorders, and the more experienced physician with a guide to less common, but still important, diseases.

The book is divided in 14 sections ranging from disorders of skin and subcutaneous tissues to infectious diseases. Each section follows a similar format, which consists of an initial description of the normal anatomy and physiology followed by diagnostic tests and procedures, and descriptions and illustrations of various disorders pertinent to that section. The format and size of this book are designed to be a handy refresher of important clinical, anatomic, laboratory and radiographic signs. There are 352 chapters, 3031 illustrations and over 100 tables, boxes and algorithms, each specifically selected to illuminate the assessment of clinical disorders. In summary, it is unlike any other existing book in both scope and content, and certainly deserves a unique place in any medical library.

I hope that this book fulfills your every expectation, provides valuable support to the learning of clinical medicine, and serves as an effective resource in daily clinical practice.

Fred F. Ferri, MD, FACP
Clinical Professor
Alpert Medical School
Brown Unversity
Providence, Rhode Island

Acknowledgments

I gratefully acknowledge the generosity of the many colleagues listed below who have lent text material to this book. It is important for me to be scrupulous in acknowledging these valuable sources of information. If I left anyone out, it is not out of immodesty or unintended claims of original material but simply an oversight given the myriad of sources involved in this project:

Sonya S. Abdel-Razeq, M.D., Philip J. Aliotta, M.D., M.S.H.A., F.A.C.S., George O. Alonso, M.D., Srividya Anandan, M.D., Gowri Anandarajah, M.D., Mel L. Anderson, M.D., F.A.C.P, Etsuko Aoki, M.D., Ph.D, Patricia Arean, Ph.D., Vasanthi Arumugam, M.D., Amaar Ashraf, M.D., Udeep Kaur Aulakh, M.D., C.M., F.R.C.P.C., Michael G. Benatar, M.B.Ch.B., D.Phil., Agnieszka K. Bialikiewicz, M.D., Jeffrey M. Borkan, M.D., Ph.D., Kelly Bossenbrok, M.D., Lynn Bowlby, M.D., Mandeep K. Brar, M.D., Joanna Brown, M.D., Robert Burd, M.D., Jonathan Burns, M.A., M.D., Steven Busselen, M.D., Gaurav Chaudhary, M.D., Kara Chew, M.D., Maria A. Corigliano, M.D., F.A.C.O.G., Karoll J. Cortez, M.D., John E. Croom, M.D., Ph.D., Alicia J., Curtin, Ph.D., G.N.P., Claudia L. Dade, M.D., George T. Danakas, M.D., F.A.C.O.G., Alexandra Degenhardt, M.D., Christine M. Duffy, M.D., M.P.H., Jeffrey S. Durmer, M.D., Ph.D., Jane V. Eason, M.D., Stuart Eisendrath, M.D., Pamela Ellsworth, M.D., Gregory J. Esper, M.D., Marilyn Fabbri, M.D., Mark J. Fagan, M.D., Gil M. Farkash, M.D., Timothy W. Farrell, M.D., Mitchell D. Feldman, M.D., M. Phil., Tamara G. Fong, M.D., Ph.D., Glenn G. Fort, M.D., M.P.H., Rebekah Leslie Gardner, M.D., Genna Gekht, M.D., Paul F. George, M.D., David R. Gifford, M.D., M.P.H., AnnGene A. Giustozzi, M.D., M.P.H., Cindy Gleit, M.D., Geetha Gopalakrishnan, M.D., Nancy R. Graff, M.D., Rebecca A. Griffith, M.D., Joseph Grillo, M.D., Mohammed Hajjiri, M.D., Michele Halpern, M.D., Mustafa A. Hammad, M.D., Sajeev Handa, M.D., Mike Harper, M.D., Taylor Harrison, M.D., Christine Hartley, M.D., Sharon S. Hartman Polensek, M.D., Ph.D., Christine Healy, D.O., Jennifer Roh Hur, M.D., Jason Iannuccilli, M.D., Richard S. Isaacson, M.D., Jennifer Jeremiah, M.D., Michael P. Johnson, M.D., Kohar Jones, M.D., Daniel Keplon, M.D., Powell H. Kazanjian, M.D., Wan J. Kim, M.D., Melvyn Koby, M.D., David Kurss, M.D., F.A.C.O.G., Cindy Lai, M.D., Suzette M. LaRoche, M.D., Joseph J. Lieber, M.D., Chun Lim, M.D., Ph.D.,Mara Linscott, M.D., Russell Linsky, M.D., Zeena Lobo, M.D., Richard Long, M.D., Michael Maher, M.D., Achraf A. Makki, M.D., M.Sc., Joseph R. Masci, M.D., Daniel T. Mattson, M.D., M.S.C. (Med.), Maitreyi Mazumdar, M.D., M.P.H., Kelly A. McGarry, M.D., Lynn McNicoll, M.D., Shalin B. Mehta, M.D., Lonnie R. Mercier, M.D., Brad Mikaelian, M.D., Dennis J. Mikolich, M.D., F.A.C.P., F.C.C.P., Michele Montandon, M.D., Takuma Nemoto, M.D., James J. Ng, M.D., Melissa Nothnagle, M.D., Judith Nudelman, M.D., Gail M. O'Brien, M.D., Carolyn J. O'Connor, M.D., Alexander B. Olawaiye, M.D., Michael K. Ong, M.D., Ph.D., Steven M. Opal, M.D., Christina A. Pacheco, M.D., Mina B. Pantcheva, M.D., Pranav M. Patel, M.D., Steven Peligian, D.O., Peter Petropoulos, M.D., F.A.C.C., Paul A. Pirraglia, M.D., M.P.H., Maurice Policar, M.D., Arundathi G. Prasad, M.D., Kittichai Promrat, M.D., Hemchand Ramberan, M.D., Chaitanya V. Reddy, D.O., Victor I. Reus, M.D., Harlan G. Rich, M.D., Luther K. Robinson, M.D., Jason M. Satterfield, Ph.D., Sean I. Savitz, M.D., Jack L. Schwartzwald, M.D., Catherine Shafts, D.O., Madhavi Shah, M.D., Harvey M. Shanies, M.D., Ph.D., Deborah L. Shapiro, M.D., Grace Shih, M.D., Mark Sigman, M.D., Joanne M. Silvia, M.D., Clifford Milo Singer, M.D.,U. Shivraj Sohur, M.D., Ph.D., Jennifer Souther, M.D., Michelle Stozek Anvar, M.D., Julie Anne Szumigala, M.D., Dominick Tammaro, M.D., Iris Tong, M.D., Margaret Tryforos, M.D., Eroboghene E. Ubogu, M.B.B.S. (Hons.), Sean H. Uiterwyk, M.D., Nicole J. Ullrich, M.D., Ph.D., Hannah Vu, D.O., Tom J. Wachtel, M.D., Marc S. Weinberg, M.D., Dennis M. Weppner, M.D., F.A.C.O.G., Laurel M. White, M.D., David P. Williams, M.D., Marie Elizabeth Wong, M.D., Wen-Chih Wu, M.D., Beth J. Wutz, M.D., John Q. Young, M.D., M.P.P., Cindy Zadikoff, M.D., Scott J. Zuccala, D.O., F.A.C.O.G.

I also extend a special thanks to the authors and contributors of the following texts who have lent multiple pictures and text material to this book:

Abeloff MD: *Clinical Oncology,* ed 3, Philadelphia, 2004, Elesevier

Besser CM, Thorner MO: *Comprehensive Clinical Endocrinology,* ed 3, St. Louis, Mosby, 2002

Crawford, MH, DiMarco JP, Paulus WJ [eds]: *Cardiology,* ed 2, St. Louis, Mosby, 2004

Cohen J, Powderly WG: *Infectious Diseases,* ed 2, St. Louis, Mosby, 2004

Ferri F: *Ferri's Clinical Advisor 2007,* St. Louis, Mosby, 2007

Grainger RG, Allison D: *Grainger & Allison's Diagnostic Radiology, a textbook of Medical Imaging,* ed 4, Philadelphia, Churchill Livingstone, 2001

Hochberg MC, Silman AJ, Smolen JS, Weinblatt ME, Weisman MH [eds]: *Rheumatology,* ed 3, St. Louis, 2003, Mosby

Johnson RJ, Feehally J: *Comprehensive Clinical Nephrology,* ed 2, St. Louis, Mosby, 2000

Mckee PH, Calonje E, Granter SR [eds]: *Pathology of the skin with clinical correlations,* ed 3, St. Louis, Mosby, 2005

Silverberg SG—*Principles and Practice of Surgical pathology and cytopathology,* ed 4, Philadelphia, Churchill Livingstone, 2006

Swartz MH: *Textbook of Physical Diagnosis,* ed 5, Philadelphia, Saunders, 2006

White GM, Cox NH [eds]: *Diseases of the skin, a color atlas and text,* ed 2, St. Louis, Mosby, 2006

Yanoff M, Duker JS: *Ophthalmology,* ed 2, St. Louis, Mosby, 2004

Young NS, Gerson SL, High KA [eds]: *Clinical Hematology,* St. Louis, Mosby, 2006

Fred F. Ferri, MD, FACP
Clinical Professor
Alpert Medical School
Brown Unversity
Providence, Rhode Island

Table of contents

SECTION 1

Skin and subcutaneous tissues   1

1. The structure and function of skin   2
2. Evaluation of skin disorders   4
3. Disorders of keratinization   14
4. Inherited and autoimmune subepidermal blistering diseases   16
5. Acantholytic disorders   21
6. Eczematous dermatoses   25
7. Psoriasis   33
8. Lichen planus   35
9. Hypersensitivity syndromes   36
10. Superficial and deep perivascular inflammatory dermatoses   39
11. Granulomatous and necrobiotic dermatoses   41
12. Porphyria cutanea tarda   44
13. Pellagra   46
14. Cutaneous adverse reactions to drugs   47
15. Neutrophilic and eosinophilic dermatoses   49
16. Vascular diseases   54
17. Disorders of pigmentation   62
18. Diseases of the hair   66
19. Acne vulgaris   72
20. Rosacea   74
21. Diseases of the nails   76
22. Tumors of the surface epithelium   84
23. Melanocytic nevi   91
24. Melanoma   98
25. Miscellaneous skin lesions   100
26. Dermatophyte infections   110
27. Viral infections   115
28. Bacterial skin infections   134
29. Infestations and bites   143
30. Decubitus ulcers   153
31. Environmental injuries   155
32. Radiation dermatitis   160

SECTION 2

Brain, peripheral nervous system, muscle   161

33. Normal anatomy   162
34. Diagnostic tests and procedures   168
35. Cerebrovascular disease   175
36. Subclavian steal syndrome   182
37. Subdural hematoma   183
38. Brain neoplasms   184
39. Dementia   192
40. Movement disorders   200
41. Developmental disorders of the spinal cord and brain   204
42. Multiple sclerosis   207
43. Amyotrophic lateral sclerosis   209
44. Neuropathies   211
45. Ataxias   214
46. Infections   216
47. Neurocutaneous syndromes   229
48. Disorders of muscle and neuromuscular junction   233
49. Bell's palsy   238
50. Cerebral palsy   239
51. Down syndrome   240
52. Normal-pressure hydrocephalus   242
53. Dandy-Walker malformation   244
54. Neuroblastoma   245
55. von-Hippel-Lindau disease   247

SECTION 3

Eyes, ears, nose, oral cavity, and neck   249

Eyes
56. Normal anatomy   250
57. Diagnostic tests and procedures   252
58. Cataracts   259
59. Conjunctivitis   261
60. Corneal ulceration (keratitis)   264
61. Scleritis   266
62. Disorders of the conjunctiva and limbus   267
63. Strabismus   270
64. Amblyopia   273
65. Entropion   274
66. Ectropion   275
67. Blepharospasm   276
68. Benign eyelid lesions   278
69. Eyelid malignancies   286
70. Retinitis pigmentosa   288
71. Retinoblastoma   289
72. Amaurosis fugax   290
73. Macular degeneration   292
74. Retinal detachment   293

Table of contents

75. Uveitis   295
76. Glaucoma, chronic open angle   297
77. Glaucoma, primary closed angle   299
78. Horner's syndrome   301
79. Optic neuritis   302

Ears
80. Normal anatomy, examination, and diagnostic testing   304
81. Hearing loss   308
82. Acoustic neuroma   311
83. Relapsing polychondritis   313
84. Otitis externa   314
85. Otitis media   316

Nose
86. Allergic rhinitis   318
87. Epistaxis   320
88. Sinusitis   322

Mouth and tongue
89. Diseases of the oral mucosa   325
90. Dental and periodontal infections   336
91. Herpangina   338
92. Stomatitis   339
93. Scarlet fever   341

Salivary glands
94. Salivary gland neoplasms   342
95. Mumps   344

Pharynx
96. Pharyngitis and tonsillitis   346
97. Epiglottitis   348

Thyroid
98. Thyroid nodule   349
99. Thyroid cancer   352
100. Thyroiditis   355

SECTION 4
Chest, mediastinum, diaphragm   357
101. Chest wall abnormalities   358
102. Mediastinal abnormalities   359
103. Superior vena cava syndrome   364
104. Diaphragm abnormalities   366

SECTION 5
Cardiovascular system   369
105. Diagnostic tests and procedures   370
106. Ischemic heart disease   382
107. Valvular disease   395
108. Infective endocarditis   406

109. Congestive heart failure   409
110. Cardiogenic pulmonary edema   413
111. Cardiomyopathies   414
112. Myocarditis   420
113. Pericarditis   422
114. Cor pulmonale   425
115. Arrhythmias   427
116. Cardiac pacemakers   440
117. Congenital heart disease   442
118. Atrial myxoma   457
119. Peripheral arterial disease   459
120. Venous ulcers and stasis dermatitis   461
121. Lymphedema   463
122. Deep vein thrombosis   465
123. Thromboangiitis obliterans (Buerger's disease)   468
124. Abdominal aortic aneurysm   470
125. Aortic dissection   472
126. Syncope   475
127. Hypertension   478

SECTION 6
Lungs   481
128. Measurement of respiratory function   482
129. Asthma   485
130. Chronic obstructive pulmonary disease   488
131. Alpha$_1$-antitrypsin deficiency   492
132. Lung neoplasms   494
133. Diseases of the pleura   500
134. Occupational lung disease   507
135. Interstitial lung disease   510
136. Idiopathic pulmonary fibrosis   512
137. Pulmonary infiltrations   514
138. Atelectasis   524
139. Respiratory infections   525
140. Acute Respiratory Distress Syndrome   547
141. Pulmonary hypertension   549
142. Altitude sickness   552
143. Pulmonary embolism   554

SECTION 7
Digestive system   559
Esophagus
144. Zenker's diverticulum   560
145. Gastroesophageal reflux   561
146. Hiatal hernia   562
147. Mallory-Weiss tear   563
148. Barrett's syndrome   564
149. Esophageal carcinoma   565

150. Rings and webs   567
151. Achalasia   568
152. Esophageal spasm   570
153. Esophageal varices   571

Stomach and duodenum
154. Gastritis   572
155. Peptic ulcer   574
156. Gastric carcinoma   576
157. Intestinal obstruction   578

Small intestine
158. Celiac disease   583
159. Meckel's diverticulum   585
160. Hernias   586
161. Appendicitis   587
162. Crohn's colitis   588

Colon
163. Ulcerative colitis   591
164. Diverticular disease   593
165. Familial polyposis syndrome   596
166. Peutz-Jegher's syndrome   597
167. Gardner's syndrome   598
168. Colorectal cancer   600

Disorders of the anus, anal canal, and perianal region
169. Hemorrhoids   603
170. Anal fissure   605
171. Perirectal abscess   606
172. Fistula   607

Pancreas
173. Acute pancreatitis   608
174. Chronic pancreatitis   612
175. Carcinoma of pancreas   613

Liver
176. Cirrhosis   616
177. Ascites   620
178. Hepatorenal syndrome   622
179. Primary biliary cirrhosis   624
180. Hemochromatosis   626
181. Non-alcoholic steatohepatitis   629
182. Hepatocellular carcinoma   631
183. Hepatic Infections   633
184. Autoimmune hepatitis   643

Gallbladder and bile ducts
185. Cholelithiasis   644
186. Cholecystitis   646
187. Cholangiocarcinoma   648

Gastrointestinal Infections
188. Viral gastroenteritis   650
189. Salmonellosis   652

190. Cholera   655
191. Whipple's disease   656
192. Mesenteric adenitis   658
193. Pseudomembranous colitis   659

Vascular
194. Mesenteric ischemia   661
195. Portal vein thrombosis   663
196. Budd-Chiari syndrome   665

Endocrine gastointestinal disorders
197. Carcinoid   667
198. Gastrinoma (Zollinger-Ellison syndrome)   671
199. Glucagonoma   673

SECTION 8
Kidneys   675
200. Normal anatomy   676
201. Diagnostic tests and procedures   678
202. Acute renal failure   691
203. Chronic renal failure   697
204. Glomerulonephritis   701
205. Acute tubular necrosis   704
206. IgA nephropathy   706
207. Nephrotic syndrome   707
208. Interstitial nephritis   709
209. Amyloidosis   711
210. Polycystic kidney disease   714
211. Renal artery stenosis and thrombosis   719
212. Neoplasms   722
213. Pyelonephritis   725
214. Hydronephrosis   727
215. Rhabdomyolysis   729

SECTION 9
Genitourinary tract   731
Ureters
216. Urolithiasis   732

Bladder
217. Bladder carcinoma   737

Prostate
218. Benign prostatic hyperplasia   739
219. Prostatitis   741
220. Prostate cancer   743

Testicles
221. Hydrocele   745
222. Varicocele   747
223. Epididymitis   748

Table of contents

224. Testicular neoplasms 750
225. Testicular torsion 752

Vulva, urethra, penis
226. Diseases of the genital skin 754
227. Urethritis, gonococcal 767
228. Urethritis, non-gonococcal 769
229. Hypospadias 771
230. Peyronie's disease 774

SECTION 10

Female reproductive system 775

231. Clinical pelvic anatomy and menstrual cycle 776
232. Diagnostic tests and procedures 782
233. Endometriosis 787
234. Contraception 789

Vulva/vagina
235. Vaginosis, bacterial 793
236. Vulvovaginitis, fungal 795
237. Vulvovaginitis, trichomonas 796
238. Vulvovaginitis, estrogen deficient 797
    (atrophic vaginitis)
239. Vulvar cancer 798

Cervix
240. Cervicitis 800
241. Cervical dysplasia 802
242. Cervical cancer 805

Uterus
243. Uterine prolapse 807
244. Uterine myomas 809
245. Uterine polyps 812
246. Endometrial cancer 813

Ovaries
247. Benign ovarian lesions 815
248. Polycystic ovary syndrome 817
249. Ovarian cancer 819

Infections
250. Pelvic inflammatory disease 820

Breasts
251. Fibrocystic breast disease 821
252. Breast abscess 824
253. Breast cancer 826
254. Paget's disease of breast 830

Pregnancy
255. Physiologic changes and prenatal monitoring 832
256. Normal labor and delivery 837
257. Abnormal labor 841
258. Ectopic pregnancy 844

259. Preeclampsia 846
260. Abruptio placentae 848
261. Placenta previa 850
262. Hydatidiform mole 852

SECTION 11

Endocrine and metabolic systems 853
and nutritional disorders

Pituitary disorders
263. Hypopituitarism 854
264. Pituitary adenoma 859
265. Diabetes insipidus 867
266. Inappropriate secretion of antidiuretic
    hormone 869

Thyroid
267. Hypothyroidism 871
268. Hyperthyroidism 875

Parathyroids
269. Hypocalcemia 878
270. Hyperparathyroidism 880

Adrenal glands
271. Cushing's syndrome 884
272. Addison's disease 887
273. Hypoaldosteronism 890
274. Hyperaldosteronism 891
275. Pheochromocytoma 894

Reproductive system and growth
276. Normal puberty 896
277. Precocious puberty 898
278. Delayed puberty 900
279. Congenital adrenal hyperplasia 903
280. Klinefelter's syndrome 906
281. Turner's syndrome 907
282. Hypogonadism 908
283. Hirsutism 910
284. Gynecomastia 912

Disorders of carbohydrate and lipid metabolism
285. Diabetes mellitus 916
286. Hypoglycemia and Insulinoma 921
287. Hyperlipidemia 923
288. Multiple endocrine neoplasia (MEN) 928

SECTION 12

Musculoskeletal system 931

289. Diagnostic tests and procedures 932
290. Osteoarthritis 949

291. Rheumatoid arthritis 952
292. Juvenile rheumatoid arthritis 957
293. Systemic lupus erythematosus 960
294. Antiphospholipid antibody syndrome 965
295. Sjögren's syndrome 967
296. Idiopathic inflammatory myopathies (dermatomyositis, polymyositis) 969
297. Raynaud's syndrome 971
298. Scleroderma 974
299. Mixed connective tissue disease 977
300. Vasculitides 978
301. Spondyloarthropathies 988
302. Crystal-related arthritis 994
303. Fibromyalgia 998
304. Regional rheumatic diseases 1000
305. Inherited connective tissue disorders 1028
306. Diseases of bone and bone metabolism 1031
307. Hypertrophic osteoarthropathy 1037
308. Infections 1038
309. Bone tumors 1047
310. Fractures 1051

SECTION 13

Blood

Blood 1059
311. Basic principles of hematology 1060
312. Anemias 1066
313. Leukemias 1084
314. Myelodysplastic syndrome 1093
315. Hodgkin's lymphoma 1095
316. Non-Hodgkin's lymphoma 1099
317. Hairy cell leukemia 1106
318. Plasma cell dyscrasias 1107
319. Polycythemia vera 1111
320. Thrombocytopenia 1114
321. Disseminated intravascular coagulation 1120
322. Hypercoagulable state 1122
323. Hemophilias 1126

324. Von Willebrand's disease 1129
325. Felty's syndrome 1131
326. Paroxysmal nocturnal hemoglobinuria 1132
327. Paroxysmal cold hemoglobinuria 1134
328. Histiocytosis X 1135
329. Kaposi's sarcoma 1137

SECTION 14

Infectious diseases

Infectious diseases 1139
330. Diagnostic tests and procedures 1140
331. Human immunodeficiency virus 1145
332. Protozoal infections 1159
333. Cestode (tapeworm) infestation 1176
334. Nematode infestation 1179
335. Filariasis 1186
336. Fungal infections 1189
337. Rheumatic fever 1211
338. Infectious mononucleosis 1214
339. Thrombophlebitis 1216
340. Leprosy 1218
341. Tetanus 1220
342. Anaerobic infections 1221
343. Diphtheria 1223
344. Listeriosis 1225
345. Yersinia pestis (plague) 1226
346. Relapsing fever 1228
347. Tularemia 1229
348. Brucellosis 1231
349. Cat-scratch disease 1233
350. Leptospirosis 1235
351. Rabies 1236
352. Toxic shock syndrome 1238

Index 1241

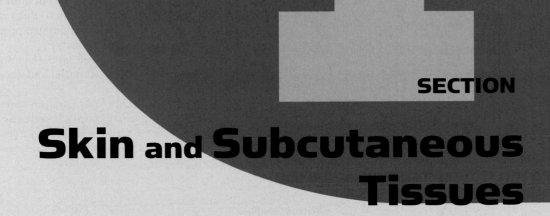

1 SECTION

Skin and Subcutaneous Tissues

Chapter 1: The structure and function of skin
Chapter 2: Evaluation of skin disorders
Chapter 3: Disorders of keratinization
Chapter 4: Inherited and autoimmune subepidermal blistering diseases
Chapter 5: Acantholytic disorders
Chapter 6: Eczematous dermatoses
Chapter 7: Psoriasis
Chapter 8: Lichen planus
Chapter 9: Hypersensitivity syndromes
Chapter 10: Superficial and deep perivascular inflammatory dermatoses
Chapter 11: Granulomatous and necrobiotic dermatoses
Chapter 12: Porphyria cutanea tarda
Chapter 13: Pellagra
Chapter 14: Cutaneous adverse reactions to drugs
Chapter 15: Neutrophilic and eosinophilic dermatoses

Chapter 16: Vascular diseases
Chapter 17: Disorders of pigmentation
Chapter 18: Diseases of the hair
Chapter 19: Acne vulgaris
Chapter 20: Rosacea
Chapter 21: Diseases of the nails
Chapter 22: Tumors of the surface epithelium
Chapter 23: Melanocytic nevi
Chapter 24: Melanoma
Chapter 25: Miscellaneous skin lesions
Chapter 26: Dermatophyte infections
Chapter 27: Viral exanthems
Chapter 28: Bacterial skin infections
Chapter 29: Infestations and bites
Chapter 30: Decubitus ulcers
Chapter 31: Environmental injuries
Chapter 32: Radiation dermatitis

1

Chapter 1   The structure and function of skin

- The skin or integument is a double-layered membrane covering the exterior of the body and is continuous with the mucous membranes lining the body's orifices. It shows a marked variation in thickness, measuring from less than 1 mm (on the eyelid) to more than 4 mm (on the back). The wide range of properties of the skin is summarized in Box 1–1.

Box 1–1   Properties of the skin
- Maintains integrity of the body
- Protects from injurious stimuli
- Absorbs and excretes liquids
- Regulates temperature
- Waterproofs
- Absorbs ultraviolet light
- Metabolizes vitamin D
- Detects sensory stimuli
- Provides cosmetic functions
- Acts as a barrier against microorganisms

From McKee PH, Calonje E, Granter SR (eds): Pathology of the Skin With Clinical Correlations, 3rd ed. St. Louis, Mosby, 2005.

- The skin can be divided into two parts, the epidermis (outer layer) and dermis (inner layer), which rests on and is attached to the subcutaneous fat (Fig. 1–1).
- The epidermis is comprised of four clearly defined layers, or strata (Fig. 1–2):
  1. Basal layer (stratum basale, stratum germinativum): mycotic activity of keratinocytes is confined to this layer, resulting in an epidermal turnover time of approximately 4 weeks. Melanocytes, which produce melanin pigment, are found in this layer.
  2. Prickle cell layer (stratum spinosum): contains polyhedral cells with intercellular attachments and Langerhans cells (specialized antigen-presenting cells involved in contact hypersensitivity)
  3. Granular cell layer (stratum granulosum): characterized by loss of cell nuclei and acquisition of dense keratohyalin granules
  4. Keratin layer (stratum corneum): acellular layer containing keratin fibrils. It serves as a protective barrier. Its thickness varies with location (maximum thickness on palms and soles, minimum thickness at flexural sites).

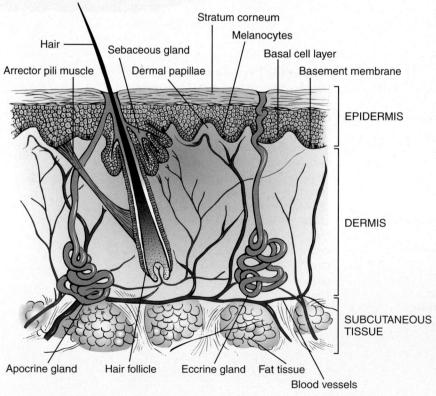

Fig 1–1

Cross section through the skin, showing the structures in the epidermis and subcutaneous tissues.

(From Swartz Swartz MH: Textbook of Physical Diagnosis, 5th ed. Philadelphia, WB Saunders, 2006.)

- The dermis is the fibrous part of the skin, which provides strength. It supports the epidermis and is composed of a fibrous connective tissue component (collagen and elastic fibers) in intimate association with ground substance. Within the dermis are the epidermal appendages (surrounded by a connective tissue sheath), blood vessels and nerves, and a cellular component, including mast cells, fibroblasts, myofibroblasts, and macrophages. Smooth muscle is also represented in the erector pili muscles.

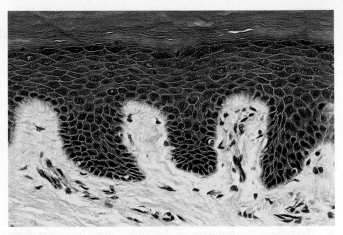

Fig 1–2
Normal skin from the fingertip showing the clearly defined layers of the epidermis.
(From McKee PH, Calonje E, Granter SR [eds]: Pathology of the Skin With Clinical Correlations, 3rd ed. St. Louis, Mosby, 2005.)

Chapter 2 Evaluation of skin disorders

A. HISTORY AND PHYSICAL EXAMINATION

- The initial step in the dermatologic evaluation involves obtaining a detailed dermatologic history. Box 2–1 lists pertinent questions.
- When examining the patient, it is essential to detail the skin lesions, their distribution, and characteristics.
- Classically, skin lesions have been classified as primary or secondary:
  - Primary lesions represent the initial basic lesion.
  - Secondary lesions may result from evolution of the primary lesions or may result from scratching or infection.
- The proper terminology for describing these lesions is given in Boxes 2–2 and 2–3.
- For diagnostic purposes, it is also important to note the distribution of the skin lesions. Figure 2–1 illustrates the classic distribution of common skin dermatoses.
- Table 2–1 describes the differential diagnosis of common maculopapular diseases.
- Table 2–2 lists common eczematous disorders and differentiates them by history and location.

- Table 2–3 provides a differential diagnosis of vesiculobullous diseases.
- Proper diagnosis will often require direct palpation of the lesion(s) and other maneuvers, such as picking the crust off moist skin lesions, scratching a scaly rash, squeezing the lesion, and applying linear pressure and rubbing to elicit a dermatologic response. Also, a scalpel is commonly used to pare keratinized lesions.

Box 2–1 Dermatologic history

A. Initial questions

1. When did the skin lesion(s) or rash start?
2. What did it look like when if first started, and how has it changed?
3. Where did it start, and where is it located now?
4. What treatments, especially over-the-counter self-remedies has the patient tried? What was the effect of each of these treatments?
5. Are there symptoms (e.g., itching, pain)?
6. What is the patient's main concern about the rash (e.g., itching, pain, cancer)?
7. How is the skin lesion(s) or rash affecting the patient's life?
8. Are other family members concerned or affected?
9. Has the patient ever had this skin lesion(s) or rash before? If so, what treatment worked?
10. What does the patient think caused the skin lesion(s) or rash?

B. Follow-up questions

1. Does the patient have a history of chronic medical problems?
2. What is the patient's social history, including occupation (chemical exposures), hobbies, alcohol and tobacco use, and any underlying interpersonal or family stress?
3. What medications is the patient taking, acutely or chronically, including birth control pills and over-the-counter medications?
4. Does the patient have any underlying allergies?
5. Is there a family history of hereditary or similar skin diseases?
6. Will the patient's education or financial status influence treatment considerations?

Modified from Goldstein BG, Goldstein AO: Practical Dermatology, 2nd ed. St. Louis, Mosby, 1997.

Box 2–2 Primary skin lesions

Macule—small spot, different in color from surrounding skin, that is neither elevated nor depressed below the skin surface

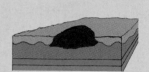

Papule—small (≤5 mm diameter) circumscribed solid elevation on the skin

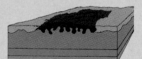

Plaque—large (≥5 mm) superficial flat lesion, often formed by a confluence of papules

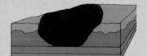

Nodule—large (5-20 mm) circumscribed solid skin elevation

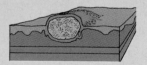

Pustule—small circumscribed skin elevation containing purulent material

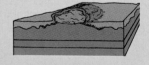

Vesicle—small (<5 mm) circumscribed skin blister containing serum

Wheal—irregular elevated edematous skin area, which often changes in size and shape

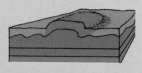

Bulla—large (>5 mm) vesicle containing free fluid
Tumor—large nodule, which may be neoplastic
Cyst—enclosed cavity with a membraneous lining, which contains liquid or semisolid matter
Telangiectasia—dilated superficial blood vessel

From Goldstein BG, Goldstein AO: Practical Dermatology, 2nd ed. St. Louis, Mosby, 1997.

Box 2–3 Secondary skin lesions

Scale—superficial epidermal cells that are dead and cast off from the skin

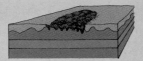

Erosion—superficial focal loss of part of the epidermis; lesions usually heal without scarring

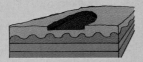

Ulcer—focal loss of the epidermis extending into the dermis; lesions may heal with scarring

Fissure—deep skin split extending into the dermis

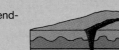

Crust—dried exudate, a "scab"

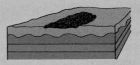

Erythema—skin redness
Hypopigmentation—decreased skin pigment
Excoriation—superficial, often linear, skin erosion caused by scratching
Depigmentation—total loss of skin pigment
Atrophy—decreased skin thickness caused by skin thinning
Lichenification—increased skin markings and thickening with induration secondary to chronic inflammation caused by scratching other irritation
Scar—abnormal fibrous tissue that replaces normal tissue after skin injury
Hyperkeratosis—abnormal skin thickening of the superficial layer of the epidermis
Edema—swelling caused by accumulation of water in tissue
Hyperpigmentation—increased skin pigment

From Goldstein BG, Goldstein AO: Practical Dermatology, 2nd ed. St. Louis, Mosby, 1997.

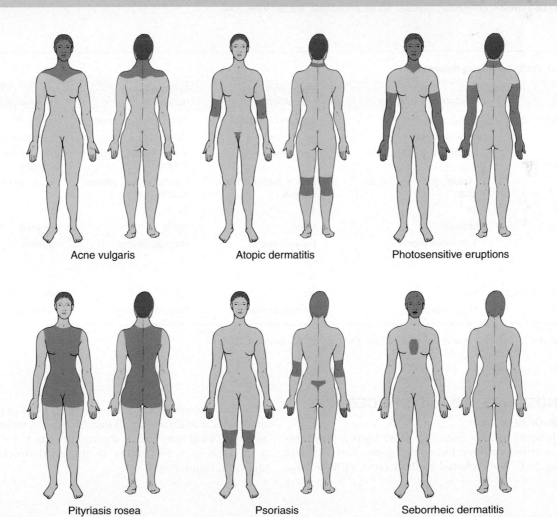

Acne vulgaris   Atopic dermatitis   Photosensitive eruptions

Pityriasis rosea   Psoriasis   Seborrheic dermatitis

Fig 2–1
Typical distributions of common skin conditions.
(From Swartz MH: Textbook of Physical Diagnosis, 5th ed. Philadelphia, WB Saunders, 2006.)

TABLE 2–1 Common maculopapular diseases

Feature	Psoriasis	Pityriasis rosea	Tinea versicolor	Seborrheic dermatitis	Lichen planus
Color	Dull red	Pinkish yellow	Reddish brown	Pinkish yellow	Violaceous
Scale	Abundant	Fine, adherent	Fine	Greasy	Shiny, adherent
Induration	1+*	0	0	1+	1+
Face lesions	Rarely	Rarely	Occasionally	Common	Rarely
Oral lesions	0	0	0	0	2+
Nail lesions	4+	0	0	0	Rarely

From Swartz MH: Textbook of Physical Diagnosis, 5th ed. Philadelphia, WB Saunders, 2006.

TABLE 2–2 Common eczematous diseases*

Parameter	Contact dermatitis	Atopic dermatitis	Neurodermatitis	Stasis dermatitis
History	Acute, localized to specific area	History in patient or family member of asthma, hay fever, or eczema	Chronic, in same areas, associated with anxiety	Varicosities, past history of thrombophlebitis or cellulitis
Location	Areas of exposure to allergen	Eyelids, groin, flexural areas	Head, lower legs, arms	Lower legs

From Swartz MH: Textbook of Physical Diagnosis, 5th ed. Philadelphia, WB Saunders, 2006.

TABLE 2–3 Vesiculobullous diseases*

Parameter	Pemphigus vulgaris	Dermatitis herpetiformis	Epidermolysis bullosa†	Bullous pemphigoid
Age of patient (yr)	40-60	Children and adults	Infants and children	60-70
Initial site	Oral mucosa	Scalp, trunk	Extremities	Extremities
Lesions	Normal skin at margins	Erythematous base	Bullae produced by trauma	Normal skin at margins
Sites	Mouth, abdomen, scalp, groin	Knees, sacrum, back, elbows	Hands, knees, elbows, mouth, toes	Trunk, extremities
Groupings	0‡	4+	1+	0
Weight loss	Marked	None	None	Minimal
Duration	1 or more years	Several years	Normal lifetime	Months to years
Pruritus	0	4+	0	±
Oral pain	4+	0	±	±
Palms, soles involved	No	No	Yes	Yes
Typical lesion	Flaccid bulla	Grouped vesicles	Flaccid vesicles	Tense bull

From Swartz MH: Textbook of Physical Diagnosis, 5th ed. Philadelphia, WB Saunders, 2006.

B. DIAGNOSTIC TESTS AND PROCEDURES

COLLECTION OF SPECIMEN

Various techniques include curettage, shave biopsy, punch biopsy, snip or scissors biopsy, incisional biopsy, and complete excision (Fig. 2–2). The preferred method varies with the location, size, and condition of the specimen to be obtained. Local anesthesia is adequate for all skin biopsies. A technique for injection of local anesthetic is shown in Figure 2–3. Collection of a nail specimen for culture in suspected onychomycosis is shown in Figure 2–4.

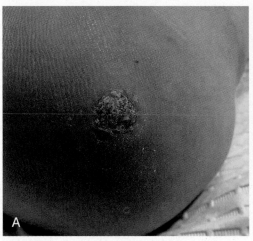 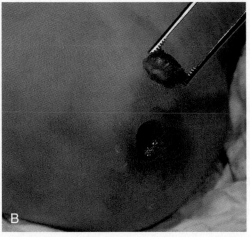

Fig 2-2
Plantar wart. **A,** Note the keratotic lesion with the yellow center and areas of hemorrhage within. **B,** After excision.
(From Swartz MH: Textbook of Physical Diagnosis, 5th ed. Philadelphia, WB Saunders, 2006.)

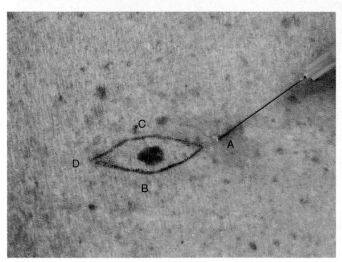

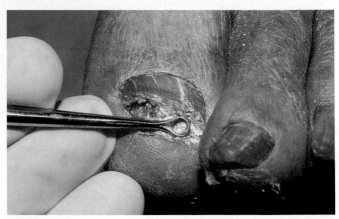

Fig 2-3
Injection of local anesthetic. Using a fine needle, local anesthetic (LA) is first infiltrated along one edge of the planned ellipse. Typically, the needle would be advanced from its insertion point A to point B, then LA is injected as the needle is slowly withdrawn but without fully removing it from the skin (thus avoiding the discomfort of a second needleprick at point A). This is repeated from point A to C to give a V- or wedge-shaped area of anesthesia. After waiting several minutes, the LA is infiltrated from B to D and then from C to D, areas B and C at this point being anesthetized.
(From White GM, Cox NH [eds]: Diseases of the Skin: A Color Atlas and Text, 2nd ed. St. Louis, Mosby, 2006.)

Fig 2-4
Collection of nail for culture. The subungual debris is the most valuable material for culture. After cutting back the nail, a curette may be used. Clippings of the nail may be added to the culture.
(From White GM, Cox NH [eds]: Diseases of the Skin: A Color Atlas and Text, 2nd ed. St. Louis, Mosby, 2006.)

Diascopy

This technique is used in the diagnosis of granulomatous disorders and to distinguish between intravascular and extravasated blood. It is performed with a strip of colorless plastic or a glass microscope slide (Fig. 2–5)

Wood's light

This is a long-wavelength ultraviolet (UV) light used to demonstrate fluorescence in skin and urine specimens to aid in the diagnosis of selected disorders. For example, urine fluorescence is reddish pink in porphyria cutanea tarda, and skin lesions in pityriasis versicolor reveal a yellow fluorescence (Fig. 2–6).

LABORATORY TESTS

- Complete blood count (CBC) with differential (blood disorders, infections)
- Antinuclear antibody (ANA; vasculitis, systemic lupus erythematosus [SLE])
- Alanine aminotransferase (ALT), aspartate transaminase (AST), bilirubin, alkaline phosphatase (liver disorders)
- Serum creatinine, urinalysis (renal disease)
- HIV (AIDS), viral hepatitis screen (viral hepatitis)
- Tzanck smear (herpes infections [herpes simplex, varicella, zoster], molluscum contagiosum) (Fig. 2–7)
- Potassium hydroxide (KOH) preparation of skin swabs or scrapings (fungus or yeast infections; Figs. 2–8 and 2–9)
- Fungal culture of nail clippings (nail infections; Fig. 2–10)
- Examination of hair with microscopy and culture
- Enzyme-linked immunosorbent assay (ELISA; herpesvirus)
- Polymerase chain reaction (PCR; human papillomavirus)
- Patch testing (type 4 hypersensitivity reactions, contact dermatitis; see Fig. 2–11), skin tests (Fig. 2–12)
- Radioallergosorbent test (RAST; blood test to detect type 1 hypersensitivity)
- Histologic examination of lesion (Fig. 2–13)

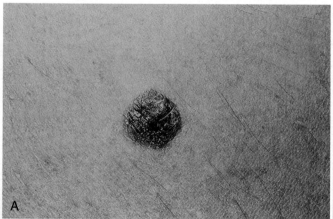
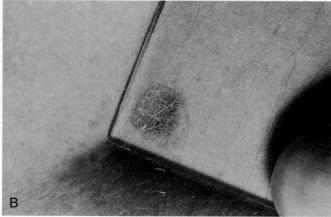

Fig 2–5

Diascopy. This technique compresses intravascular blood out of skin lesions to demonstrate other color changes or extravasated blood. It is usually performed using a glass microscope slide or, with a greater degree of safety, with a stiff strip of colorless plastic. **A, B,** In this case, diascopy of a Spitz nevus reveals the underlying brownish color or melanin that is otherwise largely obscured by the prominent vascular component. (From White GM, Cox NH [eds]: Diseases of the Skin: A Color Atlas and Text, 2nd ed. St. Louis, Mosby, 2006.)

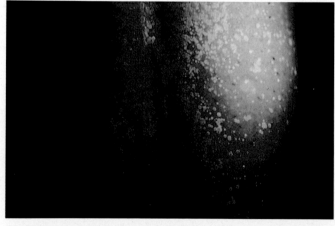

Fig 2–6

Wood's light examination. This illustration demonstrates the yellow fluorescence of pityriasis versicolor, although in normal lighting the lesions would appear pale brown.
(From White GM, Cox NH [eds]: Diseases of the Skin: A Color Atlas and Text, 2nd ed. St. Louis, Mosby, 2006.)

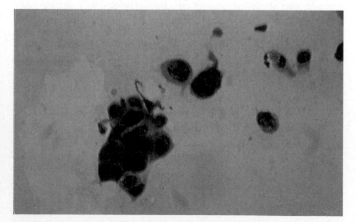

Fig 2–7

Multinucleated giant cells consistent with herpes simplex infection. (Courtesy of Dr. Paul Fischer.)

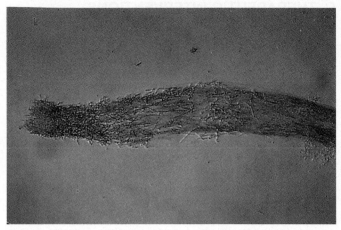

Fig 2–8
Potassium hydroxide preparation of a hair, demonstrating hyphae
and spores in a patient with tinea capitis (×10).
(From Goldstein BG, Goldstein AO: Practical Dermatology, 2nd ed.
St. Louis, Mosby, 1997.)

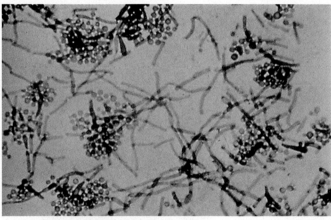

Fig 2–9
Preparation from a patient with tinea versicolor, demonstrating
pseudohyphae and spores in a spaghetti and meatball configuration.
(From Goldstein BG, Goldstein AO: Practical Dermatology, 2nd ed.
St. Louis, Mosby, 1997.)

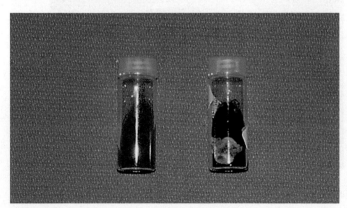

Fig 2–10
Dermatophyte test medium. Note the positive culture from a toenail
specimen (*right*), as indicated by the color change from yellow to red.
This culture took 3 weeks to become positive.
(From Goldstein BG, Goldstein AO: Practical Dermatology, 2nd ed.
St. Louis, Mosby, 1997.)

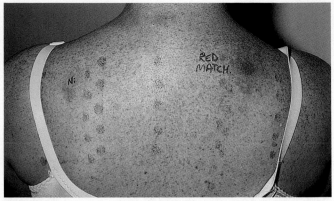

Fig 2–11
Patch testing. This patient has had test strips removed to reveal positive test results to nickel (in metal items) and phosphorus sequisulfide
(in red matchheads, a cause of facial eczema). The blue-black dots are
ink marks adjacent to the site of test application, so that any positive
reactions later can be localized and identified.
(From White GM, Cox NH [eds]: Diseases of the Skin: A Color Atlas and
Text, 2nd ed. St. Louis, Mosby, 2006.)

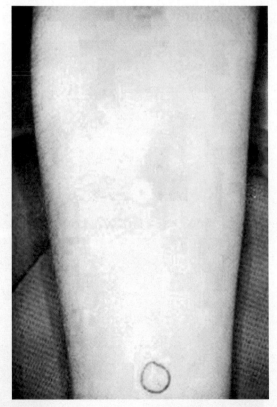

Fig 2–12
A positive prick test for *Aspergillus fumigatus* in a patient with allergic
bronchopulmonary aspergillosis. Shown are the wheal and erythema
response at 15 minutes after performing the skin test.
(From Fireman P: Atlas of Allergies and Immunology, 3rd ed. St. Louis,
Mosby, 2006.)

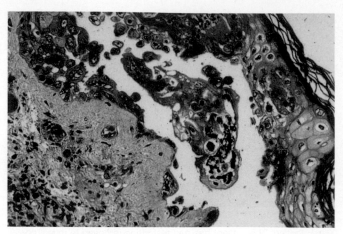

Fig 2–13
Histologic preparation of section of human skin showing typical herpes simplex virus effects—multinucleated giant cells (*arrowhead*) and intranuclear inclusion (*arrow*).
(From Cohen J, Powderly WG: Infectious Diseases, 2nd ed. St. Louis, Mosby, 2004.)

C. THERAPEUTIC INTERVENTIONS

- Surgical excision of lesion: performed following injection of local anesthetics (e.g., lidocaine, prilocaine), at times combined with vasoconstricting agents (e.g., epinephrine, vasopressin; see Fig. 2–3). The type of procedure can vary from simple curettage or shape biopsy to the removal of cysts (Fig. 2–14) and specialized excisional procedures, such as Mohs' micrographic surgery (Fig. 2–15).
- Cryotherapy: rapid freezing of lesion to induce damage and rupture of cell organelles. It is performed with the application of liquid nitrogen spray (Fig. 2–16).
- Photodynamic therapy: use of light to convert the porphyrin precursor aminolevulinic acid (ALA) into protoporphyrin IX (PPIX), which produces cytotoxic oxygen radicals and cellular damage to neoplastic cells. This technique is often used for the treatment of actinic keratosis, Bowen's disease, and basal cell carcinoma (Fig. 2–17)
- Laser therapy: use of intense light to cause cellular damage in the area of the skin lesion. This method is often used in the treatment of vascular lesions such as port-wine stains (Fig. 2–18)

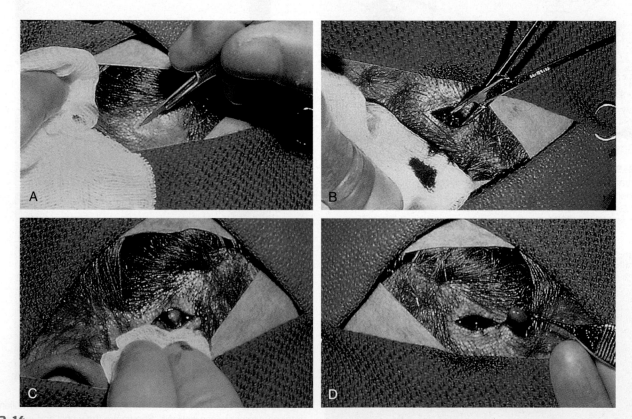

Fig 2–14
Pilar cyst removal on scalp. **A**, Elliptic excision into superficial dermis. **B**, Blunt dissection through the dermis and around the cyst. **C**, Isolated cyst. **D**, Intact cyst is removed.
(Courtesy of the Department of Dermatology, University of North Carolina at Chapel Hill.)

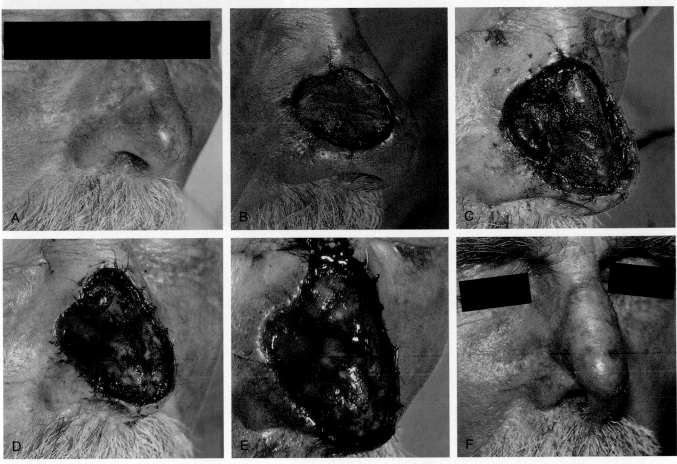

Fig 2–15
Micrographic (Mohs') surgery for a nasal basal cell carcinoma. **A**, Initial poorly defined basal cell carcinoma. **B**, Stage 1 excision. **C**, Stage 2 excision. **D**, Stage 3 excision. **E**, Stage 4 excision. **F**, After repair.
(Courtesy of Dr. C. M. Lawrence.)

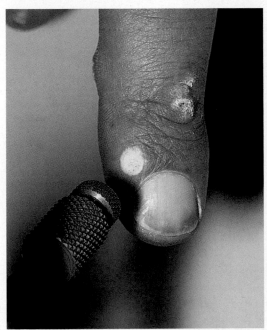

Fig 2–16
Cryotherapy for wart removal using the liquid nitrogen (LN$_2$) spray technique. For warts or actinic keratoses, it is usual to perform a single period of freezing (one freeze-thaw cycle, FTC), whereas for malignancies two FTCs are generally used to increase the degree of damage. It is routine to record the cryogen and the number and duration of treatment cycles—for example, LN$_2$, 2 × 20-second FTC.
(From White GM, Cox NH [eds]: Diseases of the Skin: A Color Atlas and Text, 2nd ed. St. Louis, Mosby, 2006.)

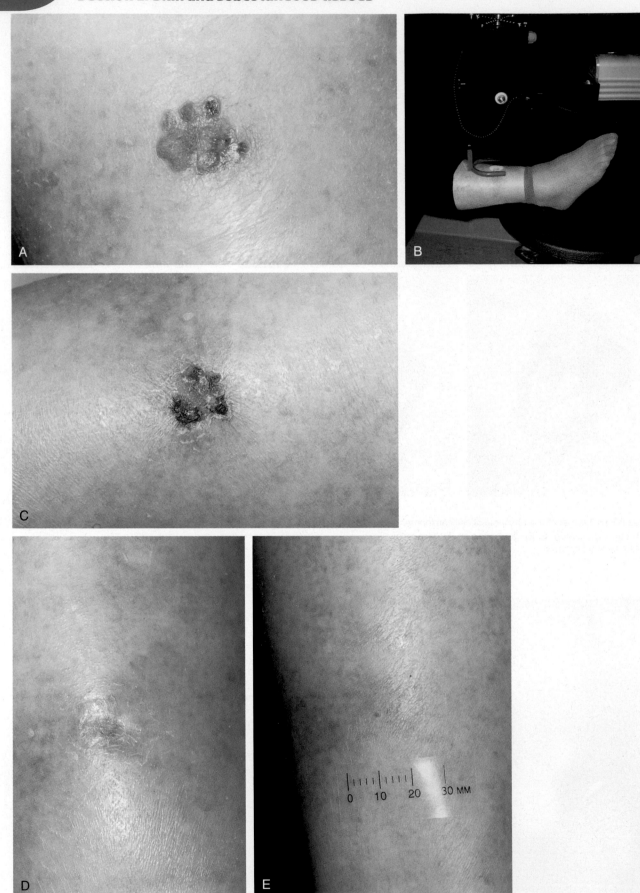

Fig 2–17
Photodynamic therapy. **A,** Lesion of Bowen's disease on the leg before treatment. **B,** Exposure to red light after pretreatment with methyl-aminolevulinic acid for 3 hours under occlusion. **C-E,** Appearance at 1 week, 1 month, and 3 months after treatment.
(From White GM, Cox NH [eds]: Diseases of the Skin: A Color Atlas and Text, 2nd ed. St. Louis, Mosby, 2006.)

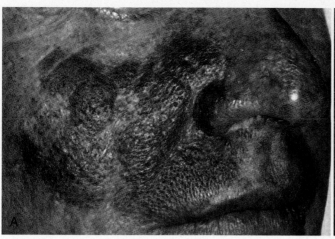
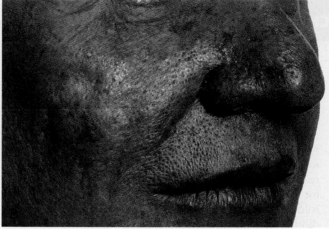

Fig 2–18
Laser therapy of a port-wine stain on the face. **A,** Before treatment. **B,** 3 years after treatment (eight sessions of treatment were required). (Courtesy of Dr. C. M. Lawrence.)

- Phototherapy: use of different wavelengths of UV light (UVB, UVA with psoralen chemical activation [PUVA]) to treat inflammatory dermatoses (e.g., psoriasis, eczema) and cutaneous lymphomas (Fig. 2–19)
- Iontophoresis: generation of hydrogen ions by using an electric current. It is used for the treatment of hyperhidrosis of the palms and soles and to enhance penetration of topically applied drugs (e.g., 5-fluorouracil, tretinoin).
- Cosmetic interventions: chemical facial peels, dermabrasion, and laser resurfacing (to smooth skin and remove blemishes and wrinkles), botulinum toxin (Botox) injections (for blepharospasm, hyperhidrosis), liposuction (to remove adipose tissue from buttocks, sides, abdomen, breasts), sclerotherapy (for varicose veins), collagen injections (to increase wrinkles, increase bulk in the lips)

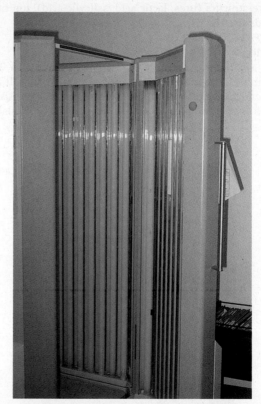

Fig 2–19
Phototherapy apparatus. Many commercial machines consist of about 40 vertically oriented fluorescent tubes in a stand-up cabinet style, as shown; the door panel includes an apparatus to set exposure doses. The main difference between a PUVA (psoralen with ultraviolet A) machine (as shown) and those for UVB is the type of fluorescent tube fitted, requiring a different output sensor and generating a different range of exposure times.
(From White GM, Cox NH [eds]: Diseases of the Skin: A Color Atlas and Text, 2nd ed. St. Louis, Mosby, 2006.)

Chapter 3   Disorders of keratinization

A. ICHTHYOSIS

- Condition characterized by abnormal keratinization
- Clinical features range from mild involvement, often passed off as dry skin (xerosis) to severe widespread scaly lesions (Fig. 3–1), causing discomfort and social embarrassment.
- Specific investigations are dictated by clinical presentation—malignancy workup, HIV, and skin biopsy to rule out sarcoidosis are indicated in acquired ichthyosis. Investigations for hereditary ichthyosis include mutational analysis, steroid sulfatase activity, (fatty alcohol [nicotinamide adenine dinucleotide [NAD] + oxidoreductase activity])
- Treatment consists of hydration (humidification of environment, bathing, soaking) and use of creams, lotions, or ointments for lubrication. Second-line therapies involve the use of keratolytics (urea, lactic acid, salicylic acid), topical retinoids (tretinoin, tazarotene), or calcipotriol.

CLASSIFICATION
(1) Ichthyosis vulgaris

This is a relatively common disorder (incidence 1 in 250 to 1000 births), with an autosomal mode of inheritance. It affects both genders equally and presents as dryness (xerosis) and slight to moderate fine, white, fishlike scaling, particularly involving the arms and legs and characteristically sparing the flexures (Fig. 3–2).

(2) Sex-linked ichthyosis

Also known as ichthyosis nigricans, this is an X-linked recessively inherited disorder with an incidence of 1 in 6000 male births (Fig. 3–3). It is associated with a deficiency of the microsomal enzyme steroid sulfatase.

(3) Acquired ichthyosis

This is an important paraneoplastic manifestation (Fig. 3–4) of a number of malignancies, most commonly Hodgkin's lymphoma. It may also accompany HIV infection, sarcoidosis, and connective tissue diseases.

B. KERATODERMA

DEFINITION AND CLINICAL CHARACTERISTICS

Diffuse palmoplantar keratoderma is an autosomal dominant disorder characterized by a diffuse, smooth hyperkeratosis involving the palms and soles as well as the ventral surfaces of the fingers and toes (Fig. 3–5). The reported incidence ranges from 1 in 12,000 to 40,000.

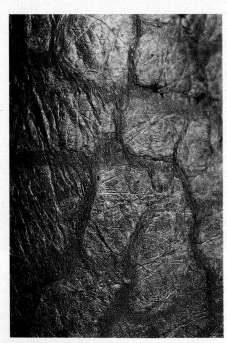

Fig 3–1
Severe generalized ichthyosis. This was an incidental postmortem finding. Ichthyosis can be very disfiguring and a considerable social disadvantage.
(From McKee PH, Calonje E, Granter SR [eds]: Pathology of the Skin With Clinical Correlations, 3rd ed. St. Louis, Mosby, 2005.)

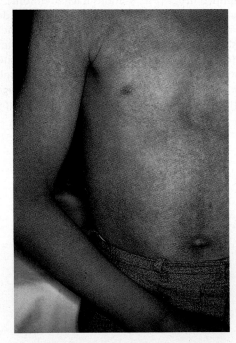

Fig 3–2
Ichthyosis vulgaris. Abdominal involvement is most noticeable in this patient. Sparing of the flexures is characteristic of this variant of ichthyosis.
(Courtesy of Dr. W. A. D. Griffiths, Institute of Dermatology, London.)

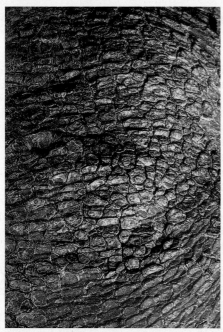

Fig 3–3
Sex-linked ichthyosis. In this example, the scales appear dirty. This can be an extremely embarrassing condition.
(Courtesy of the Institute of Dermatology, London.)

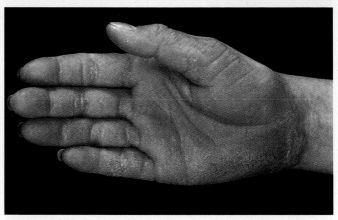

Fig 3–5
Diffuse palmoplantar keratoderma. In this patient, the palms of the hands were also affected.
(Courtesy of Dr. W. A. D. Griffiths, Institute of Dermatology, London.)

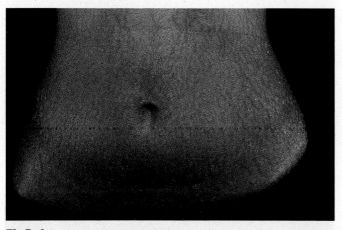

Fig 3–4
Acquired ichthyosis. Cutaneous manifestations most often resemble ichthyosis vulgaris.
(Courtesy of the Institute of Dermatology, London.)

Chapter 4   **Inherited and autoimmune subepidermal blistering diseases**

DEFINITION

Blisters, which are clinically subdivided into vesicles and bullae, are defined as accumulations of fluid either within or below the epidermis and mucous membranes.

- Although somewhat arbitrary, the term *vesicle* is applied to lesions smaller than 0.5 cm in diameter and *bulla* to those larger than 0.5 cm.
- In this section, only those conditions in which subepidermal blister formation represents an inherited or autoimmune primary event are considered. Other conditions, which may be associated with subepidermal blistering, are dealt with in other sections.

A. BULLOUS PEMPHIGOID

DEFINITION

Bullous pemphigoid refers to an autoimmune, subepidermal blistering disease seen in older adults. It is the most common of the autoimmune bullous dermatoses.

PHYSICAL FINDINGS AND CLINICAL PRESENTATION

- Bullous pemphigoid typically starts as an eczematous or urticarial rash on the extremities. Blisters form between 1 week to several months.
- Anatomic distribution involves the flexor surfaces of the arms, legs, groin, axillae, and lower abdomen. The head and neck are generally spared. The lesions are irregularly grouped but sometimes can be serpiginous. Oral lesions can be found occasionally (Fig. 4–1).
- The typical blistering bulla measures from 5 mm to 2 cm in diameter and contains clear or bloody fluid (Fig 4–2). It may arise from normal skin or from an erythematous base and will heal without scarring if denuded.

CAUSE

- Bullous pemphigoid is an autoimmune disease with an IgG and/or C3 complement component reacting with antigens in the basement membrane zone.

- Drug-induced pemphigoid, although rare, can occur in patients taking penicillamine, furosemide, captopril, penicillin, or sulfasalazine.

DIFFERENTIAL DIAGNOSIS

- Cicatricial pemphigoid (see Fig. 4–6)
- Epidermolysis bullosa acquisita (see Fig. 4–7)
- Pemphigus (see Fig. 5–1)
- Pemphigoid nodularis

LABORATORY TESTS

- Antibodies to the basement membrane zone are detected in the serum of 70% of patients with bullous pemphigoid.
- Skin biopsy staining with hematoxylin-eosin reveals subepidermal blisters.
- Direct and indirect immunofluorescence studies can detect the presence of IgG and C3 immune complexes (Fig. 4–3).
- Immunoelectron microscopy also reveals immune deposits in the basement membrane zone.

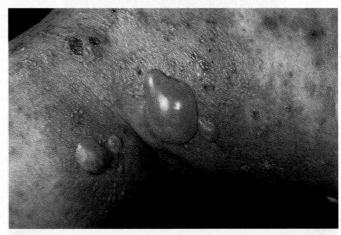

Fig 4–2
Bullous pemphigoid showing tense, dome-shaped blisters. The flexures are typically affected.
(Courtesy of the Institute of Dermatology, London.)

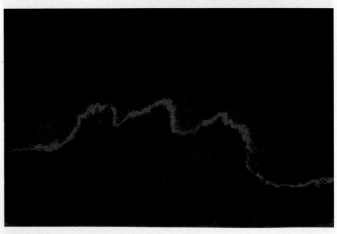

Fig 4–3
Bullous pemphigoid. Direct immunofluorescence shows C3 deposition.
(Courtesy of B. Boghal, Institute of Dermatology, London.)

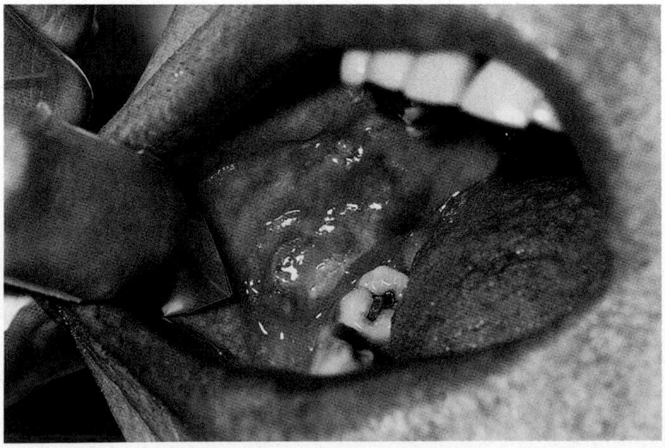

Fig 4–1
Bullous pemphigoid. Oral erosions are an occasional finding. Intact blisters are rare.
(Courtesy of Dr. R. A. Marsden, St. George's Hospital, London.)

TREATMENT

Treatment of bullous pemphigoid is based on the degree of involvement and rate of disease progression.

- Systemic corticosteroids are considered the standard treatment for more advanced bullous pemphigoid.
- Topical steroids have generally been used in patients with localized bullous pemphigoid.
- If patients cannot take corticosteroids, dapsone, combination tetracycline and nicotinamide, or azathioprine can be tried.

B. PEMPHIGOID GESTATIONIS

DEFINITION AND CLINICAL CHARACTERISTICS

This is an autoimmune bullous dermatosis of pregnancy and puerperium. Circulating antibodies are directed against the same target antigens as in bullous pemphigoid.

- It is associated with an increased risk of developing Graves' disease.
- The disease effects predominantly white women in their second or third trimester of pregnancy and is associated with intense pruritus, which may be present for days or weeks before the onset of the cutaneous manifestations.
- The dermatosis consists of erythematous or urticarial papules and plaques, with later development of vesicles and bullae at the periphery of spreading erythematous plaques.
- The umbilicus is frequently the site of initial involvement (Fig. 4–4).
- The dermatosis typically heals without scarring.
- Diagnostic investigations include a biopsy for histopathology and direct immunofluorescence, and a serum specimen for indirect immunofluorescence.
- Treatment is with topical or oral corticosteroids, antihistamines, and plasmapheresis.

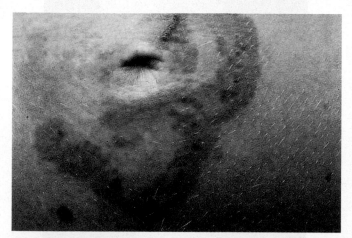

Fig 4–4
Pemphigoid gestationis. Umbilical involvement is a common mode of presentation.
(Courtesy of the Institute of Dermatology, London.)

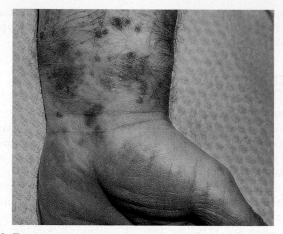

Fig 4–5
Lichen planus pemphigoides. Typical lichenoid papules are present on the anterior aspect of the wrist.
(Courtesy of Dr. M. M. Black, Institute of Dermatology, London.)

C. LICHEN PLANUS PEMPHIGOID

DEFINITION AND CLINICAL CHARACTERISTICS

This is a disorder characterized by basement membrane antibodies against a number of antigens.

- The serum contains an IgG antibasement membrane antibody in almost 60% of patients.
- It affects predominantly men in their fourth or fifth decade.
- Clinically, the pemphigoid-like lesions are usually preceded by typical lichen planus, although rarely the blisters may develop first (Fig. 4–5).
- The lichenoid lesions show the typical histopathologic and immunofluorescent changes of lichen planus, but the bullae have features more suggestive of bullous pemphigoid.
- It differs from typical bullous pemphigoid clinically by its earlier age at presentation and predilection for the lower limbs.

D. CICATRICIAL PEMPHIGOID

DEFINITION AND CLINICAL CHARACTERISTICS

This is a rare blistering disorder (incidence, 1 in 15,000) often presenting in women in their seventh decade.

- Oral lesions occur in 85% to 95% of patients and commonly follow mild trauma.
- Bullae, erosions, and erythema most commonly affect the gingival or buccal mucosa, but the hard and soft palate, tongue, and lips are also frequently involved (Fig. 4–6).
- Desquamative gingivitis is the most common manifestation.
- Patients with this condition present with painful, swollen, erythematous lesions of the gums, which may be associated with bleeding, blistering, erosions, and ulcerations.
- Ocular lesions occur in 64% of patients.
- Cicatricial pemphigoid is a chronic disease and is often associated with significant morbidity, largely because of the effects of the scarring associated with it.

- Apart from the presence of scarring in older lesions, cicatricial pemphigoid is indistinguishable from bullous pemphigoid.

E. EPIDERMOLYSIS BULLOSA ACQUISITA (DERMOLYTIC PEMPHIGOID)

DEFINITION AND CLINICAL CHARACTERISTICS

This is a rare disorder presenting in adults with the development of blisters on the hands, feet, elbows, and knees following mild trauma. It may be complicated by atrophic scarring, milia formation (Fig. 4–7), and nail dystrophy.

- Diagnosis: skin biopsy and serum for direct and indirect immunofluorescence to detect skin basement membrane–specific autoantibodies. A workup for inflammatory bowel disease and ELISA for type VII collagen-specific autoantibodies should also be considered.
- Treatment: systemic corticosteroids, dapsone, azathioprine, colchicine

F. DERMATITIS HERPETIFORMIS

DEFINITION

Dermatitis herpetiformis (DH) is a rare, chronic skin disorder characterized by an intensely burning, pruritic, vesicular rash. It is strongly associated with gluten-sensitive enteropathy. Of patients with DH, 20% to 70% will have gastrointestinal symptoms, whereas approximately 10% of patients with celiac sprue will have DH.

PHYSICAL FINDINGS AND CLINICAL PRESENTATION

- Pruritic, burning vesicles initially, frequently grouped (hence, the name "herpetiform")
- Symmetrically distributed on extensor surfaces: elbows (Fig. 4–8), knees, scalp, nuchal area, shoulders, and buttocks (Fig. 4–9); rarely found in the mouth
- May evolve in time to intensely burning urticarial papules, vesicles and, rarely, bullae
- Celiac-type permanent tooth enamel defects found in 53% of patients

DIFFERENTIAL DIAGNOSIS

- Linear IgA bullous dermatosis (not associated with gluten-sensitive enteropathy; see Fig. 4–11)
- Herpes simplex infection (see Fig. 27–4)
- Herpes zoster infection (see Fig. 27–8)
- Erythema multiforme (see Fig. 9–2)
- Bullous pemphigoid (see Fig. 4–2)

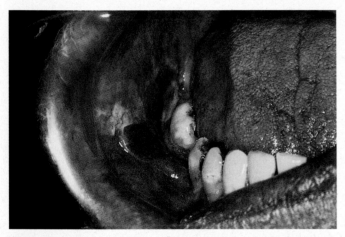

Fig 4–6
Cicatricial pemphigoid. There is erosion of the buccal mucosa.
(Courtesy of P. Morgan, London.)

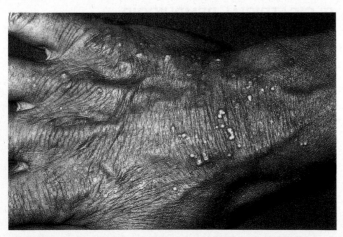

Fig 4–7
Epidermolysis bullosa acquisita. Conspicuous milia are present on the back of the hand.
(Courtesy of the Institute of Dermatology, London.)

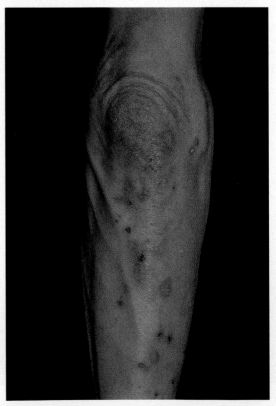

Fig 4–8
Dermatitis herpetiformis. Excoriations are present on the elbow and back of the arm. Intact blisters are uncommon in dermatitis herpetiformis because of the intense pruritus.
(Courtesy of the Institute of Dermatology, London.)

LABORATORY TESTS

- Skin biopsy for immunofluorescence studies. Diagnosis is confirmed by IgA deposits along the subepidermal basement membrane (Fig. 4–10). Biopsies should be taken from adjacent normal skin, because the diagnostic Ig deposits are usually destroyed by the blistering process.
- Circulating antibodies: IgA antiendomysial antibody, IgA antigliadin antibodies, IgA reticulin antibody, IgA antitissue transglutaminase

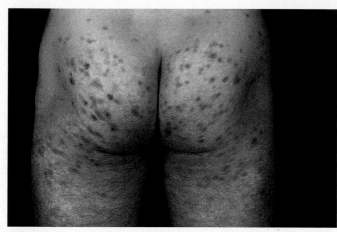

Fig 4–9
Dermatitis herpetiformis. The buttocks are frequently affected.
(Courtesy of the Institute of Dermatology, London.)

TREATMENT

- Adherence to a gluten-free diet has been associated with sustained remission of DH. Spontaneous remission of DH in patients on a normal diet can occur in up to 15% of cases.
- Medications may be helpful in resistant cases. Useful agents are dapsone, sulfapyridine, and tetracycline.

G. LINEAR IgA DISEASE

CLINICAL CHARACTERISTICS

- This disorder can occur in adults (linear IgA disease of adults) or children (childhood linear IgA disease).
- The adult form is rare and may present as a somewhat atypical bullous eruption showing features suggestive of dermatitis herpetiformis or, more commonly, bullous pemphigoid (Fig. 4–11).
- Pruritus, a burning sensation, or both are common manifestations and early lesions may include urticarial, annular, polycyclic, and targetoid lesions, often mistaken for erythema multiforme (see Fig. 9–2).

DIAGNOSIS

- Diagnosis is made histologically.
- Skin biopsy for routine microscopy and direct immunofluorescence
- Indirect fluorescence
- A homogeneous linear deposition of IgA along the basement membrane region is found by direct immunofluorescence in 100% of patients (Fig. 4–12).

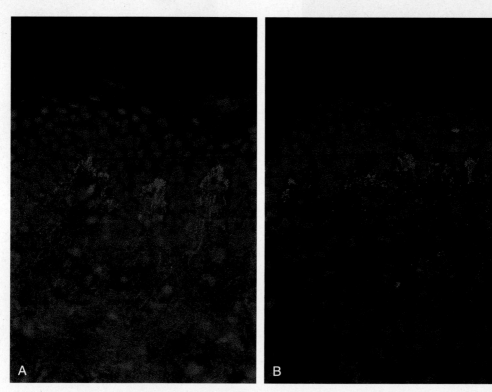

Fig 4–10
Dermatitis herpetiformis. Direct immunofluorescence showing deposits of granular IgA in the dermal papillae **(A)** and fibrin deposition in the dermal papillae **(B)**.
(Courtesy of the Department of Immunofluorescence, Institute of Dermatology, London.)

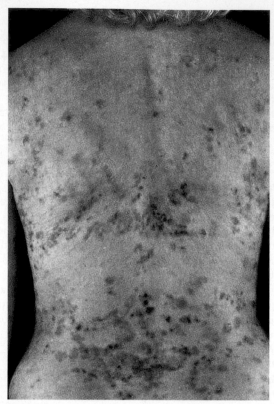

- Childhood linear IgA disease may develop after an upper respiratory illness, often following treatment with penicillin. Usually, new lesions appear around those resolving (a sign called the cluster of jewels; Fig. 4–13).
- Mucous membrane lesions are common (64%).

TREATMENT

- Dapsone, prednisone, sulfapyridine, colchicines, tetracycline

Fig 4–11
Adult linear IgA disease. In this example, the clinical appearance of excoriated lesions is suggestive of dermatitis herpetiformis. (Courtesy of the Institute of Dermatology, London.)

Fig 4–12
Linear IgA disease—direct immunofluorescence showing linear IgA deposition.
(Courtesy of the Department of Immunofluorescence, Institute of Dermatology, London.)

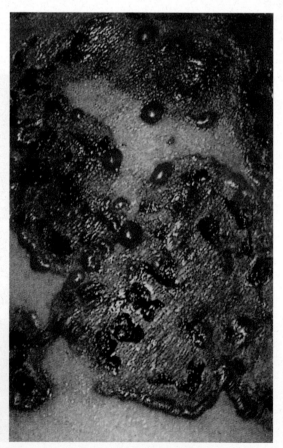

Fig 4–13
Childhood linear IgA disease. This arrangement of blisters is called the cluster of jewels.
(Courtesy of Dr. R. A. Marsden, St. George's Hospital, London.)

Chapter 5	**Acantholytic disorders**

DEFINITION

The term *acantholysis* derives from the Greek *akantha*, a thorn or prickle, and *lysis*, a loosening. In its simplest definition, the term is used to reflect a primary disorder of the skin (and sometimes the mucous membranes) characterized by separation of keratinocytes at their desmosomal junctions.

A. PEMPHIGUS

- Pemphigus (Greek *pemphix*, blister) refers to a group of chronic blistering diseases that develop as a consequence of autoantibodies directed against various desmosomal proteins.
- The clinical features and therefore classification of these disorders depend on the level of separation within the epidermis; in pemphigus vulgaris and pemphigus vegetans, the blisters are suprabasal, whereas in pemphigus foliaceus and pemphigus erythematosus the blisters are situated more superficially.
- Pemphigus vulgaris is the most common variant, accounting for 80% of cases.

(1) Pemphigus vulgaris
DEFINITION
Pemphigus vulgaris refers to an intraepidermal, blistering skin disorder characterized by the formation of a flaccid blister.
PHYSICAL FINDINGS AND CLINICAL PRESENTATION
Oral mucosa lesions typically occur first (Fig. 5–1), followed by a generalized, usually nonpruritic bullous eruption within a few months. Lesions are fragile and rupture easily, leaving painful denuded lesions (Figs. 5–2 and 5–3).

Physical findings

- Anatomic distribution: oral mucosa; can also involve the pharynx, larynx, vagina, penis, anus, and conjunctival mucosa
- Generalized cutaneous involvement may also occur.
- Lesion configuration: all stratified squamous epithelium can become involved.
- Lesion morphology: bullae. Denuded crusting and erosion (Fig 5–4) commonly occur.

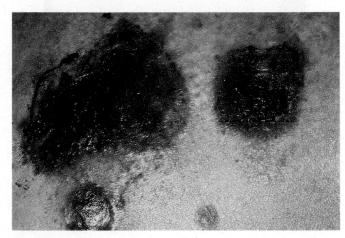

Fig 5–2
Pemphigus vulgaris. Extensive erosions and blisters are present on the skin.
(Courtesy of Dr. R. A. Marsden, St. George's Hospital, London.)

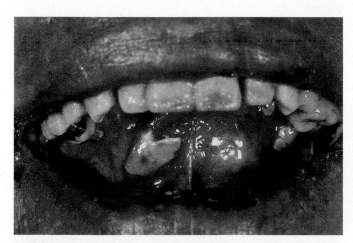

Fig 5–1
Pemphigus vulgaris. In this patient, there is an intact blister on the floor of the mouth. Pemphigus commonly appears in the mouth.
(Courtesy of the Institute of Dermatology, London.)

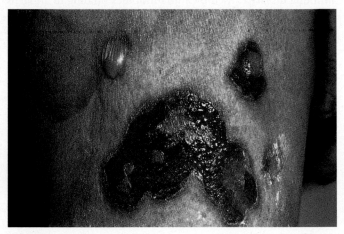

Fig 5–3
Pemphigus vulgaris—extensive trauma-induced blisters.
(Courtesy of the Institute of Dermatology, London.)

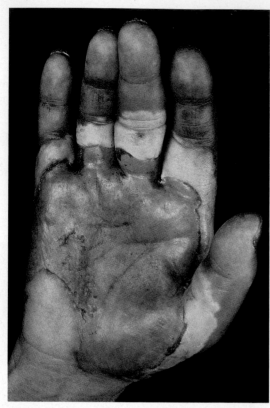

Fig 5–4
Pemphigus vulgaris. Because the blisters are superficial, erosions are more commonly encountered.
(Courtesy of the Institute of Dermatology, London.)

CAUSE

Pemphigus vulgaris, like all subtypes of pemphigus, is an auto-immune disease caused by autoantibodies binding to antigens within the epithelial layer of the skin.

DIFFERENTIAL DIAGNOSIS

- Bullous pemphigoid (see Fig. 4–2)
- Cicatricial pemphigoid (see Fig. 4–6)
- Behçet's disease (see Fig. 15–5)
- Erythema multiforme (see Fig. 9–2)
- Systemic lupus erythematosus (see Fig. 293–1)
- Aphthous stomatitis (see Fig. 89–11)
- Dermatitis herpetiformis (see Fig. 4–8)
- Drug eruptions (see Fig. 14–1)

LABORATORY TESTS

- Autoantibodies can be detected in the serum by indirect im-munofluorescence assays.
- Skin biopsy reveals intraepidermal bulla formation, also called acantholysis (loss of cell adhesion between the epi-dermal cells).
- Direct and indirect immunofluorescence studies of the le-sion show deposits of IgG and C3 in the epidermal layers of the skin (Fig. 5–5).

TREATMENT

- For mild cases, topical or intralesional steroids can be used for individual lesions.
- For more severe cases, systemic corticosteroids are indicated at high dosages.

- Adjuvant therapy is tried in patients in an attempt to de-crease the amount of steroids required.

(2) Pemphigus foliaceus

- Most often affects middle aged and older adults
- The blisters are superficial and exceedingly fragile, and therefore much less obvious; erosions and large leafy scales or crusts are often predominant (Fig. 5–6).

(3) Pemphigus vegetans

- Most often affects adults and accounts for 2% of all cases of pemphigus
- The lesions, which present as blisters and erosions, are particularly prolific in the flexures, especially the axillae, groin, inframammary region, umbilicus, and margins of the lips. Soon thereafter, patients characteristically develop hypertrophic vegetations and pustules at the blistered edges (Fig. 5–7).

Fig 5–5
Pemphigus vulgaris (direct immunofluorescence).
(Courtesy of the Institute of Dermatology, London.)

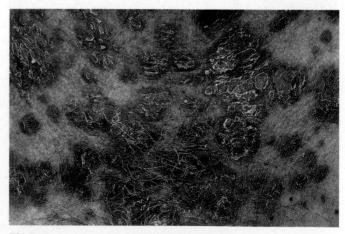

Fig 5–6
Pemphigus foliaceus—close-up view of crusted erosions.
(Courtesy of the Institute of Dermatology, London.)

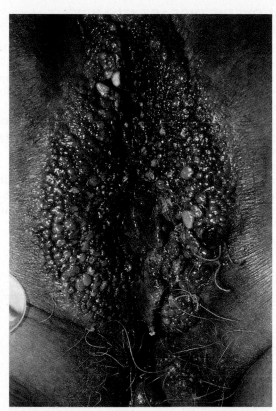

Fig 5–7
Pemphigus vegetans—perineal view showing characteristic hypertrophic flexural vegetations. Note the numerous intact vesicles.
(Courtesy of Dr. S. Dalziel, University Hospital, Nottingham, England.)

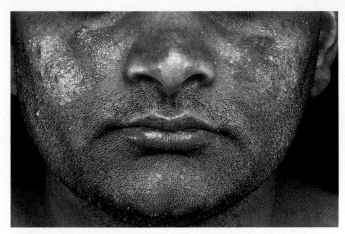

Fig 5–8
Pemphigus erythematosus. There is scarring and erythema affecting both cheeks.
(Courtesy of the Institute of Dermatology, London.)

(4) Pemphigus erythematosus

- Pemphigus erythematous is a mild localized form of superficial pemphigus with histologic and immunofluorescent findings of pemphigus foliaceus combined with features of lupus erythematosus. In general, the latter is subclinical, suggested only by laboratory findings.
- Clinically, it is commonly confined to the head, neck, and upper trunk.
- Lesions are erythematous, scaly, and crusted, with or without superficial vesicles, blisters, or erosions.
- Facial involvement often shows a butterfly distribution reminiscent of SLE (Fig. 5–8).
- Mucous membrane involvement is rare.

B. DARIER'S DISEASE

- Rare skin disorder usually transmitted in an autosomal dominant pattern
- It is characterized by abnormal keratinocyte adhesion.
- The lesions are frequently itchy and characterized by greasy, crusted, keratotic yellow-brown papules and plaques found particularly on the scalp, forehead, ears, nasolabial folds, upper chest, back, and supraclavicular fossae.
- Lesions may be induced or exacerbated by stress, heat, sweating, and maceration (Fig. 5–9).

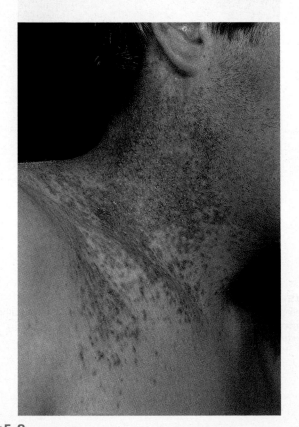

Fig 5–9
Darier's disease. Lesions may be induced by stress, heat, sweating, and maceration.
(Courtesy of the Institute of Dermatology, London.)

- Nail changes are a particularly important diagnostic feature. Longitudinal white or red streaks (often both), some of which terminate in a small nick on the free margin, are typical findings (Fig. 5–10).
- Patients with Darier's disease are susceptible to bacterial (particularly *Staphylococcus aureus*), dermatophytic, and viral infections.
- Diagnosis: skin biopsy reveals focal acantholytic dyskeratosis.
- Treatment: emollients, cool cotton clothing, topical or oral retinoids, topical 5-fluorouracil

C. GROVER'S DISEASE (TRANSIENT ACANTHOLYTIC DERMATOSIS)

- Acquired disorder affecting primarily white individuals.
- The skin lesions are usually polymorphic, consisting of 1- to 3-mm erythematous, red-brown or flesh-colored papules, vesicles, and eczematous plaques, with a predilection for the chest, back, and thighs (Fig. 5–11).
- The cause of this disorder is unknown; however, contributing factors are sun exposure, excessive heat and sweating, ionizing radiation, and adverse reaction to drugs.
- Diagnosis: skin biopsy
- Treatment: emollients, topical corticosteroids, antihistamines, avoidance of heat, sweating. Second-line therapies include systemic corticosteroids, isotretinoin, psoralen plus UVA (PUVA), and vitamin A.

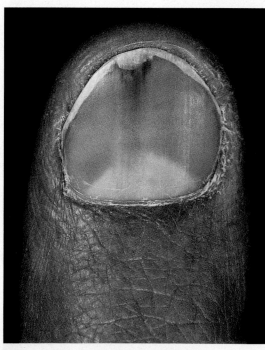

Fig 5–10
Darier's disease. Parallel white and red longitudinal streaks are pathognomonic features.
(Courtesy of the Institute of Dermatology, London.)

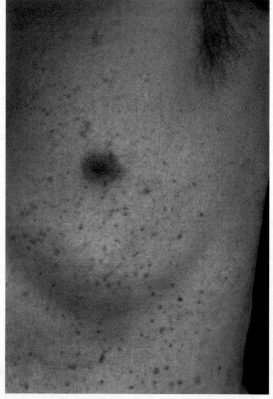

Fig 5–11
Grover's disease. Innumerable erythematous papules are present on the chest wall.
(Courtesy of the Institute of Dermatology, London.)

Chapter 6   **Eczematous dermatoses**

- The term *eczema* refers to a group of disorders that share similar clinical and histologic features but may have different causes.
- Some have objected to the term *eczema* because it does not refer to a specific disease but is a nonspecific term that simply refers to any clinical lesion that exhibits spongiosus. This is clinically manifest as moist, often "bubbly" papules or plaques superimposed on an erythematous base.
- The earliest clinical lesions are erythema and aggregates of tiny pruritic vesicles, which rupture readily, exuding clear liquid, and later become encrusted (Fig. 6–1). More chronic lesions become scaly and thickened (lichenification), especially if the skin is continually scratched or rubbed. Therefore, the clinical features of dermatitis depend on the duration of the lesions, site(s) involved, and presence of scratching.
- Eczematous dermatitis can be classified by cause as endogenous if it is related to major constitutional or hereditary factors, and exogenous if it involves environmental factors.

A. ENDOGENOUS ECZEMATOUS DERMATITIS

(1) Atopic dermatitis

DEFINITION

Atopic dermatitis is a genetically determined eczematous eruption that is pruritic, symmetrical, and associated with a personal family history of allergic manifestations (atopy). The highest incidence is in children (5% to 10%). More than 50% of children with generalized atopic dermatitis develop asthma and allergic rhinitis by the age of 13 years.

DIAGNOSIS

Diagnosis is based on the presence of three of the following major features and three minor features.

Major features
- Pruritus
- Personal or family history of atopy—asthma, allergic rhinitis, atopic dermatitis
- Facial and extensor involvement in infants and children
- Flexural lichenification in adults

Minor features
- Elevated IgE
- Eczema-perifollicular accentuation
- Recurrent conjunctivitis
- Ichthyosis
- Nipple dermatitis
- Wool intolerance
- Cutaneous *S. aureus* infections or herpes simplex infections
- Food intolerance
- Hand dermatitis (nonallergic irritant)
- Facial pallor, facial erythema
- Cheilitis
- White dermographism
- Early age of onset (after 2 months of age)

PHYSICAL FINDINGS AND CLINICAL PRESENTATION
- There are no specific cutaneous signs for atopic dermatitis and there is a wide spectrum of presentations, ranging from minimal flexural eczema to erythroderma. Inflammation in the flexural areas and lichenified skin is a common presentation in children.
- The primary lesions are a result of itching caused by severe and chronic pruritus. The repeated scratching modifies the skin surface, producing lichenification, dry and scaly skin, and redness (Fig. 6–2.)
- The lesions are typically on the neck, face, upper trunk, and bends of elbows and knees (symmetrical on flexural surfaces of extremities).
- There is dryness, thickening of the involved areas, discoloration, blistering, and oozing.
- Papular lesions are frequently found in the antecubital and popliteal fossae.

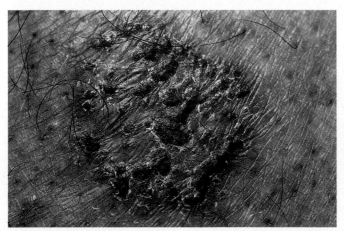

Fig 6–1
Eczema. This is a plaque of discoid eczema. Small vesicles are present at the edge of the lesion.
(Courtesy of the Institute of Dermatology, London.)

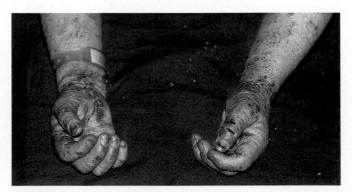

Fig 6–2
Atopic dermatitis. These crusted, exudative, and infected lesions with lichenification are characteristic.
(Courtesy of Dr. R. A. Marsden, St. George's Hospital, London.)

- In children, red scaling plaques are often confined to the cheeks and perioral and perinasal areas.
- Constant scratching may result in areas of hypopigmentation or hyperpigmentation (more common in blacks).
- In adults, redness and scaling in the dorsal aspects of the hands or about the fingers are the most common expression of atopic dermatitis; oozing and crusting may be present.
- Secondary skin infections may be present (e.g., *S. aureus*, dermatophytosis, herpes simplex).

CAUSE

Unknown; elevated T-lymphocyte activation, defective cell immunity, and B-cell IgE overproduction may play significant roles.

DIFFERENTIAL DIAGNOSIS

- Scabies (see Fig. 29–1)
- Psoriasis (see Fig. 7–2)
- Dermatitis herpetiform (see Fig. 4–9)
- Contact dermatitis (see Fig. 6–8)
- Photosensitivity (see Fig. 14–2)
- Seborrheic dermatitis (see Fig. 6–4)
- Candidiasis (see Fig. 26–9)
- Lichen simplex chronicus (see Fig. 6–15)

LABORATORY TESTS

- Laboratory tests are generally not helpful.
- Elevated IgE levels are found in 80% to 90% of atopic dermatitis cases.
- Blood eosinophilia correlates with disease severity.

TREATMENT

Avoidance of triggering factors

- Sudden temperature changes, sweating, low humidity in the winter
- Contact with irritating substance (e.g., wool, cosmetics, some soaps and detergents, tobacco)
- Foods that provoke exacerbations (e.g., eggs, peanuts, fish, soy, wheat, milk)
- Stressful situations
- Allergens and dust
- Excessive hand washing
- Clip nails to decrease abrasion of skin
- Emollients can be used to prevent dryness. Severely affected skin can be optimally hydrated by occlusion in addition to the application of emollients.
- Topical corticosteroids may be helpful.
- The topical immunomodulators pimecrolimus and tacrolimus
- Oral antihistamines
- Oral prednisone, IM triamcinolone, Goeckerman regimen, and PUVA are generally reserved for severe cases

(2) Seborrheic dermatitis

- Common dermatosis affecting up to 2% of the population
- It particularly affects areas where sebaceous glands are most numerous (scalp, forehead, eyebrows, eyelids, ears, cheeks, presternal and interscapular areas; Figs. 6–3 and 6–4).
- Often, the lesions are sharply marginated, dull red, or yellowish and covered with a greasy scale.
- They are often easily confused with psoriasis.
- Dandruff and cradle cap are also sometimes included in the spectrum of seborrheic dermatitis.

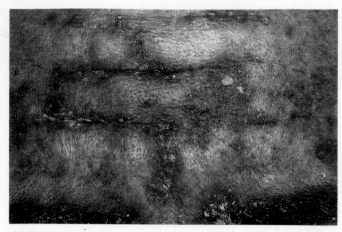

Fig 6–3
Seborrheic dermatitis. There are diffuse erythema and scaling of the forehead.
(Courtesy of the Institute of Dermatology, London.)

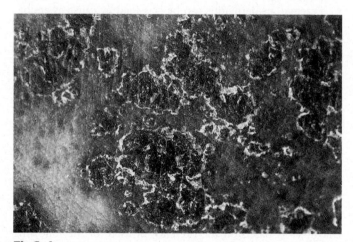

Fig 6–4
Seborrheic dermatitis. Note the marked scaling.
(Courtesy of the Institute of Dermatology, London.)

- Seborrheic dermatitis is one of the most common dermatoses seen in AIDS. It has also been associated with stress, HIV, and neurologic disorders, including Parkinson's disease.
- Treatment: topical ketoconazole, hydrocortisone. Second-line therapies include miconazole nitrate, lithium succinate, and selenium sulfide.

(3) Discoid eczema (nummular eczema)

- Dermatitis presenting clinically with single or multiple pruritic, coin-shaped, erythematous plaques with vesiculation, particularly involving the lower legs, forearms, and backs of the hands (Fig. 6–5)
- The absence of a raised border distinguishes it from ringworm.
- There are two peak ages at onset; it affects young women (15 to 30 years) and middle-aged adults of both genders.

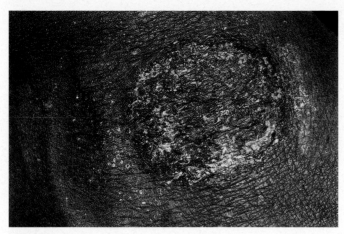

Fig 6–5
Discoid eczema. The lesion is sharply defined and there is a pronounced scale.
(Courtesy of the Institute of Dermatology, London.)

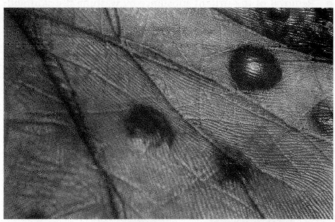

Fig 6–6
Pompholyx. Note the characterisitic tiny tense vesicles on the palm.
(Courtesy of Dr. R. A. Marsden, St. George's Hospital, London.)

B. EXOGENOUS ECZEMATOUS DERMATITIS

(1) Contact dermatitis

DEFINITION

Contact dermatitis is an acute or chronic skin inflammation, usually eczematous dermatitis, resulting from exposure to substances in the environment. It can be subdivided into irritant contact dermatitis (nonimmunologic physical and chemical alteration of the epidermis) and allergic contact dermatitis (delayed hypersensitivity reaction). Rhus dermatitis (poison ivy, poison oak, and poison sumac) is responsible for most cases of contact dermatitis. Other frequent causes of irritant contact dermatitis are soaps, detergents, and organic solvents.

PHYSICAL FINDINGS AND CLINICAL PRESENTATION

Irritant contact dermatitis

● Mild exposure may result in dryness, erythema, and fissuring of the affected area (e.g., hand involvement caused by exposure to soap, genital area involvement caused by prolonged exposure to wet diapers).

● Eczematous inflammation may result from chronic exposure.

Allergic contact dermatitis

● Poison ivy dermatitis can present with vesicles and blisters; linear lesions (as a result of dragging of the resins over the surface of the skin by scratching) are a classic presentation.

● The pattern of lesions is asymmetrical; itching, burning, and stinging may be present.

● The involved areas are erythematous, warm to the touch, swollen, and may be confused with cellulitis.

CAUSE

● Irritant contact dermatitis: cement (construction workers), rubber, ragweed, malathion (farmers), orange and lemon peel (chefs, bartenders), hair tints, shampoos (beauticians), rubber gloves (medical, surgical personnel; Fig. 6–7)

● Allergic contact dermatitis: poison ivy (Fig. 6–8), poison oak (Fig. 6–9), poison sumac (Fig. 6–10), rubber (shoe dermatitis), nickel (jewelry), balsam of Peru (hand and face dermatitis), neomycin, formaldehyde (cosmetics), acrylic in adhesive tape (Fig 6–11)

(4) Hand eczema (dyshidrotic eczema, pompholyx)

● Dermatitis characterized by a recurrent pruritic vesicular eruption of the palms, soles, or digits. Because of the increased thickness of the keratin layer at these sites, the vesicles appear as small pale papules before rupturing (Fig. 6–6).

● With the passage of time, the affected parts may show scaling and cracking. In most cases, the cause is unknown, although heat or psychological stress may precipitate attacks.

● Pompholyx is often associated with hyperhidrosis.

● Specific investigations include patch testing for contact allergens, potassium hydroxide preparation, and bacterial culture

● Treatment is aimed at control of pruritus and vesicobullous formation. Useful agents are topical or oral corticosteroids, oral antihistamines, antibiotics, PUVA, and UVA.

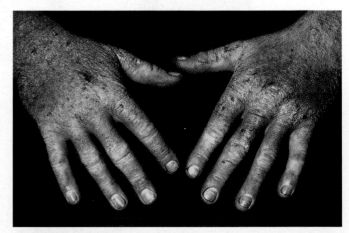

Fig 6–7
Contact dermatitis. This was caused by a reaction to rubber gloves.
(Courtesy of Dr. R. A. Marsden, St. George's Hospital, London.)

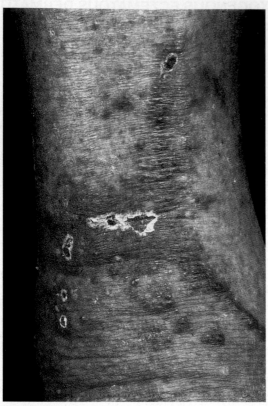

Fig 6–8
Contact dermatitis—severe reaction to poison ivy.
(Courtesy of the Institute of Dermatology, London.)

DIAGNOSIS
A diagnosis of contact dermatitis is made from the history and distribution of lesions and is confirmed by patch testing to the suspected allergen (Fig. 6–12).

DIFFERENTIAL DIAGNOSIS
- Impetigo (see Fig. 28–13)
- Lichen simplex chronicus (see Fig. 6–15)
- Atopic dermatitis (see Fig. 6–2).
- Nummular eczema (see Fig. 6–5)
- Seborrheic dermatitis (see Fig. 6–4)
- Psoriasis (see Fig. 28–13)
- Scabies (see Fig. 29–1)

LABORATORY TESTS
Patch testing is useful to confirm the diagnosis of contact dermatitis; it is indicated particularly when inflammation persists despite appropriate topical therapy and avoidance of suspected causative agent. Patch testing should not be used for irritant contact dermatitis because this is a nonimmunologically mediated inflammatory reaction.

TREATMENT
- Removal of the irritant substance by washing the skin with plain water or mild soap within 15 minutes of exposure is helpful for patients with poison ivy, poison oak, or poison sumac dermatitis.
- Cold or cool water compresses for 20 to 30 minutes five to six times daily for the initial 72 hours are effective during the acute blistering stage.
- Oral corticosteroids are generally reserved for severe, widespread dermatitis.

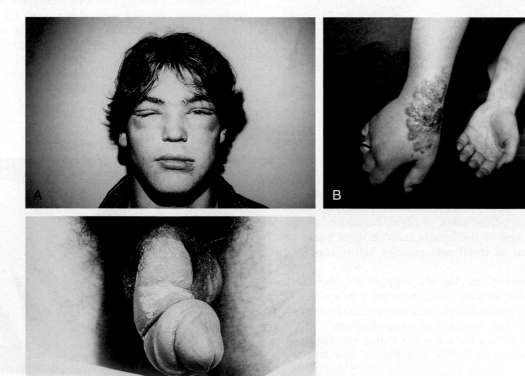

Fig 6–9
Acute poison oak dermatitis. **A**, Facial edema. **B**, Blisters. **C**, Penile edema.
(Courtesy of Axel Hoke.)

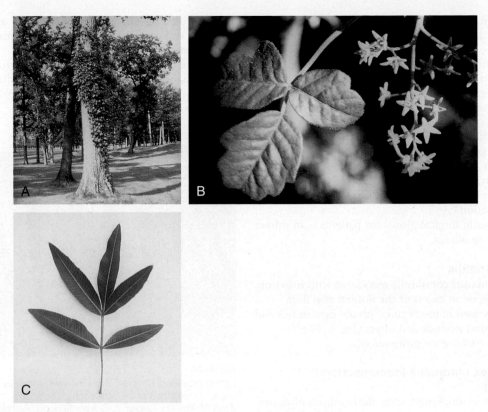

Fig 6–10
A, Poison ivy (*Toxicodendron radicans*). **B,** Poison oak (*Toxicodendron diversiloba*). **C**, Poison sumac (*Toxicodendron vernix*)
(From Auerbach P: Wilderness Medicine, 4th ed. St. Louis, Mosby, 2001.)

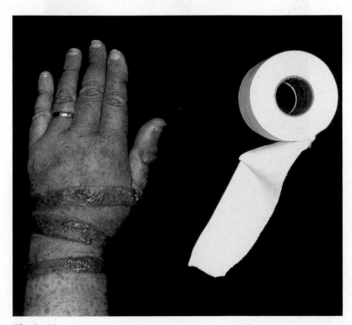

Fig 6–11
Acute allergic contact dermatitis caused by acrylic in "hypoallergenic" adhesive tape.
(From Fireman P: Atlas of Allergies and Immunology, 3rd ed. St. Louis, Mosby, 2006.)

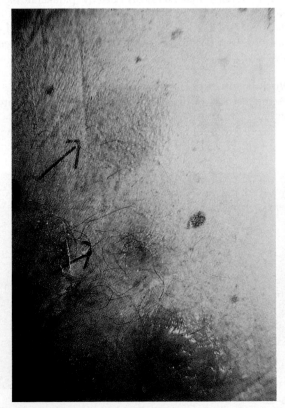

Fig 6–12
Patch test. These three positive reactions (*arrows*) were seen at 48 hours.
(Courtesy of Dr. R. A. Marsden, St. George's Hospital, London.)

- IM steroids are used for severe reactions and in patients requiring oral corticosteroids but unable to tolerate PO steroids.
- Oral antihistamines will control pruritus, especially at night; calamine lotion is also useful for pruritus but can lead to excessive drying.
- Colloidal oatmeal (Aveeno) baths can also provide symptomatic relief.
- Patients with mild to moderate erythema may respond to topical steroid gels or creams.
- Patients with a shoe allergy should change their socks at least once a day; use of aluminum chloride hexahydrate in a 20% solution (Drysol) every hour of sleep will also help control perspiration.
- Use hypoallergenic surgical gloves for patients with rubber and surgical glove allergy.

(2) Infective dermatitis

- Spongiotic dermatitis commonly associated with infection, usually *S. aureus* or an excess of the normal skin flora
- It is particularly seen in the flexures, on the ears, or feet and sometimes around wounds and ulcers (Fig. 6–13).
- Exudation and crusting are pronounced.

(3) Lichen simplex chronicus (circumscribed neurodermatitis)

- Localized areas of thickened scaly skin complicating prolonged and severe scratching in patients with no underlying dermatologic condition (Fig. 6–15)
- Biopsy reveals hyperkeratosis, patchy parakeratosis, and elongation of the rete ridges (Fig. 6–14).
- Patients present with profound pruritus and localized scaly plaques, with accentuated skin markings said to resemble tree bark.

(4) Nodular prurigo (prurigo nodularis)

- Dermatosis characterized by the development of chronic, intensely pruritic, lichenified, and excoriated nodules

- Individual lesions are often described as globular with a warty and excoriated surface and may measure up to 2 cm in diameter (Fig. 6–16).
- They are often grouped and symmetrical, occurring predominantly on extensor aspects of the distal limbs.
- The palms and soles are typically uninvolved.

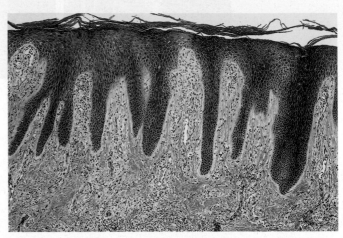

Fig 6–14
Lichen simplex chronicus. There is hyperkeratosis, patchy parakeratosis, and elongation of the rete ridges.
(From McKee PH, Calonje E, Granter SR [eds]. Pathology of the Skin With Clinical Correlations, 3rd ed. St. Louis, Mosby, 2005.)

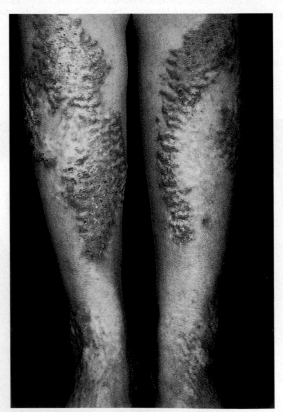

Fig 6–15
Lichen simplex chronicus. Thick, scaly erythematous plaques are present on the shins, a commonly affected site.
(Courtesy of Dr. R. A. Marsden, St. George's Hospital, London.)

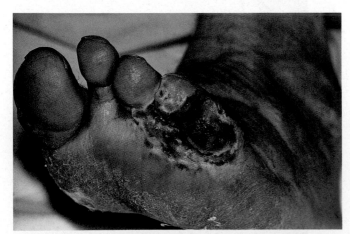

Fig 6–13
Infective dermatitis. Lesions affecting the foot web spaces are often caused by staphylococci or streptococci and are associated with excess sweating.
(Courtesy of Dr. R. A. Marsden, St. George's Hospital, London.)

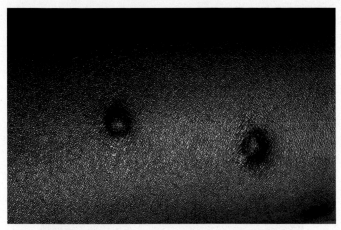

Fig 6–16
Nodular prurigo showing typical globular nodules; the intervening skin appears normal.
(Courtesy of Dr. R. A. Marsden, St. George's Hospital, London.)

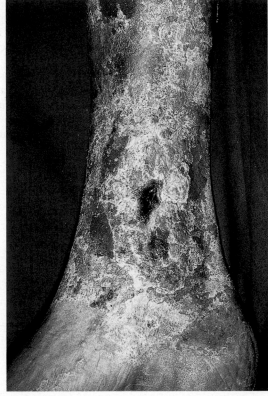

Fig 6–17
Stasis dermatitis. There are vesiculation, exudation, and crusting on the lower leg around a stasis ulcer, which were precipitated by allergy to the antibiotic dressing.
(Courtesy of Dr. R. A. Marsden, St. George's Hospital, London.)

- Psychosocial disorders have been reported in a high proportion of patients. Increased prevalence is noted with gluten enteropathy.
- Laboratory testing: HIV, ALT, AST, serum creatinine, serum IgE, histology with immunofluorescence
- Treatment: corticosteroids (PO, intralesional), occlusion, cryotherapy, UVB phototherapy, PUVA

(5) Stasis dermatitis

DEFINITION
Stasis dermatitis refers to an inflammatory skin disease of the lower extremities, commonly seen in older patients with chronic venous insufficiency.

PHYSICAL FINDINGS AND CLINICAL PRESENTATION
- Insidious onset of pruritic, erythematous, scaly, eczematous patches commonly located over the medial malleolus
- Progressive pigment changes can occur as a result of extravasation of red blood cells and hemosiderin deposition within the cutaneous tissue (Fig. 6–17).
- Secondary infections can occur.

CAUSE
Stasis dermatitis is thought to occur as a direct result from any insult or injury of the lower extremity venous system leading to venous insufficiency. Common causative factors include venous insufficiency, deep vein thrombosis, trauma, pregnancy, vein stripping, and vein harvesting in patients requiring coronary artery bypass grafting (CABG),

DIFFERENTIAL DIAGNOSIS
- Contact dermatitis (see Fig. 6–7)
- Atopic dermatitis (see Fig. 6–2)
- Cellulitis (see Fig. 28–1)
- Tinea dermatophyte infection (see Fig. 26–1)
- Pretibial myxedema

- Nummular eczema (see Fig. 6–5)
- Lichen simplex chronicus (see Fig. 6–15)
- Ichthyosis (see Fig. 21–2)
- Deep vein thrombosis (see Fig. 122–2)

TREATMENT
- Leg elevation
- Compression stocking with a gradient of at least 30 to 40 mm Hg
- For weeping skin lesions, wet to dry dressing changes are helpful.
- In patients with acute stasis dermatitis, a compression (Unna) boot can be applied. An Unna boot consists of a roll of gauze that is saturated with zinc oxide ointment supported with an elastic wrap.
- Topical corticosteroid creams or ointments are used frequently to help reduce inflammation and itching.
- Secondary infections should be treated with appropriate antibiotics. Most secondary infections are the result of *Staphylococcus* or *Streptococcus* organisms.

(6) PITYRIASIS ALBA

- Common form of chronic dermatitis usually affecting pre-adolescent children; prevalence in the U.S. population is 2%
- The skin lesions are seen most commonly on the face (Fig. 6–18).
- Early lesions present as slightly scaly, mildly pruritic, round to oval pink plaques measuring from 0.5 to more than 5.0 cm in diameter, which later appear as scaly hypopigmented lesions.
- The condition usually resolves spontaneously after months or years.

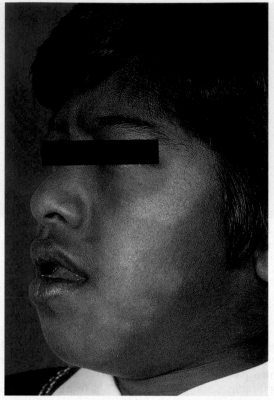

Fig 6–18
Pityriasis alba. There is striking leukoderma on the cheek and chin, which are commonly affected sites.
(Courtesy of Dr. R. A. Marsden, St. George's Hospital, London.)

Chapter 7 | Psoriasis

DEFINITION

Psoriasis is a chronic skin disorder characterized by excessive proliferation of keratinocytes, resulting in the formation of thickened scaly plaques, itching, and inflammatory changes of the epidermis and dermis. The various forms of psoriasis include guttate, pustular, and arthritis variants.

PHYSICAL FINDINGS AND CLINICAL PRESENTATION

- The primary psoriatic lesion is an erythematous papule topped by a loosely adherent scale (Fig. 7–1). Scraping the scale results in several bleeding points (Auspitz sign).
- Chronic plaque psoriasis generally manifests with symmetrical, sharply demarcated, erythematous, silver-scaled patches affecting primarily the intergluteal folds, elbows, scalp, fingernails, toenails, and knees (Fig. 7–2). This form accounts for 80% of psoriasis cases.
- Psoriasis can also develop at the site of any physical trauma (sunburn, scratching). This is known as *Koebner's phenomenon.*
- Nail involvement is common (pitting of the nail plate), resulting in hyperkeratosis, and onychodystrophy, with onycholysis .
- Pruritus is variable.
- Joint involvement can result in sacroiliitis and spondylitis.
- Guttate psoriasis is generally preceded by streptococcal pharyngitis and manifests with multiple droplike lesions on the extremities and trunk (Fig. 7–3).

CAUSE

- Unknown
- Familial clustering (genetic transmission with a dominant mode with variable penetrants)
- One third of persons affected have a positive family history.
- Within the past decade, several putative loci for genetic susceptibility to psoriasis have been reported. One locus (psoriasis susceptibility 1 [PSORS1] locus) in the major histocompatibility complex (MHC) region on chromosome 6 is considered the most important susceptibility locus.

DIFFERENTIAL DIAGNOSIS

- Contact dermatitis (see Fig. 6–7)
- Atopic dermatitis (see Fig. 6–2)
- Stasis dermatitis (see Fig. 6–17)
- Tinea (see Fig. 26–1)
- Nummular dermatitis (see Fig. 6–5)
- Candidiasis (see Fig. 26–9)
- Mycosis fungoides (see Fig. 316–11)
- Cutaneous SLE (see Fig. 293–2)
- Secondary and tertiary syphilis (see Fig. 226–14)
- Drug eruption (see Fig. 14–2)

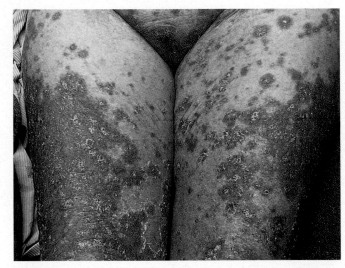

Fig 7–2
Psoriasis. Typical plaque disease shows a bilateral and fairly symmetrical distribution. In this example, the silvery scale is well demonstrated. (Courtesy of Dr. J. Kerner, Harvard Medical School, Boston.)

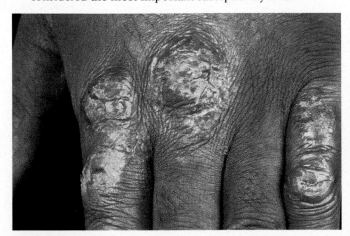

Fig 7–1
Plaque psoriasis—close-up view showing the thick scale.
(Courtesy of the Institute of Dermatology, London.)

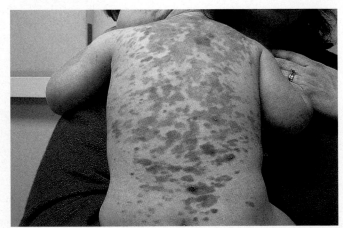

Fig 7–3
Guttate psoriasis. This infant shows a characteristic distribution over the trunk.
(Courtesy of Dr. M. Liang, Children's Hospital, Boston.)

LABORATORY TESTS
- Generally not necessary for diagnosis
- Diagnosis is clinical.
- Skin biopsy is rarely necessary.

TREATMENT
- Sunbathing generally leads to improvement.
- Eliminate triggering factors (e.g., stress, certain medications [lithium, beta blockers, antimalarials]).
- Patients with psoriasis benefit from a daily bath in warm water followed by the application of a cream or ointment moisturizer. Regular use of an emollient moisturizer limits evaporation of water from the skin and allows the stratum corneum to rehydrate itself.

- Therapeutic options vary according to the extent of disease. Approximately 70% to 80% of all patients can be treated adequately with topical therapy.
- Patients with limited disease (less than 20% of the body) can be treated with topical steroids, calcipotriene, tar products, anthralin, and retinoids.
- Therapeutic options for persons with generalized disease (affecting more than 20% of the body) include UVB light exposure three times weekly and oral PUVA. Systemic treatment includes methotrexate and cyclosporine for severe psoriasis. Chronic plaque psoriasis may be treated with alefacept, a recombinant protein that selectively targets T lymphocytes or etanercept, a tumor necrosis factor (TNF) antagonist.

Chapter 8   Lichen planus

DEFINITION

Lichen planus refers to a papular skin eruption characteristically found over the flexor surfaces of the extremities, genitalia, and mucous membranes. It is often associated with other autoimmune disorders (e.g., primary biliary cirrhosis, hepatitis C infection, myasthenia gravis, ulcerative colitis, diabetes).

PHYSICAL FINDINGS AND CLINICAL PRESENTATION

- Usually starts on an extremity and may remain localized or can spread to involve other areas over a 1- to 4-month period
- The rash is pruritic and may involve the flexor surfaces of the wrists (Fig. 8–1), forearms, shins, upper thighs, neck and back area, scalp, nails, oral mucosa, buccal mucosa, tongue, gingiva, lips (Fig. 8–2), and genital mucosa.
- Lesions may be annular (more common) or linear. A reticular pattern is often noted on oral mucosa and genital areas.
- Lesion morphology: papules (flat, smooth, and shiny) are the most common presentation. Hypertrophic, follicular, or vesicular morphology may also be found.
- Color: dark red, bluish red, purplish-violaceous color is noted in cutaneous lichen planus. Individual lesions characteristically have white lines visible *(Wickham's striae)*. Oral and genital lichen planus have a reticular network of white lines that may be raised or annular in appearance.

CAUSE

- The cause of lichen planus is unknown.

DIFFERENTIAL DIAGNOSIS

- Drug eruption (see Fig. 14–2)
- Psoriasis (see Fig. 7–2)
- Bowen's disease (see Fig. 22–15)
- Leukoplakia (see Fig. 89–36)
- Candidiasis (see Fig. 26–9)
- SLE (see Fig. 293–1)
- Secondary syphilis (see Fig. 226–14)
- Seborrheic dermatitis (see Fig. 6–4)

DIAGNOSIS

If the diagnosis is questionable, a skin biopsy is performed.

TREATMENT

Cutaneous lichen planus

- Topical steroids with occlusion twice daily
- Acitretin 30 mg/day PO for 8 week
- Systemic prednisone, 30 to 60 mg/day as a starting dose and tapered to 15 to 20 mg/day maintenance for 6 weeks
- Intradermal steroid can be tried for thick hyperkeratotic lesions.
- Hydroxyzine can be used for pruritus.
- Spontaneous remissions of cutaneous lichen planus occur in over 65% of cases within the first year.

Oral lichen planus

- Topical steroid for 9 weeks
- Topical retinoids in an adhesive base or gel
- Etretinate, 75 mg/day for 2 months
- Spontaneous remission of oral lichen planus usually occurs by 5 years.
- Approximately 10% to 20% of patients will have a recurrence.

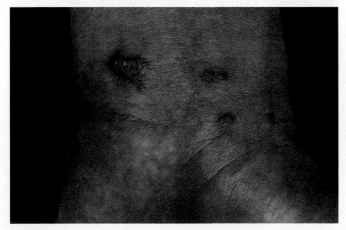

Fig 8–1
Lichen planus. There are typical flat-topped polygonal papules on the anterior aspect of the wrist.
(Courtesy of Dr. R. A. Marsden, St. George's Hospital, London.)

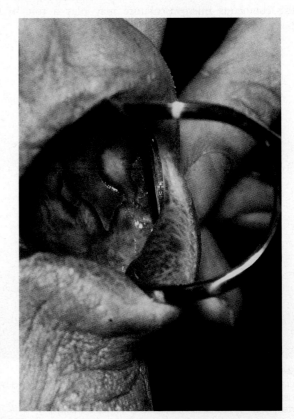

Fig 8–2
Lichen planus. There is extensive ulceration of the buccal mucosa.
(Courtesy of Dr. R. A. Marsden, St. George's Hospital, London.)

Chapter 9   Hypersensitivity syndromes

A. ERYTHEMA MULTIFORME

DEFINITION

Erythema multiforme is an inflammatory disease believed to be secondary to immune complex formation and subsequent deposition in the skin and mucous membranes. It is often associated with herpes simplex and other infectious agents (*Mycoplasma pneumoniae*), drugs (bupropion), and connective tissue diseases.

PHYSICAL FINDINGS AND CLINICAL PRESENTATION

- Symmetrical skin lesions with a classic target appearance, caused by the centrifugal spread of red macular papules to a circumference of 1 to 3 cm with a purpuric, cyanotic, or vesicular center, are present (Fig. 9–1)
- Lesions are most common on the back of the hands and feet and extensor aspects of the forearms and legs (Fig. 9–2). Trunk involvement can occur in severe cases.
- Urticarial papules, vesicles, and bullae may also be present and generally indicate a more severe form of the disease.
- Individual lesions heal in 1 or 2 weeks without scarring.
- Bullae and erosions may also be present in the oral cavity (Fig. 9–3).

CAUSE

- Immune complex formation and subsequent deposition in the cutaneous microvasculature may play a role in the pathogenesis of erythema multiforme.

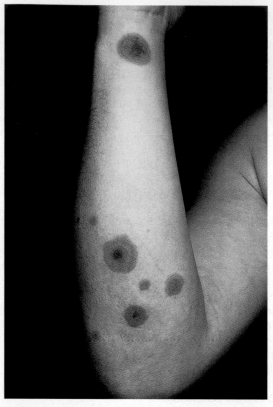

Fig 9–2
Erythema multiforme—multiple target lesions on the arm.
(Courtesy of the Institute of Dermatology, London.)

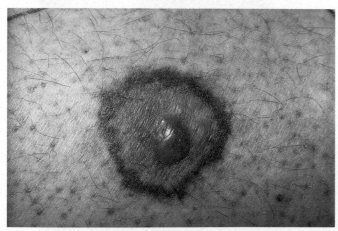

Fig 9–1
Target lesion. This is characterized by a central blister surrounded by an edematous ring and an outer erythematous border.
(Courtesy of Dr. R. A. Marsden, St. George's Hospital, London.)

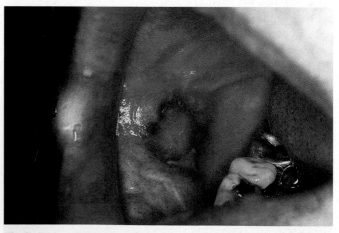

Fig 9–3
Erythema multiforme. There is a large ulcer on the buccal mucosa.
(Courtesy of Dr. P. Morgan, London.)

DIFFERENTIAL DIAGNOSIS
- Chronic urticaria (see Fig. 15–7)
- Secondary syphilis (see Fig. 226–14)
- Pityriasis rosea (see Fig. 27–34)
- Contact dermatitis (see Fig. 6–8)
- Pemphigus vulgaris (see Fig. 5–3)
- Lichen planus (see Fig. 8–1)
- Serum sickness
- Drug eruption (see Fig. 14–1)
- Granuloma annulare (see Fig. 11–5)

LABORATORY TESTS
- CBC with differential
- ANA
- Serology for *M. pneumoniae*

TREATMENT
- Mild cases generally do not require treatment; lesions resolve spontaneously within 1 month.
- Potential drug precipitants should be removed.
- Treatment of associated diseases (e.g., acyclovir for herpes simplex, erythromycin for *Mycoplasma* infection).
- Prednisone, 40 to 80 mg/day for 1 to 3 weeks may be tried for patients with many target lesions; however, the role of systemic steroids remains controversial.
- Levamisole, an immunomodulator, may be effective in the treatment of patients with chronic or recurrent oral lesions.

B. TOXIC EPIDERMAL NECROLYSIS AND STEVENS-JOHNSON SYNDROME

Toxic epidermal necrolysis (TEN, Lyell's syndrome) and Stevens-Johnson syndrome (SJS) are part of a spectrum of potentially life-threatening conditions manifesting with widespread epidermal loss and significant involvement of mucous membranes. They represent severe drug hypersensitivity reactions.
- Classification of these disorders is based on the extent of detachable skin at the worst stage of illness.
- In TEN, 30% or more of the skin is involved (Fig. 9–4), whereas in SJS less than 10% is affected.
- An intermediate category, in which 10% to 30% of the skin is involved, has also been recognized.

- Both disorders are rare (incidence is 0.5 cases/million in the United States.

DEFINITION
Stevens-Johnson syndrome is a severe vesiculobullous form of erythema multiforme.

PHYSICAL FINDINGS AND CLINICAL PRESENTATION
- The cutaneous eruption is generally preceded by vague, nonspecific symptoms of low-grade fever and fatigue occurring 1 to 14 days before the skin lesions. Cough is often present. Fever may be high during the active stages.
- Bullae generally occur on the conjunctiva (Fig. 9–5), mucous membranes of the mouth, nares, and genital regions.
- Corneal ulcerations may result in blindness.
- Ulcerative stomatitis results in hemorrhagic crusting.
- Flat, atypical target lesions or purpuric maculae may be distributed on the trunk or be widespread.
- The pain from oral lesions may compromise fluid intake and result in dehydration (Fig. 9–6).
- Thick mucopurulent sputum and oral lesions may interfere with breathing.

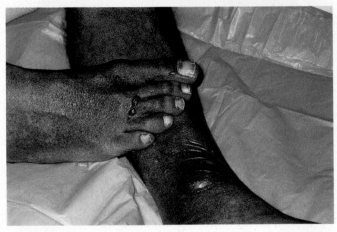

Fig 9–4
Toxic epidermal necrosis—early stage showing a large fluid-filled blister. (Courtesy of Dr. R. Reynolds, Harvard Medical School, Boston.)

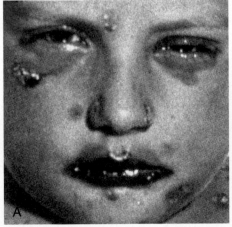
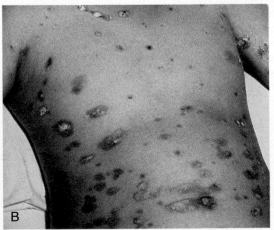

Fig 9–5
Acute phase of Stevens-Johnson syndrome. This child has the typical target-shaped macular skin lesions.
A, Lesions on the head, with an associated blepharoconjuctivitis. **B,** Lesions on the trunk.
(From Yanoff M, Duker JS: Ophthalmology, 2nd ed. St. Louis, 2004, Mosby.)

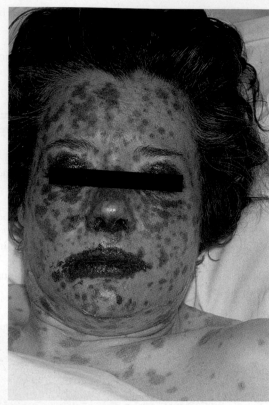

Fig 9–6
Stevens-Johnson syndrome. This patient developed Stevens-Johnson syndrome following sulfonamide therapy.
(Courtesy of Dr. R. A. Marsden, St. George's Hospital, London.)

CAUSE
- Drugs (e.g., phenytoin, penicillins, phenobarbital, sulfonamides) are the most common cause.
- Upper respiratory tract infections (e.g., *M. pneumoniae*) and herpes simplex viral infections have also been implicated in SJS.

DIFFERENTIAL DIAGNOSIS
- Pemphigus (see Fig. 5–2)
- Pemphigoid (see Fig. 4–2)
- Urticaria (see Fig. 15–7)
- Serum sickness
- Staphylococcal scalded-skin syndrome (see Fig. 28–7)
- Behçet's syndrome (see Fig. 16–14)

LABORATORY TESTS
- CBC with differential, cultures in cases of suspected infection
- Skin biopsy is generally reserved for cases in which classic lesions are absent and diagnosis is uncertain.

IMAGING STUDIES
- Chest x-ray may show patchy changes in patients with pulmonary involvement.

TREATMENT
- Withdrawal of any potential drug precipitants
- Careful skin nursing to prevent secondary infection
- Treatment of associated conditions, (e.g., acyclovir for herpes simplex virus infection, erythromycin for *Mycoplasma* infection)
- Antihistamines for pruritus
- Treatment of the cutaneous blisters with cool, wet Burow's compresses
- Relief of oral symptoms by frequent rinsing with lidocaine (Xylocaine Viscous)
- Liquid or soft diet with plenty of fluids to ensure proper hydration
- Treatment of secondary infections with antibiotics
- Corticosteroids: use remains controversial; when used, prednisone, 20 to 30 mg twice daily, until new lesions no longer appear, then rapidly tapered
- Topical steroids: may use to treat papules and plaques; however, should not be applied to eroded areas
- Vitamin A: may be used for lacrimal hyposecretion
- Prognosis varies with severity of disease. It is generally good in patients with limited disease; however, mortality may approach 10% in patients with extensive involvement.
- Oral lesions may continue for several months.
- Scarring and corneal abnormalities may occur in 20% of patients.

Chapter 10   **Superficial and deep perivascular inflammatory dermatoses**

A. ERYTHEMA ANNULARE CENTRIFUGUM

DEFINITION

This type of dermatosis is caused by a hypersensitivity reaction to various factors (e.g., infection, medication, neoplasia, autoimmune disease).

PHYSICAL FINDINGS AND CLINICAL PRESENTATION

- It is characterized by annular erythematous lesions (Fig. 10–1) that may remain stationary or gradually expand at a rate of 2 to 3 mm/day.
- The lesions are well circumscribed with raised edges and a slight scaling that tends to trail behind the advancing margin. With time, central clearing is seen.
- Some clinicians have divided the disease into two distinctive subtypes, superficial and deep gyrate erythema. The superficial variant is associated with pruritus and has a trailing scale. The deep variant is characterized by erythematous annular lesions with indurated borders but lacking a scale.

DIFFERENTIAL DIAGNOSIS

- Viral exanthemata (see Fig. 27–32)
- SLE (see Fig. 293–1)
- Pityriasis rosea (see Fig. 27–34)
- Hypersensitivity reaction (see Fig. 14–1)

LABORATORY TESTS

- Histologic examination
- KOH of lesion in suspected dermatophyte infection
- CBC, ALT, urinalysis
- PPD (purified protein derivative)

IMAGING STUDIES

- Chest x-ray

TREATMENT

- Withdrawal of any potential drug precipitants
- Therapy of underlying condition
- Antipruritics
- Corticosteroids

B. POLYMORPHOUS LIGHT ERUPTION (PHOTODERMATITIS)

DEFINITION

This dermatosis usually presents in young people with recurrent erythematous papules, vesicles, and/or plaques following exposure to UV light (Fig. 10–2). The disease is more common in people residing in northern latitudes, occurring most often in spring and summer.

PHYSICAL FINDINGS AND CLINICAL PRESENTATION

- The face, chest, upper back, and extremities are the most common sites of involvement.
- Most patients require less than 30 minutes of associated sun exposure to elicit clinical lesions. Onset of lesions following light exposure typically takes 18 to 24 hours.
- The UVA or UVB part of the light spectrum may cause lesions. In cases for which the diagnosis is in doubt, phototesting may be necessary.

DIAGNOSIS

- Skin biopsy, phototesting, ANA, lupus antibodies

DIFFERENTIAL DIAGNOSIS

- Reticular erythematous mucinosis; (clinically, polymorphous light eruption resolves once exposure to sunlight has ceased in contrast to the persistent lesions of reticular erythematous mucinosis.
- Lymphocytic infiltration; histologically, the presence of marked papillary edema favors polymorphic light eruption.
- SLE; most cases of polymorphic light eruption are negative with immunofluorescence testing.

TREATMENT

- Limitation of sun exposure, sunscreens and protective clothing, PUVA therapy, narrow band or broadband phototherapy

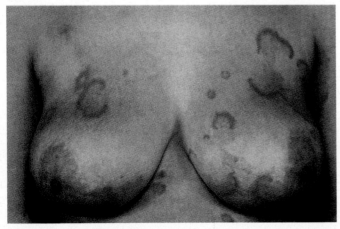

Fig 10–1
Erythema annulare centrifugum—typical bilateral annular lesions involving the chest, breasts, abdomen, and arms.
(Courtesy of Dr. R. A. Marsden, St. George's Hospital, London.)

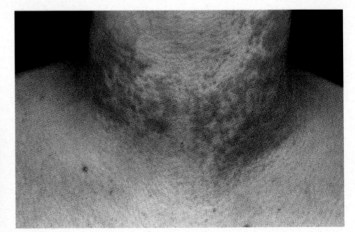

Fig 10–2
Polymorphous light eruption. The eruption is typically symmetrical and usually pruritic.
(Courtesy of the Institute of Dermatology, London.)

C. URTICARIAL VASCULITIS

- Uncommon condition characterized clinically by chronic urticaria (Fig. 10–3) and histologically by leukocytoclastic venulitis
- In addition to urticarial skin lesions, patients may have angioedema, arthralgia, gastrointestinal symptoms, and evidence of renal involvement.
- Urticarial vasculitis is often associated with or heralds the onset of several systemic disorders, including SLE, connective tissue disease, inflammatory bowel disease, interstitial lung disease, hepatitis, Wegener's granulomatosis, and hepatitis.
- Treatment: antihistamines, corticosteroids, doxepin, treatment of underlying disorder

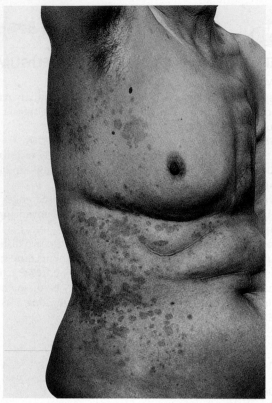

Fig 10–3
Urticarial vasculitis. Note the urticaria with a livid hue.
(Courtesy of Dr. J. Newton, St. Thomas' Hospital, London.)

| Chapter 11 | **Granulomatous and necrobiotic dermatoses** |

A. SARCOIDOSIS

- Systemic disease characterized by the presence of noncaseating granulomata, usually (but not invariably) affecting multiple organ systems. Section 6.10a describes this disorder in more detail.

- Cutaneous lesions occur in 20% to 35% of patients with systemic sarcoidosis and may be classified into nonspecific (erythema nodosum) and specific (granulomatous) subtypes.

- Cutaneous sarcoidal granulomata (Fig. 11–1) appear to be associated with a poorer prognosis and an increased incidence of pulmonary fibrosis and uveitis.

- Erythema nodosum occurs commonly in sarcoidosis (incidence, 11% to 30%). It presents as erythematous, tender, subcutaneous nodules, usually on the anterior tibial regions (Figs. 11–2 and 11–3).

- A not uncommon mode of presentation is the development of a widespread, usually asymptomatic, maculopapular eruption. Individual lesions are erythematous or violaceous, 3 to 6 mm in diameter, and most commonly seen on the face.

- Most characteristic of sarcoidosis, however, is lupus pernio (Fig. 11–4). This chronic violaceous plaque most often affects the nose, cheeks, and ears. It is a particularly disfiguring variant and resolution is especially complicated by marked scarring. *Lupus pernio* is often associated with lesions in the upper respiratory tract and can be followed by nasal obstruction and septal perforation.

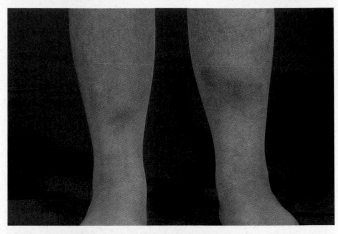

Fig 11–2
Erythema nodosum. Shown are typical erythematous nodules on the shins of a young woman.
(Courtesy of the Institute of Dermatology, London.)

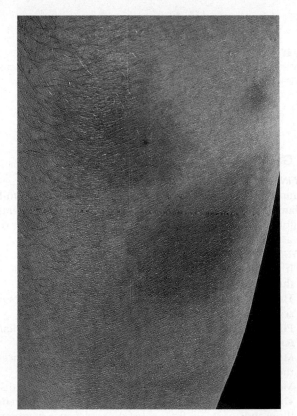

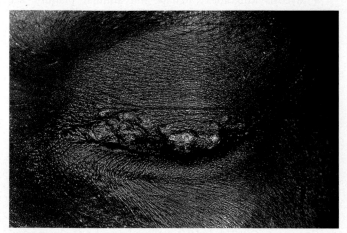

Fig 11–1
Sarcoidosis. This nodular sarcoid is producing beaded lesions on the upper eyelids. Sarcoidosis is common in blacks.
(Courtesy of Dr. R.A. Marsden, St. George's Hospital, London.)

Fig 11–3
Erythema nodosum—close-up view of the same patient as shown in Figure 11–2.
(Courtesy of the Institute of Dermatology, London.)

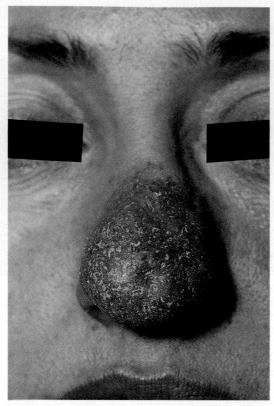

Fig 11–4
Sarcoidosis—lupus pernio. The nose shows typical scaly violaceous swelling.
(Courtesy of the Institute of Dermatology, London.)

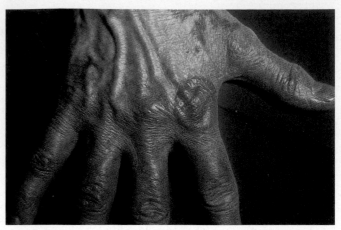

Fig 11–5
Localized granuloma annulare—a typical annular lesion over the knuckle. Stretching of the skin reveals a translucent beaded margin.
(Courtesy of Dr. R. A. Marsden, St. George's Hospital, London.)

B. GRANULOMA ANNULARE

DEFINITION
Granuloma annulare (GA) is a chronic, usually self-limited, inflammatory disorder of the dermis that classically presents as arciform to annular plaques located on the extremities. It is often associated with diabetes mellitus.

PHYSICAL FINDINGS AND CLINICAL PRESENTATION
- It often begins as small ring of colored skin or pale erythematous papules.
- The papules coalesce and evolve into annular plaques over several weeks.
- Plaques undergo central involution and increase in diameter over several months (0.5 to 5 cm).
- Most frequently found on the lateral and dorsal surfaces of the hands (Fig. 11–5) and feet
- Most lesions resolve spontaneously after several months.
- The generalized form of GA is characterized by hundreds to thousands of small, flesh-colored papules in a symmetrical distribution on the trunk and extremities.
- Deep dermal (subcutaneous GA) presents as large, painless, skin-colored nodules that are frequently mistaken for rheumatoid nodules.

CAUSE
Unknown, but may be related to vasculitis, trauma, monocyte activation, or delayed hypersensitivity

DIFFERENTIAL DIAGNOSIS
- Tinea corporis (see Fig. 26–1)
- Lichen planus (see Fig. 8–1)
- Necrobiosis lipoidica diabeticorum (see Fig. 11–6)
- Sarcoidosis (see Fig. 11–1)
- Rheumatoid nodules (see Fig. 11–7)
- Syphilis (late secondary or tertiary syphilis; see Fig. 226–14)
- Mycosis fungoides (arcuate and annular plaques; see Fig. 316–11)

LABORATORY TESTS
- There are no laboratory tests that will help confirm the diagnosis. Diagnosis is based on clinical appearance and presentation.
- Biopsy when diagnosis is unclear. Biopsy shows focal degeneration of collagen and elastic fibers, mucin deposition, and perivascular and interstitial lymphohistiocytic infiltrate in the upper and mid dermis.

TREATMENT
- Reassurance, given the self-limited and benign nature of GA
- High-potency topical corticosteroids, with or without occlusion, and intralesional steroid injection into elevated border with triamcinolone are useful first-line local therapies.
- Cryosurgery, PUVA or UVA-1 therapy, and CO_2 laser treatment can also be used.
- Systemic agents (e.g., nicotinamide, chloroquine, cyclosporine) are generally reserved for severe cases.
- Most lesions will resolve spontaneously within 2 years.

C. NECROBIOSIS LIPOIDICA

DEFINITION
This disease has a strong association with diabetes mellitus. It has been suggested that the lesions develop as a consequence of diabetic microangiopathy.

PHYSICAL FINDINGS AND CLINICAL PRESENTATION
- The characteristic lesion, sometimes referred to as a sclerodermatous plaque, is round or oval and circumscribed, and often has a slightly elevated rim. It is typically a few millimeters to several centimeters in diameter.
- Newly acquired lesions are often red-brown in color (Fig. 11–6) but, with progression, the center of the lesion becomes yellowish and the peripheral border may acquire a violaceous hue.
- Larger plaques are usually irregular and more variably shaped. Scaling and telangiectasia may become evident.
- Ulceration appears to be relatively frequent and has been reported in up to 13% of patients.

DIAGNOSIS
- Skin biopsy
- Fasting blood sugar (FBS), 2-hour postprandial glucose

TREATMENT
- Improve glycemic control
- Intralesional or topical corticosteroids under occlusion

D. RHEUMATOID NODULE

DEFINITION
Rheumatoid nodules are subcutaneous lesions that develop at sites of trauma or at pressure points in almost 30% of adults with rheumatoid arthritis.

PHYSICAL FINDINGS AND CLINICAL PRESENTATION
- They are most commonly found on the extensor aspects of the forearms and elbows (particularly the olecranon process), feet, knuckles (Fig. 11–7), buttocks, scalp, and back.
- Rheumatoid nodules are more commonly found in patients with severe rheumatoid arthritis and are associated with a high titer of rheumatoid factor, joint erosions, and an increased incidence of rheumatoid vasculitis. They are not, however, specific for rheumatoid arthritis, being found in approximately 5% to 7% of patients with SLE and occasionally in those with seronegative ankylosing spondylitis.
- Rheumatoid nodules are typically located in the subcutaneous fat or soft tissues, although they may extend into the deeper reticular dermis.

DIFFERENTIAL DIAGNOSIS
- Granuloma annulare (location is generally more superficial, tends to have more mucin deposition and less fibrin than typical rheumatoid nodule) (see Fig. 11–5)
- Necrobiosis lipoidica (location is much more superficial) (see Fig. 11–6)
- Rheumatic fever nodule (histology reveals fine fibroid strands at center)
- Epithelioid sarcoid (biopsy reveals nuclear atypia, pleomorphism)

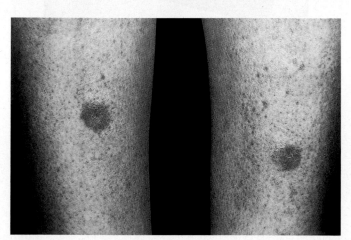

Fig 11–6
Necrobiosis lipoidica—symmetrical early lesions with erythema. (Courtesy of the Institute of Dermatology, London.)

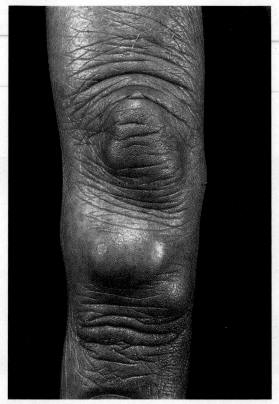

Fig 11–7
Rheumatoid nodules. Lesions on the knuckles are commonly seen in rheumatoid arthritis. (Courtesy of the Institute of Dermatology, London.)

Chapter 12   **Porphyria cutanea tarda**

DEFINITION

Porphyria cutanea tarda (PCT) is a term encompassing several related disorders caused by reduced hepatic uroporphyrinogen decarboxylase (UROD) enzyme activity. The excess porphyrins result in cutaneous photosensitivity. PCT is the most common type of porphyria. It usually manifests in middle age and shows a marked male predominance.

CAUSE

- There are two main forms, familial and sporadic.
- The familial form exhibits an autosomal dominant inheritance and its onset is earlier than the sporadic form.
- The disease is related to many different mutations in the *UROD* gene. Eighty percent of patients have the sporadic form.
- PCT may be precipitated by many exogenous factors, including alcohol abuse, iron overload, childbirth, and sun exposure. Hepatitis C and HIV infection are also often associated with PCT.

PHYSICAL FINDINGS AND CLINICAL PRESENTATION

- Typically, blisters occur on light-exposed skin and are traumatically or actinically induced (Figs. 12–1 and 12–2).
- Cutaneous fragility is usually marked. The blisters are slow to heal and leave superficial atrophic scars. Hypertrichosis and premature aging with chronic actinic damage usually occur and sclerodermatous changes may be marked (Fig. 12–3).

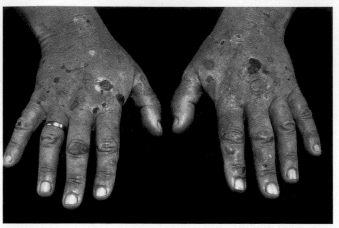

Fig 12–2

Porphyria cutanea tarda. There are numerous ruptured blisters. Milia are also evident.

(Courtesy of the Institute of Dermatology, London.)

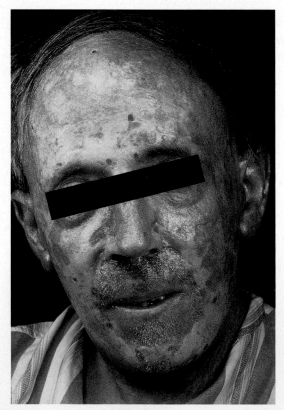

Fig 12–3

Porphyria cutanea tarda. There is marked facial scarring, with sclerodermiform features.

(Courtesy of Dr. G. Murphy, Beaumont Hospital, Dublin.)

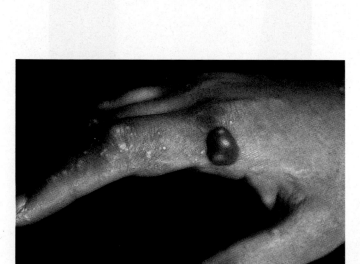

Fig 12–1

Porphyria cutanea tarda. In addition to a blood-filled vesicle, there are numerous milia.

(Courtesy of Dr. G. Murphy, Beaumont Hospital, Dublin.)

LABORATORY TESTS

- Laboratory testing includes porphyrin levels in plasma, urine and feces, ALT, AST, serum ferritin, hepatitis C serology, HIV, FBS, and ANA.
- Direct immunofluorescence of biopsy specimens reveals immunoglobulin (particularly IgG and, to a lesser extent, IgM) in the papillary dermis (Fig. 12–4).
- The diagnosis is confirmed by the presence of uroporphyrin and heptacarboxylic porphyrins in urine and plasma and by the presence of isocoproporphyrin in feces.

TREATMENT

- Protect skin from sunlight exposure and trauma.
- Ferrodepletion by serial phlebotomy or desferrioxamine chelation
- Increase porphyrin excretion with chloroquine.
- Antiviral drugs for PCT associated with hepatitis C or HIV

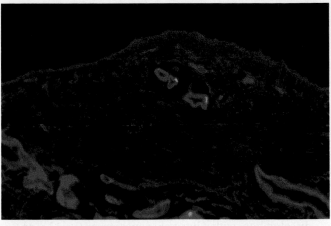

Fig 12–4
Porphyria cutanea tarda. The superficial blood vessels show striking IgG circumferential deposition (direct immunofluorescence).
(From McKee PH, Calonje E, Granter SR [eds]: Pathology of the Skin With Clinical Correlations, 3rd ed. St. Louis, Mosby, 2005.)

Chapter 13   Pellagra

DEFINITION

Pellagra is a disorder caused by deficiency of nicotinic acid (niacin, vitamin B_3) or its precursor, tryptophan.

CAUSE

- Dietary deficiency (alcoholism, malabsorption, anorexia nervosa, socioeconomic deprivation)
- Carcinoid tumors (excessive use of tryptophan, which produces serotonin)

PHYSICAL FINDINGS AND CLINICAL PRESENTATION

- The skin eruption is photosensitive. An initial, painful, sunburn-like erythema subsides to leave a dusky brownish discoloration, with a dry scaly appearance (Fig. 13–1A).
- Other features sometimes present include cheilosis, glossitis, angular stomatitis, and oral or perianal sores.

TREATMENT

- Nutritional supplementation with niacin will improve the appearance of skin lesions (see Fig. 13–1B).

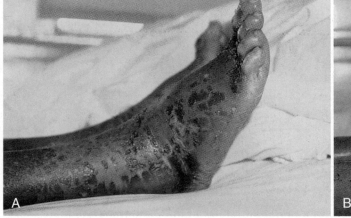 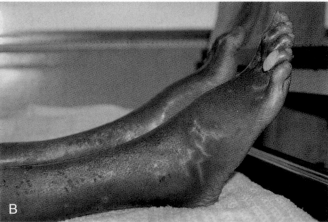

Fig 13–1
Legs and feet of a patient with niacin deficiency. **A,** Before therapy. **B,** After therapy.
(From Swartz MH: Textbook of Physical Diagnosis, 5th ed. Philadelphia, WB Saunders, 2006.)

Chapter 14 | **Cutaneous adverse reactions to drugs**

A. EXANTHEMATOUS (MORBILLIFORM, MACULOPAPULAR) REACTIONS

DEFINITION
These are the most frequently encountered adverse drug reactions. Patients who have infectious mononucleosis are particularly at risk of developing an exanthematous reaction following therapy with ampicillin or amoxicillin.

CAUSE
- They most commonly develop within 1 to 2 weeks of starting the drug.
- Penicillins, sulfonamides, trimethoprim, and phenytoin are especially incriminated.

PHYSICAL FINDINGS AND CLINICAL PRESENTATION
- Clinical presentation: patients present with erythematous macules and papules (Fig. 14–1) that with progression may become confluent or even acquire gyrate or polycyclic features.
- Pruritus, low-grade fever, and eosinophilia are sometimes present. The eruption is often symmetrical and usually presents on the trunk and extremities or sites of pressure and trauma.

DIFFERENTIAL DIAGNOSIS
- Scarlet fever (see Fig. 93–1)
- Measles (see Fig. 27–25)
- Rubella (see Fig. 27–28)

B. PHOTOTOXIC AND PHOTOALLERGIC REACTIONS

DEFINITION
Photosensitization is a process whereby a reaction to nonionizing radiation occurs because of the introduction of a radiation-absorbing reagent (the sensitizer), which induces another substance (the substrate) to undergo chemical change. Phototoxic sensitivity that does not involve an immunologic mechanism occurs as a direct consequence of cellular damage induced by the reaction between UV or visible light and the in vivo bound sensitizer.

Both UVB and UVA can produce phototoxic reactions, although the former is of greater importance.

CAUSE
- There are two basic mechanisms, phototoxic (the most common) and photoallergic. However, these are not necessarily mutually exclusive and clinically are not always distinguishable.
- Drugs frequently implicated in photosensitivity reactions are nonsteroidal anti-inflammatory drugs (NSAIDs), phenothiazines, amiodarone, antibiotics, and antifungal agents such as griseofulvin.
- Most photoallergic reactions are induced by the application of topical medications and chemicals (contact photoallergy), including antihistamines, local anesthetics, hydrocortisone sunscreens containing para-aminobenzoic acid, and halogenated phenolic compounds in soaps and fragrances.
- Photosensitivity can also occur following the administration of drugs, including tetracyclines, NSAIDs, sulfonamides, thiazides, phenothiazines, griseofulvin, and chloroquine.

PHYSICAL FINDINGS AND CLINICAL PRESENTATION
- The clinical appearance of acute phototoxic reactions mimics that of severe sunburn and include erythema, edema, and blistering, with subsequent desquamation and post-inflammatory hyperpigmentation (Fig. 14–2).

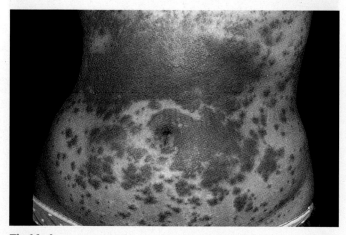

Fig 14–1
Exanthematous drug reaction. These more extensive lesions on the abdomen were associated with amoxicillin therapy.
(Courtesy of the Institute of Dermatology, London.)

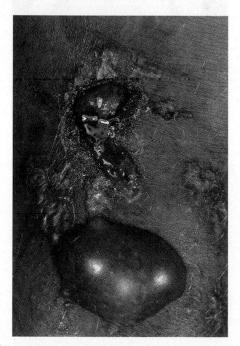

Fig 14–2
Phototoxic drug reaction. In this example, there are well-developed blisters arising on an erythematous base.
(From McKee PH, Calonje E, Granter SR [eds]: Pathology of the Skin With Clinical Correlations, 3rd ed. St. Louis, Mosby, 2005.)

- Photoallergic reactions are usually induced by UVA but not by UVB or visible light.
- The clinical appearance is variable and includes eczematous and lichenoid reactions (Fig. 14–3).
- Unlike phototoxic reactions, unexposed skin may also be affected in addition to exposed skin.
- Diagnosis is best confirmed by a photopatch test.

C. DRUG-INDUCED HYPERPIGMENTATION

DEFINITION

Cutaneous hyperpigmentation is a relatively frequent complication of drug therapy and may result from increased melanin synthesis or from the deposition of the drug or its metabolite in the skin.

CAUSE

Commonly involved agents are minocycline (Fig. 14–4) and amiodarone (Fig. 14–5).

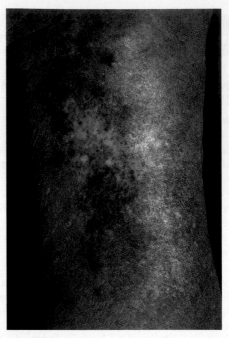

Fig 14–4
Minocycline pigmentation—typical pigmentation affecting the shin.
(Courtesy of the Institute of Dermatology, London.)

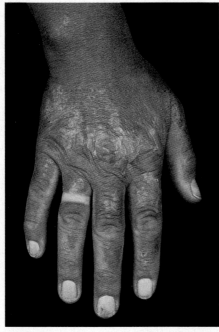

Fig 14–3
Photoallergic drug reaction. This case resulted from treatment with tetracycline.
(Courtesy of the Institute of Dermatology, London.)

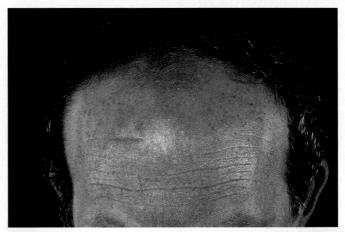

Fig 14–5
Amiodarone pigmentation. Note the slate gray discoloration on the forehead, a characteristic site.
(Courtesy of the Institute of Dermatology, London.)

| Chapter 15 | Neutrophilic and eosinophilic dermatoses |

A. PYODERMA GANGRENOSUM

DEFINITION

This clinically diagnosed entity presents as pustules and is frequently associated with various conditions, especially inflammatory bowel disease, arthritis and plasma cell dyscrasias, at times occurring at sites of prior surgery (Fig. 15–1).

PHYSICAL FINDINGS AND CLINICAL PRESENTATION

- Typically, the ulcers have undermined edges and red-purple borders (Fig. 15–2). They may be solitary or multiple, and occur most often on the lower limbs.
- The ulcers are painful and tender, and may persist for months or years.
- There is a risk of disfiguring scarring.

TREATMENT

- Treatment of associated disorders
- Topical corticosteroids, clofazimine, dapsone, intralesional steroids, minocycline, cyclosporine, systemic corticosteroids

B. SWEET'S SYNDROME (ACUTE FEBRILE NEUTROPHILIC DERMATOSIS)

DEFINITION

This disorder is characterized by multiple, painful, asymmetrically distributed red plaques or nodules, particularly on the face, neck, trunk, and upper and lower limbs (Fig. 15–3).

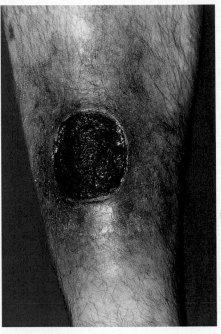

Fig 15–2
Pyoderma gangrenosum. This shows an area of ulceration with a typical undermined purplish border.
(Courtesy of Dr. R. A. Marsden, St. George's Hospital, London.)

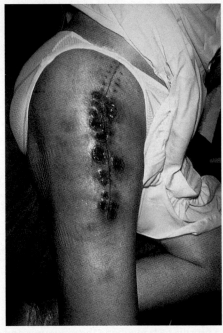

Fig 15–1
Pyoderma gangrenosum—multiple early lesions at the site of previous surgery.
(Courtesy of Dr. R. A. Marsden, St. George's Hospital, London.)

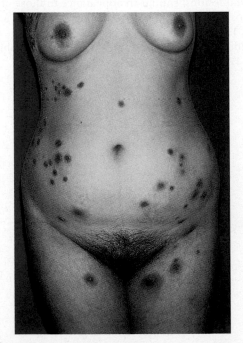

Fig 15–3
Sweet's syndrome. Shown are characteristic edematous red plaques, some showing ulceration and pustulation, that are widely distributed on the trunk and proximal limbs.
(Courtesy of Dr. R. A. Marsden, St. George's Hospital, London.)

PHYSICAL FINDINGS AND CLINICAL PRESENTATION

- The plaques vary from 1 to 4 cm in diameter (Fig. 15–4) and typically heal without scarring. Sweet's syndrome often follows an upper respiratory infection and in some cases may be a complication of drug treatment (e.g., furosemide, hydralazine, minocycline, trimethoprim-sulfamethoxazole, celecoxib, oral contraceptives).
- It may also be associated with malignancy (usually acute myelogenous leukemia [AML], lymphomas), and inflammatory bowel disease.

DIAGNOSIS

- Skin biopsy
- Laboratory findings (CBC, erythrocyte sedimentation rate [ESR], creatinine, ALT)

TREATMENT

- Oral corticosteroids
- Topical and intralesional corticosteroids

C. BEHÇET'S DISEASE

PHYSICAL FINDINGS AND CLINICAL PRESENTATION

- Papulopustular lesions are the most commonly encountered skin manifestations. Recurrent oral ulceration is an invariable feature of this condition.
- The ulcers measure up to 1 cm across and develop at any location in the oral cavity, (Fig. 15–5) pharynx, and even larynx.
- They are painful and usually regress spontaneously within 14 days. A yellow necrotic crust typically covers the ulcer floor.
- Typical of Behçet's disease and an important diagnostic clue is the development of sterile pustules at sites of mild skin trauma, such as injection sites (pathergy).
- Genital lesions, similar in appearance to those of the oral mucosa, occur on the scrotum, penis, vagina, and vulva (Fig. 15–6).
- Additional information on this disorder is available in Section 12.12e.

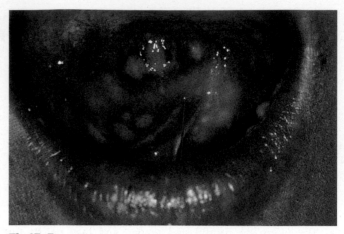

Fig 15–5
Behçet's disease. Multiple superficial ulcers are present.
(Courtesy of Dr. S. B. Woo, Brigham and Women's Hospital and Harvard Medical School, Boston.)

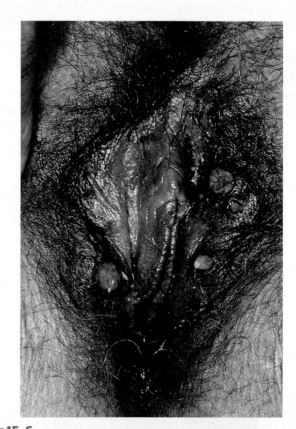

Fig 15–6
Genital lesions occur in Behcet's disease.
(From McKee PH, Calonoje E, Granter SR [eds]: Pathology of the Skin With Clinical Correlations, 3rd ed. St. Louis, Mosby, 2005.)

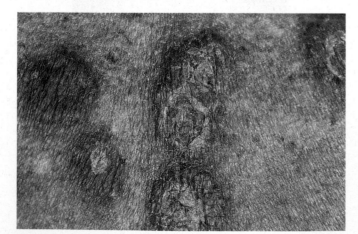

Fig 15–4
Sweet's syndrome—close-up view of typical plaques.
(Courtesy of the Institute of Dermatology, London.)

D. URTICARIA

DEFINITION

Urticaria is a pruritic rash involving the epidermis and upper portions of the dermis, resulting from localized capillary vasodilation and followed by transudation of protein-rich fluid in the surrounding tissue. It manifests clinically by the presence of hives.

PHYSICAL FINDINGS AND CLINICAL PRESENTATION

● Presence of elevated, erythematous (Fig. 15–7) , or white nonpitting plaques that change in size and shape over time; they generally last a few hours and disappear without a trace.
● Intense erythema (Fig. 15–8)
● Annular configuration with central pallor, dermatographism (Fig. 15–9)

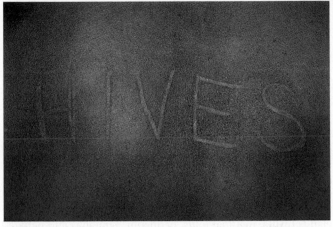

Fig 15–9
Dermatographism. Stroking the skin leads to the urticarial reaction.
(From Callen JP, Jorizzo JL, Bolognia JL, et al: Dermatologic Signs of Internal Disease, 3rd ed. Philadelphia, WB Saunders, 2003.)

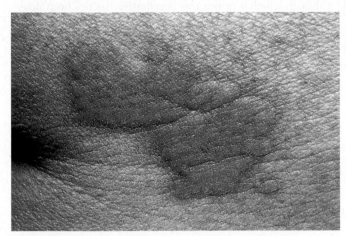

Fig 15–7
Urticaria—a typical wheal (hive). Note the edema and erythema.
(Courtesy of the Institute of Dermatology, London.)

CAUSE

● Foods (e.g., shellfish, eggs, strawberries, nuts)
● Drugs (e.g., penicillin, aspirin, sulfonamides)
● Systemic diseases (e.g., SLE, serum sickness, autoimmune thyroid disease, polycythemia vera)
● Food additives (e.g., salicylates, benzoates, sulfites)
● Infections (e.g., viral infections, fungal infections, chronic bacterial infections)
● Physical stimuli (e.g., pressure urticaria, exercise-induced, solar urticaria, cold urticaria)
● Inhalants (e.g., mold spores, animal danders, pollens)
● Contact (nonimmunologic) urticaria (e.g., caterpillars, plants)
● Other: hereditary angioedema, urticaria pigmentosa, pregnancy, cold urticaria, hair bleach, chemicals, saliva, cosmetics, perfumes, pemphigoid, emotional stress

DIFFERENTIAL DIAGNOSIS

● Erythema multiforme (see Fig. 9–2)
● Erythema marginatum
● Erythema infectiosum (see Fig. 27–1)
● Urticarial vasculitis (see Fig. 10–3)
● Drug eruption (see Fig. 14–1)
● Multiple insect bites (see Fig. 29–17)
● Bullous pemphigoid (see Fig. 4–2)

LABORATORY TESTS

● CBC with differential
● Stool for ova and parasites in patients with suspected parasitic infestations
● ANA, ESR, thyroid-stimulating hormone (TSH), liver function tests (LFTs), and eosinophil count are indicated only for select patients.
● Measurement of C_4 in patients who present only with angioedema
● Skin biopsy is helpful for patients with fever, arthralgias, and elevated ESR.

TREATMENT

● Remove suspected causative agents (e.g., stop aspirin and all nonessential drugs) and restrict diet (e.g., elimination of strawberries, nuts, eggs, shellfish).

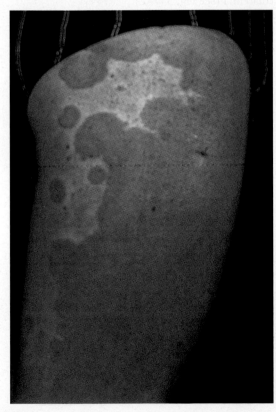

Fig 15–8
Urticaria. In this extreme example, there is intense erythema.
(Courtesy of the Institute of Dermatology, London.)

- Elimination of yeast should be attempted in patients with chronic urticaria; *Candida albicans* sensitivity may be a factor in patients with chronic urticaria.
- Oral antihistamines
- Doxepin may be effective for patients with chronic urticaria.
- Oral corticosteroids should be reserved for refractory cases.
- H_2 receptor antagonists can be added to H_1 antagonists for refractory cases.

E. HIDRADENITIS SUPPURATIVA

DEFINITION

Hidradenitis suppurativa (HS) is a chronic relapsing condition that occurs in the terminal follicular epithelium of the apocrine glands (axilla, inguinal folds, perineum, genitalia) and periareolar region, where keratinous materials occlude the follicles. This causes secondary inflammation of the apocrine glands, resulting in chronic infection and draining abscesses, which lead to scarring.

- Predisposing factors thought to be involved include hyperandrogenism, obesity, and familial predilection.
- HS has been associated with other endocrine disorders such as diabetes, Cushing's disease, and acromegaly.

PHYSICAL FINDINGS AND CLINICAL PRESENTATION

- The diagnosis is primarily clinical based on the development of typical lesions.
- Initially, there is a firm painful nodule in the groin or axilla (Fig. 15–10).
- The nodule may involute slowly or discharge pus through the skin, which is often foul smelling. In the late stages, a complex interconnecting system of sinuses extends deeply into the dermis and subcutaneous fat with extensive dense fibrosis (Fig. 15–11).

- There is a strong tendency toward relapse and recurrence.
- Other characteristics of the disease include poor response to conventional antibiotics and personal or family history of acne or pilonidal cysts.

CAUSE

- The exact cause of hidradenitis suppurativa has not been determined, although a number of theories have been proposed:

  1. Folliculitis is observed in almost all patients with HS, although whether or not this is causative has not been determined.

  2. Local friction trauma

  3. Infectious agents such as *Streptoccus*, *Staphylococcus*, and *Escherichia coli* have been identified in cultures, but it is uncertain whether these are a cause or result.

  4. Low levels of estrogen are implicated, as are high levels of androgen.

DIFFERENTIAL DIAGNOSIS

- Folliculitis and other follicular pyodermas, furuncles, pilonidal cysts (see Fig. 28–14)
- Granuloma inguinale (see Fig. 226–15)
- Crohn's disease (perianal and vulval manifestations; see Fig. 162–3)
- Bartholin's cyst infection (see Fig. 331–10)
- Actinomycosis (see Fig. 336–35)
- Lymphogranuloma venereum (see Fig. 226–21)
- Furuncle (see Fig. 28–15)
- Lymphangitis (see Fig. 28–5)
- Cat scratch disease (see Fig. 349–1)
- Tularemia (see Fig. 347–2)
- Erysipelas (see Fig. 28–2)
- Ulcerative colitis/Crohn's disease (see Fig. 171–2)

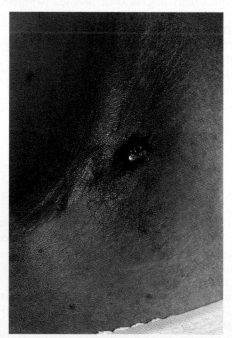

Fig 15–10
Hidradenitis suppurativa. This early lesion presented as an erythematous nodule discharging clear fluid. The axilla is a commonly affected site. (Courtesy of Dr. R. A. Marsden, St. George's Hospital, London.)

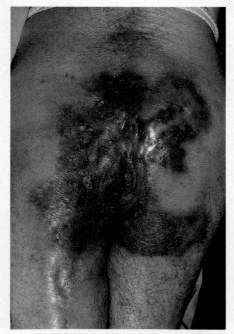

Fig 15–11
Hidradenitis suppurativa. In this very severe case, there is marked scarring, and numerous sinuses are present. (Courtesy of Dr. R. A. Marsden, St. George's Hospital, London.)

LABORATORY TESTS
- Patients with acute lesions may have an elevated ESR or white blood cell (WBC) count.
- Protein abnormalities may also be found on electrophoresis.
- Any pus should be sampled for bacterial culture and sensitivity.

TREATMENT
- Antibiotics (erythromycin, clindamycin, cephalexin)
- Surgical intervention (incision and drainage of abscess, radical excision of at risk tissue)
- Intralesional corticosteroids, hormone therapy

F. URTICARIA PIGMENTOSA (MACULOPAPULAR CUTANEOUS MASTOCYTOSIS)

- Most common manifestation of mastocytosis, with an approximate incidence of 1 in 1000 to 8000 live births.

PHYSICAL FINDINGS AND CLINICAL PRESENTATION
- Lesions, which may be present at birth or appear during the first year of life, are pruritic, erythematous, or red-brown, round to oval macules, papules, or plaques, often measuring as much as 2 to 3 cm in diameter (Figs. 15–12 and 15–13).
- Lesions occur predominantly on the trunk and gradually darken because of increased melanin pigmentation.
- The face, scalp, palms, and soles are usually spared.
- Urtication at the slightest trauma *(Darier's sign)* is characteristic (Fig. 15–14).
- Many patients show generalized dermatographism (whealing after stroking or gentle rubbing).
- In adults, small dark brown papules and macules are present, predominantly on the trunk and extremities.
- Spontaneous recovery does not occur and systemic involvement (particularly of bone marrow) is common.

DIAGNOSIS
- Skin biopsy
- Laboratory investigation: 24-hour urine histamine, histamine metabolites, prostaglandin metabolites, blood tryptase levels, bone marrow examination

TREATMENT
- H_1 and H_2 antihistamines
- Disodium cromoglycate

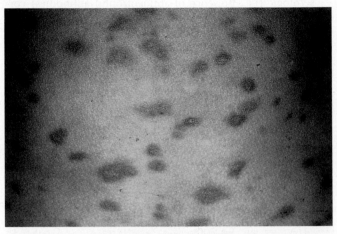

Fig 15–13
Urticaria pigmentosa—close-up view.
(Courtesy of Dr. R. A. Marsden, St. George's Hospital, London.)

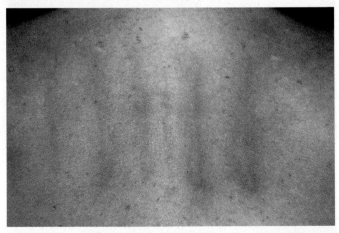

Fig 15–14
Urticaria pigmentosa. Gentle rubbing of the lesion typically results in erythema of the surrounding skin.
(Courtesy of Dr. R. A. Marsden, St. George's Hospital, London.)

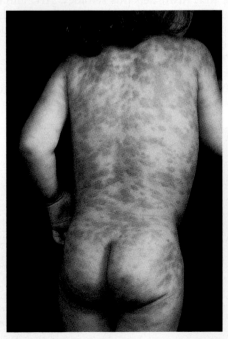

Fig 15–12
Urticaria pigmentosa. The pigmented lesions are widely distributed over the back, buttocks, and thighs of this child.
(Courtesy of Dr. R. A. Marsden, St. George's Hospital, London.)

Chapter 16 Vascular diseases

- The presence of inflammation and some evidence of vascular damage in the form of vessel wall or endothelial cell necrosis, or fibrinoid change, fulfill most criteria for a diagnosis of vasculitis.
- A specific diagnosis requires careful clinical, histologic, and serologic (i.e., presence of antineutrophil antibodies) correlation.
- A pathologic diagnosis of vasculitis may indicate a primary or secondary disease (i.e., in the setting of connective tissue disease).
- Secondary forms of vascular disease may manifest as diverse histologic patterns. The myriad schemata for the classification of the vasculitides are a reflection of the complexity of this controversial class of diseases.

A. LEUKOCYTOCLASTIC VASCULITIS (ALLERGIC VASCULITIS, HYPERSENSITIVITY VASCULITIS, LEUKOCYTOCLASTIC ANGIITIS)

- Most common form of vasculitis
- It is not a disease but represents a vascular reaction pattern caused by circulating immune complexes that may be produced by a number of disorders.

PHYSICAL FINDINGS AND CLINICAL PRESENTATION

- The skin manifestations may be associated with systemic manifestations involving the joints (Fig. 16–1), kidneys, and gastrointestinal (GI) system in 20% to 50% of patients.
- Skin manifestations are typically polymorphic, but palpable purpura (nonblanching erythematous papules) is the most common manifestation (Fig. 16–2).
- Urticarial, bullous, or vesicular ulceroinfarctive, nodular, pustular, livedoid, and annular lesions may be encountered (Fig. 16–3).
- The lesions measure from 1 mm to several centimeters in diameter.
- The lower legs are affected most often, but lesions may be present at other sites.

LABORATORY TESTS

- Skin biopsies for routine microscopy (Fig. 16–4) and direct immunofluorescence
- Immunoglobulin and complement can be identified in vitro, by immunofluorescence or immunoperoxidase techniques, and in biopsies from blood vessel wall lesions less than 24 hours old (Fig. 16–5).
- Laboratory tests should include CBC, urinalysis, serum creatinine, ALT, ANA, hepatitis serology, HIV, antineutrophil cytoplasmic antibody (ANCA), complement levels.
- Blood cultures are recommended when an infectious cause is suspected.

DIAGNOSTIC IMAGING

- Chest x-ray should be done in all patients.
- Echocardiography is indicated for suspected infections to rule out endocarditis.

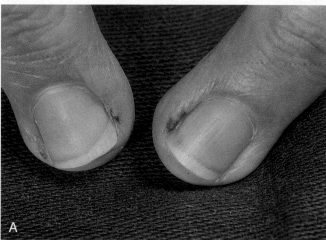

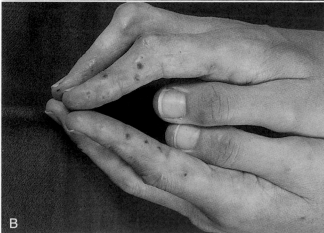

Fig 16–1
Cutaneous vasculitis. **A,** Vasculitis of the nail folds and thenar surfaces of the index fingers. **B,** Rheumatoid arthritis patient with leukocytoclastic vasculitis.
(From Hochberg MC, Silman AJ, Smolen JS, et al [eds]: Rheumatology, 3rd ed. St. Louis, Mosby, 2003.)

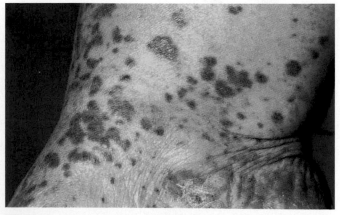

Fig 16–2
Leukocytoclastic vasculitis. Typical erythematous maculopapular lesions are present on the medial aspect of the ankle.
(Courtesy of Dr. R. A. Marsden, St. George's Hospital, London.)

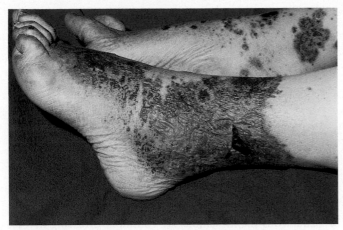

Fig 16–3
Leukocytoclastic vasculitis. Confluent purpura with ulceration is present.
(Courtesy of Dr. R. A. Marsden, St. George's Hospital, London.)

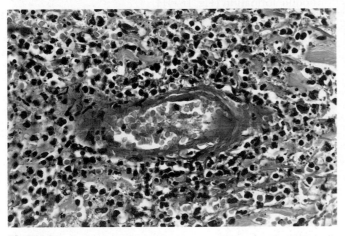

Fig 16–4
Leukocytoclastic vasculitis. This high-power view shows fibrinoid necrosis and a mixed inflammatory cell infiltrate composed of neutrophils, eosinophils, and lymphocytes. There is marked leukocytoclasis (karyorrhexis, nuclear dust).
(From McKee PH, Calonje E, Granter SR [eds]: Pathology of the Skin With Clinical Correlations, 3rd ed. St. Louis, Mosby, 2005.)

TREATMENT
- Removal (withdrawal) of causative agent
- Colchicine, dapsone, systemic corticosteroids, immunosuppressive agents

B. HENOCH-SCHÖNLEIN PURPURA

- Cutaneous lesions comprise palpable purpura predominantly affecting the lower limbs, thighs, and buttocks (Fig. 16–6).
- Targetoid lesions are often present.
- For additional information on this disorder, refer to Section 12.12f.

C. URTICARIAL VASCULITIS

DEFINITION
This disorder is characterized clinically by urticaria and histologically by leukocytoclastic venulitis.

Fig 16–5
Leukocytoclastic vasculitis. IgM is present in the blood vessel walls (direct immunofluorescence).
(Courtesy of B. Bhogal, Institute of Dermatology, London.)

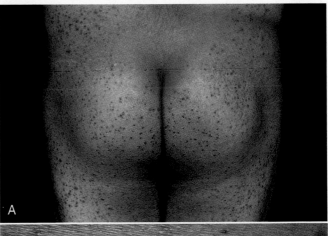

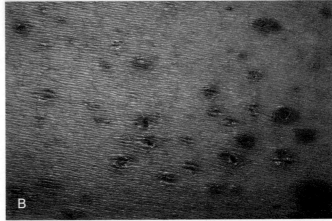

Fig 16–6
Henoch-Schönlein purpura—palpable purpura in the classic distribution on the buttocks **(A)** and thighs **(B)**.
(Courtesy of the Institute of Dermatology, London.)

PHYSICAL FINDINGS AND CLINICAL MANIFESTATIONS
- In addition to urticarial skin lesions, patients may also experience angioedema, arthralgia, GI symptoms, and evidence of renal involvement.
- Urticarial vasculitis is most often seen in the third to fifth decades and shows a female predominance.

- The cutaneus lesions are urticarial in appearance and consist of edematous, raised, erythematous plaques associated with nonblanchable purpura (Figs. 16–7 and 16–8).
- In contrast to uncomplicated urticaria, cutaneus lesions in the setting of urticarial vasculitis often last 24 to 72 hours.
- Patients often complain of pruritus, burning, or pain. The frequency of cutaneous symptoms varies considerably, from daily to monthly.
- Joint pain, stiffness and swelling, particularly of the hands, elbows, feet, ankles, and knees are seen; however, frank arthritis is extremely rare.

LABORATORY TESTS
- Complement levels (hypocomplementemia)
- Urinalysis (proteinuria, hematuria)
- ESR
- CBC, ALT, serum creatinine levels

TREATMENT
- Antihistamines, glucocorticoids, doxepin

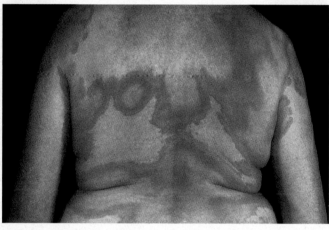

Fig 16–7
Urticarial vasculitis. This large lesion has developed a bizarre outline because of central clearing.
(Courtesy of the Institute of Dermatology, London.)

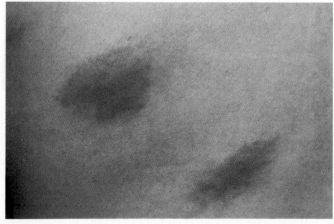

Fig 16–8
Urticarial vasculitis—close-up view.
(Courtesy of the Institute of Dermatology, London.)

D. POLYARTERITIS NODOSA
- Cutaneous lesions are common in polyarteritis nodosa.
- Palpable purpuric lesions and foci of ulceration, particularly involving the lower limbs, are most often found (Fig. 16–9).
- Livedo reticularis is also a common cutaneous manifestation (Fig. 16–10).
- Cutaneous nodules may also be seen.
- A maculopapular rash, vesiculation, and pustular lesions are occasional features.
- For additional information on this disorder, refer to Section 12.12a.

E. WEGENER'S GRANULOMATOSIS
- Cutaneous manifestations are common, occurring in 14% to 50% of patients.
- Several different types of skin lesions may be encountered, including vasculitis lesions with purpura, bruising, and nodule formation (Fig. 16–11).
- Pyoderma—gangrenous-like lesions with necrosis and ulceration that have a predilection for the lower limbs—are sometimes encountered.
- The presence of skin lesions appears to correlate with disease activity.
- Oral ulceration is common.
- For additional information on this disorder, refer to Section 6.10b.

F. ALLERGIC GRANULOMATOSIS WITH ANGIITIS (CHURG-STRAUSS SYNDROME)
- Cutaneous lesions are seen in 40% to 70% of patients and include petechiae, purpura, papules, vesicles, facial erythema, urticaria, and ulceration.
- Cutaneous infarction and bullae are less common manifestations.
- Patients may also develop tender nodules, which particularly affect the extensor aspects of the arms, legs, hands, and feet (Fig. 16–12).
- The sacrum, buttocks, and scalp may also be involved.
- The cutaneous lesions tend to appear in crops, with spontaneous relapses and remissions.
- For additional information on this disorder, refer to Section 6.10c.

G. KAWASAKI DISEASE (MUCOCUTANEOUS LYMPH NODE SYNDROME)
- The cutaneous findings are variable and include erythematous, macular (Fig. 16–13), maculopapular (morbilliform), urticarial, erythema multiforme–like (targetoid), and erythema marginatum–like lesions.
- The skin lesions show a propensity for the trunk and extremities, but may be more generalized.
- Erythema, edema, and induration of the extremities occur, followed by cutaneous desquamation of the tips of the fingers and toes.
- For additional information on this disorder, refer to Section 1.27k.

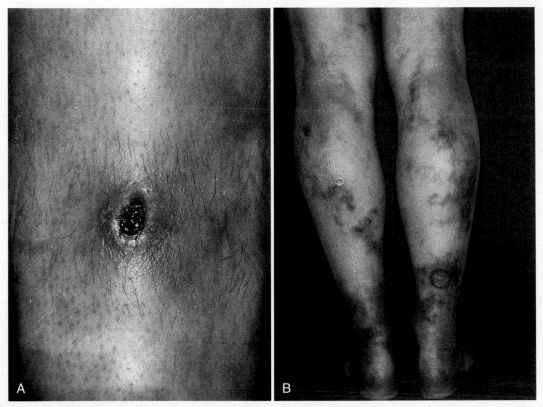

Fig 16–9
Polyarteritis nodosa. **A,** Sharply defined ulcer with an indurated purplish border on the shin. **B,** Multiple ulcers, nodules, and foci of livedo reticularis.
(Courtesy of Dr. R. A. Marsden, St. George's Hospital, London.)

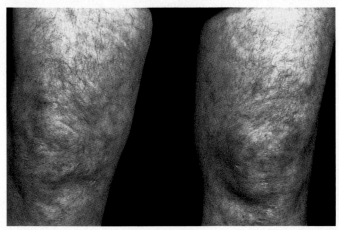

Fig 16–10
Polyarteritis nodosa. This patient exhibits florid livedo reticularis.
(Courtesy of the Institute of Dermatology, London.)

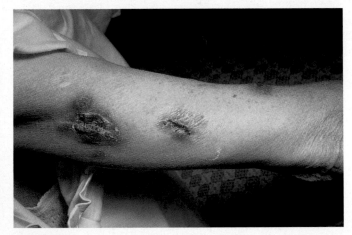

Fig 16–11
Wegener's granulomatosis This patient has ulcerating plaques and nodules.
(Courtesy of the Institute of Dermatology, London.)

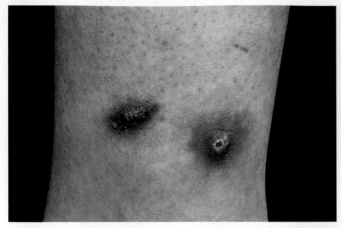

Fig 16–12
Churg-Strauss syndrome. This patient presented with painful nodes on the limbs.
(Courtesy of the Institute of Dermatology, London.)

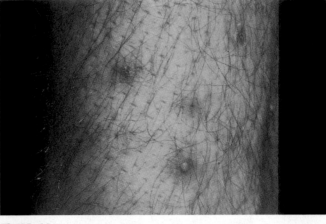

Fig 16–14
Behçet's disease—typical pustules on the lower leg.
(Courtesy of Dr. R. A. Marsden, St. George's Hospital, London.)

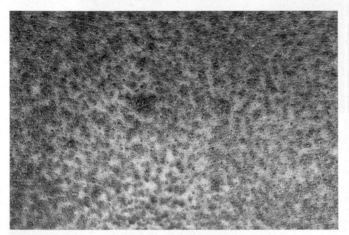

Fig 16–13
Kawasaki disease—erythematous macular eruption.
(Courtesy of Dr. W. G. Philips, Institute of Dermatology, London.)

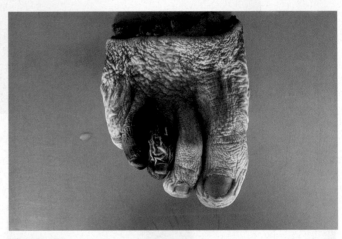

Fig 16–15
Buerger's disease. Digital gangrene is present in this amputation specimen.
(From McKee PH, Calonje E, Granter SR [eds]: Pathology of the Skin With Clinical Correlations, 3rd ed. St. Louis, Mosby, 2005.)

H. BEHÇET'S DISEASE

- Cutaneous lesions are common, recurrent, and comprise a wide variety of manifestations, including erythema-like lesions, usually on the lower extremities. Patients may also develop acneiform papules and pustules, furuncles, pyoderma, and thrombophlebitis (Fig. 16–14).
- For additional information on this disorder, refer to Section 12.12e.

I. THROMBOANGIITIS OBLITERANS (BUERGER'S DISEASE)

- Patients most often present with painful cyanotic lesions of the extremities, especially the fingers or toes, which may ulcerate and become gangrenous, often requiring amputation (Fig. 16–15).
- Lesions are characterized by thrombosis of small or medium-sized arteries and, less commonly, of veins, associated with a variable inflammatory infiltrate composed of

a mixture of neutrophils, lymphocytes, eosinophils, histiocytes, and giant cells.
- For additional information on this disorder, refer to Section 5.19.

J. GIANT CELL ARTERITIS (TEMPORAL ARTERITIS)

- Clinical examination may reveal scalp tenderness and the skin overlying the affected vessel may be erythematous, edematous, or appear bruised.
- Palpation often reveals a cordlike and nodular vessel.
- Pulsation may be diminished or absent.
- Patients may occasionally manifest ulcers, sometimes widespread, massive necrosis (Fig. 16–16), bullae, and gangrene.
- Biopsy of affected artery may reveal a dense, chronic, inflammatory cell infiltrate (Fig. 16–17).
- For additional information on this disorder, refer to Section 12.12c.

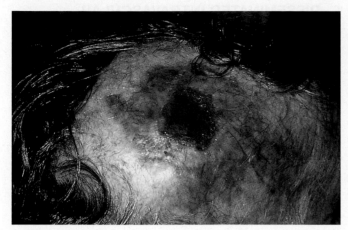

Fig 16–16
Scalp necrosis in giant cell arteritis.
(From Hochberg MC, Silman AJ, Smolen JS, et al [eds]: Rheumatology, 3rd ed. St. Louis, Mosby, 2003.)

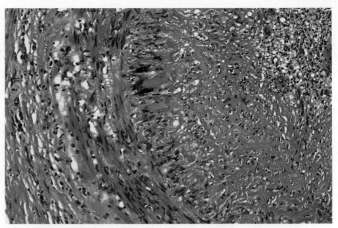

Fig 16–17
Giant cell arteritis. The intima and media are infiltrated by a dense chronic inflammatory cell infiltrate containing conspicuous Langhan's giant cells.
(Courtesy of Dr. P. A. Burton, Southmead Hospital, Bristol, England.)

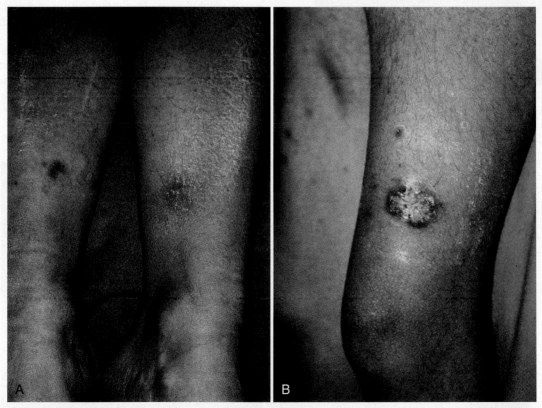

Fig 16–18
Takayasu's arteritis. **A,** This patient presented with multiple lesions as seen here on the lower legs. **B,** A large ulcerated inflammatory nodule is present on the left thigh.
(Courtesy of Drs. P. Godeau and C. Francès, Groupe Hospitalier, Pitié-Salpêtrière, Paris.)

K. TAKAYASU'S ARTERITIS

● Cutaneous manifestations have been described in up to 50% of patients; these include Raynaud's phenomenon (because of large vessel involvement), acute inflammatory nodules and erythema nodosum–like features, pyoderma gangrenosum–like lesions, superficial phlebitis, and purpura (Fig. 16–18).

● Patients may also present with cutaneous necrotizing vasculitis.

● For additional information on this disorder, refer to Section 12.12d.

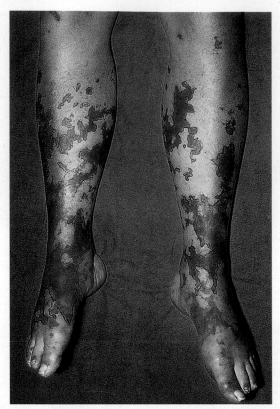

Fig 16–19
Purpura fulminans. Bilateral extensive ecchymoses are present on this child's legs.
(Courtesy of Dr. D. McGibbon, St. Thomas' Hospital, London.)

L. DISSEMINATED INTRAVASCULAR COAGULATION

- Disseminated intravascular coagulation (DIC) is a consumptive coagulopathy that is associated with a wide variety of underlying disorders, many of them life threatening.
- For additional information on this disorder, refer to Section 13.11.
- *Purpura fulminans* is a term that has been applied to infection-associated disseminated intravascular coagulation (DIC) in children. It is characterized by an acute syndrome of rapidly progressive and extensive hemorrhagic skin necrosis associated with dermal vascular thrombosis and vascular collapse caused by DIC. A common presentation is symmetrical purpura of the fingers and toes. Patients develop large confluent ecchymoses, which particularly affect the buttocks, legs, and feet, and commonly appear on the limbs (Fig. 16–19) and abdomen. The ecchymosed frequently become necrotic, and blood-filled blisters are often found.

M. CRYOGLOBULINEMIA

- Cryoglobulins are immunoglobulins that precipitate at low temperatures (4°C) and that resolve with rewarming (Fig. 16–20).
- Cryoglobulins may be divided into three classes:
  1. Type I, composed solely of monoclonal immunoglobulin (κ or λ) and usually associated with lymphoproliferative disorders (e.g., multiple myeloma, Waldenström's macroglobulinemia).

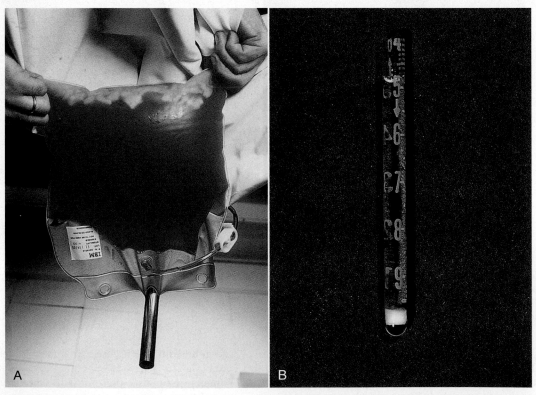

Fig 16–20
Cryoglobulinemia. **A,** There is a large quantity of precipitated cryoglobulin in this plasmapherisis specimen. **B,** A cryoprecipitate.
(Courtesy of Dr. N. Slater, St. Thomas' Hospital, London.)

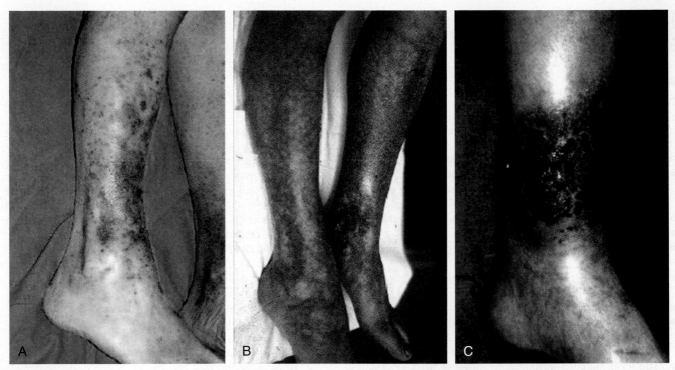

Fig 16–21
Cutaneous cryoglobulinemic vasculitis. **A,** Recent onset, palpable purpura on the legs with both isolated and confluent purpuric lesions. **B,** Ochreous coloration of the skin with stocking distribution caused by chronic hemosiderin deposits in a patient with mixed cryoglobulinemia of 15 years' duration. A residual perimalleolar scar is seen on the left leg from a healed vasculitic ulcer. **C,** Large and torpid ulcer on the left leg, with diffuse hyperpigmentation of the surrounding skin.
(From Young NS, Gerson SL, High KA [eds]: Clinical Hematology. Philadelphia, Elsevier, 2006.)

2. Type II (mixed) cryoglobulin composed of monoclonal immunoglobulin (usually IgM).
3. Type III (polyclonal) cryoglobulin composed of immunoglobulins IgG and IgM.
The last two subtypes (mixed cryoglobulins) function as immune complexes and clinical manifestations are caused, at least in part, by allergic vasculitis.
● Cryoglobulins may be associated with hepatitis C, hepatitis B, SLE, lymphoreticular neoplasms, and infective processes (e.g., infective endocarditis).

PHYSICAL FINDINGS AND CLINICAL MANIFESTATIONS
● The eponym Meltzer's triad has been applied to the combined features of purpura, arthralgias, and weakness that are often present.
● Cutaneous manifestations are common to all classes of cryoglobulinemia and are often the presenting complaint. Purpura is the most frequent initial sign.
● Type I cryoglobulinemia is usually characterized by purpuric lesions, including inflammatory macules and papules on the extremities, accompanied by foci of ulceration (Fig. 16–21). Additional features may include livedo reticularis, Raynaud's phenomenon, scarring, and infarction, which particularly affects the digits, ears, and nose.
● Mixed cryoglobulinemia is characterized by joint involvement (arthralgia and arthritis), Raynaud's phenomenon, fever, purpura, weakness, renal involvement, hepatosplenomegaly, necrosis of the extremities (Fig. 16–22), and general

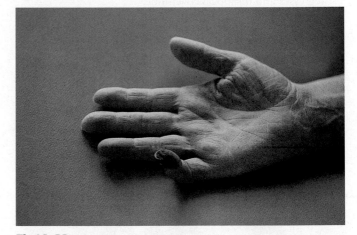

Fig 16–22
Necrosis of the distal portion of the little finger in a young woman with essential mixed cryoglobulinemia.
(From Johnson RJ, Feehally J: Comprehensive Clinical Nephrology, 2nd ed. St. Louis, Mosby, 2000.)

vasculitis. Cutaneous manifestations include palpable purpura, inflammatory macules and papules, necrotizing vasculitis, and occasionally cold urticaria. Renal involvement may be identified by proteinuria, hematuria, and red cell casts. Patients may also have polyneuropathies.
● Prognosis is variable. Renal involvement, which occurs in 50% of cases, is associated with high morbidity and mortality.

Chapter 17   Disorders of pigmentation

A. VITILIGO

DEFINITION

Vitiligo is the acquired loss of epidermal pigmentation, affecting 1% of the population and characterized histologically by the absence of epidermal melanocytes.

PHYSICAL FINDINGS AND CLINICAL PRESENTATION

- Hypopigmented and depigmented lesions (Fig. 17–1) favor sun-exposed regions, intertriginous areas, genitalia, and sites over bony prominences (type A vitiligo).
- Areas around body orifices are also frequently involved.
- The lesions tend to be symmetrical (Fig. 17–2).
- Occasionally, the lesions are linear or pseudodermatomal (type B vitiligo).
- Vitiligo lesions may occur at trauma sites (Koebner's phenomenon).
- The hair in affected areas may be white.
- The margins of the lesions are usually well demarcated and, when a ring of hyperpigmentation is seen, the term *trichrome vitiligo* is used.
- The term *marginal inflammatory vitiligo* is used to describe lesions with raised borders.
- Initially, the disease is limited, but the lesions tend to become more extensive over time.
- Type B vitiligo is more common in children.
- Vitiligo may begin around pigmented nevi, producing a halo *(Sutton's nevus)*; in such cases, the central nevus often regresses and disappears over time.

CAUSE AND PATHOGENESIS

- There are three pathophysiologic theories:
  1. Autoimmune theory (autoantibodies against melanocytes)
  2. Neural theory (neurochemical mediator selectively destroys melanocytes)
  3. Self-destructive process, whereby melanocytes fail to protect themselves against cytotoxic melanin precursors
- Although vitiligo is considered to be an acquired disease, 25% to 30% of cases are familial; the mode of transmission is unknown (polygenic or autosomal dominant, with incomplete penetrance and variable expression).

DIFFERENTIAL DIAGNOSIS

Acquired

- Chemical-induced depigmentation
- Halo nevus (see Fig. 23–12)
- Idiopathic guttate hypomelanosis (see Fig. 17–3)
- Leprosy (see Fig. 340–4)
- Pityriasis alba (see Fig. 17–4)
- Postinflammatory hypopigmentation
- Tinea versicolor (see Fig. 26–6)

Congenital

- Albinism
- Nevus anemicus
- Nevus depigmentosus
- Tuberous sclerosis (see Fig. 47–7)

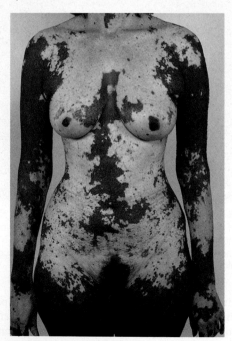

Fig 17–1
Vitiligo—symmetrical involvement of the body. Note patchy repigmentation secondary to psoralen ultraviolet A treatment.
(Courtesy of the Institute of Dermatology, London.)

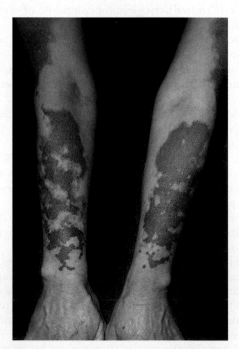

Fig 17–2
Vitiligo—symmetrical involvement of the upper limbs.
(Courtesy of the Institute of Dermatology, London.)

TREATMENT

- Treatment is indicated primarily for cosmetic purposes when depigmentation causes emotional or social distress. Depigmentation is more noticeable in those with darker complexions.
- Cosmetic masking agents
- Sunless tanning lotions
- Repigmentation—this is achieved by activation and migration of melanocytes from hair follicles; therefore, skin with little or no hair responds poorly to treatment.
- PUVA
- Topical midpotency steroids
- Intralesional steroid injection.
- Systemic steroids
- Total depigmentation (in cases of extensive vitiligo) with 20% monobenzyl ether or hydroquinone. This is a permanent procedure, and patients will require lifelong protection from sun exposure.
- Topical immunomodulators (tacrolimus, pimecrolimus) can also induce repigmentation of vitiliginous skin lesions. Their potential for systemic immunosuppression or increased risk of skin or other malignancies remains to be defined.
- Calcipotriol, a synthetic analogue of vitamin D_3, has also been used in combination with UV light or clobetasol, with limited results.

B. IDIOPATHIC GUTTATE HYPOMELANOSIS

DEFINITION

This common disorder is characterized by a few to numerous white macules developing on sun-exposed skin, particularly the forearms and legs (Fig. 17–3).

PHYSICAL EXAMINATION AND CLINICAL PRESENTATION

- Most lesions are 5 mm or less in diameter, most commonly seen in middle-aged to older patients. There may be an increased familial incidence.

CAUSE

- Unknown
- Possible factors include inheritance, actinic damage, loss of melanocytes because of aging, autoimmunity
- The main histologic feature consists of variable loss of melanin granules in epidermal keratinocytes.

DIFFERENTIAL DIAGNOSIS

- Vitiligo (see Fig. 17–2)
- Tinea versicolor (see Fig. 26–6)
- Pityriasis alba (see Fig. 17–4)
- Tuberous sclerosis (see Fig. 47–7)

TREATMENT

- Sun protection, self-tanning creams that contain dihydroxyacetone, makeup to camouflage white macules

C. PITYRIASIS ALBA

DEFINITION

This is a common localized disorder of hypopigmentation in children and young adults.

PHYSICAL EXAMINATION AND CLINICAL PRESENTATION

- It presents as ill-defined, slightly scaly macules of hypopigmentation 2 to 4 cm in diameter on the face, with a predilection for the cheeks (Fig. 17–4), lateral upper arms, and thighs.
- The condition is more obvious in darker individuals and during the summer. The loss of pigment is not permanent and the hypopigmentation usually fades with time.

TREATMENT

- None necessary other than reassurance

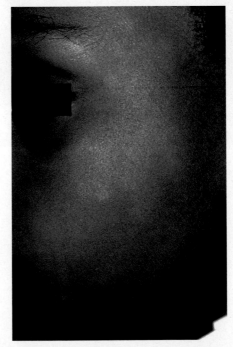

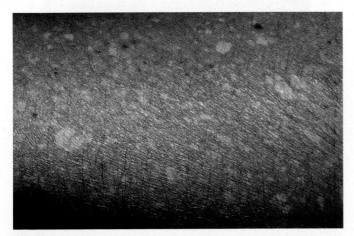

Fig 17–3
Guttate hypomelanosis—multiple small hypopigmented macules in sun-exposed skin.
(Courtesy of Dr. O. Dueñas, Bogotá, Colombia.)

Fig 17–4
Pityriasis alba—ill-defined patches of hypopigmentation on the face.
(Courtesy of the Institute of Dermatology, London.)

D. MELASMA (CHLOASMA, MASK OF PREGNANCY)

DEFINITION

This is a common, usually symmetrical, acquired hypermelanosis characterized by irregular light to dark-brown confluent or speckled macules with sharply demarcated margins involving sun-exposed skin; there is a marked predilection for the face (Fig. 17–5).

- Women, particularly Hispanic or Indian women, are more commonly affected than men. It usually develops in association with oral contraceptives and pregnancy and is worsened by sun exposure.
- An association has also been documented with cosmetics, phototoxic drugs, isotretinoin, and anticonvulsants.

CAUSE

- The exact pathogenesis is unknown but there is a clear causative link to female hormones and sun exposure.
- Histologically, there is an increase in melanin content in keratinocytes at all levels of the epidermis and an increase in the number of epidermal melanocytes.

TREATMENT

- Avoidance of sun exposure
- Sunscreens to block both UVA and UVB
- Bleaching creams that contain hydroquinone

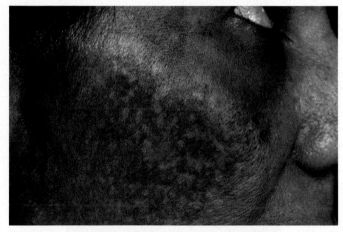

Fig 17–5
Melasma—dark-brown macular pigmentation.
(Courtesy of the Institute of Dermatology, London.)

E. PEUTZ-JEGHERS SYNDROME

DEFINITION

This autosomal dominant disease is characterized by GI polyps and pigmented macules with involvement of the perioral skin, lips (Fig. 17–6), buccal mucosa, and hands and feet, particularly the palms, soles, fingers, and toes.

- Lesions are brown or black and usually measure less than 5 mm in diameter. Skin lesions may fade at puberty but mucosal lesions tend to persist.
- The clinical appearance is almost identical to that of lentigines.
- For additional information on this disorder, refer to Section 7.28b.

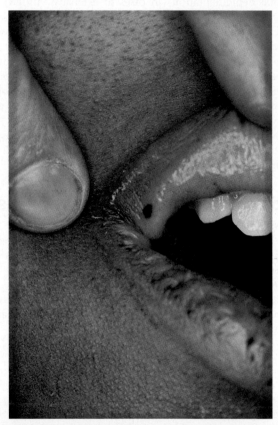

Fig 17–6
Peutz-Jeghers syndrome—darkly pigmented macular lesions on the lips.
(Courtesy of the Institute of Dermatology, London.)

F. LEOPARD SYNDROME

DEFINITION

This rare congenital autosomal dominant syndrome is referred to as the LEOPARD syndrome (*l*entiginosis [Fig. 17–7], *e*lectrocardiographic conduction abnormalities, *o*cular hypertelorism, *p*ulmonary stenosis, *a*bnormalities of the genitalia [cryptorchidism, hypospadias], growth *r*etardation, and sensorineural *d*eafness).

● The lentigines in LEOPARD syndrome are identical histologically to ordinary lentigines.

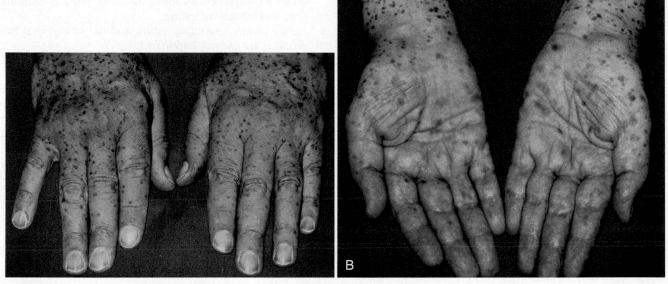

Fig 17–7
LEOPARD syndrome. Shown are prominent lentigines on the dorsa **(A)** and palms of the hands **(B)**.
(Courtesy of the Institute of Dermatology, London.)

Chapter 18   Diseases of the hair

A. NORMAL HAIR FOLLICLE AND DIAGNOSTIC EVALUATION

- Each hair follicle is composed of epithelial and mesenchymal components.
- Hair follicle development depends on the intimate association between these two elements.

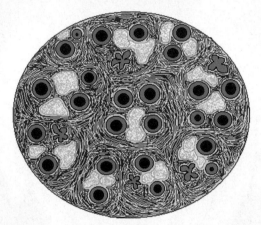

Fig 18-1
Scalp biopsy, horizontal section. numerous hair follicles are visible and quantification is easy. There are at least eight follicular units, with two to five hair follicles, including vellous and telogen hairs.
(Courtesy of Dr. M. Mejia, Universidad Pontificia Bolivariana, Medellín, Colombia.)

- The hair growth cycle is divided into three stages—active growth (anagen), involution (catagen), and a period of rest (telogen).
- Horizontal sections of the upper segment of the hair follicle show that hair follicles in the scalp are grouped, forming anatomic structures known as follicular units (Figs. 18-1 and 18-2), which are composed of terminal vellous hairs, sebaceous glands, and arrector pili muscles (Fig. 18-3).
- The evaluation of patients presenting with hair disease requires a comprehensive medical history, physical examination, and laboratory testing.
- Family history, grooming habits, and use of chemical hair products are of great importance.
- Useful laboratory tests include TSH (increase in telogen effluvium), ANA (positive in alopecia secondary to autoimmune disease), ferritin level (decreased in women with androgenetic alopecia and alopecia areata), VDRL, hormone levels (hyperandrogenism can cause hair loss in women), Gram stain and cultures, including examination of hair sample with KOH and cultures for suspected infections.
- Other useful tests are the hair pluck test (trichography), hair pull test, and scalp biopsy.

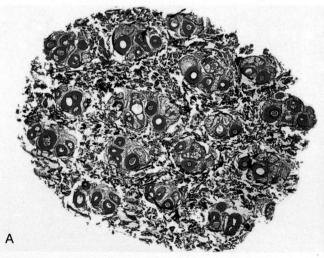
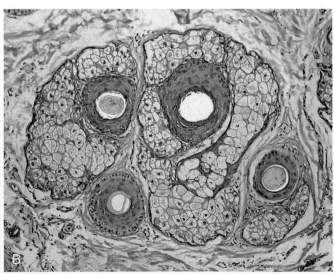

A

B

Fig 18-2
Hair biopsy, transverse section. The follicular units are clearly delineated by condensation of the adventitial collagen. **A,** Masson's trichrome stain. **B,** Hematoxylin and eosin.
(From McKee PH, Calonje E, Granter SR [eds]: Pathology of the Skin With Clinical Correlations, 3rd ed. St. Louis, Mosby, 2005.)

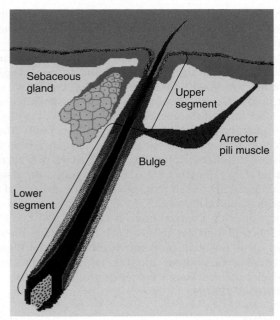

Fig 18–3
Hair biopsy, vertical section, upper and lower segments. The limit between the two segments is the insertion of the erector pili muscle (the bulge).
(Courtesy of Dr. M. Mejia, Universidad Pontificia Bolivariana, Medellín, Colombia.)

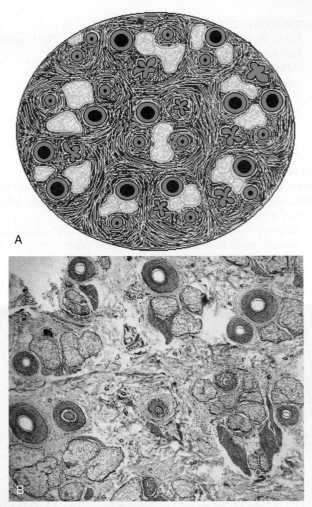

Fig 18–4
Androgenetic alopecia, horizontal section. There is an increase in the number of vellous and telogen hairs, with an apparent decrease in the total number of follicles. Compare with Figure 20–3.
(**A** courtesy of Dr. M. Mejia, Universidad Pontificia Bolivariana, Medellín, Colombia.)

B. ANDROGENETIC ALOPECIA (COMMON BALDNESS, HEREDITARY HAIR THINNING)

DEFINITION
This is a form of hair loss caused by androgens in genetically susceptible men and women.

Androgens are the main regulators of hair growth. After puberty, they promote transformation of vellous hair follicles, resulting in the production of tiny nonpigmented hairs or large pigmented terminal hairs (Fig. 18–4). However, androgens may also reverse this process, resulting in the gradual replacement of terminal hairs with vellous hairs and the onset of androgenetic alopecia. This phenomenon is the direct result of 5-alpha-reductase activity, which is mainly found on the external root sheath and hair bulb papilla. The enzyme converts testosterone into dihydrotestosterone, which has a great affinity for the androgen receptors in the hair follicle.

Androgenetic alopecia affects more than 50% of men older than 50 years and 40% of women by age 70. There is usually a familial history of baldness.

PHYSICAL EXAMINATION AND CLINICAL PRESENTATION
- In men, the condition usually starts early after puberty, mainly affecting the crown, vertex, and frontal, central, and temporal areas of the scalp *(Hamilton's male pattern)*. There is usually no involvement of the occipital and lower parietal regions (Fig. 18–5).
- In women, the hair loss is patterned and characterized by progressive thinning over the frontal parietal scalp, retention of the frontal hairline *(Ludwig's female pattern)*, and presence of miniaturized hairs (Fig. 18–6). The hair loss frequently starts around the onset of menopause.

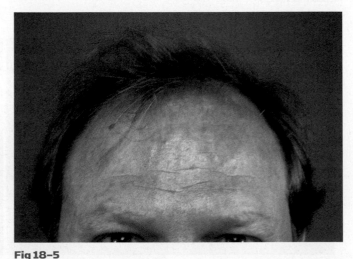

Fig 18–5
Androgenetic alopecia. This patient shows well-established male pattern baldness.
(Courtesy of the Institute of Dermatology, London.)

67

LABORATORY TESTING
- Scalp biopsy, ANA, ferritin and iron studies, TSH, serum testosterone and dihydrotestosterone levels

TREATMENT
- Topical minoxidil
- Finasteride
- Spironolactone

C. ALOPECIA AREATA

DEFINITION

This is a variant of alopecia in which large numbers of hair follicles undergo progression into catagen and telogen while smaller numbers enter an abnormal anagen stage.

- Alopecia areata is basically a disease driven by cellular immunity, with autoantibody production representing a secondary phenomenon.

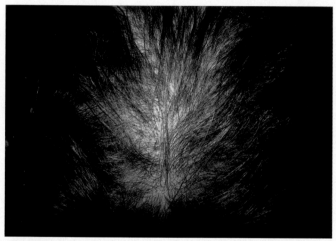

Fig 18–6
Androgenetic alopecia. This example shows the typical distribution in women, with parietal and posterior frontal hair loss. Note the sparing of the frontal hairline.
(Courtesy of Dr. A. M. Aristizábal, Instituto de Ciencias de la Salud, Medellín, Colombia.)

- The increased frequency of this disorder in genetically related individuals suggests that there is a genetic link to the disease.
- Alopecia areata affects up to 1% of the population and is more frequent in those between 15 and 40 years of age.

PHYSICAL EXAMINATION AND CLINICAL PRESENTATION
- Typically, patients present with an abrupt development of patches of nonscarring alopecia in different patterns—circumscribed, bandlike, and reticular (Fig. 18–7). The degree of involvement is variable and can range from mild disease to diffuse hair loss (Fig. 18–8), which may affect the entire scalp (alopecia totalis). Examination of the involved scalp generally reveals that, except for the absence of hair, the skin appears normal.
- Histologically, alopecia areata is characterized by normal numbers of follicular units and hair follicles (Fig. 18–9), an increase in the number of catagen and telogen follicles, and a lymphocytic infiltrate affecting the bulbs of the anagen follicles and the catagen and telogen follicular stellae

LABORATORY TESTING
- CBC, TSH, ANA

TREATMENT
- Intralesional corticosteroids

D. TRICHOTILLOMANIA

DEFINITION

This is traumatic alopecia caused by traction and pulling of hair. It represents a chronic mental illness of variable intensity and presentation.

In the most severe cases, it can be associated with trichophagia and trichobezoar. Occasionally, the compulsion to pull hair is not limited to the scalp but can involve other body sites, including the pubis, eyebrows, eyelashes, and even nostrils.

- Although some patients admit to pulling their hair, most deny it.
- Trichotillomania affects mainly young women (Fig. 18–10). Excoriations may be evident on examination of the affected areas (Fig. 18–11).
- Histologically, the most important feature is the very high percentage of catagen or telogen follicles (Fig. 18–12).

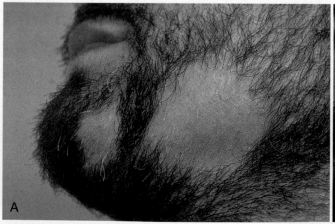

Fig 18–7
A, B, Alopecia areata—typical annular noninflammatory foci of alopecia.
(Courtesy of the Institute of Dermatology, London.)

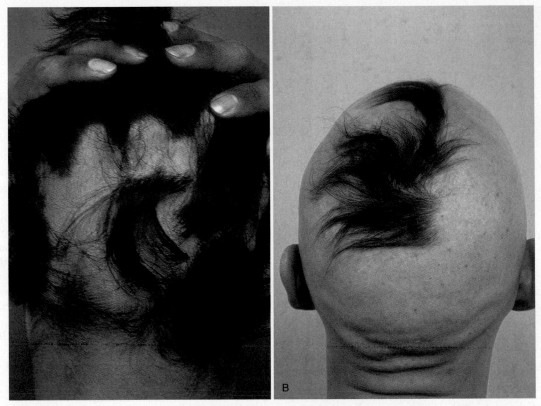

Fig 18-8
Alopecia areata. **A, B,** These patients have more severe disease, with extensive hair loss.
(Courtesy of the Institute of Dermatology, London.)

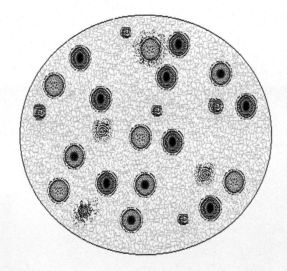

Fig 18-9
Alopecia areata. Overall, there are normal numbers of follicles with increased catagen-telogen forms and conspicuous stellae.
(Courtesy of Dr. M. Mejia, Universidad Pontificia Bolivariana, Medellín, Colombia.)

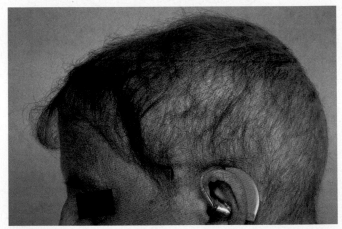

Fig 18-10
Trichotillomania. In this severely affected patient, there is obvious and extensive hair loss.
(Courtesy of the Institute of Dermatology, London.)

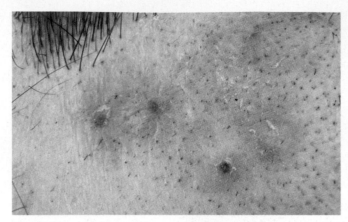

Fig 18-11
Trichotillomania. Note the excoriations.
(Courtesy of the Institute of Dermatology, London.)

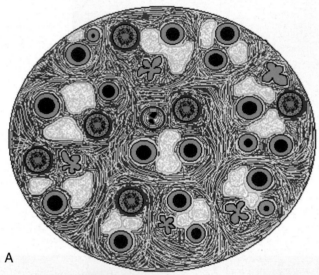

A

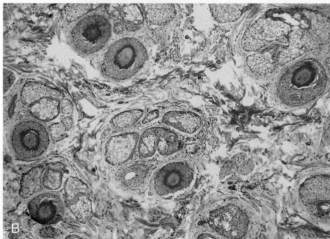

B

Fig 18-12
Trichotillomania, horizontal section. **A,** In addition to residual anagen follicles, there are conspicuous catagen follicles with a bright eosinophilic center and prominent telogen follicles. **B,** Photomicrograph taken at medium power showing several follicular units. Note that all the follicles are catagen, with a bright eosinophilic center. There is no significant inflammation.
(**A** courtesy of Dr. M. Mejia, Universidad Pontificia Bolivariana, Medellín, Colombia.)

DIAGNOSTIC INVESTIGATION
- Hair microscopy
- Scalp biopsy
- CBC, ferritin

TREATMENT
- Psychotherapy, behavioral therapy
- Selective serotonin reuptake inhibitors (SSRIs), neuroleptics

E. TELOGEN EFFLUVIUM

DEFINITION
This disorder is characterized by an early end to the anagen stage, with the progression of many hairs to catagen and subsequently telogen.

- Telogen effluvium may be precipitated by physiologic processes such as severe psychological stress, postpartum state, or crash diets or by pathologic events such as spinal cord injury, major surgery, hypothyroidism, HIV infection, septicemia, and Hodgkin's lymphoma.
- Several medications have also been implicated (e.g., lipid-lowering agents, anticoagulants, beta blockers, oral contraceptives).
- Patients show diffuse noninflammatory hair loss involving the entire scalp (Fig. 18-13).
- The loss of hair begins approximately 3 to 4 months after the precipitating event. Baldness, however, is never observed.
- Histologically, the only finding are increases in the number of telogen hair follicles and follicular stellae in the deep layers (Fig. 18-14).

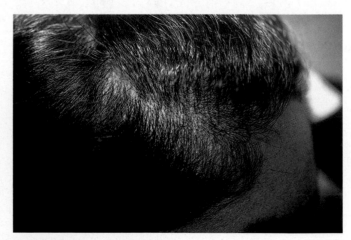

Fig 18-13
Telogen effluvium. There is diffuse hair loss without inflammation.
(From Hordinsky ME, Sawaya ME, Scher RK [eds]: Atlas of Hair and Nails. Philadelphia, WB Saunders, 2000.)

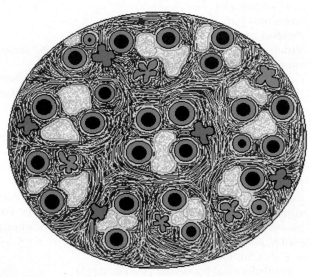

Fig 18–14
Telogen effluvium. Normal numbers of follicular units and hair follicles are present, with increased numbers of telogen follicles.
(Courtesy of Dr. M. Mejia, Universidad Pontificia Bolivariana, Medellín, Colombia.)

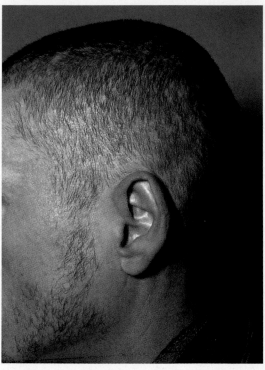

Fig 18–15
Syphilitic alopecia—typical moth-eaten pattern of alopecia.
(Courtesy of Dr. P. Reygagne, Centre Sabouraud, Paris.)

F. SYPHILITIC ALOPECIA

DEFINITION
This is a form of alopecia presenting as a manifestation of secondary syphilis.

PHYSICAL EXAMINATION AND CLINICAL PRESENTATION
- The hair loss may affect the scalp or any other hair-bearing area of the body.
- The patches of alopecia present with a characteristic moth-eaten appearance (Fig. 18–15)
- Laboratory evaluation reveals a positive VDRL.
- Histologically, the presence of plasma cells and the tendency of the infiltrate to spare the hair bulb and involve the external root sheath at a higher level are helpful diagnostic indicators.

Chapter 19   Acne vulgaris

DEFINITION

Acne vulgaris is a chronic disorder of the pilosebaceous apparatus caused by abnormal desquamation of follicular epithelium leading to obstruction of the pilosebaceous canal, resulting in inflammation and subsequent formation of papules, pustules, nodules, comedones, and scarring.

- Acne can be classified by the type of lesion (comedonal, papulopustular, nodulocystic).
- The American Academy of Dermatology classification scheme for acne has denoted the following three levels.
  1. Mild acne: characterized by the presence of comedomes (noninflammatory lesions), few papules and pustules (generally less than 10) but no nodules
  2. Moderate acne (Fig. 19-1): presence of several to many papules and pustules (10 to 40) along with comedomes (10 to 40) (Fig. 19-2). The presence of more than 40 papules and pustules along with larger, deeper nodular inflamed lesions (up to five) denotes moderately severe acne.
  3. Severe acne: presence of numerous or extensive papules and pustules as well as many nodular lesions

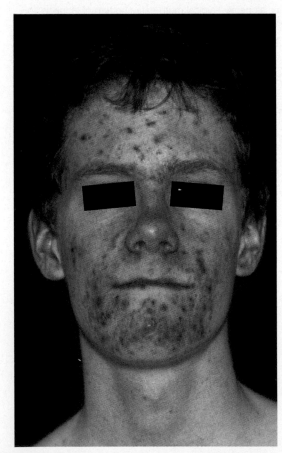

Fig 19–1
Acne vulgaris. Note the numerous papules and pustules. The chest and back are also commonly affected.
(Courtesy of Dr. R. A. Marsden, St. George's Hospital, London.)

PHYSICAL FINDINGS AND CLINICAL PRESENTATION

- Open comedones (blackheads; Fig. 19–3), closed comedones (whiteheads)
- Greasiness (oily skin)
- Presence of scars from prior acne cysts
- Various stages of development and severity may be present concomitantly.
- Common distribution of acne: face, back, and upper chest
- Inflammatory papules, pustules (Fig. 19–4), and ectatic pores

CAUSE

- Overactivity of the sebaceous glands and blockage in the ducts. The obstruction leads to the formation of comedones, which can become inflamed because of overgrowth of *Propionibacterium acnes.*
- Exacerbated by environmental factors (hot, humid tropical climate), medications (e.g., iodine in cough mixtures, hair greases), industrial exposure to halogenated hydrocarbons

DIFFERENTIAL DIAGNOSIS

- Folliculitis (see Fig. 28–14)
- Staphylococcal pyoderma (see Fig. 28–3)
- Acne rosacea (see Fig. 20–1)
- Drug eruption (see Fig. 10–2)
- Basal cell carcinoma (see Fig. 22–9)

LABORATORY TESTS

- Laboratory evaluation is generally not helpful.
- Patients who are candidates for therapy with isotretinoin (Accutane) should have baseline liver enzymes, cholesterol, and triglycerides checked, because this medication may result in elevations of lipid and liver enzyme levels.
- A negative serum pregnancy test or two negative urine pregnancy test results should also be obtained in females 1 week before the initiation of isotretinoin. It is also imperative to maintain effective contraception during and 1 month after therapy with isotretinoin is discontinued because of its teratogenic effects. Pregnancy status should be rechecked at monthly visits.
- In female patients, if hyperandrogenism is suspected, levels of dehydroepiandrosterone sulfate (DHEAS), testosterone (total and free), and androstenedione should be measured. Generally, for women with regular menstrual cycles, serum androgen measurements are not necessary.

TREATMENT

Treatment generally varies with the type of lesion (e.g., comedones, papules, pustules, cystic lesions) and the severity of the acne.

- Comedones can be treated with retinoids or retinoid analogues. Topical retinoids are comedolytic and work by normalizing follicular keratinization.
- Patients should be re-evaluated after 4 to 6 weeks. Benzoyl peroxide gel (2.5% or 5%) may be added if the comedones become inflamed or form pustules.
- Pustular acne can be treated with tretinoin and benzoyl peroxide gel applied on alternate evenings. Drying agents (sulfacetamide, sulfa lotions) are also effective when used in combination with benzoyl peroxide; oral antibiotics (doxy-

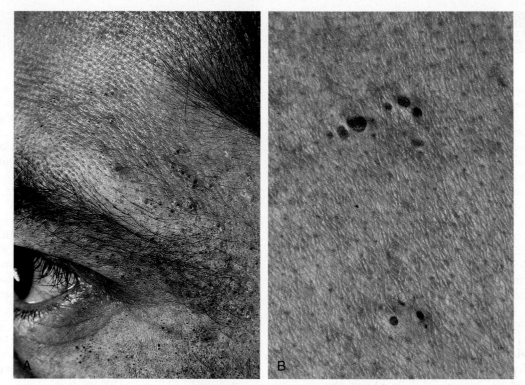

Fig 19–2
Acne vulgaris. **A,** Typical open comedones (blackheads). **B,** Close-up view.
(**A** courtesy of Dr. R. A. Marsden, St. George's Hospital, London; **B,** courtesy of the Institute of Dermatology, London.)

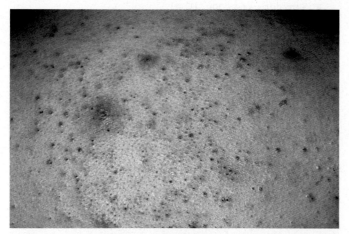

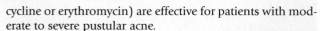

Fig 19–3
Acne vulgaris. There are widespread blackheads that develop as a result of blockage of the pilosebaceous canal by keratotic debris.
(Courtesy of Dr. R. A. Marsden, St. George's Hospital, London.)

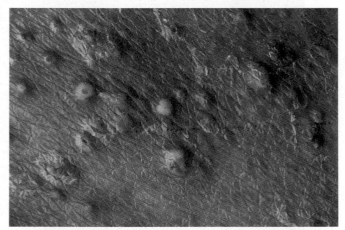

Fig 19–4
Acne vulgaris. Note the presence of multiple pustules.
(Courtesy of the Institute of Dermatology, London.)

cycline or erythromycin) are effective for patients with moderate to severe pustular acne.

- Patients with nodular cystic acne can be treated with systemic agents—antibiotics (erythromycin, tetracycline, doxycycline, minocycline), isotretinoin (Accutane), or oral contraceptives. Periodic intralesional triamcinolone (Kenalog) injections by a dermatologist are also effective. The possibility of endocrinopathy should be considered in patients responding poorly to therapy.

- Isotretinoin is indicated for acne resistant to antibiotic therapy and severe acne.
- Oral contraceptives reduce androgen levels and therefore sebum production. They represent a useful adjunctive therapy for all types of acne in women and adolescent girls.
- Blue light (ClearLight therapy system) can be used for the treatment of moderate inflammatory acne vulgaris.

Chapter 20   Rosacea

DEFINITION
Rosacea is a chronic skin disorder characterized by papules and pustules affecting the face and often associated with flushing and erythema.

PHYSICAL FINDINGS AND CLINICAL PRESENTATION
- Facial erythema, presence of papules, pustules (Fig. 20–1), telangiectasia
- Excessive facial warmth and redness are the predominant presenting complaints (Fig. 20–2).
- Itching is generally absent.
- Comedones are absent (unlike acne).
- Women are more likely to show symptoms on the chin and cheeks, whereas in men the nose is commonly involved.
- Ocular findings (mild dryness and irritation with blepharitis, conjunctival injection, burning, stinging, tearing, eyelid inflammation, swelling, and redness) are present in 50% of patients.

CLASSIFICATION
Rosacea can be classified into four major subtypes:

1. Erythematotelengiectatic: erythema in central part of the face, telangiectasia, flushing
2. Papulopustular: presence of dome-shaped erythematous papules and small pustules, in addition to facial erythema, flushing, and telangiectasia
3. Phymatous: presence of thickened skin with prominent pores that may affect the nose (rhinophyma) (Fig. 20–3), chin (gnathophyma), forehead (metophyma), eyelids (blepharophyma), and ears (otophyma)
4. Ocular: conjunctival injection, sensation of foreign body in the eye, telangiectasia and erythema of lid margins, and scaling

CAUSE
- Unknown
- Hot drinks, alcohol, and sun exposure may accentuate the erythema by causing vasodilation of the skin.
- Flare-ups may also result from reactions to medications (e.g., simvastatin, angiotensin-converting enzyme [ACE] inhibitors, vasodilators, fluorinated corticosteroids), stress, extreme heat or cold, spicy drinks, menstruation.

DIFFERENTIAL DIAGNOSIS
- Drug eruption (see Fig. 10–2)
- Acne vulgaris; distinguishing features between acne and rosacea are presence of telangiectasia, deep diffuse erythema, absence of comedones in rosacea (see Fig. 19–1)
- Contact dermatitis (see Fig. 6–8)
- SLE (see Fig. 293–1)
- Carcinoid flush (see Fig. 197–1)
- Idiopathic facial flushing
- Seborrheic dermatitis (see Fig. 6–4)
- Sarcoidosis (see Fig. 11–4)
- Photodermatitis (see Fig. 10–2)
- Urticaria pigmentosa (see Fig. 15–13)

TREATMENT
- Avoid alcohol, excessive sun exposure, and hot drinks of any type.
- Use of mild, nondrying soap is recommended; local skin irritants should be avoided.
- Reassure patient that rosacea is completely unrelated to poor hygiene.

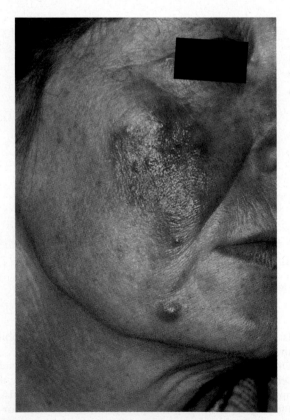

Fig 20–1
Stage 3 rosacea. Note the papules and pustules on the cheek. (Courtesy of the Institute of Dermatology, London.)

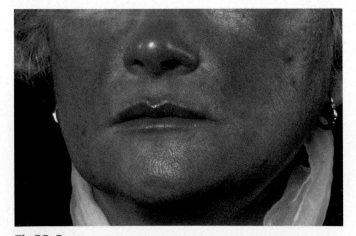

Fig 20–2
Stage 2 rosacea. There is diffuse erythema of the face, with malar telangiectasia; note the papules and pustules on the cheek (*right*). (Courtesy of the Institute of Dermatology, London.)

- Several classes of drugs are used in the treatment of rosacea, including metronidazoles, tetracyclines, and azelaic acid.
- Topical therapy with metronidazole aqueous gel applied twice daily is effective as initial therapy for mild cases or following the use of oral antibiotics.
- Systemic antibiotics: tetracycline, doxycycline, or minocycline
- Laser treatment is an option for progressive telangiectasias or rhinophyma.
- Erythema and flushing may respond to low-dose clonidine (0.1 mg daily).

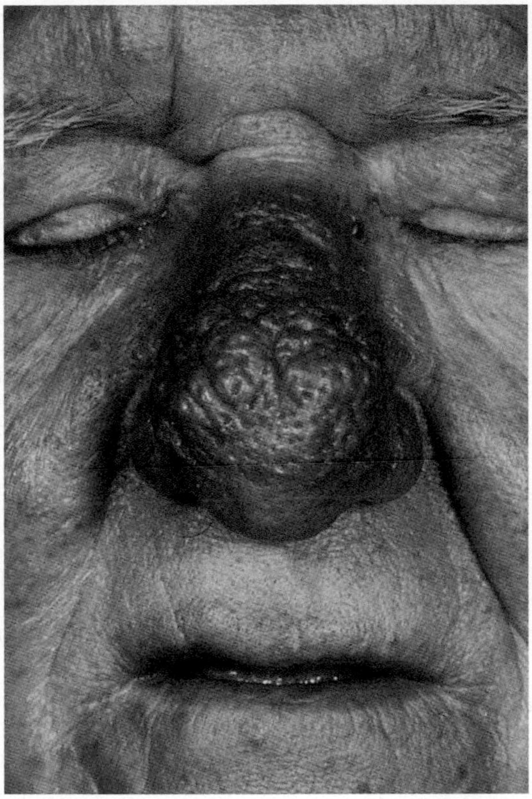

Fig 20–3
Stage 4 rosacea. This is the typical appearance of rhinophyma. Note the concomitant erythema affecting the cheeks, upper eyelids, and forehead.
(Courtesy of Dr. R. A. Marsden, St. George's Hospital, London.)

Chapter 21   **Diseases of the nails**

A. NORMAL ANATOMY

- The nail unit itself is composed of at least six specialized anatomic subunits. These include the nail folds (proximal and lateral); hyponychium at the distal end of the nail unit, which surrounds the nail plate; matrix epithelium, which produces the nail plate; nail plate, and its overlying cuticle; and structures that support the nail plate, including the underlying nail bed and ligaments (Fig. 21–1).
- The whitish nail matrix of proliferating epithelial cells grows in a semilunar pattern. It extends outward past the posterior nail fold and is called the lunula. On the average, nails grow from 0.1 to 1 mm/day, growth being faster in the summer than in the winter, and fingernails growing faster than toenails.
- Figure 21–2 illustrates structural relationship of the nail.

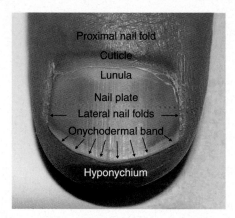

Fig 21–1
Normal nail unit. Note the nail folds, hyponychium, lunula, cuticle, and onychodermal band.
(From McKee PH, Calonje E, Granter SR [eds]: Pathology of the Skin With Clinical Correlations, 3rd ed. St. Louis, Mosby, 2005.)

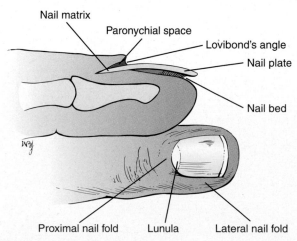

Fig 21–2
Structural relations of the nail—cross-sectional view and view from above.
(From Swartz MH: Textbook of Physical Diagnosis, 5th ed. Philadelphia, WB Saunders, 2006.)

B. ONYCHOMYCOSIS

DEFINITION
Onychomycosis is defined as a persistent fungal infection affecting the toenails and fingernails.

CAUSE
- The most common causes of onychomycosis are dermatophyte, yeast, and nondermatophyte molds. It occurs more frequently in patients with diabetes, peripheral vascular disease, and any conditions resulting in the suppression of the immune system. Occlusive footwear, physical exercise followed by communal showering, and incomplete drying of the feet predispose the individual to developing onychomycosis.
- The dermatophyte *Trichophyton rubrum* accounts for 80% of all nail infections caused by fungus.
- *T. interdigitale* and *T. mentagrophytes* are other fungi causing onychomycosis.
- The yeast *Candida albicans* is responsible for 5% of cases of onychomycosis.
- Nondermatophyte molds, *Scopulariopsis brevicaulis* and *Aspergillus niger*, although rare, can also cause onychomycosis.

PHYSICAL FINDINGS AND CLINICAL PRESENTATION
- Onychomycosis causes nails to become thick, brittle, hard, distorted, and discolored (yellow to brown color). Eventually, the nail may loosen, separate from the nail bed, and fall off.
- Onychomycosis is frequently associated with tinea pedis (athlete's foot).
- Onychomycosis is classified according to the clinical pattern of nail bed involvement. There are five main types:
  1. Distal and lateral subungual onychomycosis (DLSO) (Fig. 21–3)
  2. Superficial onychomycosis (Fig. 21–4)
  3. Proximal subungual onychomycosis
  4. Endonyx onychomycosis
  5. Total dystrophic onychomycosis

DIFFERENTIAL DIAGNOSIS
- Psoriasis (see Fig. 21–5)
- Contact dermatitis (see Fig. 6–7)
- Lichen planus (see Fig. 21–18)
- Subungual squamous cell carcinoma (see Fig. 21–22)

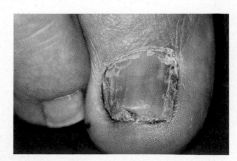

Fig 21–3
Distal subungual onychomycosis. This is the most common variant of nail dermatophyte infection.
(Courtesy of Dr. G. T. Reizner, University of Wisconsin Medical School, Madison, Wisc.)

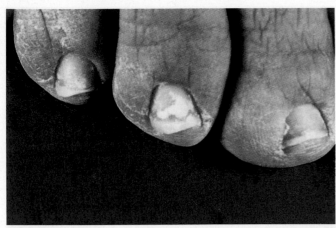

Fig 21–4
Superficial onychomycosis. In this variant, the fungi invade the dorsal aspect of the nail plate. Tinea pedis is commonly present.
(From Hordinsky ME, Sawaya ME, Scher RK [eds]: Atlas of Hair and Nails. Philadelphia, WB Saunders, 2000.)

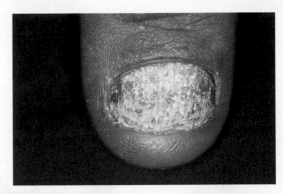

Fig 21–5
Psoriasis. This nail shows extensive pitting and onycholysis.
(Courtesy of Dr. R. K. Scher, Columbia University, New York.)

- Paronychia (see Fig. 21–6)
- Infection (e.g., *Pseudomonas*)
- Trauma
- Subungual keratoacanthoma (see Fig. 21–24)
- Yellow nail syndrome (see Fig. 21–17)

LABORATORY TESTS
- Blood tests are not specific for the diagnosis of onychomycosis. The workup of suspected onychomycosis is directed at confirming the diagnosis of onychomycosis by visualizing hyphae under the microscope or by growing the organism in culture (see Fig. 2–4).
- KOH preparation
- Fungal cultures on Sabouraud medium

TREATMENT
- Prevention of reinfection by wearing properly fitted shoes, avoiding public showers, and keeping feet and nails clean and dry
- Topical antifungal creams (miconazole, clotrimazole) are used for early superficial nail infections.
- Oral agents (terbinafine, itraconazole, fluconazole)

C. PSORIASIS
- Nails are affected in almost 80% of patients with psoriasis.
- The most common presentation is pitting of the nails, followed by discoloration (oil spots and white discoloration), onycholysis, and subungual hyperkeratosis (Fig. 21–5).

D. PARONYCHIA
- Paronychia is a bacterial infection of the proximal and lateral nail fold manifesting with pain and accumulation of pus (Fig. 21–6).
- Most commonly caused by *S. aureus*
- Treatment consists of incision and drainage. Oral antibiotics may be necessary for select patients.

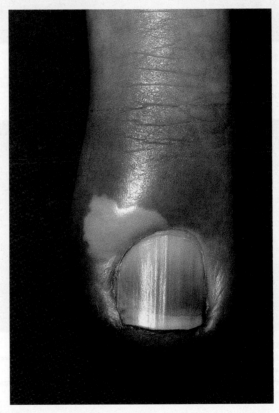

Fig 21–6
Acute paronychia. Pus and erythema are present.
(Courtesy of Dr. E. E. Gluckman, King's College Hospital, London.)

E. BEAU'S LINES
- Beau's lines are transverse grooves or depressions parallel to the lunula.
- They are caused by conditions or disorders that result in slower nail growth for a certain period.
- They are often seen following major surgery (Fig. 21–7), severe infections, chemotherapy, malnutrition, and physical and emotional stress, such as following a myocardial infarction.
- The lines progress distally and eventually disappear at the free edge.

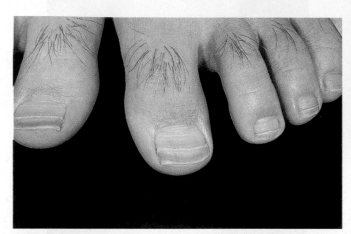

Fig 21–7
Beau's lines. This patient had major surgery 5 months earlier.
(From Callen JP, Greer KE, Paller AS, Swinyer LJ: Color Atlas of Dermatology, 2nd ed. Philadelphia, WB Saunders, 2000.)

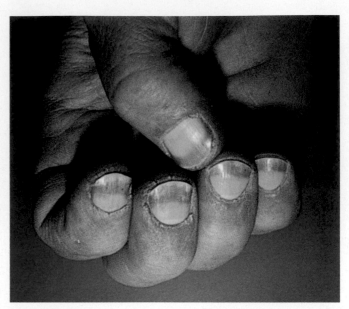

Fig 21–9
Lindsay's nails.
(From Swartz MH: Textbook of Physical Diagnosis, 5th ed. Philadelphia, WB Saunders, 2006.)

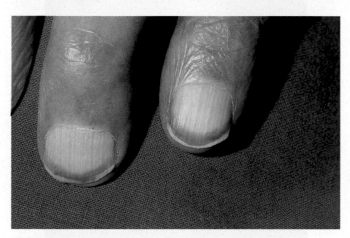

Fig 21–8
Terry nails. There is proximal pallor with distal brownish color in a patient with chronic renal failure.
(From White GM, Cox NH [eds]: Diseases of the Skin: A Color Atlas and Text, 2nd ed. St. Louis, Mosby, 2006.)

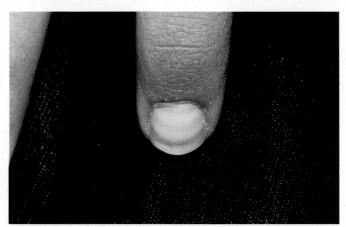

Fig 21–10
Muercke lines.
(From White GM, Cox NH [eds]: Diseases of the Skin: A Color Atlas and Text, 2nd ed. St. Louis, Mosby, 2006.)

F. TERRY NAILS

- Terry nails are white nail beds to within 1 to 2 mm of the distal border of the nail (Fig. 21–8).
- Often found in patients with liver cirrhosis
- Occasionally seen with congestive heart failure (CHF), type 2 diabetes mellitus (DM), but can also be found in normal individuals

G. LINDSAY NAILS

- Lindsay nails are nails in which the distal portion is red or pink and the proximal portion is whitish (Fig. 21–9).
- They are also called half-and-half nails because of their characteristic appearance. They are most frequently found in patients with chronic renal failure.

H. MUERCKE'S LINES

- Muercke's lines are transverse whitish bands parallel to the lunula (Fig. 21–10).
- They are commonly found in hypoalbuminemic patients (e.g., nephrotic syndrome) and in patients undergoing chemotherapy.

I. KOILONYCHIA

- Koilonychia is a thinning and cuplike depression of the nail plate (spoon nail).
- Figure 21–11 compares a nail with koilonychia with a normal one.
- It is most commonly associated with iron deficiency anemia but may occur secondary to local irritation.

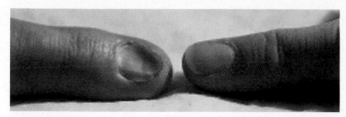

Fig 21-11
Koilonychia.
(From Swartz MH: Textbook of Physical Diagnosis, 5th ed. Philadelphia, WB Saunders, 2006.)

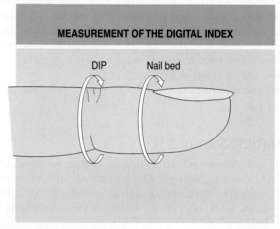

MEASUREMENT OF THE DIGITAL INDEX

DIP   Nail bed

Fig 21-12
The digital index. The perimeter of each of the 10 fingers is measured at the nail bed (NB) and at the distal interphalangeal joint (DIP). If the sum of the 10 NB:DIP ratios is more than 10, clubbing is probably present.
(From Hochberg MC, Silman AJ, Smolen JS, et al [eds]: Rheumatology, 3rd ed. St. Louis, Mosby, 2003.)

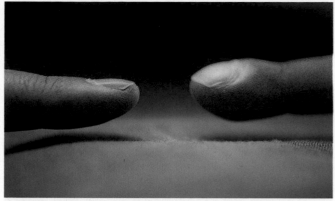

Fig 21-13
Clubbing deformity. The finger on the right is clubbed compared with the normal finger shape on the left.
(From Hochberg MC, Silman AJ, Smolen JS, et al [eds]: Rheumatology, 3rd ed. St. Louis, Mosby, 2003.)

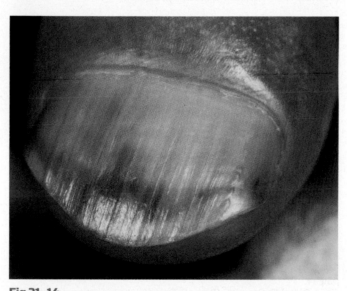

Fig 21-14
Splinter hemorrhages.
(From Swartz MH: Textbook of Physical Diagnosis, 5th ed. Philadelphia, WB Saunders, 2006.)

J. CLUBBING OF THE NAILS

- Clubbing of the nails is a disorder frequently associated with pulmonary disease (e.g., bronchogenic carcinoma, chronic obstructive pulonary disorder [COPD], cystic fibrosis, bronchiectasis) and cyanotic heart disease. It may also be inherited as an autosomal dominant trait. Measurement of the digital index is illustrated in Figure 21-12.
- The angle between the normal nail base and finger is about 160 degrees and the nail bed is firm. The angle is referred to as *Lovibond's angle*. When clubbing develops, Lovibond's angle generally exceeds 180 degrees as the base of the nail becomes swollen and the distal digit develops a fusiform enlargement.
- Figure 21-13 compares a normal with a clubbed finger.

K. SPLINTER HEMORRHAGES

- Splinter hemorrhages are the extravasation of blood from longitudinal nail bed blood vessels into adjacent troughs (Fig. 21-14).
- Although usually associated with subacute bacterial endocarditis, they may occur with various other disorders (e.g., SLE, vasculitis, infections, leukemia) and may be found in up to 20% of hospitalized patients.

L. *CANDIDA* INFECTION

- *Candida* infection of the nails usually manifests with proximal nail dystrophy and onycholysis (Fig. 21-15).
- Pigmentary changes are also common.

M. DRUG-INDUCED NAIL DISCOLORATION

- Commonly responsible agents are minocycline, antimalarials, gold, and azidothymidine (AZT) (Fig. 21-16)

N. YELLOW NAIL SYNDROME

- In yellow nail syndrome, the nail color varies from pale yellow to dark yellow-green (Fig. 21-17).
- The nails are overcurved, with disappearance of the cuticle.
- Linear nail growth is delayed.
- Onychomycosis is a frequent occurrence.

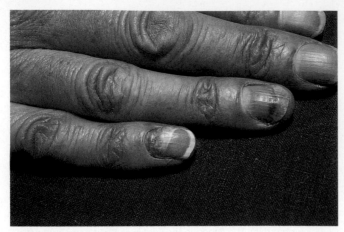

Fig 21–15
Candidiasis. There are proximal nail dystrophy and onycholysis, with pigmentary changes.
(Courtesy of the Institute of Dermatology, London.)

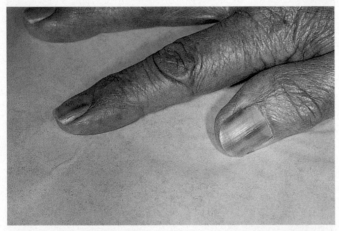

Fig 21–16
Color changes secondary to azidothymidine therapy of an HIV-infected patient.
(From Callen JP, Greer KE, Paller AS, Swinyer LJ: Color Atlas of Dermatology, 2nd ed. Philadelphia, WB Saunders, 2000.)

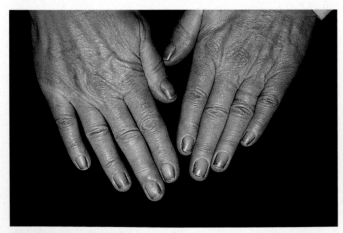

Fig 21–17
Yellow nail syndrome. These patients are commonly found to have pulmonary disease.
(From Callen JP, Greer KE, Paller AS, Swinyer LJ: Color Atlas of Dermatology, 2nd ed. Philadelphia, WB Saunders, 2000.)

- Found most often in patients with pulmonary disorders (e.g., chronic bronchitis, bronchiectasis)
- Diagnosis: rule out nail fungal infection, *Pseudomonas* infection. Laboratory tests should include CBC, TSH, ALT, creatinine, and alkaline phosphatase.
- Treatment: alpha-tocopherol, fluconazole, topical vitamin E, treatment of underlying disorder

O. LICHEN PLANUS

- Nail involvement occurs in 10% of patients with cutaneous lichen planus.
- Clinically, individually involved nails may show changes identical to those seen in trauma and other conditions that damage the matrix, such as psoriasis and eczema. The involvement of several digits helps distinguish these inflammatory processes from trauma, which is more likely to involve only a single digit (Fig. 21–18)
- Additional information on this disorder is available in Section 1.8.

P. DARIER'S DISEASE

- The nail changes in Darier's disease include longitudinal red or white streaks, or both, which terminate in a notch on the free margin of the nail plate, splitting, and subungual hyperkeratosis, with associated wedge-shaped onycholysis (Fig. 21–19).

Q. LONGITUDINAL MELANONYCHIA

- Longitudinal melanonychia refers to the presence of longitudinal bands of pigment in the nail plate caused by movement of the pigment produced in the nail plate, with the rest of the nail plate distally, to the tip of the digit (Fig. 21–20).
- The condition is rare in whites; in contrast, Hispanic, black, and Asian patients, who are particularly affected and in whom the condition may be regarded as a normal variation.

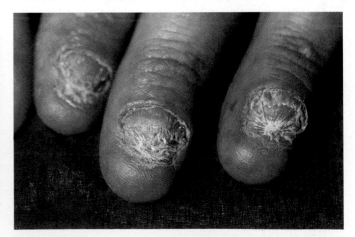

Fig 21–18
Lichen planus. In this example, there is gross nail destruction.
(Courtesy of Dr. R. K. Scher, Columbia University, New York.)

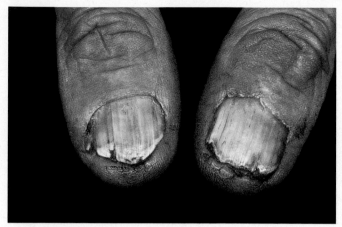

Fig 21–19
Darier's disease. Notches on the free margin of the nail are common findings.
(Courtesy of the Institute of Dermatology, London.)

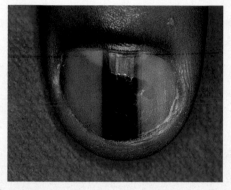

Fig 21–20
Longitudinal melanonychia. This case was caused by a melanocytic nevus of the matrix. The streak remained stable in size during observation.
(Courtesy of Dr. R. K. Scher, Columbia University, New York.)

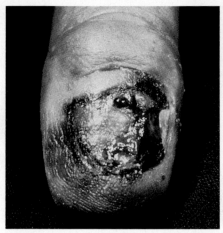

Fig 21–21
Subungual melanoma. Note the spread of pigment onto the nail folds (Hutchinson's sign).
(Courtesy of Dr. R. K. Scher, Columbia University, New York.)

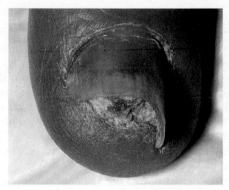

Fig 21–22
Subungual squamous cell carcinoma. This case presented as a warty tumor nodule protruding from under the nail plate.
(Courtesy of Dr. R. K. Scher, Columbia University, New York.)

R. SUBUNGUAL MELANOMA

● Subungual melanoma is a rare type of melanoma, accounting for only 2% to 3% of all melanomas in light-skinned individuals. However, it represents a significantly higher percentage of melanomas in Hispanic, black patients, and those of Asian ethnicity.
● The fingers are affected more often than the toes.
● Most tumors (more than 90%) occur on the thumb or great toe.
● The tumor may present as nail loss, nonhealing ulcer, tumor nodule, or subungual pigmentation that often extends onto the nail folds (*Hutchinson's sign, Hutchinson's melanotic whitlow*; Fig. 21–21).
● It is associated with a poor prognosis, with a mean survival of only 10 to 30 months, often caused by delay in diagnosis.

S. SQUAMOUS CELL CARCINOMA

● Squamous cell carcinoma usually grows slowly, often mimicking other chronic nail conditions (Fig. 21–22).
● The hands are affected much more often than the toes, with a predilection for the thumb and index finger (Fig. 21–23).

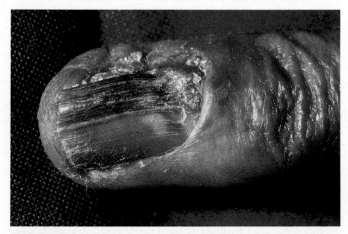

Fig 21–23
Subungual squamous cell carcinoma. There is a crusted tumor nodule elevating the proximal nail fold and extending under the lateral border of the nail plate.
(Courtesy of the Institute of Dermatology, London.)

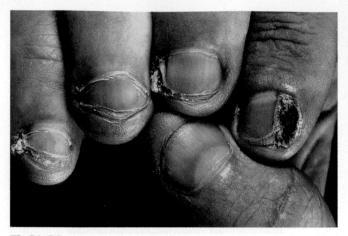

Fig 21–24
Subungual keratoaconthama. Although this lesion is pigmented because of hemorrhage, in contrast to melanoma there is no spread of pigment onto the adjacent nail folds.
(Courtesy of Dr. R. K. Scher, Columbia University, New York.)

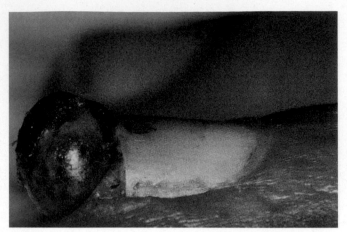

Fig 21–25
Periungual pyogenic granuloma. There is a large hemorrhagic nodule adjacent to the free edge of the nail.
(From Baran R, Dawber RPR, Levene GM: A Colour Atlas of the Hair, Scalp and Nails. London, Wolfe, 1991.)

T. SUBUNGUAL KERATOACANTHOMA

- Clinically, keratoacanthoma arising in the nail bed or matrix shows a rapid initial growth phase.
- Because the nail plate may confine the tumor, it is often characterized by early pain and bony erosion, clinical features that help differentiate it from squamous cell carcinoma, which is usually slow growing and asymptomatic.
- The thumb is most commonly affected and, at an early stage in its development, the nail plate is lifted off from the underlying bed.
- Subsequent destruction of the nail plate may occur to reveal a red keratotic nodule (Fig. 21–24).

U. PYOGENIC GRANULOMA

- Despite its name, pyogenic granuloma begins as a proliferation of vessels rather than with pyogenic or granulomatous inflammation.
- It may arise from the vasculature of the dermis of any portion of the nail unit, but the lateral nail fold is most commonly affected (Fig. 21–25).
- Lesions that occur in the dermis underlying the nail plate may be exquisitely painful. Involvement of the nail bed epithelium can cause temporary destruction of the nail plate.

V. SUBUNGUAL EXOSTOSIS

- Benign and often painful tumor-like reactive condition that arises from the bone of the distal phalanx and secondarily impinges on the overlying nail unit, with resultant distortion, subungual hyperkeratosis, and onycholysis
- As the name implies, it represents an outgrowth of bone, arising from the distal phalanx.
- The toes are most often affected and most lesions involve the great toe. Patients present with flesh-colored or erythematous, sometimes tender, hard nodules usually measuring 0.5 to 1 cm in diameter (Fig. 21–26).

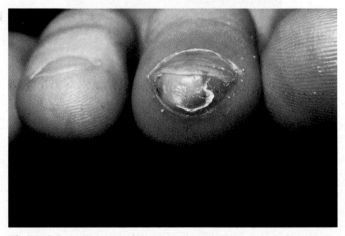

Fig 21–26
Subungual exostosis. This white nodule has elevated the nail plate.
(Courtesy of the Institute of Dermatology, London.)

- There is no evidence of destruction of the underlying phalanx.
- Treatment is surgical excision.

W. SUBUNGUAL GLOMUS TUMOR

- A subungual glomus tumor is a well-circumscribed nodule with small ectatic vascular spaces surrounded by clusters of glomus cells.
- The nodules are flesh-colored but may become purple with hemorrhage (Fig. 21–27).
- Sometimes, the nodules erode the bone of the phalanx and cause pressure dystrophy of the overlying nail.

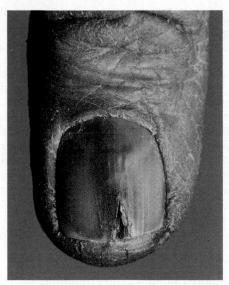

Fig 21-27
Subungual glomous tumor. There is an erythematous nodule deep to the lunula. Note the splitting of the free edge of the nail.
(From Baran R, Dawber RPR, Levene GM: A Colour Atlas of the Hair, Scalp and Nails. London, Wolfe, 1991.)

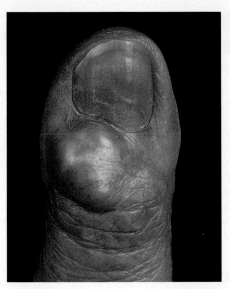

Fig 21-28
Myxoid cyst. Localization over the distal interphalangeal joint is characteristic.
(Courtesy of the Institute of Dermatology, London.)

X. MYXOID CYST

- A myxoid cyst is a soft or fluctuant cystic nodule on the dorsal aspects of the distal interphalangeal, metacarpophalangeal and, less frequently, metatarsophalangeal joints (Fig. 21-28).
- Lesions are often painful or tender.
- Myxoid cysts involving the proximal nail fold may be associated with longitudinal grooving of the nail.
- Treatment: pricking and expression of gelatinous material, cryosurgery, repeated puncture, laser therapy, use of sclerosant

Y. PERIUNGUAL FIBROMA

- Periungual fibromas are multiple asymptomatic, persistent, slowly growing, flesh-colored or reddish brown oval or filiform lesions (Fig. 21-29) located under the nail plate, with resulting onycholysis, or under the proximal or lateral nail folds, where they cause nail plate distortion.
- The fingers and toes are equally affected.
- Most lesions present around puberty.
- Periungual fibromas are a hallmark of tuberous sclerosis

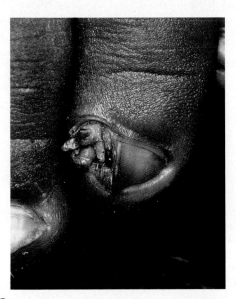

Fig 21-29
Periungual fibroma. Periungual fibromas are a hallmark of tuberous sclerosis.
(Courtesy of the Institute of Dermatology, London.)

Chapter 22 **Tumors of the surface epithelium**

A. EPIDERMAL NEVUS

- Epidermal nevi are lesions that may be present at birth or develop during childhood. They are usually yellowish-brown warty papules or plaques with irregular margins.
- They commonly affect the trunk or limbs and vary from trivial small lesions to extensive areas of involvement, which may cause the patient great cosmetic embarrassment (Fig. 22–1).
- The gender incidence is equal and there is no racial predilection.
- Familial cases may rarely be seen, with autosomal dominant transmission.

B. SEBORRHEIC KERATOSIS

- Seborrheic keratosis are common skin lesions, developing in middle-aged and older adults.

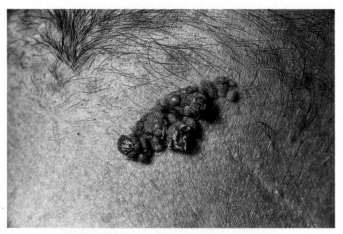

Fig 22–1
Epidermal nevus. This fairly typical lesion appeared on the chest of a young male.
(Courtesy of Dr. R. A. Marsden, St. George's Hospital, London.)

- They are frequently numerous and appear as sharply delineated, round or oval, flesh-colored or brown-black warty plaques with a rather greasy texture (Fig. 22–2). Although they may be found anywhere on the body (except palms and soles), they are particularly common on the face, chest, and back.
- A sudden onset of numerous seborrheic keratoses (*Leser-Trélat sign*) (Fig. 22–3) has been reported in association with internal malignancy, most commonly adenocarcinoma of the stomach. It has also been described after treatment with chemotherapy.
- Treatment involves curettage and cautery, cryotherapy, chemical peels, and laser therapy.

C. ACANTHOMA FISSURATUM (SPECTACLE FRAME ACANTHOMA)

- Acanthoma fissuratum is a benign epidermal tumor that develops as a result of chronic irritation from the frame of eyeglasses.
- It presents as an erythematous or flesh-colored, sometimes tender, nodule situated on the bridge of the nose or behind the ears (Fig. 22–4).
- Typically, the center of the lesion shows a linear groove.
- The importance of this entity is that clinically, it is frequently misdiagnosed as a basal cell or squamous cell carcinoma.

D. LARGE CELL ACANTHOMA

- Large cell acanthoma is a skin lesion presenting as a discrete scaly papule or plaque up to 1 cm or more in diameter.
- It is most commonly found on the head, arms, trunk, and lower limbs, in decreasing order of frequency (Fig. 22–5).
- The lesions are generally single and sharply demarcated but multiple acanthomas have occasionally been documented.

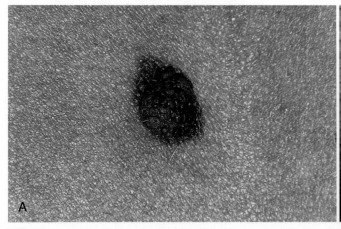
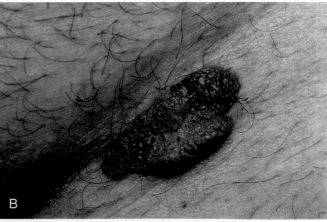

Fig 22–2
 Seborrheic keratosis. **A,** Close-up view showing the warty surface. **B,** Pigmented variants may be mistaken for malignant melanoma.
(**A** courtesy of Dr. M. Beare [deceased], Royal Victoria Hospital, Belfast, Northern Ireland; **B** courtesy of the Institute of Dermatology, London.)

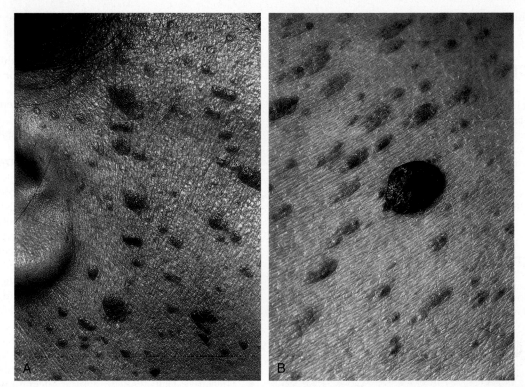

Fig 22-3
Leser-Trélat sign **(A, B)**. The sudden onset of numerous seborrheic keratoses may indicate an underlying malignant visceral neoplasm.
(Courtesy of Dr. M. M. Black, Institute of Dermatology, London.)

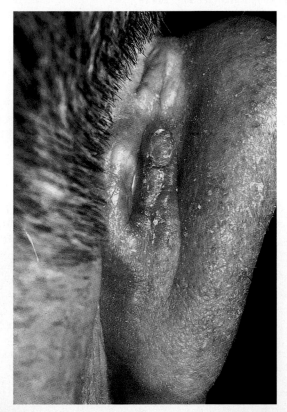

Fig 22-4
Spectacle frame acanthoma. Illustrated is a "tumor" behind the ear of a middle-aged man. Note the characteristic central groove or furrow.
(Courtesy of Dr. N. Smith [deceased], Institute of Dermatology, London.)

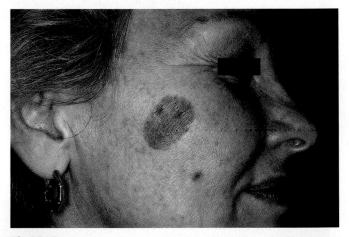

Fig 22-5
Large cell acanthoma. This pigmented lesion could be mistaken for lentigo maligna.
(Courtesy of Dr. D. Santa Cruz, MD, St. John's Mercy Medical Center, St. Louis.)

- They are often confused with seborrheic keratoses, actinic keratoses, or actinic lentigines.

E. CLEAR CELL ACANTHOMA (DEGOS)

- Clear cell acanthoma is an uncommon, usually solitary, skin tumor, generally occurring in middle-aged or older adults.
- Although variably regarded as an inflammatory epithelial hyperplasia, hamartoma, or variant of seborrheic keratosis, most believe it to be a benign neoplasm, although the cell of origin is subject to dispute.
- It is most commonly found on the lower limbs and presents as a circumscribed pink to bright red or brown oval-shaped papule or nodule, measuring 1 to 4 cm in diameter (Fig. 22–6).

F. BASAL CELL CARCINOMA

DEFINITION
Basal cell carcinoma (BCC) is a malignant tumor of the skin arising from basal cells of the lower epidermis and adnexal structures.

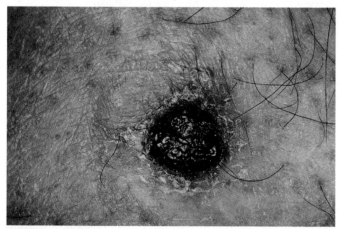

Fig 22–6
Clear cell acanthoma—typical lesion on the shin of an older woman. (Courtesy of the Institute of Dermatology, London.)

- It is the most common skin neoplasm. The most common site is on the nose (30%); 85% appear in the head and neck regions.
- It may be classified as one of six types—nodular, superficial, pigmented, cystic, sclerosing or morpheaform, and nevoid. The most common type is nodular (21%); the least common is morpheaform (1%); a mixed pattern is present in approximately 40% of cases.
- Basal cell carcinoma advances by direct expansion and destroys normal tissue.

PHYSICAL FINDINGS AND CLINICAL PRESENTATION
These vary with the histologic type:
- Nodular (Fig. 22–7): dome-shaped, painless lesion that may become multilobular and frequently ulcerates (rodent ulcer); prominent telangiectatic vessels are noted on the surface; border is translucent, elevated, pearly white; some nodular basal cell carcinomas may contain pigmentation, giving an appearance similar to a melanoma.
- Superficial (Fig. 22–8): circumscribed, scaling, black appearance, with a thin, raised, pearly white border; a crust and erosions may be present; occurs most frequently on the trunk and extremities.
- Morpheaform (Fig. 22–9): flat or slightly raised yellowish or white appearance (similar to localized scleroderma); appearance similar to scars; surface has a waxy consistency.
- Ulcerative (Fig. 22–10): central ulceration and a rolled border

DIFFERENTIAL DIAGNOSIS
- Keratoacanthoma (see Fig. 22–17)
- Melanoma (see Fig. 24–1)
- Seborrheic keratosis (see Fig. 22–2)
- Molluscum contagiosum (see Fig. 27–21)
- Psoriasis (see Fig. 7–1)

LABORATORY TESTS
- Biopsy to confirm diagnosis

TREATMENT
This varies with tumor size, location, and cell type:
- Excision surgery: preferred method for large tumors with well-defined borders on the legs, cheeks, forehead, and trunk

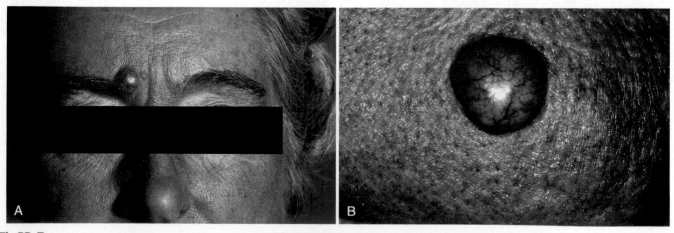

Fig 22–7
Nodular basal cell carcinoma **(A, B)**. Note the characteristic telangiectatic vessels coursing over the surface of these nodular variants. (Courtesy of Dr. R. A. Marsden, St. George's Hospital, London.)

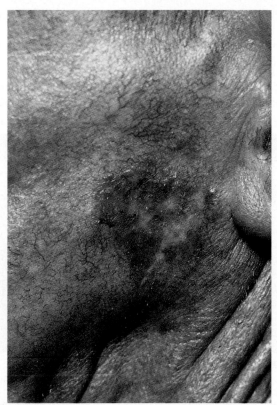

Fig 22–8
Superficial basal cell carcinoma. Note the erythema and scaling. This variant may be clinically mistaken for eczema or psoriasis. It is notoriously difficult to identify the radial border of this lesion.
(Courtesy of Dr. R. A. Marsden, St. George's Hospital, London.)

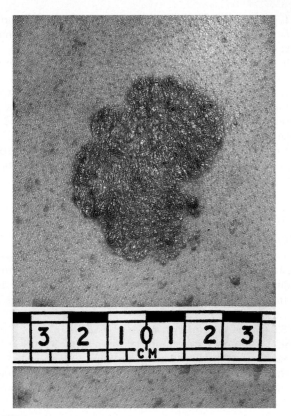

Fig 22–9
Morpheaform basal cell carcinoma. This ill-defined, white-pink, flat lesion is characteristic.
(Courtesy of Dr. R. A. Marsden, St. George's Hospital, London.)

- Mohs' micrographic surgery: preferred for lesions in high-risk areas (e.g., nose, eyelid), very large primary tumors, recurrent basal cell carcinomas, and tumors with poorly defined clinical margins
- Electrodesiccation and curettage: useful for small (less than 6 mm) nodular basal cell carcinomas
- Cryosurgery with liquid nitrogen: useful for basal cell carcinomas of the superficial and nodular types with clearly definable margins; no clear advantages over the other forms of therapy; generally reserved for uncomplicated tumors
- Radiation therapy: generally used for basal cell carcinomas in areas requiring preservation of normal surround tissues for cosmetic reasons (e.g., around lips); also useful for patients who cannot tolerate surgical procedures or for large lesions and surgical failures

G. ACTINIC (SOLAR) KERATOSIS

- Actinic keratoses are common skin lesions usually presenting as multiple, erythematous or yellow-brown, dry, scaly lesions in middle-aged or older adults. Heavily pigmented variants may be clinically mistaken for lentigo maligna.
- Actinic keratoses are more common in men than women, especially in those with fair complexions who burn rather than tan following sun exposure.
- They usually measure 1 cm in diameter or less.

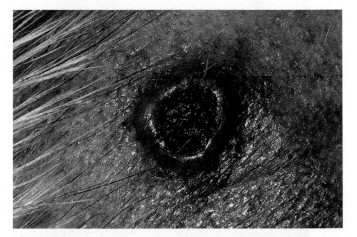

Fig 22–10
Ulcerative basal cell carcinoma. Note the central ulceration and characteristic rolled border.
(Courtesy of Dr. R. A. Marsden, St. George's Hospital, London.)

- The surrounding skin frequently shows additional features of sun damage, including atrophy, pigmentary changes, and telangiectasia.
- Actinic keratoses are of particular importance because they are a sensitive indicator of exposure to UV light and strongly predict the likelihood of developing cutaneous squamous cell carcinoma.

- Typical lesions occur on sun-damaged skin, usually on the face (Fig. 22–11) and neck and dorsal aspects of the hands and forearms (Fig. 22–12)
- It is estimated that up to 10% of actinic keratoses tend to progress to invasive carcinoma.
- The cumulative probability of the development of invasive squamous cell carcinoma in patients with 10 or more actinic keratoses has been estimated at 14% in a 5-year period.
- Diagnosis: skin biopsy
- Treatment: avoidance of sun exposure, use of sunscreens, salicylic acid, topical retinoids, cryosurgery, topical 5-fluorouracil

H. SQUAMOUS CELL CARCINOMA

DEFINITION
Squamous cell carcinoma (SCC) is a malignant tumor of the skin arising in the epithelium. SCC is the second most common cutaneous malignancy, comprising 20% of all cases of non-melanoma skin cancer. The incidence increases with age and sun exposure.

PHYSICAL FINDINGS AND CLINICAL PRESENTATION
- SCC commonly affects the scalp, neck region, backs of the hands, ears (Fig. 22–13), and lips (Fig. 22–14).
- The lesion may have a scaly, erythematous macule or plaque. Squamous cell carcinoma in situ is also known as *Bowen's disease* (Fig. 22–15).

- Telangiectasia and central ulceration may also be present (Fig. 22–16).
- Most SCCs present as exophytic lesions that grow over a period of months.

CAUSE
Risk factors include exposure to UVB light and immunosuppression; renal transplant recipients have a threefold increased risk.

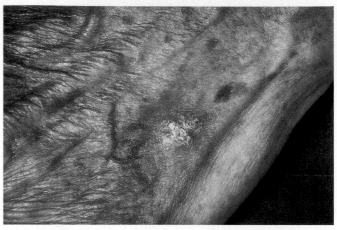

Fig 22–12
Actinic keratosis. This is a typical lesion characterized by yellow scales overlying an erythematous base. The surrounding skin is atrophic and a number of senile lentigines are present. The patient is an older man. (Courtesy of Dr. R. A. Marsden, St. George's Hospital, London.)

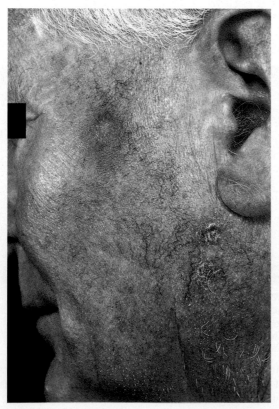

Fig 22–11
Actinic keratosis. Several lesions are present on the cheek, which is a characteristic site. Note the background telangiectasia. (Courtesy of the Institute of Dermatology, London.)

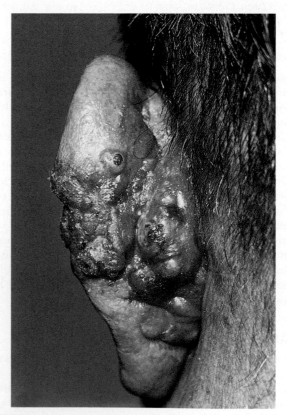

Fig 22–13
Squamous cell carcinoma. Tumors on the ear are often high-grade tumors. (Courtesy of the Institute of Dermatology, London.)

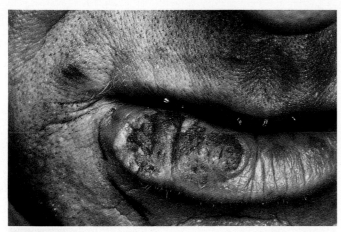

Fig 22–14
Squamous cell carcinoma. Lesions on the lip have high recurrence and metastatic rates and are associated with a poor prognosis. (Courtesy of the Institute of Dermatology, London.)

DIFFERENTIAL DIAGNOSIS
- Keratoacanthomas (see Fig. 22–17)
- Actinic keratosis (see Fig. 22–12)
- Basal cell carcinoma (see Fig. 22–9)
- Healing traumatic wounds
- Spindle cell tumors (see Fig. 23–15)
- Warts (see Fig. 27–13)

LABORATORY TESTS
Diagnosis is made with full-thickness skin biopsy (incisional or excisional).

TREATMENT
- Electrodesiccation and curettage for small SCCs (less than 2 cm in diameter), superficial tumors, and lesions located in the extremities and trunk.
- Tumors thinner than 4 mm can be managed by simple local removal.
- Lesions between 4 and 8 mm thick or those with deep dermal invasion should be excised.
- Tumors penetrating the dermis can be treated with several modalities, including excision and Mohs' surgery, radiation therapy, and chemotherapy.
- Metastatic SCC can be treated with cryotherapy and a combination of chemotherapy using 13-*cis*-retinoic acid and interferon alfa-2a.
- Survival is related to size, location, degree of differentiation, immunologic status of the patient, depth of invasion, and presence of metastases. Risk factors for metastasis include lesions on the lip or ear, increasing lesion depth, and poor cell differentiation.
- Patients whose tumors penetrate through the dermis or exceed 8 mm in thickness are at risk for tumor recurrence.
- The most common metastatic locations are the regional lymph nodes, liver, and lungs.
- Tumors on the scalp, forehead, ears, nose, and lips also carry a higher risk.
- SCCs originating in the lip and pinna metastasize in 10% to 20% of cases.
- The 5-year survival rate for metastatic squamous cell carcinoma is 34%.

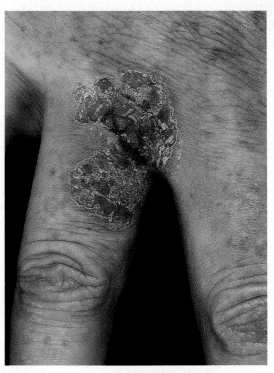

Fig 22–15
Bowen's disease—squamous cell carcinoma in situ. This example shows a sharply circumscribed irregular plaque spreading from the web space onto the dorsal surface of the adjacent proximal phalanx. (Courtesy of the Institute of Dermatology, London.)

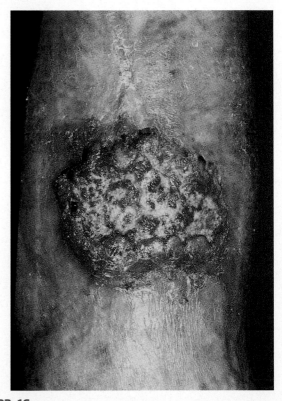

Fig 22–16
Squamous cell carcinoma. This large ulcerated tumor has arisen at the site of a previous burn (Marjolin's ulcer). (Courtesy of Dr. R. A. Marsden, St. George's Hospital, London.)

I. KERATOACANTHOMA (MOLLUSCUM SEBACEUM)

DEFINITION

- Keratoacanthoma is a rapidly growing skin tumor arising predominantly on the exposed surfaces of the body.
- Various subtypes have been recognized; most common is the solitary acanthoma. It usually appears to be related to excessive exposure to UVB. Therefore, lesions are most commonly found on sun-damaged skin, particularly of the face (Fig. 22–17), forearms, wrists, and backs of the hands.

PHYSICAL FINDINGS AND CLINICAL PRESENTATION

- Clinically, solitary keratoacanthoma presents as a smooth hemispherical papule that rapidly enlarges over the course of a few weeks to produce a 1- to 2-cm diameter, discrete, round or oval, often flesh-colored umbilical nodule, with a central keratin-filled crater.

DIAGNOSIS

- Skin biopsy

TREATMENT

- Curettage, excision, radiotherapy, intralesional fluorouracil or methotrexate

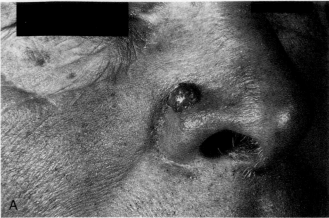

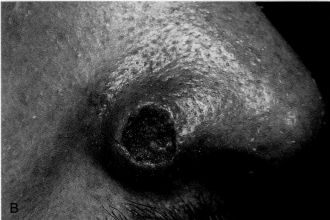

Fig 22–17
Keratoacanthoma. **A,** Typical dome-shaped lesion on the nose, a commonly affected site. **B,** In this example, the central crater is particularly well developed.
(Courtesy of the Institute of Dermatology, London.)

Chapter 23   Melanocytic nevi

A. EPHELIDES (FRECKLES)

DEFINITION

Ephelides are extremely common lesions that present as clusters of small (approximately 2 mm in diameter), uniformly pigmented macules (Fig. 23–1). They are directly related to exposure to sunlight and are much more conspicuous in summer than in winter.

PHYSICAL FINDINGS AND CLINICAL PRESENTATION

- Sites of predilection include the nose, cheeks, shoulders, and dorsal aspects of the hands and arms.
- They are more common and numerous in individuals with red hair and blue eyes, in whom there is probably an autosomal mode of inheritance.
- Ephelides present in childhood, increasing in frequency in adults and typically regressing in older adults. There is a female predilection.
- High levels of freckling may indicate a raised susceptibility to the later development of melanoma. Similarly, increasing numbers of freckles correlate with a higher frequency of acquired melanocytic nevi.
- Treatment: although a cosmetic nuisance, they are of no clinical importance and no treatment is necessary.

B. LENTIGO SIMPLEX (LENTIGINES)

DEFINITION

Lentigo simplex is a common melanocytic lesion, generally indistinguishable clinically from ephelides (Fig. 23–2).

PHYSICAL FINDINGS AND CLINICAL PRESENTATION

- Lesions are small (1 to 5 mm), uniformly pigmented, brown to black, sharply circumscribed macules that may be found anywhere on the integument.

- They often develop in childhood (juvenile lentigo) and become more conspicuous during pregnancy.
- Hyperpigmentation and increased number of lentigines are features of Addison's disease (see Section 11.10).
- Simple lentigines have no malignant potential and, in contrast to ephelides, have no connection with sunlight. They may also be associated with various inherited disorders, such as LEOPARD syndrome (Fig. 23–3; see Section 1.17f) and Peutz-Jeghers syndrome (Fig. 23–4; see Section 7.25).

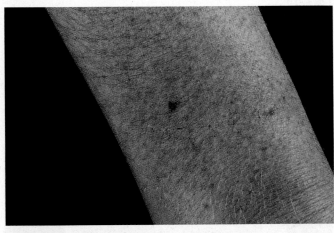

Fig 23–2
Lentigo simplex. This is a small, uniformly pigmented macule clinically indistinguishable from an ephelide. It is unrelated to sun exposure.
(From McKee PH, Calonje E, Granter SR [eds]. Pathology of the Skin With Clinical Correlations, 3rd ed. St. Louis, Mosby, 2005.)

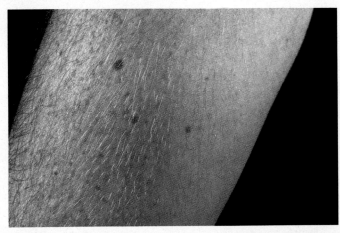

Fig 23–1
Ephelides. These present as small pigmented macules that darken on exposure to sunlight.
(From McKee PH, Calonje E, Granter SR [eds]. Pathology of the Skin With Clinical Correlations, 3rd ed. St. Louis, Mosby, 2005.)

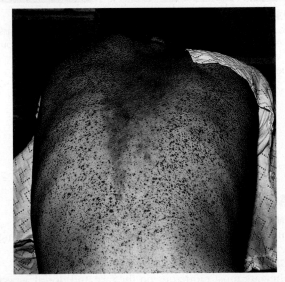

Fig 23–3
LEOPARD syndrome. This patient has an enormous number of lentigines covering the entire trunk.
(Courtesy of Dr. M. M. Black, Institute of Dermatology, London.)

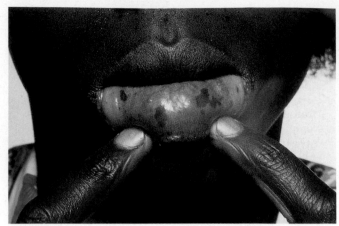

Fig 23–4
Peutz-Jeghers syndrome. Clinically extensive lentigines on the lips are characteristic. The perioral skin shows small numbers of similar lesions.
(Courtesy of Dr. M. M. Black, Institute of Dermatology, London.)

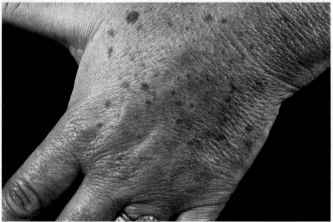
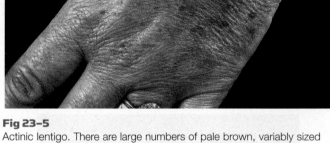

Fig 23–5
Actinic lentigo. There are large numbers of pale brown, variably sized macules on the dorsal aspect of the hand of this middle-aged woman. There was a history of excessive exposure to sunlight.
(Courtesy of Dr. R. A. Marsden, St. George's Hospital, London.)

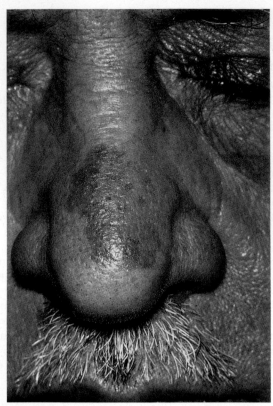

Fig 23–6
Lentigo maligna. This variably pigmented lesion was present for many years. There is no invasive component.
(Courtesy of Dr. R. A. Marsden, St. George's Hospital, London.)

C. ACTINIC (SOLAR) LENTIGO

DEFINITION
Actinic lentigines are common brown macules occurring on sun-exposed skin of white individuals.

PHYSICAL FINDINGS AND CLINICAL PRESENTATION
- They are most numerous on the face and dorsal aspects of the hands (Fig. 23–5) and forearms.
- They measure 0.1 to 1 cm or more in diameter, have a tendency to coalesce, and vary from light to dark brown in color.
- Actinic lentigines may be clinically mistaken for lentigo maligna (Fig. 23–6).

DIAGNOSIS
- Skin biopsy

TREATMENT
- Sunscreen, topical retinoids, topical 5-fluorouracil, cryosurgery, salicylic acid

D. BECKER'S NEVUS

DEFINITION
Becker's nevus is an androgen-dependent lesion that becomes more prominent after puberty.

PHYSICAL FINDINGS AND CLINICAL PRESENTATION
- It usually presents in the second decade, initially as a light to dark brown enlarging macular lesion, which subsequently shows hypertrichosis (Fig. 23–7).
- It most frequently involves the chest, shoulders, or upper arms.

DIAGNOSIS
- Skin biopsy if diagnosis is uncertain

TREATMENT
- Ruby laser

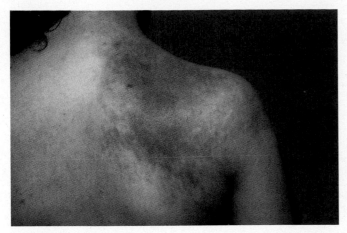

Fig 23–7
Becker's nevus.. This example shows a characteristic distribution around the shoulder region.
(Courtesy of Dr. R. A. Marsden, St. George's Hospital, London.)

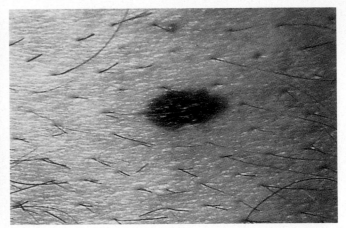

Fig 23–8
Junctional melanocytic nevus. Banal nevi are typically sharply circumscribed.
(Courtesy of Dr. M. Liang, Children's Hospital, Boston.)

E. MELANOCYTIC NEVUS (BANAL NEVI)

DEFINITION
Melanocytic nevi are skin lesions that appear initially in childhood and increase in number during the second and third decades.

An average white individual can expect to develop 15 to 40 such lesions during his or her lifetime. They generally involute during middle age and may regress completely in older adults.

PHYSICAL FINDINGS AND CLINICAL PRESENTATION
- In males, the head, neck, and trunk are particularly affected, whereas in females the upper and lower limbs are more often involved.
- Development of melanocytic nevi is related to the extent of sun exposure during the first 2 decades of life. Intermittent intense sunlight is of greater importance than chronic exposure.
- Melanocytic nevi present with various features depending on their stage of development.
- Junctional nevi are usually macular or slightly raised, up to 0.5 cm in diameter, and from light to dark brown in color (Fig. 23–8). They are well circumscribed, with a regular border, and generally are uniformly pigmented, but sometimes the central area is darker. Typically, the skin lines can be clearly discerned on the surface of the lesion (Fig. 23–9).
- The compound nevus is raised, sometimes domeshaped or warty, and often still deeply pigmented. Occasionally, there are coarse hairs projecting from its surface.
- The intradermal nevus is often devoid of pigment and may present as a dome-shaped nodule (Fig. 23–10) or a pedunculated skin tag. Malignant transformation is rare. It has been estimated that the likelihood of one nevus evolving into melanoma is roughly 1 in 100,000.

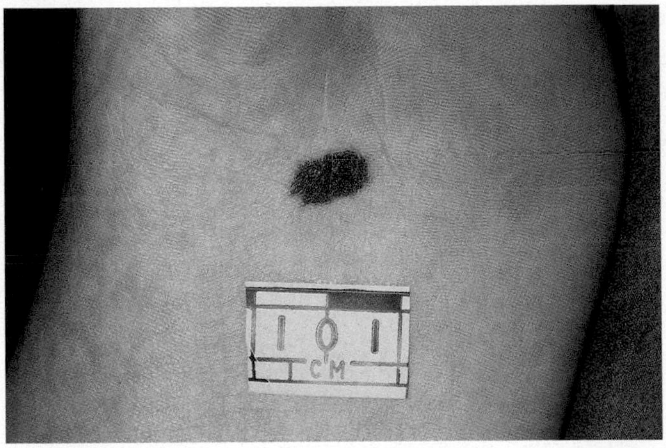

F. ACRAL NEVUS

DEFINITION
An acral nevus is a uniformly pigmented, dark brown macule or papule, with irregular and sometimes indistinct margins (Fig. 23–11), usually less than 1 cm in diameter and often found on the dorsal surfaces of the hands, feet, and digits.

Fig 23–9
Junctional nevus. The skin markings overlying the nevus are typically present in contrast to melanoma, when they are usually lost.
(Courtesy of Dr. R. A. Marsden, St. George's Hospital, London.)

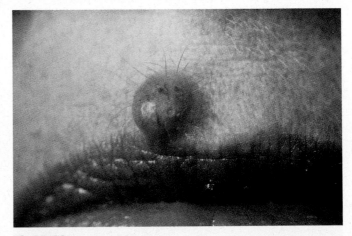

Fig 23–10
Dermal melanocytic nevus. Presentation as a pale, raised, dermal nodule is a common finding. Dermal nevi are sometimes clinically confused with nodular basal cell carcinoma.
(Courtesy of the Institute of Dermatology, London.)

PHYSICAL FINDINGS AND CLINICAL PRESENTATION

- Clinically, it is often confused with melanoma and accurate diagnosis requires biopsy.

G. HALO NEVUS

DEFINITION

A halo nevus is a skin lesion presenting clinically as a pigmented melanocytic nevus surrounded by a hypopigmented border and usually associated with regression of the nevus (Fig. 23-12).

PHYSICAL FINDINGS AND CLINICAL PRESENTATION

- It arises most frequently in the second decade, most often on the trunk, particularly the back.
- Halo nevi are sometimes multiple and occasionally exhibit a familial tendency; there is an increased incidence of associated vitiligo.

H. SPITZ NEVUS

DEFINITION

A Spitz nevus is a skin lesion presenting clinically as a rapidly growing asymptomatic, pink or reddish-brown, dome-shaped papule or nodule (Fig. 23-13).

PHYSICAL FINDINGS AND CLINICAL PRESENTATION

- Usually, the lesion is situated on the head or neck (particularly the cheek; Fig. 23-14) or the extremities.
- It is a fairly common skin lesion, accounting for approximately 1% of all nevi in children.

TREATMENT

- Reassurance, cryotherapy, curettage, cauterization

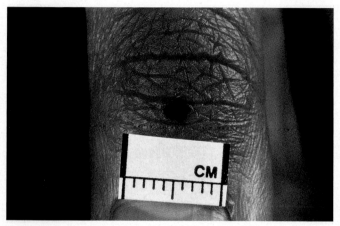

Fig 23-11
Acral nevus. Note the pigmentation and irregular border.
(Courtesy of the Institute of Dermatology, London.)

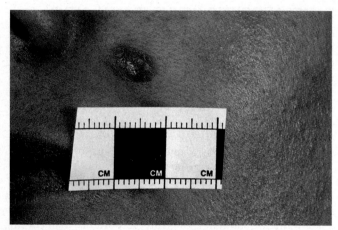

Fig 23-13
Spitz nevus. The cheek is a commonly affected site.
(Courtesy of the Institute of Dermatology, London.)

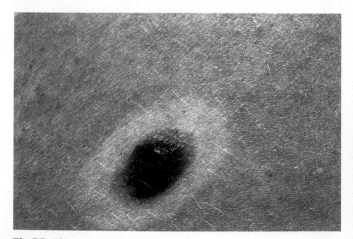

Fig 23-12
Halo nevus. Close-up view shows a heavily pigmented central nodule, with a pale-staining halo.
(Courtesy of the Institute of Dermatology, London.)

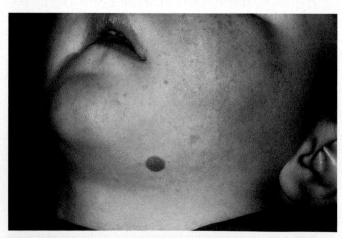

Fig 23-14
Spitz nevus. Pigmented variants overlap with a pigmented spindle cell nevus of Reed.
(Courtesy of Dr. R. A. Marsden, St. George's Hospital, London.)

I. PIGMENTED SPINDLE CELL TUMOR OF REED

DEFINITION

A pigmented spindle cell tumor of Reed is a skin lesion presenting as a dark brown or black macular or papular, often dome-shaped, lesion (Fig. 23–15).

- It is not an uncommon skin lesion and probably represents a variant of Spitz nevus.
- It is important clinically because it may easily be mistaken for melanoma.

J. DYSPLASTIC NEVUS SYNDROME (FAMILIAL ATYPICAL MULTIPLE MOLE MELANOMA SYNDROME)

DEFINITION

Dysplastic nevus syndrome is an inherited autosomal dominant syndrome with incomplete penetrance.

PHYSICAL FINDINGS AND CLINICAL PRESENTATION

- Apparently normal at birth, affected individuals develop large numbers of morphologically normal nevi in early childhood. These become more numerous and acquire atypical clinical features around puberty. New lesions continue to develop throughout life; the number of lesions per patient ranges from a few to hundreds (Fig. 23–16).
- The nevi are usually large (6 mm or more in diameter) and irregularly shaped, frequently with an uneven or ill-defined border (Fig. 23–17).
- Patients with this syndrome, particularly those with a family history of melanoma, have an increased risk of developing melanoma.
- Features suggestive of malignant transformation include the development of contour asymmetry, excessive pigment variegation, and the development of black foci or the presence of gray discoloration suggestive of regression.

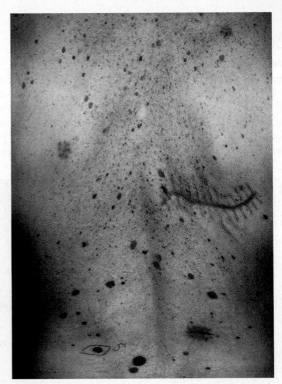

Fig 23–16
Dysplastic nevus syndrome. There are numerous large, irregular nevi. The scar marks the site of a previously excised melanoma.
(Courtesy of Dr. R. Mackie, University of Glasgow, Glasgow, Scotland.)

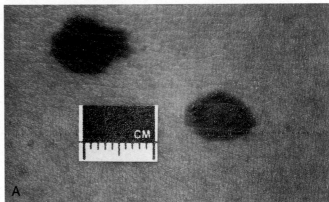

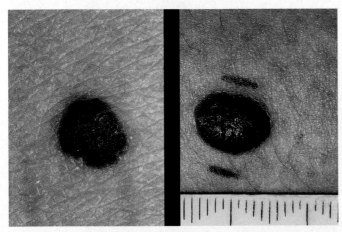

Fig 23–15
Pigmented spindle cell tumor of Reed. These lesions most often present as small, darkly pigmented circumscribed macules or papules. The thigh is a characteristic site, and females are affected more often than males.
(Courtesy of Dr. N. P Smith [deceased], St. John's Dermatology Centre, St. Thomas' Hospital, London.)

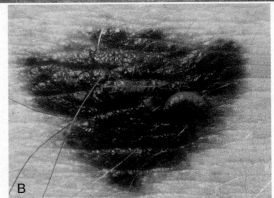

Fig 23–17
A, B, Dysplastic nevi are often larger than 6 mm in diameter. Borders are typically irregular. A small nodule is evident in B.
(Courtesy of the Institute of Dermatology, London.)

K. CONGENITAL MELANOCYTIC NEVUS

DEFINITION

A congenital melanocytic nevus is a skin lesion that may be initially flat and often pale brown, reminiscent of café au lait macules (Fig. 23–18). Occasionally, these lesions become more heavily pigmented, thicker, and hairy. They may also develop a warty surface, with discrete small nodular projections (Fig. 23–19). The incidence of malignant change in large congenital nevi ranges from 3.8% to 18%.

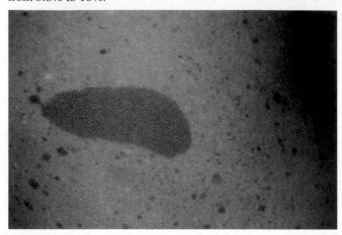

Fig 23–18
Café au lait spot in a patient with neurofibromatosis.
(From Swartz MH. Textbook of Physical Diagnosis, 5th ed. Philadelphia, WB Saunders, 2006.)

L. MONGOLIAN BLUE SPOT

DEFINITION

A mongolian blue spot is a dermal melanocytic lesion presenting as relatively uniform slate blue areas of discoloration, most often situated over the sacral region (Fig. 23–20). These skin lesions are more common in Japanese, Chinese, and pigmented races. Mongolian blue spots are believed to represent arrested transdermal migration of melanocytes from the neural crest to the epidermis.

PHYSICAL FINDINGS AND CLINICAL PRESENTATION

- The lesion is benign and characterized by variably pigmented melanocytes, which tend to be orientated parallel to the skin surface and situated predominantly in the deep reticular dermis. The overlying epithelium is normal.

M. COMMON BLUE NEVUS

DEFINITION

A common blue nevus is a skin lesion presenting typically with a dome-shaped blue or blue-black appearance (Fig. 23–21).

PHYSICAL FINDINGS AND CLINICAL PRESENTATION

- It most often involves the dorsal aspects of the hands and feet, buttocks, scalp, and face and measures about 1 cm in diameter.
- Clinically, it may be confused with melanoma.
- Diagnosis is made with biopsy.

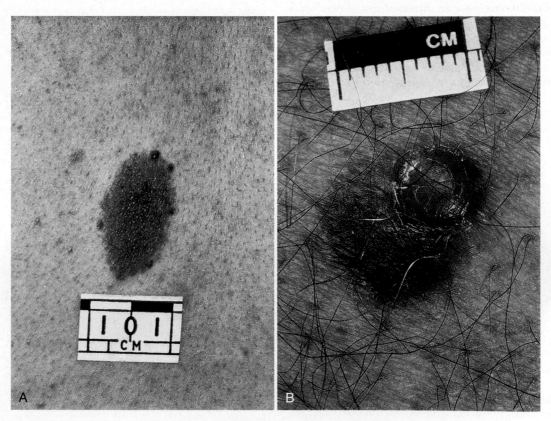

Fig 23–19
Congenital melanocytic nevus. **A,** In this example, there are scattered hyperpigmented small papules within a uniform pale brown macule.
B, A nodular component is apparent.
(**A** courtesy of Dr. R. A. Marsden, St. George's Hospital, London; **B** courtesy of the Institute of Dermatology, London.)

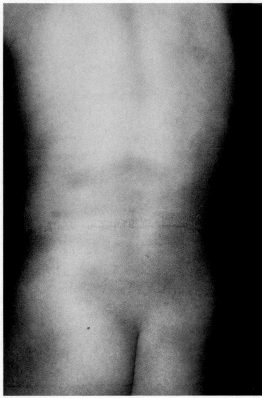

Fig 23–20
Mongolian blue spot. There is extensive pale blue discoloration on this child's trunk and buttocks.
(Courtesy of Dr. S. Bleehen, MD, Royal Hallamshire Hospital, Sheffield, England.)

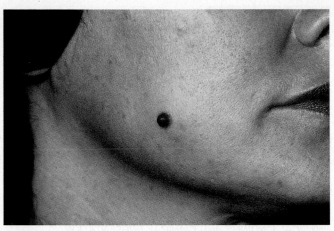

Fig 23–21
Common blue nevus. This typical dome-shaped lesion shows dark blue-black coloration.
(Courtesy of Dr. R. A. Marsden, St. George's Hospital, London.)

N. LENTIGO MALIGNA (HUTCHINSON'S MELANOTIC FRECKLE)

DEFINITION
Lentigo maligna is a relatively uncommon variant of melanoma that typically develops on chronic sun-damaged skin of older adults.

PHYSICAL FINDINGS AND CLINICAL PRESENTATION
- Sites of predilection are the malar region, nose (Fig. 23–6), temple, and forehead.
- The tumor most often presents in the sixth and seventh decades as a variably, gradually enlarging, irregular, flat macule.
- It may be brown or black and usually shows areas of hypopigmentation representing areas of regression.
- The in situ lesion is often present for 10 to 15 years before an invasive tumor develops.

DIAGNOSIS
- Skin biopsy

TREATMENT
- Excision, Mohs' micrographic surgery

Chapter 24 | Melanoma

DEFINITION

Melanoma is a skin neoplasm arising from the malignant degeneration of melanocytes. It has doubled to tripled in incidence over the past 25 years and is the most common cancer among women 20 to 29 years of age. Melanoma is the leading cause of death from skin disease. It is classically subdivided into four types:

1. Superficial spreading melanoma (70%)
2. Nodular melanoma (15% to 20%)
3. Lentigo maligna melanoma (5% to 10%)
4. Acral lentiginous melanoma (7% to 10%)

PHYSICAL FINDINGS AND CLINICAL PRESENTATION

These vary, depending on the subtype of melanoma:

- Superficial spreading melanoma is most often found on the lower legs, arms, and upper back. It may have a combination of many colors or may be uniformly brown or black (Fig. 24–1).
- Nodular melanoma can be found anywhere on the body, but it most frequently occurs on the trunk on sun-exposed areas. It has a dark-brown or red-brown appearance and can be dome-shaped or pedunculated (Fig. 24–2); it is frequently misdiagnosed because it may resemble a blood blister or hemangioma and may also be amelanotic.
- Lentigo maligna melanoma is generally found in older adults in areas continually exposed to the sun and frequently arising from lentigo maligna (Hutchinson's freckle) or melanoma in situ. It might have a complex pattern and variable shape (Fig. 24–3); the color is more uniform than in superficial spreading melanoma.
- Acral lentiginous melanoma frequently occurs on the sole of the foot, subungual mucous membranes, and palm (sole of the foot is the most prevalent site; Fig. 24–4). Unlike other types of melanoma, it has a similar incidence in all ethnic groups.

- The warning signs that the lesion may be a melanoma can be summarized with the ABCD rule:
  - A: asymmetry (e.g., lesion is bisected and halves are not identical)
  - B: border irregularity (uneven, ragged border)
  - C: color variegation (presence of various shades of pigmentation)
  - D: diameter enlargement (more than 6 mm)
- Recent data regarding small-diameter melanoma have suggested that the ABCD criteria for gross inspection of pigmented skin lesions and early diagnosis of cutaneous melanoma should be expanded to ABCDE to include evolving (i.e., lesions that have changed over time).

CAUSE

- UV light is the most important cause of malignant melanoma.
- There is a modest increase in melanoma risk in patients with small nondysplastic nevi and a much greater risk in those with dysplastic lesions.
- The *CDKN2A* gene, at the 9p21 locus, is often deleted in people with familial melanoma.

DIFFERENTIAL DIAGNOSIS

- Dysplastic nevi (see Fig. 23–17)
- Actinic keratosis (see Fig. 22–12)
- Spindle cell tumor (see Fig. 23–15)
- Blue nevus (see Fig. 23–21)
- Melanocytic nevus (see Fig. 23–8)
- Acral nevus (see Fig. 23–11)
- Junctional nevus (see Fig. 23–9)
- Halo nevus (see Fig. 23–12)
- Basal cell carcinoma (see Fig. 22–9)
- Seborrheic keratosis (see Fig. 22–2)

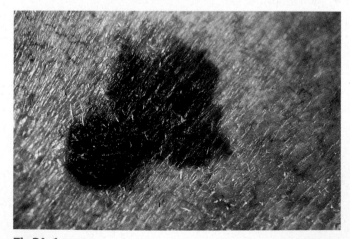

Fig 24–1
Superficial spreading melanoma. This example shows variable pigmentation and a highly irregular border. The lesion depicted is on the thigh of a young woman.
(Courtesy of R. A. Marsden, MD, St. George's Hospital, London.)

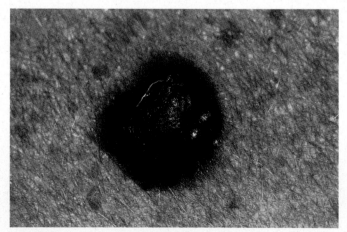

Fig 24–2
Nodular melanoma. This black, dome-shaped nodule has no adjacent macular component.
(Courtesy of the Institute of Dermatology, London.)

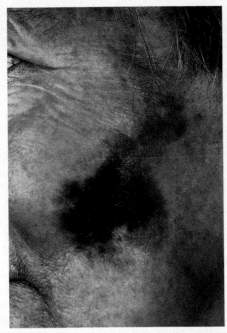

Fig 24–3
Lentigo maligna melanoma. Note the irregular border and variable
pigmentation. A small nodule of invasive tumor is apparent.
(Courtesy of the Institute of Dermatology, London.)

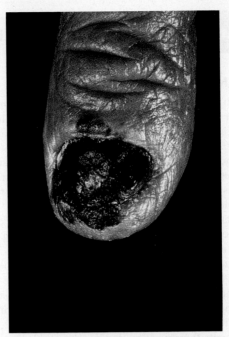

Fig 24–4
Acral lentiginous melanoma. This tumor has destroyed the entire nail.
Melanoma at this site is often thick by the time of presentation and is
therefore usually associated with a poor prognosis.
(Courtesy of the Institute of Dermatology, London.)

TREATMENT
● Excision of the melanoma
● Prognosis varies with the stage of the melanoma. The 5-year
  survival rates related to thickness are as follows: smaller
  than 0.76 mm, 99%; 0.6 to 1.49 mm, 85%; 1.5 to 2.49 mm,
  84%; 2.5 to 3.9 mm, 70%; and larger than 4 mm, 44%.
● In addition to surgical excision and lymph node dissection,
  treatment of advanced disease consists of chemotherapy,
  immunotherapy, and radiation therapy.

Chapter 25 — Miscellaneous skin lesions

A. ACANTHOSIS NIGRICANS

- Acanthosis nigricans refers to the presence of symmetrical brown velvety or verrucous plaques with a predilection for intertriginous sites as the back of the neck, groin, and axillae (Fig. 25–1).
- It is most commonly seen in individuals with insulin resistance states, internal malignancy, obesity, and certain medications (e.g., nicotinic acid, glucocorticoids, contraceptives, diethylstilbestrol).
- Laboratory evaluation often reveals elevated glucose levels. Additional useful tests are TSH follicle-stimulating hormone (FSH) and luteinizing hormone (LH).
- The sudden onset of acanthosis nigricans should be followed by investigation for internal malignancy (e.g., upper endoscopy to rule out gastric cancer) and review of new medications (e.g., nicotinic acid, contraceptives, glucocorticoids).
- Treatment: therapy of underlying cause, oral isotretinoin, topical vitamin A, dermabrasion, cyproheptadine, topical calcipotriol, carbon dioxide laser

B. CAFÉ AU LAIT SPOTS

DEFINITION

Café au lait spots are well-circumscribed brownish macules caused by an increased number of functionally hyperactive melanocytes (Fig. 25–2).

- They may be found at birth in up to 10% of the population.
- The presence of more than six macules measuring more than 5 mm in diameter is suggestive of neurofibromatosis I; see Section 2–16b.

C. TUMORS OF SWEAT GLANDS

(1) Eccrine hidrocystoma

- Eccrine hidrocystoma lesions vary in size from pinhead to pea-sized and appear as tense vesicles located predominantly on the face, particularly periorbitally (Fig. 25–3). Eccrine hydrocystomas are common and affect adults at any age.
- Typically, the lesions wax and wane with circumstances that provoke sweat production; they are therefore exacerbated in the summer, but may disappear clinically in the winter months.
- Histologically, the hidrocystoma consists of one or several partially collapsed, unilocular cysts in the dermis, which are often situated adjacent to normal eccrine glands.

(2) Eccrine poroma

- An eccrine poroma is a benign tumor generally presenting as a solitary, sessile, skin-colored to red, slightly scaly nodule on the soles or sides of the feet and on the hands (Fig. 25–4).
- Lesions may measure up to 3 cm in diameter.

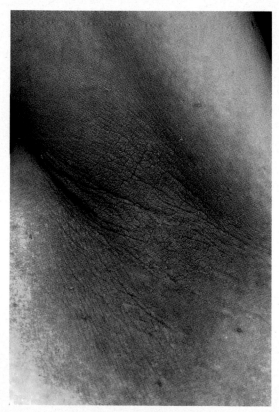

Fig 25–1
Acanthosis nigricans. There is velvety thickening of the axillary skin.
(Courtesy of the Institute of Dermatology, London.)

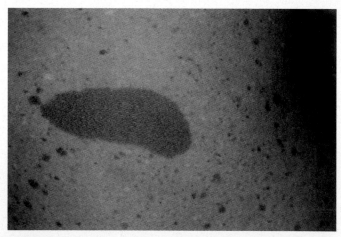

Fig 25–2
Café au lait spot in a patient with neurofibromatosis.
(From Swartz MH: Textbook of Physical Diagnosis, 5th ed. Philadelphia, WB Saunders, 2006.)

- They are usually asymptomatic, although bleeding after mild trauma is not uncommon.

(3) Syringoma
- Syringomas are common skin lesions presenting most often as multiple, symmetrically distributed, usually asymptomatic small papules (1 to 3 mm) on the lower eyelids or upper cheeks (Fig. 25–5).
- They appear at puberty or in early adult life and show a marked female predominance.
- Individual papules are firm and skin-colored or slightly yellow. Histologically, syringomas represent an adenoma of the acrosyringium, the intraepidermal eccrine sweat duct.
- Treatment: surgical excision, electrocautery, intralesional electrodesiccation, carbon dioxide laser

(4) Eccrine hidroadenoma
- Eccrine hidroadenoma lesions are sweat gland tumors usually occurring on the head and neck or limbs, and generally presenting as a solitary, slow-growing, solid or cystic nodule (Fig. 25–6).
- The overlying skin may be flesh-colored, erythematous, or blue.
- Lesions typically measure 1 to 2 cm in diameter and present most often in middle-aged or older adults, with a slight predominance in females.

(5) Dermal cylindroma
- Dermal cylindromas are one of the more common benign adnexal tumors.
- The vast majority (90%) occur on the head, neck, and scalp as slow-growing, sometimes painful, solitary pink or red dermal nodules averaging 1 cm in diameter (Fig. 25–7).
- There is a marked female preponderance.
- Scalp lesions may grow to a large size; coalescence of numerous lesions is known as a turban tumor.

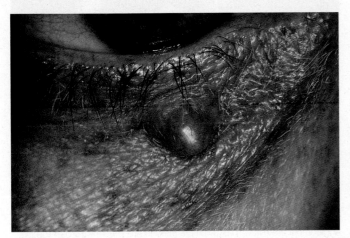

Fig 25–3
Eccrine hidrocystoma. Note the tense pea-sized swelling below the eyelid.
(Courtesy of Dr. R. A. Marsden, St. George's Hospital, London.)

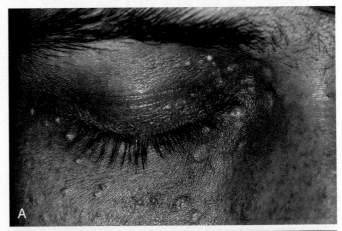

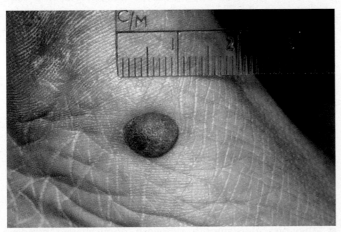

Fig 25–4
Eccrine poroma. This example is present on the palm of the hand.
(Courtesy of the Institute of Dermatology, London.)

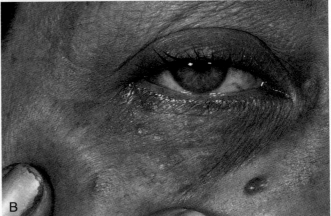

Fig 25–5
A, B, Syringoma. Note the typical periorbital distribution of these small papules.
(**A** courtesy of Dr. R. A. Marsden, St. George's Hospital, London; **B** courtesy of the Institute of Dermatology, London.)

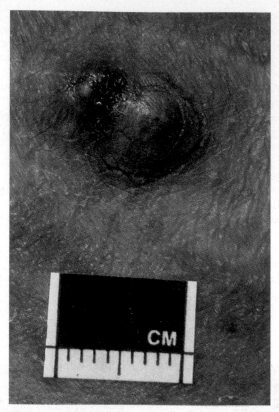

Fig 25–6
Eccrine hidradenoma. This lesion presents as a solitary nodule, most often on the head and neck or limbs.
(Courtesy of the Institute of Dermatology, London.)

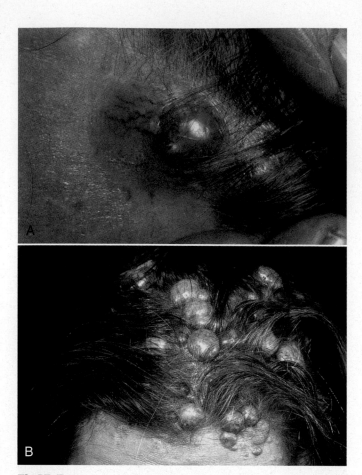

Fig 25–7
Dermal cylindroma. **A,** Two dome-shaped nodules with associated telangiectasia are evident. **B,** Multiple lesions are present (turban tumor).
(Courtesy of the Institute of Dermatology, London.)

D. CUTANEOUS CYSTS

(1) Epidermoid cyst

- An epidermoid cyst is a smooth, dome-shaped swelling occurring predominantly on the face, neck, and upper trunk resulting from damage to the pilosebaceous units. A punctum is usually present (Fig. 25–8).
- Young and middle-aged adults are most often affected.
- The presence of multiple lesions may suggest the possibility of Gardner's syndrome (see Section 7.26), which includes polyposis coli, jaw osteomas, and intestinal fibromatoses in addition to cutaneous cysts.
- Histologically, the cysts are lined by an epidermis-like epithelium, including a granular cell layer. The cysts contain laminated keratin.
- Acute inflammation, usually caused by bacteria, may result in the subsequent disruption of the cyst wall, with the development of an intense foreign body giant cell reaction.
- Epidermoid inclusion cysts may also complicate penetrating trauma to the skin, such as by a sewing needle, with resultant implantation of squamous epithelium into the dermis.

(2) Milia

- Milia are common superficial keratinous cysts that present as white or yellow dome-shaped nodules measuring 1 to 3 mm in diameter.

- They may represent primary lesions when no cause can be identified or may be secondary variants following skin trauma or other injury.
- Primary milia are seen in up to 50% of newborns and present on the face, upper trunk, and extremities. They typically regress spontaneously. Children and adults can also be affected.
- These lesions are most often apparent on the face (forehead, eyelids, and cheeks; Fig. 25–9) and the external genitalia.
- Diagnostic investigation: microbiology swab for bacteria and yeasts, histology
- Treatment: topical antiseptics, oatmeal baths, frequent showering, topical corticosteroids, systemic antibiotics

(3) Trichilemmal (pilar) cyst

- Trichilemmal cysts are lesions found on the scalp in 90% of cases (Fig. 25–10).
- They present as smooth, yellowish, dome-shaped intradermal swellings and are more common in females.
- In contrast to epidermoid cysts, they are characteristically devoid of a punctum.
- Typically, the cyst is encapsulated and uncomplicated lesions readily shell out at surgery (see Fig. 2–14).

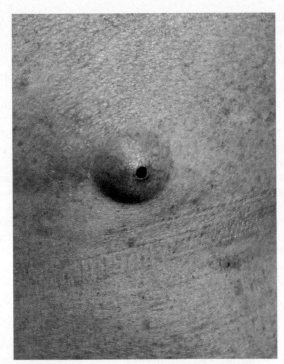

Fig 25–8
Epidermoid cyst—close-up view of a punctum.
(Courtesy of the Institute of Dermatology, London.)

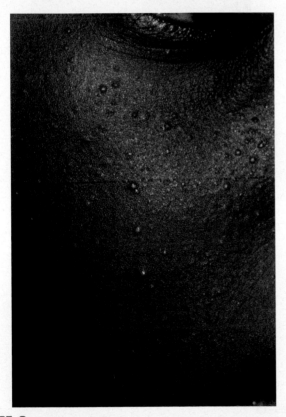

Fig 25–9
Milia. Numerous typical pale small spherical lesions are present.
The cheek is a characteristic site.
(Courtesy of Dr. R. A. Marsden, St. George's Hospital, London.)

(4) Dermoid cyst

● Dermoid cysts are lesions resulting from sequestration of cutaneous tissues along embryonal lines of closure.

● The most common clinical appearance is that of a single, nontender small subcutaneous nodule at birth on the lateral aspect of the upper eyelid (Fig. 25–11).

● Other potential sites of dermoid cysts include the midline of the neck, nasal root, forehead, mastoid area, and scalp. The latter is a particularly important site because the lesion may occasionally show intracranial extension (dumbbell dermoid).

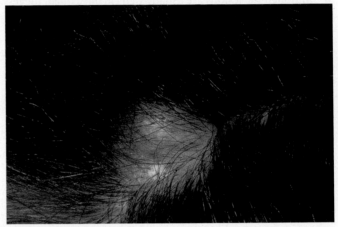

Fig 25–10
Trichilemmal cyst. Note the characteristic dome-shaped swelling on the scalp, a typical site.
(Courtesy of Dr. A. du Vivier, King's College Hospital, London.)

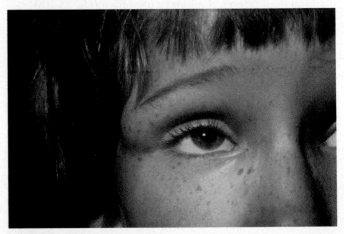

Fig 25–11
Dermoid cyst. Note the swelling adjacent to the upper eyelid, the external angular dermoid cyst.
(Courtesy of Dr. R. A. Marsden, St. George's Hospital, London.)

E. CONNECTIVE TISSUE LESIONS

(1) Lipoma

- Lipomas are the most common connective tissue tumors.
- Histologically, a lipoma is a circumscribed encapsulated tumor composed of mature adipocytes (Fig. 25–12). It may also contain foci of calcification and ossification (Fig. 25–13).
- Lipomas occur more frequently in obese individuals, usually in middle or late adult life.
- The lesions are found most often on the trunk, abdomen, neck, proximal extremities, and back (Fig. 25–14).
- Typically, they originate subcutaneously and are slow-growing, mobile, and painless.
- Although the lesions are usually well circumscribed, the less common deep variants, which arise in muscle or in association with a tendon sheath or nerve, are usually ill defined and infiltrative.
- Treatment: subcutaneous lipomas are entirely benign and local excision is almost always curative.

(2) Ganglion

- Ganglia are cystic structures thought to derive from a tendon sheath or joint capsule.
- Most ganglia occur on the dorsum of the wrist (50% to 70%; Fig. 25–15).
- Ganglia are usually solitary, firm, smooth, round, and fluctuant.
- For additional information, refer to Section 12.16b(4).

(3) Keloid

- A keloid is a reactive lesion that represents exuberant scar formation.
- It typically extends beyond the site of the original injury.
- Although keloids occasionally appear to arise spontaneously, it is believed that most develop as a direct result of local trauma, even if minor or unnoticed (Fig. 25–16).
- Keloids also develop as a result of inflammation in conditions such as acne vulgaris. The use of isotretinoin has also been linked to the development of keloids.

- Although these lesions arise at any age, they are most common in adolescents and young adults.
- They occur four times more frequently in patients of African descent and are more common in females.
- A positive family history is not uncommon and probably reflects a genetic predisposition to keloid formation.
- Keloids usually occur on the head and neck (especially the ear), upper chest, and arms.
- Characteristically they present as raised, well-circumscribed, rather smooth lesions, becoming progressively more indurated as time passes.
- They are occasionally itchy or tender and may be multiple, again reflecting individual susceptibility to their development.
- Diagnosis: skin biopsy
- Treatment: intralesional corticosteroids, occlusive dressing, compression, intralesional interferon alfa-2b. Irrespective of the treatment used, local recurrence is common.

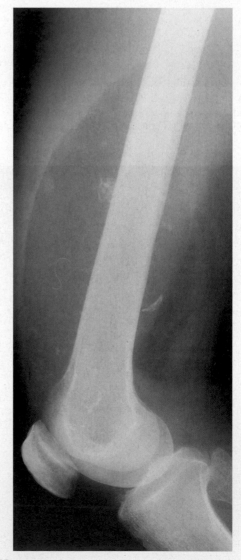

Fig 25–13
Lipoma. This lateral radiograph of the thigh shows a hypodense lipoma containing foci of calcification and ossification.
(From Grainger RG, Allison DJ, Adam A, Dixon AK [eds]: Grainger and Allison's Diagnostic Radiology: A Textbook of Medical Imaging, 4th ed. London. Harcourt, 2001.)

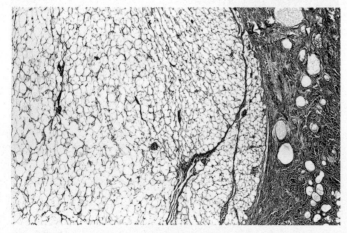

Fig 25–12
Lipoma. Low-power view showing a circumscribed encapsulated tumor composed of mature adipocytes.
(From McKee PH, Calonje E, Granter SR [eds]. Pathology of the Skin With Clinical Correlations, 3rd ed. St. Louis, Mosby, 2005.)

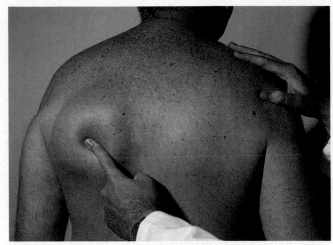

Fig 25–14
Lipoma of the back.
(From Swartz MH: Textbook of Physical Diagnosis, 5th ed. Philadelphia, WB Saunders, 2006.)

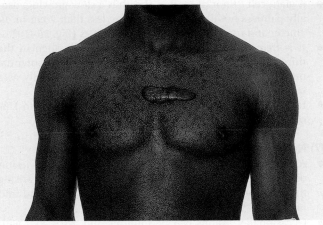

Fig 25–16
Keloid—typical raised, smooth, shiny plaque on the chest of a young African man.
(Courtesy of Dr. M. M. Black, Institute of Dermatology, London.)

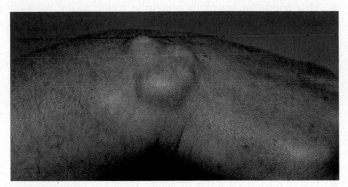

Fig 25–15
Ganglion cyst.
(From Swartz MH: Textbook of Physical Diagnosis, 5th ed. Philadelphia, WB Saunders, 2006.)

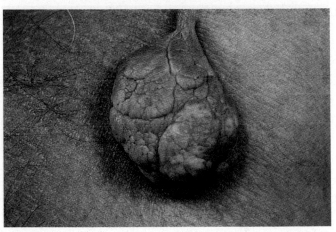

Fig 25–17
Achrochordon. Also known as a skin tag or fibroepithelial polyp, this soft polyp is exceedingly common.
(Courtesy of the Institute of Dermatology, London.)

(4) Fibroepithelial polyp (acrochordon, skin tag)

- Fibroepithelial polyps are common skin lesions typically found in adults in the neck, axillae, and groin areas.
- They are more frequent in the obese, during pregnancy, and in diabetics. Lesions are usually less than 1 cm in diameter and can be popular, filiform, or pedunculated (Fig. 25–17).
- Treatment: none necessary. Local excision when diagnosis is uncertain or for cosmetic reasons is usually curative.

(5) Knuckle pad

- A knuckle pad is an ill-defined focus of fibrous thickening over the metacarpophalangeal or proximal interphalangeal joints, occurring most often in middle age (Fig. 25–18).
- Knuckle pads may be familial, associated with Dupuytren's contracture (see Section 12.16b3), secondary to repeated trauma. or idiopathic.
- They are usually asymptomatic.
- Treatment: none necessary

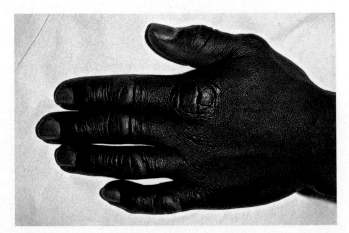

Fig 25–18
Knuckle pad. Typical thickened plaques are present over the interphalangeal joints and second metacarpophalangeal joint.
(Courtesy of Dr. M. M. Black, Institute of Dermatology, London.)

(6) Giant cell tumor of tendon sheath

- A giant cell tumor of tendon sheath is a slow-growing, usually painless nodule, often measuring less than 2 cm in diameter and usually occurring on the fingers (Fig. 25–19).
- It is frequently encountered and arises most often in the third to fifth decade. The lesion has no malignant potential but may recur locally in up to 30% of cases, usually as a consequence of incomplete excision.
- Invasion of underlying bone has been reported in up to 11% of cases.

(7) Neurilemmoma (schwannoma)

- A neurilemmoma is a solitary painless subcutaneous lesion occurring most often in the fourth or fifth decade, arising most frequently on the limbs, followed by the head and neck (Fig. 25–20).
- Occasionall,y lesions can be multiple and associated with neurofibromatosis; see Section 2.16b. Some tumors occur in other locations, including bone and the GI tract.

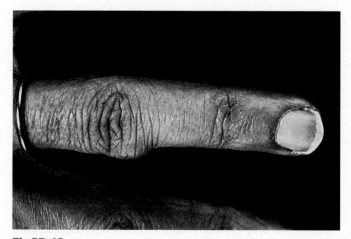

Fig 25–19
Giant cell tumor of tendon sheath. This lesion presents as a firm nodule that most often affects the finger.
(Courtesy of Dr. H. du.P. Menagé, Institute of Dermatology, London.)

- Neurologic symptoms, including pain and paresthesias, are uncommon, except in large deep-seated lesions.
- Treatment: surgical excision. Recurrence after simple excision is infrequent.

(8) Neurofibroma

- Neurofibromas are the most common tumors of nerve sheath origin.
- In most cases, neurofibromas are solitary and unassociated with any other systemic features; however, multiple lesions can occur and form the cardinal feature of neurofibromatosis type I (von Recklinghausen's disease; see Section 2.16b).
- The tumor presents as a polypoid or nodular soft lesion. It is frequently cutaneous and may arise anywhere in the integument (Fig. 25–21).
- It is essential that any patient found to have a neurofibroma be carefully examined for any other signs of neurofibromatosis.

(9) Pilar leiomyoma

- Pilar leiomyoma lesions are multiple, small, slow-growing papules, generally less than 1 cm in diameter.
- They are typically painful or tender, particularly when compressed or exposed to a cold environment.
- Pilar leiomyomas usually present in young adults, most often on the limbs or trunk (Fig. 25–22).
- Multiple leiomyomas have been described in association with HIV infection, chronic lymphocytic leukemia, and erythrocytosis.
- Treatment: local excision. Recurrence is uncommon after excision, but new lesions may continue to develop over the years.

(10) Port-wine stain

- A port-wine stain is the most common vascular malformation (0.3% of live births).
- It is characterized solely by ectatic vessels of variable caliber in the dermis; designation as a true hemangioma is therefore probably inappropriate.
- The lesion tends toward continued growth and only rarely involutes (Fig. 25–23).

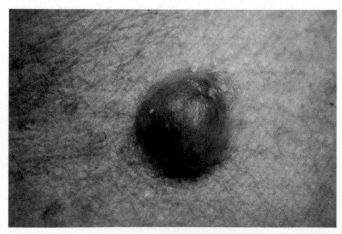

Fig 25–20
Neurilemmoma. This tumor presents as a nonspecific dermal nodule.
(Courtesy of the Institute of Dermatology, London.)

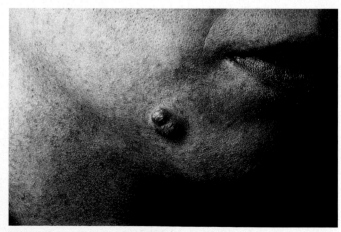

Fig 25–21
Neurofibroma. These are exceedingly common and present as dome-shaped or polypoid fleshy nodules.
(Courtesy of the Institute of Dermatology, London.)

- Familial segregation suggests genetic susceptibility and has been mapped to chromosome 5q.
- The port-wine stain may be associated with Sturge-Weber syndrome (see Section 2.16a).
- Laser therapy is an effective treatment modality (see Fig. 2–18).

(11) Spider nevus
- A spider nevus is a skin lesion consisting solely of a dilated dermal arteriole that communicates with a network of ectatic superficial capillaries.
- These lesions are extremely common and of little clinical significance.
- The lesions manifest as pinhead-sized deep red puncta from which tiny tortuous vessels radiate (Fig. 25–24).
- There is an increased frequency of these lesions with chronic liver disease, thyrotoxicosis, and pregnancy.

(12) Venous lake
- A venous lake is a fairly common vascular ectasia that presents on sun-damaged skin of older people and shows a predilection for the lip (Fig. 25–25).
- Lesions are sometimes multiple and can measure up to 1 cm in diameter. Histology shows a dilated and congested vein in the superficial dermis. There is no evidence of vascular proliferation.

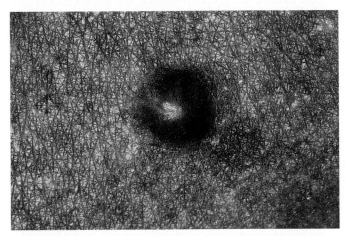

Fig 25–22
Pilar leiomyoma—close-up view of an erythematous nodule.
(Courtesy of the Institute of Dermatology, London.)

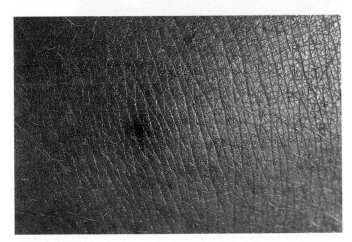

Fig 25–24
Spider nevus. Note the central macule, with radiating vessels.
(Courtesy of Dr. R. A. Marsden, St. George's Hospital, London.)

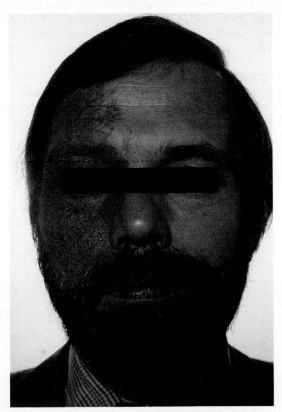

Fig 25–23
Port-wine stain. This large macular lesion was present at birth and, in contrast to the strawberry nevus, shows no tendency to regress.
(Courtesy of Dr. M. M. Black, Institute of Dermatology, London.)

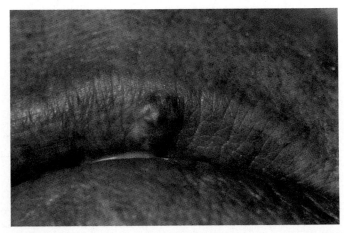

Fig 25–25
Venous lake. There is a typical blister-like vascular lesion.
(Courtesy of the Institute of Dermatology, London.)

(13) Strawberry nevus (infantile hemangioendothelioma, juvenile hemangioma)

- A strawberry nevus is a relatively common benign vascular tumor.
- These flat red or purple lesions, frequently less than 5 cm in diameter, gradually enlarge and develop a raised surface (Fig. 25–26).
- Usually, they are discrete but less often can be large, diffuse, and disfiguring. Over a period of months or years, the vast majority involute spontaneously. Strawberry nevus lesions usually occur congenitally (1 in 100 births) and affect the head and neck most commonly.

(14) Cherry angioma (capillary hemangiomas, senile angiomas, Campbell de Morgan spots)

- Cherry angiomas are common tiny red papules on the trunk and upper limbs of middle-aged and older adults (Fig. 25–27).

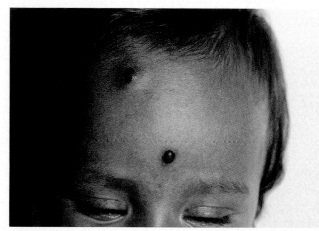

Fig 25–26
Infantile hemangioendothelioma. Two raised red nodules are present on the forehead of this infant girl.
(Courtesy of Dr. M. M. Black, St. Thomas' Hospital, London.)

- Histologically, a cherry angioma is a small polypoid lesion with an epidermal collarette and multiple lobules of dilated and congested capillaries in the papillary dermis.
- Treatment: none necessary

(15) Pyogenic granuloma (lobular capillary hemangioma

- A pyogenic granuloma is a common benign vascular lesion that was, for many years, regarded as a reactive or infective process. This assumption was based on the extensive secondary changes that are almost invariably present in these lesions. However, the underlying process is that of a lobular proliferation of capillaries and therefore it has been redesignated as lobular capillary hemangioma.
- It may arise at any age and shows a predilection for the head, neck, and limbs, particularly the arms and hands.
- Typically, the lesion evolves rapidly, reaching its maximum size (usually less than 2 cm in diameter) within a matter of months.
- It presents as a pedunculated red or bluish nodule, prone to ulceration or bleeding (Fig. 25–28).
- Treatment: surgical excision. Local recurrence after excision is relatively frequent and, in a small proportion of cases, there is a recurrence, with multiple satellite lesions. This latter phenomenon tends to occur in younger individuals who often have primary lesions on the trunk.

(16) Cavernous hemangioma

- Cavernous hemangiomas are vascular lesions composed of a nonlobular, poorly demarcated proliferation of numerous dilated vessels with flattened endothelium (Fig. 25–29).
- These lesions tend to be massive and disfiguring (Fig. 25–30).

(17) Glomus tumor

- A glomus tumor is a relatively common lesion arising from glomus bodies, which are specialized arteriovenous anastomoses usually found in the fingers and palm and

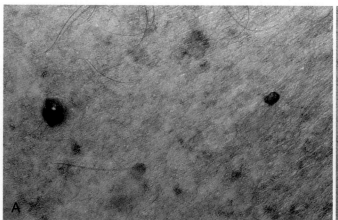
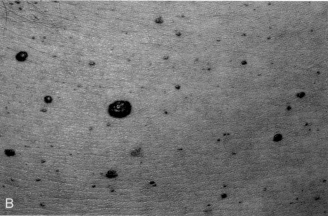

Fig 25–27
Capillary hemangiomas. **A,** The red lesion on the left contains relatively more oxygenated blood, whereas the purple lesion on the right has more venous blood. **B,** Multiple lesions, from papules to pinpoint petechia-like lesions, are present.
(From White GM, Cox NH [eds]: Diseases of the Skin: A Color Atlas and Text, 2nd ed. St. Louis, Mosby, 2006.)

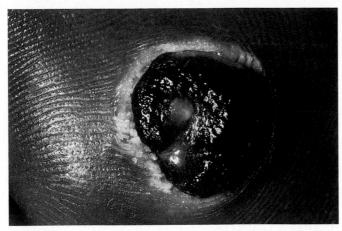

Fig 25–28
Pyogenic granuloma (lobular capillary hemangioma). These lesions are
characteristically ulcerated.
(Courtesy of the Institute of Dermatology, London.)

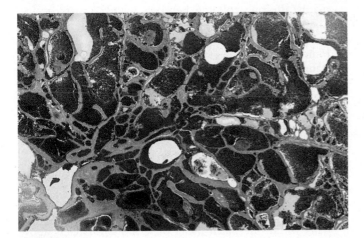

Fig 25–29
Cavernous hemangioma. Dilated thin-walled vessels are lined by flat-
tened endothelial cells.
(From Silverberg SG, DeLellis RA, Frable WJ, et al [eds]: Principles and
Practice of Surgical Pathology and Cytopathology, 4th ed. New York,
Churchill Livingstone, 2006.)

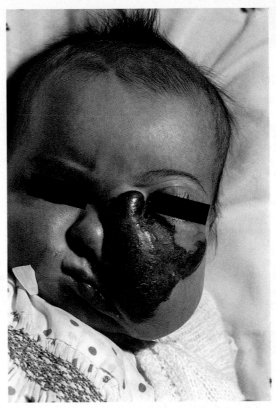

Fig 25–30
Cavernous hemangioma. This massive lesion is distorting the nose
and cheek of this infant girl. Cavernous hemangiomas often involve
the deeper tissues, with resultant pressure necrosis.
(Courtesy of Dr. M. M. Black, St. Thomas' Hospital, London.)

thought to serve as thermoregulatory receptors. Typically,
the tumors are small (less than 1 cm in diameter) reddish-
blue nodules (Fig. 25–31) and typially present with paroxysmal severe pain, which is often precipitated by cold,
pressure, or dependency.
- Treatment: surgical excision

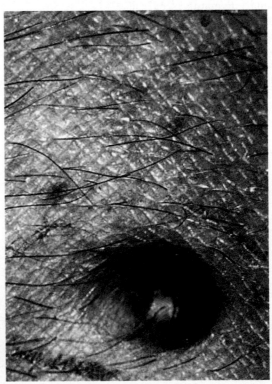

Fig 25–31
Glomus tumor, close-up view.
(Courtesy of the Institute of Dermatology, London.)

Chapter 26 | Dermatophyte infections

A. TINEA CORPORIS

DEFINITION
Tinea corporis (ringworm)is a dermatophyte fungal infection caused by the *Trichophyton* or *Microsporum* sp.

PHYSICAL FINDINGS AND CLINICAL PRESENTATION
- Typically, it appears as single or multiple annular lesions with an advancing scaly border; the margin is slightly raised and reddened (Fig. 26–1), and may be pustular.
- The central area becomes hypopigmented and less scaly as the active border progresses outward.
- The trunk and legs are primarily involved.
- Pruritus is variable.
- It is important to remember that recent topical corticosteroid use can significantly alter the appearance of the lesions.

CAUSE
- *Trichophyton rubrum* is the most common pathogen.

DIFFERENTIAL DIAGNOSIS
- Pityriasis rosea (see Fig. 20–1)
- Erythema multiforme (see Fig. 9–2)
- Psoriasis (see Fig. 7–2)
- SLE (see Fig. 293–1)
- Syphilis (see Fig. 226–12)
- Eczema (see Fig. 6–5)
- Granuloma annulare (see Fig. 11–5)
- Lyme disease (see Fig. 308–12)
- Tinea versicolor (see Fig. 26–5)
- Contact dermatitis (see Fig. 6–8)

DIAGNOSIS
- Diagnosis is usually made on clinical grounds. It can be confirmed by direct visualization under the microscope of a small fragment of the scale using wet mount preparation and KOH solution. Dermatophytes appear as translucent branching filaments (hyphae), with lines of separation appearing at irregular intervals.

LABORATORY TESTS
- Microscopic examination of hyphae
- Mycotic culture usually not necessary
- Biopsy indicated only when diagnosis is uncertain and patient has failed to respond to treatment

TREATMENT
- Antifungal creams are effective.
- Systemic therapy (terbinafine, fluconazole, or ketoconazole) is reserved for severe cases.

B. TINEA CAPITIS

DEFINITION
Tinea capitis (ringworm of the scalp) is a dermatophyte infection of the scalp.
- It is the most common dermatophytosis of childhood, primarily affecting children between 3 and 7 years of age. About 3% to 8% of U.S. children are affected, and 34% of household contacts are asymptomatic carriers.
- In urban populations, large family size, low socioeconomic status, and crowded living conditions may contribute to an increased incidence of tinea capitis.

PHYSICAL FINDINGS AND CLINICAL PRESENTATION
- Triad of scalp scaling, alopecia (Fig. 26–2), and cervical adenopathy
- Primary lesions including plaques, papules, pustules, or nodules on the scalp (usually occipital region).
- Secondary lesions include scales, alopecia, erythema, exudates, and edema.
- Two distinctly different forms:
  - Gray patch lesions are scaly and well demarcated. The hairs within the patch break off a few millimeters above the scalp. One or several lesions may be present; sometimes, the lesions join to form a larger ones.
  - Black dot: predominant form seen in the United States and most often caused by *T. tonsurans*. Early lesions with erythema

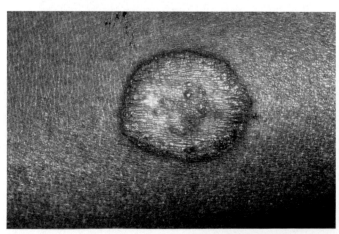

Fig 26–1
Tinea corporis. Note the annular configuration and erythematous margin.
(Courtesy of Dr. M. M. Black, Institute of Dermatology, London.)

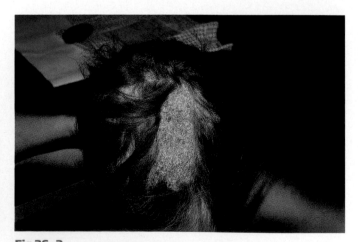

Fig 26–2
Tinea capitis. There is marked hair loss. In this example, scaling and crusting are pronounced.
(Courtesy of Dr. M. M. Black, Institute of Dermatology, London.)

and scaling patch are easily overlooked until areas of alopecia develop. Hairs within the patches break at the surface of the scalp, leaving behind a pattern of swollen black dots.
- Scalp pruritus may be present.
- Fever, pain, and lymphadenopathy (commonly postcervical) with inflammatory lesions
- Hair loss is usually reversible.
- Kerion: inflamed, exudative, pustular, boggy, tender nodules exhibiting marked edema and hair loss seen in severe tinea capitis; caused by immune response to the fungus; may lead to some scarring
- Favus: production of scutula (hair matted together with dermatophyte hyphae and keratin debris), characterized by yellow cup-shaped crusts around hair shafts. A fetid odor may be present.

CAUSE
- Most commonly caused by *Trichophyton* (80% of the cases in the United States) or *Microsporum* sp. The most common causative species for black dot tinea capitis is *T. tonsurans* and for gray patch tinea capitis are *M. audouinii* and *M. canis*.
- Transmission occurs via infected persons or asymptomatic carriers, fallen infected hairs, animal vectors, and fomites. *M. audouinii* is commonly spread by dogs and cats. Infectious fungal particles may remain viable for many months.

DIFFERENTIAL DIAGNOSIS
- Alopecia areata (see Fig. 18–6)
- Impetigo (see Fig. 28–13)
- Pediculosis (see Fig. 29–5)
- Trichotillomania (see Fig. 18–11)
- Folliculitis (see Fig. 28–14)
- Seborrheic dermatitis (see Fig. 6–4)
- Psoriasis (see Fig. 7–2)

DIAGNOSIS
- KOH testing of hair shaft extracted from the lesion, not the scale, because the *T. tonsurans* spores attach to or reside inside hair shafts and will rarely be found in the scales
- Wood's ultraviolet light reveals blue-green fluorescence on hair shafts for *Microsporum* infection but will fail to identify *T. tonsurans.*
- Fungal culture of hairs and scales on fungal medium such as Sabouraud agar may be used to confirm the diagnosis, especially if uncertain.

TREATMENT
- Griseofulvin
- New alternative treatments: oral terbinafine, itraconazole, or fluconazole are comparable in efficacy and safety with griseofulvin,

C. TINEA CRURIS

DEFINITION
Tinea cruris (jock itch) is a dermatophyte infection of the groin.

PHYSICAL FINDINGS AND CLINICAL PRESENTATION
- Erythematous plaques have a half-moon shape and scaling border.
- The acute inflammation tends to move down the inner thigh and usually spares the scrotum; in severe cases, the fungus may spread onto the buttocks.
- Itching may be severe.

- Red papules and pustules may be present (Fig. 26–3).
- An important diagnostic sign is the advancing well-defined border, with a tendency toward central clearing.

CAUSE
- Dermatophytes of the genera *Trichophyton, Epidermophyton,* and *Microsporum; T. rubrum* and *E. floccosum* are the most common causes.
- Transmission from direct contact (e.g., infected persons, animals). The patient's feet should be evaluated as a source of infection because tinea cruris is often associated with tinea pedis.

DIFFERENTIAL DIAGNOSIS
- Intertrigo (see Fig. 26–8)
- Psoriasis (see Fig. 7–2)
- Seborrheic dermatitis (see Fig. 6–3)
- Erythrasma (see Fig. 28–11)
- Candidiasis (see Fig. 26–8)
- Tinea versicolor (see Fig. 26–5)

DIAGNOSIS
- Diagnosis is based on clinical presentation and demonstration of hyphae microscopically using KOH.

LABORATORY TESTS
- Microscopic examination
- Cultures are generally not necessary.

TREATMENT
- Keep infected area clean and dry.
- Drying powders (e.g., miconazole nitrate) may be useful for patients with excessive perspiration.
- Topical antifungal agents (miconazole, terbinafine, clotrimazole).
- Oral antifungal therapy (luconazole, terbinafine, ketoconazole) is generally reserved for cases unresponsive to topical agents.

D. TINEA PEDIS

DEFINITION
Tinea pedis (athlete's foot) is a dermatophyte infection of the feet.

PHYSICAL FINDINGS AND CLINICAL PRESENTATION
- Typical presentation is variable and ranges from erythematous scaling plaques and isolated blisters to interdigital maceration (Fig. 26–4).

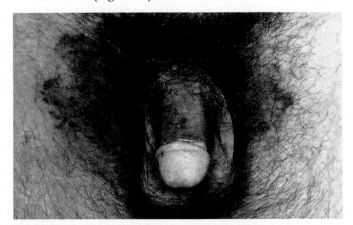

Fig 26–3
Tinea cruris. This is much more common in men than in women. In this example, pustulation is evident.
(Courtesy of Dr. R. A. Marsden, St. George's Hospital, London.)

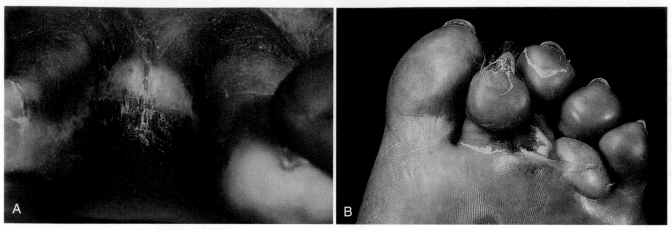

Fig 26-4
Tinea pedis. **A,** Maceration between the toes. **B,** Severe dermal edema has resulted in this bullous variant.
(**A** courtesy of Dr. A. du Vivier, King's College Hospital, London; **B** courtesy of the Institute of Dermatology, London.)

- Most common dermatophyte infection
- The infection usually starts in the interdigital spaces of the foot. Most infections are found in the toe webs or in the soles.
- Fourth or fifth toes are most commonly involved.
- Pruritus is common and is most intense following the removal of shoes and socks.
- Infection with *Tinea rubrum* often manifests with a moccasin distribution affecting the soles and lateral feet.

CAUSE
- Dermatophyte infection caused by *T. rubrum, T. mentagrophytes* or, less commonly, *E. floccosum*

DIFFERENTIAL DIAGNOSIS
- Contact dermatitis (see Fig. 6–7)
- Infective dermatitis (see Fig. 6–13)
- Cellulitis (see Fig. 28–1)
- Eczema (see Fig. 6–1)
- Psoriasis (see Fig. 7–1)

DIAGNOSIS
- Diagnosis is usually made by clinical observation.
- Laboratory testing, when performed, generally consists of a simple potassium hydroxide (KOH) preparation with mycologic examination under a light microscope to confirm the presence of dermatophytes.

LABORATORY TESTS
- Microscopic examination of a scale or the roof of a blister with 10% KOH under low or medium power will reveal hyphae.
- Mycologic culture is rarely indicated in the diagnosis of tinea pedis.
- Biopsy is reserved for when the diagnosis remains in question after testing or failure to respond to treatment.

TREATMENT
- Keep infected area clean and dry. Aerate feet by wearing sandals when possible.
- Wear 100% cotton socks rather than nylon socks to reduce moisture.
- Areas likely to become infected should be dried completely before being covered with clothing.
- Antifungal creams (clotrimazole, butenafine, naftifine).

- Oral agents (fluconazole) can be used in combination with topical agents in resistant cases.

E. TINEA VERSICOLOR

DEFINITION
Tinea versicolor is a fungal infection of the skin caused by the yeast *Pityrosporum orbiculare (Malassezia furfur)*.

PHYSICAL FINDINGS AND CLINICAL PRESENTATION
- Most lesions begin as multiple small, circular macules of various colors.
- The macules may be darker or lighter than the surrounding normal skin and will scale with scraping (Fig. 26–5).
- Most frequent site of distribution is the trunk
- Facial lesions are more common in children (forehead is the most common facial site).
- Eruption is generally of insidious onset and asymptomatic.
- Lesions may be hyperpigmented in blacks (Fig. 26–6).
- Lesions may be inconspicuous in fair-complexioned individuals, especially during the winter.
- Most patients become aware of the eruption when the involved areas do not tan.

CAUSE
- The infection is caused by the lipophilic yeast *P. orbiculare* (round form) and *P. ovale* (oval form); these organisms are normal inhabitants of the skin flora. Factors that favor their proliferation are pregnancy, malnutrition, immunosuppression, oral contraceptives, and excessive heat and humidity.

DIFFERENTIAL DIAGNOSIS
- Vitiligo (see Fig. 17–2)
- Pityriasis alba (see Fig. 6–18)
- Secondary syphilis (see Fig. 226–14)
- Pityriasis rosea (see Fig. 27–34)
- Seborrheic dermatitis (see Fig. 6–4)

DIAGNOSIS
Diagnosis is based on the clinical appearance; identification of hyphae and budding spores (spaghetti and meatballs appearance) with microscopy confirms diagnosis.

LABORATORY TESTS
- Microscopic examination using potassium hydroxide confirms the diagnosis when in doubt (Fig. 26–7).

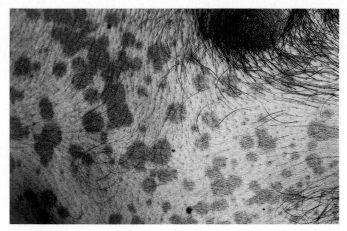

Fig 26–5
Tinea versicolor. Pale brown macules are typically seen in white individuals.
(Courtesy of Dr. R. A. Marsden, St. George's Hospital, London.)

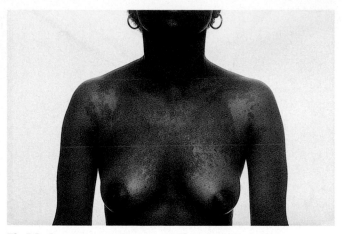

Fig 26–6
Tinea versicolor. Hyperpigmented macules, many of which have coalesced, are present on the chest, which is a commonly affected site.
(Courtesy of Dr. M. M. Black, Institute of Dermatology, London.)

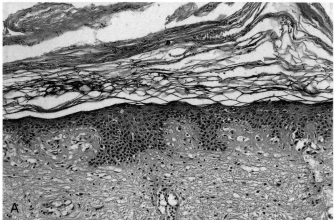

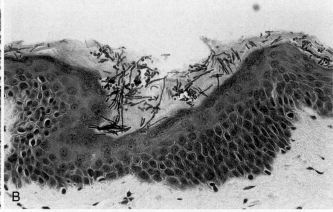

Fig 26–7
Tinea versicolor. **A,** There is hyperkeratosis and small basophilic spores are easily seen. **B,** The periodic acid–Schiff reaction reveals numerous hyphae.
(From McKee PH, Calonje E, Granter SR [eds]: Pathology of the Skin With Clinical Correlations, 3rd ed. St. Louis, Mosby, 2005.)

TREATMENT
- Topical treatment: selenium sulfide, 2.5% suspension
- Oral antifungal agents (fluconazole, ketoconazole) can be used for resistant cases.
- Sunlight accelerates repigmentation of hypopigmented areas.
- Patients should be informed that the hypopigmented areas will not disappear immediately after treatment and that several months may be necessary for the hypopigmented areas to regain their pigmentation.

F. CUTANEOUS CANDIDIASIS

DEFINITION
- Superficial mycotic infection of the skin usually caused by the yeast *Candida albicans*

PHYSICAL FINDINGS AND CLINICAL PRESENTATION
- The affected area has a red glistening surface with an advancing border and cigarette paper–like scaling.

- The intertriginous skin folds such as the inner thighs (Fig. 26–8) or other moist occluded sites such as underneath the breasts (Fig. 26–9) are most frequently affected.
- Factors that predispose to infection include diabetes mellitus, obesity, increasing moisture, use of systemic corticosteroids or antibiotics, and immunocompromised status.

DIAGNOSIS
- Diagnosis is usually made on clinical grounds.
- The presence of pseudohyphae and yeast forms on KOH preparation or other stains (Fig. 26–10) confirms the diagnosis.

LABORATORY TESTS
- Serum glucose, HIV serology (in recurrent cases)

TREATMENT
- Affected skin sites that are moist should be dried out with wet to dry soaks and exposed to air.
- Topical antifungal products (e.g., miconazole, clotrimazole, econazole) are generally effective.
- Oral therapy (e.g., fluconazole, itraconazole) is reserved for resistant cases.

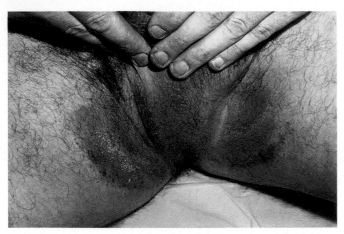

Fig 26–8
Cutaneous candidiasis. The warm moist environment of the upper thighs and scrotum predisposes to intertriginous candidiasis. Note the erythema and peripheral pustules.
(Courtesy of Dr. M. M. Black, Institute of Dermatology, London.)

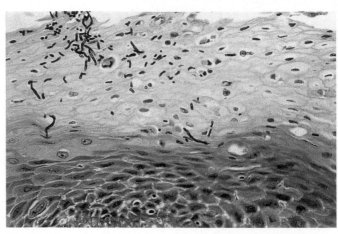

Fig 26–10
Cutaneous candidiasis. **A,** There is marked acanthosis and the superficial layers of the epithelium are infiltrated by large numbers of neutrophils. **B,** There are abundant yeastlike and pseudohyphal forms (periodic acid–Schiff.
(From McKee PH, Calonje E, Granter SR [eds]: Pathology of the Skin With Clinical Correlations, 3rd ed. St. Louis, Mosby, 2005.)

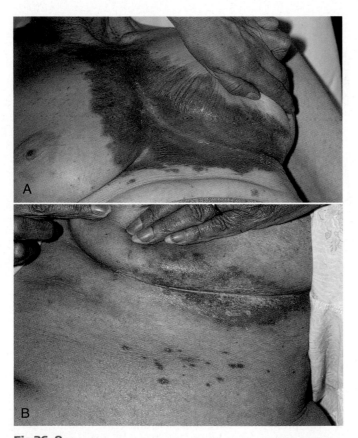

Fig 26–9
Inframammary candidiasis. The skin of the inframammary fold may become red, scaly, moist, or macerated. **A,** Obese women with large breasts exposed to hot, humid climates are most commonly affected. **B,** Candidiasis is very common, and its presence may be indicated by satellite pustules.
(From White GM, Cox NH [eds]: Diseases of the Skin: A Color Atlas and Text, 2nd ed. St. Louis, Mosby, 2006.)

A. ERYTHEMA INFECTIOSUM (FIFTH DISEASE)

DEFINITION

Fifth disease is a viral exanthem of childhood affecting primarily school-age children, and caused by parvovirus B19. Erythema infectiosum was the fifth in a series of described viral exanthems of childhood and is the most common clinical syndrome associated with parvovirus B19. Table 27–1 compares rashes associated with acute viral infections.

PHYSICAL FINDINGS AND CLINICAL PRESENTATION

- Typical bright red, nontender maxillar‚y rash with circumoral pallor over the cheeks, producing the classic "slapped cheek" appearance (Fig. 27–1)
- Reticular, nonpruritic lacy, erythematous maculopapular rash over trunk and extremities lasting up to several weeks after the acute episode; may be worsened by heat or sunlight
- Polyarthritis and arthralgias are commonly seen in older patients but are less common in children. Arthritis involves the small joints of the extremities in a symmetrical fashion.
- Mild fever seen in up to one third of patients

CAUSE

- Syndrome caused by parvovirus B19, a single-stranded DNA virus, which has been reclassified in a new genus, *Erythrovirus.*

DIFFERENTIAL DIAGNOSIS

- Juvenile rheumatoid arthritis (Still's disease; see Fig. 292–2)
- Rubella (see Fig. 27–29)
- Measles (rubeola) (see Fig. 27–25)
- Mononucleosis (see Fig. 338–2)
- Lyme disease (see Fig. 308–12)
- Acute HIV infection
- Drug eruption (see Fig. 14–1)

LABORATORY TESTS

- Human chorionic gonadotropin (hCG) in women of childbearing age. Infection during early pregnancy may result in fetal death (10%) or severe anemia but is usually asymptomatic and not associated with congenital malformations.
- CBC, Lyme titer, monospot when diagnosis is in doubt. The PCR assay has been used for early rapid diagnosis in immunocompromised patients.

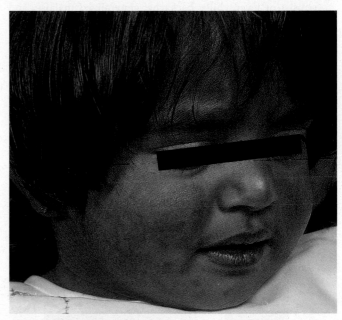

Fig 27–1
Bright red, nontender, maxillary rash, with circumoral pallor over cheeks.
(From Lebwohl MG, Heymann WR, Berth-Jones J, Coulson I [eds]: Treatment of Skin Disease. St. Louis, Mosby, 2002.)

TABLE 27–1 Rashes associated with acute viral infections

Virus	Syndrome	Comment
Measles	Measles	Maculopapular, followed by staining
Rubella	Rubella, German measles	Macular, often general facial flush
Herpesvirus 6	Roseola infantum	Macular or maculopapular after several days of fever
Parvovirus B19	Erythema infectiosum	Slapped cheeks, lacy rash on trunk and limbs, often rubelliform or hemorrhagic
Varicella-zoster	Chickenpox, shingles	Vesicular, rarely hemorrhagic; neurologic distribution, premonitory pain, erythema
Herpes simplex	Disseminated herpes, eczema herpeticum	
Epstein-Barr virus		Occasionally, macular rash; severe rashes, usually ampicillin-induced
Enteroviruses		Usually, macular or maculopapular; sometimes hemorrhagic, vesicular, or both (hand, foot, and mouth disease)
Primary HIV	Mononucleosis-like illness	Maculopapular rashes in chronic HIV infection
Viral hemorrhagic fevers		Purpura, ecchymoses

From Cohen J, Powderly WG: Infectious Diseases, 2nd ed. St. Louis, 2004.

TREATMENT
- Treatment is supportive only; NSAIDs used for arthralgias/arthritis
- Intravenous immunoglobulin and transfusion support may be used for immunocompromised patients with red cell aplasia.

B. VARICELLA (CHICKENPOX)

DEFINITION
Chickenpox is a common viral illness characterized by the acute onset of generalized vesicular rash and fever.

PHYSICAL FINDINGS AND CLINICAL PRESENTATION
- Findings vary with the clinical course. Initial symptoms consist of fever, chills, backache, generalized malaise, and headache. The incubation period of chickenpox ranges from 9 to 21 days.
- Symptoms are generally more severe in adults.
- Initial lesions generally occur on the trunk (centripetal distribution) and occasionally on the face; these lesions consist primarily of 3- to 4-mm red papules with an irregular outline and a clear vesicle on the surface (dew drops on a rose petal appearance; Fig. 27–2).
- Intense pruritus generally accompanies this stage.
- New lesion development generally ceases by the fourth day, with subsequent crusting by the sixth day.
- Lesions generally spread to the face and the extremities (centrifugal spread).
- Patients generally present with lesions at different stages at the same time.
- Crusts generally fall off within 5 to 14 days.

- Fever is usually highest during the eruption of the vesicles; temperature generally returns to normal following disappearance of vesicles.
- Signs of potential complications (e.g., bacterial skin infections, neurologic complications, pneumonia, hepatitis) may be present on physical examination.
- Mild constitutional symptoms (e.g., anorexia, myalgias, headaches, restlessness) may be present (most common in adults).
- Excoriations may be present if scratching is prominent.

CAUSE
- Varicella-zoster virus (VZV), human herpesvirus 3, can manifest with varicella or herpes zoster (i.e., shingles, which is a re-activation of varicella).

DIFFERENTIAL DIAGNOSIS
- Other viral infections (see Fig. 27–32)
- Impetigo (see Fig. 28–13)
- Scabies (see Fig. 29–1)
- Drug rash (see Fig. 14–1)
- Urticaria (see Fig. 15–8)
- Dermatitis herpetiformis (see Fig. 4–8)
- Smallpox (see Fig. 27–35)

LABORATORY TESTS
- Laboratory evaluation is generally not necessary.
- CBC may reveal leukopenia and thrombocytopenia.
- Serum varicella titers (significant rise in serum varicella IgG antibody level), skin biopsy, or Tzanck smear are used only when the diagnosis is in question.

TREATMENT
- Use antipruritic lotions for symptomatic relief.
- Avoid scratching to prevent excoriations and superficial skin infections.

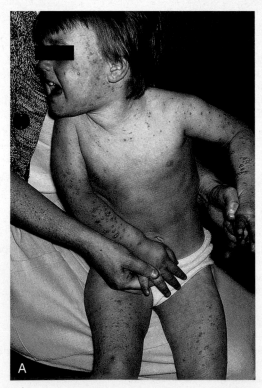
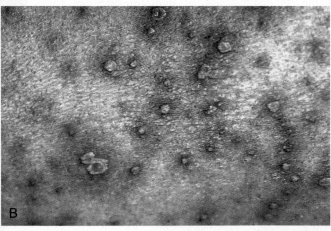

Fig 27-2
Varicella (chickenpox). **A,** Note the widespread subtribution of vesicles on the face, upper chest, arms, and legs. **B,** Close-up view.
(**A** courtesy of Dr. R. A. Marsden, St. George's Hospital, London.; **B** courtesy of the Institute of Dermatology, London.)

- Use a mild soap for bathing; hands should be washed often.
- Use acetaminophen for fever and myalgias; aspirin should be avoided because of the increased risk of Reye's syndrome.
- Oral acyclovir initiated at the earliest sign (within 24 hours of illness) is useful for healthy, nonpregnant individuals 13 years of age or older to decrease the duration and severity of signs and symptoms. Immunocompromised hosts should be treated with IV acyclovir.
- Pruritus from chickenpox can be controlled with antihistamines (e.g., hydroxyzine, 25 mg every 6 hours) and oral antipruritic lotions (e.g., calamine).

- Oral antibiotics are not routinely indicated and should be used only for patients with secondary infection and infected lesions (most common infective organisms are *Streptococcus* and *Staphylococcus* spp.).

C. HERPES SIMPLEX

DEFINITION

Herpes simplex is a viral infection caused by the herpes simplex virus (HSV; Fig. 27–3); HSV-1 is associated primarily with oral infections, whereas HSV-2 causes mainly genital infections. However, each type can infect any site. Following the primary infection, the virus enters the nerve endings in the skin directly

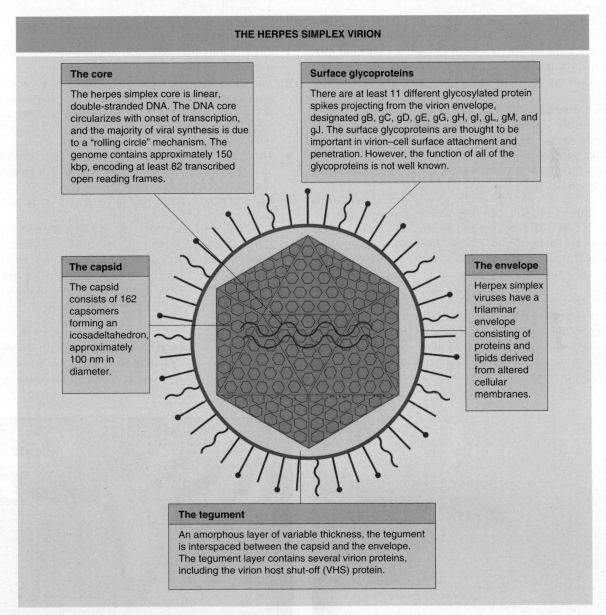

THE HERPES SIMPLEX VIRION

The core

The herpes simplex core is linear, double-stranded DNA. The DNA core circularizes with onset of transcription, and the majority of viral synthesis is due to a "rolling circle" mechanism. The genome contains approximately 150 kbp, encoding at least 82 transcribed open reading frames.

Surface glycoproteins

There are at least 11 different glycosylated protein spikes projecting from the virion envelope, designated gB, gC, gD, gE, gG, gH, gI, gL, gM, and gJ. The surface glycoproteins are thought to be important in virion–cell surface attachment and penetration. However, the function of all of the glycoproteins is not well known.

The capsid

The capsid consists of 162 capsomers forming an icosadeltahedron, approximately 100 nm in diameter.

The envelope

Herpex simplex viruses have a trilaminar envelope consisting of proteins and lipids derived from altered cellular membranes.

The tegument

An amorphous layer of variable thickness, the tegument is interspaced between the capsid and the envelope. The tegument layer contains several virion proteins, including the virion host shut-off (VHS) protein.

Fig 27–3

The herpex simplex virion. This consists of a double-stranded DNA core surrounded by a capsid, an amorphous tegument layer, and a lipid envelope, with numerous glycoprotein spikes. The overall diameter is 150 to 200 nm. Virus replication takes place within the nucleus of the infected cell. The envelope is gained as the virion passes through the nuclear membrane. Replication of virus within the host cell results in cell lysis and destruction. Latent viruses do not cause neural cell lysis within ganglia.
(From Cohen J, Powderly WG: Infectious Diseases, 2nd ed. St. Louis, Mosby, 2004.)

below the lesions and ascends to the dorsal root ganglia, where it remains in a latent stage until it is reactivated.

PHYSICAL FINDINGS AND CLINICAL PRESENTATION

Primary infection

- Symptoms occur from 3 to 7 days after contact (respiratory droplets, direct contact).
- Constitutional symptoms include low-grade fever, headache and myalgias, regional lymphadenopathy, and localized pain.
- Pain, burning, itching, and tingling last several hours.
- Grouped vesicles (Fig. 27–4), usually with surrounding erythema, appear and generally ulcerate or crust within 48 hours.
- The vesicles are uniform in size (differentiating it from herpes zoster vesicles, which vary in size).
- During the acute eruption, the patient is uncomfortable. Involvement of the lips and inside of the mouth may make it unpleasant for the patient to eat; urinary retention may complicate involvement of the genital area.
- Lesions generally last from 2 to 6 weeks and heal without scarring.

Recurrent infection

- Generally caused by alteration in the immune system; fatigue, stress, menses, local skin trauma, and exposure to sunlight are contributing factors.
- The prodromal symptoms (fatigue, burning, and tingling of the affected area) last 12 to 24 hours.
- A cluster of lesions generally evolve within 24 hours from a macule to a papule and then vesicles surrounded by erythema; the vesicles coalesce and subsequently rupture within 4 days, revealing erosions covered by crusts.
- The crusts are generally shed within 7 to 10 days, revealing a pink surface.
- The most frequent location of the lesions is on the vermilion borders of the lips (HSV-1), the penile shaft or glans penis (Fig. 27–5), and the labia (HSV-2; Fig. 27–6), buttocks (seen more frequently in women), fingertips (herpetic whitlow), and trunk (may be confused with herpes zoster).
- The rapid onset of diffuse cutaneous herpes simplex (eczema herpeticum) may occur in certain atopic infants and

adults. It is a medical emergency, especially in young infants, and should be promptly treated with acyclovir.

- Herpes encephalitis, meningitis, and ocular herpes can occur in immunocompromised patients status and occasionally in normal hosts.

CAUSE

- HSV-1 and HSV-2 are both DNA viruses.

DIFFERENTIAL DIAGNOSIS

- Impetigo (see Fig. 28–13)
- Behçet's syndrome (see Fig. 16–14)
- Syphilis (see Fig. 226–12)
- Stevens-Johnson syndrome (see Fig. 9–6)
- Herpangina (see Fig. 91–1)
- Aphthous stomatitis (see Fig. 89–11)
- Varicella (see Fig. 27–2)
- Herpes zoster. (see Fig. 27–8)

LABORATORY TESTS

- Direct immunofluorescent antibody slide tests will provide a rapid diagnosis.
- Viral culture is the most definitive method for diagnosis; results are generally available in 1 or 2 days. The lesions should be sampled during the vesicular or early ulcerative stage; cervical samples should be taken from the endocervix with a swab.
- The Tzanck smear is a readily available test; it will demonstrate multinucleated giant cells (Fig. 27–7). However, it is not a very sensitive test.
- Pap smear will detect HSV-infected cells in cervical tissue from women without symptoms.
- Serologic tests for HSV: IgG and IgM serum antibodies. Antibodies to HSV occur in 50% to 90% of adults. Routine tests do not discriminate between HSV-1 and HSV-2; the presence of IgM or a fourfold or greater rise in IgG titers indicates a recent infection (convalescent sample should be drawn 2 to 3 weeks after the acute specimen is drawn).

TREATMENT

- Application of topical cool compresses with Burow's solution for 15 minutes four to six times daily may be soothing for patients with extensive erosions on the vulva and penis

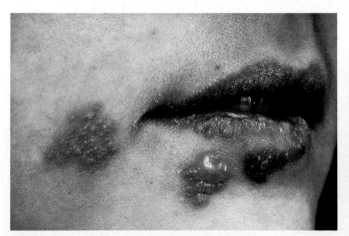

Fig 27–4
Herpes simplex 1—primary infection showing grouped vesicles on an erythematous base.
(Courtesy of Dr. R. A. Marsden, St. George's Hospital, London.)

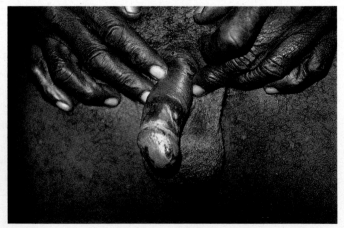

Fig 27–5
Herpes simplex 2. There is intense erythema, and multiple ulcers are present on both the glans and the shaft.
(Courtesy of Dr. C. Furlonge, Port of Spain, Trinidad.)

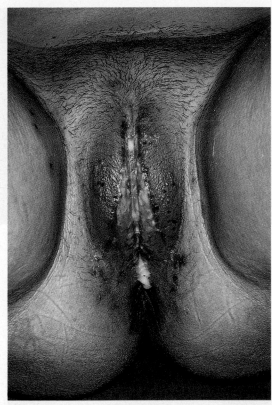

Fig 27–6
Herpes simplex 2—vulval involvement, showing erythema and crusted vesicles.
(Courtesy of Dr. R. A. Marsden, St. George's Hospital, London.)

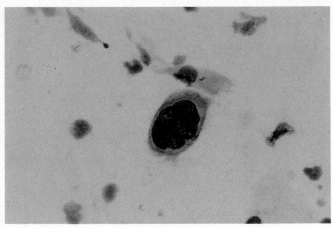

Fig 27–7
Tzanck preparation. A multinucleated giant cell is demonstrated in this scraping from the base of a vesicular lesion. Intranuclear inclusions are not readily seen, but the molding of the nuclei is clearly demonstrated. It is not possible to distinguish between herpes simplex and varicella-zoster viruses with this technique (Diff-Quik, ×1000).
(From Silverberg SG, DeLellis RA, Frable WJ, et al [eds]: Principles and Practice of Surgical Pathology and Cytopathology, 4th ed. New York, Churchill Livingstone, 2006.)

(decreased edema and inflammation, débridement of crusts and purulent material).

- Acyclovir ointment or cream applied using a finger cot or rubber glove every 3 to 6 hours (six times daily) for 7 days may be useful for the first clinical episode of genital herpes. Primary genital infections may be treated with oral acyclovir, famciclovir, or valacyclovir. Topical acyclovir, 5% cream, can also be used for herpes labialis; when started at the prodrome or papule stage, it decreases the duration of an episode by about 12 hours. Penciclovir, 1% cream, can also be used for recurrent herpes labialis on the lips and face.
- Recurrent episodes of genital herpes can be treated with acyclovir. A short course (800 mg three times daily for 2 days) is effective. Other treatment options include 800 mg PO, twice daily, for 3 to 5 days, generally started during the prodrome or within 2 days of onset of lesions. Famciclovir is also useful for the treatment of recurrent genital herpes (125 mg, every 12 hours, for 5 days for patients with normal renal function) started at the first sign of symptoms, or valacyclovir (500 mg every 12 hours for 3 days, for patients with normal renal function).
- Acyclovir-resistant mucocutaneous lesions in patients with HIV can be treated with foscarnet (40 to 60 mg/kg IV, every 8 hours, for patients with normal renal function); HPMPC has also been reported to be effective for HSV infections resistant to acyclovir or foscarnet.

- Patients with six recurrences of genital herpes annually can be treated with valacyclovir, 1 g every day, acyclovir, 400 mg twice daily, or famciclovir, 250 mg twice daily.

D. HERPES ZOSTER

DEFINITION
Herpes zoster is a disease caused by reactivation of the varicella-zoster virus. Following the primary infection (chickenpox), the virus becomes latent in the dorsal root ganglia and re-emerges when there is a weakening of the immune system (secondary to disease or advanced age).

PHYSICAL FINDINGS AND CLINICAL PRESENTATION
- Pain generally precedes skin manifestation by 3 to 5 days and is generally localized to the dermatome that will be affected by the skin lesions.
- Constitutional symptoms are often present (malaise, fever, headache).
- The initial rash consists of erythematous maculopapules generally affecting one dermatome (thoracic region in most cases; Fig. 27–8); some patients (less than 50%) may have scattered vesicles outside the affected dermatome. A hemorrhagic component to the lesions may be evident.
- The initial maculopapules evolve into vesicles and pustules by the third or fourth day.
- The vesicles have an erythematous base, are cloudy, and are of varying sizes; this is a distinguishing characteristic from herpes simplex, in which the vesicles are of uniform size.
- The vesicles subsequently become umbilicated and then form crusts that generally fall off within 3 weeks; scarring may occur.
- Pain during and after the rash is generally significant.
- Secondary bacterial infection with *S. aureus* or *S. pyogenes* may occur.
- Regional lymphadenopathy may occur.

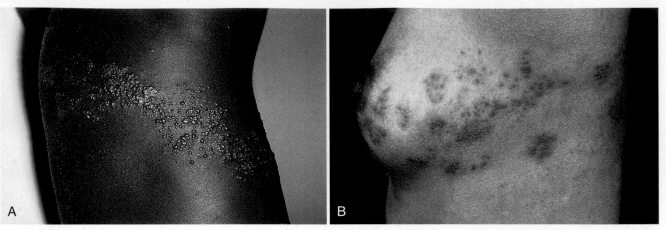

Fig 27-8
A, B, Herpes zoster (shingles)—intact vesicles in a characteristic dermatomal distribution.
(**A** courtesy of Dr. C. Furlonge, Port of Spain, Trinidad; **B** courtesy of the Institute of Dermatology, London.)

- Herpes zoster may involve the trigeminal nerve (most frequent cranial nerve involved); involvement of the geniculate ganglion can cause facial palsy and a painful ear, with the presence of vesicles on the pinna and external auditory canal (*Ramsay Hunt syndrome*).
- When the rash of herpes zoster involves the skin at the tip and side of the nose, it is known as *Hutchinson's sign* (Fig. 27–9).
- Herpes zoster ophthalmicus may manifest with third nerve palsy (Fig. 27–10)

CAUSE
- Reactivation of varicella virus (human herpesvirus 3)

DIFFERENTIAL DIAGNOSIS
- Rash: herpes simplex (see Fig. 27–4) and other viral infections (see Fig. 27–20)
- Pain from herpes zoster; may be confused with acute myocardial infarction, pulmonary embolism, pleuritis, pericarditis, renal colic

LABORATORY TESTS
- Laboratory tests are generally not necessary (viral cultures and a Tzanck smear will confirm the diagnosis in patients with an atypical presentation).

TREATMENT
- Wet compresses using Burow's solution or cool tap water, applied for 15 to 30 minutes 5 to 10 times daily, are helpful to break vesicles and remove serum and crust.
- Care must be taken to prevent any secondary bacterial infection.
- Gabapentin, pregabalin, and duloxetine are effective for the treatment of pain and sleep interference associated with postherpetic neuralgia.
- Lidocaine patch 5% (Lidoderm) is also effective in relieving postherpetic neuralgia. Patches are applied to intact skin to cover the most painful area for up to 12 hours within a 24-hour period.
- Oral antiviral agents (e.g., acyclovir, valacyclovir, or famciclovir) can decrease acute pain, inflammation, and vesicle formation when treatment is begun within 48 hours of onset of rash.
- Immunocompromised patients should be treated with IV acyclovir; IV vidarabine is also effective for the treatment of

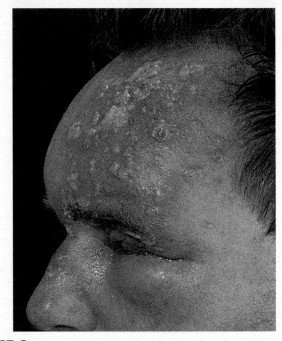

Fig 27-9
Hutchinson's sign. When the rash of herpes zoster involves the skin at the tip and side of the nose, it indicates that the nasociliary branch of the trigeminal nerve is involved and there is an increased risk of uveal tract inflammation and ocular damage.
(From Cohen J, Powderly WG: Infectious Diseases, 2nd ed. St. Louis, Mosby, 2004.)

disseminated herpes zoster in immunocompromised hosts.
- Patients with AIDS and transplant patients may develop acyclovir-resistant VZV infection; these patients can be treated with foscarnet.
- Capsaicin cream can be useful for the treatment of postherpetic neuralgia.
- Sympathetic blocks (stellate ganglion or epidural) with 0.25% bupivacaine and rhizotomy are reserved for severe cases unresponsive to conservative treatment.
- Corticosteroids should be considered for older patients if there are no contraindications.

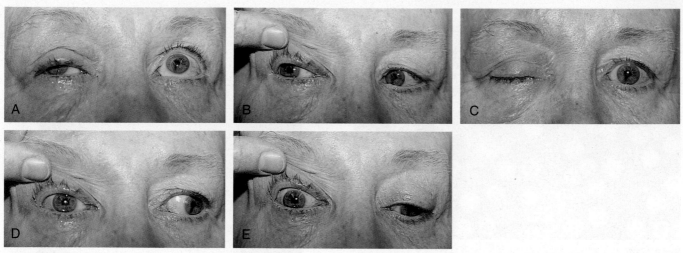

Fig 27–10
A-E, Isolated third-nerve palsy in the setting of herpes zoster ophthalmicus at the time of acute illness. Note the presence of herpes zoster lesions in the distribution of the first division of the fifth nerve. Third-nerve palsy consists of ptosis, adduction, elevation, and depression deficit, with preserved abduction.
(From Yanoff M, Duker JS: Ophthalmology, 2nd ed. St. Louis, Mosby, 2004.)

E. ROSEOLA (EXANTHEMA SUBITUM)

DEFINITION
Roseola is a benign viral illness found in infants and characterized by high fevers followed by a rash.

PHYSICAL FINDINGS AND CLINICAL PRESENTATION
- Typically, the child develops a high fever, usually up to 104° F (40° C) that lasts for 3 to 5 days.
- Fever may be associated with a runny nose, irritability, and fatigue.
- A rash appears within 48 hours of defervescence, mainly on the face, neck, trunk, arms, and legs.
- The rash is a faint pink maculopapular rash that blanches when palpated (Fig. 27–11).
- The rash usually fades away within 48 hours.
- Anorexia
- Seizures
- Cervical adenopathy
- The incubation period is between 5 and 15 days.

CAUSE
- Roseola is caused by human herpesvirus 6 (HHV-6).

DIFFERENTIAL DIAGNOSIS
  - Measles (see Fig. 27–25)
  - Rubella (see Fig. 27–28)
  - Fifth disease (see Fig. 27–1)
  - Drug eruption (see Fig. 14–1)
  - Mononucleosis (see Fig. 338–2)

LABORATORY TESTS
- CBC with differential
- Blood cultures if suspecting sepsis
- Stool cultures if diarrhea is present
- Lumbar puncture if meningitis suspected

TREATMENT
- Maintain hydration by drinking clear fluids such as water, fruit juice, and lemonade.
- Acetaminophen or ibuprofen for fever
- Avoid aspirin (increased risk of Reye's syndrome)

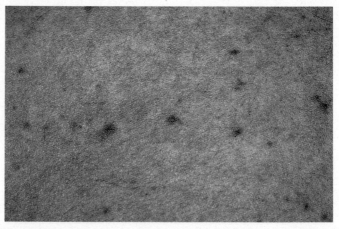

Fig 27–11
Roseola. As the fever breaks, multiple, pale pink, 1- to 5-mm macules and papules appear and last from only hours to a few days.
(From White GM, Cox NH [eds]: Diseases of the Skin: A Color Atlas and Text, 2nd ed. St. Louis, Mosby, 2006.)

F. VERRUCA (WARTS)

DEFINITION
Warts are benign epidermal neoplasms caused by human papillomavirus (HPV; Fig. 27–12). Genital warts are the most common viral sexually transmitted disease (STD) in the United States, with up to 24 million Americans carrying the causative virus.

PHYSICAL FINDINGS AND CLINICAL PRESENTATION
- Common warts (Fig. 27–13) have an initial appearance of a flesh-colored papule with a rough surface; they subsequently develop a hyperkeratotic appearance, with black dots on the surface (thrombosed capillaries). They may be single or multiple and are most common on the hands.
- Warts obscure normal skin lines (important diagnostic feature). Cylindric projections from the wart may become fused, forming a mosaic pattern.

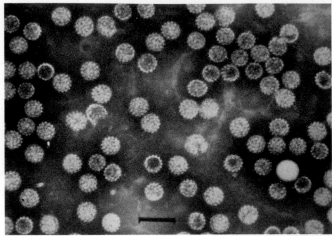

Fig 27–12
Electron photomicrograph of human paillomavirus (HPV) virions. HPVs are small, icosahedral viruses 55 nm in diameter that have a double-stranded DNA genome of approximately 8000 base pairs.
(Courtesy of A. Bennett Jenson, Georgetown University, Washington, DC.)

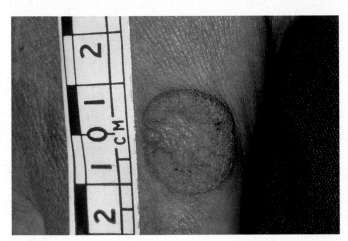

Fig 27–13
Verruca vulgaris. There is a raised, discrete scaly plaque on the dorsal aspect of the hand.
(Courtesy of Dr. R. A. Marsden, St. George's Hospital, London.)

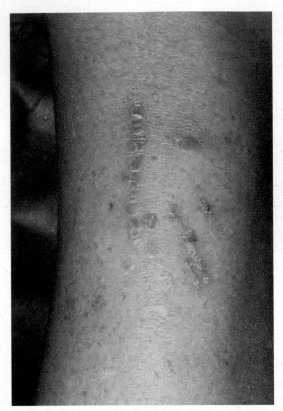

Fig 27–14
Plane wart. Note the typical flat, flesh-colored papules, which have extended in a linear distribution because of scratching (Koebner's phenomenon).
(Courtesy of Dr. R. A. Marsden, St. George's Hospital, London.)

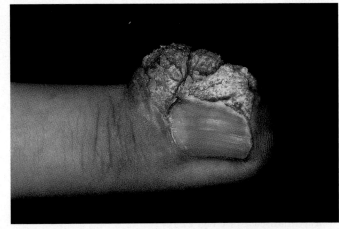

Fig 27–15
Verruca vulgaris. Verrucae are most commonly seen on the hands and fingers.
(Courtesy of the Institute of Dermatology, London.)

- Flat or plane warts (verruca plana) generally are pink or light yellow, slightly elevated (Fig. 27–14), and generally found on the forehead, backs of the hands, mouth, and beard area. They often occur in lines corresponding to trauma (e.g., a scratch) and are often misdiagnosed (particularly when present on the face) and inappropriately treated with topical corticosteroids.
- Filiform warts have a finger-like appearance with various projections (Fig. 27–15); they are generally found near the mouth, beard, or periorbital and paranasal regions.
- Plantar warts are slightly raised and have a roughened surface (Fig. 27–16). They may cause pain when walking; as they involute, small hemorrhages (caused by thrombosed capillaries) may be noted.
- Genital warts are generally pale pink with several projections and a broad base (Fig. 27–17). They may coalesce in the perineal area (Fig. 27–18) to form masses with a cauliflower-like appearance.
- Genital warts on the cervical epithelium can produce subclinical changes that may be noted on Pap smear or colposcopy.

CAUSE
- Human papillomavirus (HPV) infection; more than 60 types of viral DNA have been identified. Transmission of warts is by direct contact.
- Genital warts are usually caused by HPV type 6 or 11.

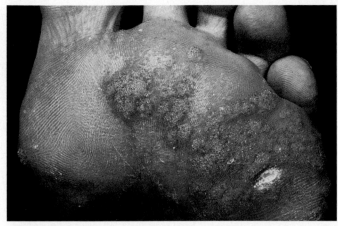

Fig 27–16
Mosaic warts. Here there is a large number of small warts. They are particularly resistant to therapy.
(Courtesy of the Institute of Dermatology, London.)

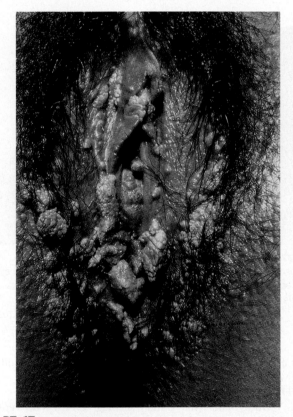

Fig 27–17
Condyloma accuminatum. In this patient, there is widespread involvement of the vulva and perineum. This patient is likely to have cervical human papilloma virus infection.
(Courtesy of Dr. R. A. Marsden, St. George's Hospital, London.)

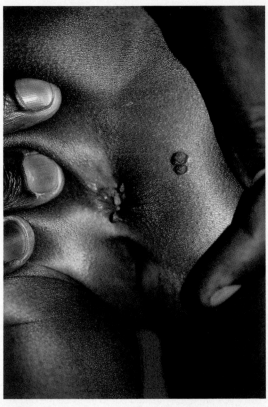

Fig 27–18
Condyloma accuminatum. Multiple perianal lesions are present.
(Courtesy of Dr. N.C. Dlova, Nelson R. Mandela School of Medicine, University of Kwazulu-Natal, South Africa.)

DIFFERENTIAL DIAGNOSIS
- Molluscum contagiosum (see Fig. 27–20)
- Condyloma latum
- Acrochordon (skin tags) (see Fig. 25–17)
- Seborrheic keratosis (see Fig. 22–2)
- Epidermal nevi (see Fig. 22–1)
- Actinic keratosis (hypertrophic; see Fig. 22–11)
- Squamous cell carcinomas (see Fig. 22–14)
- Plantar corns (may be mistaken for plantar warts)

TREATMENT
- Watchful waiting is an acceptable option for the treatment of warts because many warts will disappear without intervention over time.
- Plantar warts that are not painful do not need treatment.
- Treatment for common warts:
  - Application of topical salicylic acid
  - Liquid nitrogen, electrocautery are also common methods of removal
  - Blunt dissection can be used for large or resistant lesions.
  - Duct tape occlusion also effective
- Filiform warts: surgical removal is necessary.
- Flat warts: tretinoin cream, liquid nitrogen, 5-fluorouracil cream, electrocautery
- Plantar warts: alicyclic acid therapy, blunt dissection, laser therapy, interlesional bleomycin
- Genital warts: 20% podophyllin resin, podofilox, cryosurgery with liquid nitrogen (Fig. 27–19), carbon dioxide laser, imiquimod cream, trichloroacetic acid (TCA), or bichloroacetic acid (BCA)

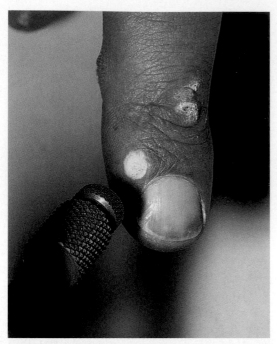

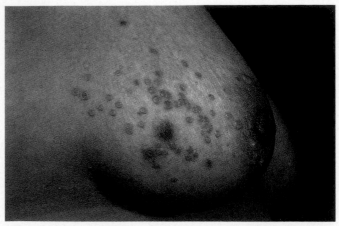

Fig 27–20
Molluscum contagiosum. This often develops as a result of sexual contact in young adults.
(Courtesy of Dr. R. A. Marsden, St. George's Hospital, London.)

Fig 27–19
Cryotherapy of warts. Cryotherapy using the liquid nitrogen (LN₂) spray technique. For warts or actinic keratoses, it is routine to perform a single period of freezing (one freeze-thaw cycle, FTC), whereas for malignancies two FTCs are usually carried out to increase the degree of damage. It is usual to record the cryogen and the number and duration of treatment cycles—for example LN₂, 2 × 20-second FTCs.
(From White GM, Cox NH [eds]: Diseases of the Skin: A Color Atlas and Text, 2nd ed. St. Louis, Mosby, 2006.)

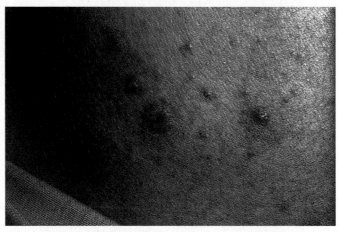

Fig 27–21
Molluscum contagiosum. Central umblication is a diagnostic clinical marker.
(Courtesy of the Institute of Dermatology, London.)

G. MOLLUSCUM CONTAGIOSUM

DEFINITION
This is a viral infection characterized by discrete skin lesions with central umbilication .

PHYSICAL FINDINGS AND CLINICAL PRESENTATION
- The individual lesion appears initially as a flesh-colored, firm, smooth-surfaced papule with subsequent central umbilication. Lesions are frequently grouped (Fig. 27–20). The size of each lesion generally varies from 2 to 6 mm in diameter.
- Typical distribution in children involves the face, extremities, and trunk. Mucous membranes are spared.
- Distribution in adults generally involves pubic and genital areas.
- Erythema and scaling at the periphery of the lesions may be present as a result of scratching or hypersensitivity reaction.
- Lesions are not present on the palms and soles.

CAUSE
- Viral infection of epithelial cells caused by a pox virus

DIAGNOSIS
Diagnosis is usually established by the clinical appearance of the lesions (distribution and central umbilication). A magnifying lens can be used to observe the central umbilication (Fig. 27–21). If necessary, the diagnosis can be confirmed by removing a typical lesion with a curette and examining it on a slide after adding KOH and gently heating. Staining with toluidine blue will identify viral inclusions.

DIFFERENTIAL DIAGNOSIS
- Verruca plana (flat warts;) see Fig. 27–14): no central umbilication, not dome-shaped, irregular surface, can involve palms and soles
- Herpes simplex (see Fig. 27–4): lesions become rapidly umbilicated
- Varicella (see Fig. 27–2): blisters and vesicles are present
- Folliculitis (see Fig. 28–14): no central umbilication, presence of hair piercing the pustule or papule
- Cutaneous cryptococcosis (see Fig. 336–23) in AIDS patients: budding yeasts present on cytologic examination of lesions
- Basal cell carcinoma (see Fig. 22–7): multiple lesions are absent

- Generally not indicated in children
- STD screening for other sexually transmitted diseases is recommended for all cases of genital molluscum contagiosum. Genital molluscum contagiosum in children may be indicative of sexual abuse.

TREATMENT
- Therapy is individualized depending on the number of lesions, immune status, and patient's age and preference.
- Observation for spontaneous resolution is reasonable for patients with few, small, nonirritated, and nonspreading lesions. Genital lesions should be treated in all sexually active patients.
- Curettage following pretreatment of the area with combination prilocaine-lidocaine 2.5% cream (EMLA) for anesthesia is useful for treatment of few lesions. Curettage should be avoided in cosmetically sensitive areas because scarring may develop.
- Treatments with liquid nitrogen therapy in combination with curettage are effective for older patients who do not object to some discomfort.
- Application of cantharidin, 0.7%, to individual lesions covered with clear tape will result in blistering over 24 hours and possible clearing without scarring. This medication should be avoided on facial lesions.
- Other treatment measures include tretinoin 0.025% gel or 0.1% cream at bedtime, salicylic acid (Occlusal) at bedtime, and laser therapy.
- Trichloroacetic acid peel, generally repeated every 2 weeks for several weeks, is useful for immunocompromised patients with extensive lesions.

H. HAND-FOOT-AND-MOUTH DISEASE

DEFINITION

Hand-foot-and-mouth (HFM) disease is a viral illness characterized by superficial lesions of the oral mucosa and the skin of the extremities. HFM is transmitted primarily by the fecal-oral route and is highly contagious. Although children are predominantly affected, adults are also at risk. The disease is usually self-limited and benign.

PHYSICAL FINDINGS AND CLINICAL PRESENTATION

Symptoms
- After a 4- to 6-day incubation period, patients may complain of odynophagia, sore throat, malaise, and fever (38.3° to 40° C).
- Characteristic oral lesions appear 1 to 2 days later.
- In 75% of cases, skin lesions on the extremities accompany these oral manifestations.
- Cutaneous findings are noted in 11% of adults.
- Lesions appear over the course of 1 or 2 days.

Physical findings
- Oral lesions, usually between five and ten, are commonly found on the tongue, buccal mucosa (Fig. 27–22), gingivae, and hard palate.
- Oral lesions initially start as 1- to 3-mm erythematous macules and evolve into gray vesicles on an erythematous base.
- Vesicles are frequently broken by the time of presentation and appear as superficial gray ulcers, with surrounding erythema.

- Skin lesions of the hands (Fig. 27–23) and feet start as linear erythematous papules (3 to 10 mm in diameter) that evolve into gray vesicles that may be mildly painful. These vesicles are usually intact at presentation and remain so until they desquamate within 2 weeks (Fig. 27–24).
- Involvement of the buttocks and perineum is present in 31% of cases.

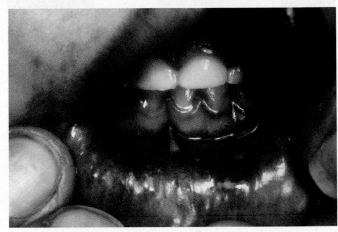

Fig 27–22
Hand-foot-and mouth disease. Multiple oral ulcers are present.
(Courtesy of the Institute of Dermatology, London.)

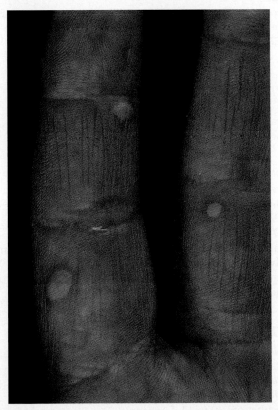

Fig 27–23
Hand-foot-and mouth disease. Note the small vesicles with surrounding erythema.
(Courtesy of E. Wilson Jones, MD, Institute of Dermatology, London.)

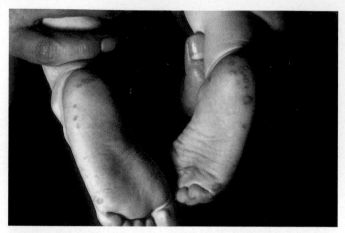

Fig 27–24
Hand-foot-and mouth disease. There are numerous erosions on the sole of the foot.
(Courtesy of Dr. R. A. Marsden, St. George's Hospital, London.)

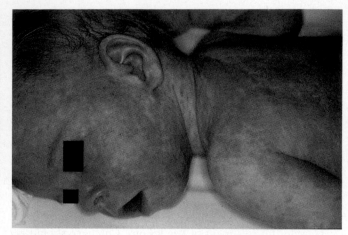

Fig 27–25
Measles. Note diffuse erythematous involvement of the face and trunk. (Courtesy Department of Dermatology, University of North Carolina at Chapel Hill.)

- In rare cases, encephalitis, meningitis, myocarditis, poliomyelitis-like paralysis, and pulmonary edema may develop. Sporadic acute paralysis has been reported with *Enterovirus* 71.
- Spontaneous abortion may occur if the infection begins early in pregnancy.

CAUSE
- Coxsackievirus group A, type 16, was the first and is the most common viral agent isolated.

DIFFERENTIAL DIAGNOSIS
- Aphthous stomatitis (see Fig. 89–11)
- Herpes simplex infection (see Fig. 27–4)
- Herpangina (see Fig. 91–1)
- Behçet's disease (see Fig. 16–14)
- Erythema multiforme (see Fig. 9–2)
- Pemphigus (see Fig. 5–1)
- Gonorrhea (see Fig. 227–1)
- Allergic contact dermatitis (see Fig. 6–9)

LABORATORY TESTS
- Not indicated unless the diagnosis is in doubt
- Throat culture or stool specimen may be obtained for viral testing.

TREATMENT
- Palliative therapy is given for this usually self-limited disease.
- Limited data have suggested that acyclovir may play a role in the treatment of certain cases.

I. RUBEOLA (MEASLES)

DEFINITION
Measles is a childhood exanthem, caused by an RNA virus called *Morbillivirus*, that belongs to the family Paramyxoviridae.

PHYSICAL FINDINGS AND CLINICAL PRESENTATION
- Incubation: 10 to 14 days (up to 3 weeks in adults)
- Prodrome: 2 to 4 days; malaise, fever, rhinorrhea, conjunctivitis, cough
- Exanthem phase: 7 to 10 days

- The fever increases and peaks at 104° to 105° F, together with the rash; it persists for 5 or 6 days. The patient's fever decreases over 24 hours.
- Rash: Erythematous maculopapular eruption begins behind the ears, progresses to the forehead and neck (Fig. 27–25), and then spreads to the face, trunk, upper extremities, buttocks, and lower extremities, in that order. After 3 days, the rash fades in the same sequence by becoming copper brown and then desquamates.
- Enanthem: *Koplik spot's* are white papules, 1 to 2 mm in diameter, on an erythematous base (Fig. 27–26). They first appear on the buccal mucosa opposite the lower molar 2 days before the rash and spread over 24 hours to involve most of the buccal and lower labial mucosa. They fade after 3 days.
- Other symptoms and signs: malaise, anorexia, vomiting, diarrhea, abdominal pain, pharyngitis, lymph adenopathy, occasional splenomegaly

CAUSE AND PATHOGENESIS
- The measles virus is transmitted through the respiratory tract by airborne droplets.
- It initially infects the respiratory epithelium; the patient becomes viremic during the prodromal phase and the virus is disseminated to the skin, respiratory tract, and other organs.
- Viral clearance is achieved via cellular immunity.

DIFFERENTIAL DIAGNOSIS
- Other viral infections by enteroviruses, adenoviruses, human parvovirus B19, rubella (see Fig. 27–29)
- Scarlet fever (see Fig. 93–1)
- Allergic reaction (see Fig. 14–1)
- Kawasaki disease (see Fig. 27–30)

LABORATORY TESTS
- CBC: leukopenia
- ELISA for measles antibodies, which appear shortly after the onset of the rash and peak 3 to 4 weeks later
- Cerebrospinal fluid (CSF) analysis in encephalitis may reveal a pleocytosis (lymphocytes) and an elevated protein level.

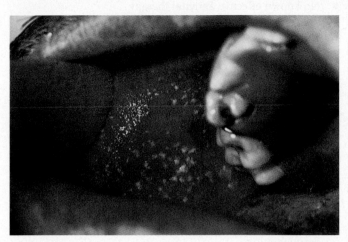

Fig 27–26
Koplik's spots, which are pathognomonic of measles. They are found on mucous membranes during the prodromal stage and are easily detected on the mucosa of the cheeks opposite the molar teeth, where they resemble coarse grains of salt on the surface of the inflamed membrane. They disappear as the rash emerges and cannot be seen after the first or second day of the exanthem. Histologically, the spots consist of small necrotic patches in the basal layers of the mucosa with exudation of serum and infiltration by mononuclear cells.
(From Emond RT, Welsby PD, Rowland HA [eds]; Color Atlas of Infectious Diseases, 4th ed. St. Louis, Mosby, 2003.)

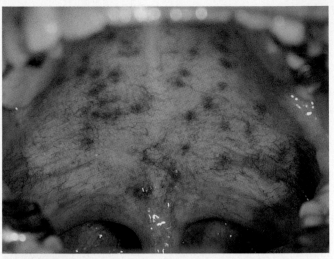

Fig 27–27
Forschheimer spots of rubella.
(From Swartz MH: Textbook of Physical Diagnosis, 5th ed. Philadelphia, WB Saunders, 2006.)

TREATMENT
- Supportive
- Ribavirin for severe measles pneumonitis

J. RUBELLA (GERMAN MEASLES)

DEFINITION
Rubella is a mild illness caused by the rubella virus; it can cause severe congenital problems via in vitro transmission to the fetus when a pregnant woman becomes infected.

PHYSICAL FINDINGS AND CLINICAL PRESENTATION

Acquired infection
- Incubation: 14 to 21 days
- Prodrome: 1 to 5 days; low-grade fever, headache, malaise, anorexia, mild conjunctivitis, coryza, pharyngitis, cough, and cervical, suboccipital, and postauricular lymphadenopathy
- Rash: 1 to 5 days
- Enanthema: palatal macules. Dusky red spots of about 1 to 3 mm on the buccal mucosa and palate are an early sign of rubella. These diffusely scattered oral lesions, known as *Forschheimer spots* (Fig. 27–27), appear on the posterior hard and soft palates and develop at the end of the prodromal stage or at the beginning of the cutaneous eruption.
- Exanthema (rash): blotchy eruption beginning on the face and neck and then spreading to the trunk and limbs (Fig. 27–28)
- Occasional splenomegaly and hepatitis (during rash)
- Complications: arthritis (15%, mostly in adult women), thrombocytopenia, myocarditis, optic neuritis, encephalitis (all less than 0.1%)

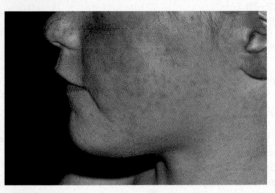

Fig 27–28
Rubella. The rash may be very mild in rubella. When present, it is similar to measles, with maculopapular erythema starting on the face and spreading to the trunk. The spots are 1 to 2 mm in diameter and slightly raised. In rubella, there is also enlargement of the cervical and occipital lymph nodes.
(From White GM, Cox NH [eds]: Diseases of the Skin: A Color Atlas and Text, 2nd ed. St. Louis, Mosby, 2006.)

Congenital infection (Fig. 27–29)
- Deafness: 85%
- Intrauterine growth retardation: 70%
- Cataracts: 35%
- Retinopathy: 35%
- Patent ductus arteriosus: 30%
- Pulmonary artery hypoplasia: 25%
- In utero death: 20%

CAUSE

Acquired infection
- Viral portal of entry is upper respiratory tract.
- Viral replication occurs in lymph nodes; hematogenous dissemination then occurs to many organs, including the placenta, if present.
- Immune complexes may be the cause of the rash and arthritis.

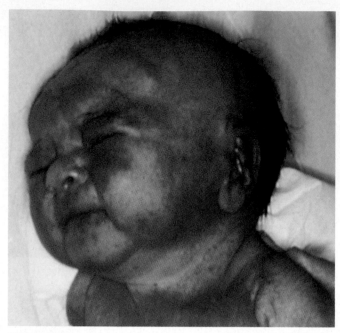

Fig 27–29
Congenital rubella.
(From Swartz MH: Textbook of Physical Diagnosis, 5th ed. Philadelphia, WB Saunders, 2006.)

Congenital infection
- Fetus is infected via the placenta during maternal acquired infection.
- Cellular damage in the fetus results from cytolysis of fetal cells, mostly via a fetal vasculitis or immune-mediated inflammation and damage.

DIFFERENTIAL DIAGNOSIS
Acquired rubella syndrome
- Other viral infections by enteroviruses, adenoviruses, human parvovirus B19 (see Fig. 27–3) measles (see Fig. 27–25)
- Scarlet fever (see Fig. 93–1)
- Allergic reaction (see Fig. 14–1)
- Kawasaki disease (see Fig. 27–30)

Congenital rubella syndrome
- Congenital syphilis
- Toxoplasmosis
- Herpes simplex (see Fig. 27–4)
- Cytomegalovirus

DIAGNOSIS
Acquired infection
- Serologic test (hemagglutination inhibition, neutralization tests, complement fixation tests, passive agglutination, enzyme immunoassay [EIA], ELISA)
- IgM antibodies (by EIA) are detected early, second to fourth week
- IgG antibodies (by ELISA) can be measured as acute phase (7 days after rash onset) and convalescent phase (14 days later)

Congenital infection
- Viral culture (from nasopharynx)
- Serologic studies: IgM antirubella virus detection by EIA is the method of choice (after the newborn is 5 months old)

TREATMENT
- No known effective antiviral therapy
- Management of specific congenital problems as appropriate

K. KAWASAKI DISEASE

DEFINITION
Kawasaki disease (KD) refers to a generalized vasculitis of unknown cause characterized by cutaneous and mucous membrane edema, rash, lymphadenopathy, and involvement of multiple organs. KD is a leading cause of acquired heart disease in children.

PHYSICAL FINDINGS AND CLINICAL PRESENTATION
A typical presentation is a young child with fever unresponsive to antibiotics for more than 5 days associated with the following:
- Bilateral conjunctivitis
- Erythema and edema of the hands and feet, desquamation
- Periungual desquamation
- Fissuring of the lips
- Erythematous pharynx
- Strawberry tongue (Fig. 27–30)
- Cervical adenopathy
- Truncal scarlatiniform rash, usually nonvesicular (see Fig. 27–30)
- Diarrhea
- Dyspnea
- Arthralgias and myalgia
- Sudden death from coronary artery involvement
- Myocardial infarction (see Fig. 27–30)
- Congestive heart failure

CAUSE
- The cause of KD is not known, although evidence substantiates an infectious cause precipitating an immune-mediated reaction. Fibrin thrombi and areas of necrosis can be found in small vessels.

DIAGNOSIS
The diagnosis of Kawasaki disease is based on a fever lasting more than 5 days, along with four of the following five features:
- Bilateral conjunctival swelling
- Inflammatory changes of the lip, tongue, and pharynx
- Skin changes of the limbs
- Rash over the trunk
- Cervical lymphadenopathy

DIFFERENTIAL DIAGNOSIS
- Scarlet fever (see Fig. 93–1)
- Stevens-Johnson syndrome (see Fig. 9–6)
- Drug eruption (see Fig. 14–1)
- Henoch-Schönlein purpura (see Fig. 300–12)
- Toxic shock syndrome (see Fig. 352–1)
- Measles (see Fig. 27–25)
- Rocky Mountain spotted fever (see Fig. 308–15)
- Infectious mononucleosis (see Fig. 338–2)

LABORATORY TESTS
- CBC commonly shows a normochromic normocytic anemia, a left shift in the white blood cell count, and an elevated platelet count
- ESR is elevated
- C-reactive protein is positive

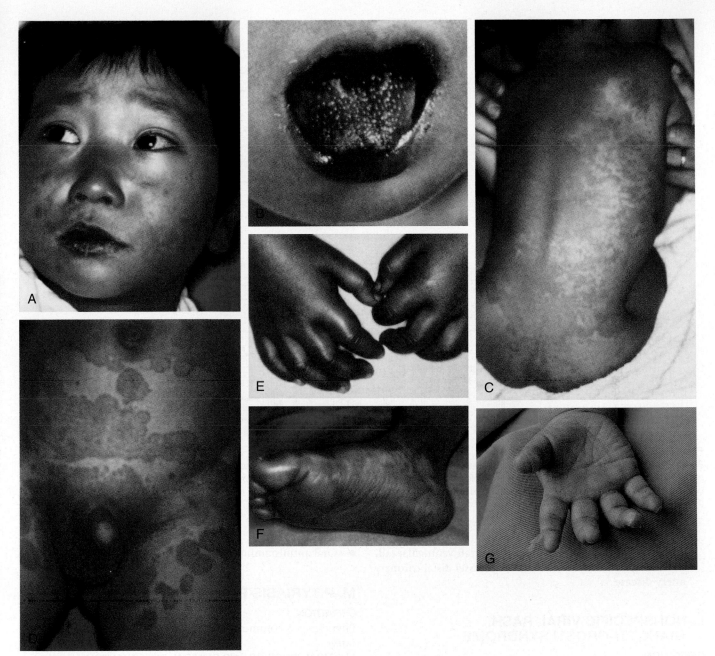

Fig 27-30
Clinical manifestations of Kawasaki disease. **A,** Typical appearance of the face, bilateral conjunctiva. **B,** strawberry tongue. **C, D,** Polymorphous exanthems. **E,** Indurative edema of the hands. **F,** Redness and swelling of the sole. **G,** Desquamation of fingers.
(From Crawford MH, DiMarco JP, Paulus WJ [eds]: Cardiology, 2nd ed. London, Mosby, 2004.)

- LFTs (e.g., elevated ALT and AST)
- Urinalysis may show sterile pyuria.

IMAGING STUDIES

- Chest x-ray may reveal pulmonary infiltrates
- Electrocardiographic abnormalities (Fig. 27–31)
- The echocardiogram is very helpful and may show depressed left ventricular function with regional wall motion abnormalities, pericardial effusions (30%), and abnormal coronary artery aneurysms. The echocardiogram is also useful for the long-term follow-up of patients with KD.
- Cardiac catheterization with coronary angiography in the proper clinical setting is done to rule out significant obstructive coronary disease

TREATMENT

- Oxygen in select patients
- Salt restriction in patients with CHF
- Intravenous immunoglobulin (IVIg), ideally given within the first 10 days of the illness.
- Aspirin, 30 to 100 mg/kg/day, in four divided doses until the patient is no longer febrile.
- In patients who do not defervesce within 48 hours or have recrudescent fever after initial IVIg treatment, a second dose of IVIg, 2 g/kg IV over 8 to 12 hours, should be considered.
- Interventional (percutaneous transluminal coronary angioplasty) and surgical procedures (coronary bypass graft surgery) can be tried for children who have developed cardiac

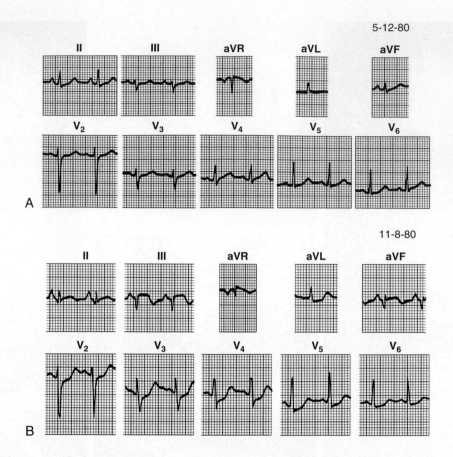

Fig 27–31
Acute inferior myocardial infarction (MI) in a 16-year-old girl with Kawasaki disease and coronary artery aneurysm. The aneurysm was demonstrated by coronary arteriography before the development of MI. These electrocardiograms were obtained before **(A)** and after **(B)** the infarction occurred. Note the appearance of Q waves with ST segment elevation and T wave inversion in the inferior leads on the tracing in **B**.
(From Chou TC: Electrocardiography in Clinical Practice, 4th ed. Philadelphia, WB Saunders, 1996.)

complications of KD. Cardiac transplantation is an option and is indicated for patients with severe left ventricular failure, malignant arrhythmias, and multivessel distal coronary artery disease.

L. NONSPECIFIC VIRAL RASH, GIANOTTI-CROSTI SYNDROME

DEFINITION
Many viral infections may be associated with a nonspecific generalized rash (Fig. 27–32). The term *Gianotti-Crosti syndrome* (GST) is used to describe viral rashes affecting the extremities presenting with papular or papulovesicular lesions (Fig. 27–33) and associated with mild constitutional symptoms (e.g., low-grade fever, generalized malaise).

PHYSICAL FINDINGS AND CLINICAL PRESENTATION
- The trunk and antecubital and popliteal surfaces are usually spared and mucous membranes are not affected.
- The lesions generally fade in 3 to 4 weeks, with mild desquamation.
- Inguinal and axillary adenopathy may be present.
- Hepatomegaly may be present when the rash is secondary to viral hepatitis or Epstein-Barr virus.

LABORATORY TESTS
- Transaminase elevations Snd leukopenia or slight leukocytosis may be present.

TREATMENT
- Oral antihistamines for severe pruritus

M. PITYRIASIS ROSEA

DEFINITION
Pityriasis is a common self-limited skin eruption of unknown cause.

PHYSICAL FINDINGS AND CLINICAL PRESENTATION
- Initial lesion (herald patch) precedes the eruption by approximately 1 to 2 weeks, typically measures 3 to 6 cm, and is round to oval in appearance and most frequently located on the trunk (Fig, 27–34).
- Eruptive phase follows within 2 weeks and peaks after 7 to 14 days.
- Lesions are most frequently located in the lower abdominal area. They have a salmon-pink appearance in whites and a hyperpigmented appearance in blacks .
- Most lesions are 4 to 5 mm in diameter; the center has a cigarette paper–like appearance and the border has a characteristic ring of scale (collarette).
- Lesions occur in a symmetrical distribution and follow the cleavage lines of the trunk (Christmas tree pattern)
- The number of lesions varies from a few to hundreds.
- Most patients are asymptomatic; pruritus is the most common symptom.

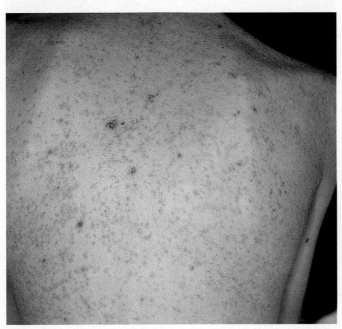

Fig 27–32
Viral exanthem as a result of an enteroviral infection.
(From Callen JP, Greer KE, Paller AS, Swinyer LJ: Color Atlas of Dermatology, 2nd ed. Philadelphia, WB Saunders, 2000.)

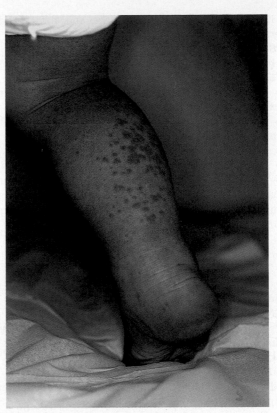

Fig 27–33
Viral rash affecting the extremities.
(From Lebwohl MG, Heymann WR, Berth-Jones J, Coulson I [eds]: Treatment of Skin Disease. St. Louis, Mosby, 2002.)

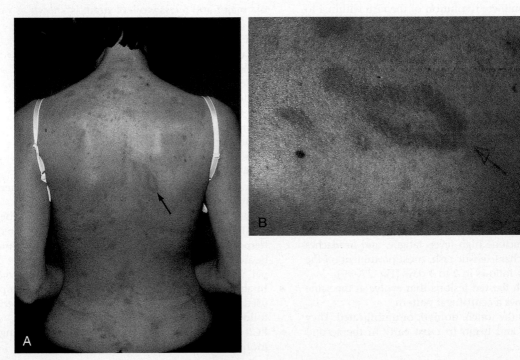

Fig 27–34
Pityriasis rosea. **A,** The herald patch marks the onset of this dermatosis (*arrow*). **B,** Close-up view.
(Courtesy of Dr. R. A. Marsden, St. George's Hospital, London.)

- History of recent fatigue, headache, sore throat, and low-grade fever is present in approximately 25% of cases.

CAUSE
- Unknown, possibly viral (picornavirus)

DIFFERENTIAL DIAGNOSIS
- Tinea corporis (can be ruled out by potassium hydroxide examination; see Fig. 26–1)
- Secondary syphilis (absence of herald patch, positive serologic test for syphilis; see Fig. 226–14)
- Psoriasis (see Fig. 7–1)
- Nummular eczema (see Fig. 6–5)
- Drug eruption. (see Fig. 14–1) Medications that may cause rashes similar to pityriasis rosea include clonidine, captopril, interferon, bismuth, barbiturates, gold, hepatitis B vaccine, and imatinib mesylate.
- Viral exanthem (see Fig. 27–32)
- Eczema (see Fig. 6–1)
- Lichen planus (see Fig. 8–1)
- Tinea versicolor (see Fig. 26–5; the lesions are more brown and the borders are not as ovoid.

DIAGNOSIS
- Presence of herald lesion and characteristic rash is diagnostic.
- Skin biopsy is generally reserved for atypical cases.

TREATMENT
The disease is self-limited and generally does not require any therapeutic intervention.
- Use oral antihistamines for patients with significant pruritus.
- Use prednisone tapered over 2 weeks for patients with severe pruritus.
- Direct sun exposure or the use of UV light within the first week of eruption is beneficial in decreasing the severity of disease.
- Spontaneous complete resolution of the rash within 4 to 8 weeks
- Recurrence rare (less than 2% of cases)

N. SMALLPOX (VARIOLA)

DEFINITION
Smallpox infection is caused by the variola virus, a DNA virus member of the genus *Orthopoxvirus*. It is a human virus with no known nonhuman reservoir of disease. Natural infection occurs following implantation of the virus on the oropharyngeal or respiratory mucosa. Smallpox infection was eliminated from the world in 1977. The last cases of smallpox, from laboratory exposure, occurred in 1978. The threat of bioterrorism has brought renewed interest in the smallpox virus.

PHYSICAL FINDINGS AND CLINICAL PRESENTATION
- Initial symptoms include high fever, fatigue, and headaches and back aches. A characteristic rash, most prominent on the face, arms, and legs, follows in 2 to 3 days (Fig. 27–35).
- The rash starts with flat red lesions that evolve at the same rate. The rash follows a centrifugal pattern.
- Lesions are firm to the touch, domed, or umbilicated. They become pus-filled and begin to crust early in the second week.

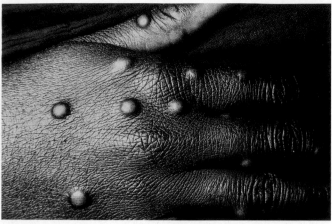

Fig 27–35
Variola (smallpox). In contrast to those of chickenpox, the lesions are larger and less superficial.
(Courtesy of Dr. H. P. Lambert, St. George's Hospital, London.)

- Scabs develop and then separate and fall off after about 3 to 4 weeks. Depigmentation persists at the base of the skin lesions for 3 to 6 months after illness. Scarring is usually most extensive on the face.
- Associated with the rash may be fever, headache, generalized malaise, vomiting, and colicky abdominal pain.
- Variola major may produce a rapidly fatal toxemia in some patients.
- Complications of smallpox include dehydration, pneumonia, blepharitis, conjunctivitis, and corneal ulcerations.

CAUSE
- Smallpox is caused by the variola virus. There are at least two strains of the virus; the most virulent is known as variola major and a less virulent strain is known as variola minor (alastrim).

DIFFERENTIAL DIAGNOSIS
- Varicella (see Fig. 27–2)
- Measles (see Fig. 27–25)
- Coxsackievirus (see Fig. 17–87)
- Meningococcemia (see Fig. 46–9)
- Insect bites (see Fig. 29–17)
- Impetigo (see Fig. 28–13)
- Dermatitis herpetiformis (see Fig. 4–9)
- Pemphigus (see Fig. 5–6)

LABORATORY TESTS
- Laboratory examination requires high-containment (BL-4) facilities.
- Electron microscopy of vesicular scrapings can be used to distinguish poxvirus particles from varicella-zoster virus or herpes simplex. To obtain vesicular or pustular fluid, it may be necessary to open lesions with the blunt edge of a scalpel. A cotton swab may be used to harvest the fluid.
- In absence of electron microscopy, light microscopy can be used to visualize variola viral particles (Guarnieri bodies) following Giemsa staining.
- PCR techniques and restriction of fragment-length polymorphisms can rapidly identify variola.

TREATMENT
- Supportive therapy
- IV hydration in severe cases
- A suspect case of smallpox should be placed in strict respiratory and contact isolation.

TREATMENT
- There is no proven treatment for smallpox. Vaccination administered within 3 to 4 days may prevent or significantly ameliorate subsequent illness. Vaccinia immune globulin can be used for the treatment of vaccine complications and for administration with vaccine to those for whom vaccine is otherwise contraindicated.

O. VACCINIA

DEFINITION
Vaccinia virus is closely related antigenically to variola (smallpox) virus, but is probably derived from cowpox. It is used for immunization against smallpox because of its similar antigenicity.

PHYSICAL FINDINGS AND CLINICAL PRESENTATION
- This skin inoculation results in a single vesicle, which becomes pustular and crusts, like variola (Fig. 27–36). It also heals similarly, leaving a scar.
- Vaccine virus in the skin lesion can be transferred to others if the skin lesion is touched directly or if the bandage is handled casually with ungloved hands.

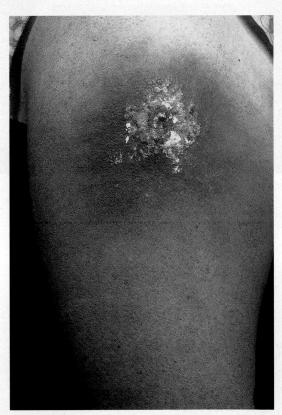

Fig 27–36
Vaccinia. Because of the eradication of smallpox, routine vaccination is no longer performed. Note the eschar, edema, and intense erythema.
(Courtesy of the Institute of Dermatology, London.)

TREATMENT
- The vaccination site is infectious until the scab falls off, approximately 21 days after vaccination.

P. COWPOX

DEFINITION
Despite the name, the reservoir for cowpox is not cattle, but wild animals such as hedgehogs and badgers. Cattle and humans are both infected accidentally, although humans may acquire the disease from cows. Cats have been identified as an additional source of infection.

PHYSICAL FINDINGS AND CLINICAL PRESENTATION
- The incubation period after inoculation is usually 5 to 7 days; a papule then develops, which rapidly becomes a pustule.
- The pustule is surrounded by a zone of erythema and edema.
- Eschars or necrotic ulcers may occur.
- The lesions are often multiple and can occur on the hands, arms, or face (Fig. 27–37).
- Lymphangitis, lymphadenitis, and fever are almost invariably present.

TREATMENT
- Healing and recovery occur in 3 to 4 weeks.

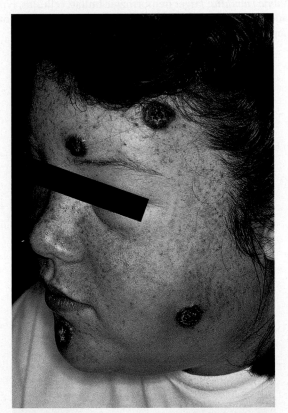

Fig 27–37
Cowpox—characteristic umbilicated, ulcerated nodules. Lesions are often multiple.
(Courtesy of Dr. M. S. Lewis Jones, Wrexham Maelor Hospital, Wrexham, England.)

Chapter 28 | **Bacterial skin infections**

A. CELLULITIS

DEFINITION

Cellulitis is a superficial inflammatory condition of the skin characterized by erythema, warmth, and tenderness of the area involved (Fig. 28–1).

PHYSICAL FINDINGS AND CLINICAL PRESENTATION

These vary with the causative organism.

- Erysipelas: superficial spreading, warm, erythematous lesion distinguished by its indurated and elevated margin (Fig. 28–2); lymphatic involvement and vesicle formation are common.
- Staphylococcal cellulites (Fig. 28–3): area involved is erythematous, hot, and swollen; differentiated from erysipelas by nonelevated, poorly demarcated margin; local tenderness and regional adenopathy are common; up to 85% of cases occur on the legs and feet (Fig. 28–4). Table 28–1 presents rashes associated with acute bacterial infections.
- *Haemophilus influenzae* cellulitis: area involved is a blue-red or purple-red color; occurs mainly in children; generally involves the face in children and the neck or upper chest in adults
- *Vibrio vulnificus:* larger hemorrhagic bullae, cellulitis, lymphadenitis, myositis; often found in critically ill patients in septic shock

CAUSE

- Group A beta-hemolytic streptococci (may follow a streptococcal infection of the upper respiratory tract). Lymphangitis may be present (Fig. 28–5)
- Staphylococcal cellulitis
- *H. influenzae*
- *Vibrio vulnificus:* higher incidence in patients with liver disease (75%) and in immunocompromised hosts (corticosteroid use, diabetes mellitus, leukemia, renal failure)
- *Erysipelothrix rhusiopathiae:* common in people handling poultry, fish, or meat
- *Aeromonas hydrophila:* generally occurring in contaminated open wound in fresh water
- Fungi *(Cryptococcus neoformans):* immunocompromised granulopenic patients
- Gram-negative rods (*Serratia, Enterobacter, Proteus, Pseudomonas* spp.): immunocompromised or granulopenic patients

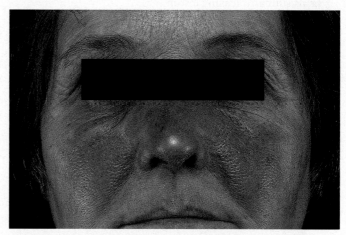

Fig 28–2
Erysipelas—characteristic sharply demarcated erythematous and edematous plaque.
(Courtesy of Dr. R. A. Marsden, St. George's Hospital, London.)

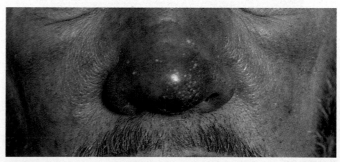

Fig 28–3
Staphylococcus aureus cellulitis of the nose. The focal lesion began in a hair follicle inside the nose, with redness, swelling, and pain. Rarely, such lesions on the nose are complicated by extension into the cavernous sinus via veins draining the central part of the face.
(From Cohen J, Powderly WG: Infectious Diseases, 2nd ed. St. Louis, Mosby, 2004.)

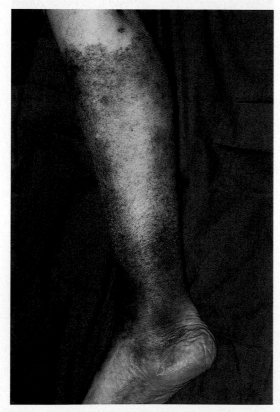

Fig 28–1
Cellulitis. Note the widespread erythema. The lower leg is a characteristic site.
(Courtesy of Dr. R. A. Marsden, St. George's Hospital, London.)

DIFFERENTIAL DIAGNOSIS

- Erythrasma (see Fig. 28–11)
- Septic arthritis (see Fig. 19–1)
- Deep venous thrombosis (DVT) (see Fig. 122–2)
- Peripheral vascular insufficiency (see Fig. 119–1)
- Paget's disease of the breast (see Fig. 254–1)
- Thrombophlebitis (see Fig. 85–8)
- Acute gout (see Fig. 18–5)
- Psoriasis (see Fig. 7–2)
- Candida intertrigo (see Fig. 26–9)
- Pseudogout (see Fig. 179–2)
- Osteomyelitis
- Insect bite (see Fig. 29–17)
- Fixed drug eruption (see Fig. 14–1)
- Lymphedema (see Fig. 121–2)

LABORATORY TESTS

- Gram stain and culture (aerobic and anaerobic; Fig. 28–6)
- Blood cultures in hospitalized patients, in patients who have cellulitis superimposed on lymphedema, in patients with buccal or periorbital cellulitis, and in patients suspected of having a saltwater or freshwater source of infection. Bacteremia is uncommon in cellulitis (positive blood cultures in only 4% of patients)

TREATMENT

- Immobilization and elevation of the involved limb; cool sterile saline dressings to remove purulence from any open lesion.
- Erysipelas: PO dicloxacillin or IV nafcillin or cefazolin
- *Staphylococcus* cellulitis: PO dicloxacillin or IV nafcillin or cefazolin

---

TABLE 28–1 Rashes associated with acute bacterial infections

Agent	Rashes	Comment
Neisseria meningitidis	Petechial, purpuric	Also, nonhemorrhagic early rashes
Neisseria gonorrhoeae	Hemorrhagic vesicles, pustules	
Staphylococcus aureus	Pyogenic skin lesions	
	Scalded skin syndrome	
	Peripheral purpura	In staphylococcal endocarditis
	Erythema	In toxic shock syndrome
Streptococcus pyogenes	Erysipelas	Local erythema, bullae
	Erythema	In toxic shock syndrome
Salmonella typhi	Rose spots	
Pseudomonas aeruginosa	Ecthyma gangrenosum; cellulitis ± blebs	Also in *Aeromonas* and other gram-negative bacillary infections
Haemophilus aegyptius	Brazilian purpuric fever	

From Cohen J, Powderly WG: Infectious Diseases, 2nd ed. St. Louis, 2004.

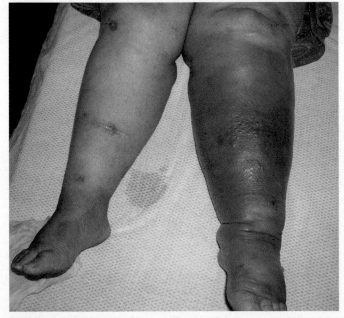

Fig 28–4
Severe recurrent cellulitis associated with obesity.
(From Cohen J, Powderly WG: Infectious Diseases, 2nd ed. St. Louis, Mosby, 2004.)

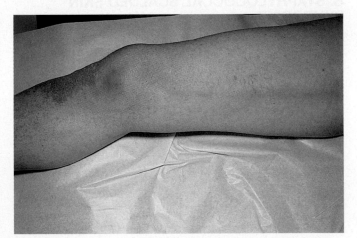

Fig 28–5
Lymphangitis. Cellulitis caused by group A streptococci began below the knee and rapidly spread; about 4 hours later, lymphangitis had spread up the inner aspect of the thigh.
(From Cohen J, Powderly WG: Infectious Diseases, 2nd ed. St. Louis, Mosby, 2004.)

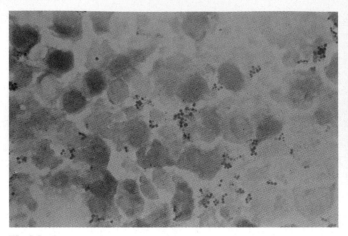

Fig 28–6
Gram stain of purulent material demonstrating *Staphylococcus aureus*. The microbial cause of cellullitis may be suspected based on signs, symptoms, and history; however, definitive diagnosis requires Gram staining and culture. If there is no portal of entry, aspiration or even punch biopsy of cellulitic skin yields a positive culture in only 20% of cases.
(From Cohen J, Powderly WG: Infectious Diseases, 2nd ed. St. Louis, Mosby, 2004.)

- *H. influenzae* cellulitis: PO dicloxacillin or IV nafcillin or cefazolin
- *Vibrio vulnificus:* Doxycycline or third-generation cephalosporin
- *Erysipelothrix:* Penicillin
- *Aeromonas hydrophila:* Aminoglycoside, chloramphenicol

B. STAPHYLOCOCCAL SCALDED SKIN SYNDROME

DEFINITION
Staphylococcal scalded skin syndrome (SSSS) is a disorder usually occurring in neonates and young children, who first develop a macular scarlatiniform eruption in association with a staphylococcal infection.

PHYSICAL FINDINGS AND CLINICAL PRESENTATION
- It is often associated with fever, irritability, and skin tenderness.
- The eruption spreads from its usual original sites on the face, axillae, and groins to involve large areas of skin surface.
- Conjunctivitis is often also present.
- Mucous membranes, however, are not affected. Traction pressure on intact skin causes bullae formation *(Nikolsky's sign)*. At the same time, the skin becomes edematous and the surface fragile so that it can be sheared off in thin wrinkled sheets, similar to peeling wet wallpaper, leaving a glistening red surface, and the child becomes sick and feverish (Fig. 28–7).
- Diagnostic investigation: CBC, blood cultures, nose and throat swabs, histologic examination of frozen section of blister roof, skin biopsy
- Treatment: IV penicillinase-resistant penicillin, IV macrolide, cephalosporins, vancomycin

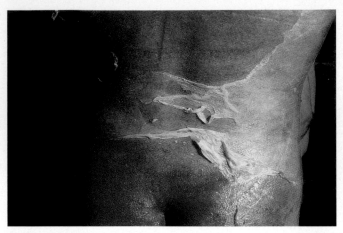

Fig 28–7
Staphylococcal scalded skin syndrome. Note the extensive blistering.
(Courtesy of Dr. A. du Vivier, King's College Hospital, London.)

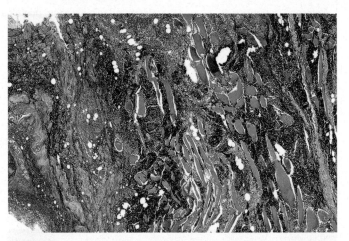

Fig 28–8
Necrotizing fasciitis. There is intense acute inflammation of the fascia, with involvement of the adjacent muscle.
(From McKee PH, Calonje E, Granter SR [eds]: Pathology of the Skin With Clinical Correlations, 3rd ed. St. Louis, Mosby, 2005.)

C. NECROTIZING FASCIITIS

DEFINITION
Necrotizing fasciitis (NF) is a bacterial infection of the subcutaneous soft tissues. There is intense acute inflammation of the fascia ,with involvement of the adjacent muscle (Fig. 28–8) and presence of bacteria (Fig. 28–9). NF may evolve following a surgical procedure (e.g., esthetic liposuction, cesarean section), with minor trauma, or even apparently in intact skin.

CAUSE
- NF is often a polymicrobial condition.
- Patients with underlying diabetes mellitus and iatrogenic immunosuppression are particularly susceptible. It can also occur as a complication of childhood varicella.

PHYSICAL FINDINGS AND CLINICAL PRESENTATION
- *Staphylococcus aureus* is the most frequently cultured organism.
- Clinical presentation: the clinical presentation may be fulminant, acute, or subacute.

- NF occurs mainly on the extremities, although almost any site can be affected.
- It usually commences as an ill-defined area of erythema and is often mistaken for cellulitis or an insignificant wound infection.
- Severe pain, indurated edema, skin necrosis, cyanosis, bullae, crepitation, muscle weakness, and malodorous exudates can develop rapidly (Fig. 28–10).

- *Fournier's gangrene* is a clinical variant of NF that involves the penis, scrotum, perineum, and abdominal wall in men and less often the vulva in women.
- Patients often have other systemic manifestations of severe sepsis, including hypotension, tachycardia, tachypnea, oliguria, and impaired mental function.
- Radiographs may reveal gas in the affected tissues.

TREATMENT
- IV antibiotics, débridement

D. ERYTHRASMA

DEFINITION

Bacterial infection caused by *Corynebacterium minutissimum*, a gram-positive bacillus.

PHYSICAL FINDINGS AND CLINICAL PRESENTATION
- It characteristically presents as symptomatic, well-defined, scaly red patches on the inguinal and intergluteal skin (Fig. 28–11).
- It has a predilection for obese and diabetic patients and is more common in regions with a humid and hot climate.

DIAGNOSIS

It is diagnosed by demonstration of coral red fluorescence under Wood's light (Fig. 28–12). It is caused by production of coproporphyrin II by the organism.

TREATMENT
- Antifungal creams (miconazole, clotrimazole, econazole)

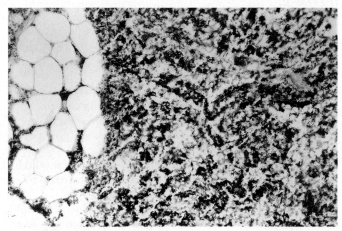

Fig 28–9
Necrotizing fasciitis. Innumerable gram-positive cocci are present. (From McKee PH, Calonje E, Granter SR [eds]: Pathology of the Skin With Clinical Correlations, 3rd ed. St. Louis, Mosby, 2005.)

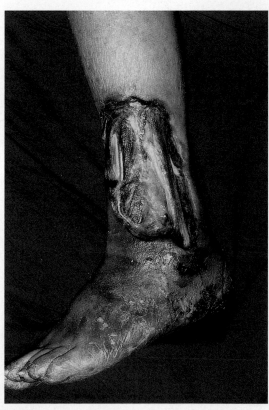

Fig 28–10
Necrotizing fasciitis. This resulted in exposure of muscle and tendons. (Courtesy of Dr. R. A. Marsden, St. George's Hospital, London.)

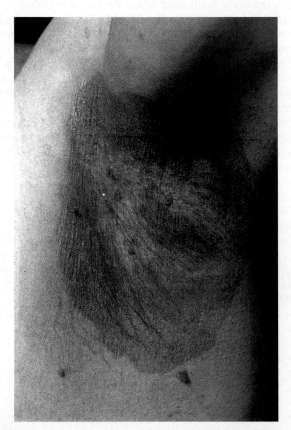

Fig 28–11
Erythrasma. Note the well-demarcated axillary scaly red patch. (Courtesy of the Institute of Dermatology, London.)

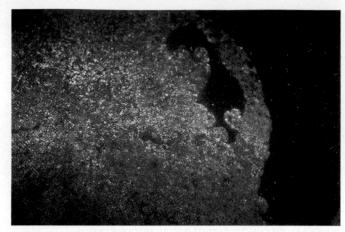

Fig 28–12
Erythrasma—typical coral red fluorescence under Wood's light.
(Courtesy of the Institute of Dermatology, London.)

E. IMPETIGO

DEFINITION
Impetigo is a superficial skin infection generally secondary to *Staphylococcus aureus* and/or *Streptococcus* spp.

PHYSICAL FINDINGS AND CLINICAL PRESENTATION
- Common presentations are bullous impetigo (generally secondary to staphylococcal disease) and nonbullous impetigo (secondary to streptococcal infection and possible staphylococcal infection); the bullous form is caused by an epidermolytic toxin produced at the site of infection.
- Multiple lesions with golden yellow crusts and weeping areas are often found on the skin around the nose, mouth, and limbs (nonbullous impetigo; Fig. 28–13).
- Presence of vesicles that enlarge rapidly to form bullae with contents that vary from clear to cloudy. There is subsequent collapse of the center of the bullae, the peripheral areas may retain fluid, and a honey-colored crust may appear in the center. As the lesions enlarge and become contiguous with the others, a scaling border replaces the fluid-filled rim (bullous impetigo); there is minimal erythema surrounding the lesions.
- Regional lymphadenopathy is most common with nonbullous impetigo.
- Constitutional symptoms are generally absent.

CAUSE
- Coagulase-positive *S. aureus* is the dominant microorganism.
- *S. pyogenes* (group A beta-hemolytic streptococci): M-T serotypes of this organism associated with acute nephritis are 2, 49, 55, 57, and 60.

DIFFERENTIAL DIAGNOSIS
- Acute allergic contact dermatitis (see Fig. 6–8)
- Herpes simplex infection (see Fig. 27–4)
- Ichthyosis (see Fig. 2–1)
- Folliculitis (see Fig. 28–14)
- Eczema (see Fig. 6–4)
- Insect bites (see Fig. 29–17)
- Scabies (see Fig. 29–1)
- Tinea corporis (see Fig. 26–1)
- Pemphigus vulgaris (see Fig. 5–3)
- Bullous pemphigoid (see Fig. 4–2)
- Varicella (see Fig. 27–2)

LABORATORY TESTS
- Generally not necessary
- Gram stain and culture and susceptibility (C&S) testing to confirm the diagnosis when the clinical presentation is unclear
- Urinalysis revealing hematuria with erythrocyte casts and proteinuria in patients with acute nephritis (most frequently occurring in children between 2 and 4 years of age in the southern United States)

TREATMENT
- Remove crusts by soaking with wet cloth compresses; crusts block the penetration of antibacterial creams.
- Application of 2% mupirocin ointment (Bactroban), three times daily for 10 days, to the affected area until all lesions have cleared
- Oral antibiotics are used in severe cases; commonly used agents are dicloxacillin, cephalexin, and azithromycin.
- Impetigo can be prevented by prompt application of mupirocin or triple-antibiotic ointment (bacitracin, polysporin, neomycin) to sites of skin trauma.
- Patients who are carriers of *S. aureus* in their nares should be treated with mupirocin ointment applied to the nares twice daily for 5 days.
- Fingernails should be kept short, and patients should be advised not to scratch any lesions to avoid spread of infection.

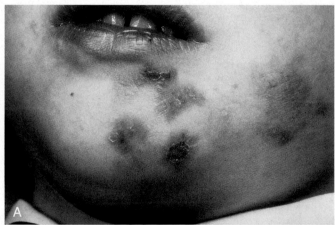
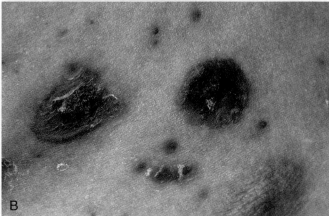

Fig 28–13
A, B, Impetigo. Note that the vesicles are covered by a golden crust. These perioral lesions are at a characteristic site.
(Courtesy of Dr. R. A. Marsden, St. George's Hospital, London.)

F. FOLLICULITIS

DEFINITION

Folliculitis is the inflammation of the hair follicle as a result of infection, physical injury, or chemical irritation. A deep folliculitis caused by *S. aureus* may affect the beard area; this form is termed *sycosis* or *folliculitis barbae*. Staphylococcal folliculitis is the most common form of infectious folliculitis; it occurs most commonly in those with diabetes.

PHYSICAL FINDINGS AND CLINICAL PRESENTATION

- The lesions generally consist of painful yellow pustules surrounded by erythema (Fig. 28–14); a central hair may be present in the pustules.
- Patients with sycosis barbae may initially present with small follicular papules or pustules that increase in size with continued shaving; deep follicular pustules may occur surrounded by erythema and swelling. The upper lip is frequently involved.
- Hot tub folliculitis occurs within 1 to 4 days following the use of a hot tub with poor chlorination; it is characterized by pustules with surrounding erythema generally affecting the torso, buttocks, and limbs.

CAUSE

- *Staphylococcus* infection (e.g., sycosis barbae), *Pseudomonas aeruginosa* (hot tub folliculitis)
- Gram-negative folliculitis (*Klebsiella, Enterobacter, Proteus* spp.) associated with antibiotic treatment of acne
- Chronic irritation of the hair follicle (use of cocoa butter or coconut oil, chronic irritation from workplace)
- Initial use of systemic corticosteroid therapy (steroid acne), eosinophilic folliculitis (AIDS patients), *Candida albicans* (immunocompromised patients)
- *Pityrosporum orbiculare*

DIFFERENTIAL DIAGNOSIS

- Acne vulgaris (see Fig. 19–1)
- Dermatophyte fungal infections (see Fig. 26–5)
- Cutaneous candidiasis (see Fig. 26–8)
- Miliaris (see Fig. 25–9)

LABORATORY TESTS

- Gram stain is useful to identify the infective organisms in infectious folliculitis and to differentiate infectious from noninfectious folliculitis.

TREATMENT

- Cleansing of the area with chlorhexidine and application of saline compresses to involved area
- Application of 2% mupirocin ointment for bacterial folliculitis affecting a limited area (e.g., sycosis barbae)
- Treatment of *Pseudomonas* folliculitis with ciprofloxacin
- Treatment of *S. aureus* folliculitis with dicloxacillin, 250 mg four times daily, for 10 days
- Chronic nasal or perineal *S. aureus* carriers with frequent folliculitis can be treated with rifampin, 300 mg, twice daily for 5 days.
- Mupirocin ointment 2% applied to the nares twice daily is also effective for nasal carriers.

G. FURUNCLE (BOIL)

DEFINITION

A furuncle is a more exuberant form of suppurative folliculitis.

PHYSICAL FINDINGS AND CLINICAL PRESENTATION

- It is more common in young adults and usually affects the skin of the face, neck, buttocks, and axillae (Fig. 28–15).
- Lesions can be up to 2 cm across and the inflammation is not confined within the follicle, but is associated with surrounding erythema (Fig. 28–16) and often systemic symptoms.
- After discharge of the pustular necrotic core, the lesion heals rapidly, but with scarring. Pseudofolliculitis (pili incarnate, shaving bumps) refers to the presence of firm skin-colored

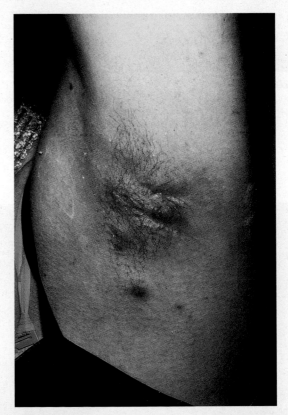

Fig 28–15
Furuncle. Shown are multiple erythematous nodules in the axilla, which is a commonly affected site. The lesions are exquisitely painful. (Courtesy of Dr. R. A. Marsden, St. George's Hospital, London.)

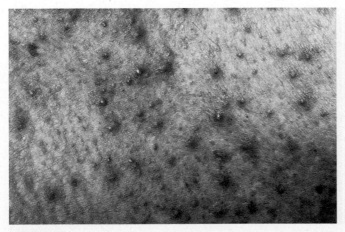

Fig 28–14
Folliculitis—characteristic small pustules with surrounding erythema. (Courtesy of Dr. R. A. Marsden, St. George's Hospital, London.)

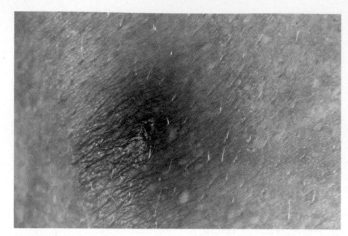

Fig 28–16
Furuncle—early lesion characterized by edema and erythema.
(Courtesy of the Institute of Dermatology, London.)

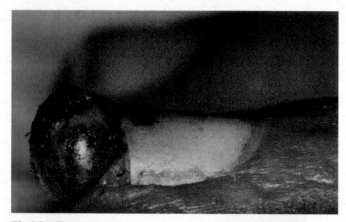

Fig 28–17
Periungual pyogenic granuloma. There is a large hemorrhagic nodule adjacent to the free edge of the nail.
(From Baran R, Dawber RPR, Levene GM: A Colour Atlas of the Hair, Scalp and Nails. London, Wolfe, 1991.)

or erythematous inflammatory papules or nodules in the shaving area of the face, often associated with postinflammatory hyperpigmentation. It may be caused by curly or kinky hair that tends to curve back directly into adjacent skin (extrafollicular penetration) or by shaving techniques that stretch the skin and result in the cut hair end retracting under the epidermis when the skin is released (transfollicular penetration).

DIAGNOSIS
- Culture and sensitivity of pus, nasal swab, CBC

TREATMENT
- Incision and drainage, systemic antibiotics, topical antibiotics
- Eradication of nasal carriage of staphylococci

H. BACILLARY ANGIOMATOSIS

DEFINITION
Vasoproliferative lesion that may be readily confused with pyogenic granuloma (Fig. 28–17) or Kaposi's sarcoma and is seen predominantly (but not exclusively) in the skin.

PHYSICAL FINDINGS AND CLINICAL PRESENTATION
- Patients present with widespread, numerous, blood-red, smooth-surfaced, superficial papules, and skin-colored or dusky subcutaneous nodules (Fig. 28–18).
- The condition may be caused by *Bartonella henselae* (the organism responsible for cat scratch disease) or, less frequently, by *B. quintana* (the cause of trench fever).
- Lesions have also been described in the bones, soft tissues, liver, lymph nodes, and spleen.
- Patients may have systemic manifestations, including fever, malaise, hepatosplenomegaly, and lymphadenopathy.
- Although it was originally thought to be a disease specific to AIDS, it has also been described in other immunocompromised states and even in apparently normal individuals.

DIAGNOSIS
- Biopsy, Warthin-Starry stain, electron microscopy, PCR of biopsy material, serology, indirect fluorescence assay (IFA), prolonged culture of blood and biopsy tissue
- CBC, HIV, ALT, CD4 lymphocyte count

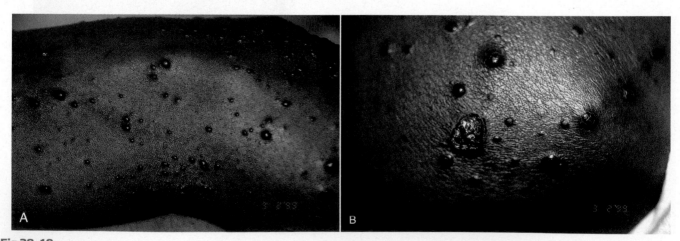

Fig 28–18
A, B, Bacillary angiomatosis. The bright red coloration is characteristic.
(Courtesy of Dr. N.C. Dlova, Nelson R. Mandela School of Medicine, University of Kwazulu-Natal, South Africa.)

TREATMENT
- Antibiotics: azithromycin, clarithromycin, erythromycin

J. BARTONELLOSIS (CARRIÓN'S DISEASE)

DEFINITION
- Infection caused by *Bartonella bacilliformis*
- This condition is endemic in the higher altitude regions of Peru.

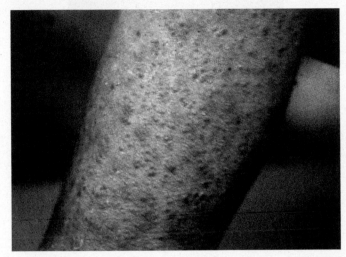

Fig 28–19
Verruga peruana. Widespread papules are present.
(Courtesy of Dr. F. von Lichtenberg, Brigham and Women's Hospital and Harvard Medical School, Boston.)

PHYSICAL FINDINGS AND CLINICAL PRESENTATION
- The initial stage of infection (hematic phase) is referred to as Oroya fever.
- Patients are acutely ill with pyrexia, rigors, myalgia, and severe hemolytic anemia.
- The latter is attributable to infection of the circulating erythrocytes and can be confirmed by a blood smear.
- Later, the disease enters an eruptive phase characterized by the evolution of numerous popular, nodular, or verrucous vascular skin lesions, referred to as *verruga peruana* (Peruvian wart, cutaneous verrucous disease). These occur predominantly on the face and extremities (Fig. 28–19).

J. YAWS (FRAMBOESIA TROPICA)

DEFINITION
This ia a tropical disease caused by infection by the spirochete *Treponema pallidum*, subsp. *pertenue* (Fig. 28–20). It is not transmitted sexually but rather by close contact—for example inoculation of skin previously traumatized by insects or scratching. Yaws is most common in children 6 to 10 years of age, who present with lesions on the feet, legs, and buttocks.

PHYSICAL FINDINGS AND CLINICAL PRESENTATION
- Generally, it is divided into early and late yaws. The initial lesion, known as a mother yaw, develops 3 to 5 weeks after inoculation.
- It starts as a nontender papilloma, which ulcerates and is then covered with a yellow crust (Fig. 28–21). It resembles a raspberry—hence, the alternative designation of framboesia (from the Dutch *framboos*, raspberry).

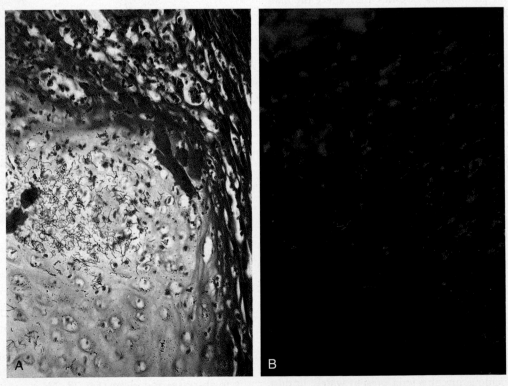

Fig 28–20
A, B, Early yaws. Note the presence of numerous spirochetes. **A,** Warthin-Starry, **B,** immunofluorescence.
(Courtesy of Drs. H. J. H. Engelkens and E. Stolz, University Hospital, Rotterdam-Dijkzigt, and Erasmus University, Rotterdam, The Netherlands.)

141

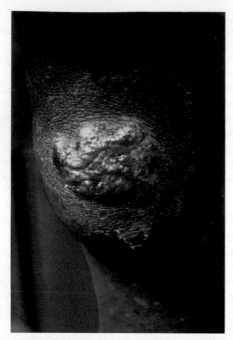

Fig 28–21
Early yaws—typical framboesiform mother yaw. Note the yellow crust and surrounding hypopigmentation.
(Courtesy of Drs. H. J. H. Engelkens and E. Stolz, University Hospital, Rotterdam-Dijkzigt, and Erasmus University, Rotterdam, The Netherlands.)

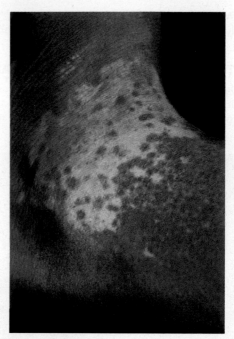

Fig 28–22
Pinta. This is a late lesion showing characteristic complete loss of pigmentation surrounded by a hyperpigmented border.
(Courtesy of Drs. R. Arenas and J. Salas, Azteca, Monterrey, Mexico.)

- Subsequently, other lesions develop daughter yaws. They eventually resolve to leave a depressed and hyperpigmented scar.
- Late lesions may develop in 10% of patients and are destructive ulcers and gummatous nodules that affect the skin, bones, and joints.

K. PINTA

DEFINITION
This is a nonsexually transmitted treponematosis characterized by depigmented skin lesions. It is caused by *Treponema pallidum*, subsp. *carateum*. Children are primarily affected and transmission is thought to be by direct cutaneous or mucous membrane contact, possibly via minute abrasions.

PHYSICAL FINDINGS AND CLINICAL PRESENTATION
- The lesions present as small, scaly, erythematous indurated papules and plaques on exposed skin, usually on the hands and feet.
- Late stages of pinta are characterized by disfiguring hyperpigmentation, achromia, hyperkeratosis, and atrophy (Fig. 28–22).
- Unlike syphilis and yaws, there is no evidence of systemic disease.

L. *MYCOBACTERIUM AVIUM-INTRACELLULARE*

DEFINITION
Mycobacterium avium-intracellulare (MAI) is a group of slow-growing nontuberculous mycobacteria present widely in dust, soil, and water. It is one of the most common causes of bacterial infection in AIDS patients.

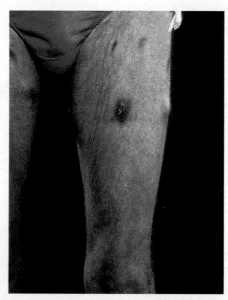

Fig 28–23
Nodules caused by *Mycobacterium avium-intracellulare*. These multiple nodules on the thighs resemble panniculitis.
(Courtesy of Dr. S. Lucas, MD, St. Thomas' Hospital, London.)

PHYSICAL FINDINGS AND CLINICAL PRESENTATION
- Cervical adenitis, disseminated infection in immunocompromised hosts
- Generally skin infections present as a panniculitis, often in relation to affected lymph nodes, or as nodules progressing to abscesses and ulcers (Fig. 28–23).
- Healing is slow, even with appropriate drug therapy, and excision may be necessary.

Chapter 29   Infestations and bites

A. SCABIES

DEFINITION

Scabies is a contagious disease caused by the mite *Sarcoptes scabiei*. It is generally acquired by sleeping with or in the bedding of infested individuals..

PHYSICAL FINDINGS AND CLINICAL PRESENTATION

- Primary lesions are caused when the female mite burrows within the stratum corneum, laying eggs within the tract she leaves behind; burrows (linear or serpiginous tracts) end with a minute papule or vesicle.
- Primary lesions are most commonly found in the web spaces of the hands (Fig. 29–1), wrists, buttocks, scrotum, penis, breasts, axillae, and knees.
- Secondary lesions result from scratching or infection.
- Intense pruritus, especially nocturnal, is common; it is caused by an acquired sensitivity to the mite or fecal pellets and is usually noted 1 to 4 weeks after the primary infestation.
- Examination of the skin may reveal burrows (Fig. 29–2), tiny vesicles, excoriations, and inflammatory papules.
- Widespread and crusted lesions (Norwegian or crusted scabies) may be seen in older and immunocompromised patients (Fig. 29–3).

CAUSE

- Human scabies is caused by the mite *S. scabiei*, var. *hominis*.

DIFFERENTIAL DIAGNOSIS

- Pediculosis (see Fig. 29–5)
- Atopic dermatitis (see Fig. 6–2)
- Flea bites (see Fig. 29–17)
- Seborrheic dermatitis (see Fig. 6–3)
- Dermatitis herpetiformis (see Fig. 4–9)
- Contact dermatitis (see Fig. 4–24)
- Nummular eczema (see Fig. 6–5)
- Syphilis (see Fig. 226–12)

DIAGNOSIS

- Diagnosis is made on the clinical presentation and on the demonstration of mites, eggs, or mite feces.

LABORATORY TESTS

- Microscopic demonstration of the organism, feces, or eggs: a drop of mineral oil may be placed over the suspected lesion before removal; the scrapings are transferred directly to a glass slide; a drop of KOH is added and a cover slip is applied.
- Skin biopsy is rarely necessary to make the diagnosis.

TREATMENT

- The following products are available for treatment of scabies mites: permethrin, lindane, ivermectin

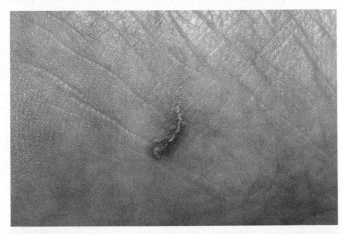

Fig 29–2
Scabies burrow on the side of the foot.
(From White GM, Cox NH [eds]: Diseases of the Skin: A Color Atlas and Text, 2nd ed. St. Louis, Mosby, 2006.)

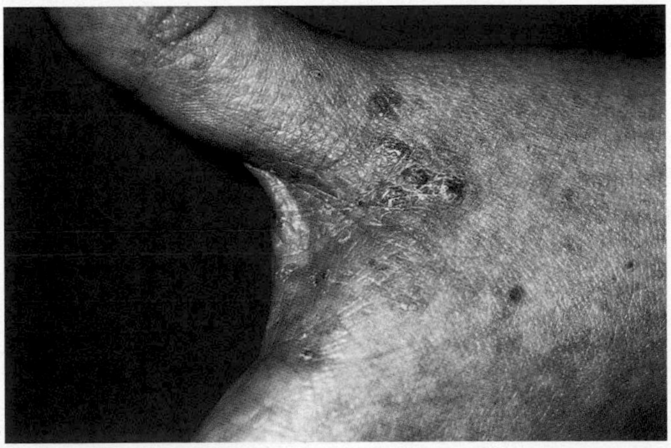

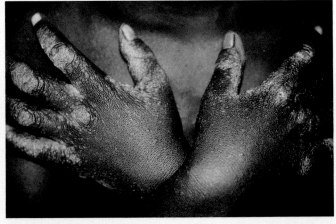

Fig 29–3
Norwegian scabies. This example, also known as the hyperkeratotic variant, may affect widespread areas of the body, and is associated with severe crusting and a heavy infestation of mites. It is exceedingly infectious.
(Courtesy of Dr. N. C. Dlova, Nelson R. Mandela School of Medicine, University of Kwazulu-Natal, South Africa.)

Fig 29–1
Scabies. The burrows are linear, slightly raised lesions. The most common sites affected include the lateral aspects of the fingers, the web between the thumb and first finger, and the wrists.
(Courtesy of Dr. R. A. Marsden, St. George's Hospital, London.)

- Clothing, underwear, and towels used in the 48 hours before treatment must be laundered.
- Sexual partners should be notified and treated.

B. PEDICULOSIS (LICE)

DEFINITION

Pediculosis is lice infestation. Humans can be infested with three types of lice—*Pediculus capitis* (head louse), *Pediculus corporis* (body louse), and *Phthirus pubis* (pubic, or crab, louse; Fig. 29-4). Lice feed on human blood and deposit their eggs (nits) on the hair shafts (head lice and pubic lice) and along the seams of clothing (body lice). Nits generally hatch within 7 to 10 days. Lice are obligate human parasites and cannot survive away from their hosts for longer than 7 to 10 days. There are 6 million to 12 million U.S. cases of head lice annually.

PHYSICAL FINDINGS AND CLINICAL PRESENTATION

- Pruritus with excoriation may be caused by hypersensitivity reaction, inflammation from saliva, and fecal material from the lice.

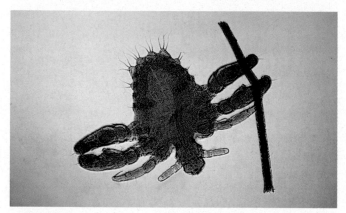

Fig 29-4
Pubic or crab louse, *Phthirus pubis*, grasping a hair.
(From Auerbach P: Wilderness Medicine, 4th ed. St. Louis, Mosby, 2001.)

- Nits can be identified by examining hair shafts (Fig. 29-5).
- The presence of nits on clothing is indicative of body lice (Fig. 29-6).
- Lymphadenopathy may be present (cervical adenopathy with head lice, inguinal lymphadenopathy with pubic lice).
- Head lice is most frequently found in the back of the head and neck, behind the ears.
- Scratching can result in pustules and crusting.
- Pubic lice may affect the hair around the anus.

CAUSE

- Lice are transmitted by close personal contact or use of contaminated objects (e.g., combs, clothing, bed linens, hats).

DIFFERENTIAL DIAGNOSIS

- Seborrheic dermatitis (see Fig. 6-3)
- Scabies (see Fig. 29-2)
- Atopic dermatitis (see Fig. 6-2)

DIAGNOSIS

- Diagnosis is made by seeing the lice or their nits. Combing hair with a fine-toothed comb is recommended because visual inspection of the hair and scalp may miss more than 50% of infestations.

LABORATORY TESTS

- Wood's light examination is useful to screen a large number of children: live nits fluoresce, empty nits have a gray fluorescence, and nits with unborn lice reveal a white fluorescence.

TREATMENT

- Patients with body lice should discard infested clothing and improve their hygiene.
- Combing out nits is a widely recommended but unproved adjunctive therapy.
- Personal items such as combs and hairbrushes should be soaked in hot water for 15 to 30 minutes.
- Close contacts and household members should also be examined for the presence of lice.
- The following products are available for treatment of lice: permethrin, lindane, pyrethrin S, malathion, ivermectin

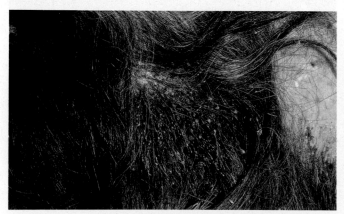

Fig 29-5
Pediculosis capitis, adult. If a patient complains of intense itching of the scalp, a close inspection for nits should always be performed. Nits are much more easily found than the lice that lay them.
(From White GM, Cox NH [eds]: Diseases of the Skin: A Color Atlas and Text, 2nd ed. St. Louis, Mosby, 2006.)

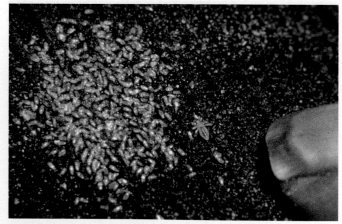

Fig 29-6
Pediculosis corporis. Inspection of the clothing allows for diagnosis. Shown here are multiple eggs and a louse. Note that the shape of the louse is very similar to that of the parasite that causes pediculosis capitis.
(From White GM, Cox NH [eds]: Diseases of the Skin: A Color Atlas and Text, 2nd ed. St. Louis, Mosby, 2006.)

C. CUTANEOUS LARVA MIGRANS (CREEPING ERUPTION)

DEFINITION
This dermatitis results from penetration of and migration through the skin by infectious nematode larvae, usually of animal origin. The condition is most prevalent in warm humid tropical regions, especially along the coastline.

CAUSE
● The larval forms of *Ancylostoma braziliensis* (the cat and dog hookworm) are the most frequent cause of cutaneous larva migrans.
● The larvae evolve in the soil from eggs passed via the feces of infested hosts. These metamorphose into infectious filariform larvae capable of penetrating human skin on contact. The larvae appear to enter the skin via the ostia of hair follicles or sweat glands, usually on the feet, buttocks, or abdomen, in decreasing order of frequency.

PHYSICAL FINDINGS AND CLINICAL PRESENTATION
● An intensely pruritic erythematous papule or vesicle develops at the site of larval penetration. Migration of the larvae commences 2 to 4 days later, and is associated with the development of a characteristic erythematous, serpiginous tract (Fig. 29–7). The larvae may migrate at a rate of 2 to 5 cm/day.

DIAGNOSIS
● Biopsy specimens obtained from the advancing tract confirm the presence of tunneling larvae. CBC reveals a high eosinophil count.
● Chest x-ray may reveal a patchy infiltrate.

TREATMENT
● Ivermectin, 200 μg/kg, single dose
● Albendazole is also effective.
● Antibiotics may be needed for secondary infection.
● Although the condition is usually self-limiting, with spontaneous resolution over a period of several weeks, secondary bacterial infection introduced by scratching is a relatively frequent complication.

D. BITE WOUNDS

DEFINITION
A bite wound can be animal or human, accidental or intentional. Infection rates are highest for cat bites (30% to 50%), followed by human bites (15% to 30%) and dog bites (5%). The extremities are involved in 75% of bites.

PHYSICAL FINDINGS AND CLINICAL PRESENTATION
● The appearance of the bite wound is variable (e.g., puncture wound, tear, avulsion; Fig. 29–8) and may be extensive (Fig. 29–9) and life-threatening.
● Cellulitis, lymphangitis, and focal adenopathy may be present in infected bite wounds.
● Patients may experience fever and chills.

CAUSE
● Increased risk of infection: human and cat bites, closed fist injuries, wounds involving joints, puncture wounds, face and lip bites, bites with skull penetration, bites in immuno-compromised hosts
● Most frequent infecting organisms:
  1. *Pasteurella* spp.: responsible for most infections within 24 hours of dog (*P. canis*) and cat (*P. multocida, P. septica*) bites
  2. *Capnocytophaga canimorsus* (formerly DF-2 bacillus): a gram-negative organism responsible for late infection, usually following dog bites
  3. Gram-negative organisms (*Pseudomonas, Haemophilus*): often found in human bites
  4. *Streptococcus* spp., *Staphylococcus aureus*
  5. *Eikenella corrodens* in human bites
  6. *Fusobacterium nucleatum* (Fig. 29–10)

DIFFERENTIAL DIAGNOSIS
  ● Bite from a rabid animal; often, the attack is unprovoked.
  ● Factitious injury

LABORATORY TESTS
● Generally not necessary
● Hematocrit if there has been significant blood loss

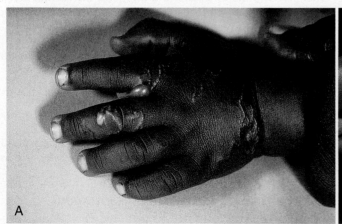
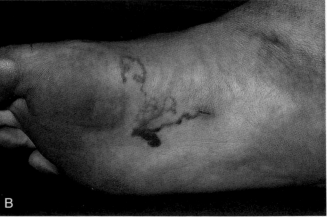

Fig 29–7
Cutaneous larva migrans. **A,** Multiple irregular tracts are present. **B,** The foot is a commonly affected site.
(**A** courtesy of Dr. N.C. Dlova, Nelson R. Mandela School of Medicine, University of Kwazulu-Natal, South Africa; **B** courtesy of Dr. R. A. Marsden, St. George's Hospital, London.)

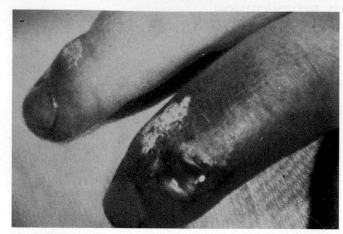

Fig 29–8
Human bite wound.
(From Cohen J, Powderly WG: Infectious Diseases, 2nd ed. St. Louis, Mosby, 2004.)

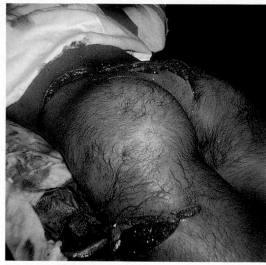

Fig 29–9
Shark bite of the buttocks.
(Courtesy of Dr. T. Hattori.)

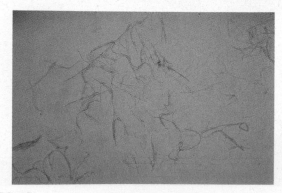

Fig 29–10
Gram stain of *Fusobacterium nucleatum.*
(Courtesy of Mike Cox.)

- Wound cultures (aerobic and anaerobic) if there is evidence of sepsis or victim is immunocompromised; cultures should be obtained before irrigation of the wound but after superficial cleaning.

IMAGING STUDIES
- X-rays are indicated when bony penetration is suspected or if there is suspicion of fracture or significant trauma; x-rays are also useful for detecting the presence of foreign bodies (when suspected).

TREATMENT
- Local care with débridement, vigorous cleansing, and saline irrigation of the wound; débridement of devitalized tissue
- High-pressure irrigation to clean bite wound and ensure removal of contaminants. For example, use saline solution with a 30- to 35-mL syringe equipped with a 20-gauge needle or catheter with the tip of the syringe placed 2 to 3 cm above the wound.
- Avoid blunt probing of wounds (increased risk of infection).
- If the animal is suspected to be rabid, infiltrate wound edges with 1% procaine hydrochloride, swab wound surface vigorously with cotton swabs and 1% benzalkonium solution or other soap, and rinse wound with normal saline.
- Avoid suturing of hand wounds and any wounds that appear infected.
- Puncture wounds should be left open.
- Give anti-rabies therapy and tetanus immune globulin and toxoid as needed
- Use empirical antibiotic therapy (amoxicillin-clavulanate or cefuroxime) for high-risk wounds (e.g., cat bite, hand bites, face bites, genital area bites, bites with joint or bone penetration, human bites, immunocompromised host).
- In hospitalized patients, the IV antibiotics of choice are cefoxitin, ampicillin-sulbactam, ticarcillin-clavulanate, and ceftriaxone.
- Prophylactic therapy for persons bitten by others with HIV and hepatitis B

E. BITES AND STINGS, ARACHNIDS

DEFINITION
There are two major classes of arthropods, insects and arachnids. This section will focus on the class Arachnida. Arachnid bites are those caused by spiders, scorpions, and ticks.

EPIDEMIOLOGY AND DEMOGRAPHICS
- Spiders: ubiquitous; only three types are potentially significantly harmful:
  - Sydney funnel-web spider: Australia
  - Black widow (Fig. 29–11): worldwide (not Alaska)
  - Brown recluse (Fig. 29–12): most common (south central United States)
- Scorpions: various warm climates—Africa, central South America, Middle East, India; in the United States—Texas, New Mexico, California, Nevada
- Ticks: woodlands

PHYSICAL FINDINGS AND CLINICAL PRESENTATION
Spiders
- Sydney funnel-web: atracotoxin; piloerection, muscle spasms leading to tachycardia, hypertension, increased intracranial pressure, coma

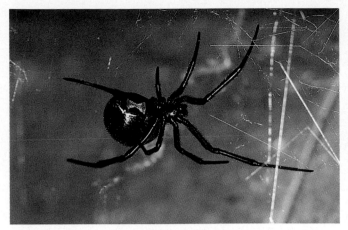

Fig 29–11
Mature female western black widow (*Latrodectus hesperus*).
(Courtesy of Michael Cardwell and Associates, 1993.)

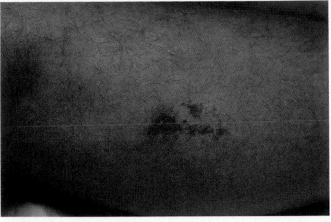

Fig 29–13
Brown recluse spider bite after 6 hours, with central hemorrhagic vesicle and gravitational spread of venom.
(Courtesy of Drs. Paul Auerbach and Riley Rees.)

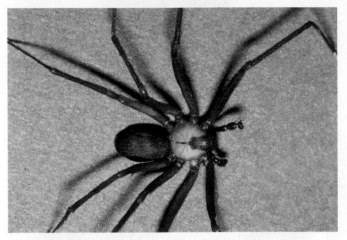

Fig 29–12
Brown recluse spider (*Loxosceles reclusa*).
(Courtesy of the Indiana University Medical Center, Bloomington. Ind.)

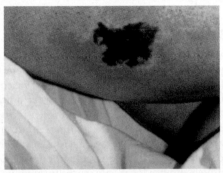

Fig 29–14
Brown recluse spider bite after 24 hours, with central ischemia and rapidly advancing cellulitis.
(Courtesy of Dr. Paul Auerbach.)

- Black widow (females toxic): initial reaction—local swelling, redness (two fang marks) leading to local piloerection, edema, urticaria, diaphoresis, lymphangitis; pain in limb leading to rest of body (chest pain, abdominal pain)
- Brown recluse: minor sting or burn; wound may become pruritic and red with a blanched center with vesicle (Fig. 29–13); can necrose, especially in fatty areas (Fig. 29–14); leaves eschar, which sloughs and leaves an ulcer, can take months to heal; systemic signs and symptoms—headache, fever, chills, GI upset, hemolysis, renal tubular necrosis, DIC possible

Scorpions
- Sting leading to sympathetic and parasympathetic stimulation: hypertension, bradycardia, vasoconstriction, pulmonary edema, reduced coronary blood flow, priapism, inhibition of insulin
- Also possible: tachycardia, arrhythmia, vasodilation, bronchial relaxation, excessive salivation, vomiting, sweating, bronchoconstriction

Ticks: United States, Europe, Asia
- Very small (smaller than 1 mm); usually must be attached longer than 36 hours to transmit disease
- Lyme disease (most common): early—erythema migrans, 60% to 80% of cases; 7 to 10 days—mild to moderate constitutional symptoms, disseminated, secondary skin lesions, fever, adenopathy, constitutional symptoms, facial palsy, peripheral neuropathy, lymphocytic meningitis, meningoencephalitis, cardiac manifestations (heart block); late—chronic arthritis, dermatitis, neuropathy, keratitis

DIFFERENTIAL DIAGNOSIS
- Cellulitis (see Fig. 28–1)
- Urticaria (see Fig. 15–7)
- Folliculitis (see Fig. 28–14)
- Other tick-borne illnesses:
  - Babesiosis
  - Tick-borne relapsing fever (see Fig. 346–1)
  - Tularemia (see Fig. 347–2)
  - Rocky Mountain spotted fever (see Fig. 308–15)

- Ehrlichiosis
- Colorado tick fever
- Tick paralysis

TREATMENT

Spiders

- Sydney funnel-web: pressure, immobilization immediately, supportive care, antivenin
- Black widow: treatment based on severity of symptoms. Bite is rarely fatal. All victims should be given oxygen, IV, cardiac monitor, tetanus prophylaxis, symptomatic supportive therapy, 10% calcium gluconate for muscle cramps (controversial)
- Brown recluse: pain management, tetanus, supportive treatment; no consensus regarding best treatment; some evidence for hyperbaric oxygen

Scorpions

- Fluids, supportive care, species-specific antivenin (equine-based, risk of serum sickness; controversial)

Ticks

- Prophylactic: after more than 36 hours, single dose of doxycycline, 200 mg
- Early localized disease: treatment of choice in children—amoxicillin for 14 days; doxycycline preferred for patients with possible concurrent ehrlichiosis

F. BITES AND STINGS, INSECTS

DEFINITION

Most stinging insects belong to the Hymenoptera order and include yellow jackets (most common cause of reactions), hornets, bumblebees, sweat bees, wasps, harvester ants, fire ants, and the African honey bee (killer bee). Brown recluse spiders, although they are not insects, are another common cause of bites (see ealier, "Bites and Stings, Arachnids"). Bedbugs (Fig. 29–15) and fleas (Fig. 29–16) are frequent offenders. The usual effect of a sting is intense local pain, some immediate erythema, and often a small area of edema caused by injecting venom. Allergic reactions can be local or generalized, leading to anaphylactic shock. Most reactions occur within the first 6 hours after the sting or bite, but a delayed presentation may occur up to 24 hours (Fig. 29–17).

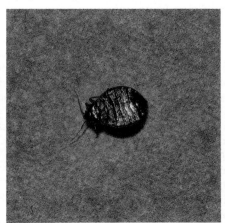

Fig 29–15
Cimex lectularius, the common bedbug.
(From White GM, Cox NH [eds]: Diseases of the Skin: A Color Atlas and Text, 2nd ed. St. Louis, Mosby, 2006.)

PHYSICAL FINDINGS AND CLINICAL PRESENTATION

Stings

- Cutaneous: the skin is the most common site of an allergic reaction. Manifestations include flushing, urticaria, pruritus, and angioedema (Fig. 29–18). Secondary infections may occur (Fig. 29–19).
- Respiratory: hoarseness, difficulty speaking, choking, throat tightness or tingling may progress to stridor, laryngeal edema, laryngospasm, bronchoconstriction. This is the leading cause of anaphylactic death.
- Cardiovascular: tachycardia, hypotension, arrhythmia, can progress to profound hypovolemic shock. Myocardial infarction is rare. Cardiac manifestations are the second leading cause of death from anaphylaxis.

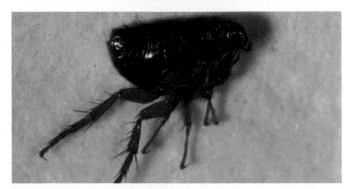

Fig 29–16
The cat flea, *Ctenocephalides felis*, under the microscope.
(From White GM, Cox NH [eds]: Diseases of the Skin: A Color Atlas and Text, 2nd ed. St. Louis, Mosby, 2006.)

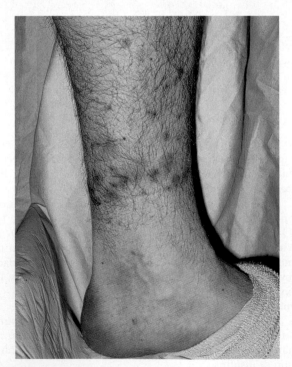

Fig 29–17
Flea bites. Multiple lesions are seen above the ankle, with sparing of the skin covered by the sock and shoe.
(From White GM, Cox NH [eds]: Diseases of the Skin: A Color Atlas and Text, 2nd ed. St. Louis, Mosby, 2006.)

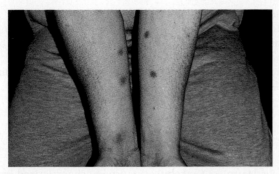

Fig 29–18
Typical lesions of papular urticaria, caused in this case by bedbug bites.
(From Cohen J, Powderly WG: Infectious Diseases, 2nd ed. St. Louis, Mosby, 2004.)

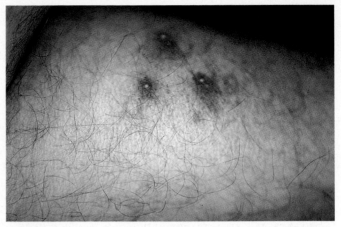

Fig 29–20
Fire ant lesions.
(From Auerbach P: Wilderness Medicine, 4th ed. St. Louis, Mosby, 2001.)

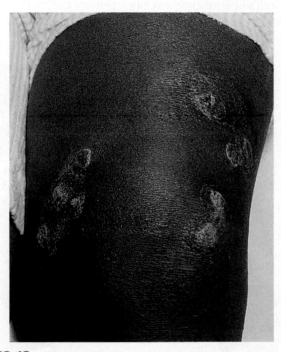

Fig 29–19
Mosquito bites with secondary staphylococcal and streptococcal infection.
(From Cohen J, Powderly WG: Infectious Diseases, 2nd ed. St. Louis, Mosby, 2004.)

- Other symptoms: abdominal pain, nausea, vomiting, and diarrhea.

Fire ants

- Initial wheal and flare reaction
- Subsequent development of circularly arrayed blisters within 24 hours (Fig. 29–20)
- Blisters may develop the appearance of pustules, but they are not infected.

CAUSE

Stings

- Most systemic reactions to insect stings are classic IgE-mediated reactions.

- Reactions occur in previously sensitized patients who have produced high titers of IgE antibody to insect venom antigens.
- Sensitization to wasp venom requires only a few stings and can occur after a single sting.
- Sensitization to bee venom occurs mainly in those who have been stung frequently by bees.

Bites

- Fire ant venom contains proteins toxic to the skin.

DIFFERENTIAL DIAGNOSIS

- Stings: cellulitis, bites
- Bites: stings, cellulitis

LABORATORY TESTS

- Skin test: skin prick test or intradermal method with fire ant or hymenoptera venom
- Measurement of serum-specific IgE measured by RAST or other assays

TREATMENT

Sting

- Stinger most easily removed with a flat tool such as a credit card, cleansing, and application of ice
- Treatment with oral antihistamines and NSAIDs for limited reactions. Topical corticosteroids may provide some relief of inflammation.
- Patients with previous reactions or multiple stings to the mouth or neck should be evaluated in an emergency department.
- Larger swellings may benefit from oral steroids.
- Anaphylaxis should be treated with epinephrine. Antihistamines, oxygen, intravenous corticosteroids, beta agonists, and IV fluids may also be beneficial.

Bite

- Supportive care
- Application of ice
- Surveillance for secondary infection

G. BITES, SNAKE

DEFINITION

This is an injury resulting from a snake biting a human. In the United States, at least one species of poisonous snake has been identified in every state except Alaska, Hawaii, and Maine. Most venomous snakes are members of the family Crotalidae, which includes rattlesnakes (Fig. 29–21), copperheads, and cottonmouths. The Elapidae family, which includes the coral snake, accounts for the remainder (Fig. 29–22).

PHYSICAL FINDINGS AND CLINICAL PRESENTATION

● In addition to local tissue injury (Fig. 29–23), envenomation may affect the renal, neurologic, gastrointestinal, vascular, and coagulation systems. Species-specific signs and symptoms include the following.

Crotalidae (pit vipers)

- Fang punctures (see "Diagnosis")
- Pain within 5 minutes
- Edema within 30 minutes
- Erythema of site and adjacent tissues, serous or hemorrhagic bullae (Fig. 29–24), ecchymosis, lymphangitis, or both over the ensuing hours

If no edema or erythema is manifested within 8 hours after a confirmed crotalid snakebite, it is safe to assume that envenomation did not occur. Approximately 25% of cases do not involve envenomation.

Systemic manifestations may include the following:
- Mild to moderate manifestations: nausea, vomiting, perioral paresthesias, metallic taste, tingling of fingers or toes (especially with rattlesnake bites), fasciculations (local or generalized).
- Severe manifestations: hypotension caused by increased vascular permeability, mental status change, respiratory distress, tachycardia, acute renal failure, rhabdomyolysis, intravascular hemolysis, DIC

Elapidae (coral snakes)

● Local symptoms are far less pronounced (little or no pain or swelling immediately after the bite).
● Systemic symptoms predominate, but onset may be delayed for up to 12 hours:
- Cranial nerve palsies—ptosis, dysphagia, dysarthria
- Tremors
- Intense salivation
- Loss of deep tendon reflexes (DTRs) and respiratory depression (late manifestations)

CAUSE

● Most victims are young men who purposefully attempt to handle or harm a snake that had no intention of biting them.
● Victims are frequently intoxicated at the time of the bite.

DIFFERENTIAL DIAGNOSIS

- Harmless snakebite
- Scorpion bite
- Insect bite (see Fig. 28–20)
- Cellulitis (see Fig. 28–1)
- Laceration or puncture wound

Note: Harmless snakebites are usually characterized by four rows of small scratches (teeth in the upper jaw) separated from two rows of scratches (teeth in lower jaw). This is in distinction to venomous snakebites, which have puncture wounds produced by the snake's fangs, regardless of whether other teeth marks are noted.

LABORATORY TESTS

● For all suspected envenomations, perform CBC (with peripheral smear and platelet count), DIC screen (prothrombin

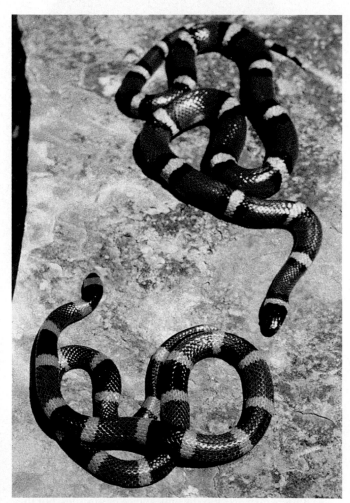

Fig 29–22
Comparison of Texas coral snake (*Micrurus fulvius tenere*) with harmless Mexican milk snake (*Lampropeltis triangulam annulata*). The coral snake (*bottom*) has contiguous red and yellow bands, whereas the milk snake has its red and yellow bands separated by black.
(Courtesy of Charles Alfaro.)

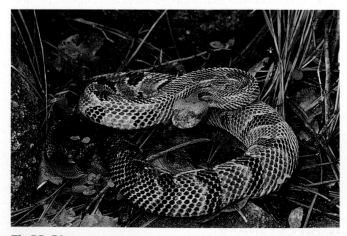

Fig 29–21
Timber rattlesnake (*Crotalus horridus*) is a large dangerous snake found in the eastern United States.
(Courtesy of Michael Cardwell, Extreme Wildlife Photography.)

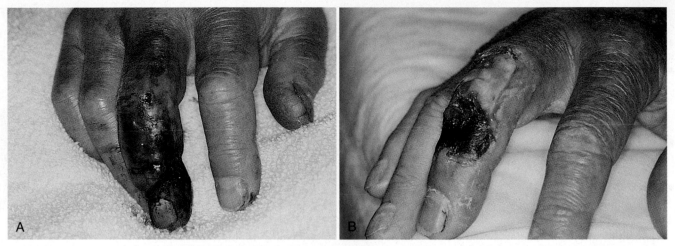

Fig 29–23
A, Soft tissue swelling, hemorrhagic blebs, and early necrosis after red diamond rattlesnake (*Crotalus ruber*) bite to the long finger (day 2). The victim received 10 vials of antivenin 6 hours after the bite and 10 more vials for severe thrombocytopenia on day 2. **B,** Seven weeks later. Note the degree of necrosis.
(Courtesy of Dr. Sean Bush.)

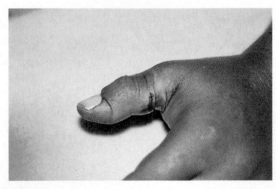

Fig 29–24
Hemorrhagic bleb at the site of a western diamondback rattlesnake (*Crotalus atrox*) bite at 24 hours.
(Courtesy of Dr. Robert Norris.)

time [PT], partial thromboplastin time [PTT], fibrinogen, fibrin degradation products, D-dimer), electrocardiography, serum electrolyte, blood urea nitrogen [BUN], and creatinine (Cr) level testing, and urinalysis.
- For more severe bites, consider LFTs, sedimentation rate, creatine kinase (rule out rhabdomyolysis), arterial blood gas (ABG) analysis, and typing and cross-matching.
- Other: consider chest x-ray in cases with severe envenomation or in patients older than 40 years with underlying cardiopulmonary disease; x-ray of bite site for retained fangs (poor sensitivity); head computed tomography (CT) scanning if concern raised for intracranial hemorrhage

TREATMENT
In the field, for a suspected snakebite:
- Immobilize affected part below heart level.
- Remove any constricting items. Local pressure has been advocated for elapid bites, particularly in Australia, as a means of delaying absorption of neurotoxins. However, crotalid bites are far more common in the United States, and these frequently have tissue-necrosing venom, which will yield

more damage with local pressure. Thus, as with incision and suction techniques, use by those without specialized training in snakebite management is discouraged.
- *Do not* apply ice; keep the victim warm.
- Avoid alcohol, stimulants (caffeine), or agents that can suppress mental status.
- Transport the victim immediately to the nearest medical facility and contact the poison control center.
In the hospital:
- Establish intravenous access.
- Initiate reconstitution of appropriate antivenin. (Antivenin is typically supplied in powder form and must be reconstituted before administration. The process can take up to 1 hour, so it is recommended that it be initiated as soon as the patient arrives in the emergency department). While this is being done:
  - Obtain time of bite and description of snake if possible.
  - Obtain past medical history; ask about allergies to horse serum in those previously treated for snakebite.
  - Record vital signs: blood pressure (BP), heart rate (HR), temperature (T), respiratory rate (RR).
  - Inspect site of bite for fang marks and local symptoms.
  - Delineate margins of erythema or edema with a marker.
  - Measure circumference of the bitten part at two or more proximal sites and compare with unaffected limb; repeat every 15 to 20 minutes; assess for extension of erythema or edema.
  - Neurologic examination
  - Gauge the severity of the bite and decide whether administration of antivenin is necessary.
- For minimal envenomation without progressive manifestations:
  - Clean and immobilize affected part.
  - Immunize against tetanus.
Observe patient for at least 8 hours. If, at the end of this interval, local and systemic sequelae are absent and laboratory values remain normal, the likelihood of significant envenomation is low, and the patient can be discharged from the acute setting.

Patients who have progressive symptoms (local or systemic) or moderate to severe envenomation should be considered for antivenin. The high incidence of allergic reactions argues against its use for less severe cases.

- Antivenin is most effective when given within 4 hours of the bite and least effective if delayed beyond 12 hours. Systemic symptoms (e.g., coagulopathy, CNS effects) respond better to treatment than local symptoms (e.g., erythema, edema, bullae).
- It is recommended that patients be monitored in an intensive care unit (ICU) setting during the administration of antivenin.
- Fasciotomy (Fig. 29–25) may be necessary in rare cases.

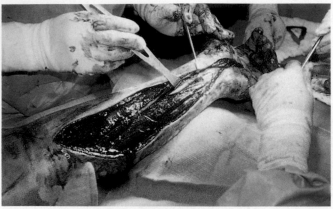

Fig 29–25
Rarely indicated fasciotomy for a victim of a severe rattlesnake bite (*Crotalus viridis helleri*). Compartment pressures were greater than 60 mm Hg, despite aggressive antivenin therapy.
(Courtesy of Dr. Robert Norris.)

DEFINITION

Decubitus ulcers (pressure ulcers) are any damage to the skin, underlying tissue, or both that results from pressure, friction, or shearing forces that usually occur over bony prominences, such as the sacrum or heels.

CLINICAL PRESENTATION

All pressure ulcers should be staged according to depth and type of tissue damage.

- Stage I—nonblanchable erythema of intact skin or boggy mushy feeling of skin
- Stage II—partial-thickness skin loss involving the epidermis, dermis, or both
- Stage III—full-thickness skin loss involving damage or necrosis of subcutaneous tissue that may extend down to, but not through, underlying fascia or muscle
- Stage IV—full-thickness skin loss with extensive destruction and tissue damage to muscle, bone, or supporting structures (e.g., tendons, joint capsule; Fig. 30–1)

LABORATORY TESTS

- Directed at identifying cause of risk factors or any complications arising from the pressure ulcer (e.g., abscess or osteomyelitis); cultures of wound bed are not helpful and should not be performed.
- Nutritional laboratory tests may reveal malnutrition, such as the presence of transthyretin (prealbumin).
- CBC if infection is suspected

IMAGING STUDIES

- Magnetic resonance imaging (MRI) or bone scans may help identify osteomyelitis when clinically suspected.

TREATMENT

- Should be cleaned at each dressing change; necrotic tissue (Fig. 30–2) should be débrided quickly because it delays wound healing (Fig 30–3).
- Wound irrigation
- No one dressing or product is superior; dressings should be used to keep ulcer bed moist and protect it from urine, stool
- Avoid agents that are cytotoxic to epithelial cells (e.g., iodine, iodophor, sodium hypochlorite, hydrogen peroxide, acetic acid, alcohol).

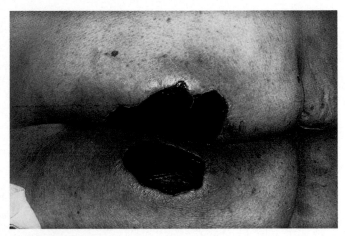

Fig 30–2
Acute pressure injury over the sacrum and buttocks in an elderly woman.
(From Tallis R, Fillit H: Brockelhurst's Textbook of Geriatric Medicine and Gerontology, 6th ed. London, Churchill Livingstone, 2003.)

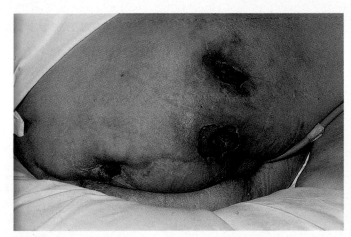

Fig 30–1
Deep pressure sore with sinuses in a patient with mutiple sclerosis.
(From Tallis R, Fillit H: Brockelhurst's Textbook of Geriatric Medicine and Gerontology, 6th ed. London, Churchill Livingstone, 2003.)

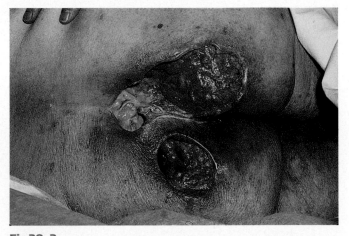

Fig 30–3
Natural débridement of the pressure injury shown in Figure 30-2 at 2 weeks.
(From Tallis R, Fillit H: Brockelhurst's Textbook of Geriatric Medicine and Gerontology, 6th ed. London, Churchill Livingstone, 2003.)

- Reduce pressure by using foam mattress, alternating pressure mattresses (Fig. 30–4), dynamic support surface (e.g., low air loss bed), and frequent repositioning (e.g., every 2 hours).
- Hyperbaric oxygen, ultrasound, UV light, and low-energy radiation are ineffective or have not been extensively evaluated for efficacy.
- Negative pressure devices (vacuum-assisted closure [VAC] devices) may be helpful for wounds that have significant drainage.
- Correct poor nutrition.
- Minimize urinary and fecal incontinence.
- Use a standardized assessment tool (e.g., PUSH tool) to monitor wound healing on a weekly basis.

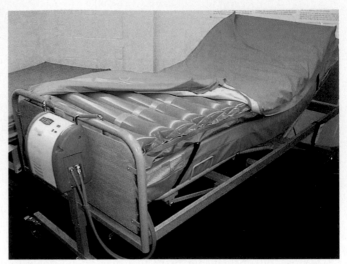

Fig 30–4
An alternating pressure mattress overlay.
(From Tallis R, Fillit H: Brockelhurst's Textbook of Geriatric Medicine and Gerontology, 6th ed. London, Churchill Livingstone, 2003.)

Chapter 31 · Environmental injuries

A. BURNS

DEFINITION

Burn injuries consist of thermal injuries (e.g., flames, scalds, cigarettes; Fig. 31–1), as well as chemical, electrical, and radiation burns.

PHYSICAL FINDINGS AND CLINICAL PRESENTATION

- Burns are defined by size (Fig. 31–2), and depth (Fig 31–3).
- First-degree burns (superficial) involve the epidermis only and appear painful and red.

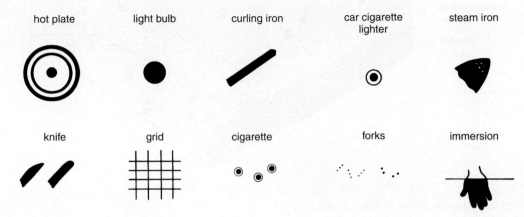

Fig 31–1
Marks from burns.
(From Swartz MH: Textbook of Physical Diagnosis, 5th ed. Philadelphia, WB Saunders, 2006.)

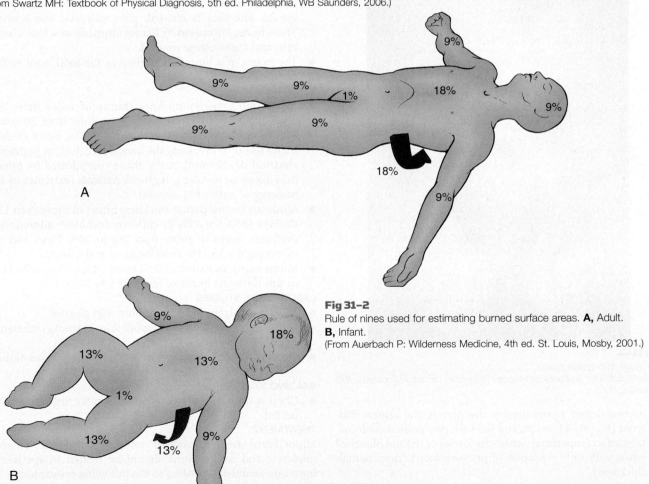

Fig 31–2
Rule of nines used for estimating burned surface areas. **A,** Adult. **B,** Infant.
(From Auerbach P: Wilderness Medicine, 4th ed. St. Louis, Mosby, 2001.)

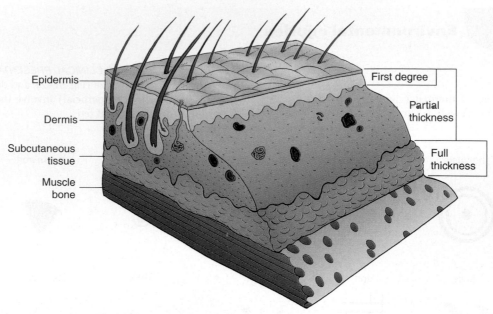

Fig 31–3
Skin anatomy.
(From Auerbach P: Wilderness Medicine, 4th ed. St. Louis, Mosby, 2001.)

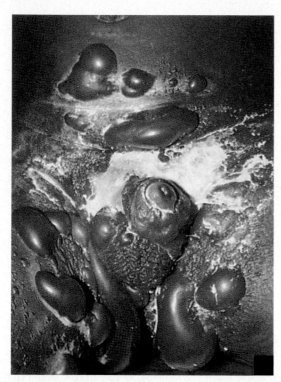

Fig 31–4
Hot water immersion burns.
(From Swartz MH: Textbook of Physical Diagnosis, 5th ed. Philadelphia, WB Saunders, 2006.)

- Second-degree burns involve the dermis and appear blistered (Fig. 31–4), moist, and red with two-point discrimination intact (superficial partial-thickness) or red and blanched white with only sensation of pressure intact (deep partial-thickness).

- Third-degree burns (full-thickness) extend through the dermis with associated destruction of hair follicles and sweat glands. The skin is charred, pale, painless, and leathery. These burns are caused by flames, immersion scalds, chemicals, and high-voltage injuries.

- The extent of a burn is described as the total burn surface area (TBSA).

CLASSIFICATION

- Major burns: partial-thickness burns of more than 25% TBSA (or 20% if younger than 10 or older than 50 years); full-thickness burns of more than 10% TBSA; burns crossing major joints or involving the hands, face, feet, or perineum; electrical or chemical burns; those complicated by inhalation injury, or involving high-risk patients (extremes of age, presence of comorbid disease)

- Moderate burns: partial-thickness burns of more than 15% to 25% TBSA (or 10% in children and older adults); full-thickness burns of more than 2% to 10% TBSA and not involving the specific conditions of major burns

- Minor burns: partial-thickness burns of less than 15% TBSA or full-thickness burns of less than 2% TBSA

LABORATORY STUDIES

- CBC, electrolytes, BUN, creatinine, and glucose
- Serial ABGs and carboxyhemoglobin if smoke inhalation suspected
- Urinalysis, urine myoglobin, and creatine phosphokinase (CPK) levels if rhabdomyolysis suspected

IMAGING STUDIES

- Chest x-ray and bronchoscopy if smoke inhalation suspected

TREATMENT

Minor burns are amenable to outpatient treatment, whereas moderate and major burns should be treated in specialized burn care facilities according to the following principles:

- Establish airway: inspect for inhalation injury and intubate for suspected airway edema (often seen 12 to 24 hours later); supplemental O_2
- Remove jewelry and clothing; place one or two large-bore peripheral IVs (if TBSA is more than 20%).
- Fluid resuscitation with Ringer's lactate solution, 2 to 4 mL/kg per percentage of TBSA/24 hours with one half the calculated fluid given in the first 8 hours
- Foley catheter and nasogastric (NG) tube (20% of patients develop an ileus)
- Tetanus update
- Pain control
- Stress ulcer prophylaxis in high-risk patients
- Prophylactic antibiotics are not recommended; however, burn victims should be considered immunosuppressed.
- High-voltage burn patients should have electrocardiographic monitoring because they are at increased risk for arrhythmia.

B. FROSTBITE

DEFINITION

Frostbite represents tissue injury (or death) from freezing and vasoconstriction induced by severe environmental cold exposure. Environmental factors include wind chill factor, temperature, duration of exposure, altitude, and degree of wetness. Hands and feet account for 90% of injuries; earlobes, nose, and male genitalia are also more susceptible. Host factors include extremes of age, immobility, history of cold injuries, skin damage, psychiatric illness, neuroleptic and sedative drugs (especially alcohol), atherosclerosis, malnutrition, tobacco use, peripheral neuropathy, hypothyroidism, fatigue, and wearing constricting clothing or footwear.

PHYSICAL FINDINGS AND CLINICAL PRESENTATION

- Frostbite may be classified into degrees of injury or, more practically, into superficial and deep groups.
- Superficial frostbite involves the skin and subcutaneous tissue. The frozen part is waxy, white, and firm but soft and resilient below the surface when gently depressed. After rewarming, the frostbitten area may appear mottled and swollen, and superficial blisters with clear or milky fluid may form within 6 to 24 hours (Fig. 31–5). There is no ultimate tissue loss.
- Deep frostbite extends into subcutaneous tissues and may involve muscles, nerves, tendons, or bones. The skin may be hard or wooden, without tissue resilience. Edema, cyanosis, hemorrhagic blisters (after 3 to 7 days), tissue necrosis, and gangrene may develop. Affected tissue has a poor prognosis and débridement or amputation is generally required (Fig. 31–6).
- Patients initially experience numbness, prickling, and itching. More severe injury can produce paresthesias and stiffness, with burning or throbbing pain on thawing.

CAUSE

Two distinct mechanisms are responsible for tissue injury in frostbite:

1. Cellular death occurring at time of exposure from ice crystal damage to cells
2. Deterioration and necrosis attributable to progressive dermal ischemia after rewarming via inflammatory mediators

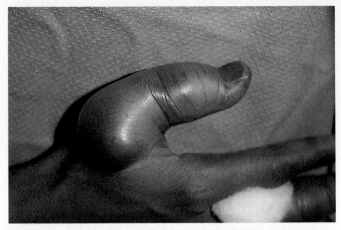

Fig 31–5
Deep second- and third-degree frostbite with hemorrhagic blebs, 1 day post-thaw.
(Courtesy of Dr. Murray P. Hamlet.)

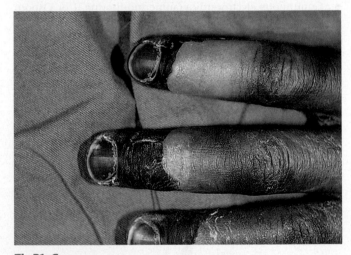

Fig 31–6
Fourth-degree frostbite, 4 weeks post-thaw. Note the sharp line of demarcation under the eschar, depigmentation of third-degree skin proximally, and indurated distal fingertips. The fingertips will autoamputate.
(Courtesy of Dr. Murray P. Hamlet.)

DIFFERENTIAL DIAGNOSIS

Other cold-induced injuries include the following:

- Frost nip: transient tingling and numbness without associated permanent tissue damage
- Pernio (chilblains): a self-limited, cold-induced vasculitis of dermal vessels associated with purple plaques or nodules, often affecting the dorsa of the hands and feet; seen with prolonged cold exposure to above-freezing temperatures
- Cold immersion (trench) foot: caused by ischemic injury resulting from sustained severe vasoconstriction in appendages exposed to wet cold at temperatures above freezing

WORKUP

- Wound and blood cultures in more severe cases.
- Technetium scintigraphy, MRI, and MR angiography (MRA) are the most promising modalities for assessment of tissue viability, but a delay of 5 days is required to distinguish the

level of débridement or amputation. (Some centers perform angiography within 24 hours and give thrombolytics to those with impaired blood flow.)

TREATMENT

- Remove constricting or wet clothing and gently insulate, immobilize, and elevate the affected area.
- Avoid thawing if there is any risk of refreezing.
- Never rub or massage the affected area. Avoid dry heat (e.g., fire, heater).
- If there is associated hypothermia, core temperature must first be stabilized with warmed, humidified oxygen, heated IV saline (45° to 65° C), and warming blankets before thawing frostbitten extremities.
- Immerse the affected area in circulating warm water bath with a mild antibacterial agent (e.g., hexachlorophene, povidone-iodine) maintained at 40° to 42° C for 15 to 30 minutes. Repeat until capillary refill returns and tissue is supple. Active motion during rewarming is advisable, but massage is not.
- IV narcotics for pain during thawing
- Continuous electrocardiographic monitoring. J or Osborn waves may be noted on the electrocardiogram (ECG; Fig. 31–7)
- Tetanus-diphtheria (Td) prophylaxis and topical antibiotics if potentially contaminated skin wound
- Streptococcal prophylaxis for 48 to 72 hours, with IV penicillin for severe cases
- Thrombolytic therapy looks promising. Multicenter trials are now underway.
- Dextran, anticoagulants, vasodilators, hyperbaric oxygen, reserpine, and sympathectomy are of unproven benefit.

C. ELECTRICAL AND LIGHTNING INJURY

DEFINITION

Electrical injuries are wounds caused by contact with an electrical current. Electrical injuries cause approximately 1000 deaths annually, with two thirds occurring in persons between 15 and 40 years of age. Lightning strikes (Fig. 31–8) kill on average 100 people annually.

PHYSICAL FINDINGS AND CLINICAL PRESENTATION

- Depending on the extent of injury, the patient may be unconscious, seizing, or confused and unable to present a history
- Extensive burns (about 10% to 25% of the body surface)
  - Located over the entry and exit sites (Fig. 31–9)
  - Most common entry sites are the hands and skull.
  - Most common exit sites are the heels.
  - "Kissing burns" over the flexor creases
  - Superficial partial-thickness burns
  - Oral burns in children
  - Bleeding from the labial artery may appear 7 to 10 days after the injury manifestations.

CAUSE

- Electricity causes tissue injury by converting electrical energy into heat.
- The higher the electrical voltage, the greater the tissue destruction.
- The longer the duration of contact with the electrical source, the greater the damage.
  - Direct current (DC) contact causes a single muscle contraction, throwing the patient away from the source.
  - Alternating current (AC) contact precipitates a tetanic contraction, not allowing the patient to withdraw from the

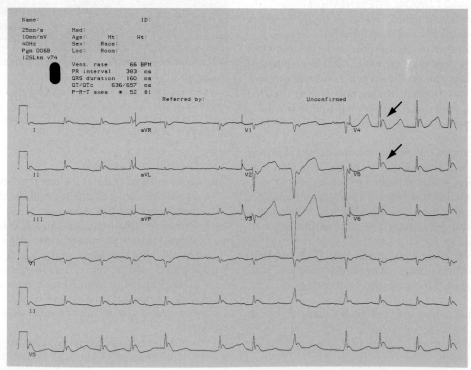

Fig 31–7

The J or Osborn wave of hypothermia.

(From Auerbach P: Wilderness Medicine, 4th ed. St. Louis, Mosby, 2001.)

source and prolonging the duration of contact. Therefore, AC contact is more harmful than DC contact.

- Electrical injuries are arbitrarily divided into high-voltage (1000 V) and low-voltage (500 V).
- The entry and exit paths through which the electrical current travels in the body determine which tissues are affected.

LABORATORY TESTS

- CBC
- Electrolytes
- BUN, creatinine
- Arterial blood gases
- Myoglobin
- Creatinine kinase, CPK, with isoenzyme fractionation
- Urinalysis, including screening for myoglobinuria
- LFTs
- Typing and cross-matching
- Electrocardiography

IMAGING STUDIES

- X-ray any suspicious area for bone fractures.
- Obtain CT scans of the head and skull in patients with major head injury.
- Technetium pyrophosphate scanning may locate areas of myonecrosis.

TREATMENT

- If present at the scene of the injury, make sure the power source is turned off before approaching the victim.
- Maintain urine output of at least 50 mL/hr with IV fluids.
- Cardiac monitoring
- Oxygen
- Tetanus prophylaxis
- Alkalinization of the urine is indicated for patients suspected of having myoglobinuria.
- Furosemide may be used to force diuresis.
- Mannitol assists in maintaining diuresis.
- Treat burns with sulfadiazine silver dressings.

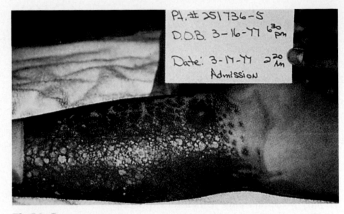

Fig 31–8
Punctate burns from lightning injury.
(Courtesy of Dr. Art Kahn.)

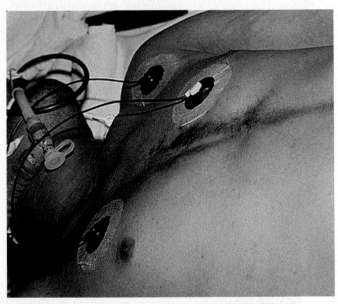

Fig 31–9
Linear burns from lightning Injury.
(From Auerbach P: Wilderness Medicine, 4th ed. St. Louis, Mosby, 2001.)

Chapter 32 Radiation dermatitis

- The clinical and pathologic features of cutaneous damage are variable and depend on the type of ionizing radiation, dosage, and individual sensitivity.
- Acute radiation dermatitis is characterized by redness, swelling, hair loss, blistering and, at times, ulceration (Fig. 32–1).
- The acute clinical effects of cutaneous radiation with UVB include erythema, edema, heat, pain, and pruritus.
- Chronic radiation dermatitis is insidious in onset and usually presents many years after exposure.
- The cutaneous manifestations include atrophy and scaling, variable hypo- and hyperpigmentation (poikiloderma), telangiectasia, and often alopecia (Fig. 32–2). It may be complicated by the development of various neoplasms (e.g., basal cell carcinoma, squamous cell carcinoma, melanoma).

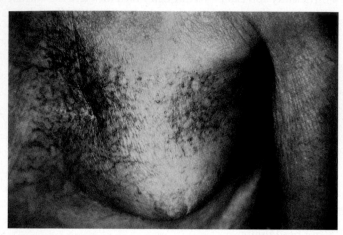

Fig 32–2
Radiation dermatitis. Note the chronic changes of atrophy, hypopigmentation, and telangiectasia-poikiloderma.
(Courtesy of Dr. A. Timothy, St. Thomas' Hospital, London.)

REFERENCES

Ferri F: Ferri's Clinical Advisor. St. Louis, Mosby, 2008.

Goldstein BG, Goldstein AO: Practical Dermatology, 2nd ed. St. Louis, Mosby, 1997.

Lebwohl MG, Heymann WR, Berth-Jones J, Coulson I (eds): Treatment of Skin Disease. St. Louis, 2002, Mosby, 2002.

McKee PH, Calonje E, Granter SR (eds): Pathology of the Skin With Clinical Correlations, 3rd ed. St. Louis, Mosby, 2005.

Swartz MH: Textbook of Physical Diagnosis, 5th ed. Philadelphia, WB Saunders, 2006.

White GM, Cox NH (eds): Diseases of the Skin: A Color Atlas and Text, 2nd ed. St. Louis, Mosby, 2006.

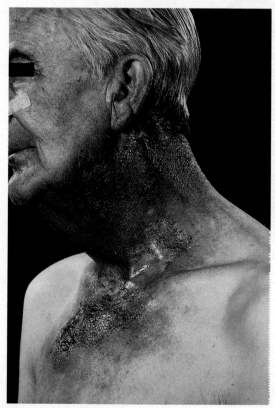

Fig 32–1
Radiation dermatitis. This patient shows severe radiation damage. Note the erythema, ulceration, and crusting. With the advent of modern techniques in radiotherapy, complications such as these are no longer seen.
(Courtesy of Dr. A. Timothy, MD, St. Thomas' Hospital, London.)

SECTION 2

Brain, Peripheral Nervous System, Muscle

Chapter 33: Normal anatomy
Chapter 34: Diagnostic tests and procedures
Chapter 35: Cerebrovascular disease
Chapter 36: Subclavian steal syndrome
Chapter 37: Subdural hematoma
Chapter 38: Brain neoplasms
Chapter 39: Dementia
Chapter 40: Movement disorders
Chapter 41: Developmental disorders of the spinal cord and brain
Chapter 42: Multiple sclerosis
Chapter 43: Amyotrophic lateral sclerosis
Chapter 44: Neuropathies

Chapter 45: Ataxias
Chapter 46: Infections
Chapter 47: Neurocutaneous syndromes
Chapter 48: Disorders of muscle and neuromuscular junction
Chapter 49: Bell's palsy
Chapter 50: Cerebral palsy
Chapter 51: Down syndrome
Chapter 52: Normal-pressure hydrocephalus
Chapter 53: Dandy-Walker malformation
Chapter 54: Neuroblastoma
Chapter 55: von Hippel-Lindau disease

- Figure 33–1 shows a midsagittal section of the brain revealing features of its major subdivisions.
- Figure 33–2 demonstrates an oblique frontal section and horizontal sections of the brain.
- The coverings of the brain are shown in Figure 33–3. The flow of cerebrospinal fluid is illustrated in Figure 33–4.
- Spinal nerves are shown in Figure 33–5 and their dermatome distribution is illustrated in Figure 33–6.

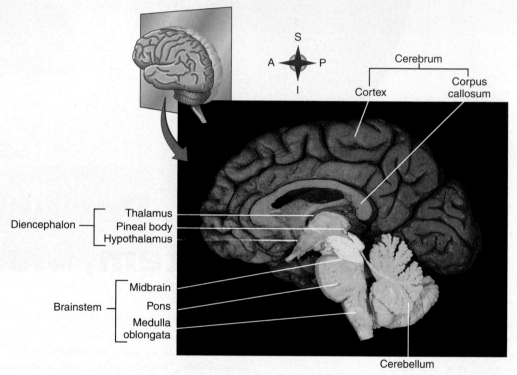

Fig 33–1
Divisions of the brain. A midsagittal section of the brain reveals features of its major divisions. A, anterior; I, inferior; P, posterior; S, superior.
(From Thibodeau GA, Patton KP: Anatomy and Physiology, 4th ed. St. Louis, Mosby, 1999.)

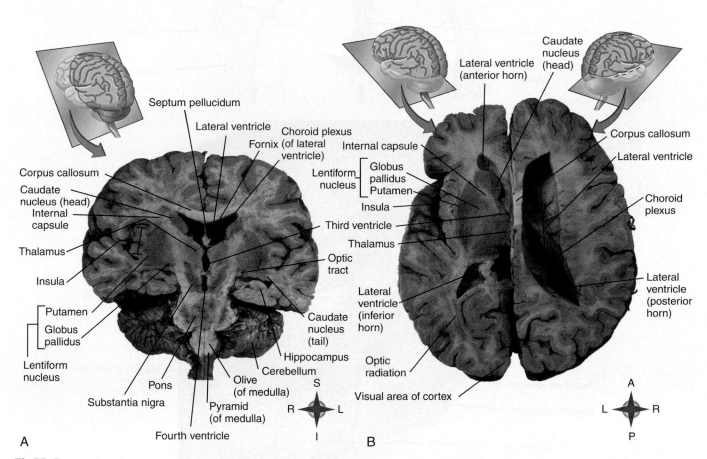

Fig 33–2

Human brain specimens. **A,** Oblique frontal section. **B,** Horizontal sections. The left section is slightly inferior to the right sections:
A, anterior; I, inferior; L, left; P, posterior; R, right; S, superior.
(From Thibodeau GA, Patton KP: Anatomy and Physiology, 4th ed. St. Louis, Mosby, 1999)

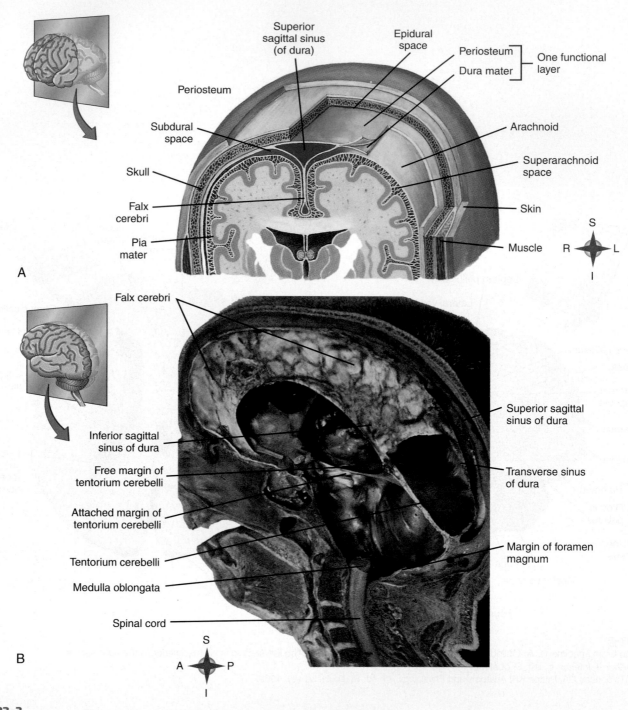

Fig 33-3
Coverings of the brain. **A**, Frontal section of the superior portion of the head, as viewed from the front. Both the bony and membranous coverings of the brain can be seen. **B**, Transverse section of the skull, viewed from below. The dura mater has been retained in this specimen to show how it lines the inner roof of the cranium and the falx cerebri extending inward. A, anterior; I, inferior; L, left; P, posterior; R, right; S, superior. (From Thibodeau GA, Patton KP: Anatomy and Physiology, 4th ed. St. Louis, Mosby, 1999.)

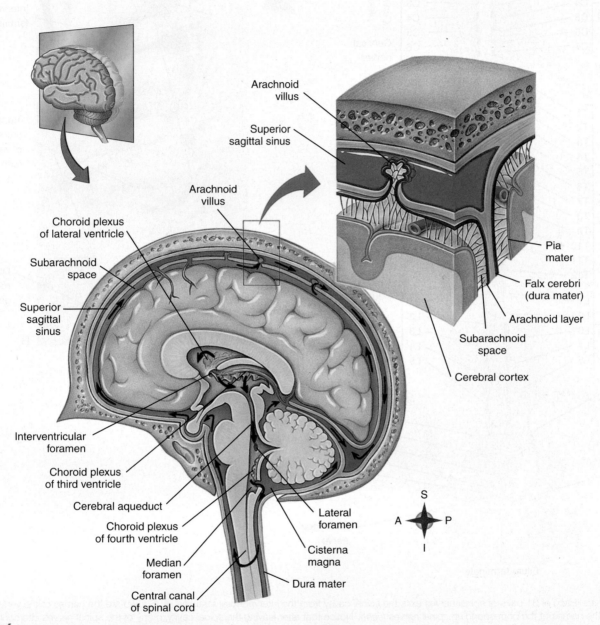

Arachnoid villus

Superior sagittal sinus

Arachnoid villus

Choroid plexus of lateral ventricle

Subarachnoid space

Superior sagittal sinus

Interventricular foramen

Choroid plexus of third ventricle

Cerebral aqueduct

Choroid plexus of fourth ventricle

Median foramen

Central canal of spinal cord

Lateral foramen

Cisterna magna

Dura mater

Pia mater

Falx cerebri (dura mater)

Arachnoid layer

Subarachnoid space

Cerebral cortex

S

A —◆— P

I

Fig 33-4
Flow of cerebrospinal fluid. The fluid produced by filtration of blood by the choroids plexus of each ventricle flows inferiorly through the lateral ventricles, interventricular foramen, third ventricle, cerebral aqueduct, fourth ventricle, and subarachnoid space and to the blood.
A, anterior; I, inferior; P, posterior; S, superior.
(From Thibodeau GA, Patton KP: Anatomy and Physiology, 4th ed. St. Louis, Mosby, 1999.)

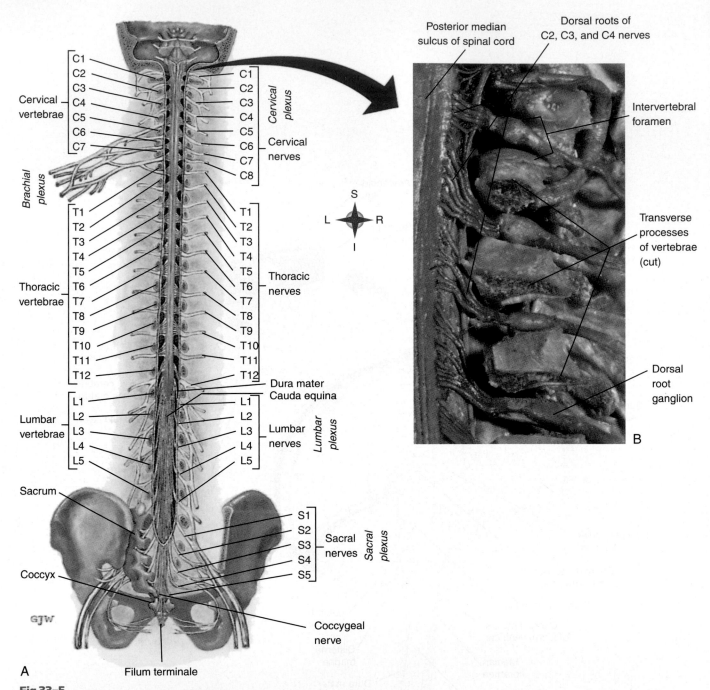

Fig 33–5

Spinal nerves. Each of 31 pairs of spinal nerves exits the spinal cavity from the intervertebral foramina. **A,** Shown are the names of the vertebrae *(left)* and the names of the corresponding spinal nerves *(right)*. Notice that after leaving the spinal cavity, many of the spinal nerves interconnect to form networks called plexuses. **B,** Dissection of the cervical region, showing a posterior view of cervical spinal nerves exiting the intervertebral foramina on the right side. I, inferior; L, left; R, right; S, superior.

(From Thibodeau GA, Patton KP: Anatomy and Physiology, 4th ed. St. Louis, Mosby, 1999.)

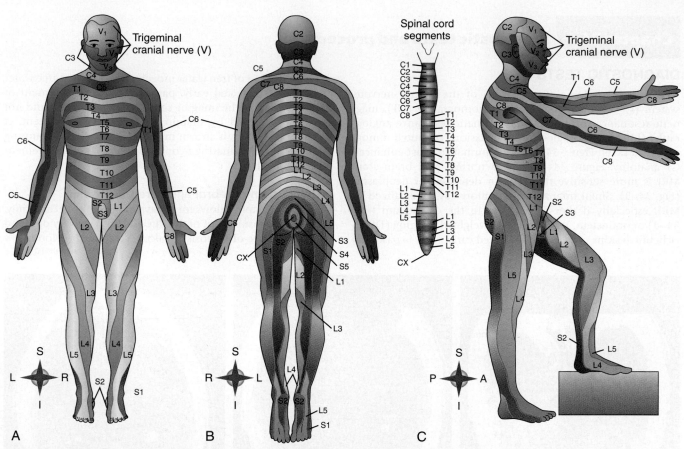

Fig 33–6
Dermatome distribution of spinal nerves. **A,** The front of the body's surface. **B,** The back of the body's surface. **C,** The side of the body's surface.
Inset, Segments of the spinal cord associated with each of the spinal nerves associated with the sensory dermatomes shown. A, anterior; I, inferior; P, posterior; S, superior.
(From Thibodeau GA, Patton KP: Anatomy and Physiology, 4th ed. St. Louis, Mosby, 1999.)

Chapter 34   Diagnostic tests and procedures

DIAGNOSTIC TESTS

Most neuroradiologic examinations of the central nervous system (CNS) consist of computed tomography (CT), magnetic resonance imaging (MRI), magnetic resonance angiography (MRA), and single-photon emission computed tomography (SPECT). Figure 34–1 shows normal contrast-enhanced CT anatomy. Figure 34–2 shows a normal MRI brain scan. MRI is more sensitive than CT for detection of neoplasms (Fig. 34–3). Small infarcts are also more easily visualized by MRI, especially if they are located in the cerebellum (Fig. 34–4) or brainstem. With diffusion-weighted imaging (DWI), ischemic lesions can be demonstrated early. DWI is based on the examination of free water movement. Restricted free water movement is detected early, paralleling the development of cytotoxic edema. The imaging sequences used are fast and not as easily disturbed by inappropriate patient movement. A normal SPECT scan is shown in Figure 34–5. SPECT scanning can be used for evaluating neoplasms (Fig. 34–6) and dementia (Fig. 34–7).

Imaging of precerebral and cerebral vessels

Duplex sonography allows for the evaluation of vessel anatomy, along with measurement of the direction and velocity of blood flow. The degree of stenosis is calculated from the blood flow

Text continued on page 172

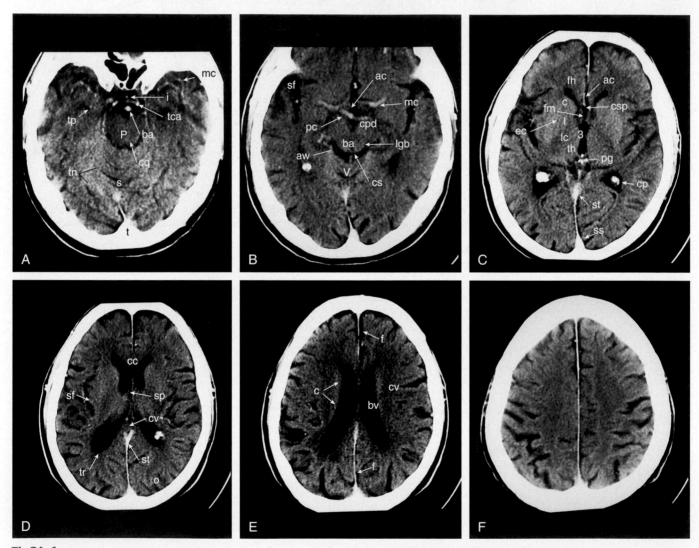

Fig 34–1

Normal contrast-enhanced CT anatomy. Figures **A** through **F** show normal CT scans at various levels in the brain. 3, 4, third and fourth ventricles; ac, anterior cerebral artery; ba, basilar artery; bv, body of lateral ventricle; c, caudate nucleus; cc, corpus callosum (genu); cp, cerebral peduncle; csp, cave of septum pellucidum; cv, internal cerebral vein; f, falx; fh, frontal horn of lateral ventricle; fm, foramen of Monro; i, infundibulum of pituitary; mc, middle cerebral artery; o, white matter tracts; p, pons; pc, posterior cerebral artery; pg, pineal gland; sf, sylvian fissure; sp, septum between lateral ventricles; th, thalamus; tp, temporal horn; tr, trigone of lateral ventricle.
(From Grainger RG, Allison DJ, Adam A, Dixon AK [eds]: Grainger and Allison's Diagnostic Radiology: A Textbook of Medical Imaging, 4th ed. London. Harcourt, 2001.)

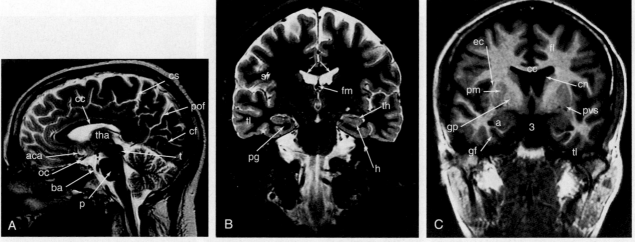

Fig 34–2
Normal MRI. **A,** T2-weighted sagittal images through the midline. **B,** Corneal T2-weighted images through the hippocampi. **C,** Coronal T1-weighted images through the level of the third ventricle. 3,4, third and fourth ventricles; a, amygdala; aca, anterior cerebral artery; ba, basilar artery; cc, corpus callosum; cf, calcarine fissure; ch, cerebellar hemisphere; cn, caudate nucleus; cs, central sulcus; ec, external capsule; fh, frontal horn; fh, frontal lobe; fm, foramen of Munro; gf, gyrus fusiformis; gp, globus pallidus; h, hippocampus; mca, middle cerebral artery; oc, optic chiasm; oh, occipital horn; p, pons; pg, parahippocampal gyrus; pm, putamen; pof, parieto-occipital fissure; pvs, perivascular spaces; sf, sylvian fissure; t, tectal plate; th, temporal horn; tha, thalamus; tl, temporal lobe.
(From Grainger RG, Allison DJ, Adam A, Dixon AK [eds]: Grainger and Allison's Diagnostic Radiology: A Textbook of Medical Imaging, 4th ed. London. Harcourt, 2001.)

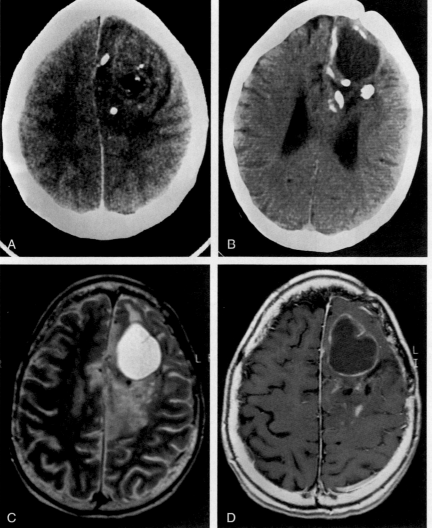

Fig 34–3
Oligodendroglioma. **A,** CT after intravenous contrast medium shows a large left frontal tumor that involves the cortex. It is predominantly solid with irregular enhancement, but there are also cysts and coarse calcification. **B,** Follow-up after 2 years with CT. T2-weighted MRI **(C)** and T1-weighted postcontrast MRI **(D)** show more extensive cyst formation and calcification than on the first scan. The calcification is much less apparent on MRI and appears as nonspecific low signal areas. Posterior infiltration of the tumor is, however, best seen on MRI **(C)**. Note that the patient had undergone a left frontal craniotomy after the first scan.
(From Grainger RG, Allison DJ, Adam A, Dixon AK [eds]: Grainger and Allison's Diagnostic Radiology: A Textbook of Medical Imaging, 4th ed. London. Harcourt, 2001.)

Section 2: Brain, peripheral nervous system, muscle

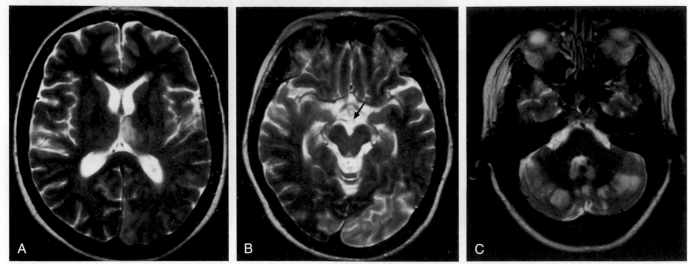

Fig 34–4
Top of the basilar syndrome. T2-weighted MRI show multiple infarcts in the basilar and posterior cerebral artery territories including the left thalamus **(A)**, both occipital lobes **(B)** and cerebellar hemispheres **(C)**. Note the absence of flow void in the distal basilar artery in **B** *(arrow)*. (From Grainger RG, Allison DJ, Adam A, Dixon AK [eds]: Grainger and Allison's Diagnostic Radiology: A Textbook of Medical Imaging, 4th ed. London. Harcourt, 2001.)

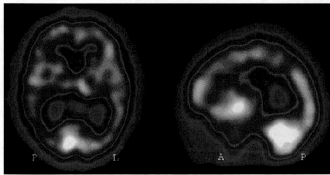

Fig 34–5
99mTcHMPAO single-photon emission computed tomography scan of the brain: axial *(left)* and sagittal *(right)* images. A, anterior; R, right; L, left; P, posterior.
(From Grainger RG, Allison DJ, Adam A, Dixon AK [eds]: Grainger and Allison's Diagnostic Radiology: A Textbook of Medical Imaging, 4th ed. London. Harcourt, 2001.)

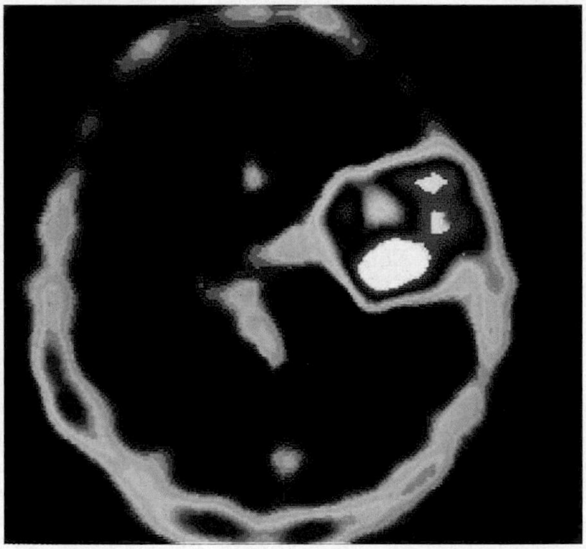

Fig 34–6
201Tl single-photon emission computed tomography scan in a 40-year-old man with a left frontotemporal mass on MRI. This reveals the high uptake typical of high-grade glioma, which was confirmed on biopsy to be a glioblastoma.
(Courtesy of Professor Donald M. Hadley, Glasgow.)

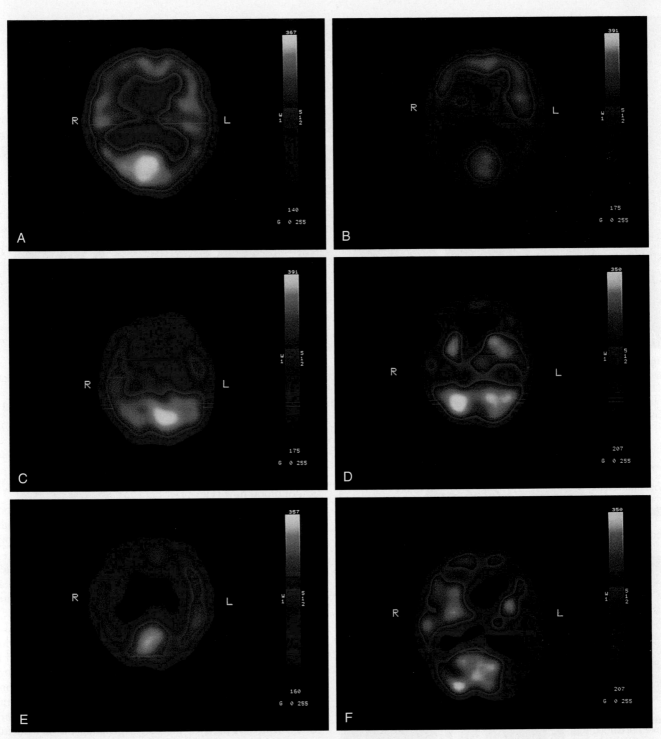

Fig 34–7
Single-photon emission computed tomography scans of normal subject **(A)**; patient with Alzheimer's disease showing bilateral parietal lobe abnormalities more marked on the right side **(B)**; patient with frontotemporal dementia, showing bilateral frontal lobe abnormalities **(C)**; patient with progressive supranuclear palsy, showing bilateral anterior abnormalities **(D)**; patient with corticobasal degeneration, showing asymmetrical right fronto-
parietal abnormality **(E)**; patient with Creutzfeldt-Jakob disease, showing multifocal cortical abnormalities **(F)**.
(From Tallis R, Fillit H: Brockelhursts's Textbook of Geriatric Medicine and Gerontology, 6th ed. London, Churchill Livingstone, 2003.)

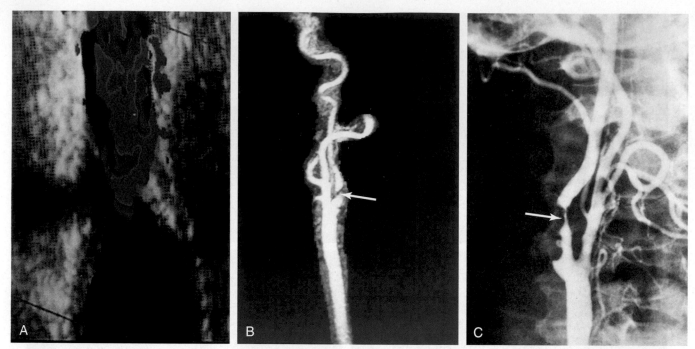

Fig 34–8

Imaging of precerebral and cerebral vessels. **A,** Color-coded Doppler sonography of the internal carotid artery close to the bifurcation in a patient with pronounced atherosclerotic changes and stenosis causing slowing of blood flow and turbulence (green and blue signals). **B,** Contrast-enhanced magnetic resonance angiography showing a tight stenosis of the internal carotid artery *(arrow)*. **C,** Conventional angiography showing a very tight stenosis of the internal carotid artery *(arrow)*.

(From Crawford, MH, DiMarco JP, Paulus WJ [eds]: Cardiology, 2nd ed. St. Louis, Mosby, 2004.)

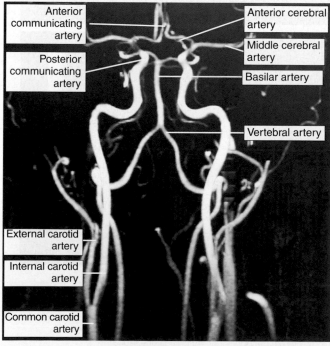

Fig 34–9

Magnetic resonance angiogram showing the arterial supply to the brain.

(From Crawford, MH, DiMarco JP, Paulus WJ [eds]: Cardiology, 2nd ed. St. Louis, Mosby, 2004.)

velocity. Color-coded Doppler signals help visualize the direction of blood flow (Fig. 34–8)

Conventional angiography (see Fig. 34–8C) allows good visualization of the aortic arch and the origins of the neck arteries but has a potential risk of nephrotoxicity, allergic reactions, and thromboembolism.

MRA (Fig. 34–9) is useful for detection of carotid artery stenosis (see Fig. 34–8B) and suspected carotid or vertebral artery dissection. MRA is also useful for evaluating the aortic arch (Fig. 34–10) and the intracranial circulation (Fig. 34–11).

ELECTROENCEPHALOGRAPHY

Electroencephalography (EEG) is a measure of the electrical activity generated by the central nervous system. It is useful to document abnormalities of the brain that are not associated with detectable structural alterations in brain tissue. It also provides a continuous measure of cerebral function over time. Electroencephalographic signals are generated by the cerebral cortex. Different parts of the cortex generate distinct fluctuations. The fluctuations also differ with eye opening and in the sleep and waking states. Figure 34–12 shows an electroencephalogram of a normal subject; an electroencephalogram of a brain-dead patient is shown in Figure 34–13.

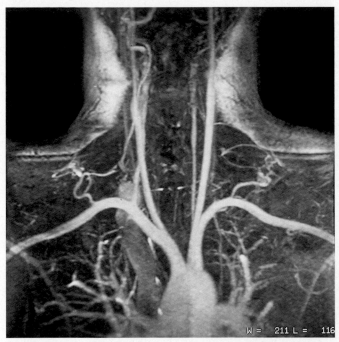

Fig 34–10
Contrast-enhanced MRA of aortic arch. A three-dimensional gradient-echo sequence has been acquired during the first pass of an intravenously injected gadolinium bolus. It shows the origins of the great vessels. Note also that there is background opacification of the pulmonary vessels.
(From Grainger RG, Allison DJ, Adam A, Dixon AK [eds]: Grainger and Allison's Diagnostic Radiology: A Textbook of Medical Imaging, 4th ed. London. Harcourt, 2001.)

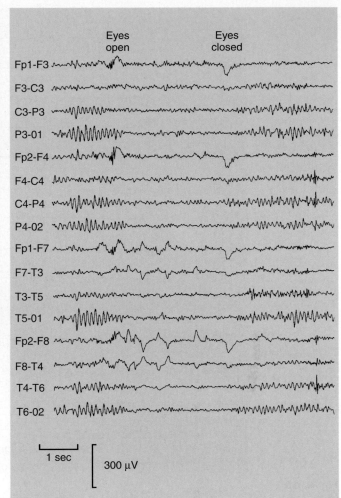

Fig 34–12
A posteriorly predominant 9-Hz alpha rhythm is present when the eyes are closed and is attenuated by eye opening in the electroencephalogram of this normal subject. Electrode placements in this and Figure 34-13 are as follows. A, earlobe; C, central; F, frontal; Fp, frontopolar; O, occipital; P, parietal; Sp, sphenoid; T, temporal. Right-sided placements are indicated by even numbers and left-sided placements by odd numbers.
(From Goetz CG, Pappert EJ: Textbook of Clinical Neurology, Philadelphia, WB Saunders, 1999)

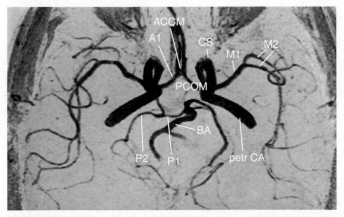

Fig 34–11
Three-dimensional TOF MRA of the intracranial circulation, axially collapsed maximum intensity projection. A1, precommunicating segment of anterior cerebral artery; ACOM, anterior communicating artery; BA, basilar artery; CS, carotid siphon; M1, first (horizontal) segment of middle cerebral artery; M2, M2 segments of middle cerebral artery; P1, precommunicating segment of posterior cerebral artery; P2, P2 segment of posterior cerebral artery; PCOM, posterior communicating artery; petr CA, petrous segment of internal carotid artery.
(From Grainger RG, Allison DJ, Adam A, Dixon AK [eds]: Grainger and Allison's Diagnostic Radiology: A Textbook of Medical Imaging, 4th ed. London. Harcourt, 2001.)

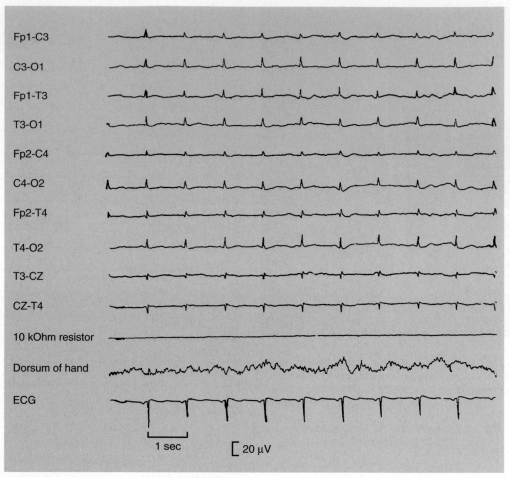

Fig 34–13
Electrocerebral silence in the electroencephalogram of a brain-dead patient following attempted resuscitation after cardiopulmonary arrest.
See Figure 34-12 for electrode placements.
(From Goetz CG, Pappert EJ: Textbook of Clinical Neurology. Philadelphia, WB Saunders, 1999.)

| Chapter 35 | **Cerebrovascular disease** |

A. TRANSIENT ISCHEMIC ATTACK

DEFINITION

Transient ischemic attack (TIA) refers to a transient neurologic dysfunction caused by focal brain or retinal ischemia, with symptoms typically lasting less than 60 minutes but always less than 24 hours. It is followed by a full recovery of function.

PHYSICAL FINDINGS AND CLINICAL PRESENTATION

- During an episode, neurologic abnormalities are confined to discrete vascular territory.
- Typical carotid artery symptoms (Box 35–1) are ipsilateral monocular visual disturbance, contralateral homonymous hemianopsia, contralateral hemimotor or sensory dysfunction, and language dysfunction (dominant hemisphere), alone or in combination.
- Typical vertebrobasilar artery symptoms (Box 35–2) are binocular visual disturbance, vertigo, diplopia, dysphagia, dysarthria, and motor or sensory dysfunction involving the ipsilateral face and contralateral body.

CAUSE

- Cardioembolic
- Large-vessel atherothrombotic disease
- Lacunar disease
- Hypoperfusion with fixed arterial stenosis
- Hypercoagulable states

DIFFERENTIAL DIAGNOSIS

- Hypoglycemia
- Seizures
- Anxiety, panic disorder
- Migraine
- Subdural hemorrhage
- Mass lesions
- Vestibular disease

LABORATORY TESTS

- Complete blood count (CBC) with platelets
- Prothrombin time (PT; international normalized ratio [INR]) and partial thromboplastin time (PTT)
- Glucose
- Lipid profile
- Erythrocyte sedimentation rate (ESR; if clinical suspicion for infectious or inflammatory process)
- Urinalysis
- Chest x-ray
- Electrocardiography (ECG); consider cardiac enzymes
- Other tests as dictated by suspected cause

IMAGING STUDIES

- Head CT scan to exclude hemorrhage including a subdural hemorrhage is often performed as the initial diagnostic imaging modality; however, it is not as sensitive as MRI.
- MRI and MRA. In several studies, MRI with diffusion-weighted imaging has identified early ischemic brain injury in up to 50% of patients with a TIA. MRA of the brain and neck can identify large-vessel intracranial and extracranial stenoses (Fig. 35–1), arteriovenous malformations, and aneurysms

---

Box 35–1 Characteristics of carotid artery syndrome

1. Ipsilateral monocular vision loss (amaurosis fugax)—the patient often feels as if "a shade" has come down over one eye.
2. Episodic contralateral arm, leg, and face paresis and paresthesias
3. Slurred speech, transient aphasia
4. Ipsilateral headache of vascular type
5. Carotid bruit may be present over the carotid bifurcation
6. Microemboli, hemorrhages, and exudates may be noted in the ipsilateral retina

Ferri F: Practical Guide to the Care of the Medical Patient, 7th ed. St. Louis, Mosby, 2007.

Box 35–2 Characteristics of vertebrobasilar artery syndrome

1. Binocular visual disturbances (blurred vision, diplopia, total blindness)
2. Vertigo, nausea, vomiting, tinnitus
3. Sudden loss of postural tone of all four extremities (drop attacks) with no loss of consciousness
4. Slurred speech, ataxia, numbness around lips or face

Ferri F: Practical Guide to the Care of the Medical Patient, 7th ed. St. Louis, Mosby, 2007.

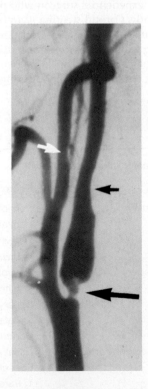

Fig 35–1
Irregular high-grade atheromatous stenosis at the origin of the internal carotid artery *(large arrow)*. Shallow atheromatous plaques are seen on the internal *(black arrow)* and external *(white arrow)* carotid arteries. (From Grainger RG, Allison DJ, Adam A, Dixon AK [eds]: Grainger and Allison's Diagnostic Radiology: A Textbook of Medical Imaging, 4th ed. London. Harcourt, 2001.)

- Carotid Doppler studies identify carotid stenosis
- Echocardiography if cardiac source is suspected
- Telemetry for hospitalized patients for at least 24 hours; may consider 24-hour Holter monitoring or event monitor post discharge if arrhythmia is suspected as cause of TIA
- Four-vessel cerebral angiogram if considering carotid endarterectomy or carotid stent

TREATMENT

- Depends on cause
- If the time of the onset of symptoms is clear, there are significant deficits on neurologic examination, and brain hemorrhage has been ruled out, then the patient may be a candidate for thrombolytic therapy, but this option should be discussed with a neurologist or specialist in cerebrovascular disease.
- Acute anticoagulation: no data supporting benefits in the acute setting. Heparin is considered for new-onset atrial fibrillation and atherothrombotic carotid disease causing recurrent transient neurologic symptoms, especially in the setting before carotid endarterectomy or carotid stenting. Also, consider basilar artery thrombosis, given concern for progression to brainstem stroke, with high morbidity and mortality.
- First-line treatment has traditionally been aspirin (81 mg/day). Other options include combination of extended-release dipyridamole and immediate-release aspirin (Aggrenox) or clopidogrel.
- Carotid endarterectomy for carotid artery TIA associated with an ipsilateral stenosis of 70% to 99%: surgery should be done by an experienced surgeon who performs this procedure frequently. Carotid stenting is an option in patients who are not surgical candidates. Trials are underway comparing stenting with surgery for carotid disease.
- Modification of risk factors, including smoking cessation, blood pressure control, and lipid lowering

B. STROKE

DEFINITION

Stroke describes acute brain injury caused by decreased blood supply or hemorrhage.

PHYSICAL FINDINGS AND CLINICAL PRESENTATION

- Motor, sensory, or cognitive deficits, or a combination, depending on distribution and extent of involved vascular arteries (Table 35–1)
- More common manifestations include contralateral motor weakness or sensory loss, as well as language difficulties (aphasia; predominantly left-sided lesions) and visuospatial neglect phenomena (predominantly right-sided lesions).
- Onset is usually sudden; however, this depends on the specific cause.
- Characteristics of cerebral thrombosis and embolism are described in Table 35–2.

CAUSE

- Of all strokes, 70% to 80% are caused by ischemic infarcts; 20% to 30% are hemorrhagic.
- Ischemic infarcts: 80% are caused by occlusion of large or small vessels because of atherosclerotic vascular disease (caused by hypertension, hyperlipidemia, diabetes, tobacco abuse), 15% are caused by cardiac embolism, and 5% are from other causes, including hypercoagulable states and vasculitis.
- Small-vessel occlusion is most often caused by lipohyalinosis precipitated by chronic hypertension.

DIFFERENTIAL DIAGNOSIS

- TIA, traditionally defined as focal neurologic deficits lasting less than 24 hours (usually lasting less than 60 minutes)
- Migraine, seizure, mass lesion

WORKUP

- Thorough history and physical examination, including detailed neurologic and cardiovascular evaluations to identify

TABLE 35–1 Select stroke syndromes	
Artery Involved	**Neurologic Deficit**
Middle cerebral artery	Hemiplegia (upper extremity and face are usually more involved than lower extremities)
	Hemianesthesia (hemisensory loss)
	Hemianopia (homonymous)
	Aphasia (if dominant hemisphere is involved)
Anterior cerebral artery	Hemiplegia (lower extremities more involved than upper extremities and face)
	Primitive reflexes (e.g., grasp and suck)
	Urinary incontinence
Vertebral and basilar	Ipsilateral cranial nerve findings, cerebellar artery findings
	Contralateral (or bilateral) sensory or motor deficits
Deep penetrating cerebral arteries	Usually seen in major hypertensive branches of older patients and diabetics
	Four characteristic syndromes (lacunar infarction) are possible:
	1. Pure motor hemiplegia (66%)
	2. Dysarthria—clumsy hand syndrome (20%)
	3. Pure sensory stroke (10%)
	4. Ataxic hemiplegia syndrome with pyramidal tract signs

Ferri F: Practical Guide to the Care of the Medical Patient, 7th ed. St. Louis, Mosby, 2007.

vascular territory and likely cause. Infectious, toxic, and metabolic causes should be excluded because each may cause clinical deterioration of old stroke symptoms.

- Cardiac: mandatory ECG, telemetry; serial cardiac enzymes, transthoracic and/or transesophageal echocardiography, Holter monitor or event monitor (should be seriously considered, especially in the setting of suspected embolic cause). Carotid Doppler should be performed in cases of embolic stroke to the anterior or middle cerebral artery region.

LABORATORY TESTS

- CBC, platelets, PT (INR), PTT, blood urea nitrogen (BUN), creatinine, glucose, electrolytes, urinalysis
- Additional tests, depending on suspected cause (e.g., coagulopathies in younger patients)

IMAGING STUDIES (FIG. 35–2)

- CT scan without contrast to distinguish hemorrhage (Fig. 35–3) from infarct (Fig. 35–4)

- MRI (Fig. 35–5) is superior to CT for identifying abnormalities in the posterior fossa and, in particular, lacunar (small-vessel) infarcts. DWI (Fig. 35–6) is best to determine hyperacute ischemia (positive within 15 to 30 minutes of symptom onset). MRA is recommended to help identify vascular pathology (e.g., extent of intracranial atherosclerosis or vascular distribution of ischemia)
- In select cases (e.g., hemorrhagic stroke), conventional angiography may identify aneurysms or other vascular malformations (Fig. 35–7).

TREATMENT

- Depends on several factors, including cause, vascular territory involved, risk factors, and elapsed time from symptom onset to arrival at hospital
- To prevent pulmonary emboli post stroke above-the-knee elastic stockings, pneumatic boots, or SC heparin if nonhemorrhagic cause and patient is immobile in bed

TABLE 35–2 **Characteristics of cerebral thrombosis and embolism**

Parameter	Thrombosis	Embolism
Onset of symptoms	Progression of symptoms over hours to days	Very rapid (seconds)
History of previous transient ischemic attack	Common	Uncommon
Time of presentation	Often, during night hours while patient is sleeping	Patient is usually awake, involved in some type of activity
	Typically, patient awakes with a slight neurologic deficit that gradually progresses in a stepwise fashion	
Predisposing factors	Atherosclerosis, hypertension, diabetes, arteritis, vasculitis, hypotension, trauma to head and neck	Atrial fibrillation, mitral stenosis and regurgitation, endocarditis, mitral valve prolapse

Ferri F: Practical Guide to the Care of the Medical Patient, 7th ed. St. Louis, Mosby, 2007.

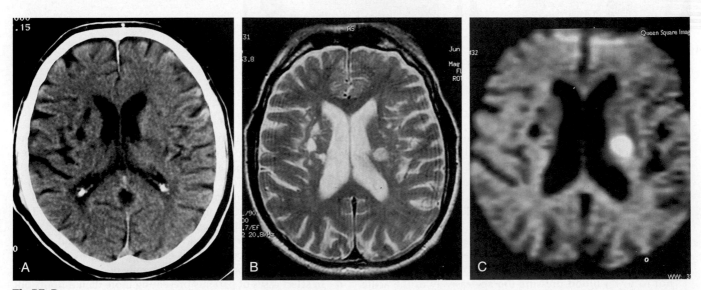

Fig 35–2

Acute lacunar infarct and small-vessel disease. **A,** CT and **B,** T2-weighted MRI show multiple low-density, high-signal foci in both hemispheres. The diffusion-weighted image **(C)** shows restricted diffusion in the left striatum, which appears as bright and unrestricted diffusion in the other lesions. This indicates that the former is acute and the latter are old.

(From Grainger RG, Allison DJ, Adam A, Dixon AK [eds]: Grainger and Allison's Diagnostic Radiology: A Textbook of Medical Imaging, 4th ed. London. Harcourt, 2001.)

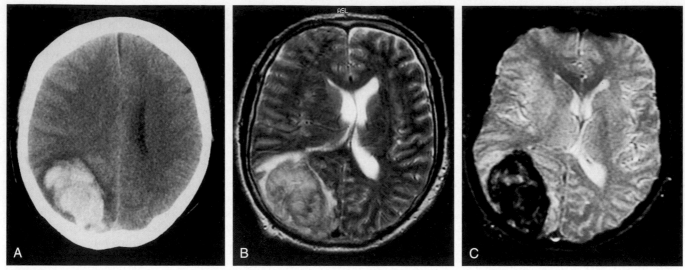

Fig 35–3
Intracranial hemorrhage in a thrombocytopenic patient. **A,** Unenhanced CT scan. **B,** T2-weighted fast spin-echo sequence (FSE). **C,** T2*-weighted gradient-echo sequence (GRE). On CT **(A)**, the high-attenuation occipitoparietal hematoma is surrounded by a low-attenuation rim, indicating clot retraction. The hematoma is of mixed signal intensity on the T2 FSE sequence **(B)** and could be mistaken for another mass lesion. It is, however, of characteristically low signal on the T2*-weighted GRE **(C)**, which is more sensitive for the detection of hemorrhage.
(From Grainger RG, Allison DJ, Adam A, Dixon AK [eds]: Grainger and Allison's Diagnostic Radiology: A Textbook of Medical Imaging, 4th ed. London. Harcourt, 2001.)

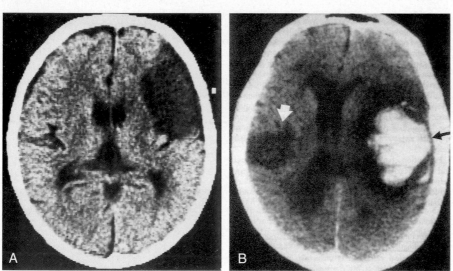

Fig 35–4
Embolic stroke. **A,** CT scan showing a large cortical infarct in the middle cerebral artery in a patient with atrial fibrillation. **B,** Embolic brain infarct in the right hemisphere *(white arrow)* treated with heparin, which has caused an intracerebral hemorrhage in the contralateral hemisphere *(black arrow)*.
(From Crawford, MH, DiMarco JP, Paulus WJ [eds]: Cardiology, 2nd ed. St. Louis, Mosby, 2004.)

- Carotid endarterectomy (CEA) is recommended for patients with carotid territory stroke associated with 70% to 99% ipsilateral carotid stenosis, performed by an experienced surgeon who has demonstrated low morbidity and mortality results.
- Modification of risk factors (e.g., smoking cessation, exercise, diet).
- Judicious control of blood pressure. Patients with chronic hypertension may extend the area of infarction if the blood pressure is lowered into the normal range. It is best not to lower blood pressure too aggressively in the acute setting unless it is markedly elevated. Adequate hydration and bed rest (e.g., head of bed down in pressure dependent ischemia vs. head of bed up if patient is an aspiration risk). Adequate glycemic control is also recommended (e.g., sliding scale insulin).

- In patients presenting less than 3 hours after onset of a non-hemorrhagic stroke—thrombolytic therapy in a specialized stroke center is beneficial in select populations.
- If atrial fibrillation, cardiac mural thrombus (or both) is found on echocardiography, heparin may be considered.
- If a subarachnoid or intracerebral hemorrhage is found on CT, MRA or cerebral angiography, or both, may be indicated to identify aneurysm. If no aneurysm is found and the clot is expanding, neurosurgical evacuation of the clot may be attempted, but outcomes are generally poor.
- In select cases of patients presenting more than 3 hours but less than 6 hours after the stroke, an interventional neuroradiologist or neurosurgeon may be able to offer direct injection of a clot-busting agent (e.g., intra-arterial tissue-type plasminogen activator, t-PA) or direct extraction of the clot (e.g., U.S. Food and Drug Administration [FDA]–approved

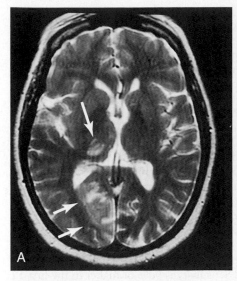

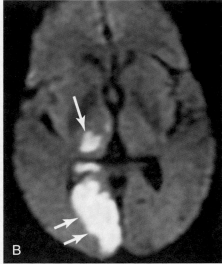

Fig 35–5
Acute right posterior cerebral artery infarct.
A, The T2-weighted fast spin-echo sequence (FSE) shows high signal in the right thalamus *(arrow)* and occipital lobe *(double arrows)*.
B, The changes are much more striking on the diffusion-weighted image, which shows a higher lesion-to-background contrast. The diffusion is restricted in the acutely infarcted tissue and appears bright.
(From Grainger RG, Allison DJ, Adam A, Dixon AK [eds]: Grainger and Allison's Diagnostic Radiology: A Textbook of Medical Imaging, 4th ed. London. Harcourt, 2001.)

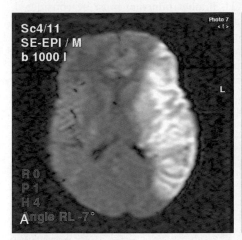

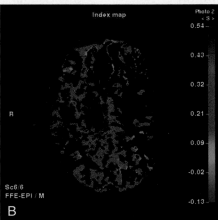

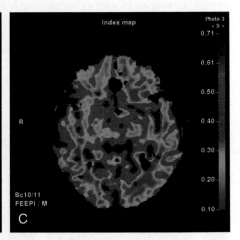

Fig 35–6
Diffusion and perfusion imaging in acute ischemic stroke. **A,** Diffusion image of a large left middle cerebral infarct. **B,** Index regional cerebral blood flow (rCBF) in the same patient showing a large nonperfused area on the left. Perfusion is also compromised in the contralateral hemisphere (diaschisis). **C,** Normal index rCBF for comparison. The patient underwent a left-sided craniectomy, resulting in restored perfusion on the right (not shown).
(From Crawford, MH, DiMarco JP, Paulus WJ [eds]: Cardiology, 2nd ed. St. Louis, Mosby, 2004.)

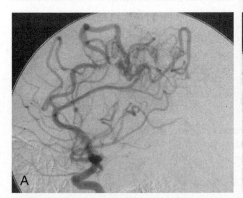

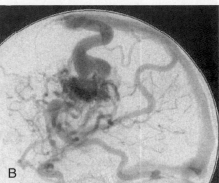

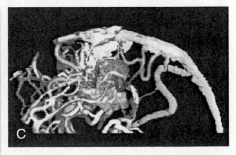

Fig 35–7
Cerebral arteriovenuous malformation (AVM). Shown are arterial **(A)** and venous **(B)** phases of digital subtraction angiography in a patient with a cerebral AVM. The AVM is fed by branches of the anterior and middle cerebral arteries and the venous drainage is predominantly superficial into the superior sagittal and transverse sinuses. **C,** Three-dimensional surface-shaded reconstruction of a CT angiogram in the same patient.
(Courtesy of Dr. Moore, National Hospital, Queen Square, England.)

Merci Retrieval System). However, this remains investigational and has yet to be well studied in the setting of a controlled trial. Intracranial angioplasty/stenting may also be a consideration.

- Antiplatelet therapy (aspirin, dipyridamole-aspirin, clopidogrel, or ticlopidine) reduces the risk of subsequent stroke.
- If patient presents with first TIA or stroke and was not on a prior antiplatelet agent, aspirin (325 mg vs. 81 mg each day) is usually chosen initially. If a TIA occurs while on aspirin, the patient should be switched to dipyridamole-aspirin.
- Warfarin is usually reserved for patients with cardioembolic stroke, as well as for patients with atrial fibrillation.

C. SUBARACHNOID HEMORRHAGE

DEFINITION

Subarachnoid hemorrhage (SAH) is the presence of active bleeding into the subarachnoid space, usually secondary to a spontaneous ruptured aneurysm or after head trauma.

PHYSICAL FINDINGS AND CLINICAL PRESENTATION

- Patients typically present with sudden onset of a severe headache, with maximal intensity at onset. Additional findings may include nuchal rigidity, nausea, and vomiting.
- Transient loss of consciousness occurs in 45% of patients.
- Focal neurologic deficits may be present.
- Funduscopic examination may reveal subhyaloid hemorrhage.

CAUSE

- Key distinction is aneurysmal (nontraumatic cause in more than 60% of cases, most commonly after rupture of saccular "berry" aneurysms) versus nonaneurysmal (traumatic) SAH
- Others: arteriovenous malformation (AVM), angioma, fusiform or mycotic aneurysm, dissecting and tumor-related aneurysms

DIFFERENTIAL DIAGNOSIS

- Intraparenchymal hemorrhage (see Fig. 35–3)
- Subarachnoid extension of an extracranial arterial dissection or intracerebral hemorrhage
- Meningoencephalitis (e.g., hemorrhagic meningoencephalitis caused by herpes simplex virus, HSV [see Fig. 46–11])
- Headache associated with sexual activity (e.g., coital or postcoital headache; usually acute onset of severe headache around time of orgasm)

WORKUP

- CT scanning (Fig. 35–8) is the initial test of choice, no contrast is necessary. Sensitivity is 90% or higher in the first 12 to 24 hours. If CT is negative and there is a high clinical suspicion for SAH, lumbar puncture must be considered, because there is an approximately 7% (or 1 in 14) chance of having a SAH. Spinal fluid is considered positive if there is xanthochromia and if there is a constant amount of red cells in each lumbar puncture (LP) tube. LP performed less than 12 hours after onset of headache may be falsely negative for xanthochromia.
- Electrocardiography (ECG): nonspecific ST and T wave changes, "cerebral T waves."

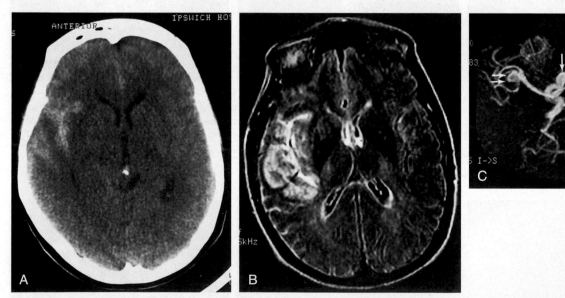

Fig 35–8
Subarachnoid hemorrhage. **A,** CT scan shows blood in the right sylvian fissure and in the interhemispheric fissure. **B,** This appears as high signal intensity on the fluid-attenuated inversion recovery (FLAIR) MRI, as opposed to the normal cerebrospinal fluid, which appears dark. **C,** A three-dimensional TOF MR angiogram shows a right middle cerebral artery aneurysm *(double arrows)*, which has bled, and an incidental ophthalmic artery aneurysm *(single arrow)*; both were confirmed with digital subtraction angiography.
(From Grainger RG, Allison DJ, Adam A, Dixon AK [eds]: Grainger and Allison's Diagnostic Radiology: A Textbook of Medical Imaging, 4th ed. London. Harcourt, 2001.)

LABORATORY TESTS

- PT (INR), PTT, platelet count at a minimum for clotting abnormality

IMAGING STUDIES

- CT scan followed by cerebral angiography if hemorrhage is confirmed
- May also use transcranial Doppler (TCD) as a baseline later to assess more adequately for vasospasm

TREATMENT

- Intubation as necessary
- Bed rest, isotonic fluids
- Short-acting analgesics (e.g., morphine 1 to 4 mg IV) and sedation (e.g., midazolam 1 to 5 mg IV); avoid oversedation and watch neurologic examination closely.
- Seizure prophylaxis controversial (consider phenytoin)
- Vasospasm prophylaxis (nimodipine)
- Blood pressure (BP) control; lower BP for unprotected aneurysms versus higher BP if protected (postcoiling, clipping)
- Stool softeners

- Neurosurgical or interventional neuroradiologic referral mandatory if aneurysm or AVM demonstrated by angiography; also, invasive intracranial pressure (ICP) monitoring, ventriculostomy may be required on an emergent basis (e.g., deteriorating level of consciousness, development of hydrocephalus); elevated ICP is associated with a worse patient outcome, particularly if ICP does not respond to treatment.
- Hypertonic saline (HS) solutions can be used in various concentrations (e.g., 7.5%, 10%, 23.5%) to treat elevated ICP and augment cerebral blood flow (CBF).
- Vasospasm occurs in 20% to 30% of patients and peaks at about 1 week; monitor closely for this. Consider TCD monitoring in high-risk patients. Triple-H therapy for prevention of vasospasm includes hemodilution, hypertension (consider pressors), and hypervolemia. Intra-arterial papaverine, balloon angioplasty, or both may be necessary in some cases.

Chapter 36   Subclavian steal syndrome

DEFINITION

Subclavian steal syndrome is an occlusion or severe stenosis of the proximal subclavian artery, leading to decreased antegrade flow or retrograde flow in the ipsilateral vertebral artery and neurologic symptoms referable to the posterior circulation.

PHYSICAL FINDINGS AND CLINICAL PRESENTATION

Symptoms

- Many patients are asymptomatic.
- Upper extremity ischemic symptoms: fatigue, exercise-related aching, coolness, numbness of the involved upper extremity
- Neurologic symptoms are reported by 25% of patients with known unilateral subclavian steal. These include brief spells of vertigo, diplopia, decreased vision, oscillopsia, and gait unsteadiness. These spells are only occasionally provoked by exercising the ischemic upper extremity (classic subclavian steal). Left subclavian steal is more common than right, but the latter is more serious.
- Posterior circulation stroke related to subclavian steal is rare.
- Innominate artery stenosis can cause decreased right carotid artery flow and cerebrovascular symptoms of the anterior cerebral circulation, but this is uncommon.

Physical findings

- Delayed and smaller volume pulse (wrist or antecubital) in the affected upper extremity
- Lower blood pressure in the affected upper extremity
- Supraclavicular bruit

Note: Inflating a blood pressure cuff will increase the bruit if it originates from a vertebral artery stenosis and decrease the bruit if it originates from a subclavian artery stenosis.

CAUSE AND PATHOGENESIS

Cause

- Atherosclerosis
- Arteritis (Takayasu's disease and temporal arteritis)
- Embolism to the subclavian or innominate artery
- Cervical rib
- Chronic use of a crutch
- Occupational (e.g., baseball pitchers, cricket bowlers)

Pathogenesis

The vertebral artery originates from the subclavian artery. For subclavian steal to occur, the occlusion must be proximal to the takeoff of the vertebral artery. On the right side, only a small distance separates the bifurcation of the innominate artery and the takeoff of the vertebral artery, explaining why the condition occurs less commonly on the right side. Occlusion of the innominate artery must affect right carotid artery flow.

DIFFERENTIAL DIAGNOSIS

- Posterior circulation TIA (and stroke)
- Upper extremity ischemia: distal subclavian artery stenosis or occlusion, Raynaud's syndrome, thoracic outlet syndrome

DIAGNOSTIC IMAGING

- Noninvasive upper extremity arterial flow studies
- Doppler sonography of the vertebral, subclavian, and innominate arteries
- Arteriography (Fig. 36–1)

TREATMENT

- In most patients, the disease is benign and requires no treatment other than atherosclerosis risk factor modification and aspirin. Symptoms tend to improve over time as collateral circulation develops.
- Vascular surgical reconstruction requires a thoracotomy; it may be indicated for innominate artery stenosis or when upper extremity ischemia is incapacitating.

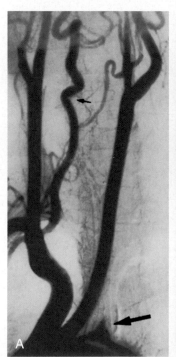 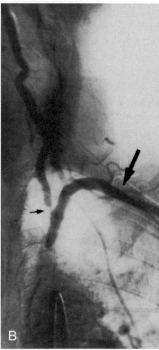

Fig 36–1

Subclavian steal, arch aortogram. **A,** Left anterior oblique projection, arterial phase, showing proximal occlusion of the left subclavian artery *(arrow)*. Note irregularity and tortuosity of the right vertebral artery, related to degenerative changes in the cervical vertebrae *(small arrow)*. **B,** Right anterior oblique projection, late phase of aortogram. The distal segment of the left subclavian artery *(arrow)* fills via retrograde flow in the left vertebral artery, despite this vessel being almost completely obstructed at its origin *(small arrow)*.
(From Grainger RG, Allison DJ, Adam A, Dixon AK [eds]: Grainger and Allison's Diagnostic Radiology: A Textbook of Medical Imaging, 4th ed. London. Harcourt, 2001.)

DEFINITION

A subdural hematoma is bleeding into the subdural space caused by rupture of bridging veins between the brain and venous sinuses.

PHYSICAL FINDINGS AND CLINICAL PRESENTATION

- Vague headache, often worse in morning than evening
- Some apathy, confusion, and clouding of consciousness are common, although frank coma may complicate late cases. Chronic subdural hematomas may cause a dementia-like clinical picture.
- Neurologic symptoms may be transient, simulating TIA.
- Almost any sign of cortical dysfunction may occur, including hemiparesis, sensory deficits, or language abnormalities, depending on which part of the cortex is compressed by the hematoma.
- New-onset seizures should raise the index of suspicion.

CAUSE

- Traumatic rupture of cortical bridging veins, especially where stretched by underlying cerebral atrophy

DIFFERENTIAL DIAGNOSIS

- Epidural hematoma
- Subarachnoid hemorrhage (see Fig. 35–8)
- Mass lesion (e.g., tumor) (see Fig. 38–1)
- Ischemic stroke (see Fig. 35–5)
- Intraparenchymal hemorrhage (see Fig. 35–3)

WORKUP

- CT scan is sensitive for diagnosis and should be performed in a timely fashion (Fig. 37–1).
- Hematocrit, platelet count, PTT, and PT/INR should be routinely checked.

TREATMENT

- Small subdural hematomas may be left untreated and the patient observed but, if there is an underlying cause, such as anticoagulation, this should be rapidly corrected to prevent further accumulation of blood.
- Neurosurgical drainage of blood from subdural space via a burr hole is the definitive procedure, although it is common for the hematoma to reaccumulate.
- There is an increased risk of seizures, which should be treated appropriately if they arise.

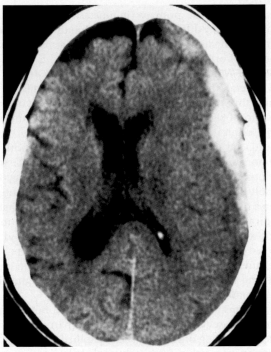

Fig 37–1

CT scan of acute subdural hematoma, 85-year-old woman. The heterogeneous density of irregular shape occupies extra-axial space overlying the left cerebral convexity. There is moderate mass effect exhibited by effacement of convexity sulci and midline shift with subfascial herniation. This required surgical decompression.
(From Grainger RG, Allison DJ, Adam A, Dixon AK [eds]: Grainger and Allison's Diagnostic Radiology: A Textbook of Medical Imaging, 4th ed. London. Harcourt, 2001.)

Chapter 38   Brain neoplasms

DEFINITION

Brain neoplasms are primary (nonmetastatic) tumors arising from one of many different cell types within the central nervous system. Specific tumor subtypes and prognosis depend on the tumor cell of origin and pattern of growth.

PHYSICAL FINDINGS AND CLINICAL PRESENTATION

- In general, the location, size, and rate of growth will determine the symptoms and signs with development of progressive focal signs and symptoms. Even within a tumor subtype, clinical presentation may vary.
- Headache is a common problem for patients with brain tumors and may be a presenting symptom in 20% and develops later in 60%. The headache can be localizing or may result from increased intracranial pressure. Concerning features of headaches include nausea and vomiting, change in typical headache pattern, and worsening with position and vertex location. Headaches with brain tumors tend to be worse during the night and may awaken the patient.
- Seizures in 33% of patients, particularly with brain metastases and low-grade gliomas. The type of seizure and clinical presentation depend on location.
- Symptoms and signs of hydrocephalus and raised intracranial pressure (e.g., headache, vomiting [particularly in children], clouding of consciousness, papilledema).
- Patients may also present with subtle behavioral changes or cognitive and visual-spatial dysfunction. These symptoms are often recognized in retrospect.
- Extremity weakness or sensory changes are common complaints in patients with brain tumors.

CAUSE

- Most cases are idiopathic, although specific chromosomal abnormalities have been implicated in some tumor types.
- Exposure to ionizing radiation has been implicated in the genesis of meningiomas, gliomas, nerve sheath tumors. No convincing evidence has linked CNS tumors with trauma, occupation, diet, or electromagnetic fields.
- The incidence of CNS lymphomas (Fig. 38–1) has increased significantly in the past 3 decades (increased incidence in AIDS patients; Fig 38–2).

DIFFERENTIAL DIAGNOSIS

- Stroke (see Fig. 35–2)
- Abscess (see Fig. 46–5), parasitic cyst (see Fig. 46–16)
- Demyelinating disease—multiple sclerosis (see Fig. 42–1), postinfectious encephalomyelitis
- Metastatic tumors
- Primary central nervous system lymphoma (see Fig. 38–2)

LABORATORY TESTS

- Cerebrospinal fluid (CSF) cytology may yield histologic diagnosis; test for tumor markers (for pineal tumors).
- LP must never be performed if there is concern for increased ICP.

IMAGING STUDIES

- A neuroradiologist is able to diagnose tumor type with considerable accuracy, but most tumors should be biopsied for 100% accuracy.
- MRI with gadolinium enhancement is highly sensitive, although CT scan is useful if calcification or hemorrhage suspected. MR imaging permits visualization of the tumor as well as the relationship to the surrounding tissue (Fig. 38–3)
- MR spectroscopy is used to define metabolic composition of an area of interest and may be useful to contrast areas of tumor progression from radiation necrosis.

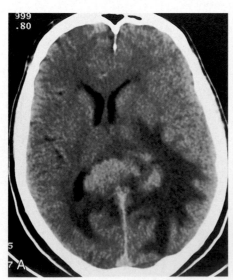
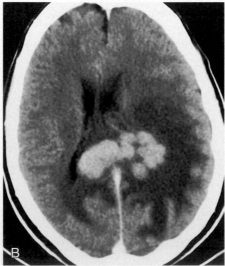

Fig 38–1
Primary cerebral lymphoma CT before **(A)** and after **(B)** intravenous contrast medium. An irregular mass that is hyperdense to gray matter expands the splenium of the corpus callosum and extends into the left hemisphere. It is surrounded by extensive white matter edema and enhances avidly with contrast.
(From Grainger RG, Allison DJ, Adam A, Dixon AK [eds]: Grainger and Allison's Diagnostic Radiology: A Textbook of Medical Imaging, 4th ed. London. Harcourt, 2001.)

- Positron emission tomography (PET; Fig. 38–4) is helpful to distinguish neoplastic lesions (with a high rate of metabolism) from other lesions, such as demyelination or radiation necrosis (with a much lower metabolic rate). It may be useful to help map functional areas of the brain before surgery or radiation.

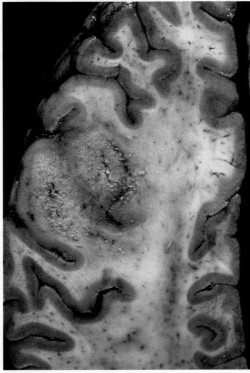

Fig 38–2
Gross appearance of central nervous system lymphoma. This ill-defined, fleshy, and partially necrotic lesion affects the gray-white matter junction.
(From Silverberg SG, DeLellis RA, Frable WJ, et al [eds]: Principles and Practice of Surgical Pathology and Cytopathology, 4th ed. New York, Churchill Livingstone, 2006.)

- Functional MRI is now used in perioperative planning for patients whose lesion is in vital regions, such as those responsible for speech, language, and motor control.

HISTOPATHOLOGY

- Ultimately, only a histologic examination can provide the exact diagnosis (Fig. 38–5).
- There are several different classification schema. Typically, diagnosis is based on histopathology, according to the predominant cell type and grading based on the presence or absence of standard pathologic features.
- Advances in molecular biology are facilitating genetic classification, because oncogenes and tumor suppressor genes play critical roles in tumor pathogenesis.

TREATMENT

- Surgical removal or debulking is generally the initial treatment of choice.
- Biopsy alone is performed if the tumor is located in eloquent regions of the brain or is inaccessible; this is essential for histopathologic diagnosis. Biopsy can be performed under CT or MRI guidance using stereotactic localization.
- If the tumor is of a benign nature (e.g., meningioma, acoustic neuroma), no further therapy is usually required.
- Corticosteroids may be used as a temporizing measure to reduce edema. In addition, steroids may be used following surgery or during radiation therapy.
- Antiseizure medications have been used perioperatively and to control seizures resulting from focal lesions. Prophylactic use of anticonvulsants is not typically recommended without clear history of seizures.
- Depending on tumor type, chemotherapy may be necessary.
- Chemotherapy (combination or single agent) may be used before, during, or after surgery and radiation therapy. In children, chemotherapy is often used to delay radiation therapy.
- Radiation is useful for certain types of tumors: conventional radiation uses external beams over a period of weeks, whereas stereotactic radiosurgery delivers a single, high dose of radiation to a well-defined area (usually smaller than 1 cm).

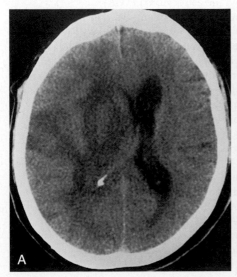

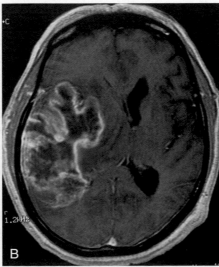

Fig 38–3
Glioblastoma multiforme unenhanced CT **(A)** and axial T1-weighted postgadolinium MRI **(B)** scans. CT shows predominantly low-density white matter in the right hemisphere that extends around but spares the basal ganglia (an important differentiation from stroke) and is compatible with edema and infiltration. Mass effect and midline shift are apparent. The postcontrast MRI **(B)** shows marked, irregular, peripheral enhancement and central low signal, implying necrosis, a hallmark of glioblastoma multiforme.
(From Grainger RG, Allison DJ, Adam A, Dixon AK [eds]: Grainger and Allison's Diagnostic Radiology: A Textbook of Medical Imaging, 4th ed. London. Harcourt, 2001.)

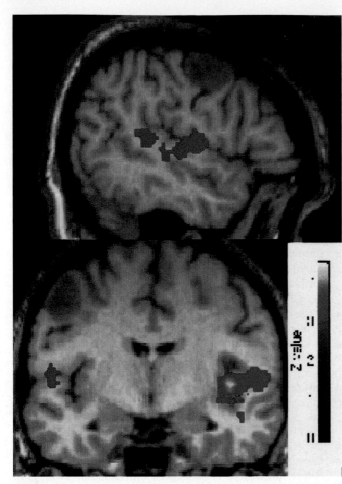

Fig 38–4

$H_2{}^{15}O$ PET activation study during a language task in a young man with a right frontal glioma, before neurosurgical resection. Language activation is seen bilaterally and is distant from the tumor.

(From Grainger RG, Allison DJ, Adam A, Dixon AK [eds]: Grainger and Allison's Diagnostic Radiology: A Textbook of Medical Imaging, 4th ed. London. Harcourt, 2001.)

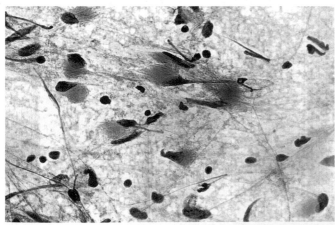

Fig 38–5

Anaplastic astrocytoma. The neoplastic astrocytes have atypical nuclei and are present in a finely granular and fibrillated background (H&E, ×400).

(From Silverberg SG, DeLellis RA, Frable WJ, et al [eds]: Principles and Practice of Surgical Pathology and Cytopathology, 4th ed. New York, Churchill Livingstone, 2006.)

A. ASTROCYTOMA

DEFINITION

Astrocytoma is a specific subtype of glioma that refers to brain neoplasia arising from glial precursor cells within the CNS (astrocytes, oligodendrocytes, ependymal cells). Astrocytoma arises from astrocytes within the CNS and can be generally subclassified as a low-grade (diffuse fibrillary astrocytoma) or high-grade (glioblastoma multiforme) tumor.

PHYSICAL FINDINGS AND CLINICAL PRESENTATION

The presenting symptoms of astrocytoma depend, in part, on the location of the lesion and its rate of growth. Astrocytomas typically present with one or more of the following features:

- Headache (less frequent)
- New-onset seizure (more than 50%)
- Nausea and vomiting
- Focal neurologic deficit (less frequent)
- Change in mental status
- Papilledema (rare)

CAUSE

- The specific cause of astrocytoma is unknown.
- Genetic abnormalities leading to defective tumor-suppressing genes or activation of proto-oncogenes has been proposed. Loss of the *CDKN2* gene on chromosome 9p has been associated with progression to higher grades in patients with low-grade astrocytomas.
- Genetic heterogeneity is common in these tumors, suggesting accumulation of genetic abnormalities and a multistep mechanism of progression to higher grades.

DIAGNOSIS

A provisional diagnosis of astrocytoma is made on clinical grounds and radiographic imaging studies. Tissue pathology is needed to establish the diagnosis and to grade the astrocytoma.

CLASSIFICATION

Astrocytomas are commonly graded by the World Health Organization (WHO) or the Saint Anne-Mayo grading system.

WHO grading system

1. Grade I: juvenile pilocytic astrocytoma, subependymal giant cell astrocytoma, and pleomorphic xanthoastrocytoma
2. Grade II: low-grade astrocytoma (LGA)
3. Grade III: anaplastic astrocytoma (see Fig. 38–5)
4. Grade IV: glioblastoma multiforme (GBM)

Saint Anne-Mayo grading system

The Saint Anne-Mayo system grades astrocytomas according to the presence or absence of four histologic features: nuclear atypia, mitoses, endothelial proliferation, and necrosis.

1. Grade I tumors have none of the features.
2. Grade II tumors have one feature.
3. Grade III tumors have two features.
4. Grade IV tumors have three or more features.

- Grades I and II astrocytomas are commonly called low-grade astrocytomas.
- Grades III and IV astrocytomas are called high-grade malignant astrocytomas.

DIFFERENTIAL DIAGNOSIS

The differential diagnosis is vast and includes any cause of headache, seizures, change in mental status, and focal neurologic deficits.

WORKUP
- A CT or MRI scan of the head essentially makes the diagnosis of an intracranial brain tumor. However, tissue is needed to establish a diagnosis of astrocytoma.
- Stereotactic biopsy under CT or MRI guidance has been shown to be a relatively safe and accurate method for the diagnosis of LGA.
- In the presence of mass effect, either clinically or radiologically, craniotomy with open biopsy and tumor debulking is more appropriate than stereotactic biopsy to establish a tissue diagnosis.

IMAGING STUDIES
- MRI is the diagnostic imaging study of choice. MRI and MRA are used to locate the margins of the tumor, distinguish vascular masses from tumors, detect low-grade astrocytomas not seen by CT, and provide clear views of the posterior fossa.
- Low-grade astrocytomas usually show mass effect and blurring of anatomic boundaries because of their infiltrative nature. Cystic changes, focal calcification, or extension into contralateral structures may also be seen.
- High-grade astrocytomas are typically associated more with enhancement after IV contrast administration because of disruption of the blood-brain barrier. Only about 8% to 15% of LGAs enhance.
- PET scanning and MR spectroscopy are newer imaging modalities that may also play a role in tumor grading and in determining an appropriate site for biopsy.

TREATMENT
- Controversy exists as to the proper management of LGA. Almost all studies to date have been retrospective and flawed by patient and treatment selection bias.
- Nonsurgical observation is one treatment option that may be justified if risks of surgical or radiation treatment are greater than risks of medical treatment of presenting symptoms. Patients who may benefit most from observation are those who are younger, with no or minimal neurologic deficit, and who present with seizures. This course of treat-

ment rests on the certainty of an accurate diagnosis on clinical and imaging grounds.
- Surgical morbidity and mortality are related to tumor location. Patients with deep tumors or tumors in eloquent cortical areas are at high risk for neurologic deterioration from surgical resection or biopsy.
- Surgery remains the initial treatment for almost all astrocytomas, particularly if the tumor is in an anatomically accessible location. Surgery helps in the following cases:
  1. Establishing a pathologic diagnosis
  2. Debulking the tumor
  3. Alleviating intracranial pressure
  4. Offering complete excision with hope for a cure
- Radiation therapy is used postoperatively in patients with low-grade astrocytoma (controversial) and in high-grade astrocytoma. Some authorities recommend waiting for symptoms to occur after surgery in patients with low-grade astrocytoma before using x-ray therapy (XRT).
- A prospective, randomized controlled trial has shown no survival benefit in treating LGA with adjuvant chemotherapy.
- Chemotherapeutic drugs have been used with some effect in patients with high-grade astrocytoma. The addition of adjuvant chemotherapy in these patients has been shown to increase the proportion of long-term survivors from less than 5% to approximately 15% to 20%.

B. MENINGIOMAS

DEFINITION
A meningioma is an intracranial tumor arising from arachnoid cells of the arachnoid villi of the meninges; 90% are benign.

PHYSICAL FINDINGS AND CLINICAL PRESENTATION
- Neurologic symptoms vary with location and size; meningiomas can arise from the dura at any site (Fig. 38–6), although they most commonly occur in the skull vault.
- May be asymptomatic and present incidentally on a neuroimaging study or at autopsy

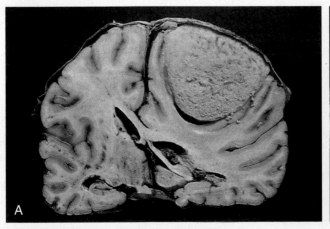
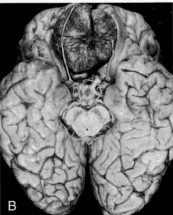

Fig 38–6
Meningioma. **A,** A large-convexity meningioma severely displaces the underlying tissue downward and laterally, creating a midline shift and marked ventricular compression. **B,** An olfactory groove meningioma bows the olfactory nerves and splays the frontal lobes.
(From Skarin AT: Atlas of Diagnostic Oncology, 3rd ed. St. Louis, Mosby, 2003.)

- Focal or generalized seizures and hemiparesis are common, as are headache, personality change or confusion, hearing loss, visual impairment, and obstructive hydrocephalus.
- Children are more likely to present with signs of increased intracranial pressure without further localizing features.

CAUSE
- Abnormalities on chromosome 22 are found in more than 50% of meningiomas. This region also contains the gene for neurofibromatosis type 2, which is a tumor suppressor gene encoding a cytoskeletal protein called merlin or schwannomin. This protein is involved in cytoskeletal organization.
- Cranial radiation may be responsible for some cases in which the tumor occurs in the irradiated field following an appropriate latency period from 10 to 20 years following radiation.
- The link with sex hormones is suggested by the increase in growth rate during the luteal phase of the menstrual cycle and during pregnancy, as well as in women who use postmenopausal hormones or in association with breast carcinoma.
- There is an increased risk in individuals after head injury (no clear causality known).

DIFFERENTIAL DIAGNOSIS
Other well-circumscribed intracranial tumors:
  - Acoustic schwannoma (see Fig. 82–1) (typically at the pontocerebellar junction)
  - Ependymoma, lipoma, and metastases within the spinal cord
  - Metastatic disease from lymphoma or adenocarcinoma, inflammatory disease, or infections such as tuberculosis

WORKUP
- Imaging studies with CT or MRI, followed by surgical removal with histologic confirmation if clinically indicated
- Meningiomas are typically benign tumors; however, they may recur after surgical resection. In addition, some tumors show histologic progression to a higher grade.

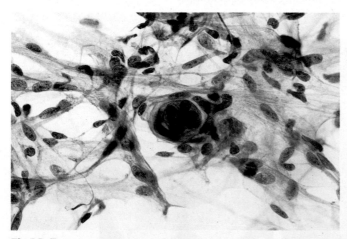

Fig 38–7
Meningioma. A small whorl is associated with a fibrillated background and free spindled meningothelial cells (H&E, ×400).
(From Silverberg SG, DeLellis RA, Frable WJ, et al [eds]: Principles and Practice of Surgical Pathology and Cytopathology, 4th ed. New York, Churchill Livingstone, 2006.)

- According to the WHO classification, there are nine benign histologic variants and four variants associated with increased recurrence and rates of metastasis. Ninety percent of meningiomas are classified as benign meningiomas or WHO grade I. The typical meningioma displays a variety of distinctive histologic patterns. Whorl formation (Fig. 38–7) is a characteristic feature of meningiomas and is usually evident, at least focally.
- Features suggesting increased rate of recurrence include the following:
  - Allelic loss of chromosome 22
  - Loss of 14q, and later losses of other chromosomes such as 1p, 2p, 6q, and 9q, which are associated with histologic and clinical progression
  - Overexpression of p53 protein
  - Brain invasion, high rate of mitosis, and highly anaplastic features

IMAGING STUDIES
- Cranial CT scanning (Fig. 38–8) or MRI can detect and determine the extent of meningiomas. MRI is preferable to show the dural origin of the tumor in most cases. Often, meningiomas show a characteristic dural tail.
- Bone windows optimally identify bone involvement.
- On nonenhanced scans, meningiomas typically are isodense to slightly hyperdense to brain and are homogeneous in appearance. With the addition of contrast, meningiomas show homogeneous enhancement; gadolinium can facilitate imaging of smaller additional lesions that are missed on nonenhanced images MRI (Fig. 38–9).
- PET scanning may help in predicting the aggressiveness of the tumor and the potential for recurrence.

TREATMENT
- The mainstay of treatment for meningiomas remains surgical removal if symptomatic.
- For lesions that cause significant mass effect, corticosteroids (e.g., dexamethasone) are sometimes used to decrease brain edema.
- Anticonvulsants to control seizures. Prophylactic anticonvulsants are generally not indicated without a history of seizures.
- Radiation therapy is the only validated form of adjuvant therapy and may be beneficial in patients with incomplete resections or inoperable tumors.
- Stereotactic radiosurgery has increasingly been used to treat meningiomas.

C. CRANIOPHARYNGIOMA

DEFINITION
Craniopharyngiomas are tumors arising from squamous cell remnants of Rathke's pouch, located in the infundibulum or upper anterior hypophysis.

PHYSICAL FINDINGS AND CLINICAL PRESENTATION
- The typical onset is insidious and a 1- to 2-year history of slowly progressive symptoms is common.
- Presenting symptoms are usually related to the effects of a sella turcica mass. Approximately 75% of patients complain of headache and have visual disturbances.

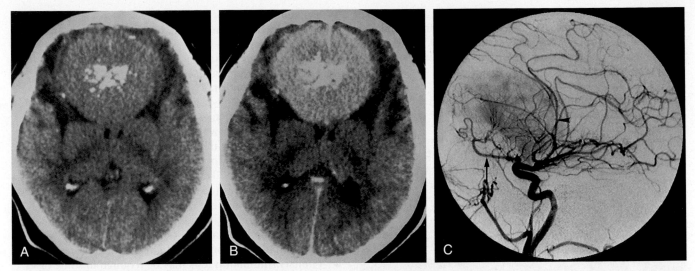

Fig 38–8
Subfrontal meningioma. CT scans before **(A)** and after **(B)** intravenous contrast medium, and lateral projection of common carotid arteriogram **(C)**. There is a large circumscribed mass in the anterior cranial fossa that is isodense to normal gray matter, contains foci of calcification centrally, and enhances homogeneously. There is edema in the white matter of both frontal lobes and posterior displacement and splaying of the frontal horns of the lateral ventricles. **C,** On the arteriogram, the mass is delineated by a tumor blush and there is posterior displacement of the anterior cerebral arteries *(arrowhead),* mirroring the mass effect see on CT. The ophthalmic artery is enlarged as its ethmoidal branches supply the tumor *(arrow).*
(From Grainger RG, Allison DJ, Adam A, Dixon AK [eds]: Grainger and Allison's Diagnostic Radiology: A Textbook of Medical Imaging, 4th ed. London. Harcourt, 2001.)

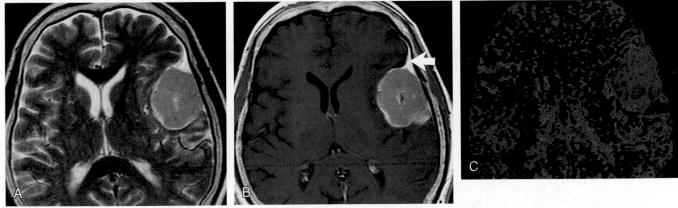

Fig 38–9
Meningioma with perfusion-weighted imaging. Shown are axial T2-weighted **(A)**, gadolinium-enhanced T1-weighted **(B)**, and perfusion-weighted **(C)** MRI scans. A gray matter isointense mass deeply indents the left cerebral convexity **(A)**. Its broad dural base, the surrounding displaced cerebral sulci, and the small pial vessel between the tumor and the brain surface *(arrowhead)* are all features of an extra-axial lesion. The tumor enhances and there is a dural tail *(arrow,* **B**), which is a frequent radiologic finding in meningioma, but is not pathognomonic. **C,** The perfusion-weighted MRI scan, a color map of the relative cerebral blood volume (rCBV), shows increased blood volume of the tumor compared with normal cortex and white matter, confirming its highly vascular nature.
(From Grainger RG, Allison DJ, Adam A, Dixon AK [eds]: Grainger and Allison's Diagnostic Radiology: A Textbook of Medical Imaging, 4th ed. London. Harcourt, 2001.)

- The usual visual defect is bitemporal hemianopsia. Optic nerve involvement with decreased visual acuity and scotomas and homonymous hemianopsia from optic tract involvement may also occur.
- Other symptoms include mental changes, nausea, vomiting, somnolence, and symptoms of pituitary failure. In adults, sexual dysfunction is the most common endocrine complaint, with impotence in males and primary or secondary amenorrhea in females. Diabetes insipidus is found in 25% of cases. In children, craniopharyngiomas may present with dwarfism.
- More than 70% of children at the time of diagnosis present with growth hormone deficiency, obstructive hydrocephalus, short-term memory deficits, and psychomotor slowing.

CAUSE

- Craniopharyngiomas are believed to arise from nests of squamous epithelial cells that are commonly found in the suprasellar area surrounding the pars tuberalis of the adult pituitary (Fig. 38–10).

DIFFERENTIAL DIAGNOSIS

- Pituitary adenoma (see Fig. 264–3)
- Empty sella syndrome

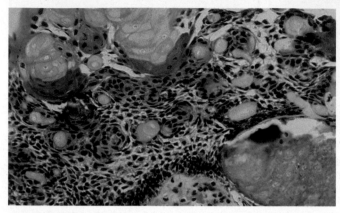

Fig 38–10
Adamantinomatous craniopharyngioma. Note the peripheral palisading of nuclei and the presence of wet keratin.
(From Silverberg SG, DeLellis RA, Frable WJ, et al [eds]: Principles and Practice of Surgical Pathology and Cytopathology, 4th ed. New York, Churchill Livingstone, 2006.)

- Pituitary failure of any cause
- Primary brain tumors (e.g., meningiomas [see Fig. 38–8], astrocytomas)
- Metastatic brain tumors
- Other brain tumors (see Fig. 34–3)
- Cerebral aneurysm IAVM (see Fig. 35–7)

LABORATORY TESTS

Abnormalities may include any of the following:

- Hypothyroidism (low free thyroxine [FT_4], free triiodothyronine [FT_3] with low thyroid-stimulating hormone [TSH]).
- Hypercortisolism (low cortisol) with low adrenocorticotropic hormone [ACTH].
- Low sex hormones (testosterone, estriol) with low follicle-stimulating hormone [FSH] and luteinizing hormone [LH].
- Diabetes insipidus (hypernatremia, low urine specific gravity, low urine osmolarity)
- Prolactin may be normal or slightly elevated.
- Pituitary stimulation tests may be required in some cases.

IMAGING STUDIES

- Visual field testing for bitemporal hemianopsia (Fig. 38–11)
- Skull film is of limited diagnostic value.
- Enlarged or eroded sella turcica (50%)
- Suprasellar calcification (50%)
- Head CT or MRI scan. MRI features include a multicystic and solid, enhancing, suprasellar mass (Fig. 38–12). Hydrocephalus may also be present if the mass is large. CT usually reveals intratumoral calcifications.

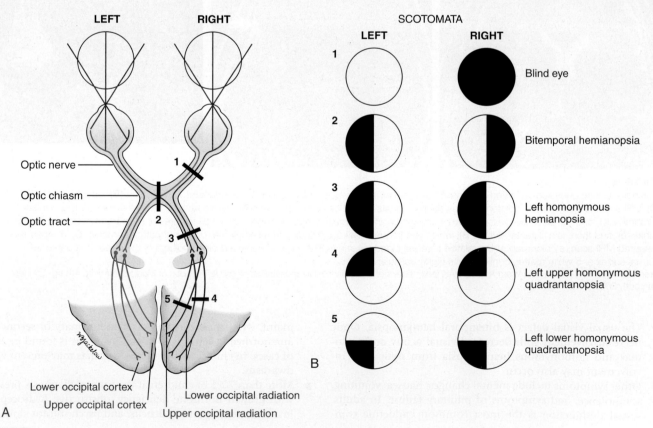

Fig 38–11
Visual field defects.
(From Swartz MH: Textbook of Physical Diagnosis, 5th ed. Philadelphia, WB Saunders, 2006.)

TREATMENT

- Surgical resection (curative or palliative)
- Trans-sphenoidal surgery for small intrasellar tumors
- Subfrontal craniotomy for most patients
- Postoperative radiation
- Intralesional irradiation or chemotherapy for unresectable tumors. Long-term complications of radiation include secondary malignancies, optic neuropathy, and vascular injury.

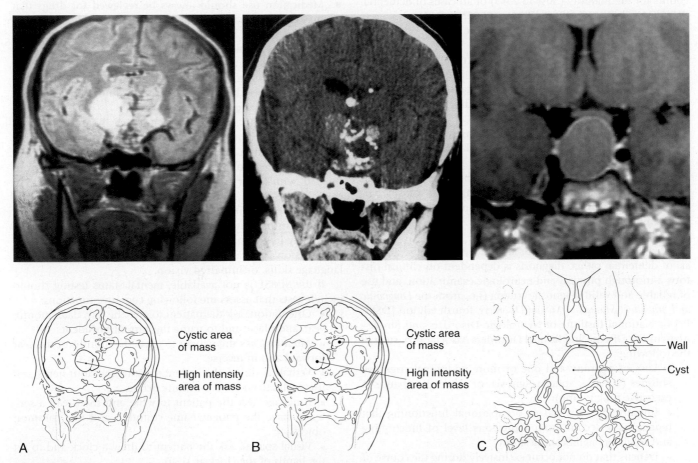

Fig 38–12

Craniopharyngioma. **A,** Proton density-weighted coronal magnetic resonance image shows a cystic area and high-intensity signal area in a large sellar-suprasellar mass, typical of craniopharyngiomas. **B,** Characteristic globular calcification is easier to identify on a coronal CT scan of the same patient. **C,** Coronal T1-weighted image of a different patient shows an intrasellar craniopharyngioma with a cyst that has intermediate signal intensity contents and a wall that enhances with intravenous contrast medium.

(From Besser CM, Thorner MO: Comprehensive Clinical Endocrinology, 3rd ed. St. Louis, Mosby, 2002.)

Chapter 39 Dementia

A. ALZHEIMER'S DISEASE

DEFINITION

Dementia is a syndrome characterized by progressive loss of previously acquired cognitive skills including memory, language, insight, and judgment. Alzheimer's disease (AD) accounts for the majority (50% to 75%) of all cases of dementia.

PHYSICAL FINDINGS AND CLINICAL PRESENTATION

- Spouse or other family member, not the patient, often notes insidious memory impairment.
- Patients have difficulties learning and retaining new information and handling complex tasks (e.g., balancing the checkbook), and have impairments in reasoning, judgment, spatial ability, and orientation (e.g., difficulty driving, getting lost away from home).
- Behavioral changes, such as mood changes and apathy, may accompany memory impairment. In later stages, patients may develop agitation and psychosis.
- Atypical presentations include early and severe behavioral changes, focal findings on examination, parkinsonism, hallucinations, falls, or onset of symptoms in those younger than 65 years.

DIAGNOSIS

There is no definitive imaging or laboratory test for the diagnosis of dementia; rather, diagnosis is dependent on clinical history, a thorough physical and neurologic examination, and use of reliable and valid diagnostic criteria (i.e., from the *Diagnostic and Statistical Manual of Mental Disorders*, fourth edition [DSM-IV] or National Institute of Neurologic Disorders and Stroke–Alzheimer's Disease and Related Disorders Association), such as the following:

- Loss of memory and one or more additional cognitive abilities (aphasia, apraxia, agnosia, or other disturbance in executive functioning)
- Impairment in social or occupational functioning that represents a decline from a previous level of functioning and results in significant disability
- Deficits that do not occur exclusively during the course of delirium
- Insidious onset and gradual progression of symptoms
- Cognitive loss documented by neuropsychological tests
- No physical signs, neuroimaging, or laboratory evidence of other diseases that can cause dementia (e.g., metabolic abnormalities, medication or toxin effects, infection, stroke, Parkinson's disease, subdural hematoma, tumors)
- Patients with isolated memory loss who lack functional impairment at home or work do not meet criteria for dementia but may have a mild cognitive impairment (MCI). Identifying patients with MCI is important because these patients may have a slightly higher rate of progression to dementia.

DIFFERENTIAL DIAGNOSIS

- Cancer (primary brain tumor, metastatic neoplasia)
- Infection (AIDS, neurosyphilis, progressive multifocal leukoencephalopathy [PML])
- Metabolic (ethanol, hypothyroidism, vitamin B_{12} deficiency)
- Organ failure (dialysis dementia, Wilson's disease)
- Normal pressure hydrocephalus (NPH)
- Vascular disorder (chronic subdural hematoma [SDH])
- Depression

WORKUP

History and general physical examination

- Medication use should always be reviewed for drugs that may cause mental status changes.
- Patients should be screened for depression, because it can sometimes mimic dementia but also often occurs as a coexisting condition and should be treated.
- On examination, look for signs of metabolic disturbance, presence of psychiatric features, or focal neurologic deficits.

Mental status testing

Brief mental status testing can be done easily and quickly in the office. Most commonly used is the Folstein Mini Mental Status Examination (MMSE). The MMSE is widely available in many reference books and on the Internet. Scores range from 0 to 30, with lower scores reflecting poorer performance. An MMSE score lower than 24 suggests dementia; however, the MMSE is not sensitive enough to detect mild dementia, or dementia in patients with a high baseline IQ. Scores may be spuriously low in patients with limited education, poor motor function, African American or Hispanic ethnicity, poor language skills, or impaired vision.

If the MMSE is not available, mental status testing should include tests that assess the following cognitive functions:

- Orientation: ask the patient to give the day, date, month, year, and place, and to name the current president.
- Attention: ask the patient to recite the months of the year forward and in reverse.
- Verbal recall: ask the patient to remember four items; test for recall after 1- and 5-minute delays.
- Language: ask the patient to write and then read a sentence; have the patient name common and less common objects.
- Visual-spatial: ask the patient to draw a clock and to set the hands of the clock at 11:10.

Patients with AD typically have trouble with verbal recall, plus visual-spatial or language deficits. Attention is usually preserved until the late stages of AD, so consider alternate diagnoses in patients who do poorly on tests of attention.

LABORATORY TESTS

- CBC
- Serum electrolytes
- Glucose
- BUN, creatinine
- Liver and thyroid function tests
- Serum vitamin B_{12} and methylmalonic acid
- Syphilis serology, if high clinical suspicion
- Lumbar puncture if history or signs of cancer, infectious process, or when the clinical presentation is unusual (i.e., rapid progression of symptoms)
- EEG if there is history of seizures, episodic confusion, rapid clinical decline, or suspicion of Creutzfeldt-Jakob disease
- Measurement of apolipoprotein E genotyping, CSF tau and amyloid; functional imaging including PET or SPECT (Fig. 39–1) are not routinely indicated.

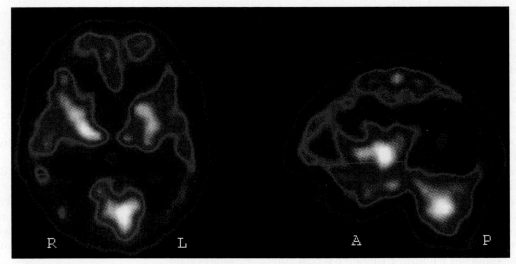

Fig 39–1
Axial (L) and sagittal (R) ^{99m}Tc HMPAO SPECT in Alzheimer's disease showing typical perfusion defects in the posterior temporal and parietal regions. A, anterior; L, left; P, posterior; R, right.
(From Grainger RG, Allison DJ, Adam A, Dixon AK [eds]: Grainger and Allison's Diagnostic Radiology: A Textbook of Medical Imaging, 4th ed. London. Harcourt, 2001.)

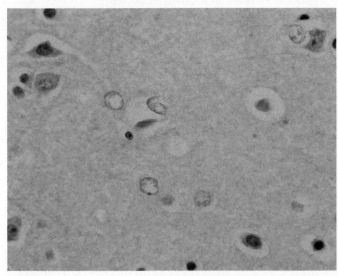

Fig 39–2
Alzheimer type II astrocytes. Note the enlarged astrocytic nuclei with ground-glass nuclei.
(From Silverberg SG, DeLellis RA, Frable WJ, et al [eds]: Principles and Practice of Surgical Pathology and Cytopathology, 4th ed. New York, Churchill Livingstone, 2006.)

- A postmortem brain biopsy slide is shown in (Fig. 39–2).

IMAGING STUDIES
- CT scan or MRI to rule out hydrocephalus and mass lesions, including chronic subdural hematoma

TREATMENT
- Patient safety, including risks associated with impaired driving, wandering behavior, leaving stoves unattended, and accidents, must be addressed with the patient and family early and appropriate measures implemented.
- Wandering, hoarding or hiding objects, repetitive questioning, withdrawal, and social inappropriateness often respond to behavioral therapies.
- Symptomatic treatment

- Memory disturbance: cholinesterase inhibitors and N-methyl-D-aspartate (NMDA) receptor antagonists (memantine) may be useful in early dementia to slow down the progression of dementia. However, they are expensive, have significant side effects, and should not be used routinely
- Neuropsychiatric and behavioral disturbances: depression, agitation, delusions, or hallucinations may respond to medications.

B. DEMENTIA WITH LEWY BODIES

DEFINITION
Dementia with Lewy bodies (DLB) is a progressive neurodegenerative disease with core features of dementia accompanied or followed by parkinsonism.

PHYSICAL FINDINGS AND CLINICAL PRESENTATION
- Usually, dementia precedes the appearance of parkinsonism by months to years. Occasionally, parkinsonism precedes dementia; in this case there is clinical overlap between DLB and Parkinson's disease with dementia (PDD). There is debate whether DLB and PDD are actually a spectrum of the same disease, because pathologic findings are similar.
- Dementia is superficially similar to Alzheimer's disease. Early visual hallucinations (outside the setting of dopaminergic therapy) occur in up to 80% and are the major differentiating feature from AD. Typically, the hallucinations are well formed and detailed.
- Fluctuations in performance, especially with regard to attention and alertness, are another key feature of the presentation. These can occur acutely, leading to misdiagnosis of vascular dementia presenting with stroke, and may last hours or days.
- Parkinsonism is typically symmetrical and axially predominant, with little tremor but prominent gait impairment and postural instability.
- Parkinsonism is not ubiquitous; up to 25% of cases diagnosed by autopsy had mild or no reported parkinsonian features.

- Rapid eye movement (REM) sleep behavior disorder and other related sleep abnormalities are common.

CAUSE

- Uncertain; it is thought that DLB probably results from abnormal handling of alpha-synuclein, with resulting aggregation of the protein inside neurons.
- Lewy bodies are eosinophilic intracellular inclusions (Fig. 39–3) that contain alpha-synuclein and ubiquitin; it is not clear whether they are pathogenic.

DIFFERENTIAL DIAGNOSIS

- PDD—differentiated from DLB in which dementia usually precedes parkinsonism. A somewhat arbitrary 1-year rule is sometimes used to differentiate DLB from PDD: if dementia presents within the first year after the parkinsonism, DLB can still be diagnosed.
- AD—differs from DLB in which visual hallucinations and parkinsonism are prominent
- Atypical parkinsonian syndromes (multiple system atrophy, progressive supranuclear palsy, corticobasal degeneration)—these syndromes have other features, such as cerebellar degeneration, supranuclear gaze palsy, or asymmetrical limb apraxia that are not seen in DLB.
- Vascular dementia—differs from DLB in that despite the fluctuations in performance seen in DLB, there is no clear history of multiple strokes.
- Frontotemporal dementia (FTD, also called Pick's disease)
- Creutzfeldt-Jakob disease (CJD)—differs from DLB in that it is usually more rapidly progressive, can have cerebellar signs and symptoms, and often has distinctive electroencephalographic abnormalities.
- Toxic, metabolic, pharmacologic-related delirium

LABORATORY TESTS

- Routine blood tests are normal but should be done to rule out treatable causes of dementia (e.g., vitamin B_{12}, TSH). In the setting of a fluctuation in performance, laboratory studies to rule out metabolic causes of delirium are appropriate.
- Spinal fluid analysis is normal; this may be helpful in more rapidly progressive cases if CJD is suspected.
- EEG may be helpful in the setting of fluctuations in performance to look for subclinical status epilepticus or other evidence of seizures, or if CJD is suspected.

IMAGING STUDIES

- Brain MRI is indicated mostly to look for multiple prior strokes suggestive of vascular dementia. In the setting of a sudden deterioration in performance, MRI with diffusion-weighted imaging may be needed to rule out acute stroke.
- Conventional neuroimaging is not diagnostic of DLB. Functional neuroimaging such as PET and SPECT show promise, but are not yet routinely indicated or available.

TREATMENT

- Dementia care education with physical and occupational therapy may be of benefit to both patients and caregivers.
- Treatment of parkinsonism with levodopa can be partially successful but, because of the risk of hallucinations, the lowest effective dose should be used.
- Cholinesterase inhibitors are modestly effective for treating cognitive impairment (possibly better than in AD), as well as hallucinations, sleep impairment, and anxiety.
- Antipsychotic medications are helpful in treating hallucinations; however, older neuroleptic agents should be avoided in favor of low doses of newer atypical antipsychotics.

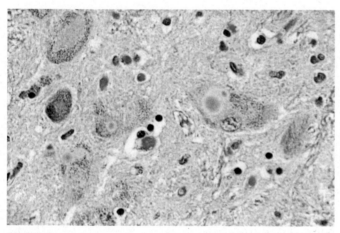

Fig 39–3
Lewy bodies in the substantia nigra. The major pathologic abnormalities in Parkinson's disease (PD) are neuronal cell loss, gliosis, and loss of pigment in the substantia nigra, especially in the ventrolateral portion projecting to the putamen, and the presence of abnormal intracytoplasmic neuronal inclusions called Lewy bodies. Lewy bodies consist of an amorphous central core with a halo of radially arranged neurofilaments measuring 10 to 20 nm in diameter. Lewy bodies stain with monoclonal antibodies to ubiquitin (a polypeptide associated with protein degradation) and to select antigens from tubulin, paired helical filaments, and neurofibrillary tangle proteins. In many patients with PD, ubiquitin staining has revealed the presence of cortical intracytoplasmic inclusions that resemble Lewy bodies but have a homogeneous structure. Dopaminergic nuclei in the ventral tegmental area also show cell loss and Lewy body formation. Other neurotransmitter systems may undergo neuronal loss and Lewy body formation in PD, including noradrenergic neurons (in the locus ceruleus and the dorsal nucleus of the vagus), cholinergic neurons (in the nucleus basalis of Meynert and the Westphal-Edinger nucleus), and serotonergic neurons (in the dorsal raphe nucleus). Damage to these systems is usually less severe than that to the substantia nigra, and some symptoms of PD that respond poorly to dopamine replacement therapy may persist because of damage to nondopaminergic systems.
(From Rosenberg RN: Atlas of Clinical Neurology. Boston, Butterworth-Heinemann, 1998.)

C. PROGRESSIVE SUPRANUCLEAR PALSY

DEFINITION

Progressive supranuclear palsy (PSP) is a progressive degenerative disease of the central nervous system particularly affecting the brainstem and basal ganglia, with core features of supranuclear ophthalmoplegia, rigidity, postural instability, and cognitive decline.

PHYSICAL FINDINGS AND CLINICAL PRESENTATION

- Common early symptoms include slowness (bradykinesia) and stiffness, as well as falls.
- Differences from PD become more pronounced with progression. Tremor is present in only 5% to 10% of patients.
- Hallmark on examination is supranuclear gaze palsy; impaired voluntary conjugate eye movements, primarily on attempted up and down gaze (Fig. 39–4).

- Predominantly axial rigidity, leading to typical neck extension. This, plus low blink rate and facial muscle contraction, give the characteristic appearance of sustained surprise.
- Limb rigidity is typically proximal in contrast to the distal rigidity seen in idiopathic PD.
- Gait is slow and stiff, with marked postural instability leading to unheralded, often backward, falls.
- Cognitive impairment is frequent and consists of mental slowness, irritability, and social withdrawal.

CAUSE
- Pathogenesis is believed to be related to the accumulation of hyperphosphorylated tau protein in neurons and glia in basal ganglia and brainstem nuclei. In this regard, PSP is thought to be pathophysiologically related to frontotemporal dementia and corticobasal degeneration.

DIFFERENTIAL DIAGNOSIS
- Parkinson's disease—differs from PSP, in which early falls are prominent, tremor is unusual, and there is very little response to levodopa.
- Cortical basal ganglionic degeneration—differentiated from PSP by presence of cortical sensory signs and asymmetrical limb apraxia
- Multiple systems atrophy—differs from PSP by the presence of prominent autonomic symptoms and/or cerebellar signs.
- DLB—in PSP, visual hallucinations typically only occur if provoked by dopaminergic therapy, whereas in DLB there are prominent visual hallucinations that may be spontaneous or provoked.

WORKUP
- Diagnosis is largely clinical. The NINDS has provided inclusion and exclusion criteria. Mandatory exclusion criteria include the following:
  1. Recent history of encephalitis
  2. Cortical sensory deficits
  3. Hallucinations or delusions unrelated to dopaminergic therapy
  4. Cortical dementia of the Alzheimer's type

LABORATORY TESTS
- There are no diagnostic laboratory tests at present.
- If there is a question of recent encephalitis, spinal fluid analysis may be indicated.

IMAGING STUDIES
- If atypical features such as unilateral symptoms or signs are present, brain MRI may be helpful in ruling out structural lesions.
- Conventional neuroimaging is not useful to differentiate PSP from the major differential diagnoses. Functional neuroimaging such as PET and SPECT show promise, but are not yet routinely indicated or available.

TREATMENT
- Physical, occupational, and speech-swallowing therapy can be helpful for patients and caregivers.
- Patients with significant dysphagia may require a feeding gastrostomy.
- Levodopa may be mildly helpful with rigidity and bradykinesia early in the disease course, but typically loses effectiveness quickly. Dopamine receptor agonists are not typically effective.
- Cholinesterase inhibitors have not been shown to help with the cognitive impairment.

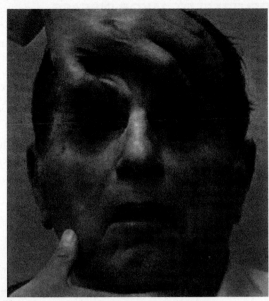

Fig 39–4
A patient with progressive supranuclear palsy (PSP) who is having his oculocephalic reflexes (doll's eyes) tested to determine whether the origin of the gaze palsy is supranuclear. The patient, who is unable to look down voluntarily, is asked to look straight ahead at an object while the examiner tilts the patient's head backward and keeps the eyelids apart to look for downward movement of the eyes. If the eyes move downward, the origin of the gaze palsy is supranuclear.
The prevalence of PSP has been estimated at 1.39 per 100,000. The mean age at onset is about 65 years, with a male preponderance in most series. Symptoms are steadily progressive, and death usually occurs 5 to 10 years after onset from aspiration or from the sequelae of multiple falls or bed sores. When supranuclear palsy (especially the loss of downward gaze) appears early in the course of an akinetic rigid syndrome, the diagnosis of PSP is likely. PSP may be suspected in the absence of supranuclear palsy when other typical features are present. Frequent or continuous square wave jerks (small saccades alternately to the left and right in the horizontal plane) are often present. Patients with PSP lose postural reflexes early in the course of disorder, and falling is an early feature. While walking, patients often assume a broad base, abduct the upper extremities at the shoulder, and flex at the elbows, producing a characteristic gait that suggests PSP. Freezing (abrupt, transient interruption of motor activity) may be severe and, in some cases, may be the major manifestation of PSP. Facial dystonia (deep nasolabial folds and furrowed brow) may create an angry or puzzled look when combined with a wide-eyed, unblinking stare. Axial rigidity is often more prominent than rigidity of the extremities and, in some cases, the limbs may have normal or reduced tone. Patients may be unable to open their lids, even in the absence of orbicularis oculi spasms. This has been termed *apraxia of eyelid opening*, but the phenomenon does not represent true apraxia. It might be the result of inappropriate inhibition of the levator palpebrae.
(From Rosenberg RN: Atlas of Clinical Neurology. Boston, Butterworth-Heinemann, 1998.)

D. CREUTZFELDT-JAKOB DISEASE

DEFINITION

Creutzfeldt-Jakob disease is a progressive, fatal, dementing illness caused by an infectious agent known as a prion.

PHYSICAL FINDINGS AND CLINICAL PRESENTATION

- All patients present with cognitive deficits (dementing illness—memory loss, behavioral abnormalities, higher cortical function impairment).
- More than 80% will have myoclonus.
- Pyramidal tract signs (weakness), cerebellar signs (clumsiness), and extrapyramidal signs (parkinsonian features) are seen in more than 50% of cases.

- Less common features include cortical visual abnormalities, abnormal eye movements, vestibular dysfunction, sensory disturbances, autonomic dysfunction, lower motor neuron signs, and seizures.

CAUSE

- Small proteinaceous infectious particle (prion).
- Noninfectious prion protein (PrP) is a cellular protein found on the surfaces of neurons. Normal function is not known.
- Protein is converted to a protease-resistant and infectious agent (PrPSc) by infectious prion protein (PrP; Fig. 39–5).

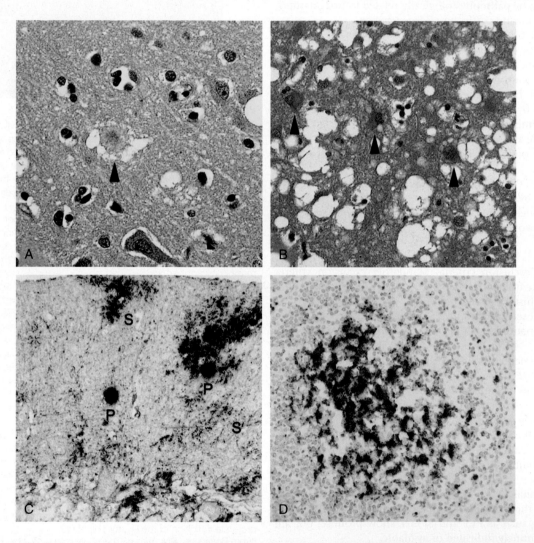

Fig 39–5

Neuropathology of prion disease—histopathologic findings in variant Creutzfeldt-Jakob disease (vCJD). **A,** Florid plaques, a characteristic feature a vCJD pathology. They consist of a round amyloid core *(arrowhead)* surrounded by a ring of vacuoles (H&E). **B,** Spongiform degeneration in prion disease. This shows severe vacuolization (spongiosus); there is severe neuronal loss and many strongly reactive astrocytes *(arrowheads).*
C, Immunostaining of the pathologic prion protein. The specimen is pretreated to denature the normal PrP and staining with a prion protein antibody reveals the presence of plaques (P) and synapses (S) staining positively for a protease-resistant and infectious agent (PrPSc). **D,** Detection of pathologic prion protein in the follicular dendritic cells in a tonsil. Accumulation of prion protein in lymphoreticular organs, such as the spleen, tonsils or appendix, is a specific finding in vCJD and is not present in other forms of CJD. Therefore, tonsillar biopsies can be used to diagnose vCJD specifically when clinical symptoms are only emerging (H&E).
(Courtesy of Dr. Sebastian Brandner.)

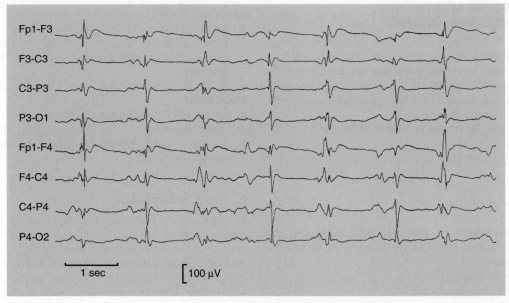

Fig 39–6
Electroencephalogram of a patient with Creutzfeldt-Jakob disease showing periodic complexes that often have a triphasic configuration.
(From Goetz CG, Pappert EJ: Textbook of Clinical Neurology, Philadelphia, WB Saunders, 1999.)

DIAGNOSIS
- Definite CJD: neuropathologically confirmed spongiform encephalopathy in a case of progressive dementia
- Probable CJD: history of rapidly progressive dementia (less than 2 years) with typical findings on EEG, with at least two of the following clinical features: myoclonus, visual or cerebellar dysfunction, pyramidal or extrapyramidal features, akinetic mutism
- Possible CJD: same as probable CJD without electroencephalographic findings

DIFFERENTIAL DIAGNOSIS
- Alzheimer's disease (see Fig. 39–2)
- Frontotemporal dementia
- Dementia with Lewy bodies (see Fig. 39–3)
- Vascular dementia
- Others (hydrocephalus, infection, vitamin deficiency, endocrine disorder)

LABORATORY TESTS
- Presence of periodic sharp wave complexes on the electroencephalogram (Fig. 39–6) in cases of rapidly progressive dementia has a sensitivity of 67% and a specificity of 86%
- Presence of the 14,3,3 protein in CSF has a 95% positive predictive value; its absence has a 92% negative predictive value in cases of probable or possible CJD.

IMAGING STUDIES
MRI scanning (Fig. 39–7) can show areas of restricted diffusion in the basal ganglia and cerebral cortex. MRI diffusion-weighted imaging has a sensitivity of 92.3% and a specificity of 93.8% in cases of rapidly progressive dementia.

TREATMENT
- Full time caregiver and/or nursing home
- Social work can be helpful with end-of-life discussions, family counseling, and optimizing appropriate home services. The disease is fatal. The mean duration of illness is 8 months.

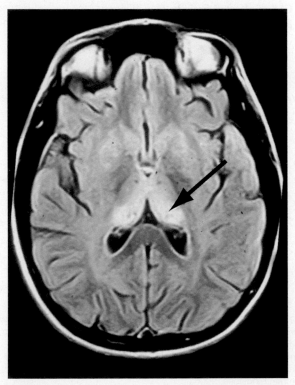

Fig 39–7
Axial T₂-weighted MRI scan of brain demonstrating high signal bilaterally in the posterior thalamus *(arrow)*, the pulvinar sign, in a patient with vCJD.
(From Cohen J, Powderly WG: Infectious Diseases, 2nd ed. St. Louis, Mosby, 2004.)

E. PROGRESSIVE MULTIFOCAL LEUKOENCEPHALOPATHY

DEFINITION

This is a degenerative brain disorder caused by a viral infection of the myelin-producing oligodendrocytes, resulting in cell destruction and demyelination and usually occurring in immunosuppressed hosts (e.g., those with AIDS, lymphomas, leukemia, systemic lupus erythematosus [SLE]).

PHYSICAL FINDINGS AND CLINICAL PRESENTATION

- Cognitive impairment
- Focal neurologic deficits
- Ataxia
- Seizures
- Psychomotor retardation

CAUSE

The JC virus is the causative agent of PML. Immunosuppression results in reactivation of the virus (believed to be in a latent phase in the kidneys)

DIFFERENTIAL DIAGNOSIS

- Encephalitis (see Fig. 46–11)
- Multiple sclerosis (see Fig. 42–1)
- CNS lymphoma (see Fig. 316–4)

LABORATORY TESTS

- Polymerase chain reaction (PCR) to detect JC virus DNA in CSF of affected patients (specificity 95%, sensitivity 75%)
- Brain biopsy of suspicious white matter lesions (Fig. 39–8)

IMAGING STUDIES

- Brain MRI (Fig. 39–9): multiple lesions, especially in the parietal-occipital regions. The lesions are nonenhancing with contrast administration and have increased signal intensity
- Brain CT: hypodense lesions in the white matter

TREATMENT

- No proved therapy. Survival from onset of symptoms is less than 6 months.
- High-dose azidothymidine (AZT) in AIDS patient may lengthen survival.

F. PICK'S DISEASE

This rare form of dementia is characterized by selective impairment of speech function (progressive aphasic dementia) and atrophy of the frontal and temporal lobes.

Pathologically, there are distinctive intraneuronal inclusions known as Pick bodies (Fig. 39–10A) and swollen, ballooned, and poorly staining neurons known as Pick cells (see Fig. 39–10B)

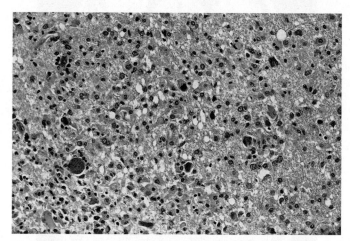

Fig 39–8
Progressive multifocal leukoencephalopathy. There is astrocytosis with bizarre astrocytes, macrophages, and several large oligodendrocytes that have ground-glass nuclei.
(From Silverberg SG, DeLellis RA, Frable WJ, et al [eds]: Principles and Practice of Surgical Pathology and Cytopathology, 4th ed. New York, Churchill Livingstone, 2006.)

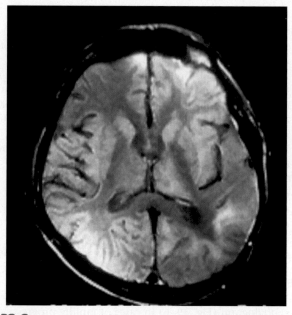

Fig 39–9
Image of progressive multifocal leukoencephalopathy (PML). PML is characterized by patchy or confluent white matter abnormalities. Note the absence of mass effect.
(From Silverberg SG, DeLellis RA, Frable WJ, et al [eds]: Principles and Practice of Surgical Pathology and Cytopathology, 4th ed. New York, Churchill Livingstone, 2006.)

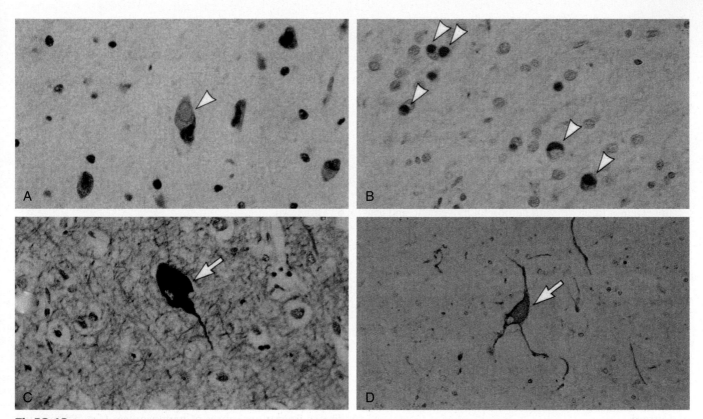

Fig 39–10
Histopathologic specimens of Pick's disease. The pathognomonic inclusions known as Pick bodies *(arrowheads)* occur in neurons of the cerebral cortex, concentrating in cortical layer II (**A**, H&E) and in the dentate gyrus of the hippocampus (**B**, tau-2 stain, counterstained with Nissl). They are argyrophilic cytoplasmic inclusions composed of straight filaments. Pale ballooned neurons *(arrows)*, sometimes called Pick cells (**C,** SMI-31 monoclonal antibody stain; **D**, crystalline stain) are also seen, typically in the frontal lobes. Note the eccentric nuclei and the large size of these neurons relative to their neighbors. Intense reactive astrocytosis is found in both the cortex and white matter. Not all cases of dementia with prominent defects in executive function share all these histopathologic features, and no criteria are universally accepted for the diagnosis. Some clinicians reserve the diagnosis of Pick's disease for those cases in which all of the classic features, including Pick bodies, are found. In this conservative scheme, as few as 10% of patients presenting with the syndrome of frontotemporal dementia would be classified as having Pick's disease. (Courtesy of Dr. Lee Reed, Department of Pathology, University of Iowa).

Chapter 40   Movement disorders

A. PARKINSON'S DISEASE

DEFINITION
Idiopathic Parkinson's disease is a progressive neurodegenerative disorder characterized clinically by rigidity, tremor, and bradykinesia.

PHYSICAL FINDINGS AND CLINICAL PRESENTATION
- Tremor—typically, a resting tremor with a frequency of 4 to 6 Hz is often first noted in the hand as a pill-rolling tremor (thumb and forefinger), and can also involve the legs and lips. Tremor improves with purposeful movement, and usually starts asymmetrically.
- Rigidity—increased muscle tone that persists throughout the range of passive movement of a joint. This is also usually asymmetrical in onset.
- Akinesia, bradykinesia—slowness in initiating movement
- Masked facies—face seems expressionless, giving the appearance of depression. There is decreased blink and often excess drooling.
- Gait disturbance (Fig. 40–1).
- Stooped posture, decreased arm swing
- Difficulty initiating the first step; small shuffling steps that increase in speed (festinating gait). Steps become progressively faster and shorter while the trunk inclines farther forward.
- Other early complaints and findings include micrographia (handwriting becomes smaller; Fig. 40–2) and hypophonia (voice becomes softer).

- Postural instability—tested by the pull test. Ask patient to stand in place with his or her back to the examiner. The examiner pulls the patient back by the shoulders; the proper response would be to take no or very few steps back without falling. Retropulsion is a positive test, as is falling straight back. This is not usually severe early. If falls and postural reflexes are greatly impaired early, then consider other disorders.

CAUSE
- Unknown
- Most cases are sporadic, with age being the most common risk factor, although there is probably a combination of environmental and genetic factors contributing to disease expression. There are rare familial forms with at least five different genes identified. The most well known is the parkin gene, which is a significant cause of early-onset autosomal recessive Parkinson's disease and isolated juvenile-onset Parkinson's disease (at or before age 20).

DIAGNOSIS
A presumptive clinical diagnosis can be made based on a comprehensive history and physical examination. The combination of asymmetrical signs, resting tremor, and good response to levodopa best differentiates idiopathic Parkinson's disease from other causes of parkinsonism (see "Differential Diagnosis" for PD).

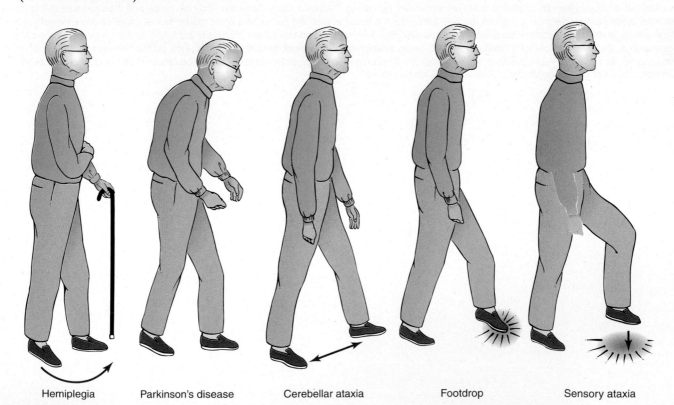

Hemiplegia   Parkinson's disease   Cerebellar ataxia   Footdrop   Sensory ataxia

Fig 40–1
Common types of gait abnormalities.
(From Swartz MH: Textbook of Physical Diagnosis, 5th ed. Philadelphia, WB Saunders, 2006.)

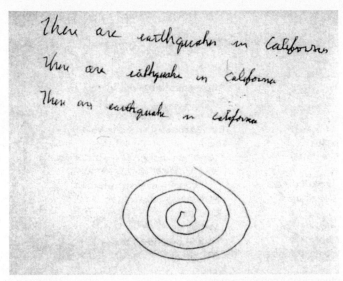

Fig 40–2
Handwriting sample of a patient with mild Parkinson's disease. The handwriting is slower and smaller, and the Archimedes spiral tends to be cramped and less open. Note the progressive shortening of the length of the sentence as it is repeatedly written. If a tremor is present, it can usually be seen in the handwriting. Bradykinesia manifests in many other ways: decreased blinking and loss of facial expression (masked facies); decreased automatic swallowing, leading to drooling; loss of arm swing while walking; and soft voice (hypophonia). During walking, some patients take faster and faster steps as the step size becomes smaller (festination).
(From Rosenberg RN: Atlas of Clinical Neurology. Boston, Butterworth-Heinemann, 1998.)

DIFFERENTIAL DIAGNOSIS

- Multisystem atrophy—distinguishing features include autonomic dysfunction, (including urinary incontinence, orthostatic hypotension, and erectile dysfunction), parkinsonism, cerebellar signs, and normal cognition.
- Diffuse Lewy body disease—parkinsonism with concomitant dementia. Patients often have early hallucinations and fluctuations in levels of alertness and mental status.
- Corticobasal degeneration—often begins asymmetrically with apraxia, cortical sensory loss in one limb, and sometimes alien limb phenomenon.
- Progressive supranuclear palsy—tends to have axial rigidity greater than appendicular (limb) rigidity. These patients have early and severe postural instability. A hallmark is supranuclear gaze palsy that usually involves vertical gaze before horizontal.
- Essential tremor—bilateral postural and action tremor.
- Secondary (acquired) parkinsonism
1. Postinfectious parkinsonism—von Economo's encephalitis
2. Parkinson's pugilistica—after repeated head trauma
3. Iatrogenic—any of the neuroleptics and antipsychotics. The high potency D_2-blocker neuroleptics are most likely to cause parkinsonism.
4. Toxins (e.g., MPTP, manganese, carbon monoxide)
- Cerebrovascular disease (basal ganglia infarcts)

IMAGING STUDIES
CT has almost no role in investigations. MRI of the head may sometimes distinguish between idiopathic Parkinson's disease and other conditions that present with signs of parkinsonism.

TREATMENT

- Physical therapy, patient education and reassurance, treatment of associated conditions (e.g., depression)
- Avoidance of drugs that can induce or worsen parkinsonism: neuroleptics (especially high potency), certain antiemetics (prochlorperazine, trimethobenzamide), metoclopramide, nonselective monoamine oxidase (MAO) inhibitors (may induce hypertensive crisis), reserpine, methyldopa
- There is persistent controversy as to whether levodopa or dopamine agonists should be the initial treatment. In younger patients, agonists are usually the drug of choice; in patients older than 70 years, levodopa is the drug of choice.
- Levodopa therapy: cornerstone of symptomatic therapy—should be used with a peripheral dopa decarboxylase inhibitor (carbidopa) to minimize side effects (nausea, lightheadedness, postural hypotension). The combination of the two drugs is marketed under the trade name Sinemet.
- Dopamine receptor agonists
- Selegiline
- Anticholinergic agents
- Pallidal (globus pallidus interna) and subthalamic deep brain stimulation are currently the surgical options of choice; thalamic deep brain stimulation (DBS) may be useful for refractory tremor. Surgery is limited to patients with disabling, medically refractory problems, and patients must still have a good response to L-dopa to undergo surgery. DBS results in decreased dyskinesias, fluctuations, rigidity, and tremor.

B. WILSON'S DISEASE

DEFINITION
Wilson's disease is a disorder of copper transport with inadequate biliary copper excretion, leading to an accumulation of the metal in the liver, brain, kidneys, and corneas.

PHYSICAL FINDINGS AND CLINICAL PRESENTATION

Hepatic presentation
- Acute hepatitis with malaise, anorexia, nausea, jaundice, elevated transaminase, prolonged prothrombin time; rarely, fulminant hepatic failure
- Chronic active (or autoimmune) hepatitis with fatigue, malaise, rashes, arthralgia, elevated transaminase, elevated serum IgG, positive antinuclear antibody (ANA) and anti–smooth muscle antibody
- Chronic liver disease, cirrhosis with hepatosplenomegaly, ascites, low serum albumin, prolonged prothrombin time, portal hypertension

Neurologic presentation
- Movement disorder: tremors, ataxia
- Spastic dystonia: masklike facies, rigidity, gait disturbance, dysarthria, drooling, dysphagia

Psychiatric presentation
- Depression, obsessive-compulsive disorder, psychopathic behaviors

Other organs
- Hemolytic anemia
- Renal disease (e.g., Fanconi's syndrome with hematuria, phosphaturia, renal tubular acidosis, vitamin D–resistant rickets)
- Cardiomyopathy
- Arthritis

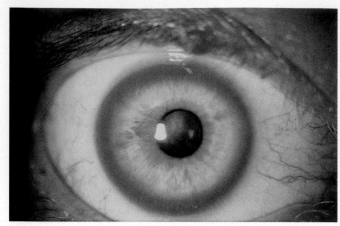

Fig 40–3
Kayser-Fleischer ring.
(From Swartz MH: Textbook of Physical Diagnosis, 5th ed. Philadelphia, WB Saunders, 2006.)

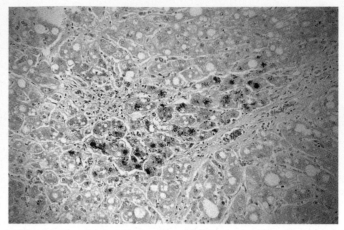

Fig 40–4
Wilson's disease, cirrhotic stage. Marked copper accumulation is demonstrated in the segment of cirrhotic nodule *(center)* as compared with other areas (rhodamine stain).
(From Silverberg SG, DeLellis RA, Frable WJ, et al [eds]: Principles and Practice of Surgical Pathology and Cytopathology, 4th ed. New York, Churchill Livingstone, 2006.)

- Hypoparathyroidism
- Hypogonadism

Physical findings
- Ocular: the Kayser-Fleischer ring is a gold-yellow ring seen at the periphery of the iris (Fig. 40–3)
- Stigmata of acute or chronic liver disease
- Neurologic abnormalities: (see p. 201)

CAUSE AND PATHOGENESIS
- Dietary copper is transported from the intestine to the liver, where normally it is metabolized into ceruloplasmin. In Wilson's disease, defective incorporation of copper into ceruloplasmin and a decrease of biliary copper excretion lead to accumulation of this mineral.
- The gene for Wilson's disease is located in chromosome 13.

DIFFERENTIAL DIAGNOSIS
- Hereditary hypoceruloplasminemia
- Menkes' disease
- Consider the diagnosis of Wilson's disease in all cases of acute or chronic liver disease in which another cause has not been established.
- Consider Wilson's disease in patients with movement disorders or dystonia, even without symptomatic liver disease.

LABORATORY TESTS
- Abnormal liver function tests (LFTs; note that AST may be higher than ALT)
- Low serum ceruloplasmin level (less than 200 mg/L)
- Low serum copper (less than 65 μg/L)
- 24-hr urinary copper excretion more than 100 μg (normal, less than 30 μg); increases to more than 1200 μg/24 hr after 500 mg of D-penicillamine (normal, less than 500 μg/24 hr)
- Low serum uric acid and phosphorus
- Abnormal urinalysis (hematuria)

BIOPSY
- Early: steatosis, focal necrosis, glycogenated hepatocyte nuclei; may reveal inflammation and piecemeal necrosis
- Late: cirrhosis (Fig. 40–4)
- Hepatic copper content (less than 250 μg/g of dry weight; normal is 20 to 50 μg/g)

TREATMENT
- Penicillamine, trientine: chelator therapy
- Zinc: inhibits intestinal copper absorption
- Ammonium tetrathiomolybdate for neurologic symptoms
- Antioxidants
- Liver transplantation (for severe hepatic failure unresponsive to chelation)

C. DYSTONIA

DEFINITION
Dystonia is characterized by involuntary muscle contractions (sustained or spasmodic) that lead to abnormal body movements or postures. Dystonia can be generalized or focal, of early (younger than 20 years of age) or late onset, and primary or secondary.

CLINICAL PRESENTATION
Focal dystonias produce abnormal sustained muscle contractions in an area of the body:
- Neck (torticollis): most commonly affected site, with a tendency for the head to turn to one side
- Eyelids (blepharospasm): involuntary closure of the eyelids
- Mouth (oromandibular dystonia): involuntary contraction of muscles of the mouth, tongue, or face
- Hand (writer's cramp)
Generalized dystonia affects multiple areas of the body (Fig. 40–5) and can lead to marked joint deformities.

CAUSE
- Exact pathophysiology is unknown but is thought to involve abnormalities of basal ganglia. Specifically, reduced and abnormal patterns of neuronal activity in the basal ganglia result in disinhibition of the motor thalamus and cortex, leading to abnormal movement.
- Hereditary forms have been described, including the severe progressive form, dystonia musculorum deformans.
- Sporadic or idiopathic forms occur.

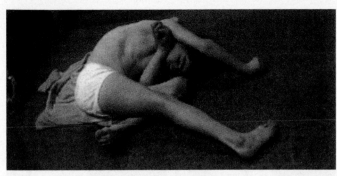

Fig 40–5
A patient with advanced childhood-onset generalized idiopathic torsion dystonia. This boy, who uses a wheelchair, is most comfortable lying on the floor in this position. The left hip, knee, elbow, and wrist are flexed; the right hip is flexed and the knee extended; and the right arm is elevated, with the elbow and wrist extended.
(From Rosenberg RN: Atlas of Clinical Neurology. Boston, Butterworth-Heinemann, 1998.)

- Dystonia can occur secondary to other diseases, such as CNS disease, hypoxia, severe head injury, kernicterus, Huntington's disease, Wilson's disease, Parkinson's disease, and lysosomal storage diseases.
- Acute dystonia can occur following treatment with drugs that block dopamine receptors, such as phenothiazines or butyrophenones.
- Tardive dyskinesia or dystonia can result from long-term treatment with antipsychotic drugs such as antiemetics (e.g., phenothiazines) or antipsychotics (e.g., butyrophenones, such as haloperidol). It can also occur with levodopa, anticonvulsants, or ergots.

DIFFERENTIAL DIAGNOSIS
- Parkinson's disease
- Progressive supranuclear palsy
- Wilson's disease
- Huntington's disease
- Drug effects

LABORATORY TESTS
- Usually not helpful for diagnosis
- Serum ceruloplasmin if Wilson's disease is suspected

IMAGING STUDIES
- Primary dystonias are generally not associated with structural CNS abnormalities; CT or MRI of brain if a CNS lesion is suspected as cause of secondary dystonia
- Electrophysiologic testing can provide diagnostic support for the diagnosis.

TREATMENT
- Heat, massage, physical therapy to relieve pain
- Splints to prevent contractures
- For acute dystonic reactions to phenothiazines or butyrophenones, use diphenhydramine, 50 mg IV, or benztropine, 2 mg IV.
- Slowly withdraw offending agents.
- Diazepam, baclofen, or carbamazepine may be helpful.
- Trihexyphenidyl may be helpful for tardive dyskinesia or dystonia.
- Injections of botulinum toxin into the affected muscles can be used for refractory cases of focal dystonias.
- Surgical procedures including myectomy, rhizotomy, thalamotomy (pallidotomy), or deep brain stimulation may be helpful for severe refractory cases.

Chapter 41   Developmental disorders of the spinal cord and brain

A. SYRINGOMYELIA

DEFINITION

Syringomyelia is a disease of the spine characterized by the formation of fluid-filled cavities in the spinal cord, sometimes extending into the brainstem.

PHYSICAL FINDINGS AND CLINICAL PRESENTATION

- Onset is usually insidious, with symptoms often not beginning until the third or fourth decade.
- Cervical spine is the most commonly affected area.
  1. Intrinsic hand atrophy, weakness, and anesthetic sensory loss may develop.
  2. The latter may lead to unnoticed burns or other injuries in the hand.
  3. Loss of pain and temperature sensation may occur, but tactile sense in the upper extremity is preserved.
  4. Sharp testing elicits no pain, but patient often perceives the sharpness of the object.
  5. A Charcot joint in the shoulder or elbow may develop.
- Reflexes are absent in the upper extremities.
- Spasticity and hyperreflexia are present in the lower extremities.
- Scoliosis is common.
- Nystagmus and Horner's syndrome may also occur.
- Trophic skin changes eventually develop in many cases.

CAUSE

- The cause is unknown, but the condition is thought to result from obstruction of the outlet of the fourth ventricle, often associated with a Chiari I malformation, which causes fluid to be diverted down the central cord.
- Often, a history of birth injury exists.
- Syringomyelia later in life may be the result of trauma or an intramedullary tumor.

DIFFERENTIAL DIAGNOSIS

- Amyotrophic lateral sclerosis (ALS)
- Multiple sclerosis (MS)
- Spinal cord tumor
- Tabes dorsalis
- Progressive spinal muscular atrophy

WORKUP

- Plain radiographs usually reveal widening of the bony canal in the region of involvement.
- Bony anomalies are often present at the base of the skull and at the C1-C2 spinal segments.
- MRI (Fig. 41–1)

TREATMENT

Drainage and operative repair of any bony anomalies are undertaken, often with decompression laminectomy of C1 and C2.

B. SPINA BIFIDA

DEFINITION

Spina bifida is a defective fusion of the vertebral arches occurring most commonly in the lumbar region.

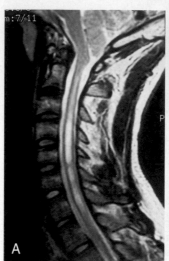
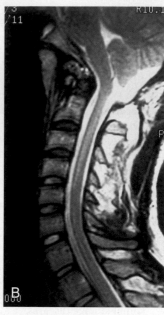

Fig 41–1
Syringomyelia. **A,** Midsagittal T2-weighted spin-echo MRI scan showing mild cerebellar ectopia and a syrinx *(white area)* in the cervical spinal cord. **B,** Same patient 1 year after foramen magnum decompression. The syrinx has partially collapsed.
(From Grainger RG, Allison DJ, Adam A, Dixon AK [eds]: Grainger and Allison's Diagnostic Radiology: A Textbook of Medical Imaging, 4th ed. London. Harcourt, 2001.)

CAUSE

The disorder is more common in females and is associated with folic acid deficiency during pregnancy and with trisomy 13 or 18.

PHYSICAL FINDINGS AND CLINICAL PRESENTATION

- In spina bifida cystica, the meninges prolapse through the bony defect (meningocele, meningomyelocele) and there is an association with hydrocephalus, kyphosis (Fig. 41–2), and Arnold-Chiari malformation.

C. MENINGOMYELOCELE

DEFINITION

Meningomyelocele is the most common type of spina bifida and is characterized by herniation of the spinal cord, nerves, or both through a bony defect of the spine (Fig. 41–3).

PHYSICAL FINDINGS AND CLINICAL PRESENTATION

- Evident at birth—a sac protruding in the lumbar region
- Severity of neurologic deficits depends on the location of the lesion along the neuraxis
- Motor dysfunction in the legs
- Lack of bladder or bowel control
- Often associated with Chiari II malformation and resulting obstructive hydrocephalus

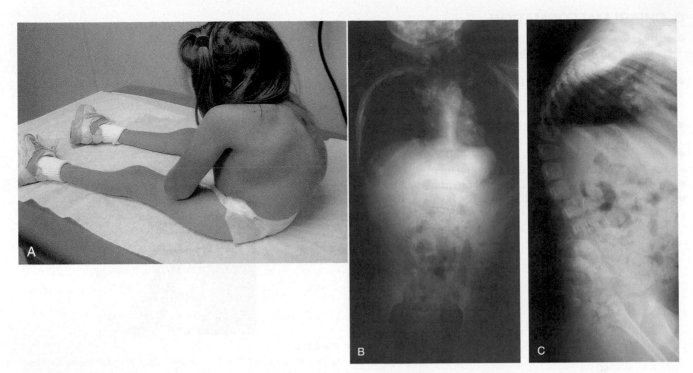

Fig 41–2
Spina bifida. **A,** This child, with thoracic level spina bifida, has an obvious kyphotic deformity. The scars on her back are from surgical closure of her myelomeningocele. **B** and **C,** Anteroposterior and lateral radiographs of the spine demonstrate that kyphosis is secondary to incomplete posterior osseous support.
(From Zitelli BJ, Davis HW: Atlas of Pediatric Physical Diagnosis, 4th ed. St. Louis, Mosby, 2002.)

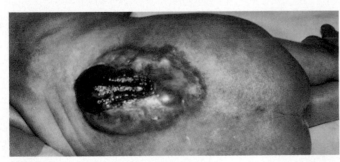

Fig 41–3
Meningomyelocele.
(From Zitelli BJ, Davis HW: Atlas of Pediatric Physical Diagnosis, 4th ed. St. Louis, Mosby, 2002.)

DIAGNOSIS
- Prenatal diagnosis through ultrasound and MRI is being made more frequently.
- MRI can provide better definition of the defect.
- Coexisting hydrocephalus is detected by measurement of head size, ultrasonography, CT, or MRI.

DIFFERENTIAL DIAGNOSIS
- Teratoma
- Meningocele

WORKUP
- Evaluate for hydrocephalus.
- Evaluate for other congenital abnormalities, such as congenital heart disease, hydronephrosis, intestinal malformation, clubfoot, and skeletal deformities.

LABORATORY TESTS
- Prenatal testing often reveals elevated alpha-fetoprotein in amniotic fluid or maternal serum.

IMAGING STUDIES
- MRI of spine
- X-ray studies of skull exhibit craniolacunia, a honeycombed pattern associated with hydrocephalus.
- CT or MRI of head may reveal hydrocephalus.

TREATMENT
- Surgical closure of myelomeningocele is performed soon after birth.
- Control of hydrocephalus (shunt)
- Management of urinary incontinence
- Counseling of parents
- Treatment of seizures, if present

D. CHIARI MALFORMATION

- Chiari malformations are hindbrain developmental abnormalities initially described by the German pathologist Hans Chiari.
- Chiari I (congenital tonsillar ectopia) consists of elongated cerebellar tonsils displaced into the upper cervical canal. It is not associated with other congenital brain malformations.
- In Chiari II, the vermis, pons, medulla, and elongated fourth ventricle are displaced inferiorly into the cervical canal.
- Chiari III consists of cervical spina bifida combined with multiple cerebellar and brainstem anomalies.
- Chiari IV is a form of severe cerebellar hypoplasia.
- MRI (Fig. 41–4) is the diagnostic imaging modality of choice.

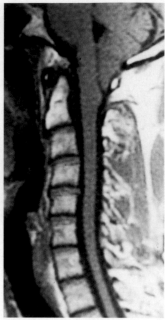

Fig 41–4

Chiari malformation. This T1-weighted sagittal image shows the cerebellar tonsils extending just below the neural arch of C1, and elongation and kinking of the medulla oblongata.
(From Grainger RG, Allison DJ, Adam A, Dixon AK [eds]: Grainger and Allison's Diagnostic Radiology: A Textbook of Medical Imaging, 4th ed. London. Harcourt, 2001.)

Chapter 42 | **Multiple sclerosis**

DEFINITION

Multiple sclerosis is a chronic demyelinating disease of unknown cause. It is characterized pathologically by zones of demyelinization (plaques) scattered throughout the white matter.

CLINICAL MANIFESTATIONS

The disease can manifest in varied patterns:

- Relapsing-remitting MS (RRMS): most common type (80% of patients at onset, 55% of all patients at any given time). Full recovery of attacks may occur early but, with subsequent attacks, recovery is incomplete.
- Secondary progressive MS (SPMS): worsening disability because of accumulating axonal loss and new inflammation. SPMS is the long-term outcome of most RRMS cases.
- Primary progressive MS (PPMS): gradual insidious worsening from onset without relapses
- Progressive-relapsing MS (PRMS): progressive course with superimposed relapses; least common form (5% of patients)

The clinical signs vary with the location of plaques. The more common manifestations are as follows:

- Weakness: usually involving the lower extremities; the patient may complain of difficulty ambulating, tendency to drop things, easy fatigability.
- Sensory disturbances: numbness, tingling, pins and needles sensation
- Visual disturbances: diplopia, blurred vision, visual loss, nystagmus, impaired visual acuity
- Incoordination: gait impairment, clumsiness of upper extremities
- Others: vertigo, incontinence, loss of sexual function, slurred speech, depression, fatigue

PHYSICAL EXAMINATION

Visual abnormalities

- Paresis of medial rectus muscle on lateral conjugate gaze (internuclear ophthalmoplegia) and horizontal nystagmus of the adducting eye
- Central scotoma, decreased visual acuity (optic neuritis)
- A *Marcus Gunn pupil* (pupil that paradoxically dilates with direct light), indicating damage to the optic nerve anterior to the chiasm, is frequently present.
- Nystagmus

Abnormalities of reflexes

- Increased deep tendon reflexes
- Positive Hoffmann's sign, positive Babinski's sign
- Decreased abdominal skin reflex, decreased cremasteric reflex
- *Lhermitte's sign:* flexion of the neck while the patient is lying down elicits an electrical sensation extending bilaterally down the arms, back, and lower trunk.
- *Charcot's triad:* nystagmus, scanning speech, and intention tremor
- Impaired recognition of objects by touch alone (astereognosis)

DIFFERENTIAL DIAGNOSIS

- Autoimmune: acute disseminated encephalomyelitis (ADEM), postvaccination encephalomyelitis
- Degenerative: subacute combined degeneration (vitamin B_{12} deficiency), inherited spastic paraparesis
- Infections: Lyme disease, progressive multifocal leukoencephalopathy, syphilis, HIV, human T-cell leukemia virus 1 (HTLV-1), Whipple's disease, expanded differential in immunocompromised patients
- Inflammatory: sarcoidosis, SLE, Sjögren's syndrome, Behçet's disease, vasculitis, celiac disease
- Spinal cord compression (cervical spondylosis, tumor, herniated disc, Chiari malformation)
- Inherited metabolic disorders: leukodystrophies, hereditary myelopathy
- Mitochondrial: Leber's hereditary optic neuropathy; mitochondrial encephalopathy, lactic acidosis, and stroke-like episodes (MELAS)
- MS variants: recurrent optic neuropathy, neuromyelitis optica (Devic disease), acute tumor-like lesion (Marburg variant), Baló's concentric sclerosis, myelinoclastic diffuse sclerosis (Schilder's disease)
- Neoplasms: metastases, CNS lymphoma
- Vascular: subcortical infarcts caused by diabetes mellitus (DM), hypertension, Binswanger's disease
- Somatoform disorders, factitious disorders

DIAGNOSTIC EVALUATION

- The diagnosis should be based on objective evidence of two or more neurologic signs occurring in different parts of the CNS more than 3 months apart (neurologic signs disseminated in time and space).
- MRI of the brain with gadolinium (Fig. 42–1) can identify lesions as small as 3 to 4 mm and is frequently diagnostic in suspected cases; it can also be used to assess disease load, activity, and progression. MRI typically reveals multiple, predominantly periventricular plaques; however, a normal MRI scan cannot be used conclusively to exclude multiple sclerosis.
- Lumbar puncture is indicated for all first-time relapses and recommended for all evaluations when the diagnosis of MS is not definite. Lumbar puncture is particularly useful when MRI is inconclusive, because Lyme disease, acute disseminated encephalopathy, and hypertensive changes may mimic multiple sclerosis.

1. In patients with multiple sclerosis, the CSF may show increased gamma globulin (mostly IgG, but often IgA and IgM).

2. Agarose electrophoresis discloses discrete oligoclonal bands in the gamma region in approximately 90% of patients, including some with normal IgG levels.

3. Other possible CSF abnormalities: increased total protein, increased mononuclear white blood cells, presence of myelin basic protein (elevated in acute attacks, indicates active myelin destruction)

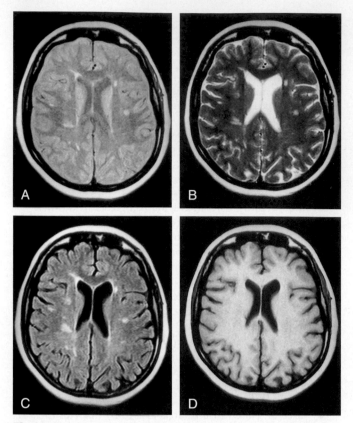

- Measurement of visual evoked response is useful to assess nerve fiber conduction (myelin loss or destruction will slow conduction velocity). It can also provide objective evidence of an optic nerve lesion that may not be evident on MRI scan.
- Serologic testing: Vitamin B_{12} level, TSH, ESR, ANA, Lyme titer, VDRL, HIV. Additional tests may include antineutrophil cytoplasmic antibody (ANCA), Sjögren's syndrome antigen A (SS-A), Sjögren's syndrome antigen B (SS-B), and acetylcholinesterase (ACE) levels.

TREATMENT

- Treatment should be given at the earliest stages, when inflammation predominates and before substantial, irreversible axonal loss occurs.
- Acute exacerbations can be treated with high-dose intravenous methylprednisolone. Corticosteroid therapy shortens the duration of acute relapses and accelerates recovery, but it does not improve the overall degree of recovery or alter the long-term course of MS.
- Disease-modifying therapies: immunomodulators have been shown to slow progression of the disease. Currently available disease-modifying drugs for multiple sclerosis are interferon beta, SC interferon beta-1a, interferon beta-1b, glatiramer acetate, and mitoxantrone.

Fig 42–1
Patient with multiple sclerosis with plaques of demyelination shown on fast spin-echo (FSE) proton density **(A)**, FSE T2 **(B)**, and FSE fluid-attenuated inversion recovery (FLAIR, **C**). In this patient, there is no discernible abnormality on T1-weighted images without contrast **(D)**. (From Grainger RG, Allison DJ, Adam A, Dixon AK [eds]: Grainger and Allison's Diagnostic Radiology: A Textbook of Medical Imaging, 4th ed. London. Harcourt, 2001.)

Chapter 43	**Amyotrophic lateral sclerosis**

DEFINITION

Amyotrophic lateral sclerosis (ALS) is a progressive, degenerative, neuromuscular condition of undetermined cause affecting corticospinal tracts and anterior horn cells (Fig. 43–1) and resulting in dysfunction of upper motor neurons (UMNs) and lower motor neurons (LMNs), respectively.

PHYSICAL FINDINGS AND CLINICAL PRESENTATION

- Lower motor neuron signs (weakness, hypotonia, wasting, fasciculations, hypoflexia or areflexia). Figure 43–2 illustrates wasting of the tongue with fasciculations in a patient with lower motor neuron bulbar palsy affecting the hypoglossal nucleus.
- Upper motor neuron signs (loss of fine motor dexterity, spasticity, extensor plantar responses, hyperreflexia, clonus).
- Preservation of extraocular movements, sensation, bowel and bladder function.
- Dysarthria, dysphagia, pseudobulbar affect, frontal lobe dysfunction.
- ALS comprises approximately 90% cases of adult-onset motor neuron disease. Other presentations of motor neuron disease include progressive muscular atrophy, primary lateral sclerosis, progressive bulbar palsy, progressive pseudobulbar palsy, and ALS-parkinsonism-dementia complex.

CAUSE

- Of all cases, 90% to 95% are sporadic; of the familial cases, approximately 20% are associated with a genetic defect in the copper-zinc superoxide dismutase enzyme (SOD1).

DIFFERENTIAL DIAGNOSIS

- Multifocal motor neuropathy with conduction block (MMN)
- Cervical spondylotic myelopathy with polyradiculopathy
- Spinal stenosis with compression of lumbosacral nerve roots
- Chronic inflammatory demyelinating polyneuropathy with CNS lesions
- Syringomyelia
- Syringobulbia
- Foramen magnum tumor
- Spinal muscular atrophy (SMA)
- Late-onset hexosaminidase A deficiency
- Bulbospinal muscular atrophy (Kennedy's disease)

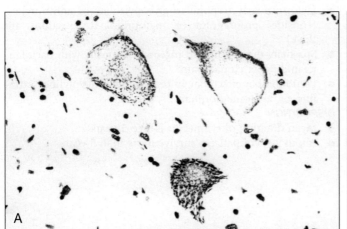
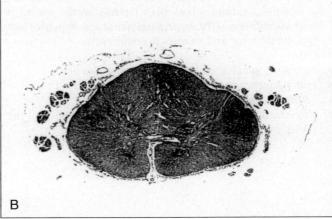
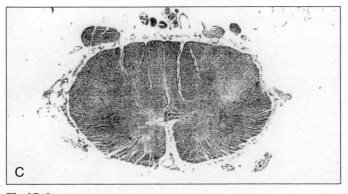

Fig 43–1
Histologic slides from patients with early-onset rapidly progressive amyotrophic lateral sclerosis (ALS). **A,** Anterior horn cells in lumbar spinal cord of a 56-year-old man showing chromatolysis of the neuron on the right (Nissl stain, ×40). **B,** Transverse section of cervical spinal cord from a 60-year-old woman from another kindred with familial ALS and **C,** her 57-year-old son, showing loss of myelin in lateral corticospinal tracts as well as posterior columns (Luxol fast blue, periodic acid–Schiff, H&E).
(**A** courtesy of Dr. D. Nochlin, University of Washington, Seattle.)

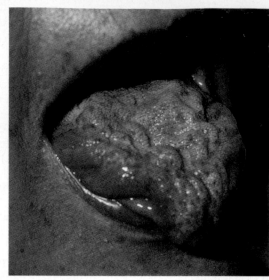

Fig 43–2
Tongue of patient with amyotrophic lateral sclerosis. Note the scalloping. (From Swartz MH: Textbook of Physical Diagnosis, 5th ed. Philadelphia, WB Saunders, 2006.)

- Monomyelic amyotrophy
- ALS-like syndromes have been reported in the setting of lead intoxication, HIV, hyperparathyroidism, hyperthyroidism, lymphoma, and vitamin B_{12} deficiency.

WORKUP

- Electromyographic and nerve conduction studies
- Lumbar puncture to assess protein
- Serum GM-1 Ab if MMN suspected
- Assessment of respiratory function (forced vital capacity [FVC], negative inspiratory force [NIF])

LABORATORY TESTS

- Vitamin B_{12}, thyroid function, serum calcium, parathyroid hormone (PTH), HIV testing may be considered.
- Serum protein and immunofixation electrophoresis
- DNA studies for SMA or bulbospinal atrophy, hexosaminidase levels in pure LMN syndrome
- 24-hour urine for lead if indicated

IMAGING STUDIES

- Craniospinal neuroimaging contingent on clinical scenario
- Modified barium swallow to evaluate aspiration risk

TREATMENT

- Noninvasive positive pressure ventilation may improve quality of life and increase tracheostomy-free survival.
- PEG tube placement improves nutritional intake, promotes weight stabilization, and eases medication administration.
- Nutrition, speech therapy, physical and occupational therapy services
- Suction device for sialorrhea
- Communication may be eased with computerized assistive devices.
- Early discussion of living will, resuscitation orders, desire for PEG and tracheostomy, potential long-term care options
- Riluzole (Rilutek), a glutamate antagonist, is an FDA-approved medication known to extend tracheostomy-free survival in patients with ALS, shown to prolong survival by 2 to 3 months.
- Sialorrhea may respond to glycopyrrolate or amitriptyline (consider propranolol or metoprolol if secretions are thick).
- Spasticity may be treated pharmacologically with baclofen, tizanidine, or clonazepam.
- Pseudobulbar effect may improve with amitriptyline, sertraline, or dextromethorphan.

DISPOSITION

- Mean duration of symptoms is 3 to 5 years
- About 20% of patients survive more than 5 years.

Chapter 44 | Neuropathies

A. GUILLAIN-BARRÉ SYNDROME

DEFINITION

Guillain-Barré syndrome (GBS) is an acute immune-mediated polyradiculoneuropathy (affects nerve roots and peripheral nerves), with predominant motor involvement. It is the most common cause of acute flaccid paralysis in the Western hemisphere and probably worldwide. By definition, maximal clinical weakness occurs within 4 weeks of disease onset.

PHYSICAL FINDINGS AND CLINICAL PRESENTATION

- Symmetrical weakness, most commonly involving proximal muscles initially, subsequently involving both proximal and distal muscles—difficulty in ambulating, getting up from a chair, or climbing stairs.
- Depressed or absent reflexes bilaterally
- Minimal to moderate glove and stocking paresthesias, dysesthesia, anesthesia, or back pain
- Pain (caused by involvement of posterior nerve roots) may be prominent.
- Autonomic abnormalities (brady- or tachyarrhythmias, hypo- or hypertension)
- Respiratory insufficiency (caused by weakness of bulbar, intercostal muscles)
- Facial paresis, ophthalmoparesis, dysphagia (secondary to cranial nerve involvement)

CAUSE

- Unknown
- Preceding infectious illness 1 to 4 weeks before disease onset in 66% of patients
- Humoral and cell-mediated immune attack of peripheral nerve myelin, Schwann cells, sometimes with axonal involvement. The histopathology is marked by demyelination associated with chronic inflammation, consisting primarily of lymphocytes and macrophages, surrounding endoneurial vessels and infiltrating into the perineurial region. Nerve roots show a predilection for inflammation (Fig. 44–1).

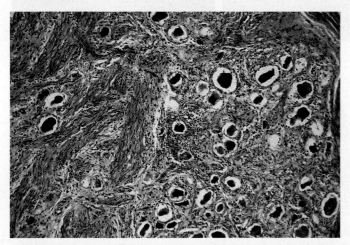

Fig 44–1
Nerve root ganglion marked by a chronic inflammatory cell infiltrate in Guillain-Barré syndrome.
(From Silverberg SG, DeLellis RA, Frable WJ, et al [eds]: Principles and Practice of Surgical Pathology and Cytopathology, 4th ed. New York, Churchill Livingstone, 2006.)

DIFFERENTIAL DIAGNOSIS

- Toxic peripheral neuropathies: heavy metal poisoning (lead, thallium, arsenic), medications (vincristine, disulfiram), organophosphate poisoning, hexacarbon (glue sniffer's neuropathy)
- Nontoxic peripheral neuropathies: acute intermittent porphyria, vasculitic polyneuropathy, infectious (poliomyelitis, diphtheria, Lyme disease, West Nile virus); tick paralysis
- Neuromuscular junction disorders: myasthenia gravis, botulism, snake envenomations
- Myopathies such as polymyositis, acute necrotizing myopathies caused by drugs
- Metabolic derangements such as hypermagnesemia, hypokalemia, hypophosphatemia
- Acute central nervous system disorders such as basilar artery thrombosis with brainstem infarction, brainstem encephalomyelitis, transverse myelitis, and spinal cord compression
- Hysterical paralysis or malingering

WORKUP

- Exclude other causes based on clinical history, examination, and laboratory tests.
- Lumbar puncture (may be normal in the first 1 to 2 weeks of the illness): typical findings include elevated CSF protein with few mononuclear leukocytes (albuminocytologic dissociation) in 80% to 90% of patients. Elevated CSF cell counts is an expected feature in cases associated with HIV seroconversion.
- Electromyography (EMG)-nerve conduction study (NCS): may be normal in the first 10 to 14 days of the disease. The earliest electrodiagnostic abnormality is prolongation or absence of H reflexes. EMG-NCS evidence of demyelination (prolonged distal latency, conduction velocity slowing, conduction block, temporal dispersion and prolonged F-waves) in two or more motor nerves confirms the diagnosis of acute inflammatory demyelinating polyradiculopathy (AIDP) in the appropriate clinical context.

LABORATORY TESTS

- CBC may reveal early leukocytosis with left shift. Monitor electrolytes to exclude metabolic causes.
- Heavy metal testing, urine porphyria screen, creatine kinase, HIV titers, neuroimaging of the brain and spinal cord if diagnosis is uncertain. Nerve root enhancement may be seen on MRI of the lumbosacral spine.
- Antibodies against ganglioside GQ_{1b} may be present in up to 90% of patients with MFS (Miller Fisher syndrome). IgG antibodies against ganglioside GM_1 may be associated with AMAN (acute motor axonal neuropathy). There are no antiganglioside antibodies commonly associated with AIDP (acute inflammatory demyelinating polyradiculoneuropathy).
- In equivocal cases (especially if peripheral nerve vasculitis is a concern), nerve biopsy may aid in confirming a diagnosis of GBS. Sensory nerve biopsy demonstrates segmental demyelination with infiltration of monocytes and T cells into the endoneurium. Axonal loss is commonly seen in sensory nerve biopsy specimens in GBS.

TREATMENT
- Close monitoring of respiratory function (frequent measurements of vital capacity, negative inspiratory force, and pulmonary toilet), because respiratory failure is the major complication in GBS
- Frequent repositioning of patient to minimize formation of pressure sores
- Prevention of thromboembolism with antithrombotic stockings and SC heparin (5000 U every 12 hours) in non-ambulatory patients
- Infusion of IV immunoglobulins
- Early therapeutic plasma exchange
- There is no proven benefit from combining IVIg and plasma exchange.
- Mechanical ventilation may be needed if FVC is less than 12 to 15 mL/kg, vital capacity is rapidly decreasing or is less than 1000 mL, negative inspiratory force 20 cm or less, H_2O, Pao_2 is less than 70 mm Hg, or the patient is having significant difficulty clearing secretions or is aspirating.

B. CHARCOT-MARIE-TOOTH DISEASE

DEFINITION

Charcot-Marie-Tooth disease is a heterogeneous group of non-inflammatory inherited peripheral neuropathies. It is the most common inherited neuromuscular disorder.

PHYSICAL FINDINGS AND CLINICAL PRESENTATION
- Variable presentation from family to family, but affected individuals in a family tend to have similar symptomatology
- Usually, gradual onset, with slowly progressive disorder
- Foot deformity producing a high arch (cavus) and hammertoes (Fig. 44–2B)
- Atrophy of the lower legs (see Fig. 44–2A), producing a storklike appearance (muscle wasting does not involve the upper legs)
- Nerve enlargement (see Fig. 44–2D)
- Sensory loss or other neurologic signs, although the sensory involvement is usually mild
- Scoliosis
- Decreased proprioception that often interferes with balance and gait
- Painful paresthesias
- In late cases, possible involvement of hands (see Fig. 44–2C)
- Absence of deep tendon reflexes (DTRs) in many cases
- Poorly healing foot ulcers in some patients

CAUSE
- Chronic segmental demyelination of peripheral nerves, with hypertrophic changes caused by remyelination

DIFFERENTIAL DIAGNOSIS
- Other inherited neuropathies
- Toxic, metabolic, and nutritional polyneuropathies

WORKUP
- The early onset, slow progression, and familial nature of the disorder are usually sufficient to establish diagnosis.
- Electrophysiologic studies are often diagnostic and may also be helpful in defining various subtypes of this group of neuropathies.
- Occasionally, muscle and nerve (sural) biopsy may be required (Fig. 44–3).

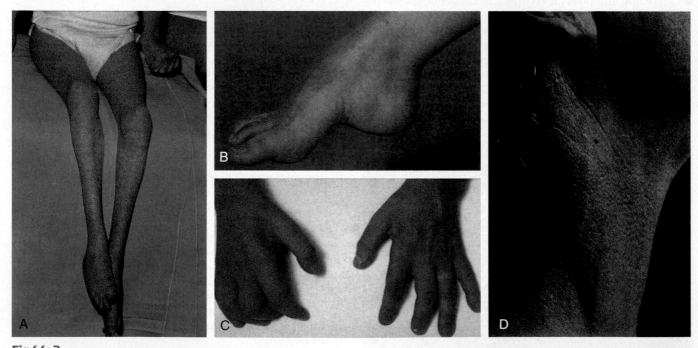

Fig 44–2
Physical manifestations of Charcot-Marie-Tooth 1 (CMT 1) disease. **A,** Marked distal atrophy of leg muscles in an unusually severe case of CMT. **B,** Typical high arch, contracted heel cord, and footdrop posture of CMT. **C,** Clawing of the fingers and interosseous muscle atrophy of the hands. **D,** Hypertrophy of the greater auricular nerve running vertically between the base of the neck and the mastoid in a man with CMT 1A. CMT 1A is associated with a DNA duplication at chromosome 17p11.2, which includes the *PMP22* (peripheral myelin protein) gene.
(From Rosenberg RN: Atlas of Clinical Neurology. Boston, Butterworth-Heinemann, 1998.)

TREATMENT
- Genetic counseling
- Supportive physical therapy and occupational therapy
- Prevention of injury to limbs with diminished sensibility
- Bracing
- Occasionally, surgery to add stability and restore a plantigrade foot

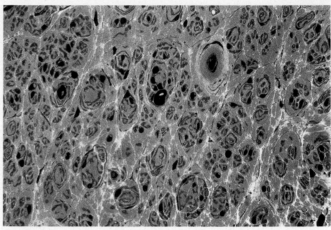

Fig 44–3
Section of sural nerve showing prominent numbers of onion bulb formations in Charcot-Marie-Tooth disease (toluidine blue).
(From Silverberg SG, DeLellis RA, Frable WJ, et al [eds]: Principles and Practice of Surgical Pathology and Cytopathology, 4th ed. New York, Churchill Livingstone, 2006.)

Chapter 45   Ataxias

A. FRIEDREICH'S ATAXIA

DEFINITION
Friedreich's ataxia is the most common neurodegenerative hereditary ataxic disorder, caused by degeneration of dorsal root ganglions, posterior columns, spinocerebellar and corticospinal tracts, and large sensory peripheral neurons (Fig. 45-1).

PHYSICAL FINDINGS AND CLINICAL PRESENTATION
- Onset of progressive appendicular and gait ataxia, with absent muscle stretch reflexes in the lower extremities.
- With disease progression (within 5 years): dysarthria, distal loss of position and vibration sense, pyramidal leg weakness, areflexia in all four limbs, extensor plantar responses
- Common findings: progressive scoliosis, distal atrophy, pes cavus, and cardiomyopathy (symmetrical concentric hypertrophic form in most cases)
- Insulin-requiring diabetes mellitus may occur in 10% of patients, with glucose intolerance occurring in an additional 10% to 20%.

CAUSE
- Genetic: frataxin gene is localized to the centromeric region of chromosome 9q13.

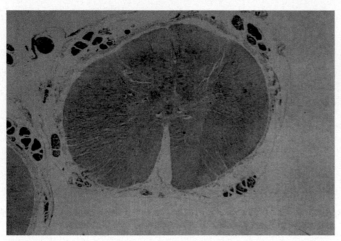

Fig 45–1
Transverse section of thoracic spinal cord from a 20-year-old man with Friedreich's ataxia who developed cardiomyopathy and diabetes. Friedreich's ataxia is an autosomal recessive disorder usually beginning in childhood and presenting with slowly progressive gait ataxia associated with depressed tendon reflexes, bilateral Babinski's reflexes, position and vibration sensory deficits, dysarthria, and nystagmus. A decreased life span is primarily the result of an associated cardiomyopathy. There is loss of myelin staining in the posterior columns and the lateral cortical spinal tracts. Of interest is the fact that Friedreich's ataxia is not associated with significant cerebellar atrophy. The gene for Friedreich's ataxia is on chromosome 9 and contains a GAA repeat in an intron. In addition, there are other autosomal causes of ataxia, one of which maps to chromosome 8 and is associated with mutations in the α-tocopherol transfer protein and is an important condition in the differential diagnosis (Luxol fast blue, periodic acid–Schiff stain, H&E). (From Rosenberg RN: Atlas of Clinical Neurology. Boston, Butterworth-Heinemann, 1998.)

- Normal sequence has 6 to 27 repeats; abnormal sequence has 120 to 1700 GAA repeats.
- Frataxin deficiency leads to impaired mitochondrial iron homeostasis.

DIFFERENTIAL DIAGNOSIS
- Charcot-Marie-Tooth disease type
- Abetalipoproteinemia
- Severe vitamin E deficiency with malabsorption
- Early-onset cerebellar ataxia with retained reflexes
- Autosomal dominant cerebellar ataxia (spinocerebellar ataxia)

WORKUP
- Diagnostic criteria include electrophysiologic evidence for a generalized axonal sensory neuropathy.
- Electrocardiography shows widespread T wave inversion and evidence of left ventricular hypertrophy in 65% of patients.
- Sural nerve biopsy shows major loss of large myelinated fibers.
- Specific gene testing for the expanded GAA trinucleotide repeat

LABORATORY TESTS
- EMG-NCS
- Electrocardiography and echocardiography
- Peripheral blood smear for acanthocytes
- Lipid profile
- Fasting glucose and two-hour glucose tolerance tests
- Vitamin E levels (if necessary)

IMAGING STUDIES
MRI of the brain and spinal cord (Fig. 45–2) may demonstrate spinal cord atrophy with essentially normal cerebrum, brainstem, and cerebellum.

TREATMENT
- Surgical correction of scoliosis and foot deformities in select patients
- Prosthetic devices as required (e.g., ankle-foot orthosis for footdrop)
- Physical therapy
- Communication devices for patients with severe dysarthria

B. ATAXIA-TELANGIECTASIA

DEFINITION
Ataxia telangiectasia (A-T) is an autosomal recessive (AR) disorder of childhood characterized by progressive cerebellar ataxia, choreoathetosis, telangiectasias of the skin and conjunctiva, frequent infections, increased sensitivity to ionizing radiation, and a predisposition to malignancies, particularly leukemia and lymphoma.

PHYSICAL FINDINGS AND CLINICAL PRESENTATION
- Children show normal early development until they start to walk, when gait and truncal ataxias become apparent. These findings are soon accompanied by polyneuropathy, progressive apraxia of eye movements, progressively slurred speech, choreoathetosis, mild diabetes mellitus, growth failure, and signs of premature aging (graying of the hair).

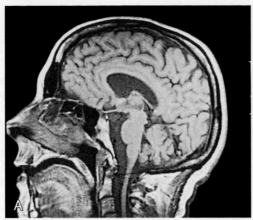 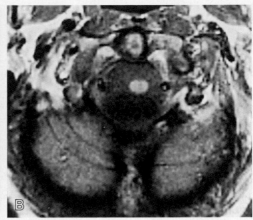

Fig 45-2

T1-weighted MRI scans of the brain and cervical spinal cord in Friedreich's ataxia. The images are the midsagittal plane of the head **(A)** and an axial slice at the level of the dens axis **(B)**. There is severe shrinkage of the cervical spinal cord. In contrast, the cerebellum and brainstem are of normal size.

(From Goetz CG, Pappert EJ: Textbook of Clinical Neurology. Philadelphia, WB Saunders, 1999.)

- Telangiectatic lesions occur in the outer parts of the bulbar conjunctivae, over the ears, on exposed parts of the neck, on the bridge of the nose, and in the flexor creases of the forearms.

- Immunodeficiencies occur in 60% to 80% of individuals with A-T, although they are seldom progressive. Recurrent sinopulmonary infections occur secondary to impaired humoral and cellular immunity in about 70% of children.

- Cancer risk in individuals with A-T is 38%, of which leukemia and lymphoma account for about 95% of malignancies. As individuals begin to have longer life spans, other malignancies are observed, such as ovarian cancer, breast cancer, melanoma, and sarcoma.

- Typically, individuals with A-T have normal intelligence. Slow motor and verbal responses may make traditional timed assessments inaccurate.

DIFFERENTIAL DIAGNOSIS

Early-onset ataxias

- Friedreich's ataxia
- Abetalipoproteinemia (Bassen-Kornzweig syndrome)
- Acquired vitamin E deficiency
- Early-onset cerebellar ataxia (EOCA) with retained reflexes
- Ataxia with biochemical abnormalities: associated with ceroid lipofuscinosis, xeroderma pigmentosa, Cockayne's syndrome, adrenoleukodystrophy, metachromatic leukodystrophy, mitochondrial disease, sialidosis, Niemann-Pick disease

WORKUP

- Patients should be evaluated for serum immunoglobulin levels (IgA, IgG, IgE, and IgG subclasses), which are decreased or absent, and alpha-fetoprotein, which is elevated in more than 95% of patients with A-T.

- Karyotype: high incidence of chromosomal breaks. A 7;14 chromosomal translocation is identified in 5% to 15% of cells in routine studies on the peripheral blood of individuals with A-T. Molecular genetic testing for the *ATM* gene is now available on a clinical basis. Carriers may have an increased risk of developing cancer. Prenatal testing is available.

- CT or MRI scans will show cerebellar atrophy, but may not be obvious in very young children.

- Immunoblotting for ATM protein. This determines whether ATM protein is present in cells; approximately 90% of individuals will have no detectable ATM protein.

- Fibroblasts can be screened in vitro for x-ray sensitivity and radioresistant DNA synthesis.

- Pathology shows cerebellar degeneration, loss of pigmented neurons, and posterior column degeneration in the spinal cord.

TREATMENT

- There is no proved treatment available to delay the progressive ataxia, dysarthria, and oculomotor apraxia. Treatment remains supportive.

- Surveillance for infections and neoplasms. Individuals with frequent and severe infections may benefit from intravenous immunoglobulin to supplement immune system.

- Antioxidant (e.g., vitamin E or alpha-lipoic acid) is recommended, although no formal testing has been done. Alpha-lipoic acid crosses the blood-brain barrier, and may therefore have some advantage.

- Minimize radiation because this may induce further chromosomal damage and lead to neoplasms.

- Physical and occupational therapy to minimize contractures

Chapter 46 | Infections

A. BRAIN ABSCESS

DEFINITION

A brain abscess is a focal intracerebral infection that begins as a localized area of cerebritis and develops into a collection of pus surrounded by a well-vascularized capsule (Fig. 46–1).

PHYSICAL FINDINGS AND CLINICAL PRESENTATION

- Classic triad: fever, headache, and focal neurologic deficit are present in 50% of cases.
- Fever is present in only 50% of patients.
- Headache is usually localized to the side of the abscess; the onset can be gradual or severe; it is present in 70% of cases.
- Focal neurologic findings (e.g., seizures, hemiparesis, aphasia, ataxia) depend on the location of the abscess and are seen in 30% to 50% of cases.
- Papilledema is present in 25% of cases.
- Presence of adjacent infections (dental abscess, otitis media, and sinusitis) may be a clue to the underlying diagnosis and should be sought in any suspected case.
- Time course from symptom onset to presentation ranges from hours in fulminant cases to more than 1 month; 75% present in the first 2 weeks.
- The nonspecific presentation of a brain abscess warrants that clinicians maintain a high index of suspicion.

CAUSE

- Brain abscesses arise from contiguous infection or hematogenous spread from a remote site.
- They are classified based on the likely portal of entry. The relationships between potential sources of infection and sites at which CNS infections may occur is illustrated in Figure 46–2.

Likely source of abscess

- Contiguous focus or primary infection (55% of all brain abscesses):

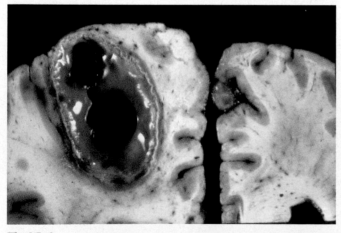

Fig 46–1

Brain abscess. Note the presence of a well-formed capsule around the necrotic center of the lesion.

(From Silverberg SG, DeLellis RA, Frable WJ, et al [eds]: Principles and Practice of Surgical Pathology and Cytopathology, 4th ed. New York, Churchill Livingstone, 2006.)

1. Paranasal sinus: occurs in frontal lobe; streptococci, *Bacteroides, Haemophilus,* and *Fusobacterium* spp.
2. Otitis media, mastoiditis: occurs in temporal lobe and cerebellum; streptococci, Enterobacteriaceae, *Bacteroides,* and *Pseudomonas* spp.
3. Dental sepsis: occurs in frontal lobe; mixed *Fusobacterium, Bacteroides,* and *Streptococcus* spp.
4. Penetrating head injury: site of abscess depends on site of wound; *Staphylococcus aureus, Clostridium* species, Enterobacteriaceae spp.
5. Postoperative: *Staphylococcus epidermidis* and *S. aureus,* Enterobacteriaceae, and Pseudomonadaceae
- Hematogenous spread, distant site of infection (25% of all brain abscesses): abscesses most commonly multiple, especially in middle cerebral artery distribution; infecting organisms depend on source
1. Congenital heart disease: *Streptococcus, Haemophilus* spp.
2. Endocarditis: *S. aureus, Viridans* streptococci
3. Urinary tract: Enterobacteriaceae, Pseudomonadaceae
4. Intra-abdominal: *Streptococcus,* Enterobacteriaceae, anaerobes
5. Lung: *Streptococcus, Actinomyces, Fusobacterium* spp.
6. Immunocompromised host: *Toxoplasma* sp., *Cryptococcus* (Fig. 46–3), fungi (Fig. 46–4), Enterobacteriaceae, *Nocardia* sp., tuberculosis, listeriosis
- Cryptogenic (unknown source): 20% of all brain abscesses

DIFFERENTIAL DIAGNOSIS

- Other parameningeal infections: subdural empyema, epidural abscess, thrombophlebitis of the major dural venous sinuses and cortical veins
- Embolic strokes in patients with bacterial endocarditis
- Mycotic aneurysms with leakage
- Viral encephalitis (usually resulting from herpes simplex)
- Acute hemorrhagic leukoencephalitis
- Parasitic infections: toxoplasmosis, echinococcosis, cysticercosis
- Metastatic or primary brain tumors
- Cerebral infarction
- CNS vasculitis
- Chronic subdural hematoma

LABORATORY TESTS

- White blood cell (WBC) counts are elevated in 60% of patients.
- ESR is usually elevated, but may be normal.
- Blood cultures are most often negative (10% positive).
- Lumbar puncture is contraindicated in patients with suspected abscess (20% die or suffer neurologic decline).
- The yield of Gram stain and culture of material aspirated at time of surgical drainage approaches 100%.

IMAGING STUDIES

- MRI is the diagnostic procedure of choice; provides superior detail compared with CT (higher sensitivity and specificity than CT, but not always immediately available)
- CT scan with intravenous contrast is still an excellent test (sensitivity, 95% to 99%; Fig. 46–5).

RELATIONSHIPS BETWEEN POTENTIAL SOURCES OF INFECTION AND SITES AT WHICH CNS INFECTIONS MAY OCCUR

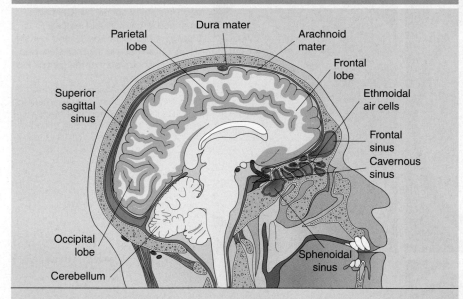

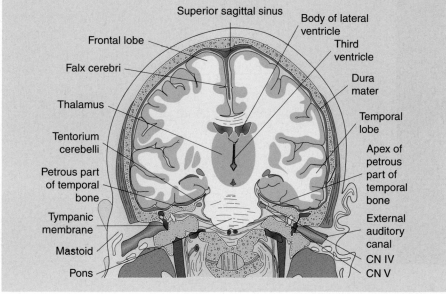

Fig 46–2
Anatomic relationships between potential contiguous sources of infection and sites at which focal pyogenic central nervous system infections may occur.
(From Cohen J, Powderly WG: Infectious Diseases, 2nd ed. St. Louis, Mosby, 2004.)

● Serial CT or MRI scanning is recommended to follow the response to therapy.

TREATMENT

● Effective treatment involves a combination of empirical antibiotic therapy and timely excision or aspiration of the abscess.
● If evidence of edema or mass effect, treatment of elevated intracranial pressure is paramount.
● Hyperventilation of mechanically ventilated patient
● Dexamethasone
● Mannitol
● Medical therapy is never a substitute for surgical intervention to relieve increased intracranial pressure. Neurologic deterioration usually mandates surgery.
● Steroids should be limited to patients with severe cerebral edema or midline shift.

Selection of empirical antibiotic therapy
● Primary infection or contiguous source:
1. Otitis media, mastoiditis, sinusitis, dental infection: third-generation cephalosporin plus metronidazole
2. Dental infection: penicillin G plus metronidazole
3. Head trauma or postcranial surgery: third-generation cephalosporin plus metronidazole and nafcillin or vancomycin
● Hematogenous spread (congenital heart disease, endocarditis, urinary tract, lung, intra-abdominal): nafcillin or vancomycin plus metronidazole plus third-generation cephalosporin
● Duration of antibiotic therapy is unclear. Most recommend parenteral treatment is for 4 to 8 weeks, with repeated neuroimaging to ensure adequate treatment. Imaging is suggested every weeks for first 2 weeks of therapy, then every

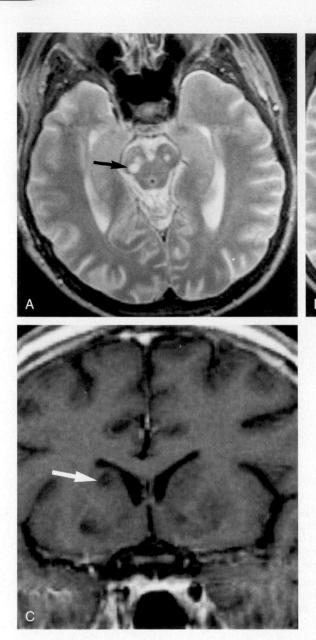

Fig 46–3
Cryptococcoma. Shown are transverse
T2-weighted spin-echo **(A, B)** and coronal T1-weighted spin-echo **(C)** images.
Expanded Virchow-Robin spaces
(arrows) of high signal on T2 and low signal on T1 are seen in the brainstem and
the basal ganglia, so that the ganglia look
like Swiss cheese.
(From Grainger RG, Allison DJ, Adam A,
Dixon AK [eds]: Grainger and Allison's Diagnostic Radiology: A Textbook of Medical Imaging, 4th ed. London. Harcourt, 2001.)

Fig 46–4
MRI scans of fungal abscess in a 48-year-old diabetic. **A,** Axial T2-
weighted image (2000/80), central hyperintense abscess cavity with
surrounding vasogenic edema. **B,** Coronal postgadolinium contrast
T1-weighted image (800/16). Large, multiloculated abscess cavity with
enhancement of the capsule and abscess wall. Note the relative thinness
of the medial wall compared with the thicker, more irregular, lateral component. Mild mass effect is evident.
(From Grainger RG, Allison DJ, Adam A, Dixon AK [eds]: Grainger and Allison's Diagnostic Radiology: A Textbook of Medical Imaging, 4th ed. London.
Harcourt, 2001.)

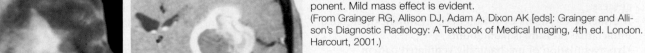

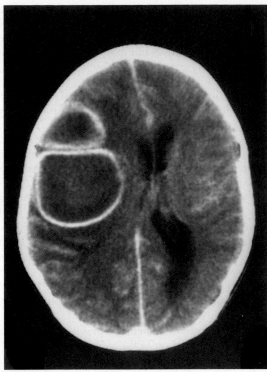

Fig 46–5
Contrast-enhanced axial CT scan demonstrating two cerebral abscesses with surrounding edema and mass effect. Thin, smooth, enhancing capsules surround the cavities of nonenhancing necrotic tissue. (Courtesy of Dr. I. Colquhoun.)

2 weeks until antibiotics are finished, and then every 2 to 4 months for 1 year to monitor for disease recurrence.

Surgical treatment
- Two indications for surgical intervention:
1. Collect specimens for culture and sensitivity.
2. Reduce mass effect.
- Stereotactic biopsy or aspirate of the abscess if surgically feasible
- Essential to selection of targeted antimicrobial coverage
- Timing and choice of surgery depend on:
  - Primary infection source
  - Numbers and locations of the abscesses
  - Whether the procedure is diagnostic or therapeutic
  - Neurologic status of the patient

B. CAVERNOUS SINUS THROMBOSIS

DEFINITION
Cavernous sinus thrombosis (CST) is an uncommon diagnosis usually stemming from infections of the face or paranasal sinuses and resulting in thrombosis of the cavernous sinus and inflammation of its surrounding anatomic structures, including cranial nerves III, IV, V (ophthalmic and maxillary branch), and VI, and the internal carotid artery.

PHYSICAL FINDINGS AND CLINICAL PRESENTATION
- The clinical presentation of CST can be varied. Both acute fulminant disease and indolent subacute presentations have been reported in the literature.

- The most common signs of CST are related to anatomic structures affected within the cavernous sinus, notably cranial nerves III to VI, as well as symptoms resulting from impaired venous drainage from the orbit and eye.
- Classic presentations are abrupt onset of unilateral periorbital edema, headache, photophobia, and proptosis. Headache is usually the presenting complaint and may precede fever and periorbital edema by several days. Older patients may present only with alterations in mental status without antecedent headache.
- Other common signs and symptoms include:
  - Ptosis
  - Chemosis
  - Cranial nerve palsies (III, IV, V, and VI)
  1. Sixth nerve palsy is the most common.
  2. Sensory deficits of the ophthalmic and maxillary branch of the fifth nerve are common. Periorbital sensory loss and impaired corneal reflex may be noted. Papilledema, retinal hemorrhages, and decreased visual acuity and blindness may occur from venous congestion within the retina.
  - Fever, tachycardia, sepsis may be present.
  - Headache with nuchal rigidity and changes in mental status, coma, and orbital swelling (Fig. 46–6) may occur.
  - Pupil may be dilated and sluggishly reactive.
- Either hypo- or hyperesthesia in the dermatomes served by the V1 and V2 branches of the trigeminal nerve may be subtle but is almost always present.
- Infection can spread to the contralateral cavernous sinus within 24 to 48 hours of initial presentation.

CAUSE
- CST most commonly results from contiguous spread of infection from the sinuses (sphenoid, ethmoid, or frontal) or middle third of the face. Nasal furuncles are the most common facial infection to produce this complication. Less common primary sites of infection include dental abscess, tonsils, soft palate, middle ear, and orbit (orbital cellulitis).
- The highly anastomotic and valveless venous system of the paranasal sinuses allows retrograde spread of infection to the cavernous sinus via the superior and inferior ophthalmic veins.
- *Staphylococcus aureus* is the most common infectious microbe, found in 50% to 60% of cases.
- *Streptococcus* is the second leading cause.
- Gram-negative rods and anaerobes may also lead to cavernous sinus thrombosis.
- Rarely, *Aspergillus fumigatus* and mucormycosis cause CST.

DIAGNOSIS
- The diagnosis of cavernous sinus thrombosis is made clinically, with imaging studies to confirm the clinical impression.
- Proptosis, ptosis, chemosis, and cranial nerve palsy beginning in one eye and progressing to the other eye establish the diagnosis.

DIFFERENTIAL DIAGNOSIS
- Orbital cellulitis
- Internal carotid artery aneurysm
- Cerebrovascular accident (CVA)
- Migraine headache
- Allergic blepharitis
- Thyroid exophthalmos
- Brain tumor

- Meningitis
- Mucormycosis
- Trauma

LABORATORY TESTS

- CBC, ESR, blood cultures, and sinus cultures help establish and identify an infectious primary source.

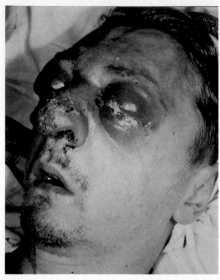

Fig 46-6
Cavernous sinus thrombosis. A patient who displays evidence of severe orbital swelling caused by obstruction of orbital veins is shown. In this patient, the originating focus was infection of the soft tissues of the nose. (Courtesy of the University of Sheffield School of Dentistry, Sheffield, England.)

- LP is necessary to rule out meningitis. LP reveals inflammatory cells in 75% of cases. The CSF profile is typically that of a parameningeal focus (high WBC, normal glucose, normal protein, culture negative) but may be similar to that of bacterial meningitis.

IMAGING STUDIES

- Sinus films are helpful in the diagnosis of sphenoid sinusitis. Opacification, sclerosis, and air-fluid levels are typical findings.
- Contrast-enhanced CT scan may reveal underlying sinusitis, thickening of the superior ophthalmic vein, and irregular filling defects within the cavernous sinus; however, findings may be normal early in the disease course.
- MRI (Fig. 46–7A) using flow parameters and MRA (Fig. 46–7B) are more sensitive than CT scanning, and are the imaging studies of choice to diagnose cavernous sinus thrombosis. Findings may include deformity of the internal carotid artery within the cavernous sinus and an obvious signal hyperintensity in thrombosed vascular sinuses on all pulse sequences.
- Cerebral angiography, can be performed, but it is invasive and not sensitive.
- Orbital venography is difficult to perform, but is excellent for diagnosing occlusion of the cavernous sinus.

TREATMENT

- Broad-spectrum intravenous antibiotics are used as empirical therapy until a definite pathogen is found. Treatment should include a penicillinase-resistant penicillin at maximum dosage plus a third- or fourth-generation cephalosporin:

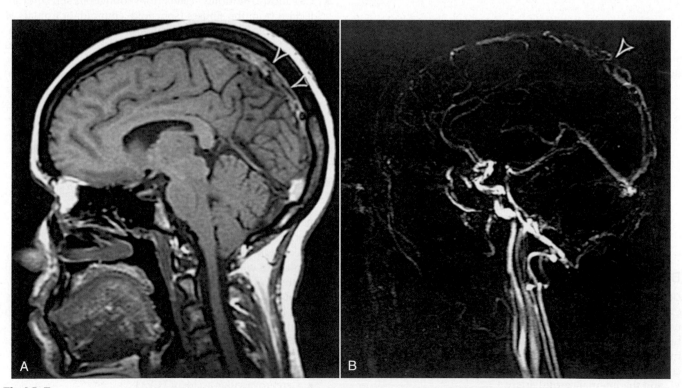

Fig 46-7
A, scan of superior sagittal sinus thrombosis. There is increased signal within the vessel on the T_2-weighted image *(arrowheads)*, indicating the presence of thrombus. **B**, MR angiogram in the same patient, showing nonfilling of the superior sagittal sinus. The sinus is surrounded by tortuous collateral vessels *(arrowhead)*.
(Courtesy of Dr. Wayne Davis, University of Utah, Utah.)

- Vancomycin may be substituted for nafcillin if significant concern exists for infection by methicillin-resistant *Staphylococcus aureus* or resistant *Streptococcus pneumoniae.*
- Appropriate therapy should take into account the primary source of infection as well as possible associated complications, such as brain abscess, meningitis, or subdural empyema.
- Anticoagulation with heparin is controversial. The current recommendation is for early heparinization in patients with unilateral cavernous sinus thrombosis. Coumadin therapy should be avoided in the acute phase of the illness, but should ultimately be instituted and continued until the infection, symptoms, and signs of cavernous thrombosis have resolved or significantly improved.
- Steroid therapy is also controversial but may prove helpful in reducing cranial nerve dysfunction. Corticosteroids should only be instituted after appropriate antibiotic coverage.
- Emergent surgical drainage with sphenoidotomy is indicated if the primary site of infection is thought to be the sphenoid sinus.
- All patients with CST are usually treated with prolonged courses (3 to 4 weeks) of IV antibiotics. If there is evidence of complications such as intracranial suppuration, 6 to 8 weeks of total therapy may be warranted.

C. BACTERIAL MENINGITIS

DEFINITION
Bacterial meningitis is an inflammation of the meninges (Fig. 46–8), with increased intracranial pressure and pleocytosis, increased WBCs in the CSF secondary to bacteria in the pia-subarachnoid space and ventricles, or both, leading to neurologic sequelae and abnormalities.

PHYSICAL FINDINGS AND CLINICAL PRESENTATION
- Fever
- Headache
- Neck stiffness, nuchal rigidity, meningismus
- Altered mental state, lethargy
- Vomiting, nausea
- Photophobia
- Seizures
- Coma, lethargy, stupor
- Rash: petechial or hemorrhagic (Fig. 46–9) associated with meningococcal infection
- Myalgia
- Cranial nerve abnormality (unilateral)
- Papilledema
- Dilated, nonreactive pupil(s)
- Posturing: decorticate, decerebrate
- Physical examination findings of Kernig's sign and Brudzinski's sign in adults with meningitis are often not helpful in determining meningeal inflammation.

CAUSE
- *Neisseria meningitidis* is now more common than *Haemophilus influenzae* as a cause of bacterial meningitis in children and adults. *H. influenzae* is the cause of more than 30% of cases of meningitis (usually in infants and children younger than 6 years old). It is associated with sinusitis and otitis media.
- Neonates: group B streptococci, *Escherichia coli*, *Klebsiella* spp., *Listeria monocytogenes*

- Infancy through adolescence:
  1. *N. meningitidis*
  2. *H. influenzae*
  3. *Streptococcus pneumoniae*
- Adults
  1. *N. meningitidis*
  2. *S. pneumoniae*

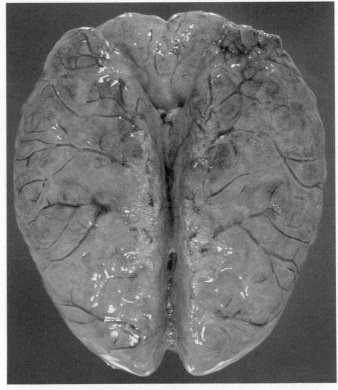

Fig 46–8
Brain with inflammatory exudate covering the cortical hemispheres in a patient with purulent meningitis.
(Courtesy of Dr. M. Tolnay, University of Basel, Basel, Switzerland,)

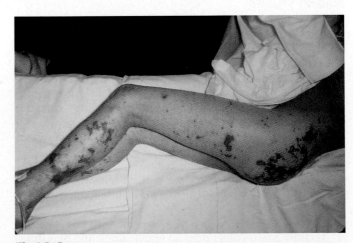

Fig 46–9
Fully developed, almost pathognomonic, hemorrhagic rash of meningococcal sepsis.
(From Cohen J, Powderly WG: Infectious Diseases, 2nd ed. St. Louis, Mosby, 2004.)

- Older adults
  1. *S. pneumoniae*
  2. *N. meningitidis*
  3. *L. monocytogenes*
  4. Gram-negative bacilli

DIAGNOSIS

The diagnostic approach is based on patient presentation and physical examination. Key elements to diagnosis are CSF evaluation and CT or MRI if the patient is in a coma or has focal neurologic deficits, pupillary abnormalities, or papilledema.

DIFFERENTIAL DIAGNOSIS

- Endocarditis, bacteremia
- Intracranial tumor
- Lyme disease
- Brain abscess
- Partially treated bacterial meningitis
- Medications
- SLE
- Seizures
- Acute mononucleosis
- Other infectious meningitides
- Neuroleptic malignant syndrome
- Subdural empyema
- Rocky Mountain spotted fever

WORKUP

CEREBROSPINAL EXAMINATION

- Opening pressure more than 100 to 200 mm Hg
- WBC, less than 5 to more than 100 mm^3
- Neutrophilic predominance: more than 80%
- Gram stain of CSF: positive in 60% to 90% patients
- CSF protein: higher than 50 mg/dL
- CSF glucose: less than 40 mg/dL
- Culture: positive in 65% to 90% cases
- CSF bacterial antigen: 50% to 100% sensitivity
- E test for susceptibility of pneumococcal isolates

LABORATORY TESTS

- Blood culturing
- WBC with differential
- CSF examination (see "Workup")

IMAGING STUDIES

- CT or MRI scanning of the head: necessary with increased intracranial pressure, coma, neurologic deficits
- Sinus CT: if sinusitis suspected

TREATMENT

- Empirical therapy is necessary with IV antibiotic treatment if patient has purulent CSF fluid at time of lumbar puncture, is asplenic, or has signs of DIC or sepsis pending Gram stain and culture results.
- Therapy after Gram stain pending cultures is recommended for the following age and patient risk groups:
  1. Neonates: ampicillin plus cefotaxime
  2. Infants, children: ampicillin or third-generation cephalosporin (plus chloramphenicol if purulent or patient is compromised)
  3. Adults (18 to 50 years): third-generation cephalosporin
  4. Older adults (older than 50 years): ampicillin plus third-generation cephalosporin
- Penicillin-resistant pneumococcus: because of an increasing incidence of this organism, empirical treatment with ceftri-axone or cefotaxime plus vancomycin has been recommended.
- Steroids: dexamethasone 0.15 mg/kg every 6 hours for first 4 days of therapy is useful in adults with bacterial meningitis and mental status changes or acute neurologic phenomena. Decreased mortality and neurologic sequelae are seen with adjunct therapy.
- Dexamethasone also benefits children with *H. influenzae* type B (Hib) or pneumococcal meningitis and should be given within the first 2 days of illness.

D. ENCEPHALITIS

DEFINITION

Acute viral encephalitis is an acute febrile syndrome with evidence of meningeal involvement and derangement of the function of the cerebrum, cerebellum, or brainstem.

CAUSE

- Can be caused by a host of viruses, with herpes simplex the most common virus identified
- Arboviruses: agents causing Eastern equine, Western equine, St. Louis, Venezuelan equine, California virus, Japanese B encephalitis, Murray Valley, West Nile, and Russian spring-summer encephalitis, as well as other lesser known agents
- Also implicated: rabies-causing agents, cytomegalovirus (CMV), Epstein-Barr, varicella-zoster, echo virus, mumps, adenovirus, Coxsackie, rubeola, and herpesviruses
- Meningoencephalitis: acute retroviral infection

PHYSICAL FINDINGS AND CLINICAL PRESENTATION

- Initially, fever and evidence of meningeal irritation
- Headache and stiff neck
- Later, development of signs of cortical dysfunction: lethargy, coma, stupor, weakness, seizures, facial weakness, and brainstem findings
- Cerebellar findings: ataxia, nystagmus, hypotonia; myoclonus, cranial nerve palsies, and abnormal tendon reflexes
- Patients with rabies: hydrophobia, anxiety, facial numbness, psychosis, coma, or dysarthria
- Rarely, movement disorders, such as chorea, hemiballismus, or dystonia
- Recall of a prodromal viral-like illness (this finding is not uniform)

DIFFERENTIAL DIAGNOSIS

- Bacterial infections: brain abscess, toxic encephalopathies, tuberculosis (TB)
- Protozoal infections
- Behçet's disease
- Lupus encephalitis
- Sjögren's syndrome
- Multiple sclerosis
- Syphilis
- *Cryptococcus*
- Toxoplasmosis
- Brucellosis
- Leukemic or lymphomatous meningitis
- Other metastatic tumors
- Lyme disease
- Cat-scratch disease
- Vogt-Koyanagi-Harada syndrome
- Mollaret's meningitis

WORKUP

- Lumbar puncture to reveal pleocytosis, usually lymphocytic, although neutrophils may be seen early
- Usually, elevated CSF protein
- Normal or low CSF glucose
- Herpes simplex encephalitis: RBCs and xanthochromia
- Electroencephalographic changes showing periodic high-voltage sharp waves in the temporal regions and slow wave complexes suggestive of herpes encephalitis (Fig. 46-10)
- CT or MRI to reveal edema and hemorrhage in the frontal and temporal lobes (Fig. 46–11)
- Arboviral infections suspected during outbreaks in specific areas
- Rising titers of neutralizing antibodies from the acute to convalescent stage demonstrated but often not helpful in the acutely ill patient
- PCR that amplifies DNA from the CSF for herpes simplex encephalitis
- Rarely, brain biopsy to assist in the diagnosis (Fig. 46–12). In herpes simplex encephalitis Cowdry A intranuclear inclusions are present (Fig. 46–13); viral culture of cerebral tissue obtained if biopsy done.
- Classic herpetic skin lesions suggestive of herpes encephalitis
- In diagnosing arboviral encephalitis:
  1. Presence of antiviral IgM within the first few days of symptomatic disease; detected and quantified by enzyme-linked immunosorbent assay (ELISA)
  2. Unusual to recover an arbovirus from the blood or CSF

LABORATORY TESTS

- Aside from the lumbar puncture, most other laboratory studies are nonspecific.
- Skin lesions and urine may be cultured for herpes simplex and CMV.

TREATMENT

- Supportive care, frequent evaluation, and neurologic examination
- Ventilatory assistance for patients who are moribund or at risk for aspiration
- Avoidance of infusion of hypotonic fluids to minimize the risk of hyponatremia
- For patients who develop seizures: anticonvulsant therapy and follow-up in a critical care setting

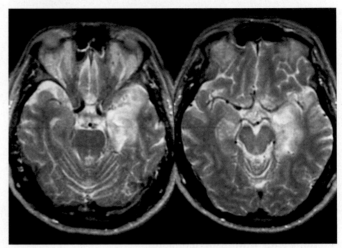

Fig 46–11
Herpes simplex encephalitis. The two contiguous axial T2-weighted MRI scans of the brain show swelling and signal change in the antero-medial parts of the left temporal lobe and minimal signal change in comparable parts of the right.
(From Grainger RG, Allison DJ, Adam A, Dixon AK [eds]: Grainger and Allison's Diagnostic Radiology: A Textbook of Medical Imaging, 4th ed. London. Harcourt, 2001.)

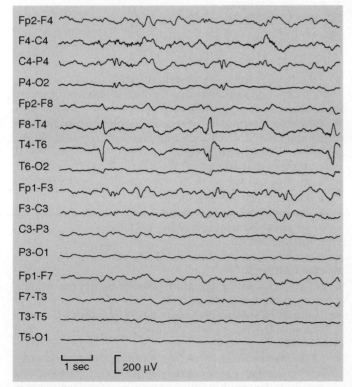

Fig 46–10
Electroencephalogram showing repetitive complexes occurring in the right temporal region of a child with herpes simplex encephalitis.
(From Goetz CG, Pappert EJ: Textbook of Clinical Neurology. Philadelphia, WB Saunders, 1999.)

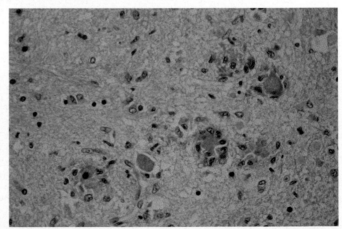

Fig 46–12
Viral encephalitis. Dead or dying neurons are surrounded by microglial cells, a process termed *neuronophagia*.
(From Silverberg SG, DeLellis RA, Frable WJ, et al [eds]: Principles and Practice of Surgical Pathology and Cytopathology, 4th ed. New York, Churchill Livingstone, 2006.)

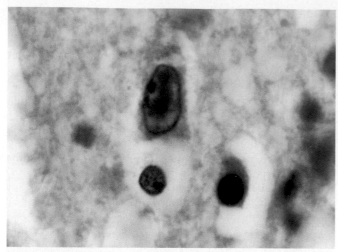

Fig 46-13
Cowdry A intranuclear inclusion in a neuron in herpes simplex encephalitis.
(From Silverberg SG, DeLellis RA, Frable WJ, et al [eds]: Principles and Practice of Surgical Pathology and Cytopathology, 4th ed. New York, Churchill Livingstone, 2006.)

- For comatose patients:
  1. Aggressive care to avoid decubiti, contractures, and DVT
  2. Close attention to weights, input and output, and serum electrolytes
- Acyclovir IV for herpes simplex encephalitis
- Short courses of corticosteroids to control brain edema and prevent herniation
- In patients with suspected rabies:
  1. Human rabies immune globulin (HRIG)
  2. Active immunization may be stimulated by a recently developed rabies vaccine, human diploid cell vaccine (HDCV), which has reduced the number of doses needed to five.
- No specific pharmacologic therapy for most other viral pathogens

E. SUBDURAL EMPYEMA, EXTRADURAL EMPYEMA, AND CRANIAL EPIDURAL ABSCESS

DEFINITION

Parameningeal pyogenic infections are defined by their location. Subdural empyema involves the space between the dura mater and the arachnoid and represents 15% to 20% of localized intracranial infections. A cranial epidural abscess occurs in the space between the dura and the inner table of the skull.

PHYSICAL FINDINGS AND CLINICAL PRESENTATION
- Headache
- Fever, lethargy
- Focal neurologic deficits
- Seizures
- Periorbital edema
- Vomiting

CAUSE
- The most common predisposing condition that leads to the development of subdural empyema and cranial epidural abscess is paranasal sinusitis.

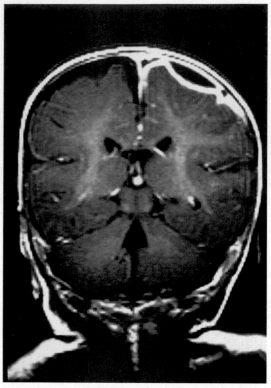

Fig 46-14
Extradural empyema. This contrast-enhanced T1-weighted coronal MRI scan demonstrates a lentiform extradural collection surrounded by enhancing dura mater.
(Courtesy of Dr. K. Chong.)

- Middle ear, orbital, or mastoid infections, and craniotomy or compound skull fractures are also risk factors for cranial epidural abscess.
- Common infecting organisms are aerobic streptococci, anaerobic and microanaerophilic streptococci, and aerobic gram-negative bacilli.

DIFFERENTIAL DIAGNOSIS
- Meningitis,
- Brain abscess (see Fig. 46-4)
- Encephalitis (see Fig 46-11)
- Subdural hematoma (see Fig 37-1)

LABORATORY TESTS
- Gram stain and culture of purulent material

IMAGING STUDIES
- MRI of brain with gadolinium enhancement is the diagnostic procedure of choice (Fig. 46-14).
- Contrast-enhanced CT of brain if MRI is contraindicated or unavailable.

TREATMENT
- High-dose broad-spectrum IV antibiotics to cover aerobic and anaerobic streptococci, staphylococci, gram-negative bacilli, and anaerobes (third-generation cephalosporin, nafcillin, metronidazole, vancomycin)
- Neurosurgical drainage

F. CYSTICERCOSIS

DEFINITION

Cysticercosis is an infection caused by the presence and accumulation of larval cysts of the pork tapeworm *Taenia solium* in tissues of the body. *T. solium* cysts, or cysticerci, may affect any area of the body including the eyes, spinal cord, skin, heart, and brain, a condition known as neurocysticercosis (Fig. 46–15). Humans acquire cysticercosis via fecal-oral transmission of *T. solium* eggs from tapeworm carriers.

PHYSICAL FINDINGS AND CLINICAL PRESENTATION

- Seizures caused by intracerebral cysts are the most common manifestation of neurocysticercosis, occurring in 70% to 90% of cases. Patients with seizures usually have a normal physical examination.
- Soft tissue deposition of cysts can cause local inflammation, which results in only minor morbidity compared with the damage possible in neurocysticercosis.
- Less common: altered mental status, including psychosis and headache, nausea and vomiting resulting from increased intracranial pressure.
- Inflammation around degenerating cysts can cause focal encephalitis, vasculitis, chronic meningitis, and cranial nerve palsies.
- Cysts can occur in the ventricles and cause hydrocephalus; more rarely, they can be found in the spinal cord and eye.

CAUSE

- *T. solium*. The presence of viable cysts in the CNS is usually asymptomatic. With time, inflammation around degenerating cysts causes symptoms, depending on the location, number, and size of the cysts. Neurocysticercosis has been reported in AIDS patients; immunosuppression does not appear to increase the incidence of the infection.

DIFFERENTIAL DIAGNOSIS

- Idiopathic epilepsy
- Migraine
- Vasculitides
- Primary neoplasia of CNS
- Toxoplasmosis
- Brain abscess
- Granulomatous disease such as sarcoidosis

LABORATORY TESTS

- Stool examination for ova if intestinal tapeworms also suspected
- CSF examination: may show pleocytosis, with lymphocytic or eosinophilic predominance, low glucose, elevated protein with neurocysticercosis
- Serum and CSF can be studied for antibodies.
- ELISA has a sensitivity and specificity of 90% when done on CSF.

IMAGING STUDIES

- Imaging studies precede laboratory tests if CNS involvement suspected:
  - Head CT
  - Sensitivity and specificity of 95%
  - Can identify living cysticerci, which appear as hypodense lesions, as well as degenerating cysts, which appear as isodense or hyperdense lesions
  - Typically, there are multiple lesions.
  - Best method for detecting calcification associated with prior infection
- Brain MRI (Fig. 46–16):
  - Most accurate technique to assess the degree of infection, location, and developmental stage of the parasites
  - Provides detailed images of living and degenerating cysts, perilesional edema, as well as small cysts or those located in the ventricles, brainstem, and cerebellum

TREATMENT

- Cysticercosis outside the nervous system is a benign disorder and does not merit specific treatment. Neurocysticercosis, however, is associated with substantial morbidity and mortality.

Inactive infection

- Patients with seizures and calcifications alone on neuroimaging studies are not thought to have viable parasites.
- Cysticidal therapy is usually not undertaken.
- Anticonvulsants can control seizures.

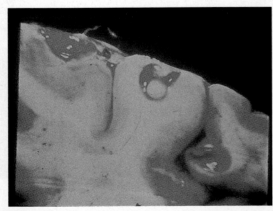

Fig 46–15
Cysticerci in the brain.
(From Cohen J, Powderly WG: Infectious Diseases, 2nd ed. St. Louis, Mosby, 2004.)

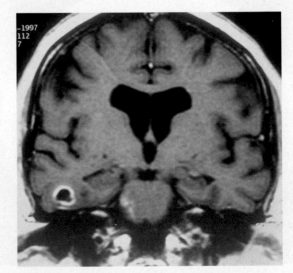

Fig 46–16
Coronal MRI brain scan showing a living cysticercus, with the scolex appearing as a hyperintense center (pea in the pod appearance). There is no visible inflammatory reaction.
(From Cohen J, Powderly WG: Infectious Diseases, 2nd ed. St. Louis, Mosby, 2004.)

• For patients with hydrocephalus, ventriculoperitoneal shunting can resolve symptoms.

Active parenchymal infection
- • Most common presentation
- • Anticonvulsants should be given to control seizures.

Cysticidal therapy
- • Praziquantel has been the mainstay of therapy and is effective.
- • Albendazole is now being used more frequently, and it may have greater efficacy at a lower cost than praziquantel.
- • Some argue that only treatment of seizures, not antiparasitic therapy, is needed.
- • Medical failures often necessitate surgical treatment. Surgical treatments may include craniotomy, cyst extraction, stereotactic cyst aspiration, and shunt placement.
- • In some cases, symptoms may worsen after surgery because of adherence of the cysts to adjacent neural and vascular structures.
- • Stereotactic aspiration of the cyst, with placement of an indwelling cyst catheter or drain for repeated aspirations, can be used.
- • Extraparenchymal neurocysticercosis requires neurosurgical intervention.
- • Ventricular: usually presents with obstructive hydrocephalus. The mainstay of therapy is the rapid correction of hydrocephalus.
- • Subarachnoid: associated with arachnoiditis. Diversion of CSF and steroid therapy may be needed.

H. TOXOPLASMOSIS

DEFINITION

Toxoplasmosis is an infection caused by the protozoal parasite *Toxoplasma gondii.*

PHYSICAL FINDINGS AND CLINICAL PRESENTATION
- • Acquired (immunocompetent host)
  1. 80% to 90% asymptomatic
  2. Adenopathy (usually cervical)
  3. Fever, myalgias, malaise,
- • Acquired (in patients with AIDS): 89% of symptomatic cases: encephalitis, intracerebral mass lesions, pneumonitis,
- • Acquired (immunocompromised patients): encephalitis, myocarditis (especially in heart transplant patients), pneumonitis
- • Ocular infection (Fig. 46–17) in the immunocompetent host
- • Congenital: results from acute infection acquired by the mother within 6 to 8 weeks before conception or during gestation: chorioretinitis, blindness, epilepsy, psychomotor or mental retardation, intracranial calcifications, hydrocephalus, microcephaly

CAUSE
- • *Toxoplasma gondii*

WORKUP

Acute infection, immunocompetent host
  1. CBC
  2. *Toxoplasma* serology (IgG, Ig) in serial blood specimens three weeks apart
  3. Lymph node biopsy if diagnosis uncertain

Immunocompromised host
  1. CNS symptoms
  - • Cerebral CT scan (Fig. 46–18) or MRI (Fig. 46–19) if CNS symptoms present
  - • Lumbar puncture if no contraindications
  - • Brain biopsy (Fig. 46–20) if no response to empirical therapy

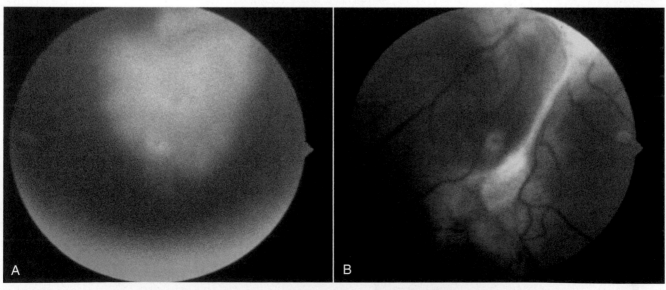

Fig 46–17
Toxoplasmic retinitis. **A,** Diagnosis from funduscopy. **B,** Evolution after antitoxoplasma therapy.
(From Cohen J, Powderly WG: Infectious Diseases, 2nd ed. St. Louis, Mosby, 2004.)

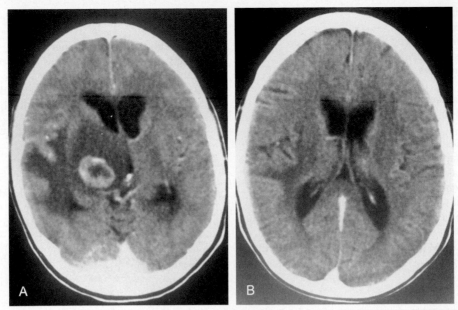

Fig 46–18
Toxoplasma abscess. **A,** This CT brain scan shows a *Toxoplasma* abscess in the left internal capsule, compressing the lateral ventricles. Contrast demonstrates a typical ring-enhancing effect. **B,** Same patient after 17 days of treatment with pyrimethamine and sulfonamide showing resolving abscess.
(From Cohen J, Powderly WG: Infectious Diseases, 2nd ed. St. Louis, Mosby, 2004.)

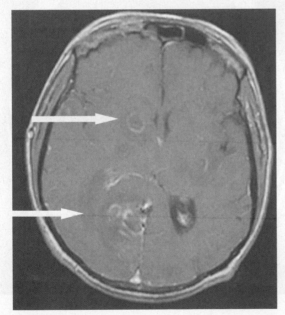

Fig 46–19
MRI scan of the brain in an autologous bone marrow transplantation patient with toxoplasmic encephalitis (TE). Enhancing lesions are shown *(arrows)*.
(From Cohen J, Powderly WG: Infectious Diseases, 2nd ed. St. Louis, Mosby, 2004.)

Fig 46–20
Cyst form of *Toxoplasma gondii* in the brain *(arrows)* (H&E).
(From Cohen J, Powderly WG: Infectious Diseases, 2nd ed. St. Louis, Mosby, 2004.)

2. Ocular symptoms
- Funduscopic examination
- Serologic studies
- Rarely, vitreous tap
3. Pulmonary symptoms
- Chest x-ray
- Bronchoalveolar lavage
- Transbronchial or open lung biopsy
4. Myocarditis
- Cardiac enzymes
- Electrocardiography
- Endomyocardial biopsy for definitive diagnosis

Toxoplasmosis in pregnancy
1. Initial maternal screening with IgM and IgG
- If negative, mother at risk of acute infection and should be retested monthly
- If both IgG and IgM positive, perform IgA and IgE ELISA and AC/HS testing.

- IgA and IgE ELISA, AC/HS test elevated in acute infection
- Ig high for 1 year or longer
- IgG repeated 3 to 4 weeks later to determine if titer is stable
2. Acute maternal infection not excluded or documented
- Fetal blood sampling (for culture, Ig, IgA, IgE)
- Amniotic fluid PCR
3. Fetal ultrasound every other week if maternal infection documented

Congenital toxoplasmosis
1. Placental histology
2. Specific IgM or IgA in infant's blood

TREATMENT
- Pyrimethamine plus leucovorin 10 to 20 mg PO every day plus sulfadiazine (Fig. 46–21)

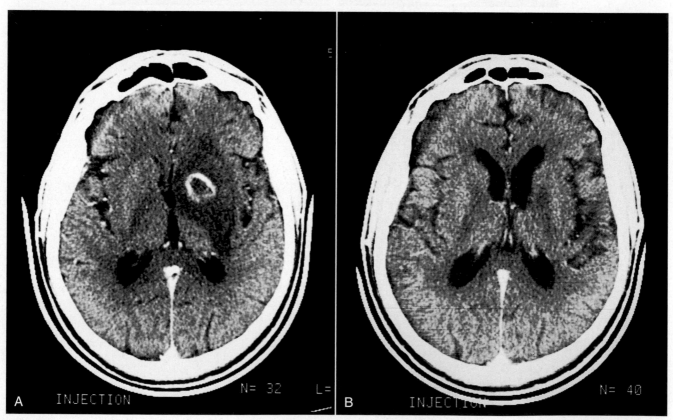

Fig 46–21
Toxoplasma abscess. **A,** This CT brain scan shows a toxoplasma abscess in the left internal capsule, compressing the lateral ventricles. Contrast demonstrates a typical ring-enhancing effect. **B.** Same patient after 17 days of treatment with Pyrimenthamine and sulfonamide showing abscess. (From Cohen, J., Powderly WG: Infectious diseases, 2nd ed. St. Louis, Mosby, 2004.)

Chapter 47 | Neurocutaneous syndromes

A. STURGE-WEBER SYNDROME

DEFINITION
Sturge-Weber syndrome (SWS) is characterized by congenital facial angioma (nevus flammeus, port-wine stain), seizures, and developmental delay

PHYSICAL FINDINGS AND CLINICAL PRESENTATION
- Congenital facial angioma, usually unilateral and generally involving the upper face, superior eyelid, or periorbital region (Fig. 47–1A). The facial angioma usually conforms to the sensory divisions of the trigeminal nerve. Episcleral telangiectasis may be present (Fig. 47–2).
- Seizures (primarily partial seizures)
- Homonymous hemianopsia (35% of patients)
- Glaucoma (25% of patients)
- Developmental delay
- Behavioral problems

CAUSE
- Unknown. SWS has no known recognized pattern of inheritance.

IMAGING STUDIES
- Brain MRI is neuroimaging study of choice.
- CT demonstrates intracerebral calcifications and cerebral atrophy.
- Skull radiograph will reveal intracranial calcifications (found in 90% of patients; see Fig. 47–1B).

- Positron emission tomography (PET) will demonstrate metabolic impairment and can be useful when considering focal resection for intractable seizures.
- Electroencephalography: decreased amplitude and frequency of activity overlying the affected hemisphere

TREATMENT
- Antiepileptic medications for seizure disorder
- Focal cerebral resection of affected lobes for refractory seizures
- Management of behavioral and emotional problems

B. NEUROFIBROMATOSIS

DEFINITION
Neurofibromatosis (NF) is an autosomal dominant inherited neurocutaneous disorder. There are two types of neurofibromatosis disorders, NF type 1 (NF1) and NF type 2 (NF2).

PHYSICAL FINDINGS AND CLINICAL PRESENTATION
Common features of NF1
1. Café au lait macules (100% of children by age 2)
- Hyperpigmented skin lesions (Fig. 47–3 occurring anywhere on the body except the face, palms, and soles
- Appear early in life and increase in size and number during puberty
- Focal or diffuse

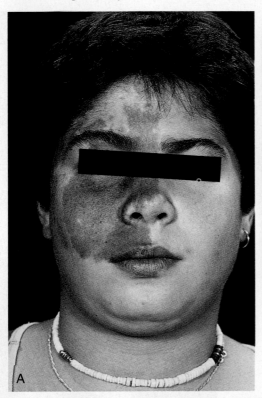
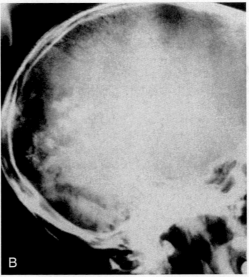

Fig 47–1
Sturge-Weber syndrome. **A,** This 12-year-old girl presented with fits, mental retardation, and a port-wine vascular nevus affecting much of the right side of her face. CT scanning showed meningeal angiomatosis. **B,** The intracranial moiety is often calcified, as in this radiograph. (**A** courtesy of Dr. D. Atherton, Institute of Dermatology and Children's Hospital at Great Ormond Street, London; **B** courtesy of Dr. I. Moseley, National Hospital for Nervous Diseases, London.)

2. Axillary and inguinal freckling (70%)

3. Multiple cutaneous and subcutaneous neurofibromas (95%)

- Firm, varying in size from millimeters to centimeters
- Vary in number from a few to thousands
- May be sessile, pedunculated, regular or irregular in shape (Fig. 47–4

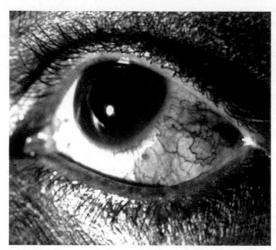

Fig 47–2
Episcleral telangiectasis ipsilateral to facial nevus flammeus and diffuse choroidal hemangioma in a patient with Sturge-Weber syndrome. (From Yanoff M, Duker JS: Ophthalmology, 2nd ed. St. Louis, Mosby, 2004.)

4. Lisch nodule (small hamartoma of the iris) found in more than 90% of adult cases

5. Visual defects possibly related to optic gliomas (2% to 5%)

6. Neurodevelopmental problems (30% to 40%)

Common features of NF2

1. Hearing loss and tinnitus related to bilateral acoustic neuromas (more than 90% of adults)

2. Cataracts (81%)

3. Headache

4. Unsteady gait

5. Cutaneous neurofibromas but less than NF1

6. Café au lait macules (1%)

CAUSE

- NF1 is caused by DNA mutations located on the long arm of chromosome 17 responsible for encoding the protein neurofibromin.
- NF2 is caused by DNA mutations located in the middle of the long arm of chromosome 22 responsible for encoding the protein merlin.

DIAGNOSIS

- NF1 is diagnosed if two or more of the following features are present:

1. Six or more café au lait macules larger than 5 mm in pre-pubertal patients and larger than 15 mm in postpubertal patients

2. Two or more neurofibromas of any type or one plexiform neurofibroma

3. Axillary or inguinal freckling

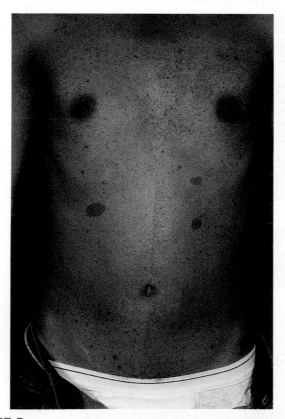

Fig 47–3
Type I neurofibromatosis. The presence of typical café au lait macules is characteristic.
(Courtesy of Dr. R. A. Marsden, St. George's Hospital, London.)

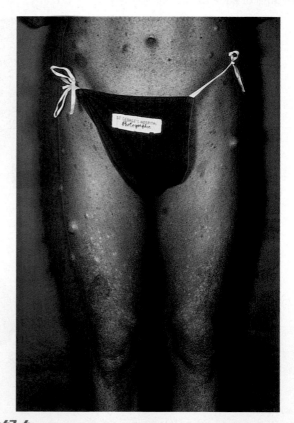

Fig 47–4
Type I neurofibromatosis. Widespread cutaneous neurofibromata are a prominent feature of the classic variant.
(Courtesy of Dr. R. A. Marsden, St. George's Hospital, London.)

4. Optic glioma

5. Two or more Lisch nodules (iris hamartomas)

6. Sphenoid wing dysplasia or cortical thinning of long bones, with or without pseudarthrosis

7. A first-degree relative (parent, sibling, or child) with NF1 based on the previous criteria

● NF2 is diagnosed if either of the following two criteria is present:

1. Bilateral eighth nerve masses seen by appropriate imaging studies

2. A first-degree relative with NF2 and either a unilateral eighth nerve mass or two of the following: neurofibroma, meningioma, glioma, schwannoma, or juvenile posterior subcapsular lenticular opacity

DIFFERENTIAL DIAGNOSIS
● Neurofibromatosis type 1
● Neurofibromatosis type 2
● Abdominal neurofibromatosis
● Myxoid lipoma
● Nodular fasciitis
● Fibrous histiocytoma

WORKUP
The diagnosis of neurofibromatosis is usually self-evident. Workup is dictated by clinical symptoms in NF1 and usually includes MRI evaluations of the head and spine in NF2.

LABORATORY TESTS
● Genetic testing is possible in individuals who desire prenatal diagnosis for NF1. There is no single standard test and multiple tests are required. Results can only reveal whether an individual is affected but cannot predict the severity of the disease.
● In NF2, linkage analysis testing provides a more than 99% certainty that the individual has NF2.

IMAGING STUDIES
● MRI with gadolinium is the imaging study of choice for NF1 and NF2 patients. MRI increases the detection of optic gliomas, tumors of the spine (Fig. 47–5), acoustic neuromas, and bright spots thought to represent hamartomas.

● MRI of the spine is recommended for all patients diagnosed with NF2 to exclude intramedullary tumors.

TREATMENT
● Counseling addressing prognosis, genetic, psychological, and social issues.
● Slit-lamp examination by an ophthalmologist searching for cataracts and hamartomas
● Hearing testing and speech pathology evaluation
● Surgery is usually not done on skin tumors unless cosmetically requested or if suspicion of malignant transformation exists.
● Surgery may be indicated for spinal or cranial neurofibromas, gliomas, or meningiomas.
● Acoustic neuromas can be treated by surgical excision.
● Radiation may be indicated for NF1 patients with optic nerve gliomas.
● Stereotactic radiosurgery using a gamma knife may be an alternative approach to surgery for acoustic neuromas.

C. TUBEROUS SCLEROSIS

DEFINITION
The tuberous sclerosis complex (TSC) consists of the following primary features: facial angiofibromas, multiple ungual fibromas, cortical tuber (Fig. 47–6) (histologically confirmed), subependymal nodule or giant cell astrocytoma (histologically confirmed), multiple calcified subependymal nodules protruding into the ventricle (radiographic evidence), and multiple retinal astrocytomas.

PHYSICAL FINDINGS AND CLINICAL PRESENTATION
● Seizures; TSC accounts for seizures in 0.3% of patients with epilepsy.
● Mental retardation (TSC accounts for 1% of the U.S. institutionalized population)
● Dysplastic or neoplastic changes of the skin, nervous system, and other organ systems
● The most common lesion is a hypopigmented macule (90% of patients), often in a polygonal or thumbprint shape, confetti-like skin lesions

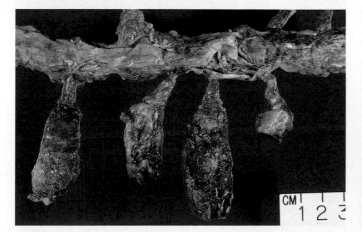

Fig 47–5

Multiple schwannomas arising off nerve roots emanating from the spinal cord in the setting of neurofibromatosis type II.
(From Silverberg SG, DeLellis RA, Frable WJ, et al [eds]: Principles and Practice of Surgical Pathology and Cytopathology, 4th ed. New York, Churchill Livingstone, 2006.)

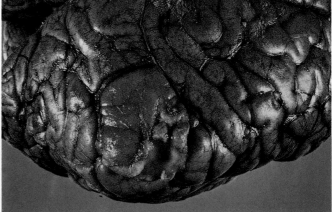

Fig 47–6

Tuberous sclerosis—a typical tuber on the cortex (lower midfield).
(Courtesy of Dr. I. Allen, Royal Victoria Hospital, Belfast, Northern Ireland.)

- Angiofibromatous lesions (adenoma sebaceum) generally found on the nose, nasolabial folds, or chin (Fig. 47–7)
- Renal tumors (mainly renal cysts or renal angiomyolipomas), hypertension
- Subungual or periungual fibromas (Koenen's tumors) can be found in 20% of patients
- Retinal tumors, cataracts, hypomelanotic macule
- Cardiac rhabdomyomas

CAUSE

- Autosomal dominant disorder with the gene located in the distal long arm of chromosome 9q34

IMAGING STUDIES

- Skull radiographs will demonstrate intracranial calcifications in 60% of patients.
- Brain CT: calcifications, calcified subependymal nodule (tuber), cerebral hamartomas, areas of demyelination, ventriculomegaly
- Brain MRI (Fig. 47–8): subependymal nodules, distorted cerebral cytoarchitecture

- Plain radiographs of hands: cystic changes of the phalanges and metacarpals
- CT (Fig. 47–9), MRI of kidneys
- Echocardiography in patients with suspected cardiac tumors

TREATMENT

- Anticonvulsant medications for seizures
- Surgical removal of adenoma sebaceum if obstructing nares
- Genetic family counseling

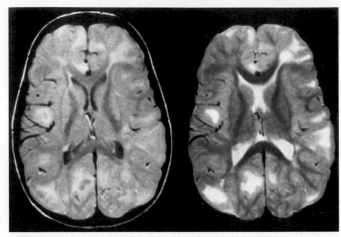

Fig 47–8
Proton density and T2-weighted images (2000/40, 2000/80) of tuberous sclerosis in a 5-year-old girl with seizures. Multiple cortical and subcortical hyperintensities represent tubers, with associated demyelination. A single hyperintense subependymal nodule is visible in the right trigone.
(From Grainger RG, Allison DJ, Adam A, Dixon AK [eds]: Grainger and Allison's Diagnostic Radiology: A Textbook of Medical Imaging, 4th ed. London. Harcourt, 2001.)

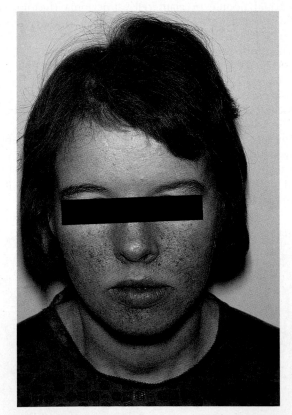

Fig 47–7
Tuberous sclerosis. The lesions of adenoma sebaceum consist of numerous papules on the nose, cheeks, and chin. Circumoral pallor is often seen in this disease.
(Courtesy of Dr. R A Marsden, St. George's Hospital, London.)

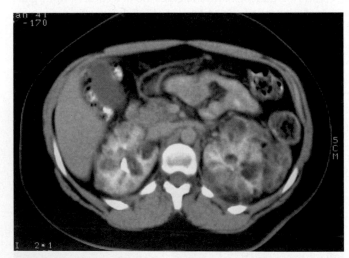

Fig 47–9
Radiologic findings associated with tuberous sclerosis complex. This contrast-enhanced CT scan shows bilateral angiomyolipomas in a 34-year-old symptomatic woman.
(From Johnson RJ, Feehally J: Comprehensive Clinical Nephrology, 2nd ed. St. Louis, Mosby, 2000.)

| Chapter 48 | **Disorders of muscle and the neuromuscular junction** |

A. MUSCULAR DYSTROPHY

DEFINITION

Muscular dystrophy (MD) refers to a heterogeneous group of inherited disorders resulting in characteristic patterns of muscle weakness, some with cardiac involvement. Only disorders with childhood or adult onset will be considered here (i.e., excluding congenital myopathies).

PHYSICAL FINDINGS AND CLINICAL PRESENTATION

Dystrophinopathies

- Proximal arm and leg weakness with hypertrophic calf muscles (Fig. 48–1), delayed motor milestones, cognitive impairment, cardiac involvement, progressive course resulting in respiratory complications and respiratory failure
- Duchenne's MD (DMD), onset 2 to 3 years old, positive Gowers' maneuver (Fig. 48–2), typically wheelchair-bound by 12 years
- Becker's MD (BMD), onset 5 to 15 years old, ambulatory beyond age 15

Myotonic dystrophy

- Variable age at onset and severity manifesting as predominantly distal weakness with long face (Fig. 48–3), percussion and grip myotonia, temporalis and masseter wasting, ptosis, hypersomnolence, cognitive impairment, and cardiac conduction defects; may be associated with frontal balding, cataracts, impaired glucose tolerance, and male infertility

Limb-girdle muscular dystrophy

- Phenotypically and genetically heterogenous, characterized by proximal hip and shoulder girdle weakness, some genotypes featuring cardiac involvement

Emery-Dreifuss muscular dystrophy

- Early adulthood onset with predominantly humeroperoneal weakness, early contractures, and cardiac dysfunction

Facioscapulohumeral muscular dystrophy

- Onset typically in late childhood or adolescence
- Weakness mostly in face and shoulder girdle musculature and possibly later, mild involvement of lower extremities

Oculopharyngeal muscular dystrophy

- Symptom onset typically in mid-adulthood
- Ptosis, dysphagia, dysarthria, and proximal muscle weakness

DIFFERENTIAL DIAGNOSIS

- Myasthenia gravis
- Inflammatory myopathy
- Metabolic myopathy
- Endocrine myopathy
- Toxic myopathy
- Mitochondrial myopathy

WORKUP

- Creatine kinase (CK)
- Electrocardiography (Fig. 48–4), Holter monitor, echocardiography
- Electromyography
- Muscle biopsy with immunohistochemistry (see Fig. 48–1) useful for diagnosis of dystrophinopathies and limb-girdle muscular dystrophy

- DNA analysis helpful if clinical suspicion is for myotonic, Emery-Dreifuss, facioscapulohumeral, and oculopharyngeal muscular dystrophies
- Assessment of respiratory parameters, including forced vital capacity (FVC)

TREATMENT

- Genetic counseling
- Physical, occupational, respiratory, speech therapy as symptoms dictate
- Screening for sleep-disordered breathing with overnight polysomnogram (PSG) if clinically indicated
- Pacemaker placement may be necessary if cardiac conduction defect present
- Prednisone may modestly prolong ambulation in Duchenne's MD
- Vigilance to avoid cardiac and respiratory complications, joint contractures

B. MYASTHENIA GRAVIS

DEFINITION

Myasthenia gravis (MG) is an autoimmune disorder of postsynaptic neuromuscular transmission usually directed against the nicotinic acetylcholine receptor (AChR) of the neuromuscular junction, resulting in a decrease in functional postsynaptic AChRs and consequent weakness.

PHYSICAL FINDINGS AND CLINICAL PRESENTATION

- The hallmark of MG is fluctuating weakness worsened with exercise and improved with rest.
- Generalized weakness involving proximal muscles, diaphragm, neck extensors in 85% of patients
- Weakness confined to eyelids and extraocular muscles in about 15% of patients
- Bulbar symptoms of ptosis (Fig. 48–5), diplopia, dysarthria, dysphagia common
- Normal reflexes, sensation, and coordination

CAUSE

- Antibody-mediated decrease in nicotinic AChRs in the postsynaptic neuromuscular junction resulting in defective neuromuscular transmission and subsequent muscle weakness and fatigue

DIFFERENTIAL DIAGNOSIS

- Lambert-Eaton myasthenic syndrome
- Botulism
- Medication-induced myasthenia
- Chronic progressive external ophthalmoplegia
- Congenital myasthenic syndromes
- Thyroid disease, basilar meningitis
- Intracranial mass lesion with cranial neuropathy
- Miller-Fisher variant of Guillain-Barré syndrome

Table 48–1 shows the differential diagnosis of neuromuscular junction disorders.

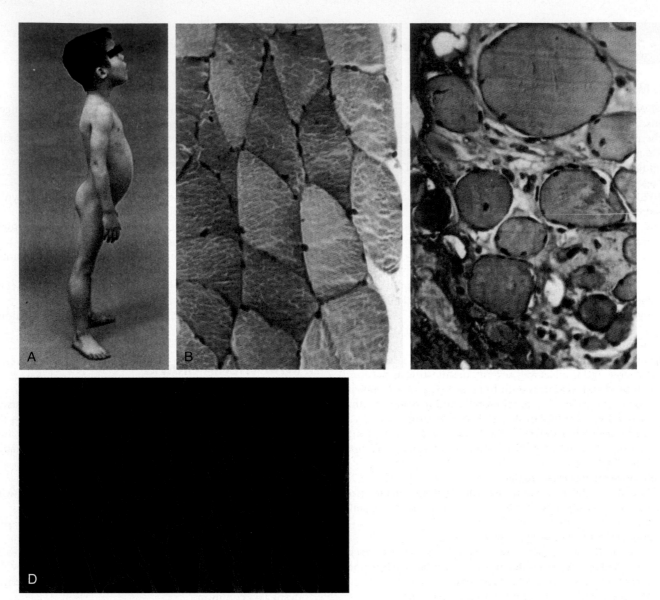

Fig 48–1
Duchenne's muscular dystrophy, an X-linked progressive myopathy of childhood caused by mutations of the dystrophia gene. **A,** Lateral photograph of a boy with Duchenne's muscular dystrophy. Note the lumbar lordosis and enlarged calves. **B,** Cross section of a normal skeletal muscle biopsy specimen (H&E). There is a similarity between muscle fibers in diameter, the presence of nuclei at the periphery of the fibers, and the lack of endomysial fibrosis. **C,** Cross section of a skeletal muscle biopsy specimen from a child with Duchenne's muscular dystrophy (H&E). There is a variation in fiber size, presence of central nuclei, and increased amounts of endomysial fibrous tissue and fat. **D,** Girls with one mutant and one normal copy of the dystrophin gene sometimes have symptoms, including elevated serum creatine kinase levels and mild weakness. This section, prepared from a skeletal muscle biopsy from a female Duchenne carrier, was immunostained with an antibody to dystrophin and then studied by indirect immunofluorescence using a rhodamine-conjugated second antibody. Most myofibers show some dystrophin staining, although some fibers (especially smaller diameter fibers) are nearly devoid of staining. In addition, the staining pattern is nonuniform along the sarcolemmal membrane in some fibers. These features indicate the presence of a reduced quantity of the normal dystrophin molecule in this patient and are typical of heterozygous, female Duchenne carriers. Dystrophin, the skeletal muscle protein mutated in Duchenne's muscular dystrophy, appears to have primarily a structural function. Mutations of other dystrophin-associated skeletal muscle structural proteins have also been found to cause muscular dystrophy phenotypes.
(From Rosenberg RN: Atlas of Clinical Neurology. Boston, Butterworth-Heinemann, 1998.)

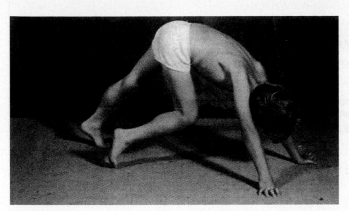

Fig 48-2

A boy with Duchenne's muscular dystrophy (DMD) demonstrating pseudohypertrophy of his calves and a positive Gower maneuver ("climbing" from a sitting position because of proximal muscle weakness). DMD is the most common inherited form of muscle disease. It is transmitted in an X-linked recessive fashion. The disease presents as a slowly progressive weakness of the proximal lower extremities, typically beginning between ages 3 and 5 years. The disease is associated with highly elevated serum creatine kinase levels, wheelchair dependence by age 12, and death, usually in the third decade from pneumonia or cardiomyopathy. Female carriers of the gene rarely have symptoms of muscle disease. However, because of random inactivation of the X chromosome, female carriers often have an elevated serum creatine kinase level (about 70% of carriers) and occasionally have enlarged calves and mild muscle weakness.
(From Rosenberg RN: Atlas of Clinical Neurology. Boston, Butterworth-Heinemann, 1998.)

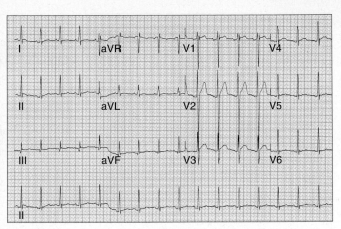

Fig 48-4

Typical electrocardiogram of a patient with Duchenne's muscular dystrophy. Note the tall precordial R waves and the deep narrow s waves in leads V1 to V3.
(From Crawford, MH, DiMarco JP, Paulus WJ [eds]: Cardiology, 2nd ed. St. Louis, Mosby, 2004.)

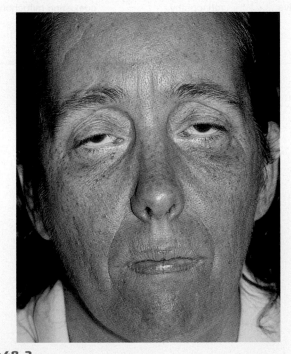

Fig 48-3

Front view of a patient who has myotonic dystrophy. The muscle wasting gives the characteristic drawn appearance of hatcher facies.
(From Yanoff M, Duker JS: Ophthalmology, 2nd ed. St. Louis, Mosby, 2004.)

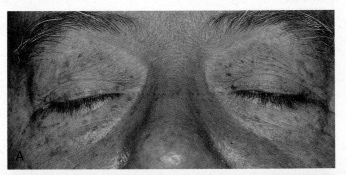
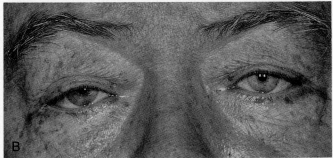

Fig 48-5

Myasthenia gravis with severe bilateral ptosis. **A,** Before treatment. **B,** The same patient after administration of intravenous edrophonium (Tensilon).
(From Yanoff M, Duker JS: Ophthalmology, 2nd ed. St. Louis, Mosby, 2004.)

TABLE 48-1 Differential diagnosis of the neuromuscular junction

Disorder	Pupils	Ocular Motility	Lids	Other Ocular Findings	Other Systemic Findings
Myasthenia gravis	Normal	Fluctuating ophthalmoparesis	Ptosis	—	Fluctuating weakness that improves with rest
			Cogan's lid twitch sign		
Graves' opthalmopathy	Normal	Restricted EOM	Lid retraction	Conjunctival infection	Symptoms of hyperthyroidism may be present
		Positive forced duction testing	Lid lag	Keratoconjunctivitis sicca	
				Exophthalmos	
				Optic neuropathy	
Botulism	Dilated, poorly reactive	Ophthalmoparesis	Ptosis	—	Limb weakness
					Bulbar signs
					Respiratory failure
	Light—near dissociation				Urinary retention
					Constipation
Lambert-Eaton myasthenic syndrome	Usually normal	Usually normal	Usually normal	Keratoconjunctivitis sicca	Autonomic and sensory symptoms
Guillain-Barré syndrome	Normal or poorly reactive	Normal or ophthalmoparesis	Ptosis	—	Facial diplegia
					Limb weakness
					Areflexia
					Respiratory failure
Progressive external ophthalmoplegia	Normal	Slowly progressive	Slowly progressive	May have pigmentary retinopathy	None unless coexisting mitochondrial disorder
		Symmetrical ophthalmoparesis	Ptosis		

EOM, extraocular movement.
From Yanoff M, Duker JS: Ophthalmology, 2nd ed. St. Louis, Mosby, 2004.

WORKUP
- Tensilon test: useful in MG patients with ocular symptoms
- Repetitive nerve stimulation (RNS): successive stimulation shows decrement of muscle action potential in clinically weak muscle; may be negative in up to 50%
- Single-fiber electromyography: highly sensitive; abnormal in up to 95% of myasthenics
- Serum AChR antibodies found in up to 80% of patients.
- A subset of patients with seronegative MG may have muscle-specific tyrosine kinase antibodies.

ADDITIONAL TESTS
- Spirometry to document pulmonary function
- CT scan of anterior chest to rule out thymoma or residual thymic tissue (Fig. 48–6)
- TSH, FT_4: to rule out thyroid disease

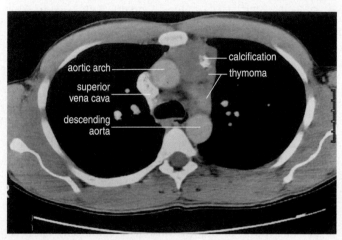

Fig 48–6
CT scan of the chest with contrast enhancement. Shown is a large, multilobulated thymoma in a 32-year-old man with ocular myasthenia gravis. The mass is in proximity to the aortic arch and the ascending aorta. A focal calcification is present anteriorly. The patient's ptosis and diplopia remitted following removal of the thymoma.
(From Yanoff M, Duker JS: Ophthalmology, 2nd ed. St. Louis, Mosby, 2004.)

TREATMENT
- Patient education to facilitate recognition of worsening symptoms and impress the need for medical evaluation at onset of clinical deterioration
- Avoidance of select drugs known to provoke exacerbations of MG (beta blockers, aminoglycoside and quinolone antibiotics, class I antiarrhythmics)
- Prompt treatment of infections, diet modification, and speech evaluation with dysphagia
- Symptomatic treatment with acetylcholinesterase inhibitors: pyridostigmine
- Immunosuppressive treatment with corticosteroids, azathioprine, mycophenolate mofetil, cyclosporine for chronic disease-modifying therapy
- Plasmapheresis and intravenous immunoglobulin are possible short-term options for immunotherapy.
- Mechanical ventilation is lifesaving in the setting of a myasthenic crisis. Consider elective intubation if forced vital capacity is lower than 15 mL/kg, maximal expiratory pressure is lower than 40 cm H_2O, or negative inspiratory pressure is lower than 25 cm H_2O.
- In thymomatous MG, thymectomy is indicated in all patients.
- For nonthymomatous autoimmune MG, thymectomy is an option for patients younger than 40 years.

Chapter 49   Bell's palsy

DEFINITION
Bell's palsy is an idiopathic, isolated, usually unilateral facial weakness in the distribution of the seventh cranial nerve; less than 1% are bilateral.

PHYSICAL FINDINGS AND CLINICAL PRESENTATION
- Unilateral paralysis of the upper and lower facial muscles (asymmetrical eye closure, brow, and smile; Fig. 49–1).
- Ipsilateral loss of taste
- Ipsilateral ear pain, usually 2 to 3 days before presentation
- Increased or decreased unilateral eye tearing
- Hyperacusis
- Subjective ipsilateral facial numbness
- In about 8% of cases, other cranial neuropathies may occur.

CAUSE
- Most cases are idiopathic, although the cause is often viral (herpes simplex).
- Herpes zoster can cause Bell's palsy in association with herpetic blisters affecting the outer ear canal or the area behind the ear (Ramsay-Hunt syndrome).
- Bell's palsy can also be one of the manifestations of Lyme disease.

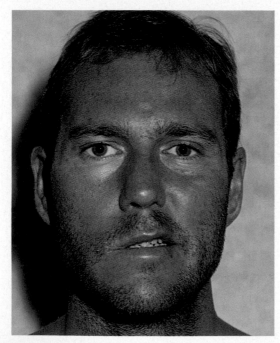

Fig 49–1
Right facial palsy.
(From Swartz MH: Textbook of Physical Diagnosis, 5th ed. Philadelphia, WB Saunders, 2006.)

DIFFERENTIAL DIAGNOSIS
- Neoplasms affecting the base of the skull or the parotid gland
- Infectious process (meningitis, otitis media, osteomyelitis of the skull base)
- Brainstem stroke
- Multiple sclerosis
- Head trauma, temporal bone fracture
- Other: sarcoidosis, Guillain-Barré syndrome, carcinomatous or leukemic meningitis, leprosy, Melkersson-Rosenthal syndrome

LABORATORY TESTS
- Consider CBC, fasting glucose, VDRL, ESR, angiotensin-converting enzyme (ACE) level in select patients.
- Lyme titer in endemic areas

IMAGING STUDIES
- Contrast-enhanced MRI to exclude neoplasms is indicated only in patients with atypical features or course.
- Chest x-ray may be useful to exclude sarcoidosis or rule out TB in select patients before treating with steroids.

TREATMENT
- Reassure patient that the prognosis is usually good and the disease is most likely a result of a virus attacking the nerve, not a stroke.
- Avoid corneal drying by patching the eye. Ophthalmic ointment at night and artificial tears during the day are also useful to prevent excessive drying.
- A short course of oral prednisone is commonly used, although the evidence from randomized controlled trials demonstrating its efficacy is inadequate. If used, prednisone therapy should be started within 24 to 48 hours of symptom onset. Optimal steroid dose is unknown.
- Combination therapy with acyclovir and prednisone may be effective in improving clinical recovery, although robust evidence from high-quality, randomized controlled trials is lacking.
- Botulinum toxin may be helpful for treatment of synkinesis and hemifacial spasm, two late sequelae of Bell's palsy.

Chapter 50   Cerebral palsy

DEFINITION
Cerebral palsy (CP) is a group of disorders of the central nervous system characterized by aberrant control of movement or posture, present since early in life and not the result of a recognized progressive or degenerative disease.

PHYSICAL FINDINGS AND CLINICAL PRESENTATION
- Monoplegia, diplegia, quadriplegia (Fig. 50–1), hemiplegia
- Often hypotonic in newborn period, followed by development of hypertonia
- Spasticity
- Athetosis
- Delay in motor milestones
- Hyperreflexia
- Seizures
- Mental retardation

CAUSE
- Multifactorial, including low birth weight, congenital malformation, asphyxia, multiple gestation, intrauterine exposure to infection, neonatal stroke, hyperbilirubinemia

DIAGNOSIS
- A motor deficit is always present.
- Usual presenting complaint is that child is not reaching motor milestones at appropriate chronologic age
- Medical history establishes that the child is not losing function. This history, combined with a neurologic examination establishing that the motor deficit is caused by a cerebral abnormality, establishes the diagnosis of CP.
- Serial examinations may be necessary if the history is unreliable.

DIFFERENTIAL DIAGNOSIS
Other causes of neonatal hypotonia include the following:
- Muscular dystrophies
- Spinal muscular atrophy
- Down syndrome
- Spinal cord injuries

LABORATORY TESTS
- Metabolic and genetic testing should be considered if, on follow-up, the child has (1) evidence of deterioration or episodes of metabolic decompensation, (2) no cause determined by neuroimaging, (3) family history of childhood neurologic disorder associated with CP, (4) developmental malformation on neuroimaging.
- If a previous stroke is seen on neuroimaging, consider evaluation for coagulopathy.
- An EEG should be obtained when a child with CP has a history suggestive of epilepsy.
- Children with CP should be screened for ophthalmologic and hearing impairments and for speech and language disorders. Nutrition, growth, and swallowing function should be monitored.

IMAGING STUDIES
- Neuroimaging is recommended if the cause has not been established previously—for example, perinatal imaging.
- MRI, when available, is preferred to CT scanning because of a higher yield in suggesting a cause and timing of the insult leading to CP.

TREATMENT
- Physical therapy, occupational therapy, speech therapy
- Orthotics and casting are used to increase musculotendinous length.
- Treatment of seizures, as directed by seizure type
- Intrathecal baclofen is used for treatment of spasticity. Indications include arm and leg spasticity interfering with function.
- Botulinum toxin A is also used for treatment of spasticity.
- Surgical reduction of spasticity by dorsal rhizotomy, tendon lengthening, and osteotomy

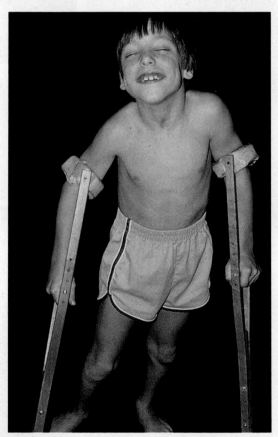

Fig 50–1
Typical cerebral palsy patient with spastic quadriplegia. Note the secondary muscle atrophy especially evident in the lower extremities. He requires crutches to ambulate, seizure medication, and a specialized educational program. His neuromuscular abnormalities are the result of a one-time central nervous system insult and are not progressive. (From Zitelli BJ, Davis HW: Atlas of Pediatric Physical Diagnosis, 4th ed. St. Louis, Mosby, 2002.)

Chapter 51 Down syndrome

DEFINITION
Down syndrome is a disorder characterized by mental retardation and multiple organ defects. It is caused by a chromosomal abnormality (trisomy 21).

PHYSICAL FINDINGS AND CLINICAL PRESENTATION (Fig. 51–1)
- Microcephaly
- Flattening of occiput and face
- Upward slant to eyes with epicanthal folds
- Brushfield spots in iris
- Broad stocky neck
- Small feet, hands, digits
- Single palmar crease
- Hypotonia
- Short stature
- Associated with congenital heart disease, malformations of the GI tract, cataracts, hypothyroidism, hip dysplasia
- About half of children with Down syndrome are born with congenital heart disease, with the most common lesions being atrial septal defect and ventricular septal defect.

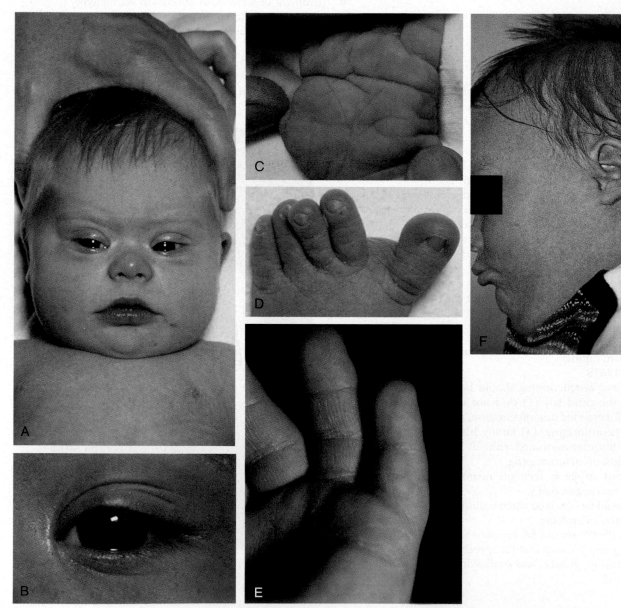

Fig 51–1
Clinical photographs of several minor anomalies associated with Down syndrome. **A,** Characteristic facial features with upward-slanting palpebral fissures, epicanthal folds, and flat nasal bridge. **B,** Brushfield spots. **C,** Bridged palmar crease, seen in some infants with Down syndrome. There are two transverse palmar creases connected by a diagonal line. **D,** Wide space between the first and second toes. **E,** Short fifth finger. **F,** Small ears and flat occiput.
(From Zitelli BJ, Davis HW: Atlas of Pediatric Physical Diagnosis, 4th ed. St. Louis, Mosby, 2002.)

- Persistent primary congenital hypothyroidism is found in 1 in 141 newborns with Down syndrome, as compared with 1 in 4000 in the general population.
- Ophthalmologic disorders increase in frequency with age. Over 80% of children aged 5 to 12 years have disorders that need monitoring or intervention, such as refractive errors, strabismus, or cataracts.

CAUSE
- Nondisjunction of chromosome 21

DIAGNOSIS
- Prenatal cytogenic diagnosis by amniocentesis or chorionic villus sampling
- Combined use of serum screening and fetal ultrasound testing for thickened nuchal fold has 80% detection rate, with 5% false-positives
- Postnatal chromosomal karyotype

DIFFERENTIAL DIAGNOSIS
- Congenital hypothyroidism
- Other chromosomal abnormalities

WORKUP
- Postnatal karyotype
- Thyroid screening at birth, at age 6 months, and yearly thereafter
- Echocardiography, usually performed in neonatal period

TREATMENT
- Treatment consists of vigilant monitoring for comorbid states, such as obesity, hypothyroidism, leukemia, hearing loss, and valvular heart disease.
- Thyroid screening at birth, at age 6 months, and yearly thereafter
- Prevention of obesity with low-calorie, high-fiber diet
- Monitoring for hematologic problems
- Auditory brainstem responses in all newborns and aggressive testing for hearing loss in children with chronic otitis media
- Echocardiography in all newborns and cardiac assessment of adolescents for development of mitral valve prolapse
- Ophthalmologic assessment by age 6 months for congenital cataracts and annual examinations for monitoring of refractive errors and strabismus
- Regular dental care
- Pelvic examination of women who are sexually active or who have menstrual problems
- Dermatologic issues such as folliculitis can become problematic in adolescents and require careful attention to hygiene and topical antibiotics.

Chapter 52   Normal-pressure hydrocephalus

DEFINITION

Normal-pressure hydrocephalus (NPH) is a syndrome of symptomatic hydrocephalus in the setting of normal CSF pressure. The classic clinical triad of NPH includes gait disturbance, cognitive decline, and incontinence.

PHYSICAL FINDINGS AND CLINICAL PRESENTATION

- Gait difficulty: patients often have difficulty initiating ambulation, and the gait may be broad-based and shuffling, with the appearance that the feet are stuck to the floor (referred to as magnetic gait or frontal gait disorder).
- Cognitive decline: mental slowing, forgetfulness and inattention without agnosia, aphasia, or other cortical disturbances.
- Incontinence: initially may have urinary urgency; later incontinence develops. Occasionally, fecal incontinence also occurs.
- On physical examination, look for signs of disease that may mimic those of NPH.

CAUSE

- Approximately 50% of cases are idiopathic; remaining cases have secondary causes, including prior subarachnoid hemorrhage, meningitis, trauma, and intracranial surgery.
- Symptoms are presumed to result from stretching of sacral motor and limbic fibers that lie near the ventricles as dilation occurs.

DIFFERENTIAL DIAGNOSIS

- Alzheimer's disease with extrapyramidal features
- Cognitive impairment in the setting of Parkinson's disease or parkinsonism-plus syndromes
- Diffuse Lewy body disease
- Frontotemporal dementia
- Cervical spondylosis with cord compromise in the setting of degenerative dementia
- Multifactorial gait disorder
- Multi-infarct dementia

WORKUP

- Large-volume lumbar puncture

  1. Mental status testing and time to walk a prespecified distance (usually 25 feet) are measured, followed by removal of 40 to 50 mL of CSF.

  2. Retest of mental status and timed walking are done at one and four hours. Patients who have significant improvement in gait or mental status tend to have better surgical outcomes; those with mild or negative response can have variable outcomes.

  3. Opening and closing pressures are measured; if pressure is elevated, alternative causes must be considered.

- Measurement of CSF outflow resistance by an infusion test, CSF pressure monitoring, or prolonged external lumbar drainage are sometimes used to help predict surgical outcome.

LABORATORY TESTS

- CSF should be sent for routine fluid analyses to exclude other pathology.

IMAGING STUDIES

- CT or MRI (Fig. 52–1) can be used to document ventriculomegaly. The distinguishing feature of NPH is ventricular enlargement out of proportion to sulcal atrophy.
- MRI has advantages over CT, including better ability to visualize structures in the posterior fossa, visualize transependymal CSF flow, and document extent of white matter lesions. On MRI, a flow void in the aqueduct and third ventricle (jet sign) may be seen.

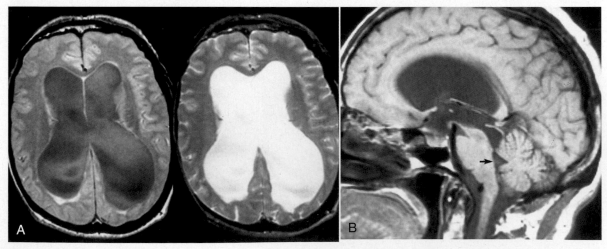

Fig 52–1

MRI scans of hydrocephalus secondary to aqueduct stenosis. **A,** Axial proton density and T2-weighted images (2674/40, 2647/80) showing marked enlargement of the lateral ventricles, with a thin halo of interstitial edema. Inhomogeneity of the fluid signal within the ventricles is caused by pulsatile artifacts. **B,** Sagittal T1-weighted image (800/20) demonstrating massive enlargement of lateral ventricles, outpouching of the suprasellar recesses of the third ventricle impinging on the sella, and ventricularization of the proximal aqueduct just above the level of obstruction and above the fourth ventricle. Note the normal size and configuration of the fourth ventricle *(arrow).*

(From Grainger RG, Allison DJ, Adam A, Dixon AK [eds]: Grainger and Allison's Diagnostic Radiology: A Textbook of Medical Imaging, 4th ed. London. Harcourt, 2001.)

- Isotope cisternography and dynamic MRI studies have not been shown to be superior in predicting shunt outcome.

TREATMENT

- Response to ventriculoperitoneal shunting is variable. Some patients (30% of those with idiopathic NPH and 60% of patients with a known cause) show significant improvement from shunting.
- Factors that may predict positive outcome with surgery:
  - NPH secondary to prior trauma, subarachnoid hemorrhage, or meningitis
  - History of mild impairment in cognition of less than 2 years' duration

- Onset of gait abnormality before cognitive decline
- Imaging demonstrates hydrocephalus without sulcal enlargement.
- Transependymal CSF flow visualized on MRI
- Large-volume tap produces dramatic but temporary relief of symptoms.
- Factors that may predict negative outcome with surgery:
  - Extensive white matter lesions or diffuse cerebral atrophy on MRI
  - Moderate to severe cognitive impairment
  - Onset of cognitive impairment before gait disorder
  - History of alcohol abuse

Chapter 53   Dandy-Walker malformation

- The Dandy-Walker complex is characterized by cystic dilation of the fourth ventricle and an enlarged posterior fossa, with upward displacement of the lateral sinuses and tentorium.
- It may also be associated with varying degrees of vermian hypoplasia corpus callosum dysgenesis and occipital cephaloceles.
- Non-CNS anomalies include polydactyly and cardiac anomalies.
- MRI is the diagnostic modality of choice (Fig. 53–1),
- In cases of hydrocephalus associated with Dandy-Walker malformation, evaluation should follow the guidelines outlined earlier for hydrocephalus.

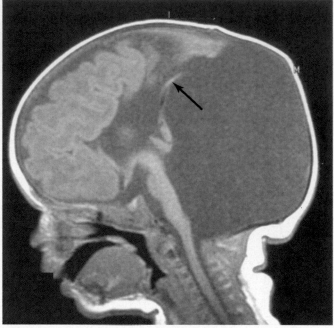

Fig 53–1
MRI scan of Dandy-Walker malformation. This female neonate was born with a large head. A midline sagittal T1 scan shows a large cystic area expanding the posterior fossa and elevating the tentorium *(arrow)*. The vermis is hypoplastic and is rotated posteriorly and upward. (From Grainger RG, Allison DJ, Adam A, Dixon AK [eds]: Grainger and Allison's Diagnostic Radiology: A Textbook of Medical Imaging, 4th ed. London. Harcourt, 2001.)

Chapter 54   Neuroblastoma

DEFINITION

Neuroblastomas are tumors of postganglionic sympathetic neurons that typically originate in the adrenal medulla or the sympathetic chain or ganglion. Neuroblastoma is often present at birth, but not diagnosed until later, when the child shows symptoms of the disease. It is almost exclusively a disease of childhood.

PHYSICAL FINDINGS AND CLINICAL PRESENTATION

- Mass in abdomen, neck, or chest. Approximately two thirds of tumors arise in the abdomen; of these, two thirds arise in the adrenal glands; 70% to 80% of children have regional lymph node involvement or distant metastases at time of presentation.
- Spinal cord, paraspinal: can present with back pain, signs of compression paraplegia, stool, urine retention
- *Horner's syndrome* (ptosis, miosis, anhidrosis; Fig. 54–1)
- Thoracic: difficulty breathing, dysphagia, infections, chronic cough
- Secondary symptoms referable to metastatic disease: fatigue, chronic pain (typically bony pain), pancytopenia, periorbital ecchymosis, proptosis, anorexia, weight loss, unexplained fever, multiple subcutaneous bluish nodules, irritability
- Paraneoplastic syndromes: opsoclonus-myoclonus syndrome is described as dancing eyes, dancing feet, which manifest as myoclonic jerks and chaotic eye movements in all directions. This may be the initial presentation before tumor diagnosis found present in 1% to 3% of patients with neuroblastoma; of all patients with opsoclonus-myoclonus, 20% to 50% have an underlying neuroblastoma. Patients who present with this syndrome often have neuroblastomas with more favorable biologic features.
- Progressive cerebellar ataxia
- Abnormal secretion of vasoactive intestinal peptide by the tumor, leading to distention of the abdomen and secretory diarrhea

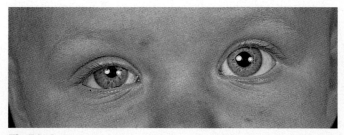

Fig 54–1

Horner's syndrome clearly acquired in infancy must be evaluated for neuroblastoma, a treatable tumor. This young girl, with a right ptosis and miosis, developed a flush during cycloplegia that made the vasomotor abnormality very clear; the Horner's side remained pale. She had no sign of Horner's syndrome during her first 8 months, but at 16 months Horner's syndrome is obvious (ptosis, miosis, and upside-down ptosis). Because the syndrome was acquired, a chest radiograph was ordered; it showed a mass in the pulmonary apex. MRI confirmed the lesion. Surgery showed it to be a neuroblastoma.
(From Yanoff M, Duker JS: Ophthalmology, 2nd ed. St. Louis, Mosby, 2004.)

LABORATORY TESTS

- Complete blood count, coagulation studies, ESR
- 24-hour urine for catecholamines: homovanillic acid (HVA) and vanillylmandelic acid (VMA) are secreted by 90% to 95% of tumors.
- Nonspecific serum markers such as neuron-specific enolase, lactate dehydrogenase, and ferritin
- Bone marrow biopsy and aspirate: karyotype, DNA index, N-MYC copy number.
- Minimum criteria for diagnosis are based on one of the following: (1) unequivocal pathologic diagnosis made from tumor tissue or (2) combination of bone marrow aspirate with unequivocal tumor cells and increased levels of serum or urinary catecholamine metabolites, as described earlier.
- Genetic and biologic variables have been studied in children with neuroblastoma, in particular the histology, aneuploidy of tumor DNA, and amplification of the N-MYC oncogene in tumor tissue, because treatment decisions may be based on these factors.
- Hyperdiploid DNA is associated with a favorable prognosis, especially in infants.
- N-MYC amplification is associated with a poor prognosis, regardless of patient age, probably because of association with deletion of chromosome 1p and gain of chromosome 17q.
- Other biologic factors studied include profile of gamma-aminobutyric (GABA)-ergic receptors, expression of neurotrophin receptors, and levels of telomerase RNA, serum ferritin, and lactate dehydrogenase.

IMAGING STUDIES

- Chest x-ray, abdominal x-ray, skeletal survey, abdominal ultrasound
- Renal, bladder ultrasound
- CT or MRI of the chest and abdomen (Fig. 54–2) to provide information about regional lymph nodes, vessel invasion, and distant metastases
- Body scan with iobenguane sulfate I 123 (Fig. 54–3), which is taken up by neuroblasts and is sensitive to metastases in the bone and soft tissue
- Bone scan with technetium Tc-99 MDP (methylenediphosphonate) to visualize lytic bone lesions and metastases

DIFFERENTIAL DIAGNOSIS

- Other small, round, blue-cell childhood tumors, such as lymphoma, rhabdomyosarcoma, soft tissue sarcoma, and primitive neuroectodermal tumors (PNETs)
- Wilms' tumor
- Hepatoblastoma

TREATMENT

- Assure patient that there is hope for recovery with aggressive treatment.
- Overall, treatment will be determined by several factors, including age at diagnosis, stage of disease, site of primary tumor and metastases, and tumor histology.
- Surgery, particularly for low-risk tumors
- Radiation therapy, often reserved for unresectable tumors or tumors unresponsive to chemotherapy

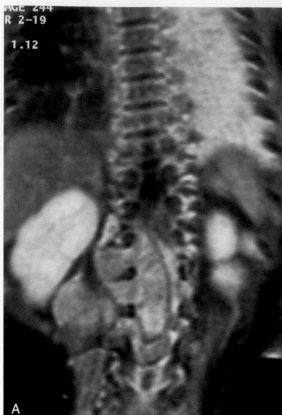

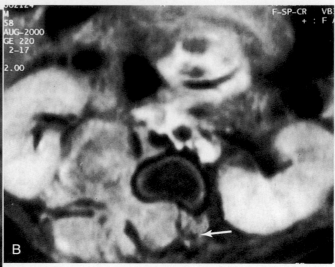

Fig 54-2
Neuroblastoma in a 5-month-old boy. **A,** Coronal T1-weighted fat-saturated MRI sequence postgadolinium contrast. There is a right paraspinal neuroblastoma with extension through the neural foramina at several levels in the lumbar spine, resulting in extensive extradural disease. A diffuse high signal in the left lung represents collapse. **B,** An axial image with the same sequence demonstrates the dumbbell configuration of the tumor with paraspinal and extradural masses. The right kidney is displaced laterally and the dural sac is displaced to the left *(arrow)*. This patient had a further mass extending posteriorly into the soft tissues on the right.
(From Grainger RG, Allison DJ, Adam A, Dixon AK [eds]: Grainger and Allison's Diagnostic Radiology: A Textbook of Medical Imaging, 4th ed. London. Harcourt, 2001.)

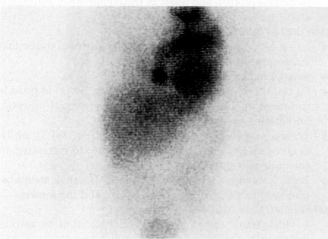

- Multiagent chemotherapy is mainstay of treatment (e.g., cisplatinum, etoposide, doxorubicin, cyclophosphamide, carboplatin).
- Autologous bone marrow transplantation following aggressive chemotherapy for stage IV disease, or patients who are at highest risk based on presence of disseminated disease or unfavorable markers such as *N-MYC* amplification
- Novel therapies include immunotherapy using monoclonal antibodies and vaccines that attempt to initiate an immune reaction against the disease; targeting of tumor cells with drugs that induce apoptosis or have antiangiogenic effect
- ACTH treatment is thought to be effective for patients with opsoclonus-myoclonus syndrome.

Fig 54-3
Neuroblastoma in a 7-year-old boy. The initial investigation was a chest radiograph, which showed a large mass within the left hemithorax. The anterior view of the thorax and abdomen on this iobenguane sulfate I 123 scan shows marked but rather patchy increased uptake in the left hemithorax. There was no evidence of any abnormal skeletal uptake. The appearances are diagnostic of a neuroectodermal tumor. Biopsy confirmed this to be a neuroblastoma.
(From Grainger RG, Allison DJ, Adam A, Dixon AK [eds]: Grainger and Allison's Diagnostic Radiology: A Textbook of Medical Imaging, 4th ed. London. Harcourt, 2001.)

Chapter 55   von Hippel-Lindau disease

DEFINITION
von Hippel-Lindau disease (VHL) is an autosomal dominant inherited disease characterized by the formation of hemangioblastomas, cysts, and malignancies involving multiple organs and systems.

PHYSICAL FINDINGS AND CLINICAL PRESENTATION
- Retinal angiomas (59%)
  1. Most common presentation usually occurs by age 25
  2. Multiple angiomas
  3. Detached retina
  4. Glaucoma
  5. Blindness
- CNS hemangioblastomas (59%)
  1. Cerebellum is the most common site followed by the spine and medulla
  2. Usually multiple; occurs by the age of 30
  3. Headache, ataxia, slurred speech, nystagmus, vertigo, nausea, and vomiting
- Renal cysts (approximately 60%) and clear cell renal cell carcinoma (25% to 45%)
  1. Usually occurs by the age of 40
  2. May be asymptomatic or cause abdominal and flank pain
  3. Renal cell carcinoma is bilateral in 75% of patients
- Pancreatic cysts
  1. Usually asymptomatic
  2. Large cysts can cause biliary obstructive symptoms.
  3. Diarrhea and diabetes may develop if enough of the pancreas is replaced by cysts.
- Pheochromocytoma (7% to 18%)
  1. Bilateral in 50% to 80% of cases
  2. Hypertension, palpitations, sweating, and headache
  3. Commonly occurs with pancreatic islet cell tumors
- Papillary cystadenoma of the epididymis (10% to 25% of men with VHL)
  1. Palpable scrotal mass
  2. May be unilateral or bilateral
- Endolymphatic sac tumors
  1. Ataxia
  2. Loss of hearing
  3. Facial paralysis

CAUSE
VHL disease is primarily caused by a mutation of the von Hippel-Lindau gene located on chromosome 3. The VHL disease gene codes for a cytoplasmic protein that functions in tumor suppression.

DIAGNOSIS
- The diagnosis of VHL disease is established if, in the presence of a positive family history, a single retinal or cerebellar hemangioblastoma is noted or a visceral lesion is found (e.g., renal cell carcinoma, pheochromocytoma, pancreatic cysts or tumor).
- If no clear family history is present, two or more hemangioblastomas or one hemangioblastoma with a visceral lesion are required to make the diagnosis.
- Screening family members is essential for the early detection of VHL disease.

LABORATORY TESTS
- CBC may reveal erythrocytosis requiring periodic phlebotomies.
- Electrolytes, BUN, and creatinine
- Urine for norepinephrine, epinephrine, and VMA, looking for pheochromocytoma

IMAGING STUDIES
- Indirect and direct ophthalmoscopy, fluorescein angioscopy, and tonometry are studies used in screening for retinal angiomas and glaucoma.
- CT of the abdomen (Fig. 55–1A) is used in the screening, detection, and monitoring of patients with renal cysts renal tumors, pheochromocytomas, pancreatic cysts, and tumors.
  1. Renal cysts grow at an average rate of 0.5 cm/yr.
  2. Renal tumors grow at an average rate of 1.5 cm/yr.
  3. CT scans are done every 6 months for the first 2 years and every year for life in patients who have had surgery for renal cell carcinoma.
- MRI with gadolinium (see Fig. 55–1B) is used for screening and evaluation of CNS and spinal hemangioblastomas, endolymphatic sac tumors, and pheochromocytomas.
- Angiography may be done before CNS surgery.

TREATMENT
- Laser photocoagulation and cryotherapy are used for patients with retinal angiomas to prevent blindness.
- For cerebellar hemangioblastomas, the treatment is surgical removal. External beam radiation and stereotactic radiosurgery can also be done.
- For renal tumors, surgery is delayed until one of the renal tumors reaches 3 cm in diameter. Nephron-sparing surgery is the preferred surgical approach.
- Nephrectomy is indicated for patients with end-stage renal disease requiring dialysis because of the malignant potential of the disease.
- Pancreatic islet cell tumors usually require surgical removal.
- Adrenalectomy for pheochromocytoma.

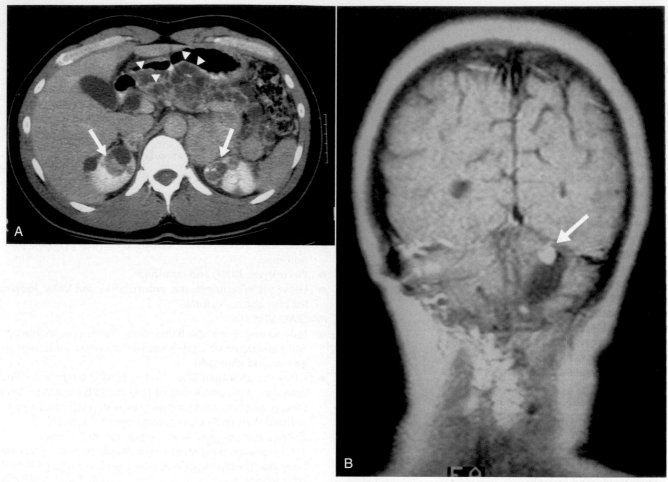

Fig 55–1
Radiologic findings associated with von Hippel-Lindau disease. **A,** Noncontrast CT scan shows massive cystic involvement of the pancreas *(arrowheads)* and bilateral renal cysts *(arrows)*. **B,** Contrast-enhanced MR image shows a right cerebellar hemangioblastoma with a small enhancing mass *(arrow)*.
(From Johnson RJ, Feehally J: Comprehensive Clinical Nephrology, 2nd ed. St. Louis, Mosby, 2000.)

REFERENCES

Ferri F: Ferri's Clinical Advisor 2007. St. Louis, Mosby, 2007.

Ferri F: Practical Guide to the Care of the Medical Patient, 7th ed. St. Louis, Mosby, 2007.

Goetz CG, Pappert EJ: Textbook of Clinical Neurology. Philadelphia, WB Saunders, 1999.

Grainger RG, Allison DJ, Adam A, Dixon AK (eds): Grainger and Allison's Diagnostic Radiology: A Textbook of Medical Imaging, 4th ed. London, Harcourt, 2001.

SECTION

Eyes, Ears, Nose, Oral Cavity, and Neck

Eyes

Chapter 56: Normal anatomy
Chapter 57: Diagnostic tests and procedures
Chapter 58: Cataracts
Chapter 59: Conjunctivitis
Chapter 60: Corneal ulceration (keratitis)
Chapter 61: Scleritis
Chapter 62: Disorders of the conjunctiva and limbus
Chapter 63: Strabismus
Chapter 64: Amblyopia
Chapter 65: Entropion
Chapter 66: Ectropion
Chapter 67: Blepharospasm
Chapter 68: Benign eyelid lesions
Chapter 69: Eyelid malignancies
Chapter 70: Retinitis pigmentosa
Chapter 71: Retinoblastoma
Chapter 72: Amaurosis fugax
Chapter 73: Macular degeneration
Chapter 74: Retinal detachment
Chapter 75: Uveitis
Chapter 76: Glaucoma, chronic open angle
Chapter 77: Glaucoma, primary closed angle
Chapter 78: Horner's syndrome
Chapter 79: Optic neuritis

Ears

Chapter 80: Normal anatomy, examination, and diagnostic testing
Chapter 81: Hearing loss
Chapter 82: Acoustic neuroma
Chapter 83: Relapsing polychondritis
Chapter 84: Otitis externa
Chapter 85: Otitis media

Nose

Chapter 86: Allergic rhinitis
Chapter 87: Epistaxis
Chapter 88: Sinusitis

Mouth and tongue

Chapter 89: Diseases of the oral mucosa
Chapter 90: Dental and periodontal infections
Chapter 91: Herpangina
Chapter 92: Stomatitis
Chapter 93: Scarlet fever

Salivary glands

Chapter 94: Salivary gland neoplasms
Chapter 95: Mumps

Pharynx

Chapter 96: Pharyngitis and tonsillitis
Chapter 97: Epiglottitis

Thyroid

Chapter 98: Thyroid nodule
Chapter 99: Thyroid cancer
Chapter 100: Thyroiditis

EYES

| Chapter 56 | **Normal anatomy** |

- The major structures of the eye are illustrated in Figure 56–1.
- Figure 56–2 shows the retina of the eye. A normal optic disc is shown in Figure 56–3.
- Sensory nerves are depicted in Figure 56–4. Diagnostic positions of gaze are shown in Figure 56–5.

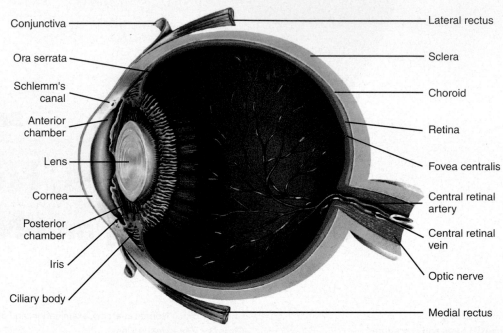

Conjunctiva — Lateral rectus
Ora serrata — Sclera
Schlemm's canal — Choroid
Anterior chamber — Retina
Lens — Fovea centralis
Cornea — Central retinal artery
Posterior chamber — Central retinal vein
Iris — Optic nerve
Ciliary body — Medial rectus

Fig 56–1
The globe, looking down on the right eye, showing major anatomic structures.
(From Palay D, Krachmer JH: Ophthalmology for the Primary Care Physician. St. Louis, Mosby, 1997.)

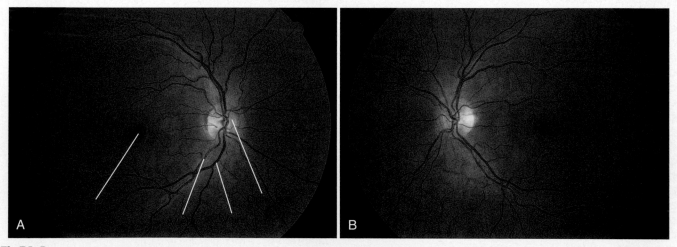

Fig 56–2
Photographs of the retinas of the right **(A)** and left **(B)** eyes.
(From Swartz MH: Textbook of Physical Diagnosis, 5th ed. Philadelphia, WB Saunders, 2006.)

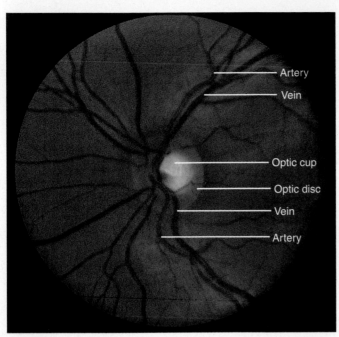

Fig 56–3
Normal optic disc, left eye.
(From Swartz MH: Textbook of Physical Diagnosis, 5th ed. Philadelphia, WB Saunders, 2006.)

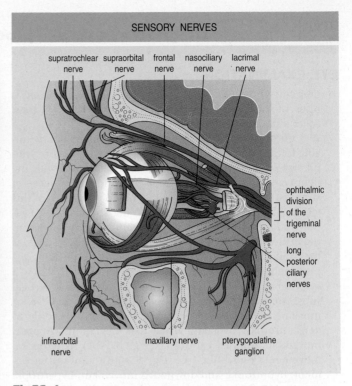

SENSORY NERVES

Fig 56–4
Sensory nerves of the orbit (lateral view).
(Adapted from Dutton JJ: Atlas of Clinical and Surgical Orbital Anatomy. Philadelphia, WB Saunders, 1994.)

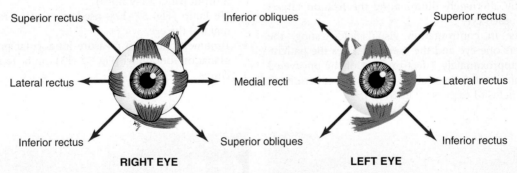

RIGHT EYE **LEFT EYE**

Fig 56–5
Diagnostic positions of gaze.
(From Swartz MH: Textbook of Physical Diagnosis, 5th ed. Philadelphia,WB Saunders, 2006.)

Chapter 57 | **Diagnostic tests and procedures**

EYE EXAMINATION

- Objective clinical methods to determine and measure deviations of the visual axes include corneal light reflex tests, cover tests, and haploscopic tests.
  - Corneal light reflexes, the oldest testing methods, are suitable for all patients. The Hirschberg method relies on a pupil size of 4 mm. The test should be performed with the light centered in each eye's pupil to detect the presence of secondary deviations (Fig. 57–1). The disadvantages of this test are the estimations necessary to measure the eye deviation and the inability to control accommodation when testing at near fixation, because the measuring light serves as the fixation target. The Krimsky test quantifies the light displacement using appropriately held prisms (Fig. 57–2).
  - Cover tests detect and measure horizontal and vertical strasbismus. The examiner observes the uncovered eye for movement as its fellow eye is covered with a paddle to detect tropias, constant visual axis deviations. A nasal movement implies exotropia (Fig. 57–3A), a temporal movement, esotropia (see Fig. 57–3B), upward movement, hypotropia, and downward movement, hypertropia (see Fig. 57–3C) of the uncovered eye. Each eye is covered in turn. Tropias detected by the cover test may be measured using the simultaneous prism and cover test; a prism of appropriate strength is introduced before one eye as the other eye is covered (Fig. 57–4).
  - Haploscopic devices present each eye with a target significantly different from that presented to the other eye. These devices measure horizontal, vertical, and torsional deviations by alternately illuminating the fixation targets presented to each eye.
- Visual fields: in confrontation visual field testing, the patient covers one eye and the examiner faces the patient, positioned approximately 3 feet in front of the uncovered eye. The examiner then moves the fingers to test peripheral and central fields of each eye (Fig. 57–5).
- Inspection of conjunctiva: eyelid inversion can be performed with the use of a small applicator stick (Fig. 57–6A).
- Snellen eye chart: standardized visual acuity chart (Fig. 57–7) or near-card (Fig. 57–8). The corresponding vision (e.g., 20/20, 20/40) is documented for each eye.
- Emmetropia, myopia, and hyperopia (Fig. 57–9):
  - Emmetropia: refractive state of the eye in which parallel rays are focused on the retina
  - Myopia: nearsightedness. The image is focused in front of the retina, because the refractive power of the eye exceeds the refraction necessary for the axial length of the eye. It may occur when the eye is abnormally long or in cataracts, or if the cornea is very steep. It can be corrected by placing a concave or minus lens in front of the eye.
  - Hyperopia: farsightedness. The image is focused posterior to the retina because the axial length of the eye is too short, the cornea is overly flat, or the lens has less refractive power. It can be corrected by placing a convex or plus lens in front of the eye.
- Astigmatism: blurring or distortion of an image (Fig. 57–10) caused by varying refractive power of the eye in different planes (meridians). It can be corrected by placing a cylindric lens in front of the eye.
- Amsler grid: used to test the central 10 degrees of the visual field of each eye (Fig. 57–11). When the patient fixates on the black central dot of the white checkerboard, the grid is projected onto the central retina (macula) and can be used to identify scotomata (blind spots) or metamorphopsia (waxy lines)
- Slit lamp (Fig. 57–12): used to examine the anterior segment of the eye
- Tonometry: used to measure intraocular pressure. The applanation tonometer (Fig. 57–13) can be found on most slit lamps.

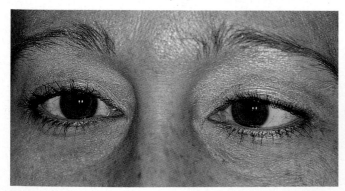

Fig 57–1
Hirschberg light reflex method. The patient has a left esotropia. Note the corneal light reflex at the temporal pupillary border of the left eye while the reflex is centered in the pupil of the right eye.
(From Yanoff M, Duker JS: Ophthalmology, 2nd ed. St. Louis, Mosby, 2004.)

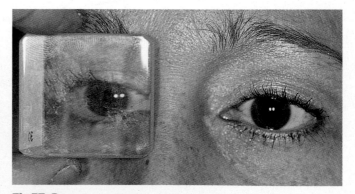

Fig 57–2
Krimsky light reflex method (same patient as in Fig. 57–1). The strength of a base-out prism over the fixing right eye sufficient to center the pupillary light reflex in the esotropic left eye is defined as the amount of left esotropia.
(From Yanoff M, Duker JS: Ophthalmology, 2nd ed. St. Louis, Mosby, 2004.)

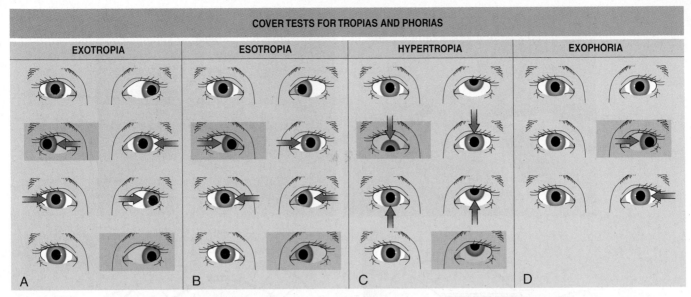

COVER TESTS FOR TROPIAS AND PHORIAS

EXOTROPIA	ESOTROPIA	HYPERTROPIA	EXOPHORIA

Fig 57–3

Cover tests for tropias. **A,** For exotropia, covering the right eye drives inward movement of the left eye to take up fixation; uncovering the right eye shows recovery of fixation by the right eye and leftward movement of both eyes; covering the left eye discloses no shift of the preferred right eye. **B,** For esotropia, covering the right eye drives outward movement of the left eye to take up fixation; uncovering the right eye shows recovery of fixation by the right eye and rightward movement of both eyes; covering the left eye discloses no shift of the preferred right eye. **C,** For hypertropia, covering the right eye drives downward movement of the left eye to take up fixation; uncovering the right eye shows recovery of fixation by the right eye and upward movement of both eyes; covering the left eye shows no shift of the preferred right eye. **D,** For exophoria, the left eye deviates outward behind a cover and returns to the primary position when the cover is removed. An immediate inward movement denotes a phoria; a delayed inward movement denotes an intermittent exotropia.

(Adapted from Diamond G, Eggers H: Strabismus and Pediatric Ophthalmology. London, Mosby, 1993.)

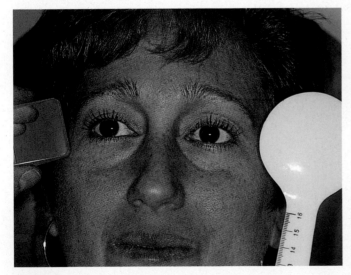

Fig 57–4

Simultaneous prism and cover test with right eye fixing. The prism is moved before the fixing right eye simultaneously with the cover held before the left eye.

(From Yanoff M, Duker JS: Ophthalmology, 2nd ed. St. Louis, Mosby, 2004.)

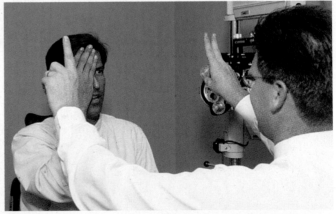

Fig 57–5

Confrontation visual fields. If the patient cannot see an object that is visualized in the examiner's field, a visual field defect is probably present.

(From Palay D, Krachmer JH: Ophthalmology for the Primary Care Physician. St. Louis, Mosby, 1997.)

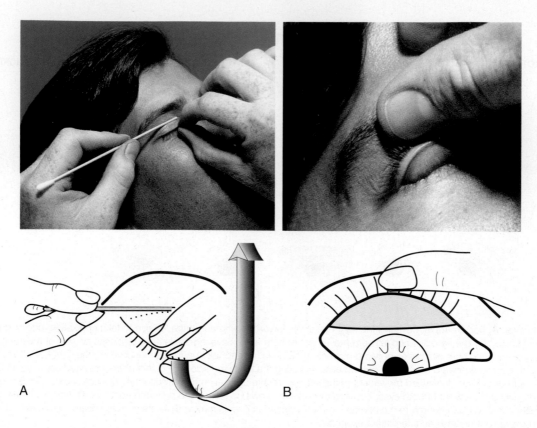

Fig 57–6

A, For eversion, the examiner places a wooden applicator stick at the superior edge of the superior tarsal plate, firmly grasps the lashes of the upper eyelid, and gently moves the applicator stick inferiorly while pulling up on the lashes slightly. **B**, The examiner removes the stick while holding the eyelid in place (often with the cotton-tipped end). Administration of a topical anesthesia (proparacaine) may make this a slightly more comfortable procedure but is not essential.

(From Palay D, Krachmer JH: Ophthalmology for the Primary Care Physician. St. Louis, Mosby, 1997.)

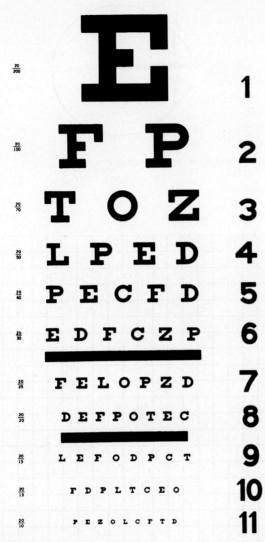

Fig 57-7
Snellen distance acuity chart.
(From Palay D, Krachmer JH: Ophthalmology for the Primary Care Physician. St. Louis, Mosby, 1997.)

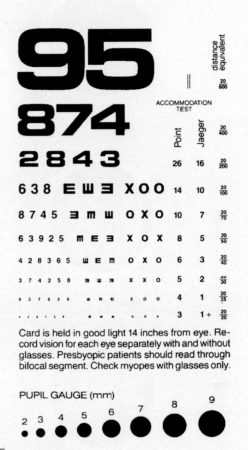

Card is held in good light 14 inches from eye. Record vision for each eye separately with and without glasses. Presbyopic patients should read through bifocal segment. Check myopes with glasses only.

Fig 57-8
Snellen distance acuity card.
(From Palay D, Krachmer JH: Ophthalmology for the Primary Care Physician. St. Louis, Mosby, 1997.)

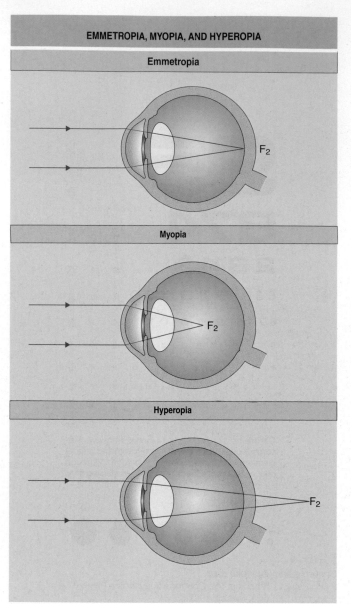

EMMETROPIA, MYOPIA, AND HYPEROPIA

Emmetropia

Myopia

Hyperopia

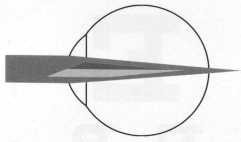

Fig 57–10
Astigmatism—blurring or distortion of an image.

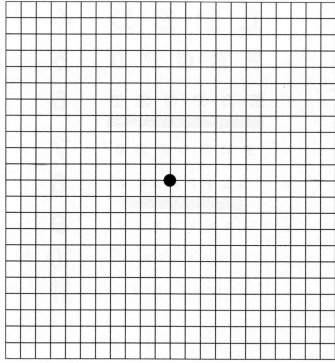

Fig 57–11
The Amsler grid.
(From Palay D, Krachmer JH: Ophthalmology for the Primary Care Physician. St. Louis, Mosby, 1997.)

Fig 57–9
Emmetropia, myopia, and hyperopia. In emmetropia, the far point is at infinity, and the secondary focal point (F_2) is at the retina. In myopia, the far point is in front of the eye, and the secondary focal point (F_2) is in the vitreous. In hyperopia, the secondary focal point (F_2) is behind the eye.
(Adapted from Azar DT, Strauss L: Principles of applied clinical optics. In Albert DM, Jakobiec FA [eds]: Principles and Practice of Ophthalmology, vol 6, 2nd ed. Philadelphia, WB Saunders, 2000, pp 5329-5340.)

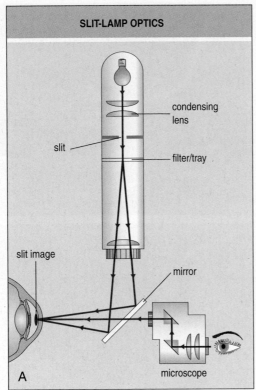

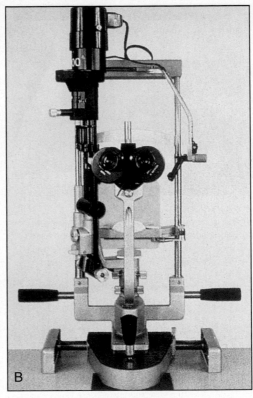

SLIT-LAMP OPTICS

condensing lens

slit

filter/tray

slit image

mirror

microscope

A

B

Fig 57–12
The slit lamp. **A**, Some slit lamps first bring the light to a sharp focus within the slit aperture, and the light within the slit is focused by the condensing lens on to the patient's eye. The observation system of a modern slit lamp has many potential faces to help reduce loss of light.
B, Slit-lamp apparatus.
(A modified from Spalton DJ, Hitchings RA, Hunter PA: Atlas of Clinical Ophthalmology. New York, Gower Medical, 1984, p 10.)

- Gonioscopy: procedure used for differentiating various forms of glaucoma and for viewing pathologic conditions in the anterior chamber of the eye (Fig. 57–14)
- LASIK
  - LASIK stands for laser-assisted in situ keratomileusis, in which an interior flap of cornea is lifted with a keratome and an excimer laser is used to sculpt the stromal bed to change the refractive error of the eye.
  - It can be used to treat wide ranges of refractive error and is the most commonly used corneal refractory procedure.
  - It can be used to treat near- and farsightedness and astigmatism.
  - Figures 57–15, 57–16, and 57–17 illustrate the surgical technique.

GOLDMANN APPLANATION TONOMETER

Fig 57–13
Photograph of a Goldmann applanation tonometer in working position on a slit-lamp microscope.
(From Yanoff M, Duker JS: Ophthalmology, 2nd ed. St. Louis, Mosby, 2004.)

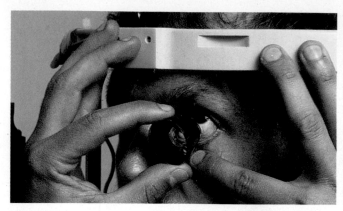

Fig 57–14
Gonioscopy. A Goldmann gonioscope lens being placed on the patient's eye. The indirect gonioscope lens is a solid contact lens within which a small mirror is mounted, allowing the anterior chamber angle structures to be easily viewed. The full circumference of the angle may be viewed by 360-degree rotation of the lens.
(From Palay D, Krachmer JH: Ophthalmology for the Primary Care Physician. St. Louis, Mosby, 1997.)

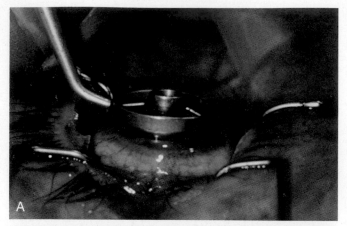

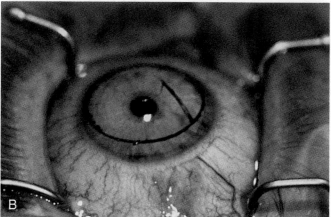

Fig 57–16
A Ruiz marker is impregnated with ink. **A,** It is used to outline a pararadial mark to enable orientation of the flap. **B,** A 9-mm optical zone is outlined to help with proper placement of the suction ring.
(From Yanoff M, Duker JS: Ophthalmology, 2nd ed. St. Louis, Mosby, 2004.)

LAMELLAR DISSECTION USING A MICROKERATOME

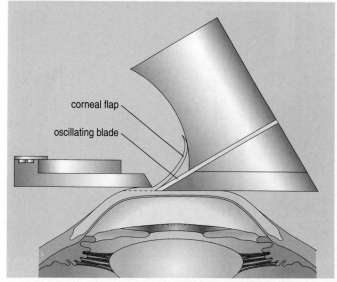

corneal flap

oscillating blade

Fig 57–15
Lamellar dissection using a microkeratome. The corneal flap is created by applanation of the cornea, which is carved in a similar fashion as when using a carpenter's plane.
(From Yanoff M, Duker JS: Ophthalmology, 2nd ed. St. Louis, Mosby, 2004.)

LASER *IN SITU* KERATOMILEUSIS

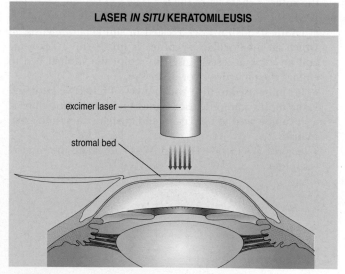

excimer laser

stromal bed

Fig 57–17
Laser in situ keratomileusis—excimer laser ablation to the stromal bed after lamellar keratectomy.
(From Yanoff M, Duker JS: Ophthalmology, 2nd ed. St. Louis, Mosby, 2004.)

Chapter 58 Cataracts

DEFINITION
Cataracts are the clouding and opacification of the normally clear crystalline lens of the eye. The opacity may occur in the cortex (Fig. 58–1), the nucleus of the lens, or the posterior subcapsular region, but it is usually in a combination of areas.

PHYSICAL FINDINGS AND CLINICAL PRESENTATION
- Cloudiness and opacification of the crystalline lens of the eye (Fig. 58–2). Complete opacification of the lens is called a mature (morgagnian) cataract (Fig. 58–3).
- Decreased vision in affected eye

CAUSE
- Heredity
- Trauma (Fig. 58–4)
- Toxins
- Age-related (Fig. 58–5)
- Drug-related
- Congenital (Fig. 58–6)
- Inflammatory
- Diabetes
- Collagen vascular disease

DIFFERENTIAL DIAGNOSIS
- Corneal lesions
- Retinal lesions, detached retina, tumors
- Vitreous disease, chronic inflammation

LABORATORY TESTS
- Rarely, urinary amino acid screening and central nervous system (CNS) imaging studies with congenital cataracts
- Fasting glucose in young adults with cataracts
- Diabetes, collagen vascular, other metabolic disease screening in younger patients with cataracts
- Genetic and hereditary evaluation screening in congenital cataracts

TREATMENT
- Surgery is indicated when corrected visual acuity in the affected eye is more than 20/30 in the absence of other ocular disease; however, surgery may be justified when visual acuity is better in specific situations (especially disabling glare, monocular diplopia). Surgery is also indicated when vision in one eye is greatly different from the other and affects the patient's life.

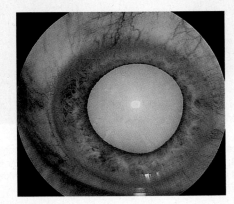

Fig 58–2
Intumescent cataract. The crystalline lens increases in volume because of swelling processes that involve the cortex.
(From Yanoff M, Duker JS: Ophthalmology, 2nd ed. St. Louis, Mosby, 2004.)

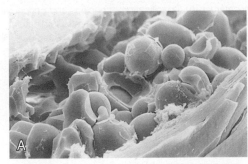

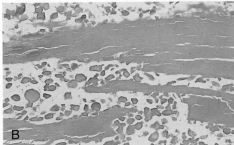

Fig 58–1
Cortical cataract. **A,** Scanning electron microscopic appearance of morgagnian globules in liquefied cortex. **B,** PAS-stained histologic section shows morgagnian globules between fragmented lens "fibers" in the cortex.
(A courtesy of Dr. R.C. Eagle, Jr; **B** from Yanoff M, Fine BS: Ocular Pathology, 5th ed. St. Louis, Mosby, 2002.)

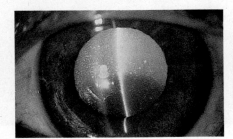

Fig 58–3
Morgagnian cataract. The nucleus is seen as a "suntan" or dark shadow in the inferior third of the pupil.
(From Yanoff M, Duker JS: Ophthalmology, 2nd ed. St. Louis, Mosby, 2004.)

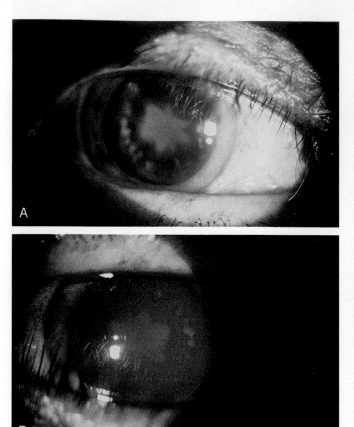

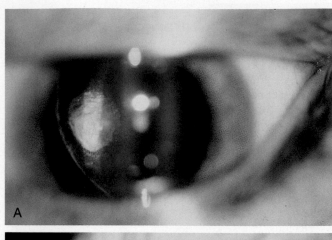

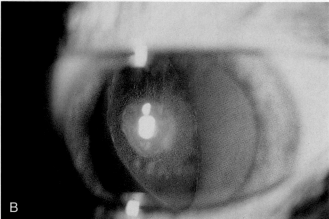

Fig 58–4
Traumatic cataract. **A,** Typical flower-shaped pattern with coronary lens opacities. **B,** Seen in retroillumination in anterior subcapsular region. (From Yanoff M, Duker JS: Ophthalmology, 2nd ed. St. Louis, Mosby, 2004.)

Fig 58–6
Congenital cataract. **A,** Opacification of nucleus and peripheral lamellae. **B,** Lamellar opacification seen with retroillumination. (From Yanoff M, Duker JS: Ophthalmology, 2nd ed. St. Louis, Mosby, 2004.)

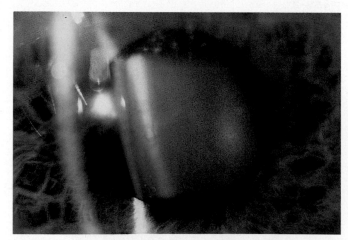

Fig 58–5
Age-related cataract. Nuclear sclerosis and cortical lens opacities are present.
(From Yanoff M, Duker JS: Ophthalmology, 2nd ed. St. Louis, Mosby, 2004.)

Chapter 59 | Conjunctivitis

DEFINITION
The term *conjunctivitis* refers to an inflammation of the conjunctiva resulting from a variety of causes, including allergies and bacterial, viral, and chlamydial infections.

PHYSICAL FINDINGS AND CLINICAL PRESENTATION
- Infection and chemosis of conjunctivae with discharge
- Cornea clear
- Vision often normal

CAUSE
- Bacterial (Fig. 59–1)
- Viral (Fig. 59–2)
- Chlamydial (Figs. 59–3 and 59–4)
- Allergic: Vernal conjunctivitis (Fig. 59–5) is a bilateral recurrent inflammation of the conjunctiva that tends to occur in children in the spring and summer. Giant papillary conjunctivitis (Fig. 59–6) is a syndrome of inflammation of the upper conjunctiva associated with contact lens wear. Infiltrates induced by contact lenses wear are accumulations of white blood cells between the corneal stroma's collagen fibers. In contact lens acute red eye (Fig. 59–7), there are larger infiltrates on various segments of the peripheral cornea, most often caused by soft, extended-wear lenses.
- Traumatic

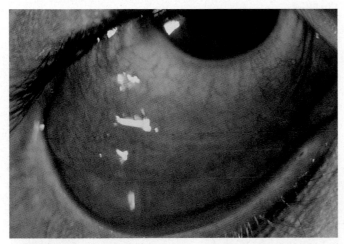

Fig 59–1
Acute bacterial conjunctivitis. This patient was culture-positive for pneumococcus.
(From Yanoff M, Duker JS: Ophthalmology, 2nd ed. St. Louis, Mosby, 2004.)

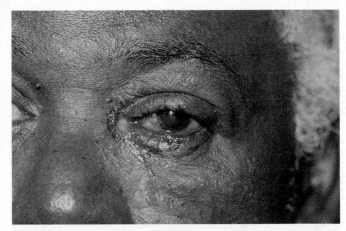

Fig 59–3
Adult inclusion conjunctivitis. This 50-year-old man had prominent follicular conjunctivitis, with a large and tender preauricular lymph node.
(From Yanoff M, Duker JS: Ophthalmology, 2nd ed. St. Louis, Mosby, 2004.)

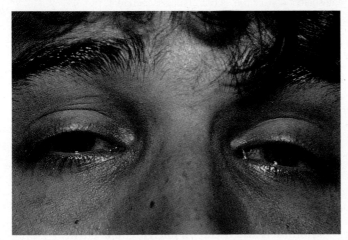

Fig 59–2
Acute bilateral viral conjunctivitis. This 22-year-old man had pharyngoconjunctival fever, and the conjunctivitis was preceded by a viral upper respiratory tract infection.
(From Yanoff M, Duker JS: Ophthalmology, 2nd ed. St. Louis, Mosby, 2004.)

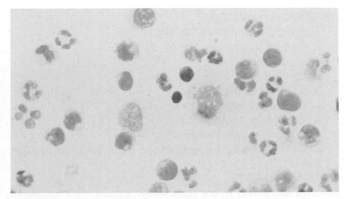

Fig 59–4
Conjunctival scraping. The epithelial cells show basophilic cytoplasmic inclusions typical of a chlamydial infection (Giemsa stain).
(From Yanoff M, Duker JS: Ophthalmology, 2nd ed. St. Louis, Mosby, 2004.)

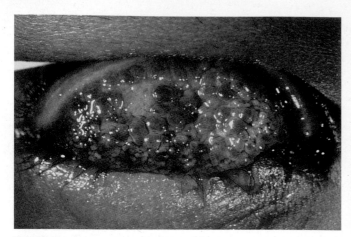

Fig 59–5
Vernal conjunctivitis. Cobblestone papillae cover the superior tarsal conjunctiva.
(From Yanoff M, Duker JS: Ophthalmology, 2nd ed. St. Louis, Mosby, 2004.)

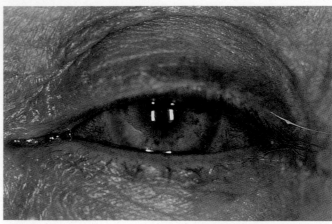

Fig 59–7
Contact lens acute red eye. This is often accompanied by pain and photophobia.
(From Yanoff M, Duker JS: Ophthalmology, 2nd ed. St. Louis, Mosby, 2004.)

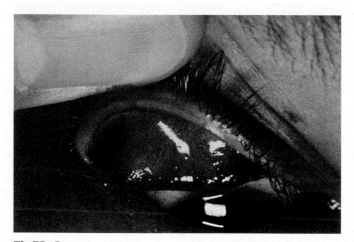

Fig 59–6
Grade one giant papillary conjunctivitis. Note the mild hyperemia and mucus.
(From Yanoff M, Duker JS: Ophthalmology, 2nd ed. St. Louis, Mosby, 2004.)

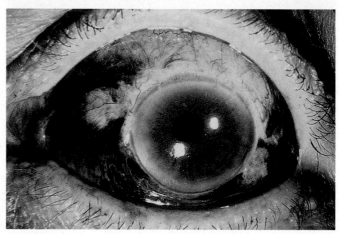

Fig 59–8
Subconjunctival hemorrhage. This small hematoma, seen through the transparent conjunctiva, is benign unless recurrent.
(From Tallis R, Fillit H: Brockelhurst's Textbook of Geriatric Medicine and Gerontology, 6th ed. London, Churchill Livingstone, 2003.)

DIFFERENTIAL DIAGNOSIS

- Acute glaucoma (see Fig. 77–2)
- Corneal lesions (see Fig. 60–2)
- Acute iritis
- Episcleritis
- Scleritis (see Fig. 61–1)
- Uveitis (see Fig. 75–1)
- Canalicular obstruction
- Subconjunctival hemorrhage
- The differential diagnosis of red eye is described in Table 59–1.

LABORATORY TESTS

Cultures are useful if not successfully treated with antibiotic medications; an initial culture is usually not necessary.

TREATMENT

- Warm compresses if infective conjunctivitis
- Cold compresses in irritative or allergic conjunctivitis
- Antibiotic drops are indicated for suspected bacterial conjunctivitis.
- Caution: be careful with opthalmic corticosteroid treatment and avoid unless sure of diagnosis; corticosteroids can exacerbate infections and have been associated with increased intraocular pressure and cataract formation.
- An oral antihistamine is effective in relieving itching.
- Mast cell stabilizers are effective for allergic conjunctivitis.
- The topical nonsteroidal anti-inflammatory drug (NSAID) ketorolac is also useful for allergic conjunctivitis.
- Antihistamine-decongestant combinations such as pheniramine-naphazoline, available over the counter (OTC), are more effective than either agent alone but have a short duration and can result in rebound vasodilation with prolonged use.

TABLE 59–1 **Differential diagnosis of red eye***

Presentation	Acute Conjunctivitis[†]	Acute Iritis	Narrow-Angle Glaucoma	Corneal Abrasion
History	Sudden onset Exposure to conjunctivitis	Fairly sudden onset	Rapid onset	Trauma pain
		Often recurrent	Sometimes history of previous attack	
			Highest incidence among Jews, Swedes, and the Inuit	
Vision	Normal	Impaired if untreated	Rapidly lost if untreated[§]	Can be affected if central
Pain	Gritty feeling	Photophobia	Severe	Exquisite
Bilaterality	Frequent	Occasional	Occasional	Usually unilateral
Vomiting	Absent	Absent	Common	Absent
Cornea	Clear (epidemic keratoconjunctivitis has corneal deposits)	Variable	"Steamy" (like looking through a steamy window)	Irregular light reflex
Pupil	Normal, reactive	Sluggishly reactive Sometimes irregular in shape	Partially dilated, oval, nonreactive	Normal, reactive
Iris	Normal	Normal[¶]	Difficult to see because of corneal edema	Shadow of corneal defect may be projected on the iris with penlight
Ocular discharge	Mucopurulent or watery	Watery	Watery	Watery or mucopurulent
Systemic effect	None	Few	Many	None
Prognosis	Self-limited	Poor if untreated	Poor if untreated	Good if not infected

[†]Can be viral, bacterial, or allergic.
[§]Seeing a "rainbow" can be an early symptom during an acute attack.
[¶]Slit-lamp examination revealing cells in anterior chamber is diagnostic.
From Swartz MH: Textbook of Physical Diagnosis, 5th ed. Philadelphia, WB Saunders, 2006.

Chapter 60   Corneal ulceration (keratitis)

DEFINITIONS

- Corneal ulceration refers to the disruption of the corneal surface and/or deeper layers caused by trauma, contact lenses infection (Fig. 60–1), degeneration, or other means.
- Noninfectious keratitis refers to corneal inflammation with no known infectious cause.
- Infectious keratitis is a corneal disease caused by bacterial (Fig. 60–2), viral (Fig. 60–5), fungal (Fig. 60–3), or parasitic organisms (Fig. 60–4).

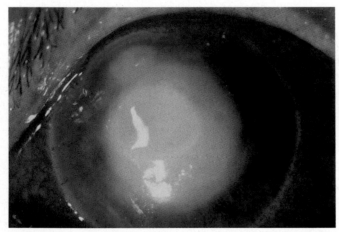

Fig 60–1
Bacterial corneal infection with dense central necrotic ulcer and infiltrate.
(From Yanoff M, Duker JS: Ophthalmology, 2nd ed. St. Louis, Mosby, 2004.)

PHYSICAL FINDINGS AND CLINICAL PRESENTATION

- Localized, well-demarcated, infiltrative lesion with corresponding focal ulcer or oval, yellow-white stromal suppuration with thick mucopurulent exudate and edema; usually red, angry-looking eye with infiltration in surrounding area of cornea
- Eye possibly painful, with conjunctival edema and infection
- Sterile neurotrophic ulcers, with tissue breakdown and no pain

CAUSE

- Complication of contact lens wear, trauma, or diseases such as herpes simplex keratitis (see Fig. 60–5), keratoconjunctivitis sicca; often associated with collagen vascular disease (Fig. 60–6) and severe exophthalmus and thyroid disease
- Viral causes often highly contagious

DIFFERENTIAL DIAGNOSIS

- *Pseudomonas*, (see Fig. 60–2) pneumococcus, other bacterial infection (see Fig. 60–1)—virulent
- *Moraxella*, *Staphylococcus*, alpha-hemolytic *Streptococcus* infection—less virulent
- Herpes simplex infection (see Fig. 60–5) or disease caused by other viruses
- Contact lens ulcers differ.

LABORATORY TESTS

- Microscopic examination and culture of scrapings

TREATMENT

- Warm compresses
- Patching
- Stop contact lens wearing.
- Remove eyelid crusting
- Intense antibiotics and antivirals
- NSAIDs
- Fungal infection: hospitalization and topical application of antifungal agents

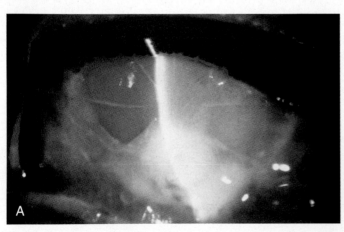

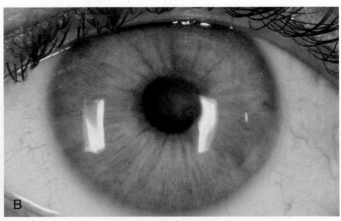

Fig 60–2
Keratitis. **A,** Severe *Pseudomonas* keratitis following radial keratotomy. **B,** Scarring at the interface of a LASIK flap and bed following *Aspergillus* infection.
(From Yanoff M, Duker JS: Ophthalmology, 2nd ed. St. Louis, Mosby, 2004.)

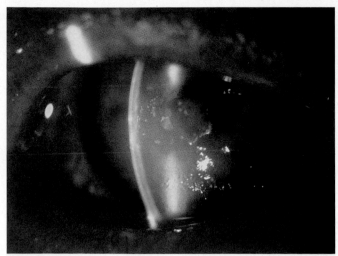

Fig 60–3
Feathery stromal infiltrates typical of fungal keratitis.
(From Yanoff M, Duker JS: Ophthalmology, 2nd ed. St. Louis, Mosby, 2004.)

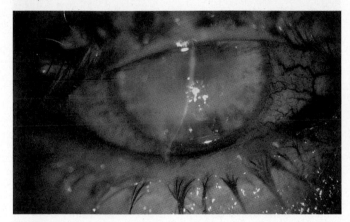

Fig 60–4
Disciform keratitis seen in *Acanthamoeba* corneal infection.
(Courtesy of Dr. Joel Sugar.)

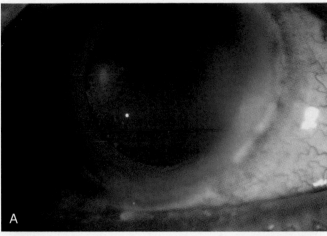

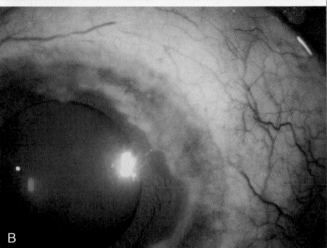

Fig 60–6
Ring corneal ulcer in a patient with rheumatoid arthritis and scleritis.
A, Note the white creamy infiltrate in the cornea, indicating active inflammation, and the lack of a lucid interval from the limbus to the ulcer.
B, Other eye of the same patient. Note the scarring and vascularization from a previous active ring ulcer.
(From Yanoff M, Duker JS: Ophthalmology, 2nd ed. St. Louis, Mosby, 2004.)

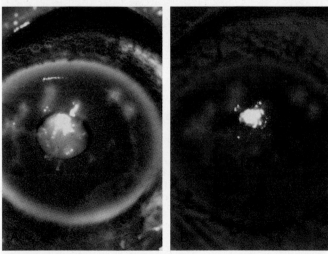

Fig 60–5
Dendritic lesions of recurrent herpes simplex epithelial disease.
A, Unstained. **B,** Stained with fluorescein and rose bengal.
(From Yanoff M, Duker JS: Ophthalmology, 2nd ed. St. Louis, Mosby, 2004.)

Chapter 61   Scleritis

DEFINITION
Scleritis is inflammation of the sclera.

PHYSICAL FINDINGS AND CLINICAL PRESENTATION
- Deep, boring eye pain
- Photophobia
- Tearing
- Conjunctival injection (Fig. 61–1)
- Thinning of the sclera
- Associated medical conditions in 44% of patients
- Infections in 7%; most common infection is herpes zoster (Fig. 61–2)
- Rheumatic disease in 37%; most common rheumatic problem is rheumatoid arthritis
- Systemic vasculitis or inflammatory bowel disease in 10% to 14% (Fig. 61–3). Most patients with systemic disease are diagnosed before the development of scleritis.

CAUSE
- Inflammatory
- Allergic
- Toxic

DIFFERENTIAL DIAGNOSIS
- Most common causes are rheumatoid arthritis and collagen-vascular disease.
- Occasionally, there are allergic, infectious, or traumatic causes.
- Conjunctivitis, iritis, and episcleritis should be considered in the differential diagnosis.

LABORATORY TESTS
- Rheumatoid factor (RF), antinuclear antibody (ANA), erythrocyte sedimentation rate (ESR) may be useful

IMAGING STUDIES
- Usually not necessary; computed tomography (CT) scan of orbit may be useful for select patients for collagen vascular disease or vasculitis
- Fluorescein angiography

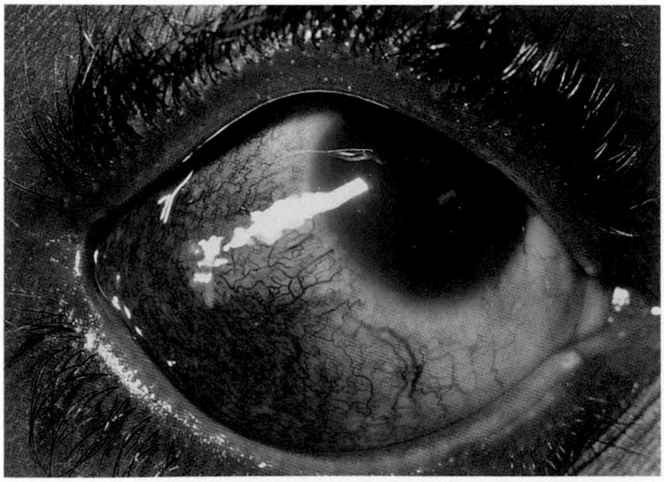

TREATMENT
- Patching
- Bandage lenses
- Surgery if thinning of the sclera is severe to prevent eye rupture
- Immunotherapy (e.g., with steroids, azathioprine)
- Steroids (topical, periocular, and systemic)
- Cycloplegic drops
- NSAIDs (topical and systemic)
- Other immunosuppressive drugs

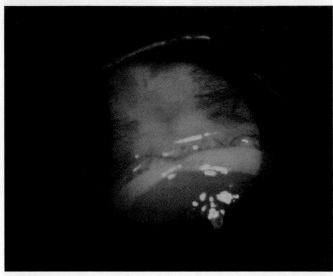

Fig 61–2
Necrotizing anterior scleritis secondary to herpes zoster. The patient underwent extracapsular cataract extraction 2 weeks earlier, which precipitated ophthalmic zoster and led to anterior segment necrosis. (From Yanoff M, Duker JS: Ophthalmology, 2nd ed. St. Louis, Mosby, 2004.)

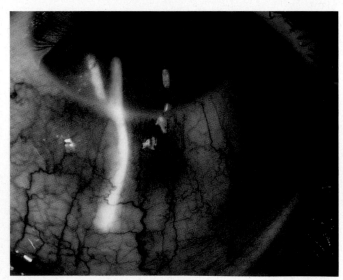

Fig 61–3
Nodular scleritis in patient who has Crohn's disease. (From Yanoff M, Duker JS: Ophthalmology, 2nd ed. St. Louis, Mosby, 2004.)

Fig 61–1
Diffuse scleritis with a violaceous hue caused by deep inflammation. Vessels do not blanch with topical phenylephrine.
(From Yanoff M, Duker JS: Ophthalmology, 2nd ed. St. Louis, Mosby, 2004.)

Chapter 62   Disorders of the conjunctiva and limbus

A. LIMBAL DERMOID

- Solid limbal dermoids are compact, pale yellow growths that typically occur unilaterally at the inferotemporal limbus (Fig. 62–1).
- Surgical excision usually involves shaving the lesion off the cornea and sclera; however, complete excision may require reconstruction.

B. EPITHELIAL INCLUSION CYSTS

- These cysts are filled with clear fluid and lined with nonkeratinized, stratified squamous epithelium (Fig. 62–2).

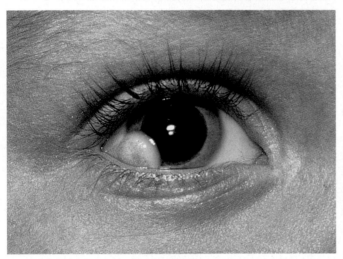

Fig 62–1
Limbal dermoid in a 5-year-old child. This is typically located at the inferotemporal limbus.
(From Yanoff M, Duker JS: Ophthalmology, 2nd ed. St. Louis, Mosby, 2004.)

- Treatment is surgical and done purely for cosmetic reasons because these cysts are asymptomatic.

C. ALLERGIC DERMATOCONJUNCTIVITIS

- Most common form of allergic reaction seen by ophthalmologists. It is a delayed, cell-mediated hypersensitivity reaction most commonly caused by eye drops and cosmetics.
- It begins with severe itching, papillary conjunctivitis and eczematous dermatitis of the periorbital skin (Fig. 62–3).
- Treatment consists of elimination of the antigenic stimulus and application of topical corticosteroids.

D. TOXIC FOLLICULAR CONJUNCTIVITIS

This disorder often follows chronic exposure of the conjunctiva to molluscum contagiosum of the lower eyelid (Fig. 62–4), infection of the eyelashes by phthirus pubis, use of eye cosmetics, and prolonged use of various eye medications. Treatment consists of discontinuation of the allergen and treatment of the infectious process.

E. LIGNEOUS CONJUNCTIVITIS

This rare disorder is characterized by induration of the conjunctiva associated with a membrane or pseudomembrane (Fig. 62–5) related to a plasminogen deficiency and often following infection or trauma of the upper respiratory tract.

The pathophysiology involves increased permeability of the conjunctival blood vessels. Treatment is difficult and consists of a combination of cyclosporine 2% and topical corticosteroids.

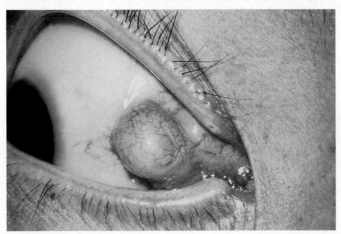

Fig 62–2
Epithelial inclusion cyst. This cyst occurred at the site of a conjunctival incision that accompanied muscle surgery.
(From Yanoff M, Duker JS: Ophthalmology, 2nd ed. St. Louis, Mosby, 2004.)

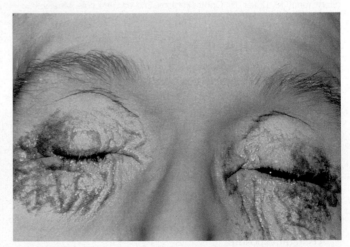

Fig 62–3
Allergic dermatoconjunctivitis. Contact allergy of the eyelids after exposure to neomycin eyedrops. The skin shows a typical eczematous dermatitis.
(From Yanoff M, Duker JS: Ophthalmology, 2nd ed. St. Louis, Mosby, 2004.)

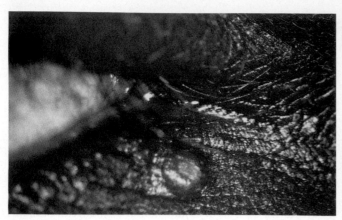

Fig 62–4
Molluscum contagiosum lesion on the lower eyelid. This patient had an accompanying chronic follicular conjunctivitis secondary to the toxic effect of viral proteins from this lesion.
(From Yanoff M, Duker JS: Ophthalmology, 2nd ed. St. Louis, Mosby, 2004.)

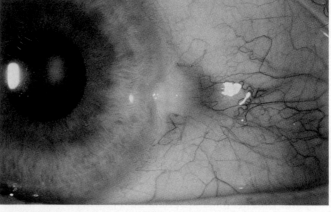

Fig 62–6
Nasal pinguecula. Elevated conjunctival lesion encroaches on a nasal limbus.
(From Yanoff M, Duker JS: Ophthalmology, 2nd ed. St. Louis, Mosby, 2004.)

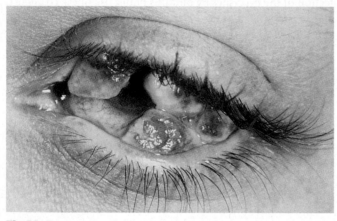

Fig 62–5
Ligneous conjunctivitis. Woody induration of the superior and inferior tarsal conjunctiva.
(From Yanoff M, Duker JS: Ophthalmology, 2nd ed. St. Louis, Mosby, 2004.)

F. PINGUECULA

- Areas of bulbar conjunctival thickening that adjoin the limbus in the palpebral fissure area (Fig. 62–6), usually associated with ultraviolet (UV) light exposure.
- Clinically, they manifest as fatty-appearing, elevated white to yellow in color, horizontally oriented conjunctival lesions (see Fig. 62–6).
- Treatment consists of topical corticosteroids or NSAIDs.

G. PTERYGIUM

- Growth onto the cornea of fibrovascular tissue that is continuous with the conjunctiva and generally associated with UV light exposure
- It may occur both on the nasal and temporal areas (double pterygium; Fig. 62–7).
- Treatment consists of simple excision, conjunctival autografting, and mitomycin C application.

H. SENILE SCLERAL PLAQUES

- Yellow, gray, or black vertebral bands found anterior to the insertion of the medial and lateral rectus muscles in older patients (Fig. 62–8)
- They are asymptomatic and do not require treatment.

I. ARCUS SENILIS (CORNEAL ARCUS)

- Deposition in the corneal periphery of a gray to white or yellow band of opacity. The deposits are made up of extracellular steroid esters of lipoproteins; it is associated with age and dyslipoproteinemia.
- Arcus senilis has a diffuse central border and a sharper peripheral border (Fig. 62–9).
- It is the most common of corneal deposits and can be found in almost 90% of normal men between 70 and 80 years of age.
- In women, a similar pattern is seen, but with a delay of about 10 years.
- Arcus senilis in older patients does not correlate with mortality and no treatment is necessary.

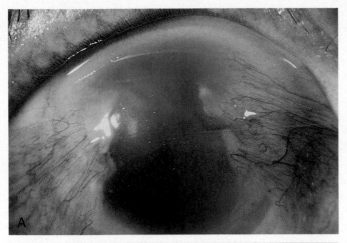

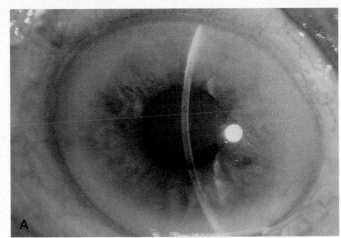

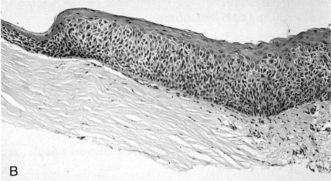

Fig 62–7
Double pterygium. **A,** Note both nasal and temporal pterygia in a 57-year-old farmer. **B,** The invasion of the cornea distinguishes a pterygium from a pinguecula.
(From Yanoff M, Duker JS: Ophthalmology, 2nd ed. St. Louis, Mosby, 2004.)

Fig 62–9
Arcus senilis, **A,** Corneal arcus in an older man. **B,** Histologic section shows that the lipid is concentrated in the anterior and posterior stroma as two red triangles, apex to apex, with the bases being Bowman's and Descemet's membranes, both of which are infiltrated heavily by fat (red staining), as is the sclera.
(From Yanoff M, Fine BS: Ocular Pathology, 5th ed. St. Louis, Mosby, 2002.)

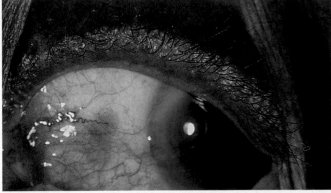

Fig 62–8
Senile scleral plaque. Calcium deposition appears as a gray scleral plaque under the medial rectus muscle insertion.
(From Yanoff M, Duker JS: Ophthalmology, 2nd ed. St. Louis, Mosby, 2004.)

Chapter 63 Strabismus

DEFINITION
Strabismus is a condition of the eyes in which the visual axes of the eyes are not straight in the primary position or in which the eyes do not follow each other in the different positions of gaze. Esotropias represent the most common forms of strasbismus and include the following:

- Congenital esotropia: inward deviation of the visual axes, with an onset before the age of 6 months (Fig. 63–1). Amblyopia occurs in 25% to 40% of patients, but the majority "cross-fixate"—use the right eye to fix across the nose to view objects to the left, and vice versa (Fig. 63–2).
- Accommodative esotropia: inward deviation of the visual axes caused by high hyperopia or high accommodative convergence-to-accomodation ratio

Exotropia is an acquired or, rarely, congenital outward deviation of the visual axis of one or both eyes, which may be constant, intermittent (Fig. 63–3), or latent.

Paralytic strasbismus is strasbismus resulting from partial or complete paralysis of the third (Fig. 63–4), fourth (Fig. 63–5), or sixth cranial nerve (Fig. 63–6).

PHYSICAL FINDINGS AND CLINICAL PRESENTATION
- Conjugate gaze loss in both eyes with the eyes focusing independently
- Amblyopia

CAUSE
- Many cases are congenital.
- Accomodative cases occur later with focusing.
- Rarely, there is neurologic disease or severe refractive errors.
- Hereditary form is common, with hyperopia (farsightedness) most common.

DIFFERENTIAL DIAGNOSIS
- Measuring eye position and movement
- Vision testing
- Refractive errors
- CNS tumors
- Orbital tumors
- Brain and CNS dysfunction

WORKUP
- Eye examination
- Visual field
- Magnetic resonance imaging (MRI) to rule out tumors when it develops later, with no apparent cause

LABORATORY TESTS
- Generally not needed

IMAGING STUDIES
- Necessary only if other neurologic findings are found

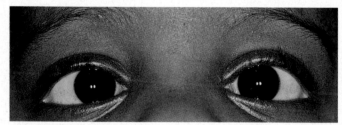

Fig 63–1
Congenital esotropia. The child is fixing with her left eye; note the decentered light reflex in the right eye.
(From Yanoff M, Duker JS: Ophthalmology, 2nd ed. St. Louis, Mosby, 2004.)

CONGENITAL ESOTROPIA AND CROSS-FIXATION

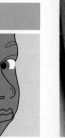

Fig 63–2
Congenital esotropia and cross-fixation. The infant uses the right eye to view left, and vice versa. Doll's head maneuver shows full abduction.
(From Yanoff M, Duker JS: Ophthalmology, 2nd ed. St. Louis, Mosby, 2004.)

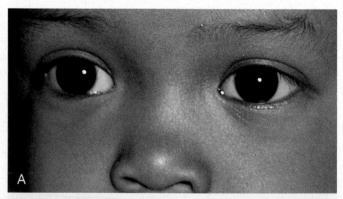

A

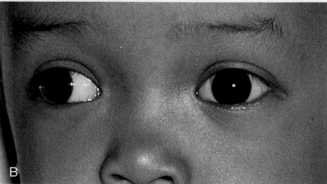

B

Fig 63–3
Intermittent exotropia. **A,** Eyes straight. **B,** A few moments later, the exotropia has become manifest.
(Courtesy of Howard Eggers.)

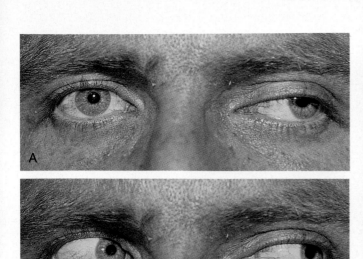

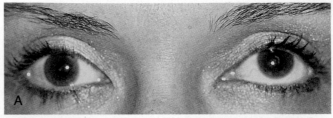

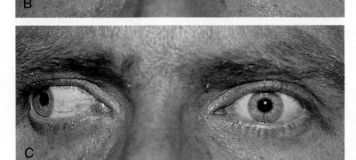

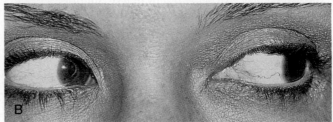

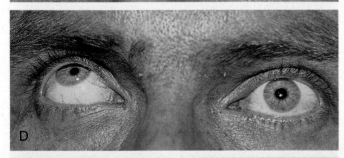

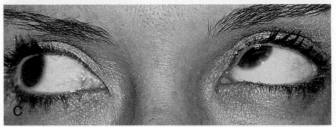

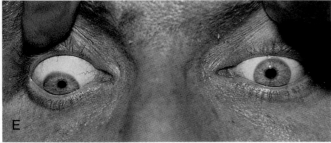

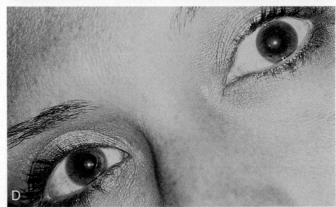

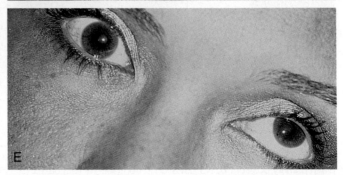

Fig 63–4

Adult who has a partial left third nerve palsy. **A,** Primary gaze showing slightly larger pupil, mild ptosis, left exotropia, and left hypotropia. **B,** Normal left gaze. **C,** No adduction of the left eye on right gaze. **D,** Poor elevation. **E,** Poor depression.

(From Yanoff M, Duker JS: Ophthalmology, 2nd ed. St. Louis, Mosby, 2004.)

Fig 63–5

Young woman who has idiopathic (presumed congenital) left fourth nerve palsy. **A,** Primary position left hypertropia from loss of the depressor effect of the paretic left superior oblique muscle. **B,** Normal motility in left gaze, away from the fields of action of the paretic left superior oblique muscle. **C,** Compensatory overaction of the antagonist left inferior oblique muscle in its field of action in right gaze. **D,** No vertical deviation on contralateral head tilt, when reflex excyclotorsion of the affected left eye is accomplished by the unaffected inferior rectus and inferior oblique muscles. **E,** Large left hypertropia on ipsilateral head tilt, when reflex cyclotorsion recruits the superior rectus muscle and the paretic superior oblique muscle, and the vertical effect of the unaffected superior rectus muscle cannot be neutralized by the paretic superior oblique muscle.

(From Yanoff M, Duker JS: Ophthalmology, 2nd ed. St. Louis, Mosby, 2004.)

TREATMENT

- Glasses (Fig. 63–7)
- Patching: best done between 3 and 7 years of age; vision most improved by 3 to 6 months of age
- Prisms
- Atropine: same as patching most of the time, although patching may give better results in resistant cases
- The earlier the condition is treated, the more likely it is that the child will have normal vision in both eyes; surgical intervention in select patients
- After age 7 years, visual loss is usually permanent from amblyopia.

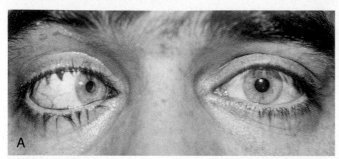

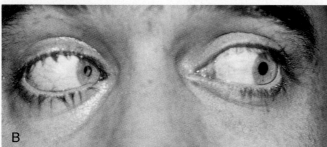

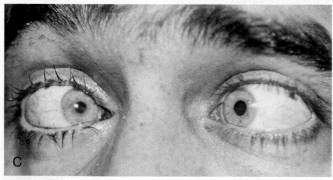

Fig 63–6
A 33-year-old man who has a right sixth nerve palsy. **A,** Right esotropia in primary position. **B,** No deviation in contralateral (left) gaze. **C,** Large esotropia in ipsilateral (right) gaze; the affected right eye cannot even get to midline position.
(From Yanoff M, Duker JS: Ophthalmology, 2nd ed. St. Louis, Mosby, 2004.)

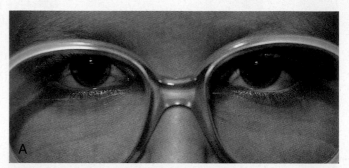

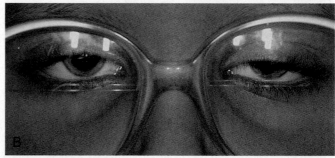

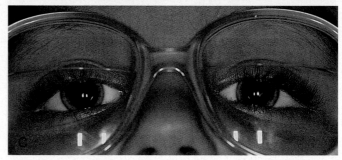

Fig 63–7
Hyperopic child with right esotropia. **A,** Esotropia controlled at distance fixation through distance (top) segment of bifocals. **B,** Esotropia near-fixation through distance segment of bifocals. **C,** Aligned eyes at near-fixation through near (bottom) segment of bifocals.
(From Yanoff M, Duker JS: Ophthalmology, 2nd ed. St. Louis, Mosby, 2004.)

Chapter 64 Amblyopia

DEFINITION
Amblyopia is a developmental defect of spatial visual processing that occurs in the central visual pathway of the eyes.

PHYSICAL FINDINGS AND CLINICAL PRESENTATION
- Amblyopia presents most dramatically as loss of visual acuity in one or, rarely, both eyes.
- Certain forms of amblyopia also present with diminished contrast sensitivity, vernier acuity (Fig. 64–1), grating acuity, and spatial localization of objects (Fig. 64–2)
- Decreased vision using best refraction in the presence of normal corneal, lens, retinal, and optic nerve appearance

CAUSE
- Visual deprivation
- Strabismus
- Occlusion with patching
- Refractive error organic lesions in the nervous system
- Toxins

DIFFERENTIAL DIAGNOSIS
- CNS disease (brainstem)
- Optic nerve disorders
- Corneal or other eye diseases

TREATMENT
- Glasses or prisms to align eyes with minor deviations and improve vision.
- Patches (Fig. 64–3), mechanical versus atropine: patching and atropine both work. Atropine 1% is used daily for 6 months; patching is used 6 hours/day for 6 months. Patching may be more effective; 50% obtain best vision improvement by 16 weeks.
- Removal of the cause of the amblyopia if possible
- Surgery to align the eyes or remove obstruction to vision

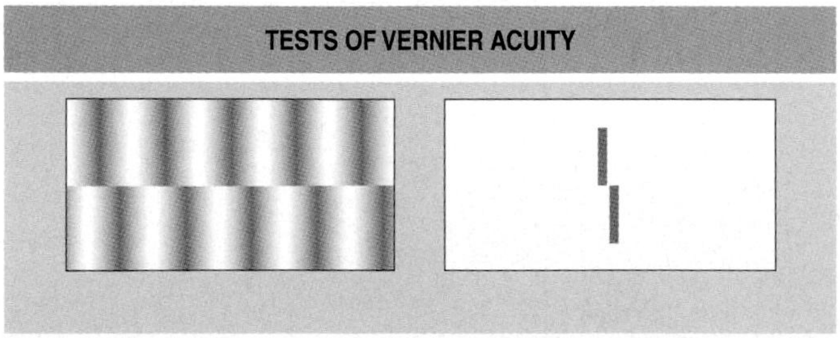

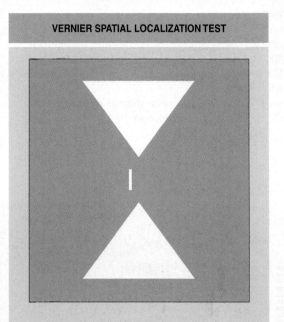

VERNIER SPATIAL LOCALIZATION TEST

Fig 64–2
Vernier spatial localization test. The goal of this test is to align the small vertical line between the triangle points.
(From Yanoff M, Duker JS: Ophthalmology, 2nd ed. St. Louis, Mosby, 2004.)

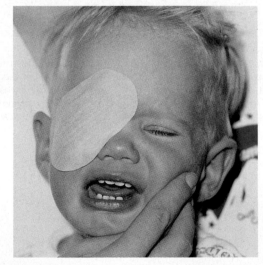

Fig 64–3
Application of a patch to the sound eye of a child. This reduces vision in proportion to the degree of amblyopia. It frequently results in crying or efforts to remove the patch, which may be used to diagnose poor vision in one eye.
(From Yanoff M, Duker JS: Ophthalmology, 2nd ed. St. Louis, Mosby, 2004.)

TESTS OF VERNIER ACUITY

Fig 64–1
Tests of vernier acuity. The vernier resolution task is to detect the offset in the grating *(left)* or line *(right)*. The smallest detectable offset (threshold) is expressed as an angle at the viewing distance used. Under optimal conditions, vernier acuity may be as good as 3 to 6 arc seconds.
(From Yanoff M, Duker JS: Ophthalmology, 2nd ed. St. Louis, Mosby, 2004.)

Chapter 65   Entropion

DEFINITION
This is an inward rotation of the tarsus and eyelid margin so that the eyelashes abrade the cornea and eyeball (Fig. 65–1).

PHYSICAL FINDINGS AND CLINICAL PRESENTATION
- The patient may experience a foreign body sensation in the affected eye.
- Secondary blepharospasm may be present.
- Ocular discharge is common.

DIFFERENTIAL DIAGNOSIS
- Epiblepharon: a horizontal fold of redundant pretarsal skin and orbicularis muscle extends beyond the eyelid margin and compresses the eyelashes against the globe (Fig. 65–2). This condition is usually bilateral, prevalent in Asian populations, and commonly involves the lower lid.
- Distichiasis: accessory row of cilia arising from the meibomian gland orifices occurring in an autosomal dominant inheritance pattern
- Trichiasis: acquired condition in which the cilia arise from their normal position and are misdirected toward the ocular surface
- Eyelid retraction: the retracted eyelid is pulled toward the orbital rim with the eyelashes obscured by the resulting fold of eyelid skin

TREATMENT
- Surgical correction

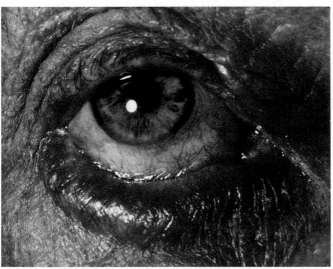

Fig 65–1
Right lower eyelid entropion. Note the inward rotation of the tarsal plate about the horizontal axis and the resultant contact between the mucocutaneous junction and ocular surface. This patient may have multiple anatomic defects contributing to the eyelid presentation.
(From Yanoff M, Duker JS: Ophthalmology, 2nd ed. St. Louis, Mosby, 2004.)

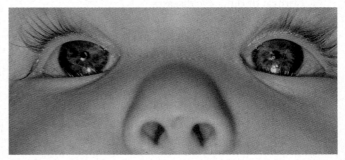

Fig 65–2
Epiblepharon. Note the bilaterality, loss of the lower eyelid skin crease, and overriding skin fold. The normal orientation of the tarsal plate distinguishes this condition from entropion.
(From Yanoff M, Duker JS: Ophthalmology, 2nd ed. St. Louis, Mosby, 2004.)

| Chapter 66 | **Ectropion** |

DEFINITION
This is an abnormal eversion of the eyelid margin away from the eye (Fig. 66–1).

PHYSICAL FINDINGS AND CLINICAL PRESENTATION
- The eyelid margin and lash are turned away from the cornea.
- Photophobia, decreased vision, ocular surface pain, and conjunctival infection may occur.
- Corneal exposure results in foreign body sensation, corneal dryness, and occasional ulceration.

TREATMENT
- Surgical correction

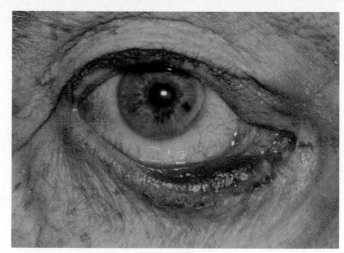

Fig 66–1
Ectropion.
(From Swartz MH: Textbook of Physical Diagnosis, 5th ed. Philadelphia, WB Saunders, 2006.)

Chapter 67   Blepharospasm

DEFINITION
This is a variable, progressive, bilateral focal dystonia characterized by contraction of the orbicularis oculi muscles, which causes spasmodic involuntary eyelid closure (Fig. 67–1) in the absence of any other ocular or adnexal causes.

PHYSICAL FINDINGS AND CLINICAL PRESENTATION
- Bilateral involuntary spasmodic closure of the eyelids
- Symptoms exacerbated by stress, fatigue, bright lights, interpersonal interactions
- Fluctuations of the symptoms marked by transient remissions and exacerbations
- Spasms absent when asleep
- Spasms improve with relaxation
- Decrease in tear production

DIFFERENTIAL DIAGNOSIS
The diagnosis of blepharospasm is one of exclusion. For this reason, a careful examination must be conducted to rule out the various causes of secondary blepharospasm. Table 67–1 describes the differential diagnosis of this disorder.

TREATMENT
- Myectomy: surgical intervention consisting of extirpation of the orbicularis, procerus, and corrugator muscles
- Pharmacologic agents: benzodiazepines
- Chemodenervation with botulinum toxin type A is the initial treatment of choice for blepharospasm. Sites of injection are illustrated in Figure 67–2.

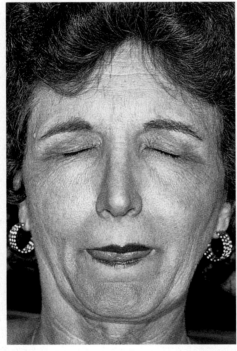

Fig 67–1
Involuntary spasms of the orbicularis and procerus muscles in essential blepharospasm. These spasms are associated with oromandibular dystonia involving the middle and lower face.
(From Yanoff M, Duker JS: Ophthalmology, 2nd ed. St. Louis, Mosby, 2004.)

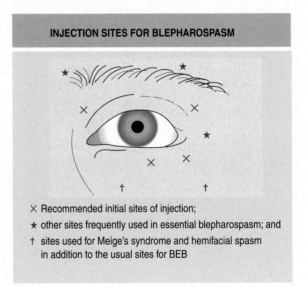

INJECTION SITES FOR BLEPHAROSPASM

✕ Recommended initial sites of injection;

★ other sites frequently used in essential blepharospasm; and

† sites used for Meige's syndrome and hemifacial spasm in addition to the usual sites for BEB

Fig 67–2
Sites of injection for botulinum toxin in the treatment of benign essential blepharospasm (BEB).
(From Yanoff M, Duker JS: Ophthalmology, 2nd ed. St. Louis, Mosby, 2004.)

TABLE 67–1 Differential diagnosis of blepharospasm

Differential Diagnosis	Gender	Age (yr)	Side	Voluntary Control	Present in Sleep	Clinical Characteristics	Diagnostic Causes	Tests
Essential blepharospasm	F > M, 2-3:1	>50	Bilateral	No	No	Isolated spasms of the orbicularis oculi	1. Uncertain 2. Basal group ganglia 3. Brainstem	None in typical cases
Meige's syndrome	F > M, 2-3:1	>50	Bilateral	No	No	Blepharospasm plus midfacial spasm	Same as for benign essential blepharospasm (BEB)	Same as for BEB
Hemifacial spasm	F > M, 3:2	>45	Unilateral, left > right	No	Yes	Tonic-clonic spasms in the distribution of the seventh cranial nerve	Usually a vascular compression of seventh cranial nerve root	CT or MRI; must rule out posterior fossa tumor
Apraxia of eyelid opening; involuntary levator inhibition	—	—	—	No	—	1. Passive involuntary closure of eyelids; raised eyebrows; relaxed eyelids 2. Occasionally seen with essential blepharospasm	Unknown; seen in extrapyramidal disease such as Parkinson's, Huntington's, and Wilson's diseases, or with supranuclear palsy, Shy-Drager syndrome	Orbicularis oculi muscle; EMG inactive; total inhibition of levator muscle
Facial myokymia	F = M	Any	Unilateral	No	Yes	Rapid undulating flicking muscles	1. Uncertain 2. Multiple sclerosis, intramedullary tumor 3. Caffeine, stress	EMG
Facial tic	F = M	Childhood	Unilateral or bilateral	Yes	Yes	Stereotypic movements, brief repetitive, suppressible	Tourette's syndrome	None
Facial seizure	F = M	Any age	Unilateral	No	—	Movements occurring with head; questionable eye deviation	Focal cortical lesion	CT, MRI
Facial synkinesis	Equally affected	Any	Unilateral	No	Yes	1. Unilateral contracture with weakness 2. Gustatory lacrimation	Prior history of facial paralysis	EMG evidence of synkinesis. fibrillation potential, reduced motor units

BEB, benign essential blepharospasm; CT, computed tomography; EMG, electromyography; MRI, magnetic resonance imaging.
From Yanoff M, Duker JS: Ophthalmology, 2nd ed. St. Louis, Mosby, 2004.

Chapter 68   Benign eyelid lesions

A. SQUAMOUS PAPILLOMA

- Most common benign lesion of the eyelid
- Also known as fibroepithelial polyp, acrochordon, or skin tag
- These lesions may be single or multiple and commonly involve the eyelid margin (Fig. 68–1).
- Treatment: simple excision at the base of the lesion

B. CUTANEOUS HORN

- Projection of packed keratin (Fig. 68–2)
- This is not a distinct pathologic entity but may develop from a variety of underlying lesions, including seborrheic keratosis, actinic keratosis, verruca vulgaris, basal cell or squamous cell carcinoma, and other epithelial tumors..
- Treatment: because definitive therapy is dependent on the underlying cause, biopsy of the cutaneous horn is required to obtain a histologic diagnosis.

C. SEBORRHEIC KERATOSIS

- These lesions are also known as senile verruca because they usually affect older adults.
- Their color varies from tan to brown (Fig. 68–3), and the surface is frequently papillomatous.
- Seborrheic keratoses are not considered premalignant lesions but a rapid increase in the size and number of these lesions (Leser-Trélat sign) may occur in patients with occult malignancy.

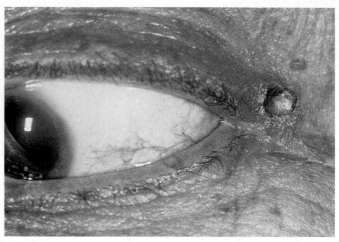

Fig 68–2
Cutaneous horn. Note the projection of packed keratin that arises from the skin in the region of the left lateral canthus.
(From Yanoff M, Duker JS: Ophthalmology, 2nd ed. St. Louis, Mosby, 2004.)

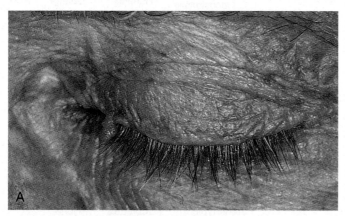

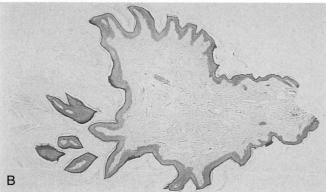

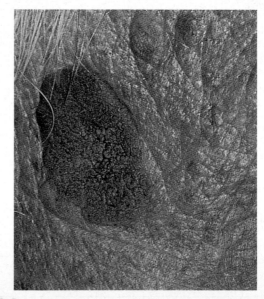

Fig 68–1
Squamous papilloma. **A,** Typical flesh-colored, pedunculated skin tag involving the left upper eyelid. **B,** Fibroepithelial papilloma consists of a narrow-based (to the right) papilloma with fibrovascular core and finger-like projections covered by acanthotic, hyperkeratotic epithelium.
(**B** from Yanoff M, Fine BS: Ocular Pathology, 2nd ed. St. Louis, Mosby, 2002.)

Fig 68–3
Seborrheic keratosis. Brown stuck-on plaque, typical of seborrheic keratosis.
(From Yanoff M, Duker JS: Ophthalmology, 2nd ed. St. Louis, Mosby, 2004.)

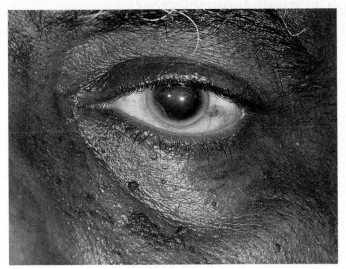

Fig 68–4
Dermatosis papulosa nigra. Multiple pigmented papules involving the malar region.
(From Yanoff M, Duker JS: Ophthalmology, 2nd ed. St. Louis, Mosby, 2004.)

- A variant of seborrheic keratosis, that shares a similar histopathologic appearance, is *dermatosis papulosa nigra*, which occurs primarily in dark-skinned individuals. These lesions usually appear on the cheeks and periorbital region as multiple pigmented papules (Fig. 68–4).
- Treatment: simple excision for biopsy, cosmesis, or to prevent irritation

D. KERATOACANTHOMA

- Keratoacanthoma most commonly appears as a solitary, rapidly growing nodule on sun-exposed areas of middle-aged and older individuals.
- The nodule is usually umbilicated, with a distinctive central crater filled with a keratin plug (Fig. 68–5).
- The lesion develops over weeks and typically undergoes spontaneous involution within 6 months to leave an atrophic scar.
- Lesions that occur on the eyelids may produce mechanical abnormalities, such as ectropion or ptosis.
- Treatment: complete excision is recommended because an invasive variant exists, with the potential for perineural and intramuscular spread. Both radiotherapy and intralesional fluorouracil have been advocated.

E. EPIDERMAL INCLUSION CYST

- Slow-growing, round, firm lesions of the dermis or subcutaneous tissue.
- Eyelid lesions are usually solitary, mobile, and less than 1 cm in diameter.
- They may be congenital in origin or may arise from traumatic implantation of surface epidermis (Fig. 68–6),
- These cysts may become infected or may rupture, producing a surrounding foreign body granulomatous reaction.
- Treatment: complete excision

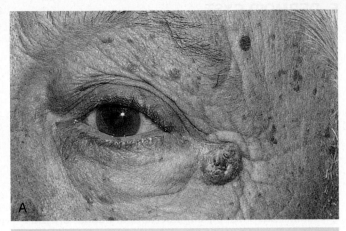

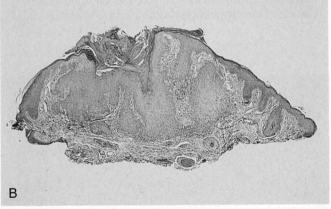

Fig 68–5
Keratoacanthoma. **A,** Lesion shows typical clinical appearance; history was also typical. **B,** The lesion that can be seen above the surface epithelium has a cup-shaped configuration and a central keratin core. The base of the acantholic epithelium is blunted (rather than invasive) at the junction of the dermis.
(From Yanoff M, Duker JS: Ophthalmology, 2nd ed. St. Louis, Mosby, 2004.)

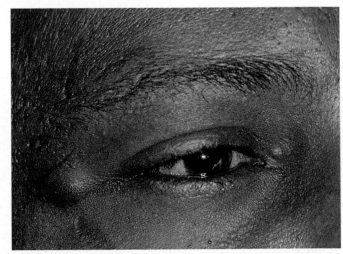

Fig 68–6
Epidermal inclusion cyst. This lesion appeared as a slow-growing cystic lesion in a region of previous penetrating trauma.
(From Yanoff M, Duker JS: Ophthalmology, 2nd ed. St. Louis, Mosby, 2004.)

279

F. DERMOID CYST

- Firm, slow-growing, nontender masses, most commonly in the lateral upper eyelid and brow region (Fig. 68–7)
- They presumably occur secondary to entrapment of skin along embryonic closure lines.
- Treatment: complete surgical excision

G. MILIA

- Milia form as multiple, firm, white lesions that range from 1 to 4 mm in diameter.
- They usually appear on the face and most commonly affect the eyelids, nose, and malar region (Fig. 68–8).
- Lesions may occur spontaneously or secondarily caused by trauma, radiotherapy, skin infection, or bullous diseases.
- Treatment: simple excision, electrodessication of the surface, or puncture and expression of the contents

H. ECCRINE HIDROCYSTOMA

- These lesions, also known as sweat gland cysts, appear as small nodules on the eyelids. The overlying skin is shiny and smooth, and the cyst usually is translucent and fluid-filled (Fig. 68–9).
- Treatment: complete excision

I. APOCRINE HIDROCYSTOMA

- Solitary, translucent cyst on the face, sometimes at the eyelid margin
- They are usually less than 1 cm in diameter and are filled with clear or milky fluid, with shiny, smooth overlying skin (Fig. 68–10).
- Treatment: complete excision

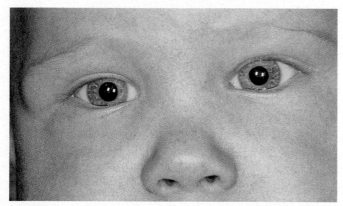

Fig 68–7
Dermoid cyst. Cystic subcutaneous lesion in the right upper lid and brow region, attached to the underlying frontozygomatic suture. (From Yanoff M, Duker JS: Ophthalmology, 2nd ed. St. Louis, Mosby, 2004.)

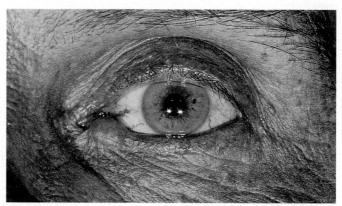

Fig 68–9
Eccrine hidrocystoma. Cystic lesion involving the left lower eyelid margin. The lesion was filled with translucent fluid. (From Yanoff M, Duker JS: Ophthalmology, 2nd ed. St. Louis, Mosby, 2004.)

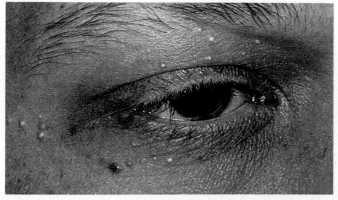

Fig 68–8
Milia. Multiple small white lesions that affect the upper and lower eyelids. (From Yanoff M, Duker JS: Ophthalmology, 2nd ed. St. Louis, Mosby, 2004.)

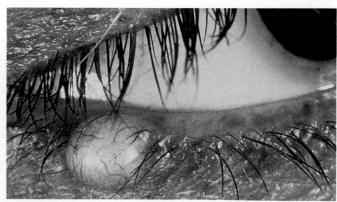

Fig 68–10
Apocrine hidrocystoma. Cystic lesion, filled with milky fluid, involving the right lower eyelid margin. (From Yanoff M, Duker JS: Ophthalmology, 2nd ed. St. Louis, Mosby, 2004.)

J. CYLINDROMA

- Dome-shaped, skin-colored, or pinkish-red dermal nodule (Fig. 68–11)
- Solitary lesions usually occur in adulthood in the head or neck region and may appear similar to a pilar or epidermal inclusion cyst.
- Treatment: surgical excision

K. CAPILLARY HEMANGIOMA

- Most common orbital tumor found in children, occurring in 1% to 2% of infants
- Approximately one third are visible at birth, with the remainder manifesting by 6 months of age.
- The classic lesion (strawberry nevus) appears as a red, raised, nodular mass that blanches with pressure (Fig. 68–12).
- The most common ocular complication is amblyopia, which may result from occlusion of the visual axis caused by eyelid involvement, or from anisometropia caused by induced astigmatism.
- Treatment: because most capillary hemangiomas undergo spontaneous regression to some extent, treatment generally is reserved for patients who have specific ocular, dermatologic, or systemic indications for intervention. Treatment modalities include intralesional corticosteroid injection, systemic corticosteroids, radiotherapy, laser therapy, systemic interferon, and surgery.

L. NEVUS FLAMMEUS

- This lesion is also known as a port-wine stain and presents as a flat, purple, vascular lesion, usually unilateral and in the distribution of the trigeminal nerve (Fig. 68–13).
- It is congenital and does not undergo spontaneous regression.
- Treatment: management is primarily with cosmetics. Tunable dye laser therapy also may be used to improve the appearance of the lesion.

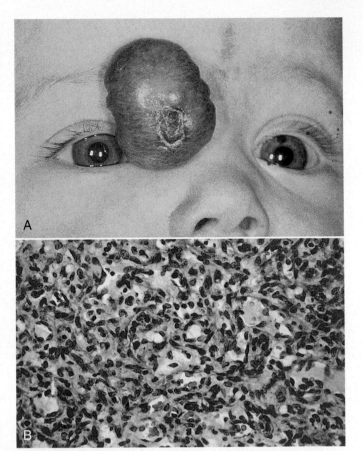

Fig 68–12
Capillary hemangioma. **A,** Superficial raised red mass involving the right upper eyelid and medial canthal region. **B,** High magnification of endothelial cells.
(**B** from Yanoff M, Fine BS: Ocular Pathology, 5th ed. St. Louis, Mosby, 2002.)

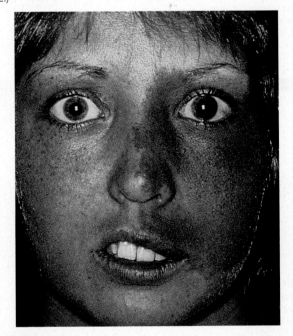

Fig 68–13
Nevus flammeus. Flat, purple, vascular lesion involving the skin of the face.
(From Yanoff M, Duker JS: Ophthalmology, 2nd ed. St. Louis, Mosby, 2004.)

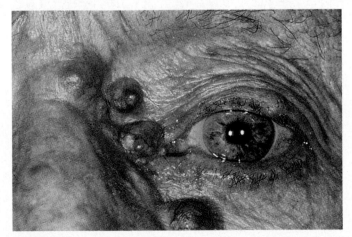

Fig 68–11
Cylindroma. Multiple pinkish-red dermal nodules involving the eyelids, forehead, nose, and malar region.
(From Yanoff M, Duker JS: Ophthalmology, 2nd ed. St. Louis, Mosby, 2004.)

M. NEUROFIBROMA

- Soft, fleshy, often pedunculated masses (Fig. 68–14)
- Plexiform neurofibroma is characteristic of type 1 neurofibromatosis and presents as a diffuse infiltration of the eyelid and orbit. The upper eyelid is usually ptotic, with an S-shaped curvature (Fig. 68–15). On palpation, it feels like a "bag of worms."
- Treatment: management depends on the site and extent of the disease. Isolated cutaneous lesions, unrelated to neurofibromatosis, may be excised surgically. However, because of the infiltrative nature of these lesions, complete excision is usually impossible and recurrences are common.

N. PYOGENIC GRANULOMA

- Most common acquired vascular lesion to involve the eyelids
- It usually occurs after trauma or surgery as a fast-growing, fleshy, red to pink mass, which readily bleeds with minor contact (Fig. 68–16). Lesions may also develop in association with inflammatory processes, including chalazia.
- Treatment: surgical excision at the base of the lesion

O. XANTHELASMA

- Most common cutaneous xanthoma, typically appearing in middle-aged and older adults as soft yellow plaques on the medial aspect of the eyelids (Fig. 68–17)
- Hyperlipidemia is present in more than 50% of patients with xanthelasma.
- Treatment: surgical excision, carbon dioxide laser ablation, topical trichloroacetic acid. Recurrence is common.

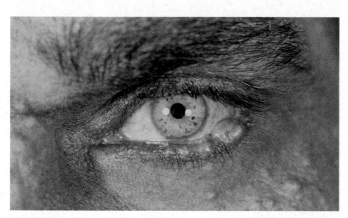

Fig 68–14
Neurofibroma. Note the fleshy mass on the eyelid of this patient, with disseminated cutaneous neurofibromas.
(From Yanoff M, Duker JS: Ophthalmology, 2nd ed. St. Louis, Mosby, 2004.)

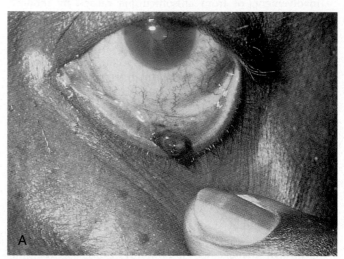

A

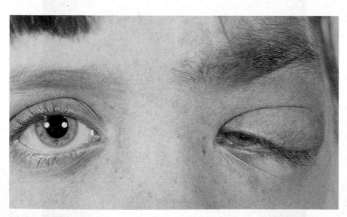

Fig 68–15
Plexiform neurofibroma. Note the ptosis and typical S-shaped curvature of the upper lid.
(From Yanoff M, Duker JS: Ophthalmology, 2nd ed. St. Louis, Mosby, 2004.)

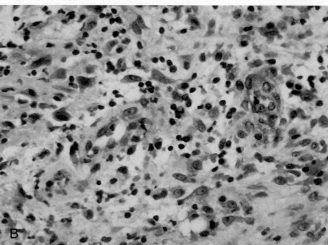

B

Fig 68–16
Pyogenic granuloma. **A,** Red mass arising from the palpebral conjunctiva and protruding over the eyelid margin. This lesion developed in association with a chalazion. **B,** Vascularized tissue (granulation tissue) that consists of inflammatory cells (polymorphonuclear lymphocytes and fibroblasts) and the endothelial cells of budding capillaries.
(From Yanoff M, Duker JS: Ophthalmology, 2nd ed. St. Louis, Mosby, 2004.)

P. FRECKLES

- These skin lesions, also known as ephelides, arise from epidermal melanocytes.
- They appear as small (less than 3-mm diameter) tan to brown macules in sun-exposed areas (Fig. 68–18).
- Treatment: no treatment is necessary but sunscreen may help prevent further darkening of the lesions.

Q. MELANOCYTIC NEVI

- Common lesions, especially in fair-complexioned individuals, occurring frequently on the eyelid skin and eyelid margin
- The histologic type may be junctional, compound, or intradermal (Fig. 68–19).
- Diagnosis is based on typical clinical appearance. Malignant transformation may occur rarely, generally in the junctional or compound stages.
- Treatment: suspicious-looking lesions that demonstrate irregular growth or appearance should be excised; otherwise, removal is not required unless desired for cosmesis or relief of mechanical irritation.

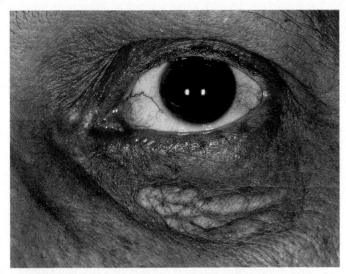

Fig 68–17
Xanthelasma. Multiple soft yellow plaques involving the lower eyelid. Lipid-laden foam cells are seen in the dermis and tend to cluster around blood vessels.
(From Yanoff M, Duker JS: Ophthalmology, 2nd ed. St. Louis, Mosby, 2004.)

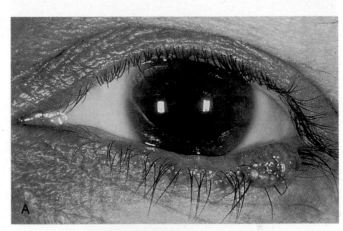

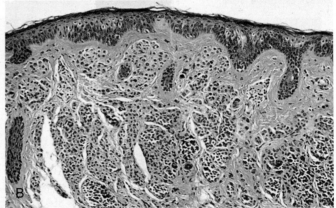

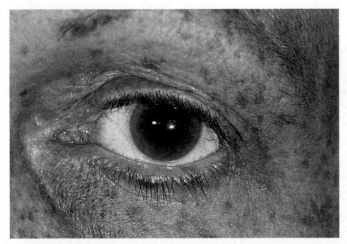

Fig 68–18
Freckles. These are multiple tan-brown small macules, involving the skin of sun-exposed areas.
(From Yanoff M, Duker JS: Ophthalmology, 2nd ed. St. Louis, Mosby, 2004.)

Fig 68–19
Intradermal nevus. **A,** Elevated papillomatous lesion, amelanotic in color, involving the eyelid margin. **B,** Nests of nevus cells fill the dermis except for a narrow area just under the epithelium. The nuclei of the nevus cells become smaller, thinner, or spindle-shaped and darker as they go deeper into the dermis (i.e., they show normal polarity).
(**B** from Yanoff M, Fine BS: Ocular Pathology, 5th ed. St. Louis, Mosby, 2002.)

R. CONGENITAL MELANOCYTIC NEVI

- These lesions are derived from nevocytes and occur in approximately 1% of newborns.
- The border is often irregular and the surface may be covered with hair. Congenital nevi that appear in a symmetrical fashion on adjacent portions of the upper and lower eyelids (Fig. 68–20) are referred to as *kissing nevi*. They are formed as a result of melanocytic migration to the lids before separation of the embryonic eyelids.
- Treatment: suspicious-looking lesions should be sampled for biopsy. Large lesions should be excised. The management of small lesions is controversial; some advocate excision of all congenital nevi.

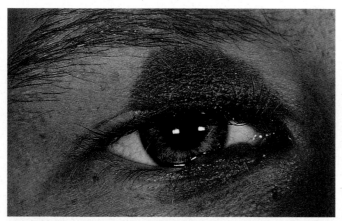

Fig 68–20
Kissing nevus. Congenital melanocytic nevus in a symmetrical fashion on adjacent portions of the upper and lower eyelids.
(From Yanoff M, Duker JS: Ophthalmology, 2nd ed. St. Louis, Mosby, 2004.)

S. CHALAZION

- Focal inflammatory lesion of the eyelid that results from obstruction of a sebaceous gland
- A chelazion may occur acutely with eyelid edema and erythema and evolve into a nodule that may point anteriorly to the skin surface or, more commonly, through the posterior surface of the lid.
- The lesion may drain spontaneously or persist as a chronic nodule. Lesions may appear insidiously as firm, painless nodules (Fig. 68–21). Large lesions on the upper lid may produce astigmatism.
- Chalazia often occurs in patients with blepharitis and rosacea.
- Treatment: variable according to the stage of the lesion. Acute lesions are treated with hot compresses to encourage localization and drainage. Chronic chelazia may be treated using intralesional corticosteroid injection or surgical drainage. Small chelazia, which may resolve spontaneously, can be removed with incision and curettage.

T. HORDOLEUM (STYE)

- Acute purulent inflammation of the eyelid. An external hordoleum (stye) results from infection of the follicle of a cilium and the adjacent glands.
- The lesion typically causes pain, edema, and erythema of the eyelid, which becomes localized and often drains anteriorly through the skin near the lash line (see Fig. 68–21).
- An anterior hordoleum occurs because of obstruction and infection of a meibomian gland. Initially, a painful edema and erythema localize as an inflammatory abscess on the posterior conjunctival surface.
- In both external and internal lesions, cellulitis of the surrounding soft tissue may develop.
- Diagnosis is based on the clinical appearance and culture, with *Staphylococcus aureus* most frequently isolated.

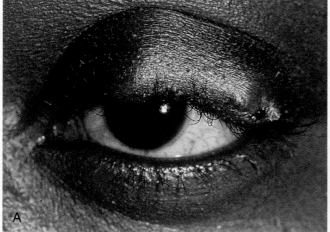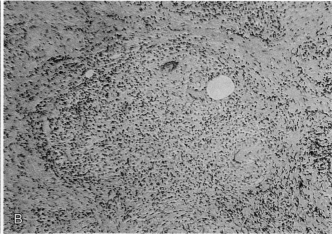

Fig 68–21
Chalazion and external hordeolum. **A,** The medial lesion of the upper eyelid appeared as a firm, painless nodule, consistent with a chalazion. The lateral lesion caused pain and eyelid erythema, subsequently becoming more localized, with drainage of purulent material through the skin surface. **B,** A clear circular area with rounded epithelioid cells and multinucleated giant cells can be seen. In processing the tissue, lipid is dissolved out, leaving a clear space.
(From Yanoff M, Duker JS: Ophthalmology, 2nd ed. St. Louis, Mosby, 2004.)

- Treatment: hot compresses, topical antibiotics. Rarely, incision and drainage are necessary.

U. MOLLUSCUM CONTAGIOUSUM

- Viral skin disease caused by a large DNA pox virus. Infection usually arises from direct contact or fomites in children and by a sexually transmitted route in adults.
- The typical lesion appears as a raised, shiny, white to pink nodule with a central umbilication filled with cheesy material.
- Patient with AIDS may present with multiple lesions on each eyelid (Fig. 68–22).
- Treatment: simple excision or incision and curettage, cryosurgery, electrodesiccation. Management is more difficult in AIDS patients because of extensive involvement and recurrences. Hyperfocal cryotherapy has been effective in these patients.

V. VERRUCA VULGARIS

- Cutaneous wart caused by epidermal infection with the human papilloma virus, which is spread by direct contact and fomites
- Lesions along the lid margin may induce a mild papillary conjunctivitis caused by shedding of virus particles.
- Treatment: observation is recommended if no ocular complications occur, because most lesions are self-limited. Treatment, if necessary, consists of cryotherapy or complete excision.

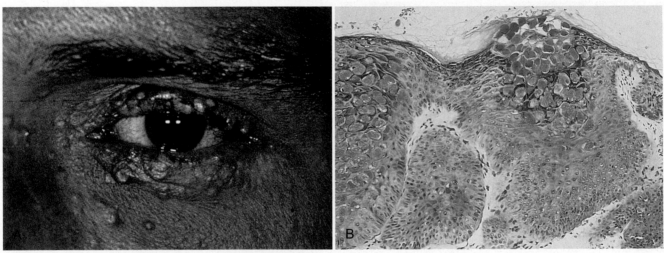

Fig 68–22
Molluscum contagiosum. **A,** Multiple raised nodules, with areas of confluent lesions, affecting the eyelids of a patient with AIDS. **B,** Intracytoplasmic, small, eosinophilic molluscum bodies occur in the deep layers of epidermis. The bodies become enormous and basophilic near the surface. The bodies may be shed into the tear film, where they cause a secondary, irritative, follicular conjunctivitis.
(From Yanoff M, Duker JS: Ophthalmology, 2nd ed. St. Louis, Mosby, 2004.)

Chapter 69   Eyelid malignancies

A. BASAL CELL CARCINOMA

- Most common malignant tumor of the eyelids
- Over 95% occur in whites over age 40; average age at diagnosis is 60 years
- 60% affect the lower eyelid.
- They can be classified into five basic types: nodular-ulcerative, pigmented, morphea or sclerosing, superficial, and fibroepithelioma. The nodular type (Fig. 69–1) is the most common lesion. It has the classic appearance of a pink or pearly papule or nodule with overlying telengiectatic vessels. As the nodule grows in size, central ulceration may occur surrounded by a rolled border. This appearance is often described as a rodent ulcer.
- Treatment: surgical excision

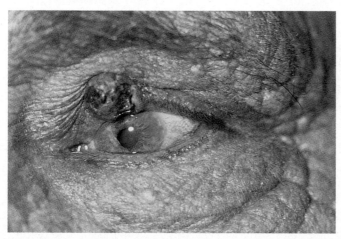

Fig 69–1
Nodular basal cell carcinoma (BCC) of the eyelid. A firm, pink-colored left upper eyelid BCC is seen with raised border, superficial telangiectatic vessels, and characteristic central ulceration. These lesions are more commonly seen on the lower eyelid.
(Courtesy of Dr. Morton Smith.)

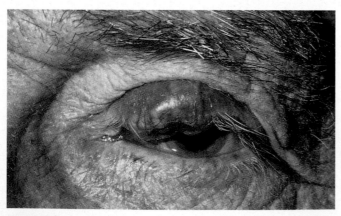

Fig 69–2
Sebaceous cell carcinoma of the eyelid. A large, firm, irregular nodule with yellowish coloration of the left upper eyelid is shown. Associated inflammation, telangiectatic vessels, and loss of cilia are observed.
(Courtesy of Dr. Morton Smith.)

B. SQUAMOUS CELL CARCINOMA

- Typically presents as an erythematous, indurated, hyperkeratotic plaque or nodule with irregular margins
- It is much less common than basal cell carcinoma but carries a much greater potential for metastatic spread.
- Treatment: wide local surgical excision

C. SEBACEOUS GLAND CARCINOMA

- Highly malignant neoplasm, accounting for 1% to 5% of all eyelid cancers
- It may present as a plaquelike thickening of the the tarsal plate with destruction of the meimobian gland orifices and tumor invasion of the eyelash follicles, leading to loss of eyelashes (Fig. 69–2).
- Treatment: wide surgical excision. Radiation therapy may be considered as an adjunct to local surgery.

D. MALIGNANT MELANOMA

- Cutaneous malignant melanoma of the eyelid accounts for 1% of all eyelid malignancies.
- Lentigo maligna melanoma and its precursor, lentigo maligna (melanotic freckle of Hutchinson), present as a flat macule with irregular borders and variable pigmentation.
- It typically occurs in sun-exposed areas and commonly involves the lower eyelid (Fig. 69–3)
- Treatment: wide surgical excision

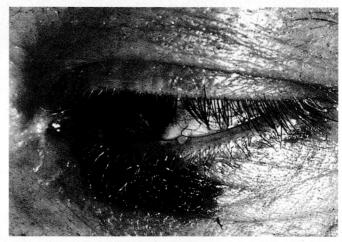

Fig 69–3
Lentigo maligna melanoma (Hutchinson freckle): clinical appearance of acquired pigmented lesion of the left lower lid.
(From Yanoff M, Duker JS: Ophthalmology, 2nd ed. St. Louis, Mosby, 2004.)

E. KAPOSI SARCOMA

- Ophthalmic involvement with Kaposi sarcoma occurs in 30% of AIDS patients.
- It usually presents as highly vascular, purple or red nodules on the cutaneous aspects of the eyelids or on the conjunctiva (Fig. 69–4).
- Treatment: cryotherapy, irradiation, surgical excision, and intralesional chemotherapy. Therapy may reduce or clear the visible lesions, but is not curative.

F. MERKEL CELL TUMOR (CUTANEOUS NEUROENDOCRINE CARCINOMA)

- Rare tumor clinically presenting on the eyelid as a solitary, vascularized, nontender, red or violaceous nodule (Fig. 69–5)
- Treatment: wide surgical excision. The possible roles of chemotherapy and radiotherapy are unclear.

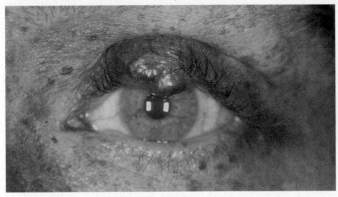

Fig 69–4
Kaposi sarcoma of the eyelid margin. Shown is a solitary, vascular reddish purple nodule of the left upper eyelid.
(Courtesy of Dr. Morton Smith.)

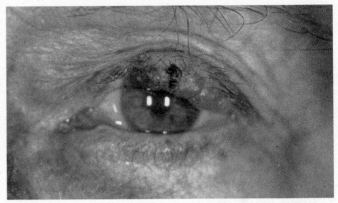

Fig 69–5
Merkel cell tumor of the eyelid. Shown is a large, firm, reddish nodule that resembles an angiomatous lesion of the left upper eyelid. Telangiectatic vessels appear on the surface of the nodule. These lesions are typically more violaceous in coloration.
(Courtesy of Dr. Morton Smith.)

Chapter 70   Retinitis pigmentosa

DEFINITION

Retinitis pigmentosa is a generalized retinal pigment degeneration associated with a variety of inheritance patterns, resulting in decreased vision. A simple recessive pattern is most severe. It may be associated with some rare neurologic syndromes.

PHYSICAL FINDINGS AND CLINICAL PRESENTATION

- Deposition of retinal pigment in midperiphery and centrally in the retina, with a pale optic nerve and narrowing of blood vessels (Fig. 70–1)
- Possible cataracts and macular edema
- Decreases in night vision and peripheral vision

CAUSE

- Usually hereditary

DIFFERENTIAL DIAGNOSIS

- Syphilis
- Old inflammatory scars
- Old hemorrhage
- Diabetes
- Toxic retinopathies (phenothiazines, chloroquine)

LABORATORY TESTS

- Usually not necessary
- Venereal Disease Research Laboratory (VDRL), glucose (select patients)

IMAGING STUDIES

- Usually not necessary

TREATMENT

- No proved effective therapy
- Sometimes vitamin E or vitamin A may be helpful.
- Rate of decline of vision for different groups cannot be accurately determined; decline rates are fastest in patients with mutations.

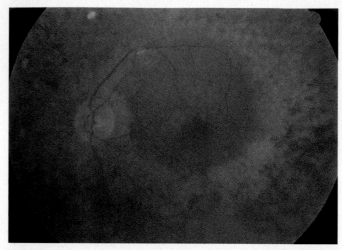

Fig 70–1

"Typical" retinitis pigmentosa changes in a 73-year-old woman who had a pro-23–His rhodopsin autosomal dominant mutation. Visible are extensive, intraneural, retinal bonespicule pigmentation, severely constricted retinal arteries, waxy pallor of the disc, and extensive retinal pigment epithelium atrophy in the macula and midperiphery (which reveals underlying choroidal vessels). Her visual acuity was 20/50 (6/15), but she made no errors on Ishihara color testing; her fields were severely constricted to 17-degree tunnel vision with the Goldmann V4e target.
(From Yanoff M, Duker JS: Ophthalmology, 2nd ed. St. Louis, Mosby, 2004.)

Chapter 71 **Retinoblastoma**

DEFINITION

Retinoblastoma is an inherited, highly malignant, congenital neoplasm arising from the neural layers of the retina.

PHYSICAL FINDINGS AND CLINICAL PRESENTATION

- White pupils (Fig. 71–1)
- White elevated retinal masses, dilated, tortuous, retinal blood vessels (Fig. 71–2)
- Strabismus
- Glaucoma
- Uveitis
- Vitreous masses and opacity

CAUSE

- Genetic

DIFFERENTIAL DIAGNOSIS

- Strabismus (see Fig. 63–1)
- Retinal detachment (see Fig. 74–2)
- Uveitis (see Fig. 75–2)
- Glaucoma (see Fig. 76–3)
- Cataract (see Fig. 58–2)

IMAGING STUDIES

- MRI: may show calcifications in the retina
- Ultrasonography: good delineation of mass

TREATMENT

Treatment depends on location and stage of tumor when diagnosed.

- Enucleation of single eye
- External beam radiation
- Chemotherapy with local vitreous injections
- Radioactive plaque brachytherapy and cryotherapy
- Surgical enucleation of the eye
- Radiation and chemotherapy

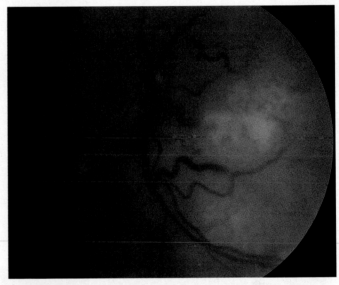

Fig 71–2
Typical appearance of intraretinal retinoblastoma. Opaque, yellow-white macular tumor fed and drained by dilated, tortuous retinal blood vessels.
(From Yanoff M, Duker JS: Ophthalmology, 2nd ed. St. Louis, Mosby, 2004.)

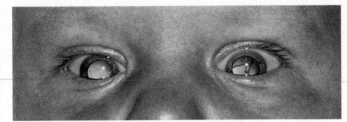

Fig 71–1
Bilateral leukokoria as a result of retinoblastoma. Note the white pupillary reflection in each eye.
(From Yanoff M, Duker JS: Ophthalmology, 2nd ed. St. Louis, Mosby, 2004.)

Chapter 72	**Amaurosis fugax**

DEFINITION

Amaurosis fugax (AF) is a temporary loss of monocular vision caused by transient retinal ischemia or occlusion (Fig. 72–1).

PHYSICAL FINDINGS AND CLINICAL PRESENTATION

- Onset is sudden, typically lasting seconds to minutes, and often accompanied by scotomas, such as a shade or curtain being pulled over the front of the eye (usually downward).
- Vision loss can be complete or quadrantic.
- There are usually no physical findings.
- Acute stage: cholesterol emboli (Fig. 72–2) may be seen in retinal artery (Hollenhorst plaque)—carotid bruits or other evidence of generalized atherosclerosis.
- If embolus is cardiac in origin, atrial fibrillation is often present.

CAUSE

- Usually embolic from the internal carotid artery or the heart
- May also be caused by vasculitis, such as giant cell arteritis (GCA), or hyperviscosity syndromes, such as sickle cell disease, that cause ischemia in the vascular territory of the ophthalmic artery

DIFFERENTIAL DIAGNOSIS

The differential diagnosis of transient monocular visual loss includes the following:

- Retinal migraine: in contrast to amaurosis fugax, the onset of visual loss develops more slowly, usually over a period of 15 to 20 minutes.
- Transient visual obscurations (TVOs) occur in the setting of papilledema; intermittent rises in intracranial pressure briefly compromise optic disc perfusion and cause transient visual loss lasting 1 to 2 seconds; the episodes may be binocular. If the visual loss persists at the time of evaluation (i.e., vision has not yet recovered), then the differential diagnosis should be broadened to include
  1. Anterior ischemic optic neuropathy—arteritic (typically GCA) or nonarteritic
  2. Central retinal vein occlusion

WORKUP

- Workup should focus on embolic sources but GCA should always be considered.
- Careful examination of retina; embolus may be visible and confirm the diagnosis.
- Auscultation of arteries for carotid bruits.
- Examination of all pulses and for temporal artery tenderness
- Inquire about symptoms of GCA (scalp tenderness, jaw claudication).
- Examine for signs of hemispheric stroke resulting from intracranial aneurysm (ICA) (e.g., contralateral limb and face weakness or sensory loss, aphasia).

LABORATORY TESTS

- Complete blood count (CBC), with ESR and C-reactive protein (CRP)
- Serum chemistries, including lipid profile
- Electrocardiography (ECG).
- Hypercoagulable workup is discretionary based on younger age and history.

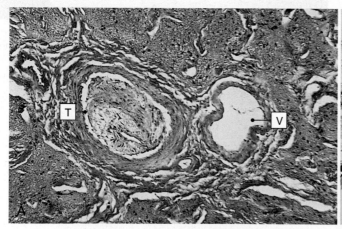 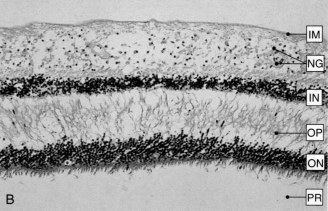

Fig 72–1

Central retinal artery occlusion. **A**, Trichrome-stained section shows an organized thrombus (T) that occludes the central retinal artery within the optic nerve (V, vein). **B**, Histologic section at the early stage shows edema of the inner neural retinal layers and ganglion cell nuclei pyknosis. The patient had a cherry-red spot in the fovea at time of enucleation. IM, internal limiting membrane; IN, inner nuclear layer; NG, swollen nerve fiber and ganglion layers; ON, outer nuclear layer; OP, outer plexiform layer; PR, photoreceptors.
(From Yanoff M, Fine BS: Ocular Pathology, 5th ed. St. Louis, Mosby, 2002.)

IMAGING STUDIES

- Carotid Doppler followed by MR or CT angiography as indicated
- Transthoracic echocardiography (TTE) is indicated to screen for embolization in patients with evidence of heart disease and in patients without an evident source for their transient neurologic deficit. Transesophageal echocardiography (TEE) is more sensitive for detecting cardiac sources of embolization (e.g., ventricular mural thrombus, atrial appendage, patent foramen ovale, aortic arch).
- Consider MRI of the brain with diffusion-weighted imaging to look for infarcts.

TREATMENT

- Give aspirin if cause is presumed embolic.
- If GCA is suspected, start prednisone and refer for temporal artery biopsy within 48 hours.
- Reduce risks by carotid endarterectomy or stent if stenosis more than 70%.
- Control hypertension and manage vascular risk factors.
- Antiplatelet therapy
- Consider initiation of statin therapy.

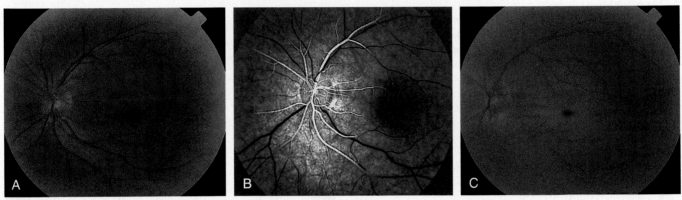

Fig 72–2

Left eye of a healthy 37-year-old man. The patient had a 3-hour history of visual loss and a visual acuity of 20/60 (6/18). **A,** Retinal whitening is very subtle and the retinal vessels appear normal. **B,** Fluorescein angiography reveals abnormal arterial filling with a leading edge of dye that confirms central retinal artery obstruction. **C,** The same eye 24 hours later. Despite intravenous urokinase, visual acuity dropped to hand movements, and intense retinal whitening with a cherry-red spot is present. Note the interruption in the blood column of the retinal arteries.
(From Yanoff M, Duker JS: Ophthalmology, 2nd ed. St. Louis, Mosby, 2004.)

Chapter 73 | Macular degeneration

DEFINITION

Macular degeneration refers to a group of diseases associated with loss of central vision and damage to the macula. Degenerative changes occur in the pigment, neural, and vascular layers of the macula. Dry macular degeneration is usually ischemic in cause, and wet macular degeneration is associated with leakage of fluid from blood vessels, usually referred to as age-related macular degeneration (ARMD).

PHYSICAL FINDINGS AND CLINICAL PRESENTATION

- Decreased central vision
- Macular hemorrhage, pigmentation, edema, atrophy
- The most common abnormality seen in ARMD is the presence of drusen, or yellowish deposits deep to the retina (Fig. 73–1); this may be early in the course of the disease.

CAUSE

- Subretinal neovascular membrane early
- Pigmentary and vascular changes with exudate, edema, and scar tissue development
- Early in the course of disease, possible subretinal neovascularization
- Dry-type atrophy of macular pigment epithelium

DIFFERENTIAL DIAGNOSIS

- Diabetic retinopathy (Fig. 73–2)
- Hypertension (Fig. 73–3)
- Histoplasmosis
- Trauma with scar

LABORATORY TESTS

- Evaluate for diabetes and other metabolic problems, as well as vascular diseases.

IMAGING STUDIES

- Optical coherence tomography (OCT)
- Fluorescein angiography

TREATMENT

- Intravitreous steroids, photodynamic treatment (PDT) with laser
- Intravitreous injections of pegaptanib (Macugen), an antivascular endothelial growth factor, have been reported as effective therapy for slowing vision loss in neovascular ARMD. Pegaptanib is administered once every 6 weeks by intravitreous injection into one eye.
- Antioxidants and zinc may slow the progression of ARMD.

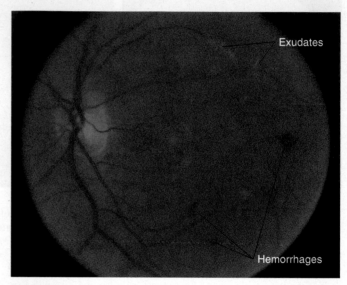

Fig 73–2
Nonproliferative diabetic retinopathy.
(From Swartz MH: Textbook of Physical Diagnosis, 5th ed. Philadelphia, WB Saunders, 2006.)

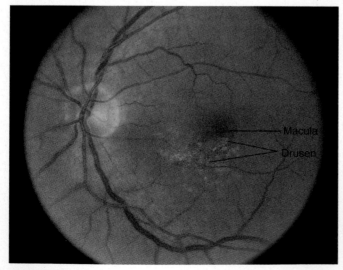

Fig 73–1
Age-related macular degeneration.
(From Swartz MH: Textbook of Physical Diagnosis, 5th ed. Philadelphia, WB Saunders, 2006.)

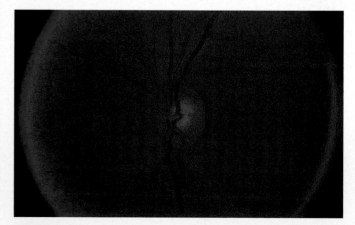

Fig 73–3
Mild to moderate chronic hypertensive retinopathy. Note the color change in the retinal arterioles and the early arteriovenous crossing changes.
(From Yanoff M, Duker JS: Ophthalmology, 2nd ed. St. Louis, Mosby, 2004.)

Chapter 74 Retinal detachment

DEFINITION
Retinal detachment is a retinal separation in which the inner or neural layer of the retina separates from the pigment epithelial layer. It results from numerous causes.

PHYSICAL FINDINGS AND CLINICAL PRESENTATION
- Elevation of retina and vessels associated with tears in the retina, with fluid and/or hemorrhage beneath the retina and changes in the vitreous
- Complaints of flashing lights and floaters.

CAUSE
- Trauma
- Tears in the retina (Fig. 74–1)
- Uveitis
- Fluid accumulation beneath the retina
- Tumors
- Scleritis
- Inflammatory disease
- Diabetes
- Collagen-vascular disease
- Vascular abnormalities

DIFFERENTIAL DIAGNOSIS
- Hemorrhage (see Fig. 59–8)
- Tumors (see Fig. 71–1)

IMAGING STUDIES
- B-scan of the eye
- Evaluation of visual field defect (Fig. 74–2)

TREATMENT
- Early surgery to repair the detachment
- Treatment of the underlying disorder

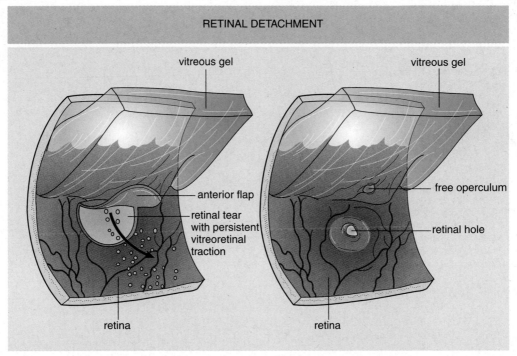

RETINAL DETACHMENT

Fig 74–1
Retinal detachment. Retinal tears are caused by vitreoretinal traction. Persistent traction frequently causes extensive retinal detachment (*left*). If the traction results in a break that is not associated with persistent vitreoretinal traction (*right*), the tear is a retinal hole and detachment is unlikely. (From Yanoff M, Duker JS: Ophthalmology, 2nd ed. St. Louis, Mosby, 2004.)

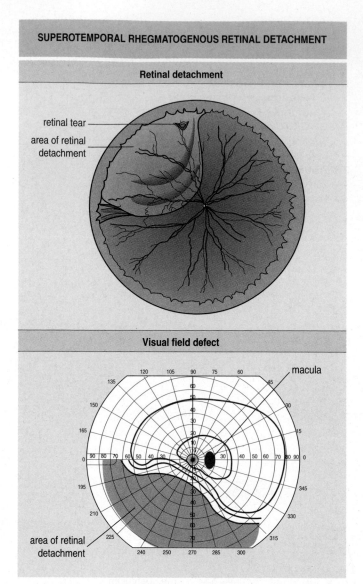

SUPEROTEMPORAL RHEGMATOGENOUS RETINAL DETACHMENT

Retinal detachment

retinal tear

area of retinal detachment

Visual field defect

macula

area of retinal detachment

Fig 74-2

Superotemporal rhegmatogenous retinal detachment. The neural retina is elevated in the area of detachment and the macula remains uninvolved. A visual field defect associated with retinal detachment shows that peripheral vision is lost inferonasally, corresponding to the area of detachment. The visual defect is an inverted image of the retinal detachment.

(From Yanoff M, Duker JS: Ophthalmology, 2nd ed. St. Louis, Mosby, 2004.)

Chapter 75   Uveitis

DEFINITION

Uveitis is an inflammation of the uveal tract, including the iris, ciliary body, and choroid. It may also involve other closed structures, such as the sclera, retina, and vitreous humor.

PHYSICAL FINDINGS AND CLINICAL PRESENTATION

- Symptoms of uveitis depend on the site of involvement and whether the process is acute or insidious.
  - Acute anterior uveitis: pain and photophobia. Vision may not be affected initially.
  - Posterior uveitis: floaters, hazy vision. Involvement of the retina may produce blind spots or flashing lights.
  - Insidious anterior uveitis: symptoms may not be present until scarring cataracts and loss of vision occur.
- Photophobia
- Blurred visual acuity
- Irregular pupil
- Hazy cornea
- Abnormal cells (Fig. 75–1) and flare in anterior chamber or vitreous humor
- Retinal hemorrhage, vascular sheathing
- Conjunctival injection
- Ciliary flush
- Keratitic precipitates (precipitates on the cornea; Fig. 75–2)
- Hazy vitreous
- Retinal inflammation
- Iris nodules (Fig. 75–3)
- Glaucoma
- Rheumatoid arthritis
- Scleritis
- Systemic symptoms related to cause

CAUSE

- Infections: herpes simplex virus, cytomegalovirus, toxoplasmosis, tuberculosis, syphilis, HIV
- Systemic disorders: sarcoidosis, Behçet's syndrome, HLA-B27–associated diseases (e.g., ankylosing spondylitis, reactive arthritis), inflammatory bowel disease, juvenile idiopathic arthritis
- Idiopathic
- A comprehensive history (Box 75–1) is essential for determining the cause of uveitis.

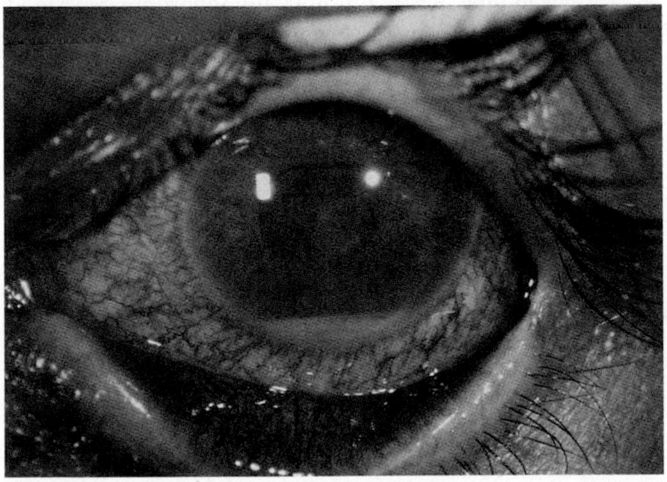

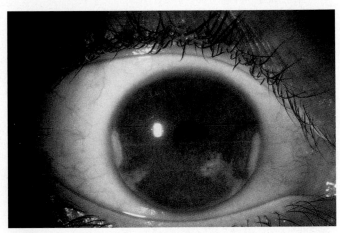

Fig 75–2
Slit-lamp photograph of the right eye of a patient with chronic anterior uveitis related to juvenile idiopathic arthritis. As is typical of this condition, the eye appears uninflamed. Band keratopathy is present.
(From Yanoff M, Duker JS: Ophthalmology, 2nd ed. St. Louis, Mosby, 2004.)

Fig 75–1
HLA-B27–related acute anterior uveitis. This severe case of anterior uveitis demonstrates fibrin clot formation and hypopyon in the anterior chamber.
(From Yanoff M, Duker JS: Ophthalmology, 2nd ed. St. Louis, Mosby, 2004.)

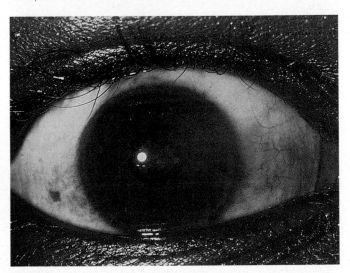

Fig 75–3
Typical appearance of chronic sarcoid uveitis. Note the multiple Busacca iris nodules and posterior synechiae.
(From Yanoff M, Duker JS: Ophthalmology, 2nd ed. St. Louis, Mosby, 2004.)

Box 75–1 History taking in uveitis*

Present illness

Onset, course, symptoms, laterality, treatment

Past ocular history

Previous episodes, past therapy and response, previous or antecedent ocular trauma or surgery

Medical history

Systemic illnesses (especially sarcoidosis, juvenile rheumatoid arthritis, AIDS, tuberculosis, syphilis), prodromal syndromes, medications (especially immunosuppressive agents)

Social history

Dietary habits, sexual history, intravenous drug abuse

Demographic data

Age, race, gender

Geographic history

Birthplace, previous locations (e.g., Mississippi River valley for ocular histoplasmosis), foreign travel

Family history

Medical illnesses, contagious diseases (e.g., tuberculosis), maternal infections, history of uveitis

Review of systems

General—fever, weight loss, malaise, night sweats
Rheumatologic—arthralgias, lower back pain, joint stiffness
Dermatologic—rashes, sores, alopecia, vitiligo, poliosis, tick/insect bites
Neurologic—tinnitus, headache, meningism, paresthesias, weakness/paralysis
Respiratory—shortness of breath, cough, sputum production
Gastrointestinal (GI)—diarrhea, bloody stools, oral aphthous ulcers
Genitourinary (GU)—dysuria, discharge, genital ulcers, balanitis

---

*A comprehensive history and review of systems is critical for the evaluation of the uveitis patient.
From Yanoff M, Duker JS: Ophthalmology, 2nd ed. St. Louis, Mosby, 2004.

DIFFERENTIAL DIAGNOSIS

- Glaucoma (see Fig. 77–2)
- Conjunctivitis (see Fig. 59–1)
- Retinal detachment
- Retinopathy (see Fig. 73–2)
- Keratitis (see Fig. 60–2)
- Scleritis (see Fig. 61–1)
- Episcleritis
- Masquerading syndromes: lymphoma, uveal melanoma, metastases (breast, lung, renal), leukemia, retinitis pigmentosa (see Fig. 70–1), retinoblastoma (see Fig. 71–2)

LABORATORY TESTS

- CBC
- Laboratory tests for specific inflammatory causes (e.g., ANA, ESR, VDRL, HLA-B27, purified protein derivative [PPD], Lyme titer)
- Visual field testing; slit-lamp examination, indirect ophthalmoscopy

IMAGING STUDIES

- Chest x-ray in suspected sarcoidosis, tuberculosis (TB), histoplasmosis
- Sacroiliac x-ray in suspected ankylosing spondylitis

TREATMENT

- Treat the underlying disease. Treatment is often multidisciplinary (ophthalmologist, internist, rheumatologist, infectious disease [ID] specialist).
- Treat photophobia and local pain.
- Acute general medical therapy
  - Corticosteroids are the mainstay of therapy for noninfectious causes.
  - Antibiotics for bacterial infections and antiviral agents, when viral infection is suspected, should be started to prevent retinal damage.
- Systemic steroids, if appropriate for the underlying disease. Systemic corticosteroid therapy is generally reserved for patients with systemic disorders and those with bilateral disease refractory to local medication or those with major ocular disability or retinitis.
- Antimetabolites, when indicated. Immunosuppressive medications used in steroid-dependent or refractory uveitis include methotrexate, sulfasalazine, azathioprine, cyclosporine, and tacrolimus. These medications can have significant toxicity and should be prescribed only by physicians experienced with their use.

Chapter 76   Glaucoma, chronic open angle

DEFINITION

Chronic open-angle glaucoma refers to optic nerve damage often associated with elevated intraocular pressure; it is a chronic, slowly progressive, usually bilateral disorder associated with visual loss, eye pain, and optic nerve damage. It is now thought to be a primary disease of the optic nerve, with high pressure a high risk factor for glaucoma. Table 76–1 compares characteristics of glaucoma.

PHYSICAL FINDINGS AND CLINICAL PRESENTATION

- High intraocular pressures and large optic nerve cup. Figure 76–1 shows glaucoma cupping. Optic cup asymmetry in glaucoma is illustrated in Figure 76–2.
- Cornea thickens faster in vision loss
- Abnormal visual fields
- Open-angle gonioscopy
- Red eye
- Restricted vision and field

CAUSE

- Uncertain hereditary tendency. Congenital glaucoma is defined as glaucoma that arises in children younger than 2 years. Primary infantile glaucoma (Fig. 76–3) is the result of isolated abnormal development of the anterior chamber angle structures
- Topical steroids

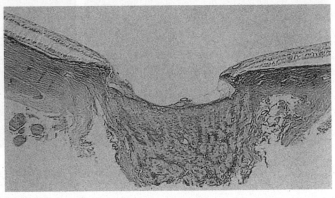

Fig 76–1

Glaucoma cupping. The optic nerve head is deeply cupped. Atrophy of the optic nerve is determined by comparing the diameter of the optic nerve at its internal surface and posteriorly, where it should double in size. Here it is the same size because of a loss of axons and myelin, which also causes an increase in size of the subarachnoid space and a proliferation of glial cells, resulting in an increased cellularity of the optic nerve.

(From Yanoff M, Duker JS: Ophthalmology, 2nd ed. St. Louis, Mosby, 2004.)

TABLE 76–1 Characteristics of glaucoma

Parameter	Primary Open-Angle Glaucoma	Narrow-Angle Glaucoma
Occurrence	85% of all glaucoma cases	15% of all glaucoma cases
Cause	Unclear*	Closed angle prevents aqueous drainage
Age at onset	Variable	50–85 yr
Anterior chamber	Usually normal	Shallow
Chamber angle	Normal	Narrow
Symptoms	Usually none	Headache
	Decreased vision, late	Halos around lights
		Sudden onset of severe eye pain
		Vomiting during attack
Cupping of disc	Progressive if not treated	After untreated attack(s)
Visual fields	Peripheral fields involved early	Involvement is late sign
	Central involvement a very late sign	
Ocular pressure	Progressively higher if not medically controlled	Early: detected with provocative tests only
	Late: high	
Other signs		Fixed, partially dilated pupil
		Conjunctival injection
		"Steamy" cornea†
Treatment	Medical laser surgery	Surgical
Prognosis	Good if recognized early	Good
	Very dependent on patient compliance	

*Thought to be a defect in the trabecular network ultrastructure.
†Like looking through a steamy window.
From Swartz MH: Textbook of Physical Diagnosis, 5th ed. Philadelphia, WB Saunders, 2006.

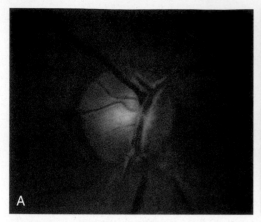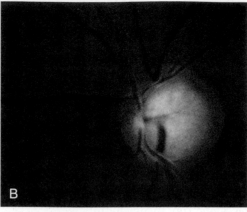

Fig 76–2
Optic cup asymmetry in glaucoma. The cup-to-disc ratio is approximately 30% in **A** and 70% in **B**.
(From Swartz MH: Textbook of Physical Diagnosis, 5th ed. Philadelphia, WB Saunders, 2006.)

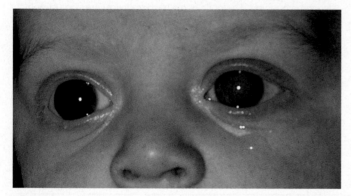

Fig 76–3
Clinical appearance of primary infantile glaucoma. This 8-month-old boy had an acute (3-day) history of corneal edema in the left eye. Note the enlarged corneas in both eyes and the epiphora. Intraocular pressure at examination under anesthetic was more than 35 mm Hg (more than 4.7 kPa) in the right eye. Trabeculotomy ab externo was carried out bilaterally.
(From Yanoff M, Duker JS: Ophthalmology, 2nd ed. St. Louis, Mosby, 2004.)

- Trauma
- Inflammatory
- High-dose oral corticosteroids taken for prolonged periods

DIFFERENTIAL DIAGNOSIS
- Other optic neuropathies
- Secondary glaucoma from inflammation and steroid therapy
- Red eye differential (see Table 59–1)
- Trauma
- Contact lens injury (see Fig. 59–7)

WORKUP
- Intraocular pressure
- Slit-lamp examination
- Visual fields
- Gonioscopy
- Nerve fiber analysis: laser scanning of nerve fiber layer using a glaucoma imaging device.
- Corneal thickness: important in prognosis

LABORATORY TESTS
- Blood sugar

IMAGING STUDIES
- Optic nerve photography: stereo photographs
- Visual field testing
- GDx

TREATMENT
- Beta blockers (e.g., timolol)
- Acetazolamide or pilocarpine
- Hyperosmotic agents (mannitol) in acute treatment
- Prostaglandins
- Laser trabeculoplasty as needed
- Pilocarpine four times daily

Chapter 77   **Glaucoma, primary closed angle**

DEFINITION

Primary closed-angle glaucoma occurs when elevated intraocular pressure is associated with closure of the filtration angle or obstruction in the circulating pathway of the aqueous humor. Potential sites of increased resistance to aqueous flow are illustrated in Figure 77–1.

PHYSICAL FINDINGS AND CLINICAL PRESENTATION

- Hazy cornea
- Narrow angle
- Red eyes
- Pain
- Injection of conjunctiva
- Shallow anterior chamber
- Thick cataract
- Old trauma
- Chronic eye infections

CAUSE

- Narrow angles with acute closure or blockage of circulatory path of the aqueous humor, causing increase in interior ocular pressure (Fig. 77–2)

DIFFERENTIAL DIAGNOSIS

- High pressure
- Optic nerve cupping (see Fig. 76–1)
- Field loss
- Shallow chamber
- Open-angle glaucoma (see Fig. 76–2)
- Conjunctivitis (see Fig. 59–1)

- Corneal disease: keratitis (see Fig. 60–4)
- Uveitis (see Fig. 75–1)
- Scleritis (see Fig. 61–1)
- Allergies, viral conjunctivitis (see Fig. 59–2)
- Contact lens wearing with irritation (see Fig. 59–7)

WORKUP

- Intraocular pressure
- Gonioscopy
- Slit-lamp examination
- Visual field examination
- GDx examination (laser scan of nerve fiber layer)
- Optic nerve evaluation
- Anterior chamber depth
- Cataract evaluation
- High hyperopia

LABORATORY TESTS

- Blood sugar and CBC (if diabetes or inflammatory disease is suspected)
- Visual field
- GDx nerve fiber analysis

IMAGING STUDIES

- Fundus photography
- Fluorescein angiography for neurovascular disease

TREATMENT

- Primary angle closure attack is an ophthalmologic emergency. Figure 77–3 illustrates initial management.
- Argon laser iridoplasty (Fig. 77–4)

POTENTIAL SITES OF INCREASED RESISTANCE TO AQUEOUS FLOW

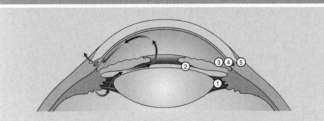

1 Ciliary body processes (when ciliary body swollen by congestion), fibrin debris, vitreous face against the lens equator
2 Pupillary block by anterior position of lens or swollen lens
3 Pretrabecular by neovascular or cellular membranes
4 Trabecular by abnormal accumulation of extracellular matrix
5 Post-trabecular by increased episcleral venous pressure

Fig 77–1
Potential sites of increased resistance to aqueous flow.
(From Yanoff M, Duker JS: Ophthalmology, 2nd ed. St. Louis, Mosby, 2004.)

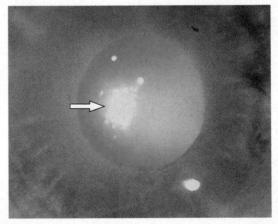

Fig 77–2
Acute attack of angle-closure glaucoma. The central anterior chamber is deep, intraocular pressure is elevated, and corneal edema is present. Epithelial edema is outlined by the irregular slit reflex (*arrow*).
(From Yanoff M, Duker JS: Ophthalmology, 2nd ed. St. Louis, Mosby, 2004.)

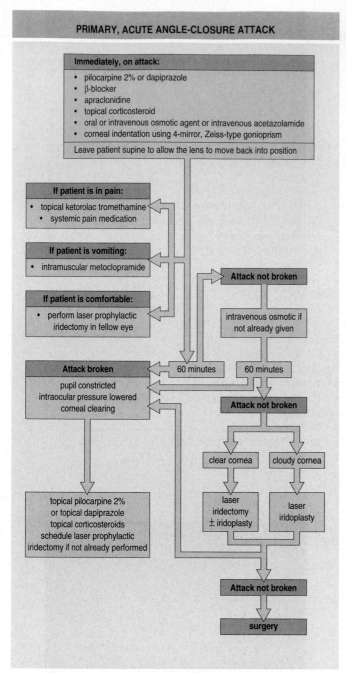

Fig 77–3
Initial management of a primary acute angle-closure attack.
(From Yanoff M, Duker JS: Ophthalmology, 2nd ed. St. Louis, Mosby, 2004.)

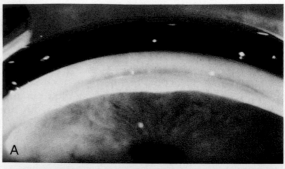
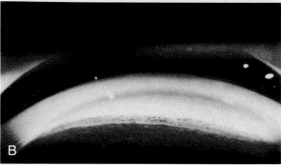

Fig 77–4
Angle-closure glaucoma with pupillary block component. **A,** No angle structures are visible in the primary position. **B,** After iridectomy, the iris curvature is less pronounced, and the trabecular meshwork can be visualized.
(From Yanoff M, Duker JS: Ophthalmology, 2nd ed. St. Louis, Mosby, 2004.)

Chapter 78	Horner's syndrome

DEFINITION
Horner's syndrome is the clinical triad of ipsilateral ptosis, miosis, and sometimes anhidrosis. These findings result from the disruption of the cervical sympathetic pathway along its course from the hypothalamus to the eye. Disruption of any of the three neurons in the pathway (central, preganglionic, or postganglionic) can cause Horner's syndrome.

PHYSICAL FINDINGS AND CLINICAL PRESENTATION
- Ptosis results from loss of sympathetic tone to eyelid muscles.
- Miosis results from loss of sympathetic pupillodilator activity (Fig. 78–1). The affected pupil reacts normally to bright light and accommodation. Anisocoria is greater in darkness.
- Dilation lag: The Horner's pupil dilates more slowly than the normal pupil when lights are dimmed (20 vs. 5 seconds), because Horner's pupil is dilating passively because of relaxation of the iris sphincter.
- Presence of anhidrosis is variable and depends on site of injury in pathway. Anhidrosis may occur with lesions affecting central or preganglionic neurons.
- Conjunctival or facial hyperemia may occur on affected side because of loss of sympathetic vasoconstriction.
- In congenital Horner's syndrome, the iris on the affected side may fail to become pigmented, resulting in heterochromia of the iris, with the affected iris remaining blue-gray.

CAUSE
Lesions affecting any neuron in the sympathetic pathway can cause Horner's syndrome.

Mechanical
- Syringomyelia
- Trauma
- Benign tumors
- Malignant tumors (thyroid, Pancoast)
- Metastatic tumor
- Lymphadenopathy
- Neurofibromatosis
- Cervical rib
- Cervical spondylosis

Vascular (ischemia, hemorrhage, or arteriovenous malformation [AVM])
- Brainstem lesion: commonly occlusion of the posterior inferior cerebellar artery but almost any of the vessels may be responsible (vertebral; superior, middle, or inferior lateral medullary arteries; superior or anterior inferior cerebellar arteries)
- Internal carotid artery aneurysm or dissection. Injury of other major vessels (carotid artery, subclavian artery, ascending aorta) can also cause Horner's syndrome.
- Cluster headache, migraine

Miscellaneous
- Idiopathic
- Congenital
- Demyelination (multiple sclerosis)
- Infection (apical TB, herpes zoster)
- Pneumothorax
- Iatrogenic (angiography, internal jugular or subclavian catheter, chest tube, surgery, epidural spinal anesthesia)
- Radiation

DIFFERENTIAL DIAGNOSIS
- Causes of anisocoria (unequal pupils)
  - Normal variant
  - Mydriatic use
  - Prosthetic eye
  - Unilateral cataract
  - Iritis
- Causes of ptosis

IMAGING STUDIES
Imaging the entire three neuron sympathetic pathway is usually warranted.
- MRI of the head and neck to identify lesions affecting the central and cervical sympathetic pathways
- Ultrasound, CT angiography, or MR angiography to assess the vessels in the head and neck
- Chest CT scan to rule out lung tumors

TREATMENT
- Treatment depends on underlying cause.

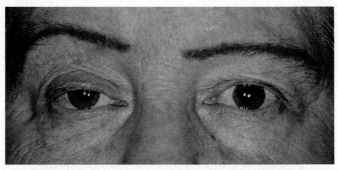

Fig 78–1
Horner's syndrome, with ipsilateral right upper eyelid ptosis and pupillary miosis.
(From Yanoff M, Duker JS: Ophthalmology, 2nd ed. St. Louis, Mosby, 2004.)

Chapter 79 | Optic neuritis

DEFINITION
Optic neuritis is an inflammation of the optic nerve resulting in a reduction of visual function.

PHYSICAL FINDINGS AND CLINICAL PRESENTATION
- Presents with acute or subacute (days) visual loss and most often tenderness with movement of affected eye.
- *Marcus Gunn pupil* (RAPD, relative afferent pupillary defect): direct and consensual response is normal; however, when swinging flashlight from eye to eye, the affected eye's pupil dilates to direct light.
- Decreased visual acuity.
- Unilateral visual field abnormalities; often, a central scotoma
- Color desaturation, red most affected
- Normal orbit and fundus; occasionally, there is optic disc swelling (Fig. 79–1), optic disc edema and macular star formation (Fig. 79–2), uveitis, or periphlebitis.
- May have movement or light-induced phosphenes (flashes of light lasting 1 to 2 seconds)
- Many have *Uhthoff's phenomenon* (benign exercise or heat-induced deterioration of vision). Vision may also worsen in bright sunlight.
- After several months, the optic disc may atrophy and become pale.

CAUSE
- An inflammatory response associated with an infection, autoimmune disease (e.g., multiple sclerosis [MS]) or, rarely, a mitochondrial disorder

DIFFERENTIAL DIAGNOSIS
- Inflammatory: multiple sclerosis, neuromyelitis optica, sarcoidosis, systemic lupus erythematosus (SLE), Sjögren's syndrome, Behçet's disease, postinfection, postvaccination
- Infectious: syphilis, TB, Lyme disease, *Bartonella*, HIV, cytomegalovirus (CMV), herpesvirus, orbital infection
- Ischemic: giant cell arteritis, anterior and posterior ischemic optic neuropathies, diabetic papillopathy, branch or central retinal artery or vein occlusion
- Mitochondrial: Leber's hereditary optic neuropathy
- Mass lesion: pituitary tumor, aneurysm, meningioma, glioma, metastases, sinus mucocele
- Ocular: optic drusen, retinal detachment, vitreous hemorrhage, uveitis, posterior scleritis, neuroretinitis, maculopathies and retinopathies
- Toxic: vitamin B_{12} deficiency, tobacco-ethanol amblyopia, methanol or ethambutol intoxication (painless, most bilateral, slowly progressive)
- Other: acute papilledema, retinal migraine, factitious visual loss
- Box 79–1 describes the differential diagnosis of acute unilateral optic neuropathy.

Box 79–1 Differential diagnosis of acute unilateral optic neuropathy

Anterior ischemic optic neuropathy
Tumor
Aneurysm
Vasculitis
Neuroretinitis
Metastatic carcinoma
Lymphoreticular disorder
Sinusitis
Granulomatous inflammation
Leber's hereditary optic neuropathy (always bilateral, but frequently presents initially with visual loss in only one eye)

From Yanoff M, Duker JS: Ophthalmology, 2nd ed. St. Louis, Mosby, 2004.

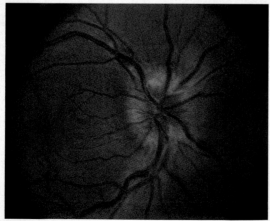

Fig 79–1
Optic disc swelling (papillitis) associated with acute optic neuritis. (From Yanoff M, Duker JS: Ophthalmology, 2nd ed. St. Louis, Mosby, 2004.)

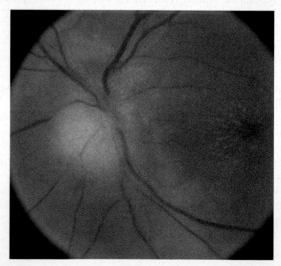

Fig 79–2
Optic disc edema and macular star formation. This color fundus photograph is from a 13-year-old girl who came to medical attention with counting finger acuity secondary to cat scratch (*Bartonella*) neuroretinitis. (From Yanoff M, Duker JS: Ophthalmology, 2nd ed. St. Louis, Mosby, 2004.)

WORKUP

A thorough neurologic examination should otherwise be normal. Dilated ophthalmoscopy is recommended.

LABORATORY TESTS

- Recommend: CBC, ANA, ESR
- Consider: HIV Ab, Lyme titer, angiotensin-converting enzyme (ACE), rapid plasma reagin (RPR), Leber's hereditary optic neuropathy (LHON), mitochondrial DNA (mtDNA) mutations.

IMAGING STUDIES

- MRI of the brain and orbits (thin section, fat-suppressed, T2-weighted) with gadolinium is needed to rule out compressive and infiltrative causees. Often, enhancement of the optic nerve is seen. The risk for developing MS can also be assessed.

TREATMENT

- Not all ophthalmologists and neurologists recommend treatment, but treatment is indicated if the visual loss is severe or if there is an abnormal MRI scan (higher risk of MS). Consider methylprednisolone IV, followed by an oral prednisone taper.

EARS

Chapter 80   Normal anatomy, examination, and diagnostic testing

- Figure 80–1 illustrates the normal ear anatomy.
- The proper technique for an adult otoscopic examination is shown in Figure 80–2. The normal landmarks of the tympanic membrane are shown in Figure 80–3. Common abnormalities seen with an otoscopic examination are noted (see later).
- Ear wax (Figs. 80–4 and 80–5). The equipment used for removal of cerumen is shown in Figure 80–6.

- Otitis media (Fig. 80–7)
- Bullous myringitis (Fig. 80–8)
- Tympanic membrane perforation (Fig. 80–9)
- Ear canal hematoma (Fig. 80–10)
- Cholesteatoma (Fig. 80–11)

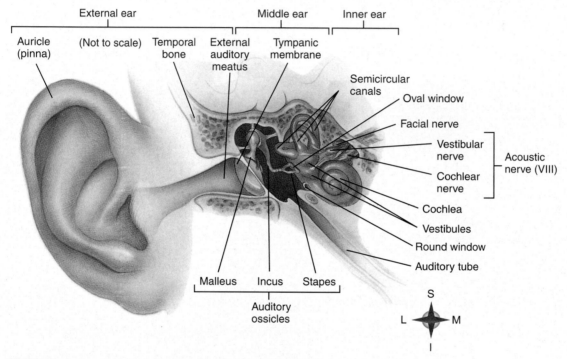

Fig 80–1

The ear: external, middle, and inner ears. (Anatomic structures are not drawn to scale.) I, inferior; L, lateral; M, medial; S, superior.
(From Thibodeau GA, Patton KP: Anatomy and Physiology, 4th ed. St. Louis, Mosby, 1999.)

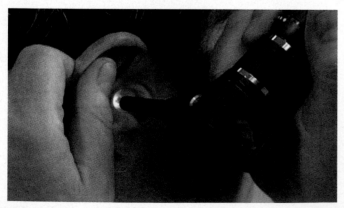

Fig 80–2

Technique for otoscopic examination. Note that the ear is pulled up, out, and back.
(From Swartz MH: Textbook of Physical Diagnosis, 5th ed. Philadelphia, WB Saunders, 2006.)

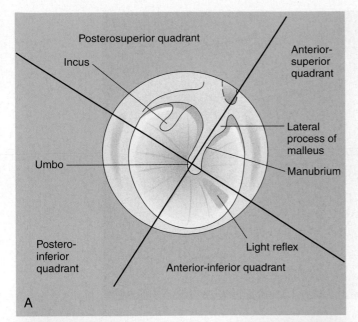

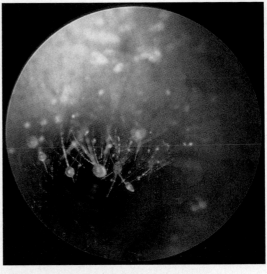

Fig 80–4
Ear wax on the bases of hairs.
(From Swartz MH: Textbook of Physical Diagnosis, 5th ed. Philadelphia, WB Saunders, 2006.)

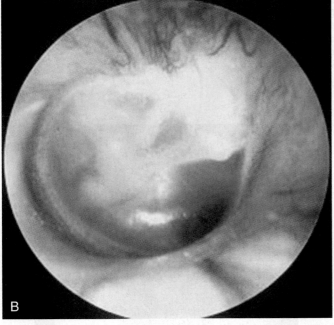

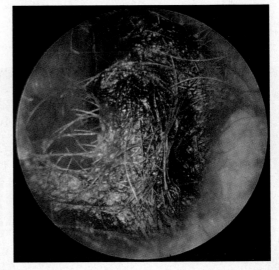

Fig 80–3
A, The normal landmarks of the tympanic membrane. **B,** Photograph of a normal tympanic membrane.
(From Fireman P: Atlas of Allergies and Immunology, 3rd ed. St. Louis, Mosby, 2006.)

Fig 80–5
Ear wax in the external ear canal.
(From Swartz MH: Textbook of Physical Diagnosis, 5th ed. Philadelphia, WB Saunders, 2006.)

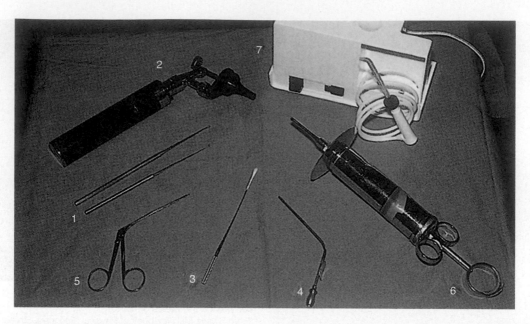

Fig 80–6
Equipment for cleaning the external auditory canal. The curette (1) is the implement most commonly used to remove cerumen. Use of a surgical otoscope head (2) makes the process considerably easier. Additional implements include cotton wicks (3) and a suction tip (4) for removal of discharge or moist wax, alligator forceps (5) for the removal of foreign bodies, an ear syringe (6), and a motorized irrigation apparatus (7) for the removal of firm objects or impacted cerumen. Lavage is contraindicated when there is a possible perforation of the tympanic membrane. If the motorized apparatus is used for irrigation, it must be kept on the lowest power setting to avoid traumatizing the eardrum.
(From Fireman P: Atlas of Allergies and Immunology, 3rd ed. St. Louis, Mosby, 2006.)

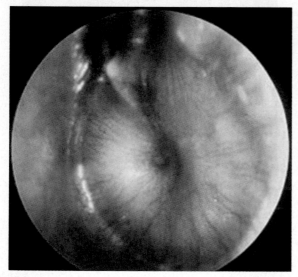

Fig 80–7
Acute otitis media. This is a typical erythematous, bulging tympanic membrane as seen by otoscopy. Mobility and light reflex are reduced, and landmarks are partially obscured.
(From Fireman P: Atlas of Allergies and Immunology, 3rd ed. St. Louis, Mosby, 2006.)

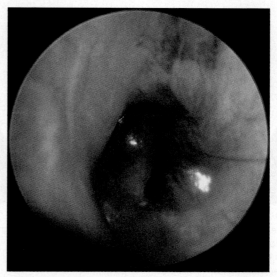

Fig 80–8
Bullous myringitis.
(From Swartz MH: Textbook of Physical Diagnosis, 5th ed. Philadelphia, WB Saunders, 2006.)

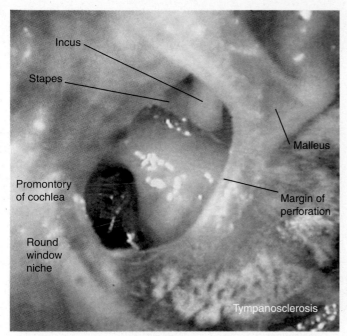

Fig 80-9
Chronic tympanic membrane perforation.
(From Swartz MH: Textbook of Physical Diagnosis, 5th ed. Philadelphia, WB Saunders, 2006.)

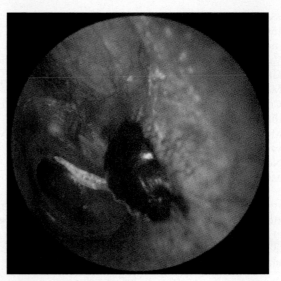

Fig 80-10
External ear canal with large hematoma.
(From Swartz MH: Textbook of Physical Diagnosis, 5th ed. Philadelphia, WB Saunders, 2006.)

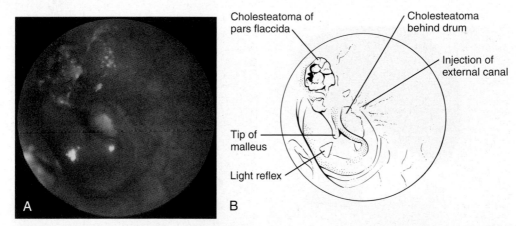

Fig 80-11
Photograph **(A)** and labeled schematic **(B)** showing a cholesteatoma of the left ear that resulted from a marginal perforation of the tympanic membrane. Note the injection of the distal external canal.
(From Swartz MH: Textbook of Physical Diagnosis, 5th ed. Philadelphia,WB Saunders, 2006.)

Chapter 81	**Hearing loss**

CAUSE

- Infections: mumps, herpes simplex, herpes zoster, cytomegalovirus, syphilis
- Vascular: sickle cell disease, Berger's disease, polycythemia, fat emboli, hypercoagulable states
- Metabolic: diabetes, hyperlipoproteinemia
- Conductive: cerumen impaction, foreign bodies, otitis media, otitis externa, barotrauma, trauma
- Medications: aminoglycosides, antineoplastics, salicylates, vancomycin
- Neoplasm: acoustic neuroma, metastatic neoplasm
- Meniere's disease

EVALUATION

- Comparative features of conductive and sensorineural hearing loss are described in Table 81–1.
- Commonly performed bedside tests includes the Rinne test (Fig. 81–1) and Weber test (Fig. 81–2).
- Figure 81–3 and Box 81-1 describe testing for the evaluation of hearing loss.

TABLE 81–1 Comparative features of conductive and sensorineural hearing loss

Feature	Conductive Hearing Loss	Sensorineural Hearing Loss
Pathologic process	External canal	Cochlea
	Middle ear	Cochlear nerve
		Brainstem
Loudness of speech	Softer than normal	Louder than normal
External canal	May be abnormal	Normal
Tympanic membrane	Usually abnormal	Normal
Rinne test	Negative	Positive
Weber test	Heard on "deaf" side	Heard on better side (only in severe unilateral loss)

From Swartz MH: Textbook of Physical Diagnosis, 5th ed. Philadelphia, WB Saunders, 2006.

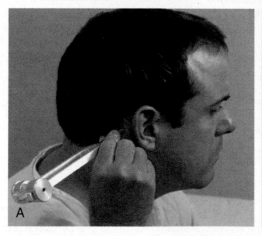 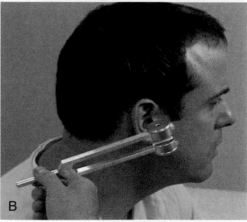

Fig 81–1
The Rinne test. **A,** The tuning fork is first placed on the mastoid process. **B,** When the sound can no longer be heard, the tuning fork is placed in front of the external auditory meatus. Normally, air conduction is better than bone conduction (AC > BC).
(From Swartz MH: Textbook of Physical Diagnosis, 5th ed. Philadelphia,WB Saunders, 2006.)

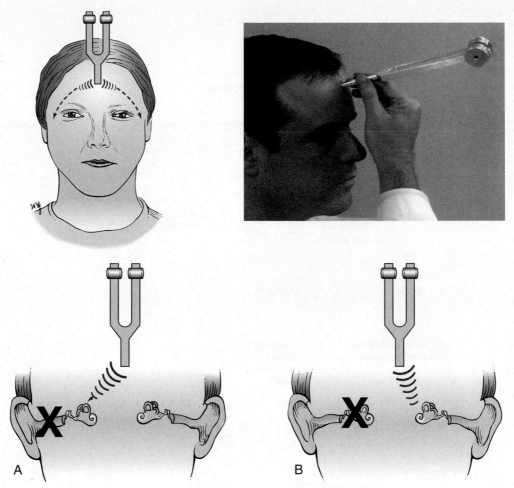

Fig 81–2

The Weber test. When a vibrating tuning fork is placed on the center of the forehead, the normal response is for the sound to be heard in the center, without lateralization to either side. **A,** In the presence of a conductive hearing loss, the sound is heard on the side of the conductive loss. **B,** In the presence of a sensorineural loss, the sound is heard better on the opposite (unaffected) side.
(From Swartz MH: Textbook of Physical Diagnosis, 5th ed. Philadelphia, WB Saunders, 2006.)

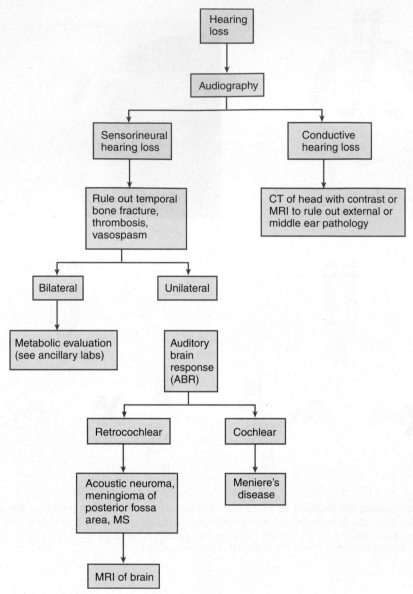

Fig 81-3
Evaluation of hearing loss. CT, computed tomography; MRI, magnetic resonance imaging; MS, multiple sclerosis.
(From Ferri FF: Ferri's Best Test: A Practical Guide to Clinical Laboratory Medicine and Diagnostic Imaging. Philadelphia, Elsevier Mosby, 2004.)

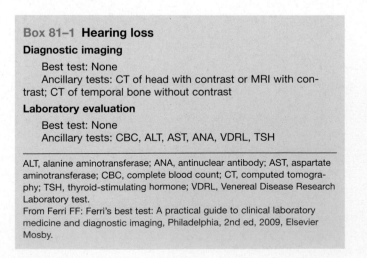

Box 81-1 Hearing loss

Diagnostic imaging

Best test: None
Ancillary tests: CT of head with contrast or MRI with contrast; CT of temporal bone without contrast

Laboratory evaluation

Best test: None
Ancillary tests: CBC, ALT, AST, ANA, VDRL, TSH

ALT, alanine aminotransferase; ANA, antinuclear antibody; AST, aspartate aminotransferase; CBC, complete blood count; CT, computed tomography; TSH, thyroid-stimulating hormone; VDRL, Venereal Disease Research Laboratory test.
From Ferri FF: Ferri's best test: A practical guide to clinical laboratory medicine and diagnostic imaging, Philadelphia, 2nd ed, 2009, Elsevier Mosby.

DEFINITION

Acoustic neuroma is a benign proliferation of the Schwann cells that cover the vestibular branch of the eighth cranial nerve (CN VIII). Symptoms are commonly a result of compression of the acoustic branch of CN VIII, the facial nerve (CN VII), and the trigeminal nerve (CN V). The glossopharyngeal nerve (CN IX) and vagus nerve (CN X) are less commonly involved. In extreme cases, compression of the brainstem may lead to obstruction of cerebrospinal fluid (CSF) outflow and elevated intracranial pressure (ICP).

PHYSICAL FINDINGS AND CLINICAL PRESENTATION

- Most frequently, unilateral hearing loss, tinnitus, or both; also balance problems, vertigo, facial pain (trigeminal neuralgia) and weakness, difficulty swallowing, fullness or pain of the involved ear. Headache may occur.
- With elevated ICP, patients may also suffer from vomiting, fever, and visual changes.
- Hearing loss is the most common presenting complaint and is usually of high frequency.

CAUSE

The cause is incompletely understood, but long-term exposure to acoustic trauma has been implicated. Bilateral acoustic neuromas may be inherited in an autosomal dominant manner as part of neurofibromatosis type 2. This disease is associated with a defect on chromosome 22q1.

DIFFERENTIAL DIAGNOSIS

- Benign positional vertigo
- Meniere's disease
- Trigeminal neuralgia
- Cerebellar disease
- Normal-pressure hydrocephalus
- Presbycusis
- Glomus tumors
- Vertebrobasilar insufficiency
- Ototoxicity from medications
- Other tumors
  1. Meningioma, glioma
  2. Facial nerve schwannoma
  3. Cavernous hemangioma
  4. Metastatic tumors

LABORATORY TESTS

- Audiometry is useful; often shows asymmetrical, sensorineural, high-frequency hearing loss
- CSF protein may be elevated.

IMAGING STUDIES

- MRI with gadolinium is the preferred test (Fig. 82–1). It can detect tumors as small as 2 mm in diameter.
- CT scan with contrast can detect tumors 1 cm in diameter or larger.
- Treatment decisions should be based on the size of the tumor, rate of growth (older patients tend to have slower growing tumors), degree of neurologic deficit, desire to preserve hearing, life expectancy, age of the patient, and surgical risk. A combination of treatments can also be used.

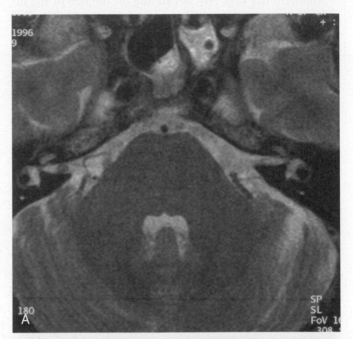

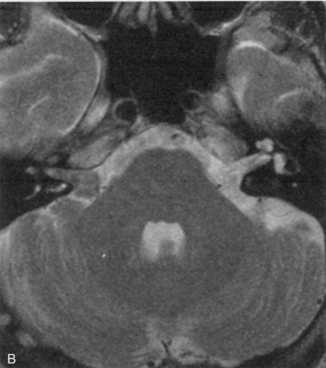

Fig 82–1

Two T2-W MRI scans showing a small intracanalicular **(A)** and a larger cerebellopontine angle acoustic neuroma **(B)**.
(From Grainger RG, Allison D: Grainger & Allison's Diagnostic Radiology: A Textbook of Medical Imaging, 4th ed. London, Churchill Livingstone, 2001.)

TREATMENT

- Surgery is the definitive treatment. Choice of approach (middle cranial fossa, translabyrinthine, or retromastoid suboccipital) may vary, depending on the size of the tumor, amount of residual hearing desired, and degree of surgical risk that can be tolerated. Partial resection is sometimes undertaken to minimize the risk of injury to nearby structures. Intraoperative facial nerve monitoring is recommended.
- Radiation therapy (stereotactic radiotherapy, stereotactic radiosurgery, or proton beam radiotherapy) is useful for tumors less than 3 cm in diameter or for those in whom surgery is not an option. Radiotherapy following partial resection has also been used to minimize complications.

Chapter 83 Relapsing polychondritis

DEFINITION

- Rare autoimmune disease of unknown cause with episodic but potentially progressive inflammatory manifestations.
- It involves primarily cartilaginous structures throughout the body, including the ears, nose, eyes, laryngobronchial and costal cartilage, and joints in a heterogeneous pattern and sequence.
- It may be associated with other autoimmune diseases (e.g., rheumatoid arthritis [RA], SLE, scleroderma, Sjögren's syndrome) and neoplastic disorders (e.g., myelodysplastic syndrome, lymphoma)

EPIDEMIOLOGY

- Rare disorder (3.5 per million); peak age at onset is between 40 and 50 years of age.
- Over 30% of cases are associated with existing or autoimmune diseases.

CLINICAL PRESENTATION

- The classic clinical manifestation is acute unilateral or bilateral auricular chondritis.
- The onset is characteristic, with redness or violaceous discoloration, warmth and swelling involving the cartilaginous portion of the pinna, and sparing of the lobe (Fig. 83–1).
- The episode lasts days to weeks and resolves with or without treatment. Over time, and with repeated attacks, the pinna loses its firmness and becomes soft and flops over or assumes a knobby, cauliflower-like appearance.

DIAGNOSIS

- Biopsy will confirm the diagnosis (Fig. 83–2).

TREATMENT

- NSAIDs and prednisone

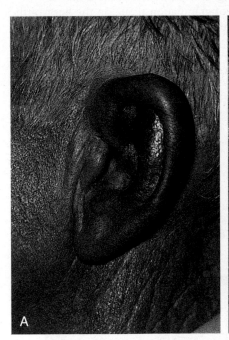
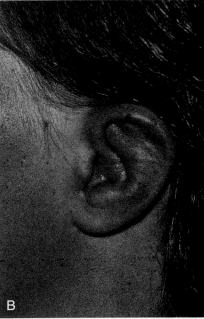

Fig 83–1
Otorhinolaryngeal disease in relapsing polychondritis. **A,** The pinna of the ear becomes inflamed. Note the sparing of the noncartilaginous portion of the ear. **B,** Recurrent attacks cause loss of cartilage, with the ear flopping over.
(From Hochberg MC, Silman AJ, Smolen JS, et al [eds]: Rheumatology, 3rd ed. St. Louis, Mosby, 2003.)

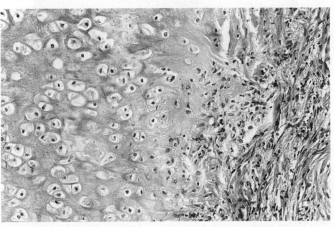

Fig 83–2
Biopsy of auricular chondritis. The ear shows perichondritis with the presence of mononuclear cells and occasional polymorphonuclear leukocytes at the fibrochondral junction (H&E, ×200).
(Courtesy of Dr. Lester E. Wold.)

Chapter 84 — Otitis externa

DEFINITION

Otitis externa is a term encompassing a variety of conditions causing inflammation and/or infection of the external auditory canal (or of the auricle, tympanic membrane, or both). There are six subgroups of otitis externa:

- Acute localized otitis externa (furunculosis)
- Acute diffuse bacterial otitis externa (swimmer's ear)
- Chronic otitis externa
- Eczematous otitis externa
- Fungal otitis externa (otomycosis)
- Invasive or necrotizing (malignant) otitis externa

PHYSICAL FINDINGS AND CLINICAL PRESENTATION

The two most common symptoms are otalgia, ranging from pruritus to severe pain exacerbated by motion (e.g., chewing), and otorrhea. Patients may also experience aural fullness and hearing loss secondary to swelling, with occlusion of the canal. More intense symptoms may occur with bacterial otitis externa, with or without fever, and lymphadenopathy (anterior to tragus). There are also findings unique to the various forms of the infection:

- Acute localized otitis externa (furunculosis)
  1. Occurs from infected hair follicles, usually in the outer third of the ear canal, forming pustules and furuncles
  2. Furuncles are superficial and pointing or deep and diffuse.
- Impetigo:
  1. In contrast to furunculosis, this is a superficial spreading infection of the ear canal that may also involve the concha and the auricle.
  2. Begins as a small blister that ruptures, releasing straw-colored fluid that dries as a golden crust
- Erysipelas
  1. Caused by group A streptococcus
  2. May involve the concha and canal
  3. May involve the dermis and deeper tissues
  4. Area of cellulitis, often with severe pain
  5. Fever chills, malaise
  6. Regional adenopathy
- Eczematous otitis externa
  1. Stems from a variety of dermatologic problems that can involve the external auditory canal
  2. Severe itching, erythema, scaling, crusting, and fissuring possible
- Acute diffuse otitis externa (swimmer's ear):
  1. Begins with itching and a feeling of pressure and fullness in the ear that becomes increasingly tender and painful
  2. Mild erythema and edema of the external auditory canal, which may cause narrowing and occlusion of the canal, leading to hearing loss
  3. Minimal serous secretions (Fig. 84–1), which may become profuse and purulent
  4. Tympanic membrane may appear dull and infected.
  5. Usually absence of systemic symptoms such as fever, chills
- Otomycosis
  1. Chronic superficial infection of the ear canal and tympanic membrane

2. In primary fungal infection, major symptom is intense itching
3. In secondary infection (fungal infection superimposed on bacterial infection), major symptom is pain
4. Fungal growth in a variety of colors
- Chronic otitis externa
  1. Dry and atrophic canal
  2. Typically, lack of cerumen
  3. Itching, often severe, and mild discomfort, rather than pain
  4. Occasionally, mucopurulent discharge
  5. With time, thickening of the walls of the canal, causing narrowing of the lumen
- Necrotizing otitis externa (also known as malignant otitis externa); typically seen in older patients with diabetes or in patients who are immunocompromised (Fig. 84–2)
  1. Redness, swelling, and tenderness of the ear canal
  2. Classic finding of granulation tissue on the floor of the canal and the bone-cartilage junction
  3. Small ulceration of necrotic soft tissue at bone-cartilage junction
  4. Most common complaints: pain (often severe) and otorrhea
  5. Lessening of purulent drainage as infection advances
  6. Facial nerve palsy often the first and only cranial nerve defect
  7. Possible involvement of other cranial nerves

CAUSE

- Acute localized otitis externa: *Staphylococcus aureus*
- Impetigo
  1. *S. aureus*
  2. *Streptococcus pyogenes*
- Erysipelas: *S. pyogenes*

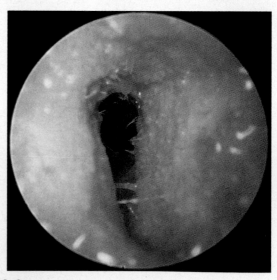

Fig 84–1
Acute otitis externa.
(From Swartz MH: Textbook of Physical Diagnosis, 5th ed. Philadelphia, WB Saunders, 2006.)

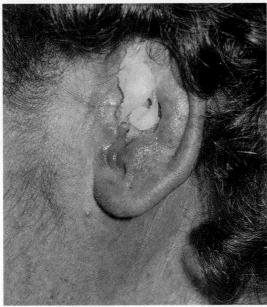

Fig 84–2
Malignant otitis externa in a diabetic woman. This is an aggressive infection caused by *Pseudomonas aeruginosa*.
(From White GM, Cox NH [eds]: Diseases of the Skin: A Color Atlas and Text, 2nd ed. St. Louis, Mosby, 2006.)

- Eczematous otitis externa
  1. Seborrheic dermatitis
  2. Atopic dermatitis
  3. Psoriasis
  4. Neurodermatitis
  5. SLE
- Acute diffuse otitis externa
  1. Swimming
  2. Hot, humid climates
  3. Tightly fitting hearing aids
  4. Use of earplugs
  5. *Pseudomonas aeruginosa*
  6. *S. aureus*
- Otomycosis
  1. Prolonged use of topical antibiotics and steroid preparations
  2. *Aspergillus* (80% to 90%)
  3. *Candida*
- Chronic otitis externa: persistent low-grade infection and inflammation
- Necrotizing otitis externa (NOE)
  1. Complication of persistent otitis externa
  2. Extends through Santorini's fissures, small apertures at the bone-cartilage junction of the canal, into the mastoid and along the base of the skull
  3. *P. aeruginosa*

DIFFERENTIAL DIAGNOSIS
- Acute otitis media (see Fig. 80–7)
- Bullous myringitis (see Fig. 80–8)
- Mastoiditis
- Foreign bodies, earwax (see Fig. 80–5)
- Neoplasms

LABORATORY TESTS
- Cultures from the canal are usually not necessary unless the patient is refractory to treatment.
- Leukocyte count normal or mildly elevated
- ESR is often markedly elevated in malignant otitis externa.

IMAGING STUDIES
- CT scan is the best technique for defining bone involvement and extent of disease in malignant otitis externa.
- MRI is slightly more sensitive in evaluation of soft tissue changes.
- Gallium scans are more specific than bone scans in diagnosing NOE.
- Follow-up scans are helpful in determining efficacy of treatment.

Note: Expert opinion supports history and physical examination as the best means of diagnosis. Persistent pain that is constant and severe should raise the question of NOE, particularly in older patients, diabetics, and immunocompromised individuals.

TREATMENT
- Cleansing and débridement of the ear canal with cotton swabs and hydrogen peroxide or other antiseptic solution allow for a more thorough examination of the ear.
- If the canal lumen is edematous and too narrow to allow adequate cleansing, a cotton wick or gauze strip inserted into the canal serves as a conduit for topical medications to be drawn into the canal (usually remove wick after 2 days).
- Local heat is useful for treating deep furunculosis.
- Incision and drainage are indicated for treatment of superficial pointing furunculosis.
- Medications

Topical medications
- An acidifying agent, such as 2% acetic acid, inhibits growth of bacteria and fungi.
- Topical antibiotics (in the form of otic or ophthalmic solutions) or antifungals, often in combination with an acidifying agent and a steroid preparation

Systemic antibiotics
- Reserved for severe cases, most often infections with *P. aeruginosa* or *S. aureus*

Chapter 85   Otitis media

DEFINITION

Otitis media is the presence of fluid in the middle ear accompanied by signs and symptoms of infection.

PHYSICAL FINDINGS AND CLINICAL PRESENTATION

- Fluid in the middle ear along with signs and symptoms of local inflammation
  1. Erythema with diminished light reflex (Fig. 85–1)
- Erythema of the tympanic membrane without other abnormalities is not a diagnostic criterion for acute otitis media because it may occur with any inflammation of the upper respiratory tract, crying, or nose blowing.
- As infection progresses, middle ear exudation occurs (exudative phase); the exudate rapidly changes from serous to purulent (suppurative phase).
- Retraction and poor motility of the tympanic membrane, which then becomes bulging and convex. Air bubbles may be seen (Fig. 85–2).
- At any time during the suppurative phase, the tympanic membrane may rupture (see Fig. 80–9), releasing the middle ear contents.
- Symptoms
  1. Otalgia, ranging from slight discomfort to severe, spreading to the temporal region
  2. Ear stuffiness and hearing loss may precede or follow otalgia.
  3. Otorrhea
  4. Vertigo, nystagmus, tinnitus, fever, lethargy, irritability, nausea, vomiting, anorexia
- After an episode of acute otitis media
  1. Persistence of effusion for weeks or months (called secretory, serous, or nonsuppurative otitis media)

2. Fever and otalgia usually absent
3. Hearing loss possible (10 to 50 dB, with predominant involvement of the low frequencies)

CAUSE

- Most common causative factor is an upper respiratory tract infection (often viral), which causes inflammation and obstruction of the eustachian tube. Bacterial colonization of the nasopharynx in conjunction with eustachian tube dysfunction leads to infection.
- May occasionally develop as a result of hematogenous spread or via direct invasion from the nasopharynx
- Most common bacterial pathogens
  1. *Streptococcus pneumoniae* causes 40% to 50% of cases and is the least likely of the major pathogens to resolve without treatment.
  2. *Haemophilus influenzae* causes 20% to 30% of cases.
  3. *Moraxella catarrhalis* causes 10% to 15% of cases.
  4. Of increasing importance, infection caused by penicillin-nonsusceptible *S. pneumoniae* (PNSSP).
- Viral pathogens
  1. Respiratory syncytial virus
  2. Rhinovirus
  3. Adenovirus
  4. Influenza
- Others
  1. *Mycoplasma pneumoniae*
  2. *Chlamydia trachomatis*

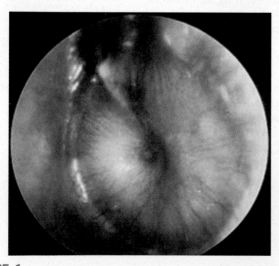

Fig 85–1
Acute otitis media. This is a typical erythematous bulging tympanic membrane as seen by otoscopy. Mobility and light reflex are reduced, and landmarks are partially obscured.
(From Fireman P: Atlas of Allergies and Immunology, 3rd ed. St. Louis, Mosby, 2006.)

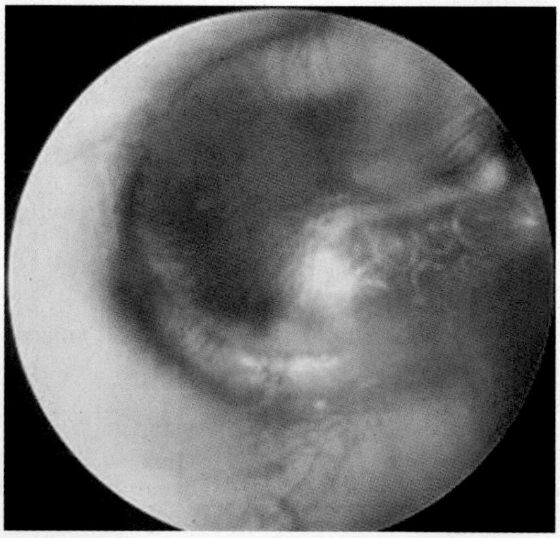

Fig 85–2
Obvious air bubbles seen on otoscopy lead to the diagnosis of otitis media with effusion. There is a loss of normal landmarks.
(From Fireman P: Atlas of Allergies and Immunology, 3rd ed. St. Louis, Mosby, 2006.)

DIFFERENTIAL DIAGNOSIS
- Otitis externa
- Referred pain
  1. Mouth
  2. Nasopharynx
  3. Tonsils
  4. Other parts of the upper respiratory tract

WORKUP
- Thorough otoscopic examination; adequate visualization of the tympanic membrane requires removal of cerumen and debris.
- Tympanometry
  1. Measures compliance of the tympanic membrane and middle ear pressure
  2. Detects the presence of fluid
- Acoustic reflectometry
  1. Measures sound waves reflected from the middle ear
  2. Useful for infants older than 3 months
  3. Increased reflected sound correlated with the presence of effusion

LABORATORY TESTS
- Tympanocentesis
  1. Not necessary in most cases, because the microbiology of middle ear effusions has been shown to be quite consistent
  2. May be indicated for:
     a. Highly toxic patients
     b. Patients who fail to respond to treatment in 48 to 72 hours
     c. Immunocompromised patients
- Cultures of the nasopharynx: sensitive but not specific
- Blood counts: usually show a leukocytosis with polymorphonuclear elevation
- Plain mastoid radiographs: generally not indicated; will reveal haziness in the periantral cells that may extend to entire mastoid
- CT or MRI may be indicated if serious complications suspected (meningitis, brain abscess)

TREATMENT
Most uncomplicated cases of acute otitis media resolve spontaneously, without complications.

Medications
Studies have demonstrated limited therapeutic benefit from antibiotic therapy. However, when opting to use antibiotic therapy, consider the folllowing:
- Amoxicillin remains the drug of choice for first-line treatment of uncomplicated acute otitis media, despite increasing prevalence of drug-resistant *S. pneumoniae*.
- Treatment failure is defined by lack of clinical improvement of signs or symptoms after 3 days of therapy.
- With treatment failure, in the absence of an identified causative pathogen, therapy should be redirected to cover these:
  1. Drug-resistant *S. pneumoniae*
  2. Beta-lactamase–producing strains of *H. influenzae* and *M. catarrhalis*
- Agents fulfilling these criteria include amoxicillin-clavulanate, second-generation cephalosporins (e.g., cefuroxime axetil, cefaclor), and ceftriaxone (given IM). Cefaclor, cefixime, loracarbef, and ceftibuten are active against *H. influenzae* and *M. catarrhalis*, but less active against pneumococci, especially drug-resistant strains, than the agents listed previously.
- Trimethoprim-sulfamethoxazole (TMP-SMZ) and macrolides have been used as first- and second-line agents, but pneumococcal resistance to these agents is rising (up to 25% resistance to TMP-SMZ, and up to 10% resistance to erythromycin).
- Cross-resistance between these drugs and the beta-lactams exist; therefore, patients who are treatment failures on amoxicillin are more likely to have infections resistant to TMP-SMZ and macrolides.
- Newer fluoroquinolones (levofloxacin, moxifloxacin) have enhanced activity against pneumococci compared with older agents (ciprofloxacin, ofloxacin).
- Treatment should be modified according to cultures and sensitivities.

Note: Effusions may persist for 2 to 6 weeks or longer in many patients with adequately treated otitis media.

Surgical therapy
- No evidence to support the routine of myringotomy, but in severe cases it provides prompt pain relief and accelerates resolution of infection
- Purulent secretions retained in the middle ear lead to increased pressure that may lead to spread of infection to contiguous areas. Myringotomy to decompress the middle ear is necessary to avoid complications.
- Complications include mastoiditis, facial nerve paralysis, labyrinthitis, meningitis, and brain abscess.
- Other procedures used for drainage of the middle ear include insertion of a ventilation tube and simple mastoidectomy.

Chronic therapy
- Myringotomy and tympanostomy tube placement for persistent middle ear effusion unresponsive to medical therapy for 3 months or longer if bilateral or 6 months or longer if unilateral
- Adenoidectomy, with or without tonsillectomy, often advocated for treatment of recurrent otitis media, although indications for this procedure are controversial
- Chronic complications include tympanic membrane perforations, cholesteatoma, tympanosclerosis, ossicular necrosis, toxic or suppurative labyrinthitis, and intracranial suppuration.

NOSE

Chapter 86   Allergic rhinitis

DEFINITION

Allergic rhinitis is an IgE-mediated hypersensitivity response to nasally inhaled allergens that causes sneezing, rhinorrhea, nasal pruritus, and congestion.

PHYSICAL FINDINGS AND CLINICAL PRESENTATION

- Pale or violaceous mucosa of the turbinates (Fig. 86–1) caused by venous engorgement (this can distinguish it from erythema present in viral rhinitis [Fig. 86–2])
- Nasal polyps (Fig. 86–3)
- Lymphoid hyperplasia in the posterior oropharynx, with cobblestone appearance
- Erythema of the throat, conjunctival and scleral infections
- Clear nasal discharge

- Clinical presentation: usually consists of sneezing, nasal congestion, cough, postnasal drip, loss of or alteration of smell, and sensation of plugged ears
- The fiberoptic rhinoscope can be used in select patients for a more thorough examination of the nares (Fig. 86–4).

CAUSE

- Pollens in spring, ragweed in fall, grasses in summer
- Dust, dust mites, animal allergens
- Smoke or any irritants
- Perfumes, detergents, soaps
- Emotional stress, changes in atmospheric pressure or temperature

DIFFERENTIAL DIAGNOSIS

- Infections (sinusitis; viral, bacterial, or fungal rhinitis)
- Rhinitis medicamentosa (cocaine, sympathomimetic nasal drops)
- Vasomotor rhinitis (e.g., secondary to air pollutants)
- Septal obstruction (e.g., deviated septum), nasal polyps, nasal neoplasms
- Systemic diseases (e.g., Wegener's granulomatosis, hypothyroidism [rare])

WORKUP

- The initial strategy should be to determine whether patients should undergo diagnostic testing or receive empirical treatment.
- Workup is often unnecessary if the diagnosis is apparent. A detailed medical history is useful in identifying the culprit allergen.
- Select patients with allergic rhinitis that is not controlled with standard therapy may benefit from allergy testing to target

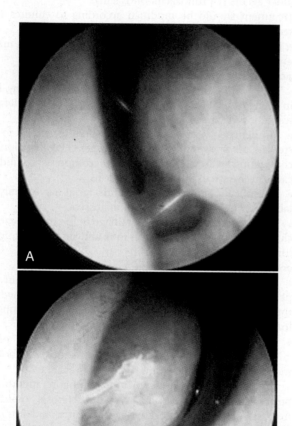

Fig 86–1

The inferior nasal turbinate of a patient with allergic rhinitis as seen through a fiberoptic rhinoscope. **A,** The mucosa are swollen, pale, and edematous, with increased nasal secretions, which may be watery to mucoid. **B,** Nasal obstruction caused by the engorged and swollen nasal mucosa.
(From Fireman P: Atlas of Allergies and Immunology, 3rd ed. St. Louis, Mosby, 2006.)

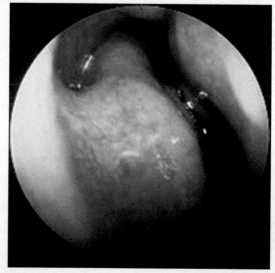

Fig 86–2

Clear, watery nasal secretions with swollen, reddish turbinates seen via fiberoptic rhinoscopy in a patient during the first few days of viral rhinitis. Often, the secretions become mucopurulent after several days.
(From Fireman P: Atlas of Allergies and Immunology, 3rd ed. St. Louis, Mosby, 2006.)

allergen avoidance measures or guide immunotherapy. Allergy testing can be performed using a skin test or radioallergosorbent test (RAST). In vitro tests also can assess serum levels of specific IgE antibodies. Overall, skin tests show greater sensitivity than serum assays. In vitro tests should be considered in rare patients who fear skin tests, must take medication that interferes with skin testing, or have generalized dermatographism.

- Examination of nasal smears for the presence of neutrophils to rule out infectious causes and the presence of eosinophils (suggestive of allergy) may be useful in select patients.
- Peripheral blood eosinophil counts are not useful in allergy diagnosis.

TREATMENT

- Maintain allergen-free environment by covering mattresses and pillows with allergen-proof casings, eliminating carpeting and animal products, and removing dust-collecting fixtures.
- Use of air purifiers and dust filters is helpful.
- Maintain humidity in the environment below 50% to prevent dust mites and mold.
- Use air conditioners, especially in the bedroom.
- Remove pets from homes of patients with suspected sensitivity to animal allergens.
- Determine whether the patient is troubled by swollen turbinates (best treated with decongestants) or blockages secondary to mucus (effectively treated by antihistamines).
- Most first-generation antihistamines can cause considerable sedation and anticholinergic symptoms. The second-generation antihistamines (loratadine, fexofenadine, cetirizine, desloratadine) are preferred because they do not have any significant anticholinergic or sedative effects; however, they are more expensive.

- Montelukast, a leukotriene receptor antagonist commonly used for asthma, is also effective for allergic rhinitis.
- Azelastine is an antihistamine nasal spray effective for seasonal allergic rhinitis.
- Topical nasal steroids are effective and are preferred by many as first-line treatment for allergic rhinitis in adults.
- Cromolyn sodium can be used for prophylaxis (mast cell stabilizer).
- Immunotherapy is generally reserved for patients responding poorly to these treatments.

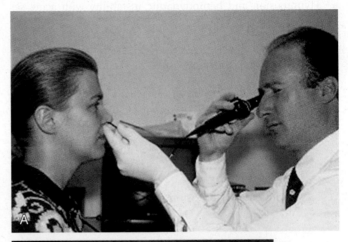

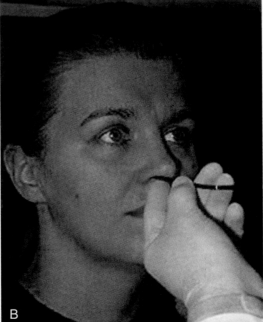

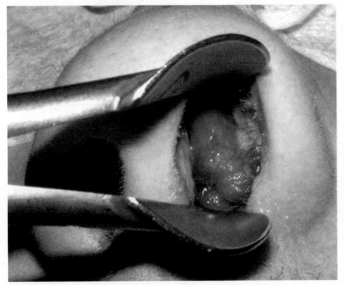

Fig 86–3
Nasal polyps.
(From Swartz MH: Textbook of Physical Diagnosis, 5th ed. Philadelphia, WB Saunders, 2006.)

Fig 86–4
Lateral **(A)** and frontal **(B)** views of the fiberoptic rhinoscopic procedure that can be used for a more thorough examination of the nares, especially the anterior and posterior nasopharynx, which cannot be seen with a speculum. This examination also provides magnification of the nasal structures.
(From Fireman P: Atlas of Allergies and Immunology, 3rd ed. St. Louis, Mosby, 2006.)

Chapter 87   Epistaxis

DEFINITION

Epistaxis is defined as bleeding from the nose or nasal hemorrhage and is classified as anterior or posterior.

EPIDEMIOLOGY AND DEMOGRAPHICS

- Up to 60% of the population experiences at least one episode over a lifetime, and 6% of these patients will seek professional health care assistance to control the bleeding.
- Over 80% of cases of epistaxis are anterior in origin (Little's area) and occur from Kiesselbach's plexus (Fig. 87–1)

PHYSICAL FINDINGS AND CLINICAL PRESENTATION

- Nosebleed
- Hypotension and hemodynamic instability with acute severe epistaxis

CAUSE

- Approximately 90% of epistaxes presenting to primary care physicians, emergency departments, and otolaryngologists are idiopathic.
- Other common causes of epistaxis can be local or systemic in nature. Many cases of epistaxis are multifactorial in cause.
  1. Cold, dry environment
  2. Trauma (nose picking, accidents, physical altercations)
  3. Structural deformities (septal deviations or spurs, chronic perforations)
  4. Inflammatory (rhinosinusitis, nasal polyposis)
  5. Allergies
  6. Foreign bodies in the nasal cavity
  7. Tumors (juvenile angiofibroma)
  8. Irritants
  9. Hypertension
  10. Coagulopathy (hemophilia, von Willebrand's disease, thrombocytopenia)
  11. Osler-Weber-Rendu disease
  12. Renal failure
  13. Drugs: aspirin, NSAIDs, warfarin, alcohol
  14. Blood vessel disorders (connective tissue disease, hereditary hemorrhagic telangiectasia)

DIFFERENTIAL DIAGNOSIS

- Pseudoepistaxis must be ruled out. Common extranasal sites of bleeding that can present with epistaxis include the following:
  1. Pulmonary hemoptysis
  2. Bleeding esophageal varices
  3. Tumor bleeding from the pharynx, larynx, or trachea

LABORATORY TESTS

- Hemoglobin and hematocrit
- Platelet count
- Blood urea nitrogen (BUN), creatinine
- Coagulation studies (prothrombin time [PT], partial thromboplastin time [PTT])
- Typing and cross-matching of blood products when there is significant blood loss

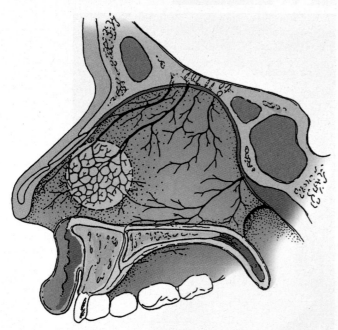

Fig 87–1
Nasal anatomy. Kiesselbach's plexus is the most common site of anterior epistaxis. The sphenopalatine artery is the most common site of posterior epistaxis. Tubes and instruments should be inserted in the direction of the nasopharynx, not the cribriform plate.
(From Fleisher GR, Ludwig S: Textbook of Pediatric Emergency Medicine. Philadelphia, Lippincott, Williams & Wilkins, 1999.)

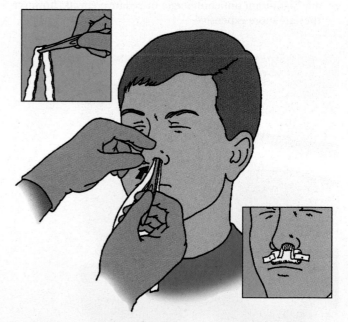

Fig 87–2
Anterior epistaxis from one side of the nasal cavity can be treated using nasal packing soaked in a vasoconstrictor. Vaseline-impregnated gauze or strips of nonadherent dressing can be packed in the nose so that both ends of the gauze remain outside the nasal cavity.
(From Auerbach P: Wilderness Medicine, 5th ed. St. Louis, Mosby, 2006.)

TREATMENT

- Digital compression or pinching of the lower soft cartilaginous part of the nose for 10 minutes is the method of choice.
- Cotton or tissue plug
- The patient should be sitting and leaning forward, breathing through the mouth, allowing blood to flow out of the nostrils as opposed to bending backward, which would allow the blood to flow down the throat.
- Application of cold compresses to the bridge of the nose, causing a vasoconstrictive effect; the patient may also suck on ice to achieve this effect.

Anterior epistaxis

- Local vasoconstriction is performed by moistening a cotton pledget with one of the following:
  1. 4% lidocaine with 1:1000 epinephrine
  2. 4% lidocaine with 1% phenylephrine (Neo-Synephrine)
  3. 4% lidocaine with 0.05% oxymetazoline (Afrin)
  4. 4% cocaine or cocaine 25% in paraffin base ointment, inserting the pledget into the nasal cavity with bayonet forceps
- Cauterization with silver nitrate or trichloroacetic acid is performed once hemostasis is achieved.
- Anterior nasal packing is needed when local measures are unsuccessful in controlling hemostasis. Nasal packing is performed under local anesthesia and is done by inserting petroleum jelly (Vaseline) gauze strips in layers from the floor of the nasal cavity to the front entrance of the nasal orifice (Fig. 87–2). Enough pressure is placed to tamponade the epistaxis.
- Other commercially available nasal packing, using sponge packs that expand when exposed to blood or moisture, can be used for anterior epistaxis.

Posterior epistaxis

- Posterior nasal packing
1. Commercially available nasal sponge packing can be applied.
2. Rolled gauze technique (Fig. 87–3)
- Foley catheter balloon insertion into the nasopharynx can be tried in patients with posterior epistaxis.
- If acute treatment fails to stop the bleeding or the site of bleeding cannot be located, electrocautery or endoscopic cauterization can be used.

- Electrocautery is performed after suitable anesthesia, such as application of a topical anesthetic followed by a local anesthetic injection. Only one side of the nasal septum should be cauterized at a time because perforation can result from bilateral cauterization.
- Arterial ligation or embolization has been used in refractory posterior epistaxis.
- For cases involving irritated or inflamed mucosa, a conservative regimen of triamcinolone 0.025%, neomycin undecenoate with bacitracin zinc (Nemdyn), chlorhexidine gluconate–phenylephrine hydrochloride (Nasalate), or equivalent cream should be applied once a week, combined with nightly application of a small quantity of petroleum jelly to the septum before bedtime.

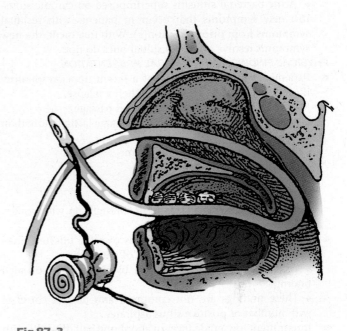

Fig 87–3
Inserting a posterior nasal pack.
(From Fleisher GR, Ludwig S: Textbook of Pediatric Emergency Medicine, Philadelphia, Lippincott, Williams & Wilkins, 1999.)

Chapter 88   **Sinusitis**

DEFINITION
Sinusitis is inflammation of the mucous membranes lining one or more of the paranasal sinuses. The various presentations are as folllows:

- Acute sinusitis: infection lasting less than 30 days, with complete resolution of symptoms
- Subacute infection: lasts from 30 to 90 days, with complete resolution of symptoms
- Recurrent acute infection: episodes of acute infection lasting less than 30 days, with resolution of symptoms, which recur at intervals of at least 10 days apart
- Chronic sinusitis: inflammation lasting more than 90 days, with persistent upper respiratory symptoms
- Acute bacterial sinusitis superimposed on chronic sinusitis: new symptoms that occur in patients with residual symptoms from prior infection(s). With treatment, the new symptoms resolve but the residual ones do not.

PHYSICAL FINDINGS AND CLINICAL PRESENTATION
- Patients often give a history of a recent upper respiratory illness with some improvement, then a relapse.
- Mucopurulent secretions in the nasal passage
  - Purulent nasal and postnasal discharge lasting more than 7 to 10 days
  - Facial tightness, pressure, or pain
  - Nasal obstruction
  - Headache
  - Decreased sense of smell
  - Purulent pharyngeal secretions, brought up with cough, often worse at night
- Erythema, swelling, and tenderness over the infected sinus (Fig. 88–1) in a small proportion of patients
  - Diagnosis cannot be excluded by the absence of such findings.
  - These findings are not common, and do not correlate with number of positive sinus aspirates.
- Intermittent low-grade fever in about one half of adults with acute bacterial sinusitis

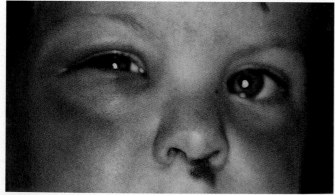

Fig 88–1
Acute sinusitis with facial swelling and periorbital edema.
(From Cohen J, Powderly WG: Infectious Diseases, 2nd ed. St. Louis, Mosby, 2004.)

- Toothache is a common complaint when the maxillary sinus is involved.
- Periorbital cellulitis and excessive tearing with ethmoid sinusitis
  - Orbital extension of infection: chemosis, proptosis, impaired extraocular movements
- Characteristics of acute sinusitis in children with upper respiratory tract infections:
  - Persistence of symptoms
  - Cough
  - Bad breath
- Symptoms of chronic sinusitis (may or may not be present)
  - Nasal or postnasal discharge
  - Fever
  - Facial pain or pressure
  - Headache
- Nosocomial sinusitis is typically seen in patients with nasogastric tubes or nasotracheal intubation.

CAUSE
- Each of the four paranasal sinuses is connected to the nasal cavity by narrow tubes (ostia), 1 to 3 mm in diameter; these drain directly into the nose through the turbinates. The sinuses are lined with a ciliated mucous membrane (mucoperiosteum).
- Acute viral infection
  - Infection with the common cold or influenza
  - Mucosal edema and sinus inflammation
  - Decreased drainage of thick secretions, obstruction of the sinus ostia
  - Subsequent entrapment of bacteria
    a. Multiplication of bacteria
    b. Secondary bacterial infection
- Other predisposing factors
  - Tumors
  - Polyps
  - Foreign bodies
  - Congenital choanal atresia
  - Other entities that cause obstruction of sinus drainage
  - Allergies
  - Asthma
- Dental infections lead to maxillary sinusitis.
- Viruses recovered alone or in combination with bacteria (in 16% of cases):
  - Rhinovirus
  - Coronavirus
  - Adenovirus
  - Parainfluenza virus
  - Respiratory syncytial virus
- The principal bacterial pathogens in sinusitis are *Streptococcus pneumoniae*, nontypeable *Haemophilus influenzae*, and *Moraxella catarrhalis*.
- In the remainder of cases, findings include *Streptococcus pyogenes*, *Staphylococcus aureus*, alpha-hemolytic streptococci, and mixed anaerobic infections (*Peptostreptococcus, Fusobacterium, Bacteroides, Prevotella*).

- Infection is polymicrobial in about one third of cases.
- Anaerobic infections seen more often in cases of chronic sinusitis and in cases associated with dental infection; anaerobes are unlikely pathogens in sinusitis in children.
- Fungal pathogens are isolated with increasing frequency in immunocompromised patients but remain uncommon pathogens in the paranasal sinuses. Fungal pathogens include *Aspergillus, Pseudallescheria, Sporothrix,* phaeohyphomycoses, Zygomycetes.
- Nosocomial infections occur in patients with nasogastric tubes, nasotracheal intubation, cystic fibrosis, or those who are immunocompromised.
  - *S. aureus*
  - *Pseudomonas aeruginosa*
  - *Klebsiella pneumoniae*
  - *Enterobacter* spp.
  - *Proteus mirabilis*
- Organisms typically isolated in chronic sinusitis:
  - *S. aureus*
  - *S. pneumoniae*
  - *H. influenzae*
  - *P. aeruginosa*
  - Anaerobes

DIFFERENTIAL DIAGNOSIS
- Migraine headache
- Cluster headache
- Dental infection
- Trigeminal neuralgia

WORKUP
- Water's projection: sinus radiograph (Fig. 88–2)
- CT scan (Fig. 88–3)
  - Much more sensitive than plain radiographs in detecting acute changes and disease in the sinuses
  - Recommended for patients requiring surgical intervention, including sinus aspiration; it is a useful adjunct to guide therapy.
- Transillumination (Fig. 88–4)
  - Used for diagnosis of frontal and maxillary sinusitis
  - Place transilluminator in the mouth or against cheek to assess maxillary sinuses, and under the medial aspect of the supraorbital ridge to assess frontal sinuses.
  - Absence of light transmission indicates that sinus is filled with fluid.
  - Dullness (decreased light transmission) is less helpful in diagnosing infection.
- Endoscopy
  - Used to visualize secretions coming from the ostia of infected sinuses
  - Culture collection via endoscopy often contaminated by nasal flora; not nearly as good as sinus puncture
- Sinus puncture
  - Gold standard for collecting sinus cultures
  - Generally reserved for treatment failures, suspected intracranial extension, nosocomial sinusitis

TREATMENT
Nonpharmacologic therapy
- Sinus drainage
- Nasal vasoconstrictors, such as phenylephrine nose drops, 0.25% or 0.5%

- Topical decongestants should not be used for more than a few days because of the risk of rebound congestion.
- Systemic decongestants
- Nasal or systemic corticosteroids, such as nasal beclomethasone, short-course oral prednisone
- Nasal irrigation, with hypertonic or normal saline (saline may act as a mild vasoconstrictor of nasal blood flow)
- Use of antihistamines has no proved benefit, and the drying effect on the mucous membranes may cause crusting, which blocks the ostia, thus interfering with sinus drainage.
- Analgesics, antipyretics

Antimicrobial therapy
- Most cases of acute sinusitis have a viral cause and will resolve within 2 weeks without antibiotics.
- Current treatment recommendations favor symptomatic treatment for those with mild symptoms.
- Antibiotics should be reserved for those with moderate to severe symptoms who meet the criteria for diagnosis of bacterial sinusitis.

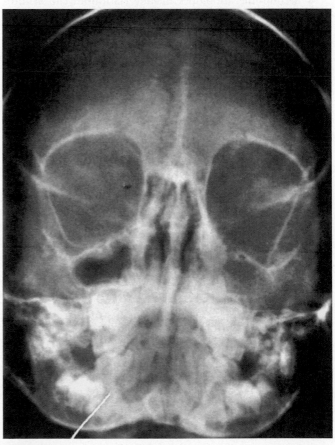

Fig 88–2
Sinus radiograph showing maxillary sinus opacification, Water's projection.
(From Wald ER: Rhinitis and acute and chronic sinusitis. In Bluestone CD, Stool SE, Kenna MA [eds]: Pediatric Otolaryngology, 3rd ed., Philadelphia, WB Saunders, 1996.)

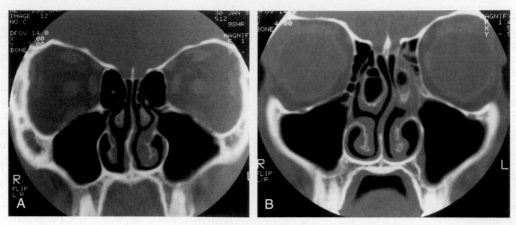

Fig 88-3
Coronal computed tomography scans of sinuses. **A,** Normal findings. **B,** Cancha bullosa and ethmoid sinusitis.
(From Woodson GE: Ear, Nose and Throat Disorders in Primary Care. Philadelphia, WB Saunders, 2001.)

- Antibiotic therapy is usually empirical, targeting the common pathogens.
- First-line antibiotics include amoxicillin, TMP-SMZ.
- Second-line antibiotics include clarithromycin, azithromycin, amoxicillin-clavulanate, cefuroxime axetil, loracarbef, ciprofloxacin, levofloxacin.
- For patients with uncomplicated acute sinusitis, the less expensive first-line agents appear to be as effective as the costlier second-line agents.

Surgery
- Surgical drainage indicated
- If intracranial or orbital complications suspected
- For many cases of frontal and sphenoid sinusitis
- For chronic sinusitis recalcitrant to medical therapy
- Surgical débridement imperative for treatment of fungal sinusitis

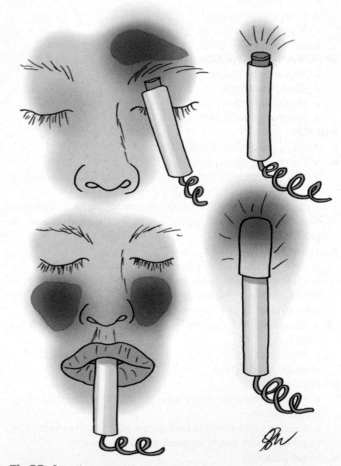

Fig 88-4
Technique of sinus transillumination. **Upper panel,** Frontal sinus.
Lower panel, Maxillary sinus. Dotted lines indicate transilluminated areas; light sources are shown at right.
(From Woodson GE: Ear, Nose and Throat Disorders in Primary Care. Philadelphia, WB Saunders, 2001.)

MOUTH AND TONGUE

Chapter 89 | **Diseases of the oral mucosa**

- Figure 89–1 shows a normal mouth. A normal palate histology is seen in Figure 89–2, and the normal buccal mucosa epithelium can be seen in Figure 89–3.

A. TUMOR-LIKE LESIONS

(1) Oral lymphoepithelial cyst: painless yellowish nodules usually less than 1 cm in diameter most commonly affecting the floor of the mouth, posterior ventral tongue, soft palate, and tonsillar fauces (Fig. 89–4). They are commonly filled with cheesy keratinoceous material and occur generally in the fourth decade of life, with an equal gender distribution.

DIAGNOSIS
- Biopsy

TREATMENT
- Surgical removal

(2) Congenital granular cell epulis: soft tissue tumor presenting as a pink, pedunculated mass, usually on the anterior alveolar ridge, with an intact surface (Fig. 89–5). There is a 10:1 female predilection and it is three times more common in the maxilla. Approximately 9% of patients have multiple nodules and some may have concurrent tongue lesions.

DIAGNOSIS
- Biopsy

TREATMENT
- Surgical removal

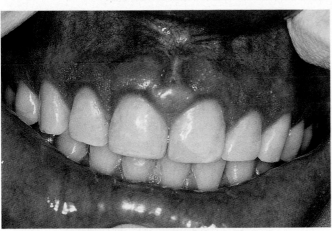

Fig 89–1
Normal mouth. Note the maxillary sulcus, attached, and nonattached gingiva and teeth.
(From McKee PH, Calonje E, Granter SR [eds]: Pathology of the Skin With Clinical Correlations, 3rd ed. St. Louis, Mosby, 2005.)

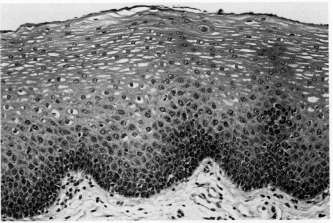

Fig 89–3
Normal buccal mucosa. The epithelium is nonkeratinized and is 12 to 25 cells thick.
(From McKee PH, Calonje E, Granter SR [eds]: Pathology of the Skin With Clinical Correlations, 3rd ed. St. Louis, Mosby, 2005.)

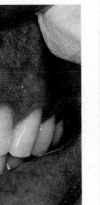

Fig 89–2
Normal palate. The palate and gingiva are thinly keratinized. The dense fibrous tissue beneath is normal for these sites.
(From McKee PH, Calonje E, Granter SR [eds]: Pathology of the Skin With Clinical Correlations, 3rd ed. St. Louis, Mosby, 2005.)

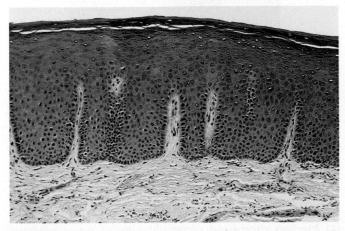

Fig 89–4
Oral lymphoepithelial cyst. Note the yellow nodule located behind the anterior faucial pillar.
(From McKee PH, Calonje E, Granter SR [eds]: Pathology of the Skin With Clinical Correlations, 3rd ed. St. Louis, Mosby, 2005.)

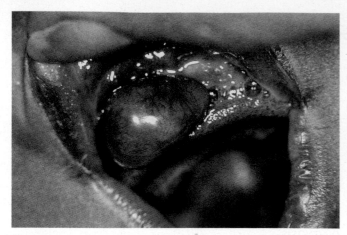

Fig 89–5
Congenital granular cell epulis. The maxillary alveolus is a typical location for this tumor.
(Courtesy of Dr. B. Padwa, DDS, Boston.)

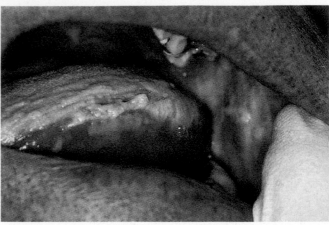

Fig 89–7
Chronic bite injury. Note the macerated shaggy plaques on the buccal mucosa and lateral border of the tongue.
(From McKee PH, Calonje E, Granter SR [eds]: Pathology of the Skin With Clinical Correlations, 3rd ed. St. Louis, Mosby, 2005.)

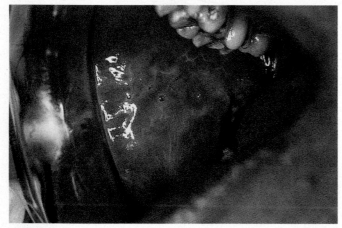

Fig 89–6
Leukoedema. Note the pale milky film on the buccal mucosa.
(From McKee PH, Calonje E, Granter SR [eds]: Pathology of the Skin With Clinical Correlations, 3rd ed. St. Louis, Mosby, 2005.)

B. REACTIVE CONDITIONS

(1) Leukoedema: benign, painless condition usually affecting the buccal mucosa bilaterally. The mucosa has a diffuse gray-white opalescent hue with vertical wrinkles and streaks (Fig. 89–6) that usually disappear on stretching. There is an increased incidence of this condition in users of tobacco, cannabis, and coca leaves.

(2) Chronic bite injury: lesions occurring as a result of cheek, lip, or tongue biting habits as part of a neurosis or as a conscious habit or self-mutilating behavior. The site of injury exhibits shaggy white plaques that have a peeling, desquamative surface; erosions are often present, and occasionally ulcers are seen (Fig. 89–7).

(3) Benign migratory glossitis: these tongue lesions appear as recurrent, erythematous, and atrophic areas with a serpiginous white, slightly raised border that may appear annular or scalloped (Fig. 89–8). These "maplike" areas migrate and change shape over the tongue dorsum as the condition resolves

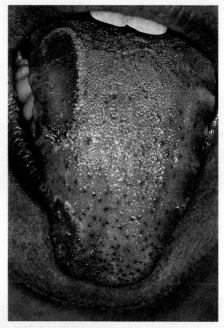

Fig 89–8
Benign migratory glossitis. Note the erythematous depapillated area rimmed by a white margin.
(From McKee PH, Calonje E, Granter SR [eds]: Pathology of the Skin With Clinical Correlations, 3rd ed. St. Louis, Mosby, 2005.)

at one edge and involves another. Some lesions are, however, stationary. Pain, in the form of a burning or sensitivity, may or may not be present. One fifth of patients have a concurrent fissured tongue.

(4) Median rhomboid glossitis: form of oral candidiasis that occurs specifically in the midline of the tongue just anterior to the circumvallate papillae (Fig. 89–9). Diagnosis depends on the presence of psoriasiform mucositis, with spongiolitic pustules associated with candidal hyphae.

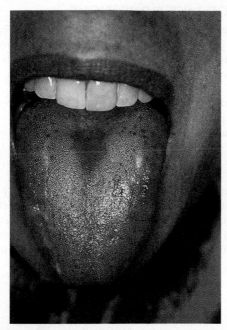

Fig 89–9
Median rhomboid glossitis. There is a typical rhomboid-shaped area in the posterior midline of the tongue.
(From McKee PH, Calonje E, Granter SR [eds]: Pathology of the Skin With Clinical Correlations, 3rd ed. St. Louis, Mosby, 2005.)

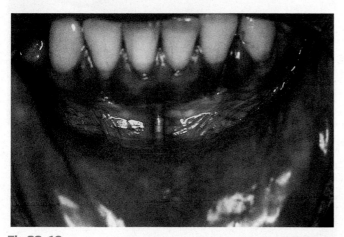

Fig 89–10
Smokeless tobacco keratosis. Note the milky white, pale, wrinkled mandibular sulcular mucosa.
(From McKee PH, Calonje E, Granter SR [eds]: Pathology of the Skin With Clinical Correlations, 3rd ed. St. Louis, Mosby, 2005.)

(5) Smokeless tobacco keratosis: the severity of oral lesions is proportionate to the duration of use and the amount of smokeless tobacco in contact with the mucosa. Early and mild lesions show slight wrinkling and pallor of the mucosa, whereas more advanced lesions show deep furrows and thickened white mucosa, more typical of leukoplakia (Fig. 89–10)

C. ULCERATIVE CONDITIONS

(1) Recurrent aphthous stomatitis: disorder occurring in 15% to 20% of the adult population, generally younger than 40 years. It is a chronic, painful, relapsing ulcerative condition of

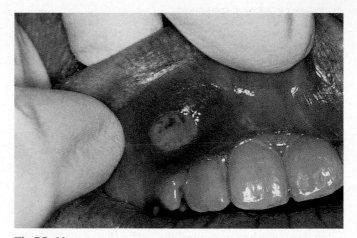

Fig 89–11
Recurrent aphthous ulcer. A typical aphthous ulcer is noted on the upper labial mucosa.
(From McKee PH, Calonje E, Granter SR [eds]: Pathology of the Skin With Clinical Correlations, 3rd ed. St. Louis, Mosby, 2005.)

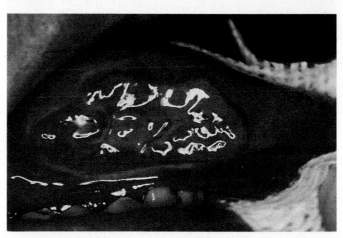

Fig 89–12
Traumatic ulcerative granuloma. This patient had bitten her tongue during a seizure and the indurated mass developed over a few days.
(From McKee PH, Calonje E, Granter SR [eds]: Pathology of the Skin With Clinical Correlations, 3rd ed. St. Louis, Mosby, 2005.)

the nonkeratinized mucosa (Fig. 89–11). There are three variants: minor, major, and herpetiform. Ulcers of the minor form (the most common variant) are less than 1 cm, last 7 to 14 days, and heal without scarring. Ulcers of the major form are usually >1 cm, last many weeks, and heal with scarring. Ulcers of the herpetiform variety occur in small crops of 10 to 100 ulcers in any one episode. Some conditions frequently associated with the minor variant include Behçet's disease, inflammatory bowel disease, and gluten sensitivity.

(2) Traumatic ulcerative granuloma: lesion affects the lateral tongue (64% of cases), followed by the buccal mucosa, and manifests as an ulcer or indurated area persisting for weeks or months (Fig. 89–12). The lack of pain, often a feature of this condition, raises the clinical suspicion of squamous cell carcinoma. A history of trauma is elicited in only 50% of cases.

D. PAPILLARY LESIONS

(1) Squamous papilloma: generally present in adults in the second to fourth decades and manifests as a white or erythematous lesion with a warty, finger-like, or cauliflower-like appearance (Fig. 89–13). Sites of predilection include the soft palate–uvula complex and the tongue, although any region in the oral cavity may be affected. Differential diagnosis includes verruca vulgaris and oral condyloma acuminatum (Fig. 89–14). The latter occurs most commonly in patients who are on long-term immunosuppression, such as organ transplant patients.

(2) Verruciform xanthoma: most frequently affects adults in the fourth and fifth decades. It presents with a well-circumscribed rough, granular or pebbly, raised or depressed, yellowish, reddish, or gray plaque. Seventy percent occur primarily on the keratinized attached mucosa of the palate (Fig. 89–15) or gingival or alveolar ridge mucosa, which are areas constantly traumatized by mastication. It also occurs in association with lichen planus, pemphigus vulgaris, discoid lupus erythematosus, and following bone marrow transplantation.

E. TUMOR-LIKE CONDITIONS

(1) Fibroma: most common tumor-like condition in the mouth. It is usually located at sites of trauma. It presents as a fleshy, pedunculated, or sessile dome-shaped nodule that may be mucosa-colored, ulcerated, or hyperkeratotic (Fig. 89–16).

(2) Lipoma: presents as a yellowish, soft and doughy, painless, sessile or pedunculated nodule that generally occurs on the buccal mucosa or sulcus (Fig. 89–17). Some lipomas of the buccal mucosa are not true tumors but represent herniation of the buccal fat pad.

(3) Denture-associated fibrous hyperplasia: presents as a linear mass of tissue arising in the mucobuccal sulcus around the flange of poorly fitting dentures. The anterior maxillary and mandibular sulci are the preferred sites of involvement (Fig. 89–18). There is a 3:1 female predisposition and most commonly occurs in the sixth decade.

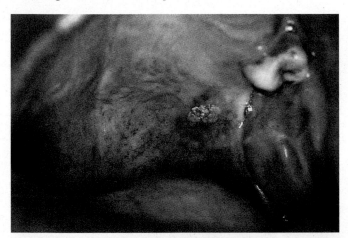

Fig 89–13
Squamous papilloma. There is a rough, warty lesion of the soft palate.
(From McKee PH, Calonje E, Granter SR [eds]: Pathology of the Skin With Clinical Correlations, 3rd ed. St. Louis, Mosby, 2005.)

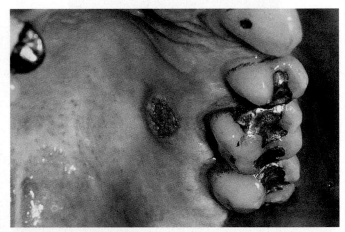

Fig 89–15
Verruciform xanthoma. Note the warty sessile lesion on the left hard palate.
(Courtesy of Dr. C. Allen, DDS, Columbus, Ohio.)

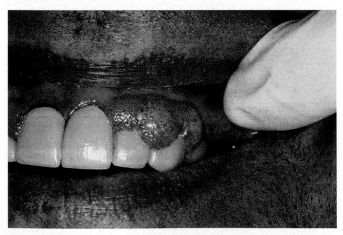

Fig 89–14
Condyloma acuminatum. This larger warty lesion on the gingiva occurred in a patient on long-term immunosuppression to prevent organ rejection.
(From McKee PH, Calonje E, Granter SR [eds]: Pathology of the Skin With Clinical Correlations, 3rd ed. St. Louis, Mosby, 2005.)

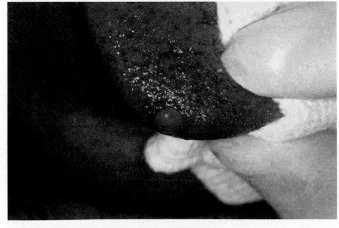

Fig 89–16
Fibroma. The lateral border of the tongue is a common site for a fibroma.
(From McKee PH, Calonje E, Granter SR [eds]: Pathology of the Skin With Clinical Correlations, 3rd ed. St. Louis, Mosby, 2005.)

(4) Gingival nodules: most solitary gingival nodules represent one of the following conditions: reactive tumor-like proliferations (most common), odontogenic cysts, primary odontogenic and nonodontogenic tumors, and metastatic tumors. These lesions are located on the attached or marginal gingiva adjacent to teeth. Depending on the degree of vascularity, inflammation, and/or ulceration present, they may be mucosa-colored, erythematous, or ulcerated and painful (Fig. 89–19).

(5) Pyogenic granuloma: these nodules tend to be dark red and bleed readily. One variant of this lesion, granuloma gravidarum, occurs during pregnancy, usually in the second or third trimester, probably as a consequence of the neovascularizing effects of estrogen (Fig. 89–20). The majority present in the second or third trimester. Histologically, gingival pyogenic granulomas are characterized by a lobular or diffuse proliferation of endothelial cells, many of which form canalized and congested capillaries. Pyogenic granulomas occurring outside of the buccal mucosa are described in Section 1.

(6) Generalized gingival hyperplasia: in this condition initially there is nodular hyperplasia in the interdental areas, which then coalesces to form diffuse nodular or papillary masses. The gingiva may be edematous and boggy, or can be firm, fibrotic and so proliferative as to reach the biting surfaces. Provoking factors include poor oral hygiene (Fig. 89–21), ingestion of medications (e.g., phenytoin, valproic acid, cyclosporine, calcium channel blockers), and hormonal influences (e.g., puberty, pregnancy) (Fig. 89–22).

(7) Varix (venous lake): dilation of an endothelium-lined blood vessel with a very thin muscular wall. These are bluish-purple blebs that may become firm if thrombosed (Fig. 89–23). They are found most frequently on the ventral surfaces of the tongue and on the lower lip and buccal mucosa, usually in older individuals.

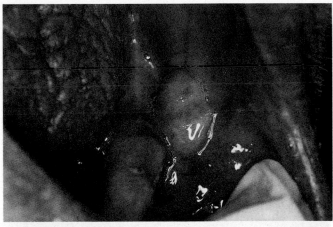

Fig 89–17
Lipoma. Note the yellowish nodule on the buccal mucosa.
(From McKee PH, Calonje E, Granter SR [eds]: Pathology of the Skin With Clinical Correlations, 3rd ed. St. Louis, Mosby, 2005.)

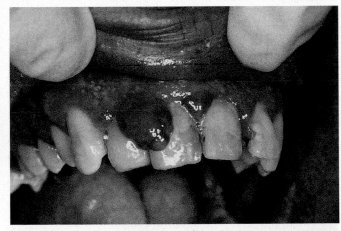

Fig 89–19
Gingival nodule. Note how the nodule arises from the gingival margin and hangs down onto the tooth.
(From McKee PH, Calonje E, Granter SR [eds]: Pathology of the Skin With Clinical Correlations, 3rd ed. St. Louis, Mosby, 2005.)

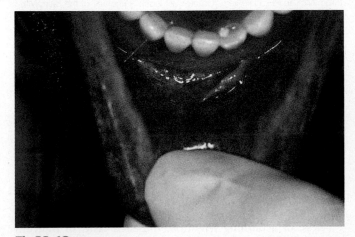

Fig 89–18
Denture-induced fibrous hyperplasia. The denture flange (edge) fits into the fissure.
(From McKee PH, Calonje E, Granter SR [eds]: Pathology of the Skin With Clinical Correlations, 3rd ed. St. Louis, Mosby, 2005.)

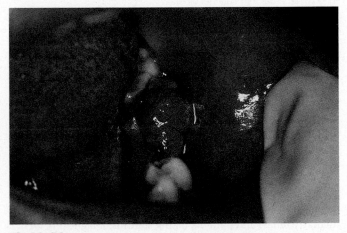

Fig 89–20
Granuloma gravidarum. This nodule occurred in an edentulous part of the mandible.
(From McKee PH, Calonje E, Granter SR [eds]: Pathology of the Skin With Clinical Correlations, 3rd ed. St. Louis, Mosby, 2005.)

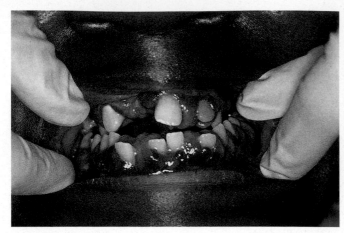

Fig 89–21
Generalized gingival hyperplasia. This overgrowth of gingiva was caused by poor oral hygiene.
(From McKee PH, Calonje E, Granter SR [eds]: Pathology of the Skin With Clinical Correlations, 3rd ed. St. Louis, Mosby, 2005.)

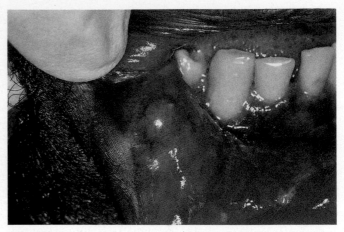

Fig 89–23
Varix. Note the blue bleb on the lower labial mucosa.
(From McKee PH, Calonje E, Granter SR [eds]: Pathology of the Skin With Clinical Correlations, 3rd ed. St. Louis, Mosby, 2005.)

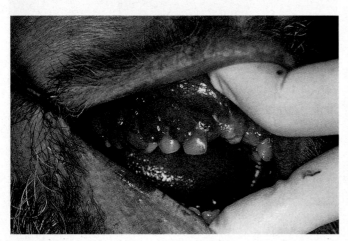

Fig 89–22
Cyclosporine-induced gingival hyperplasia. This patient was taking cyclosprine to prevent rejection of a renal allograft; he was also taking nifedipine, a calcium channel blocker.
(From McKee PH, Calonje E, Granter SR [eds]: Pathology of the Skin With Clinical Correlations, 3rd ed. St. Louis, Mosby, 2005.)

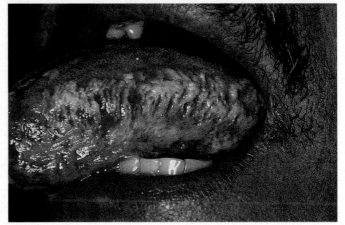

Fig 89–24
Hairy leukoplakia. The thick white plaque on the lateral border of the tongue has typical vertical fissures.
(From McKee PH, Calonje E, Granter SR [eds]: Pathology of the Skin With Clinical Correlations, 3rd ed. St. Louis, Mosby, 2005.)

F. INFECTIONS

(1) Hairy leukoplakia

DEFINITION
Oral hairy leukoplakia (OHL) is a painless, white, nonremovable, plaquelike lesion, typically located on the lateral aspect of the tongue.

RISK FACTORS
OHL is usually found in human immunodeficiency virus (HIV) seropositive individuals but may also be identified in other immunocompromised patients, such as transplant recipients (particularly renal) and patients taking steroids. Diagnosing OHL is an indication to institute a workup to evaluate for HIV infection and immunosuppressed stable.

PHYSICAL FINDINGS AND CLINICAL PRESENTATION
- Varying morphology and appearance
- May be unilateral or bilateral

- White plaque can be small, with fine vertical corrugations on the lateral margin of the tongue (Fig. 89–24)
- Irregular surface; may have prominent folds or projection, occasionally markedly resembling hairs (Fig. 89–25)
- May spread to cover the entire dorsal surface or spread onto the ventral surface of the tongue, where they usually appear flat
- Rarely, lesions manifest on the soft palate, buccal mucosa, and posterior oropharynx
- Usually asymptomatic, but some have mouth pain, soreness, or a burning sensation, impaired taste, or difficulty eating; others complain of its unsightly appearance.
- OHL may progress to oral squamous cell carcinoma, which has a poor prognosis.

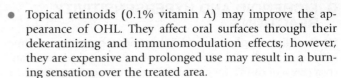
CAUSE

- Epstein-Barr virus (EBV) is implicated in its cause, and OHL is a result of replication of EBV in the epithelium of keratinized cells. OHL differs from most EBV-related diseases in that infection is predominantly lytic rather than latent.

DIFFERENTIAL DIAGNOSIS

- *Candida albicans* (see Fig. 89–28)
- Focal epithelial hyperplasia (Fig. 89–26)
- Lichen planus (Fig. 89–27)
- Idiopathic leukoplakia (see Fig. 89–37)
- White sponge nevus
- Squamous cell carcinoma (see Fig. 89–38)

TREATMENT

- OHL is usually asymptomatic and requires no specific therapy. It may resolve spontaneously and has no known premalignant potential.
- Highly active antiretroviral therapy (HAART) has considerably changed the frequency of oral lesions caused by opportunistic infections in HIV-seropositive individuals.

- Topical retinoids (0.1% vitamin A) may improve the appearance of OHL. They affect oral surfaces through their dekeratinizing and immunomodulation effects; however, they are expensive and prolonged use may result in a burning sensation over the treated area.
- Surgical excision and cryotherapy may help, but the lesions may recur.
- High-dose acyclovir, ganciclovir, or foscarnet will cause lesions to resolve only temporarily.

(2) Focal epithelial hyperplasia (Heck's disease): benign epithelial hyperplasia appearing as mucosa-colored papules or nodules that sometimes appear papillary (see Fig. 89–26). Lesions are almost always multiple and multifocal, favoring the labial mucosa, lips, buccal mucosa, and lateral tongue. Females are affected twice as often as males. The condition tends to regress over time. Human papilloma virus (HPV) has been identified in almost 50% of cases. It also occurs in patients infected with HIV.

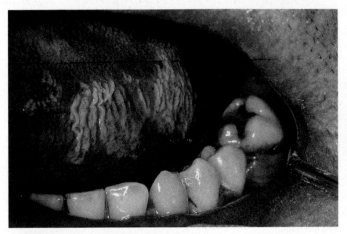

Fig 89-25
Oral hairy leukoplakia. Shown are the characteristic delicate linear white lesions on the tongue.
(Courtesy of Dr. P.R. Morgan, Institute of Dermatology, London.)

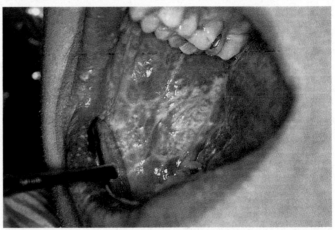

Fig 89-27
Oral lichen planus. Shown are Wickham's striae of reticular lichen planus with mild erythema.
(From McKee PH, Calonje E, Granter SR [eds]: Pathology of the Skin With Clinical Correlations, 3rd ed. St. Louis, Mosby, 2005.)

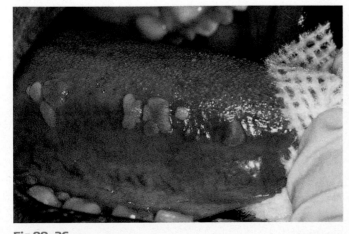

Fig 89-26
Focal epithelial hyperplasia (Heck's disease). The lesions are pale fleshy papules.
(From McKee PH, Calonje E, Granter SR [eds]: Pathology of the Skin With Clinical Correlations, 3rd ed. St. Louis, Mosby, 2005.)

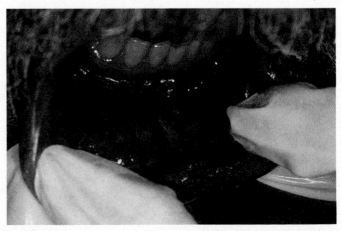

Fig 89-28
Oral Crohn's disease. Note the fissures and cobblestoning of the lower labial mucosa.
(From McKee PH, Calonje E, Granter SR [eds]: Pathology of the Skin With Clinical Correlations, 3rd ed. St. Louis, Mosby, 2005.)

G. LICHENOID AND HYPERSENSITIVITY REACTIONS

(1) Oral lichen planus and lichenoid stomatitis: chronic inflammatory condition of the mouth affecting the buccal mucosa (85% of cases), tongue, and gingiva. It occurs in 1% to 2% of the population, more commonly in women, and in the sixth decade. Clinically, it can present with three main variants: reticular and/or papular form in which lesions have classic lacy white keratotic striations (Wickham's striae; see Fig. 89–27), erythematous (or erosive) form in which lesions consist of reddened mucosa, and ulcerative form which presents with a yellow painful fibrinous exudates on the surface.
DIAGNOSIS
● Biopsy and direct immunofluorescence studies

(2) Oral Crohn's disease: presents usually with swelling of the face or lips. Additionally, there may be linear vestibular aphtheiform ulcers, angular cheilitis, papulous and polypoid masses, mucosal tags, gingival erythema, and cobblestoning of the mucosa (see Fig. 89–28). In 22% to 60% of cases, oral symptoms precede intestinal symptoms.
DIAGNOSIS
● Biopsy and direct immunofluorescence studies
For additional information on this disorder, see Section 7.

(3) Wegener's granulomatosis: oral involvement occurs in 5% of patients. The gingival is hyperplastic, often with a friable, granular, erythematous to magenta appearance, so-called "strawberry gingivitis" (Fig. 89–29). For additional information on this disorder, see Section 6.

H. AUTOIMMUNE CONDITIONS

(1) Cicatricial pemphigoid: most common autoimmune subepithelial blistering disease presenting in the mouth. The oral cavity is affected in 90% of cases and the conjunctiva in 70%. Other sites of involvement include the upper airway (45%), skin (30%), and genitalia (15%). In the mouth, the gingiva is most frequently affected. Lesions present as painful areas of erosion, erythema, and ulceration. Desquamative gingivitis (Fig. 89–30) may be the sole manifestation of cicatricial pemphigoid in 60% of cases.
DIAGNOSIS
● Biopsy and direct immunofluorescence studies

(2) Pemphigus: oral pemphigus typically begins in the sixth decade of life. Lesions in the oral cavity precede those at other sites in most cases. The buccal mucosa, tongue, palate and floor of mouth are most often affected (Fig. 89–31).
DIAGNOSIS
● Biopsy and direct immunofluorescence studies
For additional information on this disorder, see Section 1.

(3) Linear IgA disease: oral mucosal lesions associated with linear IgA disease occur in 26% to 100% of cases and present as vesicles, bullae, erosions, or ulcerations. The condi-

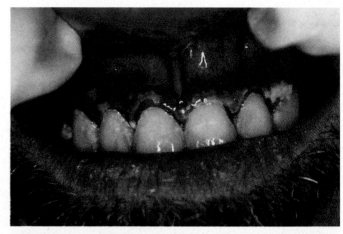

Fig 89–30
Cicatricial pemphigoid. This typical case presented with erythematous gingiva and white epithelial sloughs.
(From McKee PH, Calonje E, Granter SR [eds]: Pathology of the Skin With Clinical Correlations, 3rd ed. St. Louis, Mosby, 2005.)

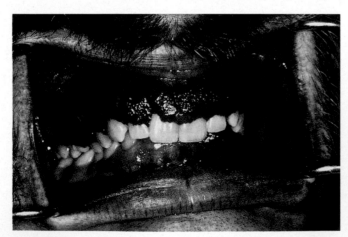

Fig 89–29
Oral Wegener's granulomatosis. Note the typical "strawberry gingivitis."
(Courtesy of Dr. S. Zunt, DDS, Indianapolis.)

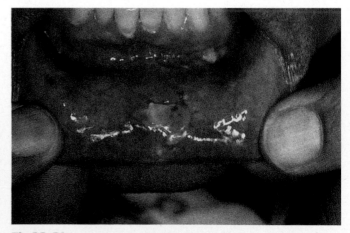

Fig 89–31
Pemphigus vulgaris. This patient presented with an ulcer on the lower labial mucosa.
(From McKee PH, Calonje E, Granter SR [eds]: Pathology of the Skin With Clinical Correlations, 3rd ed. St. Louis, Mosby, 2005.)

tion sometimes manifests as desquamative gingivitis and erosive cheilitis (Fig. 89–32).

DIAGNOSIS
● Biopsy and direct immunofluorescence studies

I. REACTIVE SALIVARY DISEASE

(1) Mucocele (ranula, salivary gland cyst): dome-shaped fluctuant, bluish (Fig. 89–33) and sessile lesion, which often increases or decreases in size. The most frequent variant is the mucous extravasation type, caused by a tear in the excretory duct and spillage of mucin into the connective tissue. This usually arises in children and young adults and the most common location is the lower labial mucosa (Fig. 89–34).

(2) Nicotinic stomatitis: early lesions appear as small red punctuate areas sometimes associated with whitening of the surrounding mucosa on the posterior half of the palate. Involvement is usually symmetrical, As the lesions progress, the palate may take on a cobblestone appearance, with raised white papules having slightly umbilicated central puncta (Fig. 89–35). The red puncta represent the inflamed ostia of the excretory salivary ducts. Nicotinic stomatitis is associated with pipe smoking. Its severity is proportional to the duration of the habit. It is reversible after cessation of pipe smoking. It is caused by the heat of the pipe smoke and not the nicotine itself. The condition has also been noted in patients who consume hot beverages.

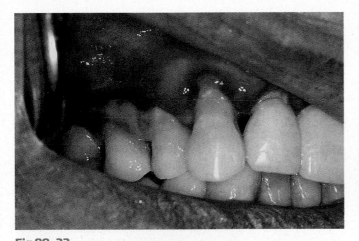

Fig 89–32
Linear IgA disease. This erythema and ulceration of the gingiva is clinically considered a desquamative gingivitis.
(From McKee PH, Calonje E, Granter SR [eds]: Pathology of the Skin With Clinical Correlations, 3rd ed. St. Louis, Mosby, 2005.)

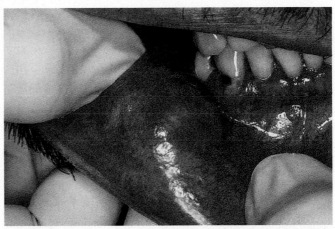

Fig 89–34
Mucocele. Note the bluish sessile nodule on the lower labial mucosa, a typical site.
(From McKee PH, Calonje E, Granter SR [eds]: Pathology of the Skin With Clinical Correlations, 3rd ed. St. Louis, Mosby, 2005.)

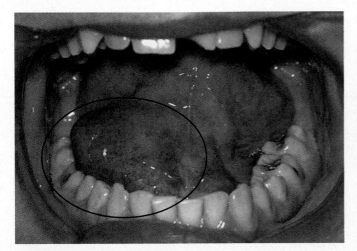

Fig 89–33
Mucocele (Ranula, salivary gland cyst).
(From Swartz MH: Textbook of Physical Diagnosis, 5th ed. Philadelphia, WB Saunders, 2006.)

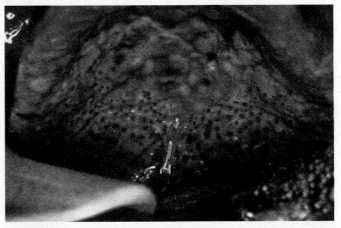

Fig 89–35
Nicotinic stomatis. Note the cobblestone appearance of the hard palate in a smoker.
(Courtesy of Dr. L. Lee, DDS, Toronto, Canada.)

J. LEUKOPLAKIA

This oral lesion is defined as a white plaque that does not wipe off and cannot be characterized clinically or pathologically as any other disease; it is not associated with any physical or chemical agent, except tobacco. Clinically, lesions may appear homogeneous (in color and texture; Fig. 89–36) or nonhomogeneous (known as erythroleukoplakia; Fig. 89–37). The most common sites are the buccal mucosa, gingival-alveolar mucosa, and palate. Dysplasia, carcinoma in situ, or invasive squamous cell carcinoma is present in 9% to 34% of leukoplakias overall.

K. SQUAMOUS CELL CARCINOMA

The most common malignancy in the oral cavity, accounting for more than 90% of all oral cancers. In the United States, it constitutes 3% of all malignancies and accounts for 30,000 cancer cases diagnosed annually. The two most significant risk factors are cigarette smoking and excessive alcohol consumption. Other risk factors include HPV infection, history of previous oral squamous carcinoma, history of cancer elsewhere in the body, and history of immunosuppression. The tumor may present initially as plaque lesions of leukoplakia or nonhealing ulcers, masses, or nodules (Fig. 89–38). For additional information on this disorder, see Section 1.22h.

L. BENIGN PIGMENTED LESIONS

(1) Amalgam tattoo: asymptomatic gray, bluish, black, or slate-colored macules that generally occur on the gingival-alveolar ridge (Fig. 89–39) or buccal mucosa. Particles of amalgam restorations may be traumatically implanted into the mucosa by the dentist during placement or removal of a restoration,

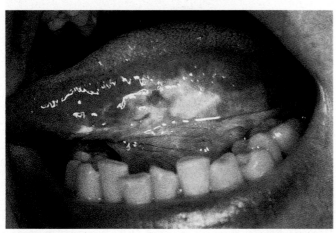

Fig 89–36
Leukoplakia. This leukoplakia exhibited severe epithelial dysplasia.
(From McKee PH, Calonje E, Granter SR [eds]: Pathology of the Skin With Clinical Correlations, 3rd ed. St. Louis, Mosby, 2005.)

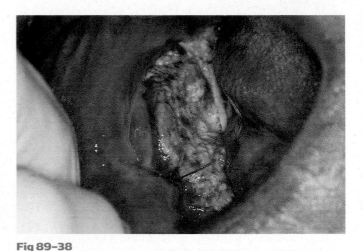

Fig 89–38
Squamous cell carcinoma. There is a fungating mass on the buccal mucosa.
(From McKee PH, Calonje E, Granter SR [eds]: Pathology of the Skin With Clinical Correlations, 3rd ed. St. Louis, Mosby, 2005.)

Fig 89–37
Leukoplakia. There is an area of nonhomogenous leukoplakia on the buccal mucosa. This exhibited moderate dysplasia.
(From McKee PH, Calonje E, Granter SR [eds]: Pathology of the Skin With Clinical Correlations, 3rd ed. St. Louis, Mosby, 2005.)

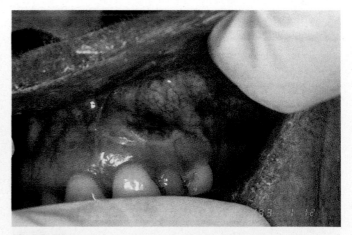

Fig 89–39
Amalgam tattoo. There is a blue-black macule on the attached gingiva superior to a semilunar scar. This tattoo is caused by a root canal–related surgical procedure.
(From McKee PH, Calonje E, Granter SR [eds]: Pathology of the Skin With Clinical Correlations, 3rd ed. St. Louis, Mosby, 2005.)

by the patient from bite injury, from leakage and disintegration of a restoration (or root canal filling material), or from a restoration falling into a tooth socket after extraction.

(2) Oral melanocytic macule: well-defined, brown to black macules measuring less than 1.5 cm and occurring on the lips (usually lower; Fig. 89–40), palate, or gingival or buccal mucosa. Biopsy is usually performed to exclude a melanoma.

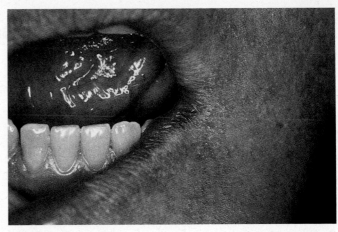

Fig 89–40
Oral melanotic macule. Note the typical dark brown to black macule on the vermillion.
(From McKee PH, Calonje E, Granter SR [eds]: Pathology of the Skin With Clinical Correlations, 3rd ed. St. Louis, Mosby, 2005.)

Chapter 90   Dental and periodontal infections

CAUSE

- Most periodontal disease arises from an anti-inflammatory response to the accumulation of dental plaque in the gingival margin.
- Plaque contains mainly *Streptococcus* and *Actinomyces* spp., which generate an early gingivitis leading ultimately to periodontitis.
- The indigenous oral flora includes aerobic and anaerobic bacteria.
- Dental caries are usually polymicrobial, whereas gingivitis has microbial specificity.
- When abscesses form, the flora is always polymicrobial (*Fusobacteria, Bacteroides, Peptostreptococcus, Actinomyces, Streptococcus*).
- Dental pulp infections can lead to involvement of the maxillary and mandibular spaces (Fig. 90–1)
- Spread of the infection from maxillary (upper) teeth most commonly leads to vestibular abscesses (Fig. 90–2).

CLINICAL MANIFESTATIONS

- In simple gingivitis, there is usually discoloration of the gum margin, with occasional bleeding after brushing of the teeth.
- Halitosis may be present.
- Peridontal tissue destruction and loosening of the teeth are present with chronic gingivitis.
- Canine space abscesses can produce swelling lateral to the nose, which usually obliterates the nasolabial fold.

- Buccal space abscesses can result when pulp abscesses of the molar teeth erode above or below the attachment of the buccinator muscle. These abscesses point below the zycomatic arch and above the inferior border of the mandible (Fig. 90–3).
- Deeper abscesses may point into the sublingual and submandibular spaces.

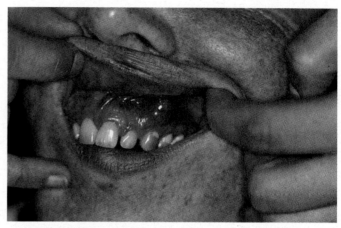

Fig 90–2
Painful vestibular abscess.
(Courtesy of Professor I. Brook.)

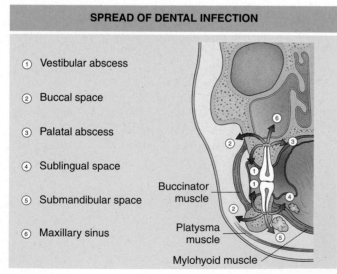

SPREAD OF DENTAL INFECTION

1. Vestibular abscess
2. Buccal space
3. Palatal abscess
4. Sublingual space
5. Submandibular space
6. Maxillary sinus

Buccinator muscle
Platysma muscle
Mylohyoid muscle

Fig 90–1
Spread of dental infection. A spreading tooth abscess will encroach on the nearest cortical plate and its subsequent spread depends on the relationship of that site to muscle attachment.

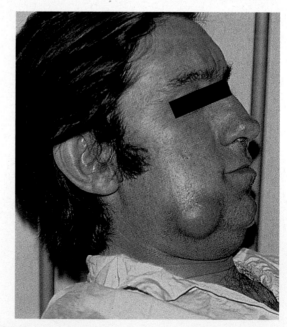

Fig 90–3
Buccal space abscess originating from right lower molar infection. The buccal space lies between the buccinator muscle and the overlying skin and fascia.
(Courtesy of Professor I. Brook.)

- Occasionally, abscesses may point spontaneously and rupture (Fig. 90–4).
- Erythema and swelling of the face may mimic periorbital cellulitis (Fig. 90–5).

TREATMENT:
- Antibiotics
- Surgical drainage
- Treatment of periodontal disease

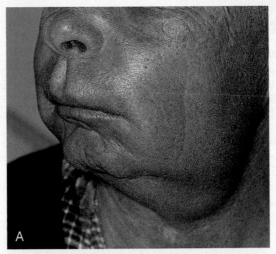

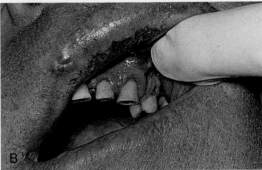

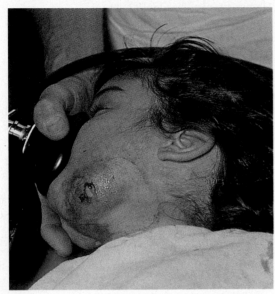

Fig 90–4
Submandibular abscess originating from a second molar tooth infection.
(Courtesy of the University of Sheffield School of Dentistry, Sheffield, England.)

Fig 90–5
Erythema and swelling of the face caused by a tooth abscess.
A, Swelling of the face. On examination, this resembled periorbital cellulitis. **B,** Further examination reveals a gingival abscess above the patient's left upper canine tooth.
(From Cohen J, Powderly WG: Infectious Diseases, 2nd ed. St. Louis, Mosby, 2004.)

Chapter 91 Herpangina

DEFINITION

Herpangina is a self-limited upper respiratory tract infection associated with a characteristic vesicular rash on the soft palate.

PHYSICAL FINDINGS AND CLINICAL PRESENTATION

- Characterized by ulcerating lesions typically located on the soft palate (Fig. 91–1)
- Usually fewer than six lesions that evolve rapidly from a diffuse pharyngitis to erythematous macules and subsequently to vesicles that are moderately painful
- Fever, vomiting, and headache in the first few days of illness but these subside spontaneously
- Pharyngeal lesions typical for several more days

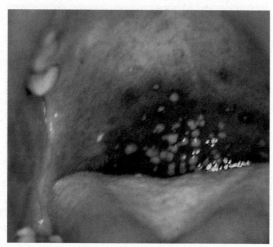

Fig 91–1
Herpangina in a teenager with severe throat pain.
(From Cohen J, Powderly WG: Infectious Diseases, 2nd ed. St. Louis, Mosby, 2004.)

CAUSE

- Most caused by coxsackie A viruses (A2, A4, A5, A6, and A10)
- Occasional cases caused by other enteroviruses (echovirus and enterovirus 71)

DIFFERENTIAL DIAGNOSIS

- Herpes simplex (see Fig. 92–1)
- Bacterial pharyngitis (see Fig. 96–3)
- Tonsillitis/pharyngitis (see Fig. 96–2)
- Aphthous stomatitis (see Fig. 89–1)
- Hand-foot-and-mouth disease (see Fig. 27–22)
- Viral pharyngitis (see Fig. 96–2)

LABORATORY TESTS

- Viral and bacterial cultures of the pharynx to exclude herpes simplex infection and streptococcal pharyngitis if the diagnosis is in doubt

TREATMENT

- Symptomatic treatment for sore throat, saline gargles, analgesics, encourage oral fluids.
- No antiviral therapy indicated; avoid antibacterial agents because they are ineffective, increase cost, might result in side effects, and promote antibiotic resistance.

DEFINITION

Stomatitis is inflammation involving the oral mucous membranes.

PHYSICAL FINDINGS AND CLINICAL PRESENTATION

White lesions

- Candidiasis (thrush)
  - Caused by yeast infection *(Candida albicans)*
  - Examination: white, curdlike material that when wiped off leaves a raw bleeding surface
  - Epidemiology: seen in the very young and the very old, those with immunodeficiency (AIDS, cancer), persons with diabetes, and patients treated with antibacterial agents
- Other
  - Leukoedema: filmy opalescent-appearing mucosa, which can be reverted to normal appearance by stretching (see Fig. 89–6). This condition is benign.
  - White sponge nevus: thick, white corrugated folds involving the buccal mucosa. Appears in childhood as an autosomal dominant trait; benign condition
  - Darier's disease (keratosis follicularis): white papules on the gingivae, alveolar mucosa, and dorsal tongue. Skin lesions also present (erythematous papules); inherited as an autosomal dominant trait
  - Chemical injury: white sloughing mucosa
  - Nicotine stomatitis: whitened palate with red papules (see Fig. 89–35)
  - Lichen planus: linear, reticular, slightly raised striae on buccal mucosa (see Fig. 89–27). Skin is involved by pruritic violaceous papules on forearms and inner thighs.
  - Discoid lupus erythematosus: lesion resembles lichen planus
  - Leukoplakia: white lesions that cannot be scraped off (see Fig. 89–37); 20% are premalignant epithelial dysplasia or squamous cell carcinoma.
  - Hairy leukoplakia: shaggy white surface that cannot be wiped off (see Fig. 89–25); seen in HIV infection, caused by EBV.

Red lesions

- Candidiasis may present with red instead of the more frequent white lesion (see "White Lesions"). Median rhomboid glossitis is a chronic variant.
- Benign migratory glossitis (geographic tongue): area of atrophic depapillated mucosa surrounded by a keratotic border (see Fig. 89–8); benign lesion, no treatment required
- Hemangiomas
- Histoplasmosis: ill-defined irregular patch with a granulomatous surface, sometimes ulcerated
- Allergy
- Anemia: atrophic reddened glossal mucosa seen with pernicious anemia
- Erythroplakia: red patch usually caused by epithelial dysplasia or squamous cell carcinoma
- Burning tongue (glossopyrosis): normal examination; sometimes associated with denture trauma, anemia, diabetes, vitamin B_{12} deficiency, psychogenic problems

Dark lesions (brown, blue, black)

- Coated tongue: accumulation of keratin; harmless condition that can be treated by scraping
- Melanotic lesions: freckles, lentigines, lentigo, melanoma, Peutz-Jeghers syndrome (see Fig. 17–6), Addison's disease
- Varices
- Kaposi sarcoma: red or purple macules that enlarge to form tumors; seen in patients with AIDS

Raised lesions

- Papilloma (see Fig. 89–13)
- Verruca vulgaris
- Condyloma acuminatum (see Fig. 89–14)
- Fibroma (see Fig. 89–16)
- Epulis (see Fig. 89–5)
- Pyogenic granuloma (see Fig. 89–20)
- Mucocele (see Fig. 89–34)
- Retention cyst (see Fig. 89–33)

Blisters

- Primary herpetic gingivostomatitis (Fig. 92–1)
- Caused by herpes simplex virus type 1 or, less frequently, type 2
- Course: day 1—malaise, fever, headache, sore throat, cervical lymphadenopathy; days 2 and 3—appearance of vesicles that develop into painful ulcers (see Fig. 92–1) of 2 to 4 mm in diameter; duration of up to 2 weeks
- Recurrent intraoral herpes: rare, recurrences typically involve only the keratinized epithelium (lips).
- Pemphigus and pemphigoid (see Figs. 89–30, 89–31)
- Hand-foot-and-mouth disease (see Fig. 27–22): caused by coxsackievirus group A
- Erythema multiforme (see Fig. 8–3)
- Herpangina: caused by echovirus (see Fig. 91–1)
- Traumatic ulcer (see Fig. 89–12)
- Primary syphilis (see Fig. 226–12)
- Perlèche (or angular cheilitis)
- Recurrent aphthous stomatitis (canker sores)

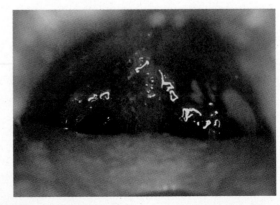

Fig 92–1
Primary herpes simplex virus 1 (HSV-1) stomatitis.
(From Cohen J, Powderly WG: Infectious Diseases, 2nd ed. St. Louis, Mosby, 2004.)

- Behçet's syndrome (see Fig. 15–5) (aphthous ulcers, uveitis, genital ulcerations, arthritis, aseptic meningitis)
- Reiter's syndrome (conjunctivitis, urethritis, arthritis, with occasional oral ulcerations)
- Unknown cause
- Course: solitary or multiple painful ulcers may develop simultaneously and heal over 10 to 14 days. The size of the lesions and the frequency of recurrences are variable.

DIAGNOSTIC WORKUP
White lesions

- Candidiasis (thrush) diagnosis: ovoid yeast and hyphae seen in scrapings treated with KOH culture

Blisters

- Exfoliative cytology
- Viral culture
- Immunofluorescence for herpes antigen

TREATMENT
White lesions

- Candidiasis (thrush) treatment: topical with nystatin or clotrimazole; systemic with ketoconazole or fluconazole

Blisters

- Supportive
- Consider acyclovir

Recurrent intraoral herpes

- Topical corticosteroids or systemic steroids for severe cases

Chapter 93 | Scarlet fever

DEFINITION
Scarlet fever is a rash involving the skin and tongue and complicating a streptococcal group A pharyngitis.

PHYSICAL FINDINGS AND CLINICAL PRESENTATION
- Diffuse erythema, beginning on the face and spreading to the neck, back, chest, rest of trunk, and extremities; most intense on inner aspects of arms and thighs
- Erythema blanches, but nonblanching petechiae may be present or produced by a tourniquet.
- Strawberry or raspberry tongue (Fig. 93–1)
- Rash lasts about 1 week and then desquamates
- Febrile illness with headache, malaise, anorexia, and pharyngitis begins after a 2- to 4-day incubation period
- Scarlatinal rash begins 1 or 2 days after the onset of pharyngitis.

CAUSE
Caused by group A beta-hemolytic *Streptococcus* infection, which produces one of three erythrogenic toxins. *Note:* Some streptococcal species have the ability to cause both scarlet fever and rheumatic fever.

DIFFERENTIAL DIAGNOSIS
- Viral exanthems (see Fig. 27–33)
- Kawasaki disease (see Fig. 27–32)
- Toxic shock syndrome (see Fig. 352–1)
- Drug rashes (see Fig. 14–1)

LABORATORY TESTS
- Identification of group A *Streptococcus* by throat culture
- SLO antibody titers

TREATMENT
- Penicillin

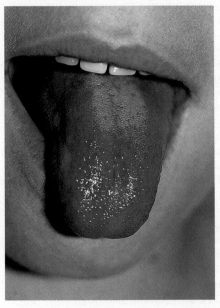

Fig 93–1
Mucosal lesions of scarlet fever.
(From Callen JP, Jorizzo JL, Bolognia JL, et al: Dermatological Signs of Internal Disease, 3rd ed. Philadelphia, WB Saunders, 2003.)

SALIVARY GLANDS

Chapter 94 | **Salivary gland neoplasms**

DEFINITION

Salivary gland neoplasms are benign or malignant tumors of a salivary gland (parotid, submandibular, or sublingual).

PHYSICAL FINDINGS AND CLINICAL PRESENTATION

- Parotid gland
- Painless swelling overlying the masseter muscle (under the temporomandibular joint; Fig. 94–1A)
- Pain
- Facial nerve palsy
- Cervical lymph nodes
- Mass in oral cavity
- Submandibular gland: swelling under anterior portion of the mandible
- Sublingual gland: intraoral swelling under the tongue, medial to the mandible
- Salivary gland neoplasms most often present as slow-growing, well-circumscribed masses. Pain, rapid growth, nerve weakness, fixation to skin or underlying muscle, and paresthesias usually are indicative of malignancy.

DIFFERENTIAL DIAGNOSIS

Benign tumors

- Mixed tumor (usually parotid)
- Adenolymphoma (Warthin's tumor)
- Pleomorphic adenoma
- Capillary hemangioma, lymphangioma (in children)
- Intraductal papilloma
- Other (e.g., myoepithelioma, canalicular adenoma, basal cell adenoma)

Malignant tumors

- Mucoepidermoid carcinoma (most common malignant tumor of the parotid gland)
- Adenoid cystic carcinoma
- Adenocarcinoma
- Malignant mixed tumor
- Squamous cell carcinoma
- Other

WORKUP

- Fine-needle aspiration. The sensitivity, specificity, and accuracy of parotid gland aspirates are approximately 92%, 100%, and 98%, respectively
- Imaging by CT scan (see Fig. 94–1B) or MRI
- Open biopsy (rarely indicated; see Fig. 94–1C)

TREATMENT

Malignant tumors

- Surgery is the mainstay of treatment; gland resection and neck dissection if lymph nodes are involved
- A lateral lobectomy with preservation of facial nerve should be considered for tumors confined to the superficial lobe of the parotid gland. Gross tumor should not be left in situ, but if the facial nerve is able to be preserved by "peeling" the tumor off the nerve, it should be attempted, followed by radiation therapy for microscopic disease.
- Postoperative radiation is indicated for high-grade malignancies demonstrating extraglandular disease, perineural invasion, direct invasion of surrounding tissues, or regional metastases.
- Chemotherapy

Benign tumors

- Surgery for tumor resection

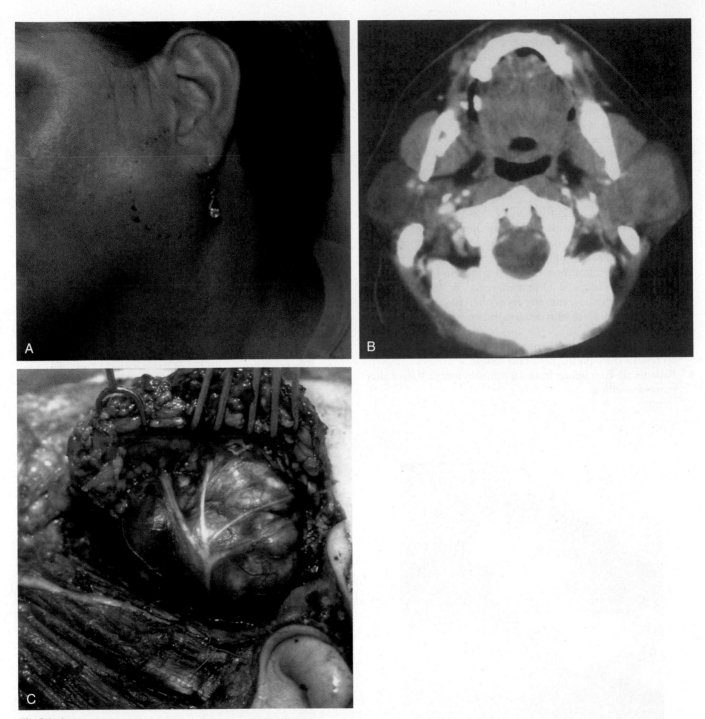

Fig 94-1
A, 34-year old woman with an asymptomatic left parotid mass. B, CT scan demonstrating a rim of normal parotid tissue superficial to a deeper, heterogeneous mass. C, The facial nerve stretched over the deep lobe pleomorphic adenoma with preservation of the superficial lobe. This was raised, along with the skin flap, by better postoperative cosmesis and prevention of postoperative Frey's syndrome or gustatory sweating. (From CM, Beauchamp RD, Evers BM, Mattox KL [eds]: Sabiston Textbook of Surgery, 17th ed. Philadelphia, WB Saunders, 2004.)

Chapter 95   Mumps

DEFINITION

Mumps is an acute generalized viral infection usually characterized by nonsuppurative swelling and tenderness of one or both parotid glands. It is caused by mumps virus, a paramyxovirus and member of the Paramyxoviridae family.

PHYSICAL FINDINGS AND CLINICAL PRESENTATION

- Prodromal period: low-grade fever, malaise
- Parotid swelling and tenderness are often first signs of infection.
- Redness of the parotid papilla (Fig. 95–1)
- Considerable pain with parotid swelling, causing trismus and difficulty with mastication and pronunciation (Fig. 95–2). Parotid swelling usually resolves within 1 week.
- Epididymo-orchitis: most common extra salivary gland complication of mumps in adult men; occurs in 38% of postpubertal men who have mumps; most often unilateral but bilateral in 30% of those who develop this complication

CAUSE

- Virus is spread via direct contact, droplet nuclei, fomites, or secretions through the nose and mouth.
- Patients are contagious from 48 hours before to 9 days after parotid swelling.

DIFFERENTIAL DIAGNOSIS

- Other viruses that may cause acute parotitis
1. Parainfluenza types 1 and 3
2. Coxsackie viruses
3. Influenza A
4. Cytomegalovirus
- Suppurative parotitis (Fig. 95–3)
1. Most often caused by *Staphylococcus aureus*
2. May be differentiated from mumps
   a. Extreme indurations, tenderness, and erythema overlying the gland
   b. Ability to express pus from Stensen's duct or massage of parotid
- Other conditions that may occur with parotid enlargement or swelling: Sjögren's syndrome, drugs (e.g., phenothiazines, phenylbutazone), tumors, cysts, stones causing obstruction, strictures causing obstruction

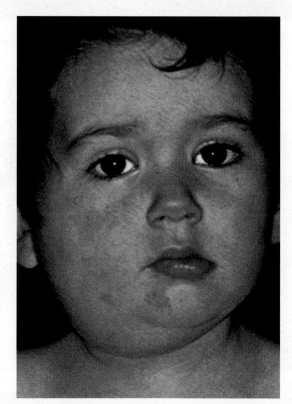

Fig 95–2
Parotitis in a child. Mumps is a generalized infection with a wide range of clinical manifestations. Parotitis is common and may be accompanied by inflammation of other structures. Both parotid glands are involved in 70% of patients with parotitis. The illness begins with fever and malaise, quickly followed by trismus and pain behind the angle of the jaw. Within 24 hours, the parotid gland begins to swell, the hollow behind the angle of the mandible fills, and the swelling extends over the ramus. Confusion sometimes arises with enlarged lymph nodes, but these are usually located below the parotid gland and the posterior border of the ramus can be sharply defined.
(From Emond RT, Welsby PD, Rowland HA [eds]: Colour Atlas of Infectious Diseases, 4th ed. St. Louis, Mosby, 2003.)

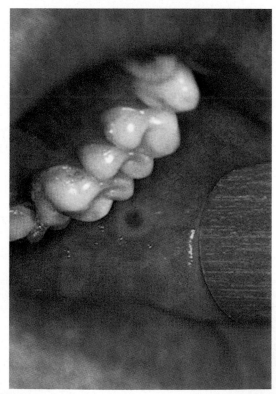

Fig 95–1
Parotid papilla in mumps. Redness of the parotid papilla is a helpful early sign. Any fluid discharged from the parotid duct is clear.
(From Emond RT, Welsby PD, Rowland HA [eds]: Colour Atlas of Infectious Diseases, 4th ed. St. Louis, Mosby, 2003.)

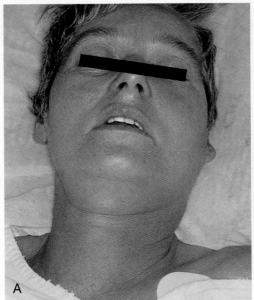 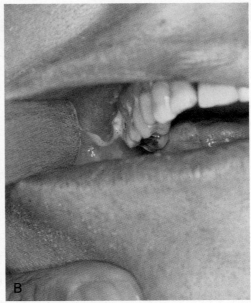

Fig 95-3
Suppurative parotitis. **A,** In a diabetic patient who had a recent history of dehydration secondary to diabetic ketoacidosis. **B,** Pus was manually expressed from Stensen's duct, from which *Staphylococcus aureus* was cultured. (Courtesy of Dr. E. Ridgway.)

LABORATORY TESTS

- Diagnosis is confirmed by a fourfold rise between acute and convalescent sera by CF, enzyme-linked immunosorbent assay (ELISA), or neutralization tests.
- Virus can be isolated from the saliva, usually from 2 to 3 days before to 4 to 5 days after the onset of parotitis.
- Serum amylase: elevated in the presence of parotitis

TREATMENT

- Analgesics and antipyretics to relieve pain and fever
- Narcotic analgesics, along with bed rest, ice packs, and a testicular bridge, to relieve pain associated with mumps orchitis
- IV fluids for patients with frequent vomiting associated with mumps pancreatitis or meningitis

PHARYNX

| **Chapter 96** | **Pharyngitis and tonsillitis** |

DEFINITION
Pharyngitis or tonsillitis is inflammation of the pharynx or tonsils.

PHYSICAL FINDINGS AND CLINICAL PRESENTATION
- Pharynx
  1. May appear normal to severely erythematous
  2. Tonsillar hypertrophy and exudates commonly seen but do not indicate cause
- Viral infection
  1. Rhinorrhea
  2. Conjunctivitis
  3. Cough
- Bacterial infection, especially group A *Streptococcus* (Fig. 96–1)
  1. High fever
  2. Systemic signs of infection
- Herpes simplex or enterovirus infection: vesicles
- Streptococcal infection
  1. Rare complications:
     a. Scarlet fever
     b. Rheumatic fever
     c. Acute glomerulonephritis
  2. Extension of infection: tonsillar, parapharyngeal, or retropharyngeal abscess presenting with severe pain, high fever, trismus

CAUSE
- Viruses
  1. Respiratory syncytial virus
  2. Influenza types A and B
  3. Epstein-Barr virus
  4. Adenovirus (Fig. 96–2)
  5. Herpes simplex
- Bacteria
  1. *Streptococcus* (Fig. 96–3)
  2. *Neisseria gonorrhoeae*
  3. *Arcanobacterium haemolyticum*
- Other organisms
  1. *Mycoplasma pneumoniae*
  2. *Chlamydia pneumoniae*

DIFFERENTIAL DIAGNOSIS
- Sore throat associated with granulocytopenia, thyroiditis
- Tonsillar hypertrophy associated with lymphoma
- Section II describes the differential diagnosis of sore throat.

WORKUP
- Throat swab for culture to exclude *S. pyogenes*, *N. gonorrhoeae* (requires specific transport medium)
- Rapid streptococcal antigen test (culture should be performed if rapid test negative and diagnosis suspected)
- Monospot

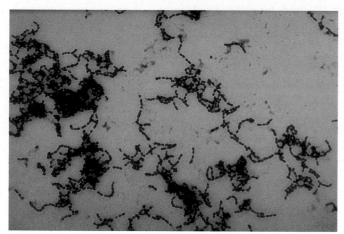

Fig 96–1
Gram stain of beta-hemolytic streptococci group A.
(From Cohen J, Powderly WG: Infectious Diseases, 2nd ed. St. Louis, Mosby, 2004.)

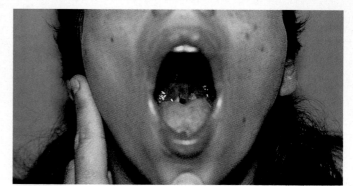

Fig 96–2
Adenoviral pharyngitis.
(From Cohen J, Powderly WG: Infectious Diseases, 2nd ed. St. Louis, Mosby, 2004.)

LABORATORY TESTS
- CBC with differential
  1. May help support diagnosis of bacterial infection
  2. Streptococcal infection suggested by leukocytosis of more than $15,000/mm^3$
- Viral cultures, serologic studies rarely needed

IMAGING STUDIES
- Seldom indicated

TREATMENT
- If streptococcal infection proved or suspected:
  1. Penicillin
  2. Erythromycin if penicillin allergic
- If gonococcal infection proved or suspected: ceftriaxone
- Tonsillopharyngitis is generally managed in an outpatient setting with follow-up arranged in a week or two. Admission to the hospital is indicated for local suppurative complications (peritonsillar abscess, lateral pharyngeal or posterior pharyngeal abscess, impending airway closure, or inability to swallow food, medications, or water).

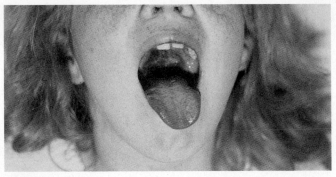

Fig 96–3
Pharyngitis associated with GAS (Group A strep) infection. Exudates are not always present.
(From Cohen J, Powderly WG: Infectious Diseases, 2nd ed. St. Louis, Mosby, 2004.)

Chapter 97　Epiglottitis

DEFINITION
Epiglottitis is a rapidly progressive cellulitis of the epiglottis and adjacent soft tissue structures with the potential to cause abrupt airway obstruction.

PHYSICAL FINDINGS AND CLINICAL PRESENTATION
- Irritability, fever, dysphonia, dysphagia
- Respiratory distress, with child tending to lean up and forward
- Often, drooling or oral secretions
- Often, presence of tachycardia and tachypnea
- On visualization, edematous and cherry red epiglottis (Fig. 97–1)
- Often, no classic barking cough as seen in croup
- Possibly fulminant course (especially in children), leading to complete airway obstruction

CAUSE
- In children, *Haemophilus influenzae* type B is usual.
- In adults, *H. influenzae* can be isolated from blood, epiglottis (about 26% of cases), or both.
- Pneumococci, streptococci, and staphylococci are also implicated.
- Role of viruses in epiglottitis unclear

DIFFERENTIAL DIAGNOSIS
- Croup
- Angioedema
- Peritonsillar abscess
- Retropharyngeal abscess
- Diphtheria (see Fig. 343–1)
- Foreign body aspiration
- Lingual tonsillitis

WORKUP
- Cultures of blood and urine
- Lateral neck radiograph to show an enlarged epiglottis, ballooning of the hypopharynx, and normal subglottic structures (Fig. 97–2)
  1. Radiographs are of only moderate sensitivity and specificity and take time to perform.
  2. Visualization of the epiglottitis may be safer in adults than in children. In children, visualization and intubation are best done in the most controlled environment.
- Cultures of the epiglottitis

LABORATORY TESTS
- CBC: may reveal a leukocytosis, with a shift to the left
- Chest x-ray examination: may reveal evidence of pneumonia in almost 25% of cases
- Cultures of blood, urine, and epiglottis, as noted

TREATMENT
- Maintenance of adequate airway is critical.
- Early placement of an endotracheal or nasotracheal tube in a child is advised.
- Closely follow adult patient and defer intubation, provided the airway reveals no signs of obstruction.
- *H. influenzae* in children may be less common because of the availability of the Hib vaccine.
- Use antibiotics such as ceftriaxone, cefotaxime.

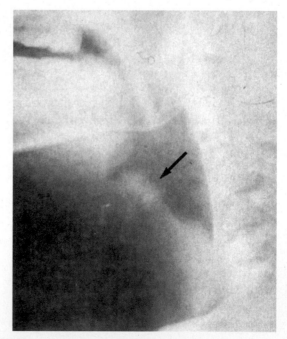

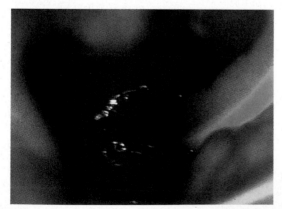

Fig 97–1
Acutely inflamed epiglottis associated with *Haemophilus influenza* type B (HIB). The epiglottis protrudes upward and is cherry red from the bottom of the figure.
(Courtesy of the Intensive Care Unit, Royal Children's Hospital, Melbourne, Australia.)

Fig 97–2
Lateral neck radiograph of a child with acute epiglottitis demonstrating an enlarged hypopharynx caused by forward neck extension and an enlarged thumb-shaped epiglottis (*arrow*).
(Courtesy of Dr. Donald Frush.)

THYROID

Chapter 98   Thyroid nodule

DEFINITION

A thyroid nodule is an abnormality found on physical examination of the thyroid gland; nodules can be benign (70%) or malignant.

PHYSICAL FINDINGS AND CLINICAL PRESENTATION

- Palpable, firm, and nontender nodule in the thyroid area should prompt suspicion of carcinoma. Signs of metastasis are regional lymph adenopathy and inspiratory stridor.
- Signs and symptoms of thyrotoxicosis can be found in functioning nodules.

CAUSE

- History of prior head and neck irradiation
- Family history of pheochromocytoma, carcinoma of the thyroid, and hyperparathyroidism (medullary carcinoma of the thyroid is component of multiple endocrine neoplasia, type II [MEN-II])

DIFFERENTIAL DIAGNOSIS

- Thyroid carcinoma (Fig. 98–1)
- Multinodular goiter (Figs. 98–2 and 98–3)
- Thyroglossal duct cyst (Fig. 98–4)
- Epidermoid cyst
- Laryngocele
- Nonthyroid neck neoplasm
- Branchial cleft cyst

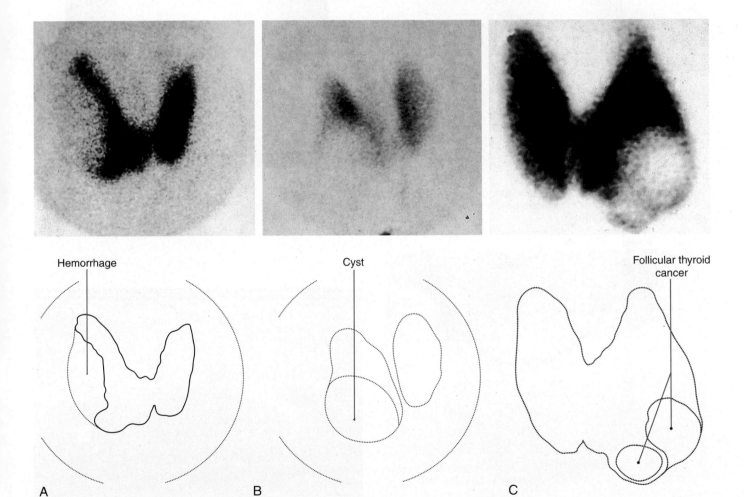

Fig 98–1

Thyroid images in patients with palpable solitary nodules in their thyroid glands. Note that the appearances of the scans are similar; each shows an area of deficient or reduced uptake, whereas the rest of the gland shows a homogenous normal uptake. It is not possible to distinguish among the causes of a solitary nodule. **A,** Hemorrhage. **B,** Cyst. **C,** Follicular thyroid cancer. Ultrasound should be combined with thyroid imaging to demonstrate the simple cyst for aspiration cytology and to enable fine-needle biopsy for the echogenic (solid) nodule, which is nonfunctional in a thyroid scan. If the mass in the gland is solitary and solid, about 12% of these cases prove to be malignant.

(From Besser CM, Thorner MO: Comprehensive Clinical Endocrinology, 3rd ed. St. Louis, Mosby, 2002.)

WORKUP

- Fine-needle aspiration (FNA) biopsy is the best diagnostic study; the accuracy can be more than 90%, but it is directly related to the level of experience of the physician and cytopathologist interpreting the findings.
- FNA biopsy is less reliable with thyroid cystic lesions; surgical excision should be considered for most thyroid cysts not abolished by aspiration.

LABORATORY TESTS

- Thyroid-stimulating hormone (TSH), thyroxine (T_4), and serum thyroglobulin levels should be obtained before thyroidectomy in patients with confirmed thyroid carcinoma on FNA biopsy.

- Serum calcitonin at random or after pentagastrin stimulation is useful when suspecting medullary carcinoma of the thyroid and in anyone with a family history of medullary thyroid carcinoma.
- Serum thyroid autoantibodies are useful when suspecting thyroiditis.

IMAGING STUDIES

- Thyroid ultrasound (Fig. 98–5) is done in some patients to evaluate the size of the thyroid and the number, composition (solid vs. cystic), and dimensions of the thyroid nodule; solid thyroid nodules have a higher incidence of malignancy, but cystic nodules can also be malignant.

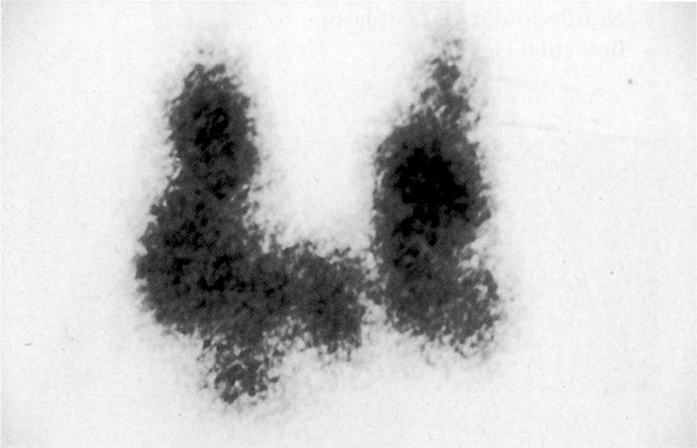

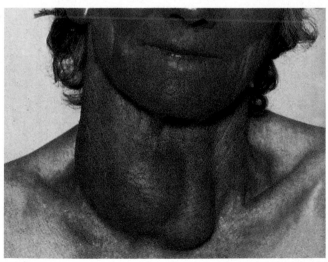

Fig 98–2
Technetium-99m thyroid scan of a multinodular goiter.
(From Besser CM, Thorner MO: Comprehensive Clinical Endocrinology, 3rd ed. St. Louis, Mosby, 2002.)

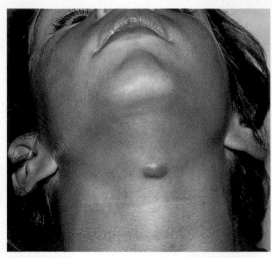

Fig 98–4
Thyroglossal cyst.
(From Swartz MH: Textbook of Physical Diagnosis, 5th ed. Philadelphia, WB Saunders, 2006.)

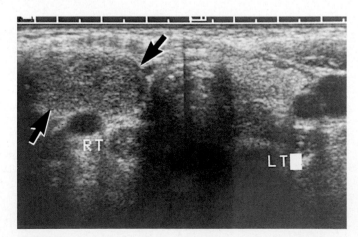

Fig 98–3
A large multinodular goiter with a dominant nodule in the right lobe.
(From Besser CM, Thorner MO: Comprehensive Clinical Endocrinology, 3rd ed. St. Louis, Mosby, 2002.)

Fig 98–5
Preoperative ultrasound of a patient with a 4- × 2-cm homogeneous right thyroid (RT) mass (*arrows*). Resection demonstrated a follicular adenoma. LT, left thyroid.
(From CM, Beauchamp RD, Evers BM, Mattox KL [eds]: Sabiston Textbook of Surgery, 17th ed. Philadelphia, WB Saunders, 2004.)

- Thyroid scan (see Fig. 98–1) can be performed with technetium-99m pertechnetate, iodine-123, or iodine-131. Iodine isotopes are preferred because 35% to 38% of nodules that appear functioning on pertechnetate scanning may appear nonfunctioning on radioiodine scanning. A thyroid scan:
  1. Classifies nodules as hyperfunctioning (hot), normally functioning (warm), or nonfunctioning (cold); cold nodules have a higher incidence of malignancy
  2. Has difficulty evaluating nodules near the thyroid isthmus or at the periphery of the gland
  3. Normal tissue over a nonfunctioning nodule may mask the nodule as "warm" or normally functioning
- Both thyroid scan and ultrasound provide information about the risk of malignant neoplasia based on the characteristics of the thyroid nodule, but their value in the initial evaluation of a thyroid nodule is limited because neither provides a definite tissue diagnosis.

TREATMENT
- Evaluation of results of FNA
  1. Normal cells: may repeat biopsy during present evaluation or re-evaluate patient after 3 to 6 months of suppressive therapy (L-thyroxine, prescribed in doses to suppress the TSH level to 0.1 to 0.5 mU/L)
    a. Failure to regress indicates increased likelihood of malignancy.
    b. Reliance on repeat needle biopsy is preferable to routine surgery for nodules not responding to thyroxine.
  2. Malignant cells: surgery
  3. Hypercellularity: thyroid scan
    a. Hot nodule: ^{131}I therapy if the patient is hyperthyroid
    b. Warm or cold nodule: surgery (rule out follicular adenoma vs. carcinoma)

Chapter 99 | Thyroid cancer

DEFINITION

Thyroid carcinoma is a primary neoplasm of the thyroid. There are four major types of thyroid carcinoma—papillary, follicular, anaplastic, and medullary.

PHYSICAL FINDINGS AND CLINICAL PRESENTATION

- Presence of thyroid nodule
- Hoarseness and cervical lymphadenopathy
- Painless swelling in the region of the thyroid

CAUSE

- Risk factors: prior neck irradiation
- MEN-II (medullary carcinoma)

DIFFERENTIAL DIAGNOSIS

- Multinodular goiter
- Lymphocytic thyroiditis
- Ectopic thyroid

WORKUP

The workup of thyroid carcinoma includes laboratory evaluation and diagnostic imaging. However, diagnosis is confirmed with FNA or surgical biopsy (Fig. 99–1). The characteristics of thyroid carcinoma vary with the type.

- Papillary carcinoma
    1. Most frequently occurs in women during the second or third decade

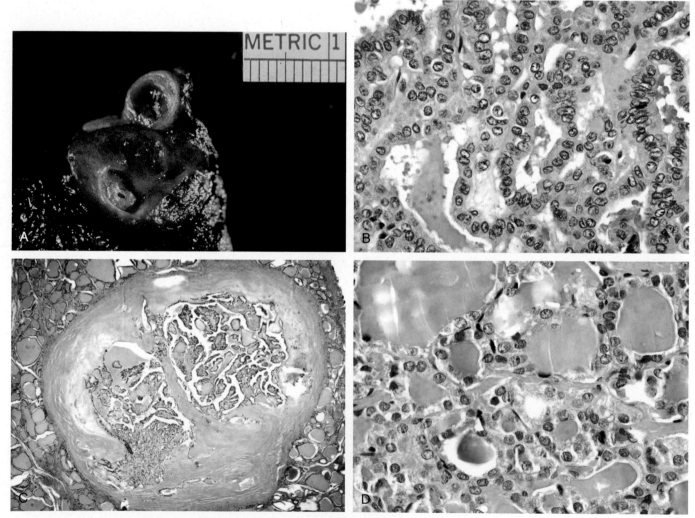

Fig 99–1

A, Papillary thyroid carcinoma with focal cystic change. **B,** Papillary thyroid carcinoma, classic variant. Papillae are lined by tumor cells, with nuclear features of papillary carcinoma. **C,** Encapsulated papillary microcarcinoma. **D,** Follicular variant of papillary thyroid carcinoma. This follicular patterned tumor has nuclear features of papillary thyroid carcinoma (**B–D,** H&E, ×150.)
(From Silverberg SG, WJ Frable, Wick MR, et al [eds]: Principles and Practice of Surgical Pathology and Cytopathology, 4th ed. Philadelphia, Elsevier, 2006.)

2. Histologically, *psammoma bodies* (calcific bodies present in papillary projections) are pathognomonic; found in 35% to 45% of papillary thyroid carcinomas
3. Majority are not papillary lesions but mixed papillary follicular carcinomas
4. Spread is via lymphatics and by local invasion
- Follicular carcinoma
  1. More aggressive than papillary carcinoma
  2. Incidence increases with age
  3. Tends to metastasize hematogenously to bone, producing pathologic fractures

4. Tends to concentrate iodine (useful for radiation therapy)
- Anaplastic carcinoma
  1. Very aggressive neoplasm
  2. Two major histologic types: small cell (less aggressive, 5-year survival approximately 20%) and giant cell (death usually within 6 months of diagnosis)
- Medullary carcinoma
  1. Unifocal lesion: found sporadically in older patients
  2. Bilateral lesions: associated with pheochromocytoma and hyperparathyroidism; this combination is known as MEN-II and is inherited as an autosomal dominant disorder.

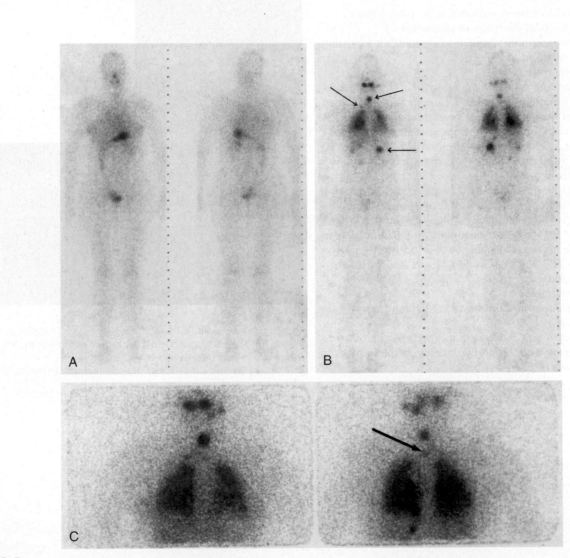

Fig 99–2
Whole-body ^{131}I scan. **A,** Whole-body scan 1 day after treatment with 179 mCi of ^{131}I for recurrent metastatic papillary carcinoma. Uptake is initially seen only in the nasopharyngeal, salivary, and gastrointestinal tissues. **B,** Whole-body scan 1 week after treatment now shows marked diffuse uptake in the lungs, with locally recurring disease at the base of the neck (*arrow*) and right supraclavicular region (*arrow*). A metastatic lesion is also seen in the superior region of the left kidney (*arrow*). **C,** Close-up image of the 7-day post-treatment scan also suggests the presence of mediastinal disease (*arrow*).
(From Besser CM, Thorner MO: Comprehensive Clinical Endocrinology, 3rd ed. St. Louis, Mosby, 2002.)

LABORATORY TESTS

- Thyroid function studies are generally normal. TSH, T_4, and serum thyroglobulin levels should be obtained before thyroidectomy in patients with confirmed thyroid carcinoma.
- Increased plasma calcitonin assay in patients with medullary carcinoma (tumors produce thyrocalcitonin)

IMAGING STUDIES

- Thyroid scanning can identify hypofunctioning (cold) nodules, which are more likely to be malignant. However, warm nodules can also be malignant.
- Thyroid ultrasound can detect solitary solid nodules that have a high risk of malignancy. However, a negative ultrasound does not exclude diagnosis of thyroid carcinoma.

TREATMENT

- Papillary carcinoma

    1. Total thyroidectomy is indicated if the patient has:

    a. Extrapyramidal extension of carcinoma

    b. Papillary carcinoma limited to thyroid but a positive history of irradiation to the neck

    c. Lesion larger than 2 cm

    2. Lobectomy with isthmectomy may be considered for patients with intrathyroid papillary carcinoma smaller than 2 cm and no history of neck or head irradiation; most follow surgery with suppressive therapy with thyroid hormone because these tumors are TSH-responsive. The accepted practice is to suppress serum TSH concentrations to lower than 0.1 μU/mL.

    3. Radiotherapy with iodine-131 (after total thyroidectomy), followed by thyroid suppression therapy with triiodothyronine, can be used in metastatic papillary carcinoma. Whole-body iodine-131 scan post-treatment for identification of metastases is shown in Figure 99–2. A positron emission tomography (PET) scan (Fig. 99–3) can also be used to identify metastases.

- Follicular carcinoma

    1. Total thyroidectomy followed by TSH suppression (see earlier)

    2. Radiotherapy with iodine-131 followed by thyroid suppression therapy with triiodothyronine is useful for patients with metastasis.

- Anaplastic carcinoma

    1. At diagnosis, this neoplasm is rarely operable; palliative surgery is indicated for an extremely large tumor compressing the trachea.

    2. Management is usually restricted to radiation therapy or chemotherapy (combination of doxorubicin, cisplatin, and other antineoplastic agents); these measures rarely provide significant palliation.

- Medullary carcinoma

    1. Thyroidectomy should be performed.

    2. Patients and their families should be screened for pheochromocytoma and hyperparathyroidism.

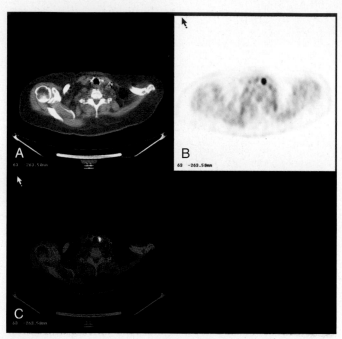

Fig 99–3

Thyroid cancer. Positron emission tomography and CT scans show an intense ^{18}F-fluorodeoxyglucose uptake focus near clips in the left thyroid bed, consistent with recurrent thyroid cancer.

(From Abeloff MD: Clinical Oncology, 3rd ed. Philadelphia, Elsevier, 2004.)

DEFINITION

Thyroiditis is an inflammatory disease of the thyroid. It is a multifaceted disease with varying causes, different clinical characteristics (depending on the stage), and distinct histopathology. Thyroiditis can be subdivided into three common types (Hashimoto's, painful, painless) and two rare forms (suppurative, Riedel's). To add to the confusion, there are various synonyms for each form, and there is no internationally accepted classification of autoimmune thyroid disease.

SYNONYMS

- Hashimoto's thyroiditis: chronic lymphocytic thyroiditis, chronic autoimmune thyroiditis, lymphadenoid goiter
- Painful subacute thyroiditis: subacute thyroiditis, giant cell thyroiditis, de Quervain's thyroiditis, subacute granulomatous thyroiditis, pseudogranulomatous thyroiditis
- Painless postpartum thyroiditis: subacute lymphocytic thyroiditis, postpartum thyroiditis
- Painless sporadic thyroiditis: silent sporadic thyroiditis, subacute lymphocytic thyroiditis
- Suppurative thyroiditis: acute suppurative thyroiditis, bacterial thyroiditis, microbial inflammatory thyroiditis, pyogenic thyroiditis
- Riedel's thyroiditis: fibrous thyroiditis

PHYSICAL FINDINGS AND CLINICAL PRESENTATION

- Hashimoto's: patients may have signs of hyperthyroidism (tachycardia, diaphoresis, palpitations, weight loss) or hypothyroidism (fatigue, weight gain, delayed reflexes) depending on the stage of the disease. Usually, there is diffuse, firm enlargement of the thyroid gland; the thyroid gland may also be of normal size (atrophic form with clinically manifested hypothyroidism).
- Painful subacute: exquisitely tender, enlarged thyroid, fever; signs of hyperthyroidism are initially present; signs of hypothyroidism can subsequently develop.
- Painless thyroiditis: clinical features are similar to subacute thyroiditis except for the absence of tenderness of the thyroid gland.
- Suppurative: patient is febrile with severe neck pain, focal tenderness of the involved portion of the thyroid, erythema of the overlying skin.
- Riedel's: slowly enlarging hard mass in the anterior neck; often mistaken for thyroid cancer; signs of hypothyroidism occur in advanced stages.

CAUSE

- Hashimoto's: autoimmune disorder that begins with the activation of CD4 (helper) T lymphocytes specific for thyroid antigens. The causative factor for the activation of these cells is unknown.
- Painful subacute: possibly postviral; usually follows a respiratory illness. It is not considered to be a form of autoimmune thyroiditis.
- Painless thyroiditis: it frequently occurs postpartum.
- Suppurative: infectious cause, generally bacterial, although fungi and parasites have also been implicated. It often occurs in immunocompromised hosts or following a penetrating neck injury.

- Riedel's: fibrous infiltration of the thyroid; cause is unknown.
- Drug-induced: lithium, interferon alfa, amiodarone, interleukin-2

DIFFERENTIAL DIAGNOSIS

- The hyperthyroid phase of Hashimoto's, subacute, or silent thyroiditis can be mistaken for Graves' disease.
- Riedel's thyroiditis can be mistaken for carcinoma of the thyroid.
- Painful subacute thyroiditis can be mistaken for infections of the oropharynx and trachea or for suppurative thyroiditis.
- Factitious hyperthyroidism can mimic silent thyroiditis.

LABORATORY TESTS

- TSH, free T_4: may be normal or indicative of hypo- or hyperthyroidism, depending on the stage of the thyroiditis.
- WBC with differential: increased WBC with shift to the left occurs with subacute and suppurative thyroiditis.
- Antimicrosomal antibodies: detected in more than 90% of patients with Hashimoto's thyroiditis and 50% to 80% of patients with silent thyroiditis.
- Serum thyroglobulin levels are elevated in patients with subacute and silent thyroiditis; this test is nonspecific but may be useful in monitoring the course of subacute thyroiditis and distinguishing silent thyroiditis from factitious hyperthyroidism (low or absent serum thyroglobulin level).
- Biopsy of thyroid (Fig. 100–1)

IMAGING STUDIES

24-hour radioactive iodine uptake (RAIU) is useful to distinguish Graves' disease (increased RAIU) from thyroiditis (normal or low RAIU; Fig. 100–2).

TREATMENT

- Treat hypothyroid phase with levothyroxine, 25-50 μg/day initially; monitor serum TSH initially every 6 to 8 weeks.
- Control symptoms of hyperthyroidism with beta blockers (e.g., propranolol, 20 to 40 mg PO every 6 hours).
- Control pain in patients with subacute thyroiditis with NSAIDs. Prednisone, 20 to 40 mg daily, may be used if NSAIDs are insufficient, but should be gradually tapered over several weeks.
- Use IV antibiotics and drain abscess (if present) in patients with suppurative thyroiditis.

DISPOSITION

- Hashimoto's thyroiditis: long-term prognosis is favorable; most patients recover their thyroid function.
- Painful subacute thyroiditis: permanent hypothyroidism occurs in 10% of patients.
- Painless thyroiditis: 6% of patients have permanent hypothyroidism.
- Suppurative thyroiditis: there is usually full recovery following treatment.
- Riedel's thyroiditis: hypothyroidism occurs when fibrous infiltration involves the entire thyroid.

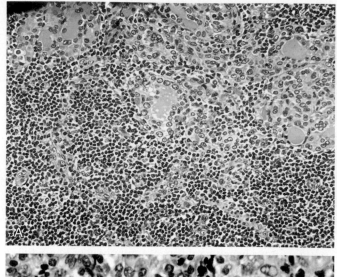

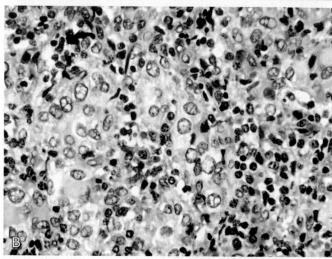

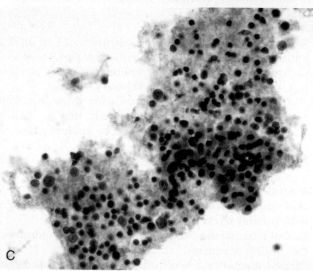

Fig 100–1

A, Hashimoto's thyroiditis. Note the extensive replacement of the thyroid parenchyma (*top*) by lymphoid infiltrate (H&E, ×100). **B,** Marked reactive nuclear chromatin clearing in Hashimoto's thyroiditis. This nuclear change can be mistaken for papillary thyroid carcinoma (H&E, ×200). **C,** Cytology of lymphocytic thyroiditis. Clusters of follicular cells are infiltrated by lymphocytes (Papanicolaou, ×150).
(From Silverberg SG, WJ Frable, Wick MR, et al [eds]: Principles and Practice of Surgical Pathology and Cytopathology, 4th ed. Philadelphia, Elsevier, 2006.)

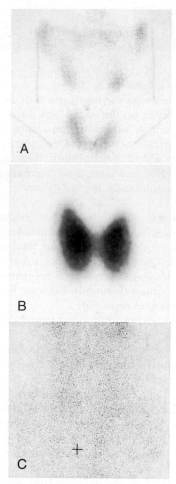

Fig 100–2

Technetium-99m thyroid scans. **A,** Normal. **B,** Graves' disease, showing enlarged thyroid with increased uptake. **C,** Low patchy uptake in destructive thyroiditis.
(From Besser CM, Thorner MO: Comprehensive Clinical Endocrinology, 3rd ed. St. Louis, Mosby, 2002.)

REFERENCES

Besser CM, Thorner MO: Comprehensive Clinical Endocrinology, 3rd ed. St. Louis, Mosby, 2002.

Bryan CS: Infectious Diseases in Primary Care, Philadelphia, WB Saunders, 2002.

Cohen J, Powderly WG: Infectious Diseases, 2nd ed. St. Louis, Mosby, 2004.

Ferri F: Ferri's Clinical Advisor, 2008. St. Louis, Mosby, 2008.

Ferri F: Practical Guide to the Care of the Medical Patient, 7th ed, St. Louis, Mosby, 2008.

Fireman P: Atlas of Allergies and Immunology, 3rd ed. St. Louis, Mosby, 2006.

Hochberg MC, Silman AJ, Smolen JS, et al (eds): Rheumatology, 3rd ed. St. Louis, Mosby, 2003.

McKee PH, Calonje E, Granter SR (eds): Pathology of the Skin With Clinical Correlations, 3rd ed. St. Louis, Mosby, 2005.

Yanoff M, Duker JS: Ophthalmology, 2nd ed. St. Louis, Mosby, 2004.

4

SECTION

Chest, Mediastinum, and Diaphragm

Chapter 101: Chest wall abnormalities
Chapter 102: Mediastinal abnormalities

Chapter 103: Superior vena cava syndrome
Chapter 104: Diaphragm abnormalities

Chapter 101   Chest wall abnormalities

Commonly encountered chest wall abnormalities include pectus excavatum (funnel chest), manifested by a depression of the sternum (Fig. 101–1) and often associated with mitral valve prolapse and pectus carinatum (pigeon chest), manifested by an anterior protrusion of the sternum (Fig. 101–2). The former may interfere with breathing, resulting in a restrictive lung problem, whereas the latter is rarely of clinical significance.

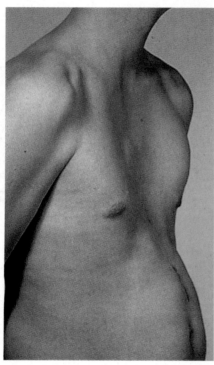

Fig 101–1
Pectus excavatum.
(From Swartz MH: Textbook of Physical Diagnosis, 5th ed. Philadelphia, WB Saunders, 2006.)

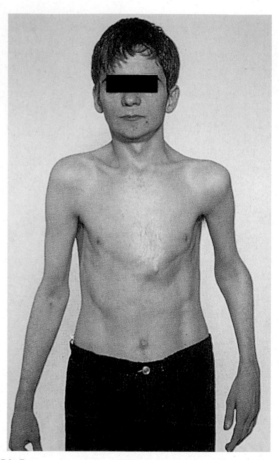

Fig 101–2
Pectus carinatum.
(From Swartz MH: Textbook of Physical Diagnosis, 5th ed. Philadelphia, WB Saunders, 2006.)

Chapter 102 Mediastinal abnormalities

DIAGNOSIS

The mediastinum is an anatomic division of the thorax extending from the diaphragm to the thoracic inlet (Fig. 102–1). Mediastinal abnormalities can be initially detected with chest radiographs, but chest CT is generally necessary for localizing and demonstrating the extent of mediastinal masses, as well as providing important diagnostic information about their nature.

CLASSIFICATION

Mediastinal masses are conventionally classified by location into anterior, middle, or posterior mediastinal compartments. Table 102–1 describes the most frequent causes of mediastinal masses.

Characteristics of mediastinal masses

- Most thyroid masses in the mediastinum represent downward extensions of a multinodular goiter (Fig.102–2) or, occasionally, an adenoma or carcinoma.

TABLE 102–1 Most frequent causes of mediastinal masses

Anterior	Middle	Posterior
Thymoma	Lymphoma	Neurogenic tumors
Lymphoma	Cancer	Enteric cysts
Teratogenic tumors	Cysts	Esophageal lesions
Thyroid aneurysms	Aneurysms	Diaphragmatic hernias (Bochdalek)
Parathyroid aneurysms.	Hernia (Morgagni)	

From Goldman L, Ausiello D: Cecil Textbook of Medicine, 22nd ed, Philadelphia, WB Saunders, 2004.

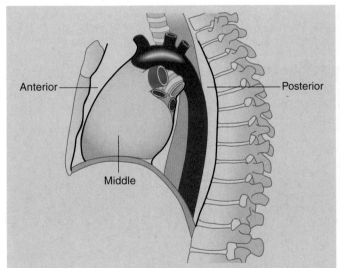

Fig 102–1

Anatomic compartments of the mediastinum. The anterior compartment is bound posteriorly by the pericardium, ascending aorta, and brachiocephalic vessels and anteriorly by the sternum. The middle compartment extends from the posterior limits of the anterior compartment to the posterior pericardial line. The posterior compartment extends from the pericardial line to the dorsal chest wall.
(From Goldman L, Ausiello D: Cecil Textbook of Medicine, 22nd ed. Philadelphia, WB Saunders, 2004.)

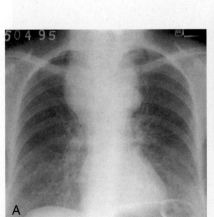
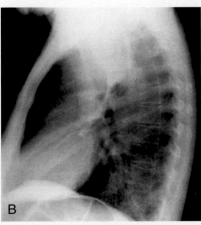

Fig 102–2

Intrathoracic thyroid mass. This benign multinodular goiter is predominantly posterior to the trachea with components to either side, resulting in forward displacement and narrowing of the trachea. **A,** AP view. **B,** lateral view.
(From Grainger RG, Allison DJ, Adam A, Dixon AK [eds]: Grainger & Allison's Diagnostic Radiology, 4th ed. Philadelphia, Churchill-Livingstone, 2001.)

- Thymic masses may be simple thymic cysts (Fig. 102–3) that occur in an otherwise normal gland, may lie within a thymoma, or may follow thymic irradiation for Hodgkin's disease. Thymomas are lymphoepithelial neoplasms that may be benign or malignant (10% to 40%). The average age at diagnosis is approximately 50 years, or somewhat earlier in those who present with myasthenia gravis (Fig. 102–4).

- Teratomas or germ cell tumors (Fig. 102–5) can present as mediastinal masses. They can be divided into benign forms (also known as dermoid cysts) and malignant forms, which may secrete human chorionic gonadotropin-beta and alpha-fetoprotein (Fig. 102–6)

- Mediastinal lymphadenopathy can be initially detected by plain chest radiography but is best appreciated with chest

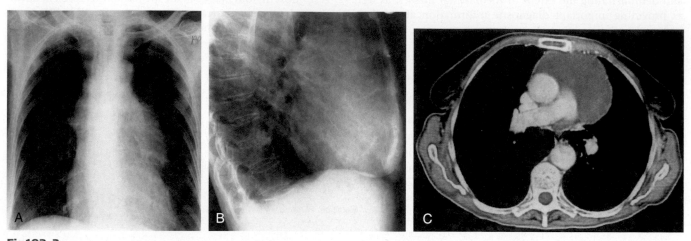

Fig 102–3
Thymic cyst producing an anterior mediastinal mass on anteroposterior **(A)** and lateral **(B)** chest radiographs, filling in the normal retrosternal window and widening the mediastinum. **C,** Its cystic nature is best demonstrated by CT.
(From Grainger RG, Allison DJ, Adam A, Dixon AK [eds]: Grainger & Allison's Diagnostic Radiology, 4th ed. Philadelphia, Churchill-Livingstone, 2001.)

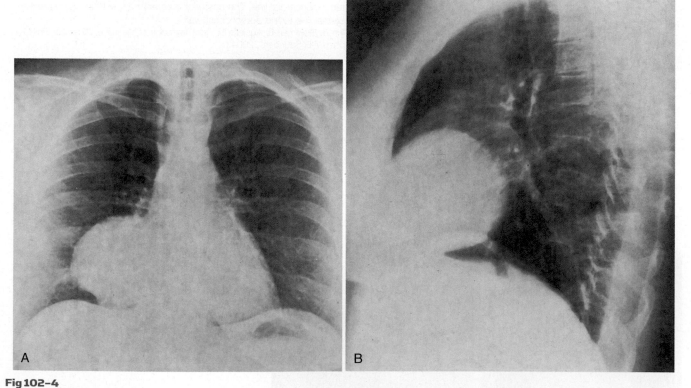

Fig 102–4
Thymoma situated low in the anterior mediastinum adjacent to the right-heart border in a 35-year-old woman with myasthenia gravis. **A,** AP view. **B,** lateral view.
(From Grainger RG, Allison DJ, Adam A, Dixon AK [eds]: Grainger & Allison's Diagnostic Radiology, 4th ed. Philadelphia, Churchill-Livingstone, 2001.)

computed tomography (CT). Lymphadenopathy can occur with malignant lymphomas (Fig. 102–7) , leukemias, metastatic neoplasms, sarcoidosis (Fig. 102–8), and infectious diseases, such as tuberculosis (Fig. 102–9) and histoplasmosis.

● Bronchogenic cysts (Fig.102–10) represent a common cause of mediastinal masses. Typically, they are thinwalled, with a respiratory or enteric mucosal lining, which often contains cartilage and mucous glands. The contents usually consist of thick mucoid material. The cysts can grow large without causing symptoms, but may compress surrounding structures, particularly the airway, and give rise to symptoms.

● Lymphagiomas (cystic hygromas) (Fig. 102–11), are benign, tumor-like congenital malformations of the lymphatic system comprised of complex lymph channels or cystic spaces containing clear or straw-colored fluid.

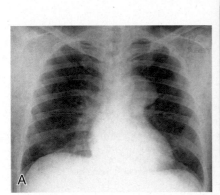
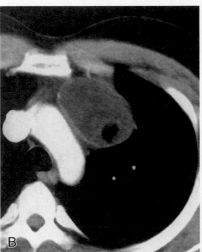

Fig 102–5
Teratoma in a young man undergoing an immigration chest radiograph. **A,** There are no specific features on the plain film to indicate the nature of the mass. **B,** CT scan demonstrates that the opacity visible on the chest radiograph is well-defined and contains soft tissue and fat densities.
(From Grainger RG, Allison DJ, Adam A, Dixon AK [eds]: Grainger & Allison's Diagnostic Radiology, 4th ed. Philadelphia, Churchill-Livingstone, 2001.)

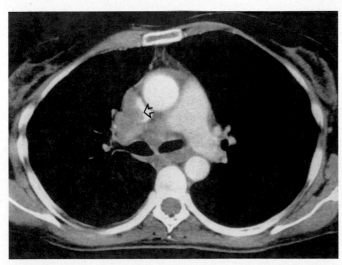

Fig 102–6
Metastatic malignant teratoma involving mediastinal nodes and directly invading the lumen of the superior vena cava (*arrow*), where it is outlined by intravenous contrast medium.
(From Grainger RG, Allison DJ, Adam A, Dixon AK [eds]: Grainger & Allison's Diagnostic Radiology, 4th ed. Philadelphia, Churchill-Livingstone, 2001.)

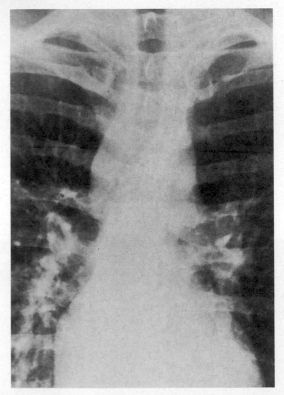

Fig 102–7
Right paratracheal lymphadenopathy caused by malignant lymphoma.
(From Grainger RG, Allison DJ, Adam A, Dixon AK [eds]: Grainger & Allison's Diagnostic Radiology, 4th ed. Philadelphia, Churchill-Livingstone, 2001.)

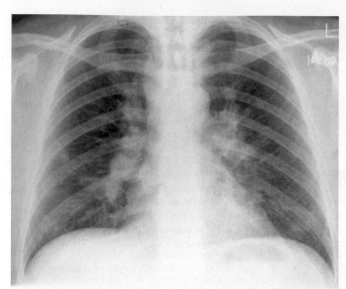

Fig 102–8
Bilateral hilar lymph node enlargement caused by sarcoidosis.
(From Grainger RG, Allison DJ, Adam A, Dixon AK [eds]: Grainger & Allison's Diagnostic Radiology, 4th ed. Philadelphia, Churchill-Livingstone, 2001.)

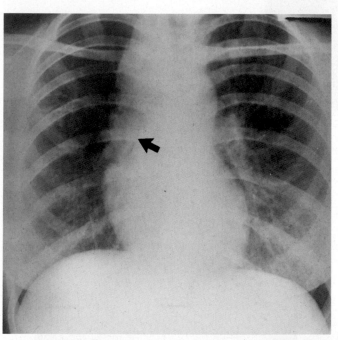

Fig 102–9
Primary tuberculosis in an adult. There is massive paratracheal and tracheobronchial adenopathy, with the latter compressing the right intermediate-stem bronchus (*arrow*). Minor parenchymal changes (mainly acinar nodules) are present in the right upper zone.
(From Grainger RG, Allison DJ, Adam A, Dixon AK [eds]: Grainger & Allison's Diagnostic Radiology, 4th ed. Philadelphia, Churchill-Livingstone, 2001.)

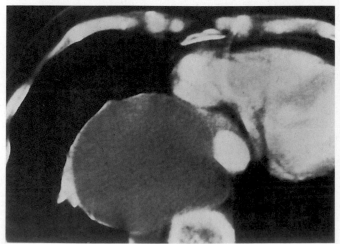

Fig 102–10
Bronchogenic cyst in an older asymptomatic woman. This contrast-enhanced CT scan shows the uniform water density contents of the cyst and the uniformly thin smooth wall. The slightly thicker irregular density at the lateral bounadry of the cyst is caused by the lung compressed by the cyst.
(From Grainger RG, Allison DJ, Adam A, Dixon AK [eds]: Grainger & Allison's Diagnostic Radiology, 4th ed. Philadelphia, Churchill-Livingstone, 2001.)

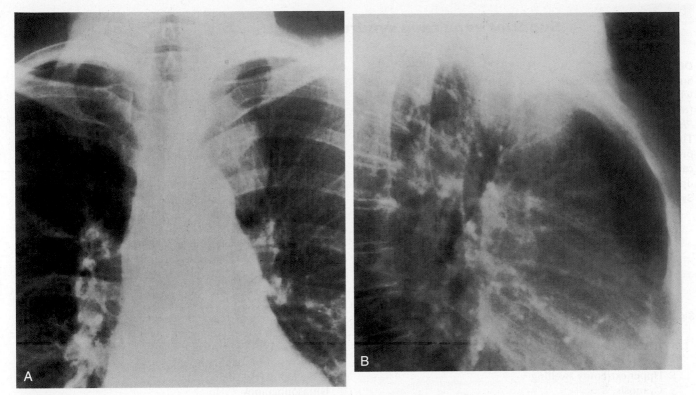

Fig 102–11
Cystic hygroma showing a smooth mass in contact with the neck in an asymptomatic 52-year-old woman. The tumor was surgically resected.
A, Posteroanterior projection. **B,** Lateral projection.
(From Grainger RG, Allison DJ, Adam A, Dixon AK [eds]: Grainger & Allison's Diagnostic Radiology, 4th ed. Philadelphia, Churchill-Livingstone, 2001.)

Chapter 103 Superior vena cava syndrome

DEFINITION
Superior vena cava syndrome is a set of symptoms that results when a mediastinal mass compresses the superior vena cava (SVC) or the veins that drain into it.

PHYSICAL FINDINGS AND CLINICAL PRESENTATION
The pathophysiology of the syndrome involves increased pressure in the venous system draining into the superior vena cava (Fig. 103–1), producing edema of the head, neck, and upper extremities.

Symptoms
- Shortness of breath
- Chest pain
- Cough
- Dysphagia
- Headache
- Syncope
- Visual trouble

Signs
- Chest wall vein distention
- Neck vein distention
- Facial edema
- Upper extremity swelling
- Cyanosis

CAUSE
- Lung cancer (80% of all cases, of which half are small cell lung cancer)
- Lymphoma (15%)
- Tuberculosis
- Goiter
- Aortic aneurysm (arteriosclerotic or syphilitic)
- SVC thrombosis
  1. Primary: associated with a central venous catheter
  2. Secondary: as a complication of SVC syndrome associated with one of the above mentioned causes

DIFFERENTIAL DIAGNOSIS
The syndrome is characteristic enough to exclude other diagnoses. The differential diagnosis concerns the underlying causes listed.

WORKUP
- Chest x-ray
- Chest CT scan or magnetic resonance imaging (MRI; Fig. 103–2) is usually adequate to establish the diagnosis of superior vena cava obstruction and to assist in the differential diagnosis of probable cause.
- Venography (Fig. 103–3)
- Ultrasonography

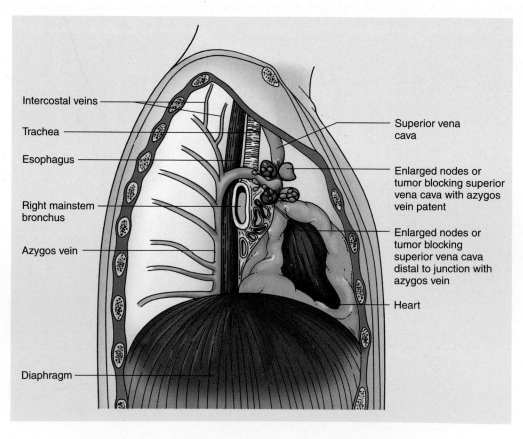

Fig 103–1
Lateral view of the thorax, with superior vena cava obstruction.
(From Abeloff MD: Clinical Oncology, 3rd ed. Philadelphia, Elsevier, 2004.)

- Percutaneous needle biopsy (generally the initial diagnostic modality used to establish a histologic diagnosis)
- Bronchoscopy
- Mediastinoscopy
- Thoracotomy

TREATMENT

- Emergency empirical radiation is indicated in critical situations such as respiratory failure or central nervous system signs associated with increased intracranial pressure.
- Treatment of the underlying malignancy—radiation, chemotherapy
- Anticoagulant or fibrinolytic therapy in patients who do not respond to cancer treatment within a week or if an obstructing thrombus has been documented

- Diuretics, upright positioning, and fluid restriction until collateral channels develop and allow for clinical regression are useful modalities for superior vena cava (SVC) syndrome secondary to benign disease.
- Corticosteroids
- Percutaneous self-expandable stents that can be placed under local anesthesia with radiologic manipulation are useful in the treatment of SVC syndrome, especially in cases associated with malignant tumors.

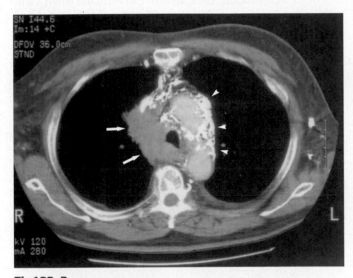

Fig 103–2

Obstruction of the superior vena cava caused by mediastinal adenopathy. In this 55-year-old man with lung carcinoma, a lymph node mass (*arrows*) is obstructing the superior vena cava. Multiple collateral vessels are demonstrated (*arrowheads*).
(From Crawford MH, DiMarco JP, Paulus WJ [eds]: Cardiology, 2nd ed. St. Louis, Mosby, 2004.)

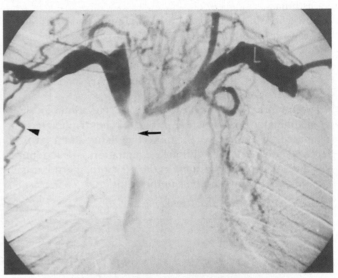

Fig 103–3

Upper limb venography. Bilateral arm venography reveals obstruction of the superior vena cava (SVC) by tumor in the mediastinum (*arrow*). This was a case of SVC syndrome secondary to lung carcinoma metastatic disease. Note the collateral venous channels that have opened up (*arrowhead*).
(From Grainger RG, Allison DJ, Adam A, Dixon AK [eds]: Grainger & Allison's Diagnostic Radiology, 4th ed. Philadelphia, Churchill-Livingstone, 2001.)

Chapter 104	Diaphragm abnormalities

DIAGNOSIS

Chest x-ray

- Normally, each hemidiaphragm is seen on the posteroinferior (PA) chest film as a smooth, curved line that is upwardly convex. The lateral attachment of the diaphragm to the ribs is represented by the lateral costophrenic abscess, a sharply refined acute angle (Fig. 104–1).

CAUSE

- The most common cause of a flat diaphragm is emphysema (Fig. 104–2).
- Depression of the diaphragm can also occur with severe asthma.
- Inversion of the diaphragm is sometimes seen with a tension pneumothorax (Fig. 104–3) and with large basal bullae. It is also a common accompaniment of pleural effusions (Fig.104–4). Elevation of a single hemidiaphragm is usually secondary to adjacent pleural, pulmonary, or subphrenic disease, or to a phrenic nerve palsy.
- Eventration (Fig.104–5) can also cause elevation of a single diaphragm. In eventration, a part of the diaphragm is replaced by a thin layer of connective tissue and a few scattered muscle fibers. Although eventration is a recognized cause of respiratory distress in the newborn, it is not usually associated with symptoms in the adult.

- Intrathoracic herniation of abdominal content occurs through congenital defects in the muscle, through traumatic tears or, most commonly, through acquired areas of weakness at the central esophageal hiatus. Bochdalek defects through the pleuroperitoneal canal occur along the posterior aspect of the diaphragm, and the hernia usually contains retroperitoneal fat and a portion of kidney or spleen.
- Asymptomatic *Bochdalek hernias* (Fig. 104–6) are present in 6% of otherwise normal adults. These hernias appear on a lateral chest film as a focal bulge centered approximately 4 to 5 cm anterior to the posterior diaphragmatic insertion. On CT or MRI scans, the diagnosis can be made when a soft tissue or fatty mass is seen protruding through a small defect in the posteromedial aspect of either hemidiaphragm.
- A *Morgagni hernia* presents in adulthood as an opacity at the right cardiophrenic angle (Fig. 104–7). It frequently contains omentum and may contain gut. Its smooth, well-defined margin and soft tissue radiodensity usually allow its differentiation from the much more common fat pad collection at this site. The diagnosis is easily established with CT or MRI.

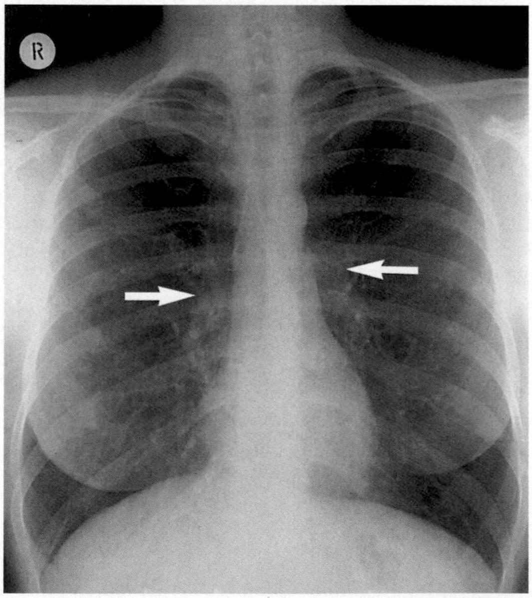

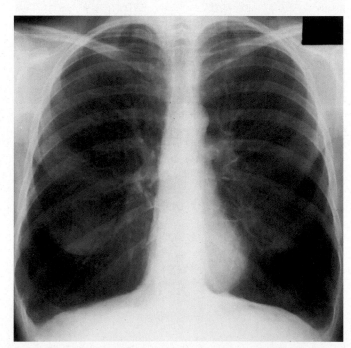

Fig 104–1

Normal digital posteroanterior chest radiograph demonstrating position and density of the hilar structures. *Arrows* indicate the hilar points, where the superior pulmonary vein crosses the descending lower lobe artery, the left normally being level with or slightly higher than the right. (From Grainger RG, Allison DJ, Adam A, Dixon AK [eds]: Grainger & Allison's Diagnostic Radiology, 4th ed. Philadelphia, Churchill-Livingstone, 2001.)

Fig 104–2

Severe diffuse emphysema. The posteroanterior chest radiograph shows the right hemidiaphragm to be flattened and located below the anterior aspect of the eighth rib. Left lung parenchyma is seen between the heart and the left hemidiaphragm. Arterial depletion is present in the lung bases. (From Grainger RG, Allison DJ, Adam A, Dixon AK [eds]: Grainger & Allison's Diagnostic Radiology, 4th ed. Philadelphia, Churchill-Livingstone, 2001.)

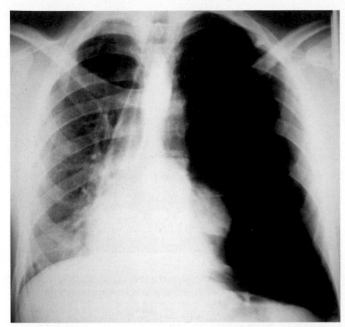

Fig 104-3
Tension pneumothorax. In this chest radiograph, a left-sided pneumothorax is accompanied by a mediastinal shift to the right and striking depression of the left hemidiaphragm. The right lung is partially collapsed.
(From Grainger RG, Allison DJ, Adam A, Dixon AK [eds]: Grainger & Allison's Diagnostic Radiology, 4th ed. Philadelphia, Churchill-Livingstone, 2001.)

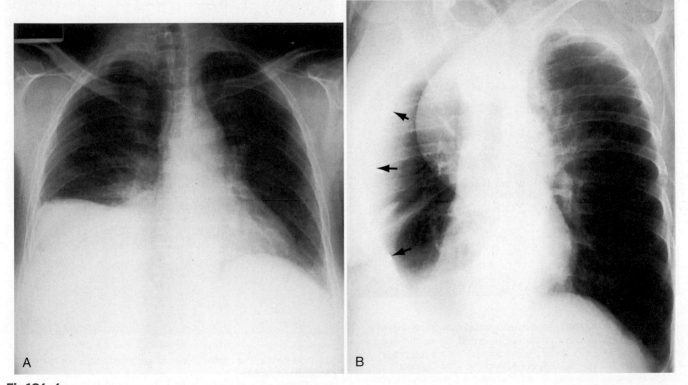

Fig 104-4
Subpulmonary pleural effusion. **A,** On the erect posteroanterior film, the effusion stimulates a high hemidiaphragm. **B,** A right lateral decubitus view demonstrates the fluid (*arrows*).
(From Grainger RG, Allison DJ, Adam A, Dixon AK [eds]: Grainger & Allison's Diagnostic Radiology, 4th ed. Philadelphia, Churchill-Livingstone, 2001.)

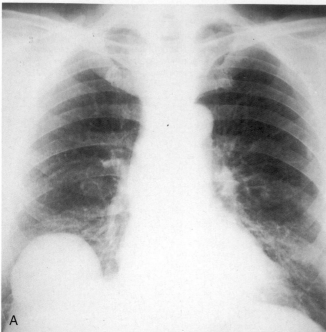

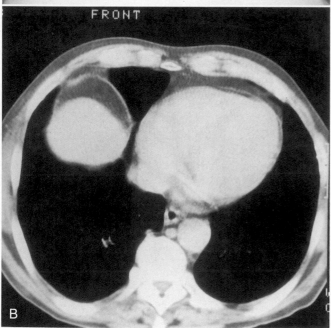

Fig 104–5
Focal eventration. **A,** The posteroanterior chest radiograph reveals a soft tissue opacity arising from the diaphragm. **B,** CT scan shows the presence of fat and liver under the elevated part of the diaphragm.
(From Grainger RG, Allison DJ, Adam A, Dixon AK [eds]: Grainger & Allison's Diagnostic Radiology, 4th ed. Philadelphia, Churchill-Livingstone, 2001.)

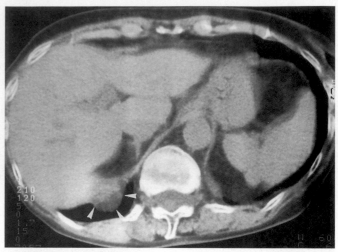

Fig 104–6
Bochdalek hernia. The CT scan shows a fatty mass abutting the upper surface of the posteromedial aspect of the right hemidiaphragm *(arrowheads)*.
(From Grainger RG, Allison DJ, Adam A, Dixon AK [eds]: Grainger & Allison's Diagnostic Radiology, 4th ed. Philadelphia, Churchill-Livingstone, 2001.)

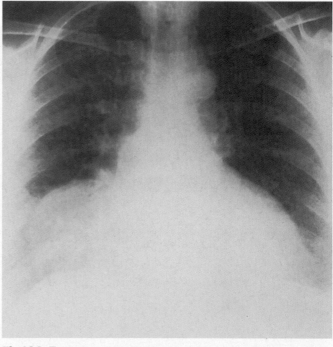

Fig 104–7
Morgagni hernia. The hernia is seen as an opacity adjacent to the right cardiophrenic angle.
(From Grainger RG, Allison DJ, Adam A, Dixon AK [eds]: Grainger & Allison's Diagnostic Radiology, 4th ed. Philadelphia, Churchill-Livingstone, 2001.)

REFERENCES

Ferri F: Ferri's Clinical Advisor 2007. St. Louis, Mosby, 2007

Grainger RG, Allison D: Grainger & Allison's Diagnostic Radiology: A Textbook of Medical Imaging, 4th ed. Philadelphia, Churchill-Livingstone, 2001.

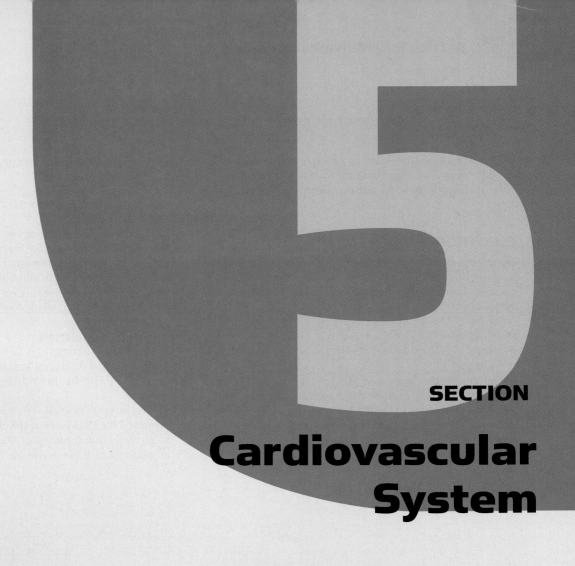

SECTION

Cardiovascular System

Chapter 105: Diagnostic tests and procedures
Chapter 106: Ischemic heart disease
Chapter 107: Valvular disease
Chapter 108: Infective endocarditis
Chapter 109: Congestive heart failure
Chapter 110: Cardiogenic pulmonary edema
Chapter 111: Cardiomyopathies
Chapter 112: Myocarditis
Chapter 113: Pericarditis
Chapter 114: Cor pulmonale
Chapter 115: Arrhythmias
Chapter 116: Cardiac pacemakers

Chapter 117: Congenital heart disease
Chapter 118: Atrial myxoma
Chapter 119: Peripheral arterial disease
Chapter 120: Venous ulcers and stasis dermatitis
Chapter 121: Lymphedema
Chapter 122: Deep vein thrombosis
Chapter 123: Thromboangiitis obliterans (Buerger's disease)
Chapter 124: Abdominal aortic aneurysm
Chapter 125: Aortic dissection
Chapter 126: Syncope
Chapter 127: Hypertension

Chapter 105 — Diagnostic tests and procedures

Symptoms from heart disease are nonspecific and in addition to a detailed history and physical examination will often require many of the diagnostic tests and procedures described in this section.

A. ELECTROCARDIOGRAM

- The electrocardiogram (ECG) provides information on the heart rhythm and underlying cardiac morphology and represents a fundamental component of the cardiovascular assessment.
- A normal ECG is described in Figure 105–1. Positions of leads and electrodes in the ECG are shown in Figure 105–2.
- Proper ECG evaluation requires the following systematic approach:
  - **Determine the heart rate (HR).** If the heart rhythm is regular, the heart rate can be determined by dividing 300 by the number of boxes in the R-R interval (e.g., if the R-R interval contains four large boxes, the heart rate is 75 beats/min [HR = 300/4]).
  - **Determine the heart rhythm.**
  1. Is the rhythm regular?
  2. Are there P waves?
  3. Is the P wave related to the QRS (i.e., are P waves "married" to the QRS)?
  4. The P wave should always be upright in lead II if there is sinus rhythm (unless there is reversal of leads or dextrocardia). If the rhythm is irregular, the P wave can help with the diagnosis (e.g., with sinus arrhythmia, the P waves will be identical; with wandering pacemaker, the P waves will have different shapes; with atrial fibrillation, the P waves are not discernible).
  - **Evaluate the intervals.**
  1. PR interval: normal is 0.12 to 0.21 second (for practical purposes, the PR interval is normal if it does not exceed a large box). The PR interval becomes shorter as the rate increases.
  2. QRS interval: normal is 0.04 to 0.10 second (for practical purposes, the QRS interval should not be greater than half a large box). Interruptions of the bundle branches produce a bundle branch block pattern.

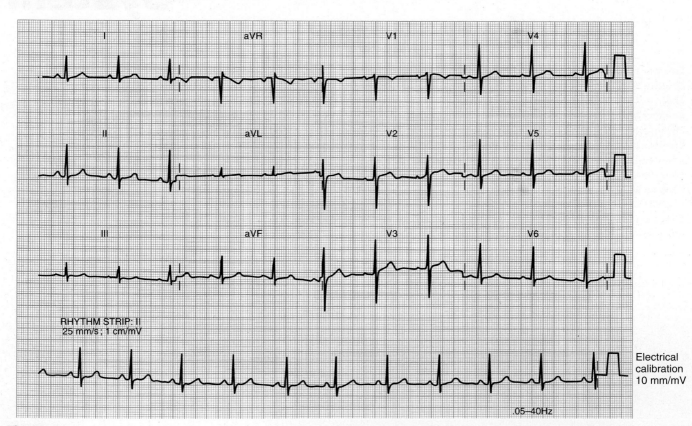

Fig 105–1
Normal electrocardiogram.
(From Souhami RL, Moxham J: Textbook of Medicine, 4th ed. London, Churchill Livingstone, 2002.)

RHYTHM STRIP: II
25 mm/s ; 1 cm/mV

Electrical calibration 10 mm/mV

.05–40Hz

If the QRS is wide, evaluate for bundle-branch block:

a. Left bundle branch block (LBBB) (Fig. 105–3). The following may be seen:

(1) Wide slurred R in V_{5-6}

(2) QRS prolonged 0.12 second or more, lengthened ventricular time, or intrinsicoid deflection

(3) Lead aVL similar to V_{5-6}, lead I similar to aVL and V_{5-6} (with depression of the ST segments and inversion of the T waves).

b. Right bundle branch block (RBBB) (Fig. 105–4)

(1) QRS 0.12 second or more

(2) Wide slurred S waves in V_{5-6}, rsR′ complexes in V_3R and V_{1-2}, with absent Q waves

(3) VAT prolonged in in V_3R and V_{1-2}; wide S wave in lead I

3. Q–T interval: the normal Q–T interval should be less than half the R-R interval (if the heart rate is less than 100 beats/min).

c. Determine the axis deviation: look at the net QRS deflection in leads I and aVF.

(1) Normal axis: net QRS deflection is positive in leads I and aVF.

(2) Right axis deviation (RAD): net QRS deflection negative in lead I, positive in lead aVF

(3) Left axis deviation (LAD): net QRS deflection positive in lead I, negative in lead aVF

(4) Indeterminate axis: net QRS deflection negative in leads I and aVF

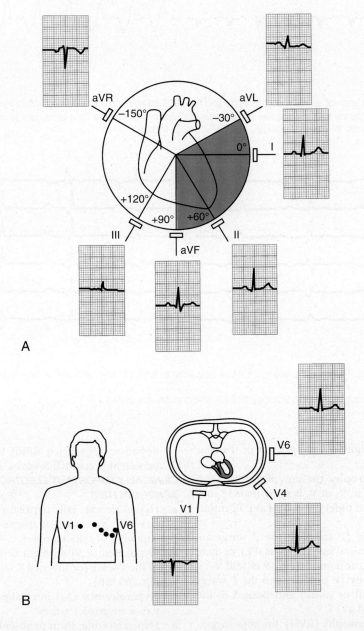

Fig 105–2

Positions of leads and electrodes in the electrocardiogram. **A,** Frontal plane. **B,** Horizontal plane. Four limb leads and six precordial leads are routinely used. The anatomic landmarks are V1, right sternal edge, fourth intercostal space; V2, complementary position to left of sternum; V3, between V2 and V4; V4, midclavicular line, fifth space; V5, anterior axillary line; V6, midaxillary line, horizontally in line with V4.

(From Souhami RL, Moxham J: Textbook of Medicine, 4th ed. London, Churchill Livingstone, 2002.)

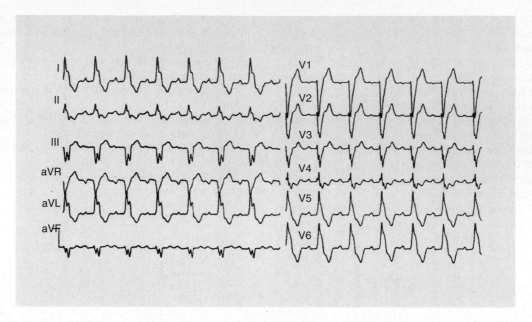

Fig 105–3
Left bundle branch block. The P–R interval is within normal limits and the QRS complexes are wide and without marked axis deviation.
Note the typical QRS-T axis discordance and the atypical persistence of a small r wave in the right precordial leads.
(From Crawford, MH, DiMarco JP, Paulus WJ [eds]: Cardiology, 2nd ed. St. Louis, Mosby, 2004.)

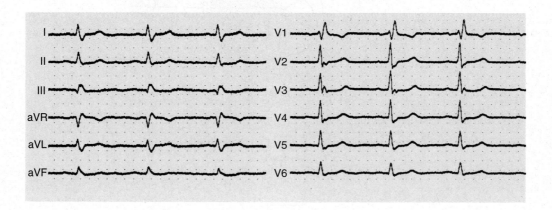

Fig 105–4
Complete right bundle branch block. The typical pattern of rSR is best seen in lead V1. The QRS axis is slightly deviated on the right
(at 90 degrees).
(From Crawford, MH, DiMarco JP, Paulus WJ [eds]: Cardiology, 2nd ed. St. Louis, Mosby, 2004.)

4. **Hypertrophy:** look for signs of enlargement of the four chambers.

    a. Left ventricular hypertrophy: the sum of the deepest S in V_1 or V_2 and the tallest R in V_5 or V_6 is more than 35 mm (in patients 35 years of age or older); R in lead aVL 12 mm or more; "strain" pattern

    b. Left atrial hypertrophy (P mitrale): the P waves are notched (M-shaped) in the mitral leads (I, II, or aVL), or there is a deep terminal negative component to the P in lead V_1

    c. Right atrial hypertrophy (P pulmonale): the P waves are prominent (2.5 mm tall or more) and peaked in the pulmonary leads (II, III, and aVF).

    d. Right ventricular hypertrophy (RVH): findings suggestive of RVH in adults are right atrial enlargement, right axis deviation, incomplete RBBB, low voltage, tall R wave in V_1, persistent precordial S waves, and right ventricular strain.

CLINICALLY IMPORTANT ELECTROCARDIOGRAPHIC ABNORMALITIES

- Hyperkalemia: tall, narrow, or tent-shaped T waves (Fig. 105–5A), decreased or absent P waves, short Q–T intervals, widening of QRS complex
- Hypokalemia: ST segment depression, decreased amplitude of the T wave (or inverted T waves), prominent U waves (see Fig. 105–5B)
- Hypocalcemia: Q–T interval prolongation (see Fig. 105–6), flat or inverted T waves
- Hypercalcemia: short or absent ST segment (see Fig. 105–6), decreased Q–Tc interval.

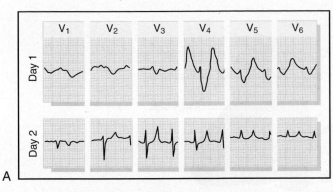

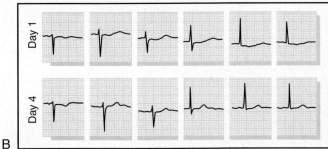

Fig 105–5
Electrocardiographic changes in hyperkalemia **(A)** and hypokalemia **(B)**. **A**, On day 1, at a K^+ level of 8.6 mEq/liter, the P wave is no longer recognizable and the QRS complex is diffusely prolonged. Initial and terminal QRS delay is characteristic of K^+-induced intraventricular conduction slowing and is best illustrated in leads V_2 and V_6. On day 2, at a K^+ level of 5.8 mEq/liter, the P wave is recognizable with a P–R interval of 0.24 second; the duration of the QRS complex is approximately 0.10 second, and the T waves are characteristically "tented." **B**, On day 1, at a K^+ level of 1.5 mEq/liter, the T and U waves are merged. The U wave is prominent and the QU interval is prolonged. On day 4, at a K^+ level of 3.7 mEq/liter, the tracing is normal. (Courtesy of Dr. C. Fisch.)

B. CHEST X-RAY

- Figure 105–7 illustrates the composition of the normal cardiac silhouette on a chest x-ray.
- Examination of a chest x-ray requires a logical approach. The following is a short guide to reading a chest x-ray:
  - Check exposure technique for lightness or darkness.
  - Verify left and right by looking at stomach bubble and heart shape.
  - Check for rotation: does the thoracic spine shadow align in the center of the sternum between the clavicles?
  - Make sure the x-ray is taken in full inspiration (10 posterior or 6 anterior ribs should be visible).
  - Is the film a portable, anteroposterior (AP), or posteroanterior film (PA)? (The heart size cannot be accurately judged from an AP film.)
- Check the soft tissues for foreign bodies or subcutaneous emphysema.
- Check all visible bones and joints for osteoporosis, old fractures, metastatic lesions, rib notching, or presence of cervical ribs.
- Look at diaphragm for tenting, free air, and position.
- Check hilar and mediastinal areas for the following: size and shape of aorta, presence of hilar nodes, prominence of hilar blood vessels, elevation of vessels (left normally slightly higher), elevation of left mainstem bronchus indicating left atrial enlargement.
- Look at heart for size, shape, calcified valves, and enlarged atria.
- Check costophrenic angles for fluid or pleural scarring.
- Check pulmonary parenchyma for infiltrates, increased interstitial markings, masses, absence of normal margins, air bronchograms, or increased vascularity, and silhouette signs.
- Look at lateral film for the following: confirmation and position of questionable masses or infiltrates, size of retroster-

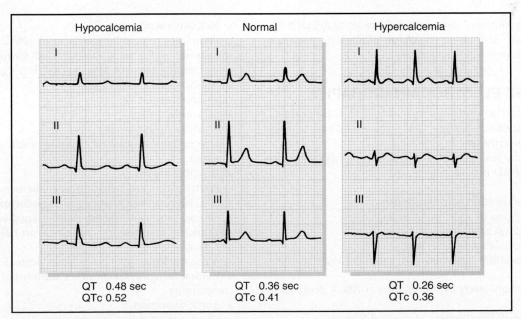

Fig 105–6
Prolongation of the Q–T interval (ST segment portion) is typical of hypocalcemia. Hypocalcemia may cause abbreviation of the ST segment and shortening of the Q–T interval.
(From Goldberger AL: Clinical Electrocardiography: A Simplified Approach. 6th ed. St. Louis, Mosby, 1999.)

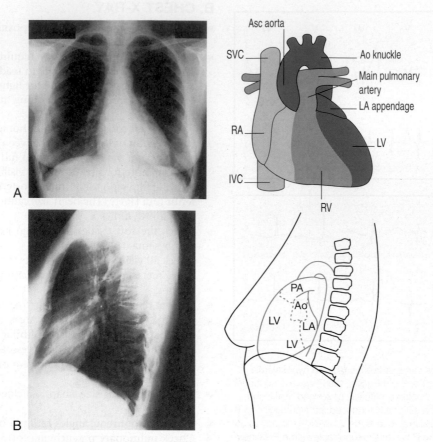

Fig 105–7
Composition of the normal cardiac silhouette on chest X-rays. **A,** Posteroanterior view. **B,** Lateral view. Ao, aorta; LA, left atrium; RA, right atrium; RPA and LPA, right and left pulmonary arteries; RV and LV, right and left ventricles; SVC, superior vena cava.
(From Souhami RL, Moxham J: Textbook of Medicine, 4th ed. London, Churchill Livingstone, 2002.)

nal air space, anteroposterior chest diameter, vertebral bodies for bony lesions or overlying infiltrates, posterior costophrenic angle for small effusion.

C. EXERCISE ELECTROCARDIOGRAPHY

- Treadmill exercise tolerance test is useful to identify patients with coronary artery disease (CAD) who would benefit from cardiac catheterization.
- The sensitivity and specificity of treadmill exercise testing in diagnosing CAD is 65% to 80%.
- Indications
  - Evaluation of chest pain syndromes
  - Typical angina or effort-induced angina
  - Atypical chest pain
  - Evaluation of exercise tolerance
  - Post–myocardial infarction (MI; modified exercise tolerance test)
  - Post–coronary artery bypass grafting (CABG), postangioplasty
  - Evaluation of effectiveness of medical therapy
  - Evaluation of arrhythmias

- Sick sinus syndrome
- Premature ventricular contractions (PVCs); benign PVCs usually disappear with exercise, and frequent ventricular ectopy during recovery after exercise is a significant predictor of increased risk of death.
- Contraindications
  - MI within 2 days
  - Aortic stenosis (severe)
  - Hypertrophic obstructive cardiomyopathy (HOCM; symptomatic)
  - Unstable angina
  - Poorly controlled arrhythmias, malignant PVCs
  - ECG suggestive of active or recent ischemia
  - Severe chronic obstructive pulmonary disease (COPD)
  - Clinically manifested congestive heart failure (CHF)
  - Endocarditis
  - Atrioventricular (AV) block (high degree)
  - Cardiac arrhythmias causing symptoms of hemodynamic compromise
  - Aortic dissection
  - Severe uncontrolled hypertension
  - Recent or active cerebral ischemia

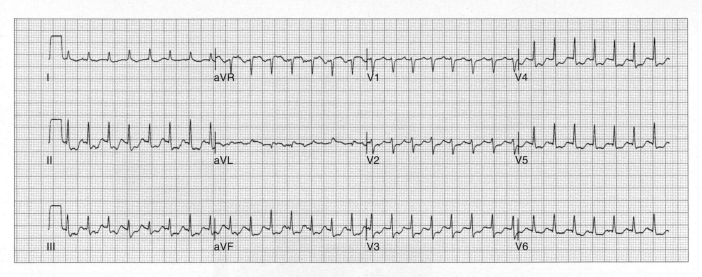

Fig 105–8

The baseline electrocardiogram is essentially normal. During exercise and recovery, the patient developed ST segment depression in the inferolateral leads, reaching 2 mm. This exercise test suggests multivessel coronary artery disease.
(From Crawford, MH, DiMarco JP, Paulus WJ [eds]: Cardiology, 2nd ed. St. Louis, Mosby, 2004.)

- Choice of protocols:
  - Bruce protocol is preferred for patients with minimum symptomatic limitation; it entails a higher initial workload and greater work increments.
  - Low-level or symptom-limited test is preferred for post-MI, post-CABG, and more debilitated patients; it entails a lower initial workload and smaller increments than the Bruce protocol.
- Interpretation: both protocols aim at eliciting a diagnostic response within 6 to 15 minutes. Exercise duration is one of the strongest independent prognostic indicators and correlates well with outcome. A stress test is generally considered positive for ischemia if the following occur:
  - ST segment depression (Fig. 105–8)
  - Patient develops chest pain.
  - Patient develops hypotension (normally during exercise, there is an increase in systolic blood pressure because of an increase in stroke volume).
  - Patient develops significant arrhythmias. Frequent ventricular ectopy during recovery after exercise is a better predictor of an increased risk of death than ventricular ectopy occurring only during exercise.
  - ST segment elevation during exercise, although uncommon, provides reliable information about the location of the underlying coronary lesion (e.g., anterior ST segment elevation generally indicates left anterior descending coronary disease, whereas inferior ST segment elevation is suggestive of a lesion in or proximal to the posterior descending artery).

D. ECHOCARDIOGRAPHY

Echocardiography is an excellent diagnostic tool in cardiology because of its noninvasive nature, relatively low cost, superb special and temporal resolutions, and ability to image cardiovascular anatomy and to evaluate physiology in real time. To obtain an echocardiographic image, a burst of ultrasound energy is generated by a transducer and travels through the soft tissue. When the propagating ultrasound wave encounters an interface between tissues with different acoustic properties, some of the energy is reflected back toward the transducer and some of the energy is refracted and continues to travel in the medium until it encounters the next interface. The returning ultrasound energy is then converted into an electrical energy that goes through a series of electronic processes, including amplification, postprocessing, and display (Fig. 105–9). The use of Doppler ultrasound to assess normal and abnormal hemodynamics has become an integral part of the echocardiographic examination. Spectral and color-coded Doppler flow mapping is used extensively to measure velocity and direction of blood flow (Fig. 105–10). Calculations based on Doppler-derived measurements allow quantitative estimation of flow volume (e.g., cardiac output), pressure gradient across a stenotic region, cross-sectional flow area, and prediction of intracardiac pressures. Doppler echocardiography also provides qualitative and semiquantitative assessment of valve regurgitation, intra- and extracardiac shunts, and myocardial motion.

Echocardiography is indicated in patients with systolic murmur suggestive of aortic stenosis, mitral valve prolapse, or hypertrophic cardiomyopathy. It is also useful in the detection of ischemia-induced regional wall motion abnormalities or mitral regurgitation. Figure 105–11 shows the diagnosis of a mitral valve abnormality. Doppler ultrasound can be used to measure pressure gradients and to demonstrate the degree of valvular regurgitation.

- Echocardiography combined with treadmill exercise (stress echo) or pharmacologic stress with dobutamine can be used to detect regional wall abnormalities that occur during myocardial ischemia associated with CAD.
- Stress echocardiography: can be used in place of nuclear testing. Decrements in contractile function are directly related to decreases in regional subendocardial blood flow.

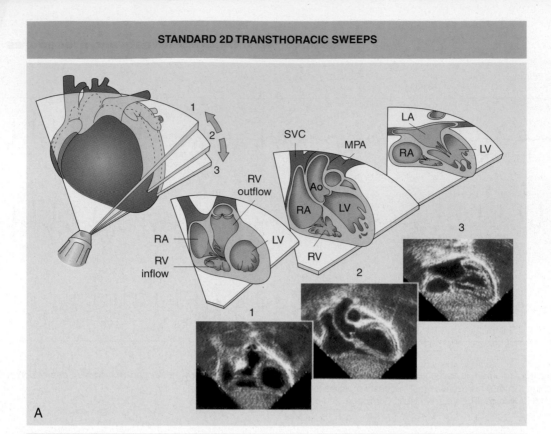

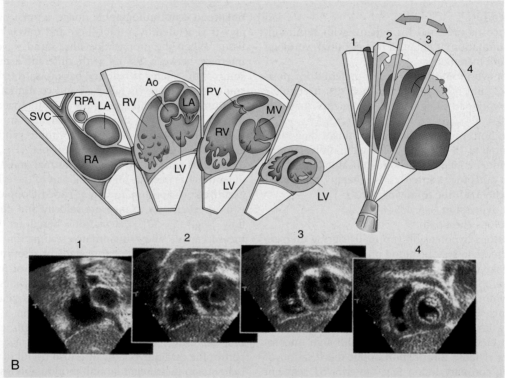

Fig 105–9

Standard two-dimensional transthoracic imaging sweeps. **A,** Subxiphoid long-axis sweep. Slow gradual sweep starting at the level of the upper abdomen will show the connection of the inferior vena cava to the right atrium (RA). The left atrium (LA) is seen next. The connection of the pulmonary veins and the atrial septum can be demonstrated from this view. The left ventricle (LV) is seen along its long axis. Further superior angulation of the transducer depicts the left ventricular outflow tract, aortic valve, and ascending aorta (Ao). The superior vena cava (SVC) is seen to the right of the ascending aorta and the main pulmonary artery (MPA) is seen to the left of the aorta. Further superior tilt of the transducer shows the right ventricular inflow (RV inflow) and outflow (RV outflow) and the pulmonary valve. The sweep ends with the anterior free wall of the right ventricle. **B,** Subxiphoid short-axis sweep. From the subxiphoid long-axis view, the transducer is rotated clockwise by approximately 90 degrees. The sweep begins at the rightward-most aspect of the heart and progresses from right to left through the cardiac apex. The superior vena cava (SVC) and inferior vena cava are seen entering the right atrium (RA). The right pulmonary artery (RPA) is seen in cross section behind the SVC and above the left atrium (LA). The atrial septum is well seen in this plane. Sweeping the transducer leftward will show the base of the left ventricle (LV) and right ventricle (RV) and the atrioventricular valves. The aortic valve is seen in cross section at this level. Further leftward tilt of the transducer depicts a cross-sectional view of the LV and mitral valve (MV), in addition to the right ventricular outflow tract and pulmonary valve (PV). The sweep ends with imaging of the midmuscular septum, the papillary muscles, and the apical portions of both ventricles.

(From Crawford, MH, DiMarco JP, Paulus WJ [eds]: Cardiology, 2nd ed. St. Louis, Mosby, 2004.)

Pharmacologic agents can also be used to induce stress in select patients. For example, dobutamine echocardiography is preferable to dipyridamole or adenosine scintigraphy in patients with moderate or severe bronchospastic disease. On the other hand, advantages of stress perfusion imaging are its higher sensitivity, especially for one-vessel CAD, and better accuracy in evaluating possible ischemia when multiple left ventricular wall motion abnormalities are present. Table 105–1 describes risk stratification based on stress testing modalities.

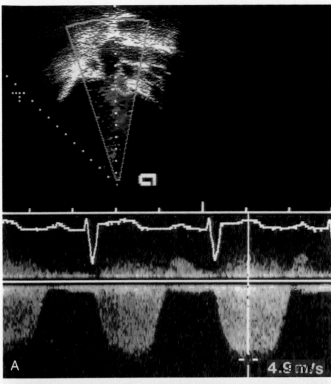

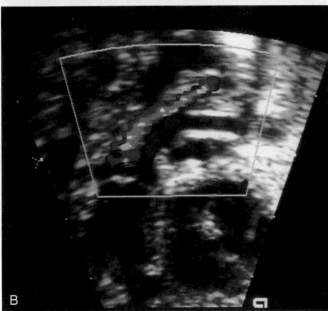

Fig 105–10

Doppler echocardiography. **A,** Visualization of a high-velocity jet by color Doppler aids in aligning the continuous-wave Doppler cursor in a patient with SLL transposition of the great arteries (visceroatrial situs solitus [S], L-ventricular loop [L], and L-transposition [L]), with severe subpulmonary stenosis (predicted maximal instantaneous gradient, approximately 96 mm Hg.) **B,** Imaging of a left-to-right flow jet through a patent ductus arteriosus by color Doppler flow mapping from the subxiphoid, short-axis view.
(From Crawford, MH, DiMarco JP, Paulus WJ [eds]: Cardiology, 2nd ed. St. Louis, Mosby, 2004.)

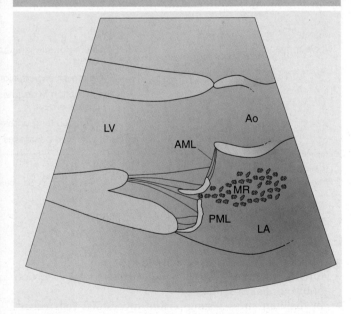

Fig 105–11

Echocardiographic diagnosis of mitral valve abnormality. There is severe posterior mitral leaflet (PML) prolapse into the left atrium (LA), producing loss of coaptation with the anterior mitral leaflet (AML) and allowing severe mitral regurgitation (MR). Ao, aorta; LV, left ventricle.
(From Crawford, MH, DiMarco JP, Paulus WJ [eds]: Cardiology, 2nd ed. St. Louis, Mosby, 2004.)

TABLE 105–1 Characterization of low-risk and high-risk stress test results

Test	Low likelihood of future events	High likelihood of future events
Standard exercise ECG	No more than 1-mm ST segment depression at moderate to high workload	≥2-mm ST segment depression
	No or minimal chest discomfort with adequate stress (not all studies agree; diabetics excluded)	Positive ECG at low level of exercise stress
		Decrease in blood pressure during exercise
		Low or poor functional capacity
		ST depression documented in multiple ECG leads
		Prolonged (≥2-3 min) ST depression
		Severe chest pain and/or ST depression, with slow resolution
Dipyrimadole or adenosine study	Chest pain not helpful	Appearance of ST depression
	Segment depression uncommon and, if absent, not helpful; positive ST response implies an adverse prognosis	
Stress echo: exercise, dobutamine, or butamine	Single region of stress-induced abnormal wall motion	Wall motion defect(s) appear at low level of stress
	Mild degree of stress-induced abnormality (e.g., hypokinesis)	Multiple (two or more) wall motion abnormalities
	Abnormality occurs at high level of exercise or dobutamine infusion	Development of akinesis or dyskinesis
		Decrease in global LV ejection fraction
		LV cavity dilation
Nuclear imaging	Small area of stress-induced isotope defect	Multiple (two or more) regions of isotope uptake
	Single region of perfusion deficit	Large area(s) of reversible ischemia
	Mild reduction in degree of isotope uptake at peak stress	Moderate to severe reduction in degree of isotope uptake
	No increased lung uptake	Lung uptake
	LV cavity size decreases	LV cavity size increases

LV, left ventricular.
From Crawford, MH, DiMarco JP, Paulus WJ (eds): Cardiology, 2nd ed. St. Louis, Mosby, 2004.

E. NUCLEAR IMAGING

- Radionuclide testing (e.g., thallium, dipyramidole [Persantine], dobutamine) is useful and sensitive in the detection of myocardial ischemia.
- In thallium stress testing, viable myocardial cells extract thallium-201 from the blood (Fig. 105–12).
- An absent thallium uptake (cold spot on thallium scan) is an indicator of an absence of blood flow to an area of the myocardium (Fig. 105–13).
- A fixed defect on thallium scanning indicates MI at that site, whereas a defect that reperfuses suggests myocardial ischemia.
- Increased uptake of thallium by the lungs during exercise predicts myocardial ischemia and risk of subsequent cardiac events.

F. CARDIAC CATHETERIZATION

Coronary angiography is performed to define the location and extent of coronary disease; it is indicated in select patients who are candidates for coronary graft bypass surgery, angioplasty, or stent placement and in patients with suspected syndrome X. Coronary arteriography with ergonovine provocation may be indicated in patients with suspected vasospastic angina and inconclusive noninvasive studies. Figure 105–14 illustrates a normal left coronary angiogram, and Figure 105–15 shows stenotic coronary lesions.

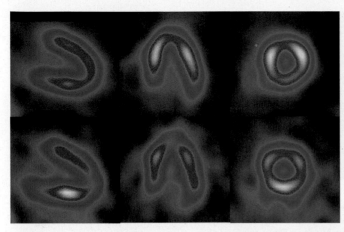

Fig 105–12
Normal thallium myocardial perfusion tomograms in vertical long axis (*left*), horizontal long axis (*center*), and short-axis planes (*right*); stress images (*top*) and redistribution (*bottom*). There is homogeneous uptake of tracer throughout the myocardium and hence no coronary obstruction. (From Grainger RG, Allison DJ, Adam A, Dixon AK [eds]: Grainger & Allison's Diagnostic Radiology, 4th ed. London, Harcourt, 2001.)

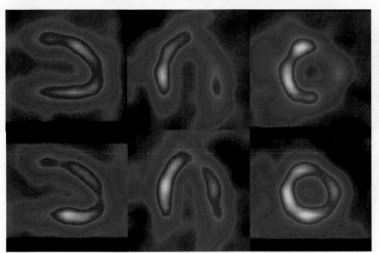

Fig 105–13
Left circumflex stenosis-inducible ischemia—stress (*top*) and redistribution (*bottom*) thallium tomograms in the vertical long-axis (*left*), horizontal long-axis (*center*), and short-axis (*right*) planes in a patient with left circumflex stenosis. There is inducible ischemia of moderate extent and severity in the lateral wall, as seen in stress images.
(From Grainger RG, Allison DJ, Adam A, Dixon AK [eds]: Grainger & Allison's Diagnostic Radiology, 4th ed. London, Harcourt, 2001.)

NORMAL LEFT CORONARY ANGIOGRAPHY

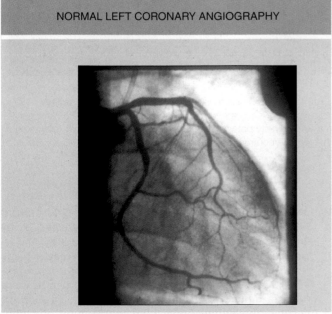

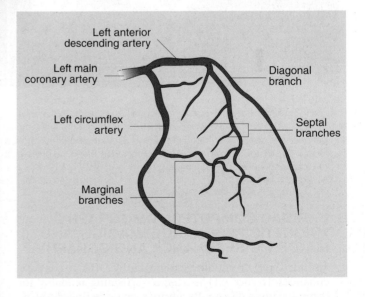

Fig 105–14
Normal left coronary angiography, right anterior oblique projection.
(From Crawford, MH, DiMarco JP, Paulus WJ [eds]: Cardiology, 2nd ed. St. Louis, Mosby, 2004.)

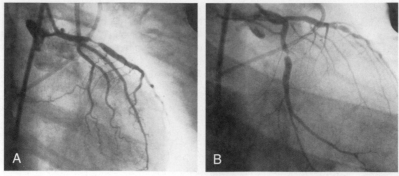

Fig 105–15
Stenotic coronary lesions. **A,** Discrete stenosis in the proximal portion of the left anterior descending artery. **B,** Discrete stenosis in the midportion of the left anterior descending artery and discrete stenosis in the midportion of the left circumflex artery.
(From Crawford, MH, DiMarco JP, Paulus WJ [eds]: Cardiology, 2nd ed. St. Louis, Mosby, 2004.)

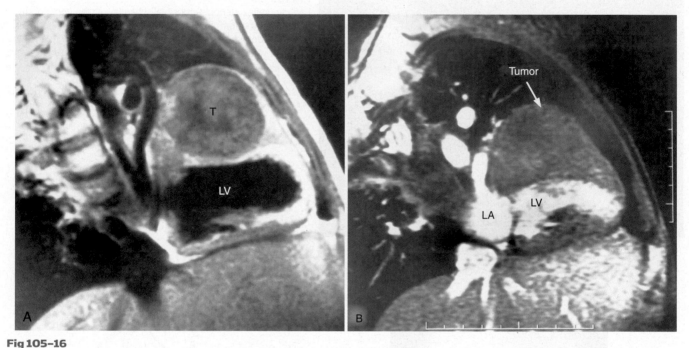

Fig 105–16
Spin-echo and gradient echo magnetic resonance imaging (MRI) sequences in a 4-year-old boy with large fibroma of the left ventricle.
A, Fast spin-echo with double-inversion recovery showing the left ventricle (LV) and tumor (T) in the long axial oblique plane. Note the clear definition between the dark blood pool and the myocardium, and the difference in signal intensity between the tumor and the myocardium (dark blood sequence). **B,** Diastolic frame of cine MRI obtained in the same plane as in **A**. Note the contrast between the bright signal from the myocardium (bright blood sequence). LA, left atrium.
(From Crawford, MH, DiMarco JP, Paulus WJ [eds]: Cardiology, 2nd ed. St. Louis, Mosby, 2004.)

G. CARDIAC COMPUTED TOMOGRAPHY, MAGNETIC RESONANCE IMAGING, AND MAGNETIC RESONANCE ANGIOGRAPHY

- Multidetector computed tomography (CT; contrast-enhanced 16-slice CT) is a newer screening modality for coronary artery disease. Its advantages are its speed, safety, and low cost when compared with angiography. Its limitations are as follows: limited to patients with a regular rhythm and slow rates, poor image in morbidly obese patients, inaccurate visualization of the coronary artery within a stent, decreased diagnostic accuracy in older patients because of the prevalence and severity of coronary calcifications with increasing age.

- Cardiac magnetic resonance imaging (MRI) is a sophisticated noninvasive imaging modality that overcomes many of the limitations of echocardiography and cardiac catheterization. High-resolution static and dynamic images of the heart, blood vessels, and other thoracic structures are obtained, regardless of body size and acoustic barriers. Current MRI is a modality capable of real-time imaging, succinct, dynamic, three-dimensional (3D) visualization of cardiovascular anatomy, and accurate quantification of blood flow and myocardial function. Cine MRI is used to delineate cardiovascular anatomy and function (Fig. 105–16).

- Magnetic resonance angiography: gadolinium-enhanced 3D magnetic resonance angiography (MRA) is useful to delineate extracardiac vascular anatomy. This technique produces a 3D data set in which the signal from blood is particularly high and strongly contrasts with nonvascular structures (Figs. 105–17 and 105–18). It can be used to detect coronary artery disease of the proximal and middle segments and can be used to identify (or rule out) left main coronary artery or three-vessel disease reliably.

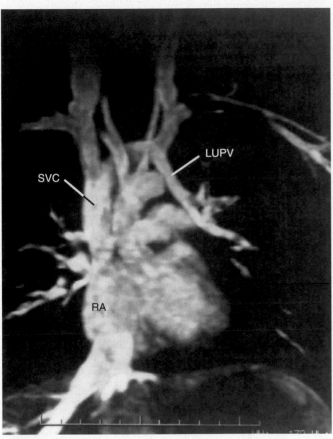

Fig 105–17
Gadolinium-enhanced 3D magnetic resonance angiography in a 9-year-old girl with partially anomalous pulmonary venous connection of the left upper pulmonary vein (LUPV) to the left innominate vein. The course of the anomalous pulmonary vein, its connection to the systemic vein, and its distance from the left atrium are seen on this maximal intensity projection image. The 3D data set was acquired during a 21-second period of breath holding. RA, right atrium; SVC, superior vena cava.
(From Crawford, MH, DiMarco JP, Paulus WJ [eds]: Cardiology, 2nd ed. St. Louis, Mosby, 2004.)

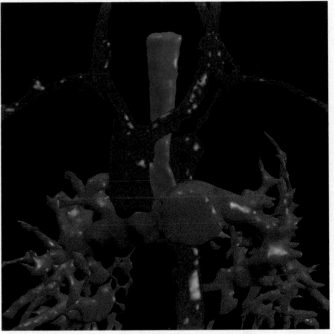

Fig 105–18
3D surface reconstruction from gadolinium-enhanced 3D magnetic resonance angiography data set in a patient with a right aortic arch and an aberrant origin of the left subclavian artery from the descending aorta. This frontal view shows the ascending aorta (red) and the aortic arch to the right of the trachea (purple). The pulmonary arteries are seen in yellow. The caliber of the left subclavian artery increases at its junction with the left vertebral artery. Phase velocity flow mapping (not shown) demonstrated retrograde flow in the left vertebral artery, which supplies the left subclavian artery.
(From Crawford, MH, DiMarco JP, Paulus WJ [eds]: Cardiology, 2nd ed. St. Louis, Mosby, 2004.)

Chapter 106 | Ischemic heart disease

A. ANGINA PECTORIS

DEFINITION

Angina pectoris is characterized by discomfort that occurs when myocardial oxygen demand exceeds the supply. Myocardial ischemia can be asymptomatic (silent ischemia), particularly in diabetics. Angina can be classified as follows.

(1) Chronic (stable)

- Usually follows a precipitating event (e.g., climbing stairs, sexual intercourse, a heavy meal, emotional stress, cold weather)
- Generally same severity as previous attacks; relieved by rest or by the customary dose of nitroglycerin
- Caused by a fixed coronary artery obstruction secondary to atherosclerosis. An ECG taken during the acute episode may show transient T wave inversion or ST segment depression

or elevation, but more than 50% of patients with chronic stable angina have normal results on resting ECG. Figure 106–1 illustrates significant ECG findings. The presence of one or more obstructions in major coronary arteries is likely; the severity of stenosis is usually more than 70%.

(2) Unstable (rest or crescendo, coronary syndrome)

- Recent onset
- Increasing severity, duration, or frequency of chronic angina
- Occurs at rest or with minimal exertion. ECG abnormalities are described in Figure 106–2.

(3) Prinzmetal's variant

- Occurs at rest
- Manifests electrocardiographically as episodic ST segment elevations (Fig. 106–3)
- Caused by coronary artery spasms (Fig. 106–4), with or without superimposed coronary artery disease
- Patients also more likely to develop ventricular arrhythmias.

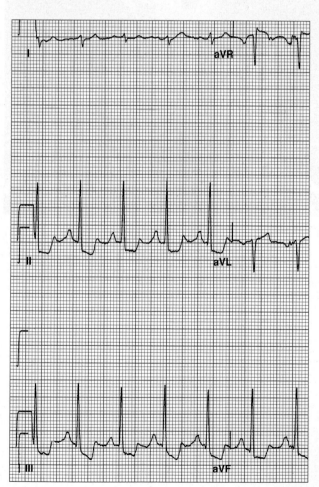

Fig 106–1

Flat (horizontal) and down-sloping ST segment depression greater than 1 mm in a patient with proven angina and obstructive coronary artery disease.

(From Kahn MG: Rapid ECG Interpretation, 2nd ed. Philadelphia, WB Saunders, 2003.)

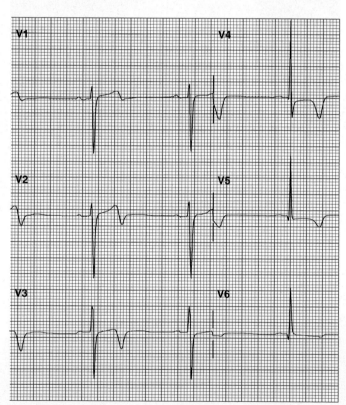

Fig 106–2

V leads in a patient with unstable angina. ST-T segment abnormalities seen in V_1 through V_4. The tracing was taken when the patient was pain-free. Note the "hitched up" ST segment in V_2 and V_3 with deep T inversion. The pattern is typical of significant proximal left anterior descending coronary artery stenosis.

(From Kahn MG: Rapid ECG Interpretation, 2nd ed. Philadelphia, WB Saunders, 2003.)

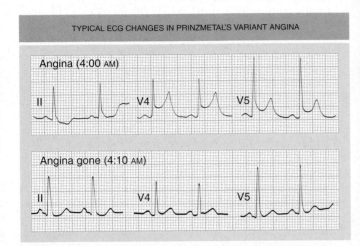

Fig 106-3

Typical ECG changes in Prinzmetal's variant angina. This man had completely normal coronary arteriograms. The vasospastic episode recorded here occurred while the patient was asleep. He was awakened by angina, which subsided after the administration of sublingual nitrate, and the ST segment returned to baseline within minutes after the nitrate treatment.
(From Crawford, MH, DiMarco JP, Paulus WJ [eds]: Cardiology, 2nd ed. St. Louis, Mosby, 2004.)

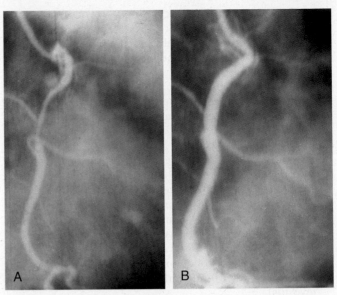

Fig 106-4

Segmental coronary artery spasm. **A,** The spasm involves the proximal segment of the right coronary artery. **B,** Administration of intracoronary nitrate resulted in significant vasodilation of the coronary artery and abolished the spasm.
(From Crawford, MH, DiMarco JP, Paulus WJ [eds]: Cardiology, 2nd ed. St. Louis, Mosby, 2004.)

(4) Microvascular angina (syndrome X)

- Refers to patients with normal coronary angiograms and no coronary spasm but chest pain resembling angina and positive exercise test
- Defective endothelium-dependent dilation in the coronary microcirculation contributing to the altered regulation of myocardial perfusion and the ischemic manifestations in these patients
- Patients with chest pain and normal or nonobstructive coronary angiograms are predominantly women, and many have a prognosis that is not as benign as commonly thought (2% risk of death or MI at 30 days of follow-up).
- Useful therapeutic agents for symptom relief are beta blockers, angiotensin-converting enzyme (ACE) inhibitors, and tricyclic agents. Aggressive antiatherosclerotic therapy with statins should also be undertaken.

(5) Other

- Angina caused by aortic stenosis and idiopathic hypertrophic subaortic stenosis, cocaine-induced coronary vasoconstriction

(6) Refractory angina

- Refers to patients who, despite optimal medical therapy, have both angina and objective evidence of ischemia and are not considered candidates for revascularization.
- Current FDA-approved therapies consist of enhanced external counterpulsation (EECP), transcutaneous electrical nerve stimulation (TENS), and invasive therapies, such as spinal cord stimulation, transmyocardial revasculariza-

tion, and percutaneous myocardial revascularization. Although some of these therapies may improve symptoms and quality of life, they have not been shown to improve mortality rates.

FUNCTIONAL CLASSIFICATION

- New York Heart Association functional classification of angina:
  - Class I—angina only with unusually strenuous activity
  - Class II—angina with slightly more prolonged or rigorous activity than usual
  - Class III—angina with usual daily activity
  - Class IV—angina at rest.
- Grading of angina by the Canadian Cardiovascular Society classification system:
  - Class I—ordinary physical activity does not cause angina, such as walking, climbing stairs. Angina occurs with strenuous, rapid, or prolonged exertion at work or recreation.
  - Class II—slight limitation of ordinary activity. Angina occurs on walking or climbing stairs rapidly; walking uphill; walking or stair climbing after meals, in cold, in wind, or under emotional stress; or only during the few hours after awakening. Angina occurs on walking more than two blocks on level ground and climbing more than one flight of ordinary stairs at a normal pace and in normal condition.
  - Class III—marked limitations of ordinary physical activity. Angina occurs on walking one to two blocks on level ground and climbing one flight of stairs in normal conditions and at a normal pace.
  - Class IV—inability to carry on any physical activity without discomfort; anginal symptoms may be present at rest.

383

PHYSICAL FINDINGS AND CLINICAL PRESENTATION

- Although there is significant individual variation, most patients complain of substernal chest pain (pressure, tightness, heaviness, sharp pain, sensation similar to intestinal gas or dysphagia).
- The pain is of short duration (30 seconds to 30 minutes), nonpleuritic, and often accompanied by shortness of breath, nausea, diaphoresis, and numbness or pain in the left arm, jaw, or shoulder.

DIFFERENTIAL DIAGNOSIS

Noncardiac pain mimicking angina may be caused by:
- Pulmonary diseases (pulmonary hypertension, pulmonary embolism, pleurisy, pneumothorax, pneumonia)
- Gastrointestinal (GI) disorders (peptic ulcer disease, pancreatitis, esophageal spasm or spontaneous esophageal muscle contraction, esophageal reflux, cholecystitis, cholelithiasis)
- Musculoskeletal conditions (costochondritis, chest wall trauma, cervical arthritis with radiculopathy, muscle strain, myositis)
- Acute aortic dissection
- Herpes zoster
- Anxiety disorder

HISTORY AND PHYSICAL EXAMINATION

- The most important diagnostic factor is the history. Chest pain or left arm pain or discomfort reproducing previously documented angina and a known history of CAD or MI are indicative of a high likelihood of acute coronary syndrome.
- The physical examination is of little diagnostic help and may be totally normal in many patients, although the presence of an S_4 gallop is suggestive of ischemic chest pain. Transient mitral regurgitation, hypotension, diaphoresis, and rales indicate a high likelihood of acute coronary syndrome.

LABORATORY TESTS

- Initial laboratory tests in patients with chronic stable angina should include hemoglobin, fasting glucose, and fasting lipid panel.

- Cardiac isoenzymes (creatine kinase [CK]-MB, every 8 hours twice) should be obtained to rule out MI in patients presenting with acute chest pain.
- Cardiac troponins I and T are specific markers of myocardial necrosis and are useful in evaluating patients with acute chest pain. Elevation of either of these proteins in the setting of an acute coronary syndrome identifies patients with a several-fold increased risk of death in subsequent weeks.
- Measurement of total cholesterol, low-density lipoprotein (LDL) cholesterol (LDL-C), high-density lipoprotein cholesterol (HDL-C), and fasting serum triglycerides are recommended for cardiovascular screening.
- A single measurement of brain-type natriuretic peptide (BNP), a natriuretic and vasodilative peptide regulated by ventricular wall tension and stored mainly in the ventricular myocardium, obtained in the first few days after the onset of ischemic symptoms, provides predictive information for risk stratification in acute coronary syndromes. N-terminal (NT)–pro-BNP is also a marker of long-term mortality in patients with stable coronary disease and provides prognostic information beyond that provided by conventional cardiovascular risk factors and the degree of left ventricular systolic dysfunction.

TREATMENT

- Aggressive modification of preventable risk factors (weight reduction in obese patients, regular aerobic exercise program, low-cholesterol and low-sodium diet, cessation of tobacco use)
- Diets using nonhydrogenated unsaturated fats as the predominant form of dietary fat, whole grains as the main form of carbohydrates, an abundance of fruits and vegetables, and adequate omega-3 fatty acids are optimal for prevention of coronary heart disease.
- Correction of possible aggravating factors (e.g., anemia, hypertension, diabetes mellitus, hyperlipidemia, thyrotoxicosis, hypothyroidism)

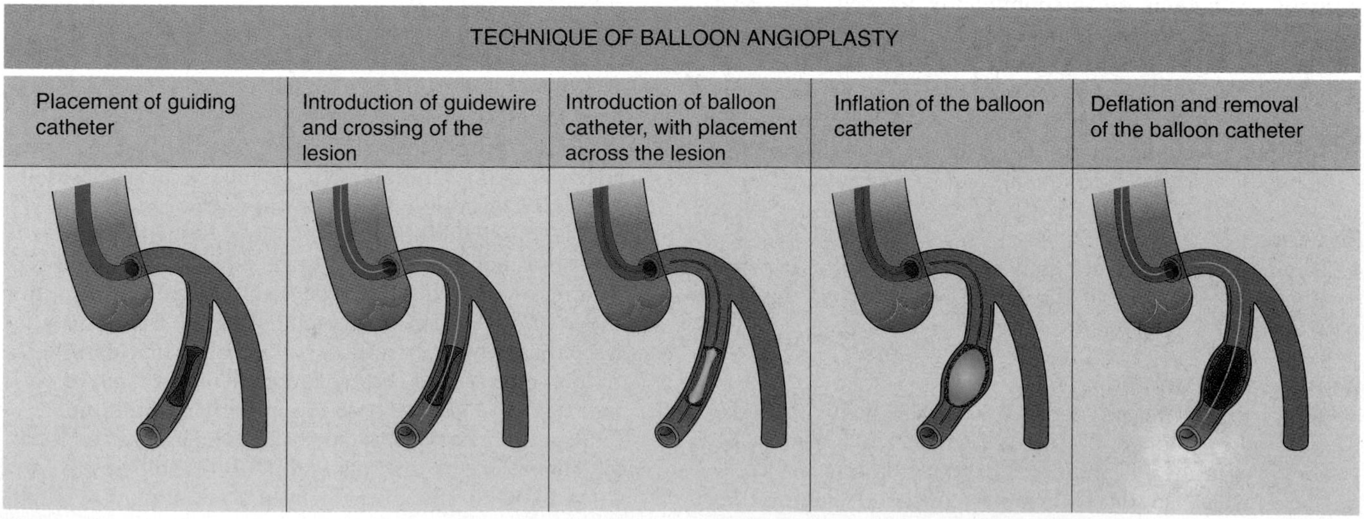

TECHNIQUE OF BALLOON ANGIOPLASTY				
Placement of guiding catheter	Introduction of guidewire and crossing of the lesion	Introduction of balloon catheter, with placement across the lesion	Inflation of the balloon catheter	Deflation and removal of the balloon catheter

Fig 106–5
Technique of balloon angioplasty.
(From Crawford, MH, DiMarco JP, Paulus WJ [eds]: Cardiology, 2nd ed. St. Louis, Mosby, 2004.)

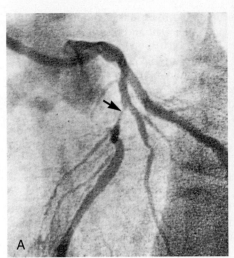 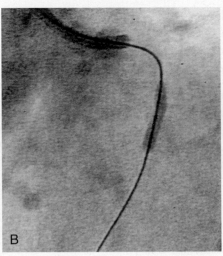 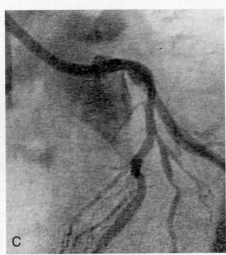

Fig 106–6
Left anterior oblique views of localized stenosis *(arrow)* of mid–left anterior descending artery, treated by balloon angioplasty. **A,** Before balloon angioplasty. **B,** Balloon-dilating stenosis. **C,** After balloon angioplasty—no residual stenosis.
(From Grainger RG, Allison DJ, Adam A, Dixon AK [eds]: Grainger & Allison's Diagnostic Radiology, 4th ed. London, Harcourt, 2001.)

DELIVERY OF A BALLOON EXPANDABLE STENT

Deflated balloon with premounted stent

Stent

Balloon

Delivery of stent with inflation of balloon

Stent

Inflated balloon

Fig 106–7
Delivery of a balloon-expandable stent. When the stent is delivered, the balloon is inflated so that the stent is pushed against the wall of the artery. The stent does not recoil after the balloon is deflated and removed.
(From Crawford, MH, DiMarco JP, Paulus WJ [eds]: Cardiology, 2nd ed. St. Louis, Mosby, 2004.)

- The major classes of anti-ischemic agents are nitrates, beta-adrenergic blockers, calcium channel blockers, aspirin, and heparin; they can be used alone or in combination.
- Aspirin: use of aspirin reduces cardiovascular mortality and morbidity by 20% to 25% in patients with coronary artery disease..
- CABG is recommended for patients with left main coronary disease, for those with symptomatic three-vessel disease, and for those with a left ventricular ejection fraction (EF) less than 40% and critical stenosis (more than 70%) in all three major coronary arteries. Surgical therapy improves prognosis, particularly in diabetic patients with multivessel disease.
- Percutaneous coronary intervention (PCI) (Figs. 106–5 and 106–6) should be considered for patients with one- or two-vessel disease that does not involve the main left coronary artery and in whom ventricular function is normal or near-normal.
- The development of coronary stents (Fig. 106–7) has broadened the number of patients who can be treated in the cardiac laboratory. Cardiac stents are currently used in almost 95% of all percutaneous interventional lesions. Drug-eluting stents are shown in Figure 106–8.

B. MYOCARDIAL INFARCTION

DEFINITION
Acute coronary syndromes are manifestations of ischemic heart disease and represent a broad clinical spectrum that includes non–ST segment elevation acute coronary syndrome (NSTEACS) (collectively unstable angina [UA]/non–ST elevation MI [NSTEMI]), and ST elevation MI [STEMI]).
- Myocardial infarction is characterized by necrosis resulting from an insufficient supply of oxygenated blood to an area of the heart. According to the joint European Society of Cardiology/American College of Cardiology guidelines, either one of the following criteria for acute evolving or recent MI satisfies the diagnosis:
  - Typical rise and gradual fall (troponin) or more rapid rise and fall (CK-MB) of biochemical markers of myocardial necrosis with at least one of the following:
  1. Ischemic symptoms
  2. Development of pathologic Q waves on ECG
  3. ECG changes indicative of ischemia (ST segment elevation or depression)
  4. Coronary artery intervention (e.g., coronary angioplasty)
- Pathologic findings of acute MI (Fig. 106–9)

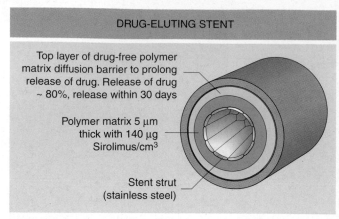

DRUG-ELUTING STENT

Top layer of drug-free polymer matrix diffusion barrier to prolong release of drug. Release of drug ~ 80%, release within 30 days

Polymer matrix 5 μm thick with 140 μg Sirolimus/cm³

Stent strut (stainless steel)

Fig 106–8
Drug-eluting stent.
(From Crawford, MH, DiMarco JP, Paulus WJ [eds]: Cardiology, 2nd ed. St. Louis, Mosby, 2004.)

- STEMI: area of ischemic necrosis that penetrates the entire thickness of the ventricular wall and results in ST segment elevation
- Unstable angina: coronary arterial plaque rupture with fragmentation and distal arterial embolization resulting in myocardial necrosis;.usually occurs without ST elevation and is thus called NSTEMI

PHYSICAL FINDINGS AND CLINICAL PRESENTATION

Clinical presentation

- Crushing substernal chest pain usually lasting longer than 30 minutes.
- Pain is unrelieved by rest or sublingual nitroglycerin or is rapidly recurring.
- Pain radiates to the left or right arm, neck, jaw, back, shoulders, or abdomen and is not pleuritic in character.
- Pain may be associated with dyspnea, diaphoresis, nausea, or vomiting.

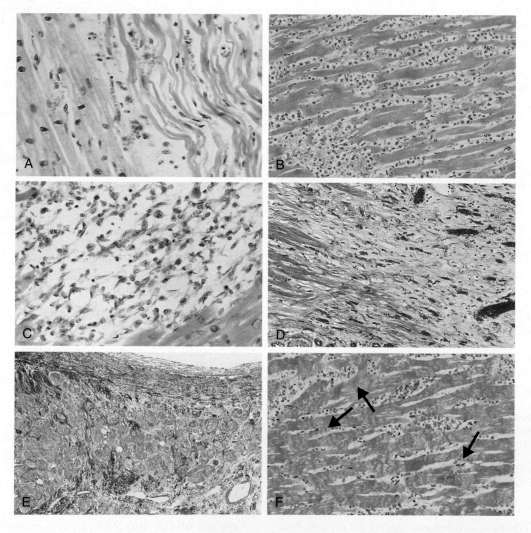

Fig 106–9
Microscopic features of myocardial infarction. **A,** One-day-old infarct showing coagulative necrosis, wavy fibers with elongation, and narrowing, compared with adjacent normal fibers (lower right). Widened spaces between the dead fibers contain edema fluid and scattered neutrophils. **B,** Dense polymorphonuclear leukocytic infiltrate in an area of acute myocardial infarction of 3 to 4 days' duration. **C,** Almost complete removal of necrotic myocytes by phagocytosis (approximately 7 to 10 days). **D,** Granulation tissue with a rich vascular network and early collagen deposition, approximately 3 weeks after infarction. **E,** Well-healed myocardial infarct, with replacement of the necrotic fibers by dense collagenous scar. A few residual cardiac muscle cells are present. (In **D** and **E,** collagen is highlighted as blue color in this Masson trichrome stain.) **F,** Myocardial necrosis with hemorrhage and contraction bands, visible as dark bands spanning some myofibers (arrows). This is the characteristic appearance of markedly ischemic myocardium that has been reperfused.
(From Schoen FJ: The heart. In Cotran RS, Kumar V, Collins T [eds]: Pathologic Basis of Disease, 6th ed. Philadelphia, WB Saunders, 1999, pp 560-561.)

- There is no pain in approximately 20% of infarctions (usually in diabetic or older patients).

PHYSICAL FINDINGS
- Skin may be diaphoretic, with pallor (because of decreased oxygen).
- Rales may be present at the bases of lungs (indicative of CHF).
- Cardiac auscultation may reveal an apical systolic murmur caused by mitral regurgitation secondary to papillary muscle dysfunction; S_3 or S_4 may also be present.
- Physical examination may be completely normal.

CAUSE
- Coronary atherosclerosis and thrombosis (Fig. 106–10)
- Coronary artery spasm (Fig. 106–11)
- Coronary embolism (caused by infective endocarditis, rheumatic heart disease, intracavitary thrombus)
- Periarteritis and other coronary artery inflammatory diseases
- Dissection into coronary arteries (aneurysmal or iatrogenic)
- Congenital abnormalities of coronary circulation
- MI with normal coronaries (MINC syndrome): more frequent in younger patients and cocaine addicts. The risk of acute MI is increased by a factor of 24 during the 60 minutes after the use of cocaine in persons who are otherwise at relatively low risk. Most patients with cocaine-related MI are young, nonwhite, male cigarette smokers without other risk factors for arteriosclerotic heart disease (ASHD) who have a history of repeated cocaine use. Blood and urine toxicology screen for cocaine is recommended in all young patients who present with acute MI.

- Hypercoagulable states, increased blood viscosity (polycythemia vera)

LABORATORY TESTS
- Table 106–1 describes characteristics of commonly used markers of myocardial injury. Figure 106–12 illustrates typical cardiac marker diagnostic window curves and serum levels after acute MI.
- Cardiac troponin levels: cardiac-specific troponin T (cTnT) and cardiac-specific troponin I (cTnI) are generally indicative of myocardial injury.
- CK-MB isoenzyme is a useful marker for MI. It is released in the circulation in amounts that correlate with the size of the infarct.
- Neither CK-MB nor troponin consistently appears in the blood within 6 hours after an ischemic event; therefore, serial testing (e.g., on presentation and after 8 hours) is necessary to rule out MI definitely.
- ECG (Fig. 106–13):
  - In STEMI, there is development of:
  1. Inverted T waves, indicating an area of ischemia.
  2. Elevated ST segment, indicating an area of injury (Fig. 106–14). Significant ST segment elevation of 0.10 mV or more measured 0.02 second after the J point is evident in two contiguous leads. The presence of this finding in leads V_1-V_6 indicates anterior or anterolateral MI, in leads I and aVL a lateral MI, and in leads II, III, or aVF is diagnostic of inferior wall MI.
  3. Q waves, indicating an area of infarction (usually develop over 12 to 36 hours).

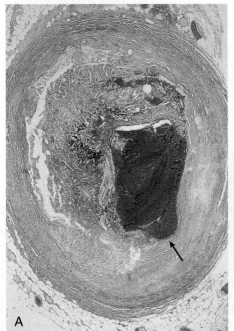 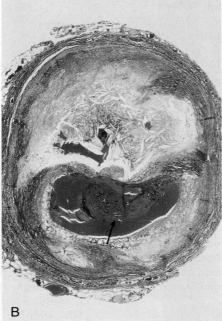 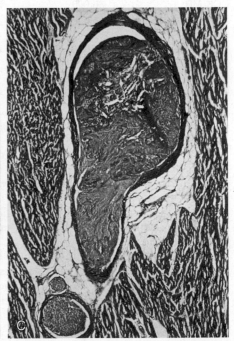

Fig 106–10
Coronary thrombosis. Coronary thrombosis is a dynamic process that is usually superimposed on a disrupted plaque. **A,** Lipid-rich plaque with ruptured surface and occlusive luminal thrombosis *(arrow)* superimposed. **B,** Disrupted plaque with platelet-rich nonocclusive thrombosis *(arrow)* superimposed. **C,** Small artery occluded by aggregated platelets (microembolus) found in the myocardium downstream of an evolving coronary thrombus. Such downstream embolization is often associated with microinfarcts in the myocardium.
(Courtesy of Professor Erling Falk, Aarhus, Denmark. From Crawford, MH, DiMarco JP, Paulus WJ [eds]: Cardiology, 2nd ed. St. Louis, Mosby, 2004.)

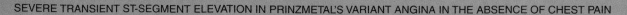

SEVERE TRANSIENT ST-SEGMENT ELEVATION IN PRINZMETAL'S VARIANT ANGINA IN THE ABSENCE OF CHEST PAIN

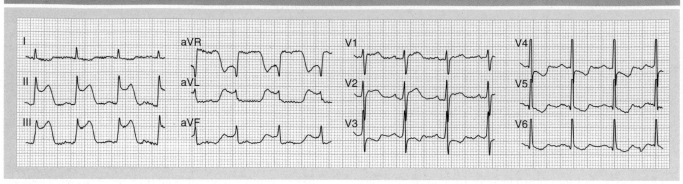

Fig 106–11

Severe transient ST segment elevation in Prinzmetal's variant angina in the absence of chest pain (silent myocardial ischemia). This episode was recorded at 9:28 AM. In a sizable proportion of patients, occlusive coronary spasm and ST segment elevation develop in the absence of chest pain (silent ischemia).

(From Crawford, MH, DiMarco JP, Paulus WJ [eds]: Cardiology, 2nd ed. St. Louis, Mosby, 2004.)

TABLE 106–1   Characteristics of commonly used markers of myocardial injury

Marker	Molecular weight (Da)	Range of times to initial elevation (hr)	Mean time to peak elevations without recanalization (hr)	Time to return to normal range	Most common sampling schedule
HFABP	14,000-15,000	1.5	5-10	24 hr	Admission and 4 hr
Myoglobin	17,800	1-4	6	24 hr	Admission and every 2 hr
cTnI	23,500	6-12	24	5-10 days	Admission and 6-9 hr
cTnT	33,000	3-12	12-48	5-14 days	Admission and 6-9 hr
CK-MB	86,000	3-12	24	48-72 hr	Admission and 6-9 hr
CK-MM tissue isoform	86,000	1-6	18	38 hr	Admission and every 2 hr
CK-MB tissue isoform	86,000	6-10	24	?	Admission and every 2 hr
LDH	135,000	10	24-48	10-14 days	24 hr after onset

CK, creatine kinase; cTnI, cardiac troponin I; cTnT, cardiac troponin T; HFABP, heart fatty acid binding protein; LDH, lactate dehydrogenase.
From Crawford, MH, DiMarco JP, Paulus WJ (eds): Cardiology, 2nd ed. St. Louis, Mosby, 2004.

● In NSTEMI:

1. History and myocardial enzyme elevations are compatible with MI.

2. ECG shows no ST segment elevation and sometimes shows a small depression of the ST segment (Fig. 106–15).

IMAGING STUDIES

● Chest radiography is useful to evaluate for pulmonary congestion and exclude other causes of chest pain.

● Echocardiography can evaluate wall motion abnormalities and identify mural thrombus or mitral regurgitation, which can occur acutely after MI.

RISK ASSESSMENT

Several risk assessment models are available. The TIMI risk score uses the following seven variables: age 65 years or older, at least three conventional risk factors for coronary artery disease, prior coronary stenosis 50% or more, ST segment deviation on ECG at presentation, two or more anginal events in the preceding 24 hours, use of aspirin in the prior 7 days, and elevated serum cardiac markers.

TREATMENT

● Any patient with suspected acute MI should immediately receive the following:

1. Antiplatelet therapy: aspirin, 160 to 325 mg PO unless true aspirin allergy is suspected. Clopidogrel 75 mg daily may be substituted if true allergy is present or given in addition to aspirin.

2. Nitrates: they increase the supply of oxygen by reducing coronary vasospasm and decrease consumption of oxygen by reducing ventricular preload.

3. Adequate analgesia: morphine sulfate, 2 to 4 mg IV initially, with increments of 2 to 8 mg IV at 5- to 15-minute intervals can be given for severe pain unrelieved by nitroglycerin.

4. Nasal oxygen: administer at 2 to 4 L/min.

● Prompt myocardial reperfusion can be accomplished with PCI, fibrinolytic therapy, or CABG. If readily available without delay, PCI is superior to thrombolytic therapy for treating patients with ST segment elevation MI. It is effective and generally results in more favorable outcomes than thrombolytic therapy.

- Beta-adrenergic blocking agents should generally be given to all patients with evolving acute MI.
- ACE inhibitors reduce left ventricular dysfunction and dilation and slow the progression of CHF during and after acute MI. They should be initiated within hours of hospitalization, provided the patient does not have hypotension or a contraindication (bilateral renal stenosis, renal failure, or history of angioedema caused by previous treatment with ACE inhibitors).

COMPLICATIONS OF POST–MYOCARDIAL INFARCTION

- <u>Arrhythmias</u>:
  High-grade ventricular arrhythmias occurring after thrombolytic therapy for acute MI are often attributed to successful reperfusion; however, they generally indicate a worsened

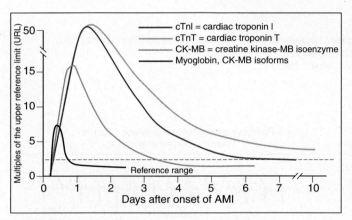

Fig 106–12
Typical cardiac marker: diagnostic window curves and serum levels, post–acute myocardial infarction (AMI).
(From Lehman CA [ed]: Saunders Manual of Clinical Laboratory Science. Philadelphia, WB Saunders, 1998.)

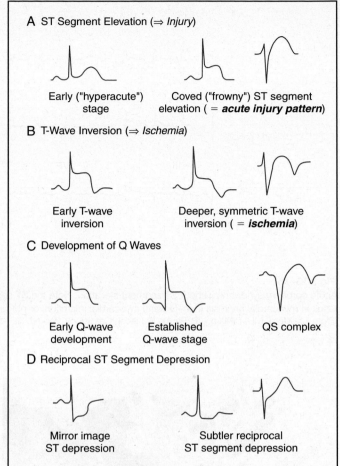

Fig 106–13
Principal electrocardiographic indicators of acute infarction.
(From Grauer K: ECG Interpretation Pocket Reference. St. Louis, Mosby-Year Book, 1992.)

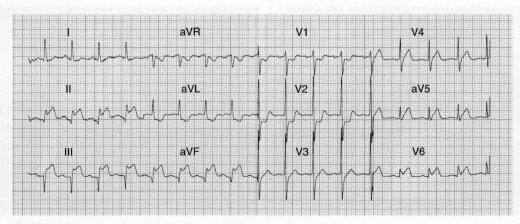

Fig 106–14
Acute transmural myocardial infarction. Note the ST segment elevation in the inferior leads.
(From Crawford, MH, DiMarco JP, Paulus WJ [eds]: Cardiology, 2nd ed. St. Louis, Mosby, 2004.)

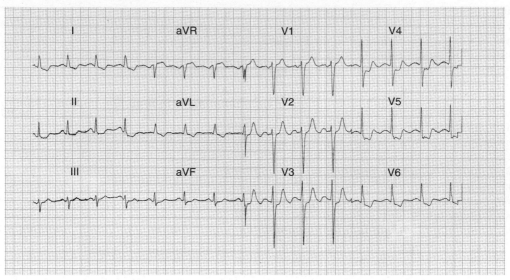

Fig 106–15
Acute coronary syndrome without ST segment elevation. Note the ST segment depression without Q wave formation. This condition may result in myocardial necrosis (non–Q wave myocardial infarction) or not (unstable angina)
(From Crawford, MH, DiMarco JP, Paulus WJ [eds]: Cardiology, 2nd ed. St. Louis, Mosby, 2004.)

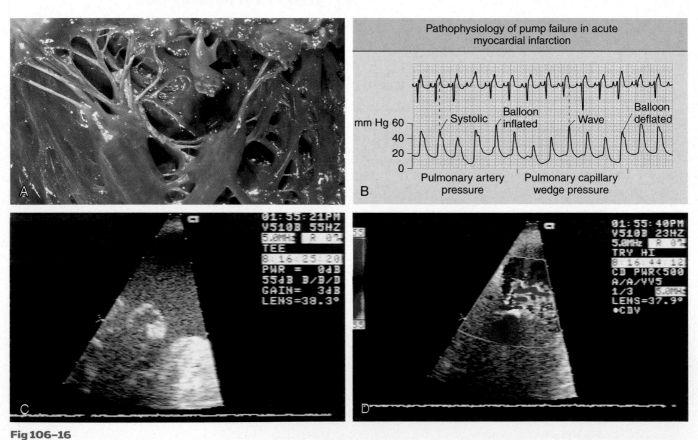

Fig 106–16
Papillary muscle rupture. **A,** Pathology specimen showing a ruptured papillary muscle. **B,** Hemodynamic findings in acute severe mitral regurgitation showing a large V wave in the wedge pressure tracing and reflected onto the pulmonary artery pressure tracing. Transesophageal echo-Doppler findings in papillary muscle rupture, showing the triangular head of the papillary muscle attached to the flail mitral leaflet **(C)**, and anteriorly directed color flow jet of severe mitral regurgitation **(D)**.
(From Crawford, MH, DiMarco JP, Paulus WJ [eds]: Cardiology, 2nd ed. St. Louis, Mosby, 2004.)

prognosis and should call into question the success of thrombolysis. Electrophysiologically guided antiarrhythmic therapy with implantable defibrillators has been shown to reduce the risk of sudden death in select survivors of acute MI who have sustained significant left ventricular dysfunction.

● **Mitral regurgitation:**
Characterized by the sudden appearance of an apical systolic murmur with radiation to the axilla; a loud first heart sound is often associated with the murmur.

CAUSE
● Papillary muscle dysfunction (Fig. 106–16) or left ventricular aneurysm (Fig. 106–17); it occurs primarily in inferior, lateral, and subendocardial infarcts.

CLINICAL PRESENTATION
● The classic clinical manifestation is acute onset of hypotension and respiratory distress caused by pulmonary edema, occurring 2 to 7 days after MI.

DIAGNOSTIC STUDIES
● Doppler echocardiography: establishes the diagnosis and assesses the severity of regurgitant flow
● Swan-Ganz catheterization: may reveal elevated mean pulmonary capillary wedge pressures (PCWPs) and large V waves
● Cardiac catheterization: defines the coronary anatomy and provides an opportunity to intervene to revascularize the infarct-related artery

TREATMENT
● IV nitroprusside is used to decrease PCWP.
● If the patient is hypotensive, dopamine or dobutamine combined with nitroprusside (combined use of inotropic and vasodilator agents) is needed.
● Intra-aortic balloon counterpulsation: (Fig. 106–18) provides lifesaving physiologic support by facilitating ventricular

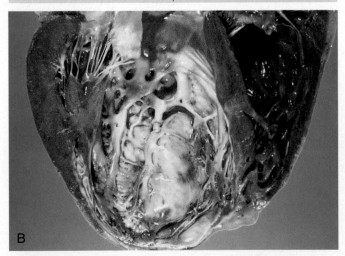

Fig 106–17
Pseudoaneurysm and true aneurysm. **A,** The features of a true ventricular aneurysm as compared with those of a false ventricular aneurysm. **B,** A pathologic specimen of a true ventricular aneurysm.
(From Crawford, MH, DiMarco JP, Paulus WJ [eds]: Cardiology, 2nd ed. St. Louis, Mosby, 2004.)

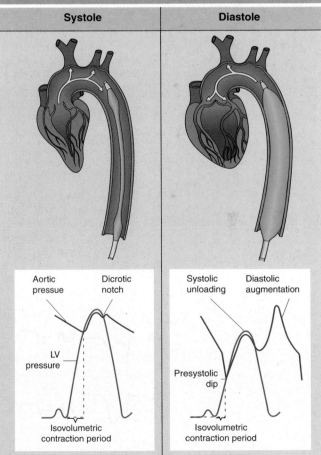

Fig 106–18
The principle of the intra-aortic balloon pump. Initiation of balloon inflation is timed to the arterial dicrotic notch, producing an augmentation in proximal aortic diastolic pressure. Deflation of the balloon is timed to begin just before the onset of the next ventricular systole, which produces the systolic unloading effect (presystolic dip). LV, left ventricular.
(From Crawford, MH, DiMarco JP, Paulus WJ [eds]: Cardiology, 2nd ed. St. Louis, Mosby, 2004.)

emptying during systole and increasing retrograde coronary perfusion during diastole.

- Emergency percutaneous coronary intervention to open the infarct-related artery may improve valvular function and should be considered in hemodynamically unstable patients.

- Surgical repair or replacement of the mitral valve after stabilization of the patient with significant persistent regurgitation

Note: Despite the preceding measures, the mortality rate of these patients remains extremely high.

Right ventricular infarct

- Generally caused by thrombotic occlusion of atherosclerotic plaque in the right coronary artery. It is characterized by jugular venous distention, *Kussmaul's sign* (a steady or rising jugular venous pulse on inspiration), and hypotension without pulmonary congestion (clear lung fields). It is usually seen in patients with coexistent left ventricular infarction.

- It should be suspected when ECG changes suggesting an acute inferior wall MI (changes in leads II, III, aVF) are observed.

DIAGNOSTIC STUDIES

- Hemodynamic monitoring shows right atrial pressure/PCWP higher than 0.8.
- Right precordial ECG leads reveal ST segment elevation in V_4R (Fig. 106–19).
- Bedside echocardiography may reveal right ventricular enlargement and hypokinesia.

TREATMENT

- Vigorous IV hydration to maintain left ventricular preload while attempting to re-establish blood flow with thrombolysis, angioplasty, or CABG.
- Normal saline, 40 mL/min IV, up to total of 2 liters, keeping right atrial pressure lower than 18 mm Hg or PCWP approximately 15 is advisable.
- Administration of diuretic therapy or preload-reducing drugs (nitrates, ACE inhibitors) can be fatal in these patients.
- When volume loading alone is insufficient, inotropic support with dobutamine may be added.

Ventricular septal defect

- Characterized by a new pansystolic murmur at the lower left sternal border and a parasternal thrill. It usually occurs within 2 weeks after acute MI in 2% of patients and causes 5% of peri-infarction mortality.

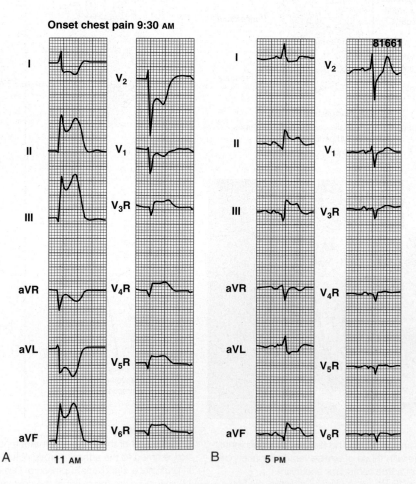

Onset chest pain 9:30 AM

A   11 AM   B   5 PM

Fig 106–19

A, Serial tracing (from a patient with acute inferoposterior and right ventricular infarction. **B,** Note that the diagnostic changes of right ventricular infarction seen in lead V_4R have disappeared 7.5 hours after the onset of pain.
(From Wellens JJH, Conover MB: The ECG in Emergency Decision Making, Philadelphia, WB Saunders, 1992.)

DIAGNOSTIC STUDIES

- An increase in oxygen content in blood samples from the pulmonary artery when compared with blood flow from the right atrium (a step-up in oxygen saturation from the right atrium to the right ventricle)
- Bedside echocardiography with color flow imaging is useful to visualize the ventricular septal defect and the resultant left-to-right shunting through the defect.

TREATMENT

- Same as for acute mitral regurgitation (see earlier); early surgical repair is usually necessary.

Myocardial rupture

Myocardial rupture (Fig. 106–20): usually seen in older patients 2 to 4 days after MI and accounts for 10% of acute MI-induced mortality. It is characterized by sudden hypotension and loss of consciousness, followed by electromechanical dissociation and generally death. Incomplete rupture may result in the formation of a pseudoaneurysm (see Fig. 106–17) (pericardium and mural thrombus from the outer walls). Bedside echocardiography may be useful in demonstrating the pseudoaneurysm. Surgical resection is recommended for these patients because of the high risk of spontaneous rupture.

Systemic embolism

This is characterized by sudden onset of neurologic deficit or pain in the involved area (e.g., flank pain and tenderness in renal artery embolism).

CAUSE

- Mural thrombi occur most frequently with anterior wall MI.

DIAGNOSTIC STUDIES

- Echocardiography may reveal the presence of mural thrombi. Transesophageal echocardiography is highly accurate for identifying left atrial and ventricular thrombi.
- Perform arteriography if peripheral embolism is suspected.
- Perform renal computed tomography or scintigraphy if renal embolism is suspected.

TREATMENT

- IV heparinization
- Embolectomy if the clot is accessible (e.g., in femoral artery)

Pericarditis (see Chapter 113)

Dressler's syndrome

- Characterized by fever, pleurisy, pericarditis, friction rub, pericardial and pleural effusions, and joint pain; usually occurs between 1 week and 6 months after MI

CAUSE

- Autoimmune disorder secondary to previous damage to the myocardium and pericardium

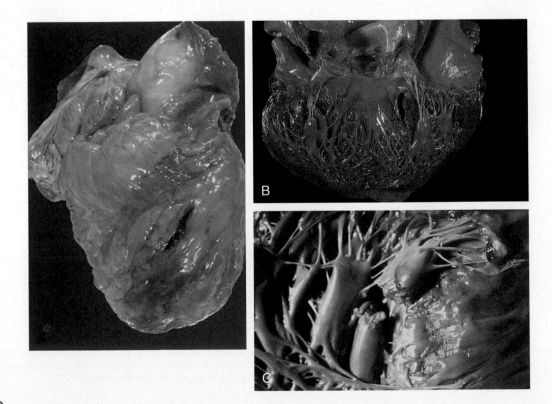

Fig 106–20
Cardiac rupture syndromes complicating ST elevation myocardial infarction.
A, Anterior myocardial rupture in an acute infarct *(arrow).* **B,** Rupture of the ventricular septum *(arrow).* **C,** Complete rupture of a necrotic papillary muscle.
(From Schoen FJ: The heart. In Cotran RS, Kumar V, Collins T [eds]: Pathologic Basis of Disease, 6th ed. Philadelphia, WB Saunders, 1999, p 562.)

TREATMENT

- Indomethacin, 50 mg PO every 6 hours or other nonsteroidal anti-inflammatory drugs (NSAIDs); if no improvement, consider prednisone, 30 mg PO twice daily initially, tapered off over several weeks.

Left ventricular aneurysm

DIAGNOSTIC STUDIES

- Echocardiography
- ECG shows persistent ST elevations 3 to 4 weeks after MI (Fig. 106–21).
- Chest x-ray may show a "squared-off" shape of the left ventricle (Fig. 106–22)

TREATMENT

- Surgical excision if the aneurysm is associated with recurrent ventricular tachycardia, intractable CHF, recurrent embolization, or persistent angina despite intensive medical treatment
- Chronic anticoagulation is usually indicated if the aneurysm is not excised.

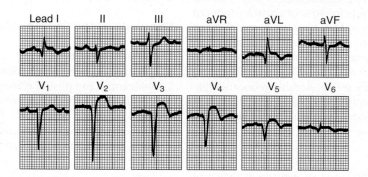

Fig 106–21

Ventricular aneurysm. This 52-year-old man had an acute extensive anterior myocardial infarction 5 months before the recording of this ECG. Note the persistent ST segment elevation in the precordial leads and in leads I and aVL. Left anterior hemiblock also is present.
(From Chou TC: Electrocardiography in Clinical Practice, 4th ed. Philadelphia, WB Saunders, 1996.)

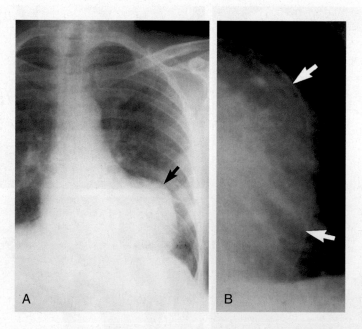

Fig 106–22

Chest radiograph in left ventricular aneurysm. **A,** Chest radiograph showing characteristic squared-off shape *(arrow)* of the left ventricle in a large left ventricular aneurysm. **B,** Spot view of the aneurysm shows a thin line of calcification *(arrows)* in the wall of the left ventricular aneurysm.
(From Grainger RG, Allison DJ, Adam A, Dixon AK [eds]: Grainger & Allison's Diagnostic Radiology, 4th ed. London, Harcourt, 2001.)

Chapter 107 Valvular disease

A. MITRAL STENOSIS

DEFINITION

Mitral stenosis is a narrowing of the mitral valve orifice. The cross section of a normal orifice measures 4 to 6 cm². A murmur becomes audible when the valve orifice becomes smaller than 2 cm². When the orifice approaches 1 cm², the condition becomes critical, and symptoms become more evident. Figure 107–1 describes anatomic and functional features of mitral stenosis.

PHYSICAL FINDINGS AND CLINICAL PRESENTATION

- Exertional dyspnea initially, followed by orthopnea and paroxysmal nocturnal dyspnea (PND)
- Acute pulmonary edema (may develop after exertion)
- Systemic emboli (caused by stagnation of blood in the left atrium; may occur in patients with associated atrial fibrillation)

ANATOMIC AND FUNCTIONAL FEATURES OF MITRAL STENOSIS

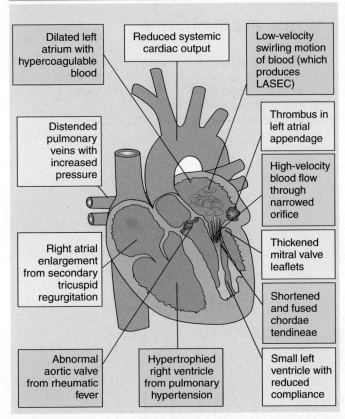

Fig 107–1
Anatomic and functional features of mitral stenosis. The heart undergoes a variety of anatomic and physiologic modifications from the initial rheumatic insult and the subsequent development of hemodynamically important mitral stenosis. LASEC, left atrial spontaneous echo contrast.
(From Crawford, MH, DiMarco JP, Paulus WJ [eds]: Cardiology, 2nd ed. St. Louis, Mosby, 2004.)

- Hemoptysis (may be present as a result of persistent pulmonary hypertension)
- Prominent jugular A waves are present in patients with normal sinus rhythm.
- Opening snap occurs in early diastole; a short (less than 0.07 second) A_2 to opening snap interval indicates severe mitral stenosis.
- Apical mid-diastolic or presystolic rumble that does not radiate is present.
- Accentuated S_1 (because of delayed and forceful closure of the valve) is present.
- If pulmonary hypertension is present, there may be an accentuated P_2 and/or a soft, early diastolic decrescendo murmur (Graham Steell's murmur) caused by pulmonary regurgitation (it is best heard along the left sternal border and may be confused with aortic regurgitation).
- A palpable right ventricular heave may be present at the left sternal border.
- Patients with mitral stenosis usually have symptoms of left-sided heart failure: dyspnea on exertion, PND, orthopnea.
- Right ventricular dysfunction (in late stages) may be manifested by peripheral edema, enlarged and pulsatile liver, and ascites.

CAUSE

- Progressive fibrosis, scarring, and calcification of the valve
- Rheumatic fever (still a common cause in underdeveloped countries); heart valves most frequently affected in rheumatic heart disease (in descending order of occurrence)—mitral, aortic, tricuspid, and pulmonary
- Congenital defect (parachute valve)
- Rare causes: endomyocardial fibroelastosis, malignant carcinoid syndrome, systemic lupus erythematosus (SLE)

DIFFERENTIAL DIAGNOSIS

- Left atrial myxoma
- Other valvular abnormalities (e.g., tricuspid stenosis, mitral regurgitation)
- Atrial septal defect

IMAGING STUDIES

- Echocardiography:
  - The characteristic finding on the echocardiogram is a markedly diminished E to F slope of the anterior mitral valve leaflet during diastole; there is also fusion of the commissures, resulting in anterior movement of the posterior mitral valve leaflet during diastole (calcification in the valve may also be noted).
  - Two-dimensional echocardiography can accurately establish valve area.
- Chest x-ray:
  - Straightening of the left cardiac border caused by dilated left atrial appendage (Fig. 107–2)
  - Left atrial enlargement on lateral chest x-ray (appearing as double density of PA chest x-ray)
  - Prominence of pulmonary arteries
  - Possible pulmonary congestion and edema (Kerley B lines)

- ECG (Fig. 107–3):
  - Right ventricular hypertrophy, right axis deviation caused by pulmonary hypertension
  - Left atrial enlargement (broad, notched, P waves)
  - Atrial fibrillation
- Cardiac catheterization to help establish the severity of mitral stenosis and diagnose associated valvular and coronary lesions. Findings on cardiac catheterization include:
  - Normal left ventricular function
  - Elevated left atrial and pulmonary pressures

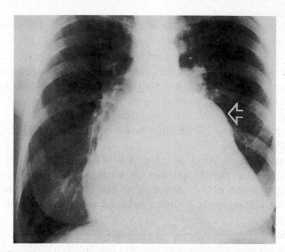

Fig 107–2

Severe mitral valve disease. The left atrial appendage is large, producing a convex bulge *(arrow)*. The heart is considerably enlarged. (From Grainger RG, Allison DJ, Adam A, Dixon AK [eds]: Grainger & Allison's Diagnostic Radiology, 4th ed. London, Harcourt, 2001.)

TREATMENT

Medical

- If the patient is in atrial fibrillation, control the rate response with diltiazem, digitalis, or esmolol. Although digitalis can be used for chronic heart rate control, IV diltiazem or esmolol may be acutely preferable when a rapid decrease in heart rate is required.
- If the patient has persistent atrial fibrillation (because of a large left atrium), permanent anticoagulation is indicated to decrease the risk of serious thromboembolism.
- Treat CHF with diuretics and sodium restriction.

Surgical

- Valve replacement is indicated when the valve orifice is smaller than 0.7 to 0.8 cm^2 or if symptoms persist despite optimal medical therapy; commissurotomy may be possible if the mitral valve is noncalcified and if there is pure mitral stenosis without significant subvalvular disease.
- Percutaneous transvenous mitral valvotomy (PTMV) is an option for many patients with mitral stenosis responding poorly to medical therapy, particularly those who are poor surgical candidates and whose valve is not heavily calcified; balloon valvotomy (Fig. 107–4) gives excellent mechanical relief, usually resulting in prolonged benefit.

B. MITRAL REGURGITATION

DEFINITION

Mitral regurgitation (MR) is retrograde blood flow through the left atrium secondary to an incompetent mitral valve. Eventually, there is an increase in left atrial and pulmonary pressures, which may result in right ventricular failure.

PHYSICAL FINDINGS AND CLINICAL PRESENTATION

- Patients with MR generally present with the following symptoms:
  - Fatigue, dyspnea, orthopnea, frank CHF
  - Hemoptysis (caused by pulmonary hypertension)

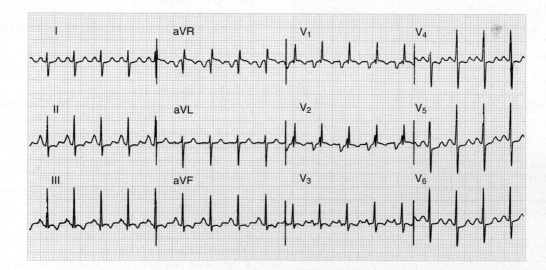

Fig 107–3

This electrocardiogram from a 45-year-old woman with severe mitral stenosis shows multiple abnormalities. The rhythm is sinus tachycardia. Right axis deviation and a tall R wave in lead V$_1$ are consistent with right ventricular hypertrophy. The very prominent biphasic P wave in lead V$_1$ indicates left atrial abnormality–enlargement. The tall P waves in lead II suggest concomitant right abnormality. Nonspecific ST-T changes and incomplete right bundle branch block are also present. The combination of right ventricular hypertrophy and marked left or biatrial abnormality is highly suggestive of mitral stenosis. (From Goldberger AL: Clinical Electrocardiography: A Simplified Approach, 6th ed. St. Louis, Mosby, 1999.)

- Possible systemic emboli in patients with left atrial mural thrombi associated with atrial fibrillation
- Hyperdynamic apex, often with palpable left ventricular lift and apical thrill
- Holosystolic murmur at apex with radiation to base or to left axilla; poor correlation between the intensity of the systolic murmur and the degree of regurgitation
- Apical early to mid-diastolic rumble (rare)

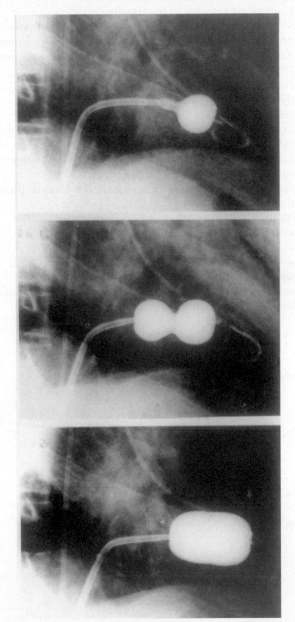

Fig 107–4

Mitral valvuloplasty performed by the Inoue technique. The catheter is placed in the mitral valve and the distal part of the Inoue balloon is inflated *(top)*. The balloon is then pulled back in the mitral valve and is inflated for 10 to 15 seconds under fluoroscopic control *(middle)* until the waist of the balloon is no longer visible *(bottom)* and the balloon falls back into the left atrium.

(From Crawford, MH, DiMarco JP, Paulus WJ [eds]: Cardiology, 2nd ed. St. Louis, Mosby, 2004.)

CAUSE

- Papillary muscle dysfunction (as a result of ischemic heart disease)
- Ruptured chordae tendineae
- Infective endocarditis
- Calcified mitral valve annulus
- Left ventricular dilation
- Rheumatic valvulitis
- Primary or secondary mitral valve prolapse
- Hypertrophic cardiomyopathy
- Idiopathic myxomatous degeneration of the mitral valve
- Myxoma
- SLE
- Fenfluramine, dexfenfluramine

DIFFERENTIAL DIAGNOSIS

- Hypertrophic cardiomyopathy
- Pulmonary regurgitation
- Tricuspid regurgitation
- Ventricular septal defect (VSD)

IMAGING STUDIES

- Echocardiography (Fig. 107–5): enlarged left atrium, hyperdynamic left ventricle (erratic motion of the leaflet is seen in patients with ruptured chordae tendineae). Doppler electrocardiography will show evidence of MR. The most important aspect of the echocardiographic examination is the quantification of left ventricular systolic performance.

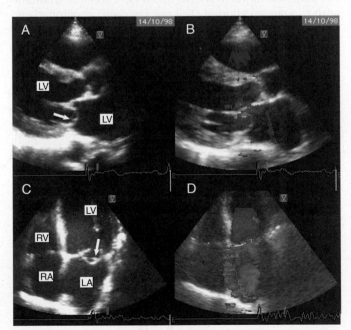

Fig 107–5

Echocardiographic studies in mitral regurgitation. **A, B,** Parasternal long-axis views show prolapse of the posterior mitral leaflet *(arrow)* with corresponding flow directed along the anterior mitral leaflet toward the atrial septum. Apical four-chamber views show the prolapse more clearly (**C,** *arrow*), and the extension of the regurgitation is more clearly visualized **(D)**. The jet is spoon-shaped, broad, and thin along the wall, and therefore easily underestimated. LA, left atrium; LV, left ventricle; RA, right atrium; RV, right ventricle.

(From Crawford, MH, DiMarco JP, Paulus WJ [eds]: Cardiology, 2nd ed. St. Louis, Mosby, 2004.)

- Chest x-ray
  - Left atrial enlargement (usually more pronounced in mitral stenosis)
  - Left ventricular enlargement
  - Possible pulmonary congestion
- ECG
  - Left atrial enlargement
  - Left ventricular hypertrophy
  - Atrial fibrillation

TREATMENT
Medical
- Medical therapy is primarily directed toward treatment of complications (e.g., atrial fibrillation).
  - Digitalis may be used for inotropic effect and to control ventricular response if atrial fibrillation with fast ventricular response is present.
  - Afterload reduction (to decrease the regurgitant fraction and to increase cardiac output): may be accomplished with nifedipine, hydralazine plus nitrates or ACE inhibitors
  - Anticoagulants if atrial fibrillation occurs

Surgical
- Surgery is the only definitive treatment for MR. Figure 107–6 shows mitral valve repair with mitral annuloplasty.

C. MITRAL VALVE PROLAPSE

DEFINITION
Mitral valve prolapse (MVP) is the posterior bulging of interior and posterior leaflets in systole. Mitral valve prolapse syndrome refers to a constellation of MVP and associated symptoms (e.g., autonomic dysfunction, palpitations) or other physical abnormalities (e.g., pectus excavatum). Increased incidence of MVP is seen with autoimmune thyroid disorders, Ehlers-Danlos syndrome, Marfan's syndrome, pseudoxanthoma elasticum, pectus excavatum, anorexia nervosa, and bulimia.

PHYSICAL FINDINGS AND CLINICAL PRESENTATION
- Usually, young female patient with narrow AP chest diameter, low body weight, low blood pressure
- Mid to late click, heard best at the apex
- Crescendo mid to late diastolic murmur
- Findings accentuated in the standing position
- Most patients with MVP are asymptomatic; symptoms (if present) consist primarily of chest pain and palpitations
- Neurologic abnormalities (e.g., transient ischemic attack [TIA] or stroke) are rare.
- Patients may also complain of anxiety, fatigue, and dyspnea.

CAUSE
- Myxomatous degeneration of connective tissue of mitral valve
- Congenital deformity of mitral valve and supportive structures
- Secondary to other disorders (e.g., Ehlers-Danlos, pseudoxanthoma elasticum)

DIFFERENTIAL DIAGNOSIS
- Other valvular abnormalities
- Constrictive pericarditis
- Ventricular aneurysm

IMAGING STUDIES
Echocardiography (Fig. 107–7) shows the anterior and posterior leaflets bulging posteriorly in systole.

Reduction excision of posterior leaflet

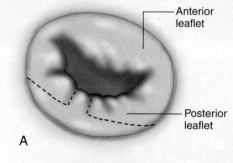

Anterior leaflet

Posterior leaflet

A

Re-attach posterior leaflet (sliding valvuloplasty)

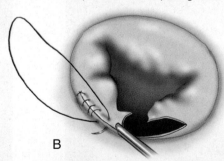

B

Repair posterior leaflet

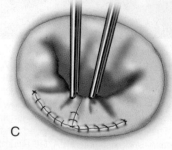

C

Completed supported repair

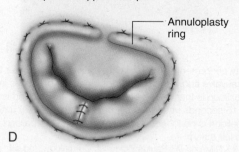

Annuloplasty ring

D

Fig 107–6

A to D, Mitral valve repair using reduction excision and re-attachment of the posterior leaflet with implantation of an annuloplasty ring.
(From Doty DB [ed]: Cardiac Surgery: Operative Technique. St. Louis, Mosby-Year Book, 1997, p 259.)

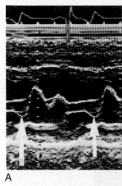
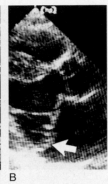
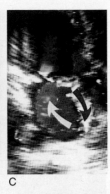

Fig 107–7
Mitral valve prolapse. **A,** M-mode echo shows late systolic prolapse of the posterior mitral leaflet *(arrows)*. **B,** Two-dimensional echo (parasternal long axis) in the same patient shows posterior mitral leaflet prolapse *(arrow)* convex into left atrium. **C,** Color Doppler (apical four chamber) in the same patient shows an eccentric jet of mitral regurgitation (following direction of *arrows*).
(From Grainger RG, Allison DJ, Adam A, Dixon AK [eds]: Grainger & Allison's Diagnostic Radiology, 4th ed. London, Harcourt, 2001.)

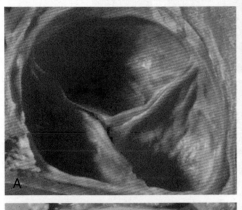
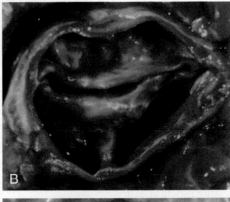
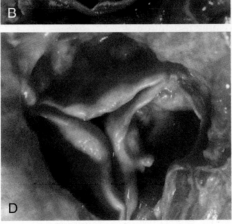

Fig 107–8
Major types of aortic valve stenosis. **A,** Normal aortic valve. **B,** Congenital bicuspid aortic stenosis. A false raphe is present at 6 o'clock. **C,** Rheumatic aortic stenosis. The commissures are fused with a fixed central orifice. **D,** Calcific degenerative aortic stenosis.
(**A** and **D,** from Manabe H, Yutani C [eds]: Atlas of Valvular Heart Disease. Singapore, Churchill Livingstone, 1998, pp 6, 131; **B** and **C,** Courtesy of Dr. William C. Roberts.)

TREATMENT

- The empirical use of antiarrhythmic drugs to prevent sudden death in patients with uncomplicated MVP is not advisable; beta blockers may be tried in symptomatic patients (e.g., palpitations, chest pain); they decrease the heart rate, thus decreasing the stretch on the prolapsing valve leaflets.

D. AORTIC STENOSIS

DEFINITION

Aortic stenosis is obstruction to systolic left ventricular outflow across the aortic valve. Symptoms appear when the valve orifice decreases to less than 1 cm^2 (normal orifice is 3 cm^2). The stenosis is considered severe when the orifice is less than 0.5 cm^2 or the pressure gradient is 50 mm Hg or higher.

PHYSICAL FINDINGS AND CLINICAL PRESENTATION

- Rough, loud systolic diamond-shaped murmur, best heard at base of heart and transmitted into neck vessels; often associated with a thrill or ejection click; may also be heard well at the apex
- Absence or diminished intensity of sound of aortic valve closure (in severe aortic stenosis)
- Late, slow-rising carotid upstroke with decreased amplitude
- Strong apical pulse
- Narrowing of pulse pressure in later stages of aortic stenosis
- Some patients with aortic stenosis experience bleeding into their GI tract or skin. This is caused by an acquired defect in von Willebrand's factor. Aortic valve replacement restores normal hemostasis.

CAUSE

- Rheumatic inflammation of aortic valve (Fig. 107–8)
- Progressive stenosis of congenital bicuspid valve (found in 1% to 2% of population)
- Idiopathic calcification of the aortic valve
- Congenital (major cause of aortic stenosis in patients younger than 30 years)

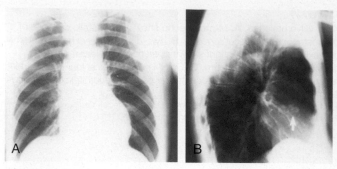

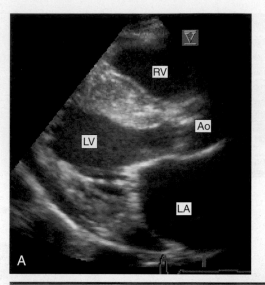

Fig 107–9

Aortic stenosis. The heart is normal in the frontal view **(A)**, but the ascending aorta shows slight poststenotic dilation. **B,**The lateral view shows aortic valve *(arrow)* and posterior displacement of the calcification left ventricle behind the line of the inferior vena cava.
(From Grainger RG, Allison DJ, Adam A, Dixon AK [eds]: Grainger & Allison's Diagnostic Radiology, 4th ed. London, Harcourt, 2001.)

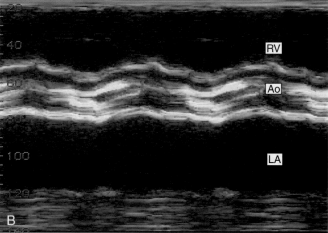

DIFFERENTIAL DIAGNOSIS
- Hypertrophic cardiomyopathy
- Mitral regurgitation
- Ventricular septal defect
- Aortic sclerosis. Aortic stenosis is distinguished from aortic sclerosis by the degree of valve impairment. In aortic sclerosis, the valve leaflets are abnormally thickened but obstruction to outflow is minimal.

IMAGING STUDIES
- Chest x-ray (Fig. 107–9)
  - Poststenotic dilation of the ascending aorta
  - Calcification of aortic cusps
  - Pulmonary congestion (in advanced stages of aortic stenosis)
- ECG
  - Left ventricular hypertrophy (found in more than 80% of patients)
  - ST-T wave changes
  - Atrial fibrillation: frequent
- Echocardiography(Fig. 107–10): thickening of the left ventricular wall; if the patient has valvular calcifications, multiple echoes may be seen from within the aortic root and there is poor separation of the aortic cusps during systole. Gradient across the valve can be estimated but is less precise than with cardiac catheterization.
- Cardiac catheterization: indicated in symptomatic patients; it confirms the diagnosis and estimates the severity of the disease by measuring the gradient across the valve, allowing calculation of the valve area. It also detects coexisting coronary artery stenosis that may need bypass at the same time as aortic valve replacement.

TREATMENT
Medical
- Strenuous activity should be avoided.
- Diuretics and sodium restriction are needed if CHF is present; digoxin is used only to control rate of atrial fibrillation.

Fig 107–10

Echocardiography of aortic stenosis. **A,** Parasternal long-axis view of a stenotic aortic valve in systole. The valve is thickened, with a reduced opening. The walls, in particular the interventricular septum, are hypertrophic. **B,** Corresponding M-mode study through the stenotic valve. Ao, aorta; LA, left atrium; LV, left ventricle; RV, right ventricle.
(From Crawford, MH, DiMarco JP, Paulus WJ [eds]: Cardiology, 2nd ed. St. Louis, Mosby, 2004.)

- ACE inhibitors are relatively contraindicated.
- Calcium channel blocker verapamil may be useful only to control rate of atrial fibrillation.

Surgical
- Valve replacement is the treatment of choice in symptomatic patients, because the 5-year mortality rate after onset of symptoms is extremely high, even with optimal medical therapy; valve replacement is indicated if cardiac catheterization establishes a pressure gradient higher than 50 mm Hg and valve area less than 1 cm^2.
- Balloon aortic valvotomy for adult acquired aortic stenosis is useful only for palliation.

E. AORTIC REGURGITATION

DEFINITION

Aortic regurgitation is retrograde blood flow into the left ventricle from the aorta secondary to an incompetent aortic valve.

PHYSICAL FINDINGS AND CLINICAL PRESENTATION

The clinical presentation varies, depending on whether aortic insufficiency is acute or chronic. Chronic aortic insufficiency is well tolerated (except when secondary to infective endocarditis), and patients can remain asymptomatic for years. Common manifestations after significant deterioration of left ventricular function are dyspnea on exertion, syncope, chest pain, and CHF. Acute aortic insufficiency manifests primarily with hypotension caused by a sudden fall in cardiac output. A rapid rise in left ventricular diastolic pressure results in a further decrease in coronary blood flow.

Physical findings in chronic aortic insufficiency include the following:

- Widened pulse pressure (markedly increased systolic blood pressure, decreased diastolic blood pressure) is present.
- Bounding pulses, head bobbing with each systole *(de Musset's sign)* are present; water hammer or collapsing pulse *(Corrigan's pulse)* can be palpated at the wrist or on the femoral arteries (pistol shot femorals), caused by rapid rise and sudden collapse of the arterial pressure during late systole; capillary pulsations *(Quincke's pulse)* may occur at the bases of the nail beds.
- A to-and-fro *double-Duroziez* murmur may be heard over the femoral arteries with slight compression.
- Popliteal systolic pressure is increased over brachial systolic pressure 40 mm Hg or more *(Hill's sign)*.
- Cardiac auscultation reveals:
1. Displacement of cardiac impulse downward and to the patient's left

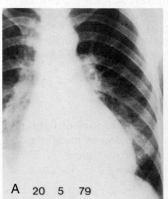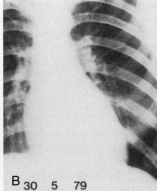

A 20 5 79   B 30 5 79

Fig 107–11
Acute aortic regurgitation in an infant caused by bacterial endocarditis. **A,** 3 months after delivery by cesarean section. There were repeated febrile episodes, treated by short courses of antibiotics. Ultimately, the murmur of aortic regurgitation was heard. The film shows a large heart with left ventricular configuration, and pulmonary oedema. **B,** 10 days later, the infection and the cardiac failure have been controlled. The heart size is reduced and the lungs are clear.
(From Grainger RG, Allison DJ, Adam A, Dixon AK [eds]: Grainger & Allison's Diagnostic Radiology, 4th ed. London, Harcourt, 2001.)

2. S_3 heard over the apex
3. Decrescendo, blowing diastolic murmur heard along left sternal border
4. Low-pitched apical diastolic rumble (Austin Flint murmur) caused by contrast of the aortic regurgitant jet with the left ventricular wall
5. Early systolic apical ejection murmur

In patients with acute aortic insufficiency, both the wide pulse pressure and the large stroke volume are absent. A short blowing diastolic murmur may be the only finding on physical examination.

CAUSE

- Infective endocarditis
- Rheumatic fibrosis (most common cause in developing countries)
- Trauma with valvular rupture
- Congenital bicuspid aortic valve (most common cause in the United States)
- Myxomatous degeneration
- Annuloaortic ectasia
- Syphilitic aortitis
- Rheumatic spondylitis
- SLE
- Aortic dissection
- Fenfluramine, dexfenfluramine
- Takayasu's arteritis, granulomatous arteritis

DIFFERENTIAL DIAGNOSIS

- Patent ductus arteriosus, pulmonary regurgitation, and other valvular abnormalities

IMAGING STUDIES

- Chest x-ray (Fig. 107–11)
  - Left ventricular hypertrophy (chronic aortic regurgitation)
  - Aortic dilation
  - Normal cardiac silhouette with pulmonary edema: possible in patients with acute aortic regurgitation
- ECG: left ventricular hypertrophy (LVH)
- Echocardiography: coarse diastolic fluttering of the anterior mitral leaflet; LVH in patients with chronic aortic regurgitation. Use of Doppler echo can quantify regurgitant orifice (severe if more than 0.30 cm²) and regurgitant volume (severe if more than 60 mL/beat) (Fig. 107–12).
- Cardiac catheterization in select patients to assess degree of left ventricular dysfunction, confirm the presence of a wide pulse pressure, assess surgical risk, and determine if there is coexistent coronary artery disease

TREATMENT

Salt restriction

- ACE inhibitors, diuretics, and sodium restriction for CHF; nitroprusside in patients with acute aortic regurgitation
- Long-term vasodilator therapy with ACE inhibitors or nifedipine for reducing or delaying the need for aortic valve replacement in asymptomatic patients with severe aortic regurgitation and normal left ventricular function

Surgical

This is reserved for:

- Symptomatic patients with chronic aortic regurgitation despite optimal medical therapy
- Patients with acute aortic regurgitation (i.e., infective endocarditis) producing left ventricular failure

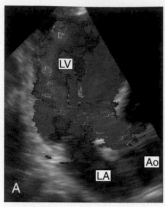 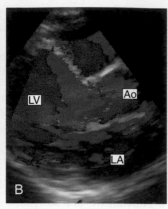

Fig 107–12
Severe aortic regurgitation. **A,** Apical view showing a wide jet reaching to the apex. **B,** Parasternal long-axis view, showing a wide origin of the jet, although this view does not demonstrate that the jet extends far into the ventricle. Ao, aorta; LA, left atrium; LV, left ventricle.
(From Crawford, MH, DiMarco JP, Paulus WJ [eds]: Cardiology, 2nd ed. St. Louis, Mosby, 2004.)

F. TRICUSPID STENOSIS

DEFINITION

Tricuspid stenosis (TS) is a very uncommon valvular pathology caused by the narrowing of the orifice of the tricuspid valve resulting in restriction of the right atrial emptying. This in turn causes a diastolic pressure gradient between the right atrium and right ventricle. TS is mostly rheumatic in origin. Rheumatic TS seldom occurs alone; it is usually associated with mitral or aortic valve disease.

PHYSICAL FINDINGS AND CLINICAL PRESENTATION

- Symptoms of right heart failure: fatigue, abdominal swelling, right upper quadrant abdominal pain secondary to passive congestive hepatomegaly, peripheral edema
- Jugular venous distention with a prominent a wave is noted, along with a palpable hepatic pulsation.
- Right atrial pulsation may be palpated to the right of the sternum and a diastolic thrill may be felt over the left sternal edge that is increased with inspiration.
- An opening snap and diastolic murmur are best heard along the left sternal border of the fourth intercostal space and is augmented by inspiration.
- Ascites or anasarca

CAUSE

- Rheumatic heart disease is the primary cause of TS, resulting in scarring of the valve leaflets and fusion of the commissures. This, along with shortening of the chordae tendineae and immobility of the valve leaflets, results in narrowing of the tricuspid valve orifice.
- Other causes of TS are congenital TS, right atrial myxoma, metastatic tumor (e.g., lymphoma), metabolic or enzymatic abnormalities (carcinoid syndrome, Whipple's disease, Fabry's disease), systemic lupus endocarditis, and tricuspid valve bacterial endocarditis.

DIFFERENTIAL DIAGNOSIS

- Congenital tricuspid atresia
- Endomyocardial fibrosis
- Right atrial thrombi or tumors
- Constrictive pericarditis
- Tricuspid valve vegetation

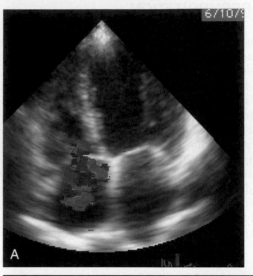

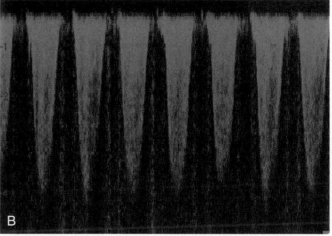

Fig 107–13
Echocardiography of tricuspid regurgitation. **A,** Apical four-chamber view with color Doppler through a tricuspid valve with a medium to severe regurgitation. **B,** Corresponding continuous Doppler recording through the jet, demonstrating a peak velocity of 4 m/sec, which indicates a systolic pressure in the right ventricle of at least 64 mm Hg (plus the pressure in the right atrium).
(From Crawford, MH, DiMarco JP, Paulus WJ [eds]: Cardiology, 2nd ed. St. Louis, Mosby, 2004.)

- Other pathologies that cause obstruction of right atrial emptying, such as extrinsic compression by massive ascites, pleural effusion, pericardial effusion, or tumor

WORKUP

- Echocardiography (Fig. 107–13)
- Chest x-ray (Fig. 107–14)
- ECG
- Cardiac angiography in select patients

IMAGING STUDIES

- Echocardiography reveals thickening and shortening of tricuspid valve leaflets. There is doming of the anterior leaflet with restriction of movement of the leaflet tip, along with reduced excursion of the posterior and septal leaflets. Also, evidence of right atrial enlargement is present in most of these patients.
- Demonstration of a diastolic gradient across the tricuspid valve is possible through Doppler echocardiography or car-

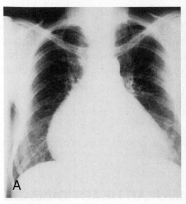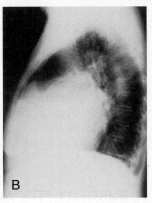

Fig 107–14
Tricuspid stenosis leading to right atrial enlargement. **A,** In the frontal view, the right heart border bulges to the right and forms a segment of a circle of increased curvature. **B,** In the lateral view, there is increased application of the heart shadow to the sternum, in this case caused by a large right atrial appendage filling in the gap superiorly. (From Grainger RG, Allison DJ, Adam A, Dixon AK [eds]: Grainger & Allison's Diagnostic Radiology, 4th ed. London, Harcourt, 2001.)

diac catheterization (normal gradient, less than 1 mm Hg), along with estimation of the tricuspid valve area (severe, less than 1 cm^2).
- Chest x-ray reveals an enlarged right atrium and pulmonary oligemia.
- ECG in many cases will show atrial fibrillation secondary to an enlarged right atrium. However, in patients who are in normal sinus rhythm, the ECG will show criteria for right atrial enlargement (tall P waves more than 2.5 mm in height in leads II, III, or aVF).

TREATMENT
- Diuretics
- Salt and fluid restrictions are essential to decrease peripheral edema.
- Balloon valvotomy or dilation of the stenosed tricuspid valve has been described in both rheumatic and congenital TS with some success, but experience is limited and complications may occur (e.g., advanced heart block, significant tricuspid regurgitation).
- Because rheumatic TS is usually associated with mitral disease or aortic disease, the decision to proceed with surgery for TS typically occurs in the setting of significant symptomatic mitral or aortic valve disease requiring surgery, and a concomitant mean diastolic gradient across the tricuspid valve of more than 5 mm Hg with a tricuspid valve area less than 2 cm^2.
- Surgical procedures for significant tricuspid stenosis include closed commissurotomy, open commissurotomy, and tricuspid valve replacement. This is usually determined during surgery.

G. TRICUSPID REGURGITATION

DEFINITION
Tricuspid regurgitation (TR) refers to flow of blood from the right ventricle to the right atrium during systole

EPIDEMIOLOGY AND DEMOGRAPHICS
- TR is much more common than TS.

- In patients with rheumatic heart disease, TR rarely occurs alone and is usually associated with mitral or aortic valve disease.
- Trivial TR is frequently detected by echocardiography and is considered a normal variant.

PHYSICAL FINDINGS AND CLINICAL PRESENTATION
- Isolated TR can cause nonspecific symptoms, such as exercise intolerance.
- Signs and symptoms in the presence of TR are usually a result of the underlying cause.
- Signs and symptoms may be caused by accompanying right-sided heart failure (e.g., jugular venous distention [JVD], peripheral edema, ascites, hepatomegaly, right-sided S$_3$).
- Holosystolic murmur, heard best along the left sternal border in the fourth intercostal space. The murmur becomes louder during inspiration and during maneuvers that increase venous return.
- Prominent V waves in the jugular venous waveform
- Pulsatile liver

CAUSE
- TR is usually functional rather than structural.
- Functional TR refers to conditions leading to dilation of the tricuspid annulus or right ventricle, including:
  - Any cause of pulmonary hypertension (e.g., COPD, pulmonary embolism, restrictive lung disease, collagen vascular disease, and primary pulmonary hypertension)
  - Right ventricular infarction
  - Left-sided heart failure leading to right-sided heart failure
  - Dilated cardiomyopathy
- Structural TR refers to conditions directly affecting the tricuspid valve, including the following:
  - Iatrogenic damage to the valve (e.g., pacemaker or implantable cardioverter-defibrillator [ICD] insertion, endocardial biopsy)
  - Rheumatic fever
  - Endocarditis
  - Congenital (e.g., Ebstein's anomaly)
  - Carcinoid syndrome
  - Marfan's syndrome
  - Tricuspid valve prolapse (Fig. 107–15)
  - External trauma (deceleration injury)
  - Right atrial myxoma
  - Collagen-vascular disease (e.g., SLE)
  - Radiation injury

DIAGNOSIS
The diagnosis of TR is made by clinical history, physical examination, and adjunctive studies including ECG, chest x-ray, echocardiography, and right-sided heart catheterization in select patients.

DIFFERENTIAL DIAGNOSIS
The systolic murmur associated with TR could be mistaken for:
  - Mitral regurgitation
  - Aortic stenosis
  - Pulmonic stenosis
  - Ventricular septal defect
  - Innocent murmur
  - Hypertrophic cardiomyopathy

WORKUP
- Any patient suspected of having significant TR should undergo the following:

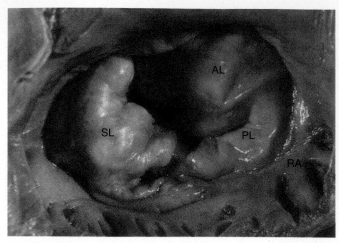

Fig 107–15
Tricuspid valve prolapse, viewed from the right atrium (RA). AL, anterior leaflet; PL, posterior leaflet; SL, septal leaflet.
(From Virmani R, Burke AP, Farb A: Pathology of valvular heart disease. In Rahimtoola SH [ed]: Vavular Heart Disease. In Braunwald E [series ed]: Atlas of Heart Diseases, vol 11. Philadelphia, Current Medicine, 1997, pp 1-17.)

- Chest x-ray
- Electrocardiography
- Echocardiography (confirmatory)
- Right-sided cardiac catheterization (in select cases)

LABORATORY TESTS

- Electrocardiogram may show evidence of:
  - Right atrial enlargement (e.g., P wave amplitude in leads II, III, aVF more than 2.5 mV)
  - Right ventricular enlargement or hypertrophy (e.g., R wave more than S wave in lead V_1)
  - Right axis deviation more than 100 degrees
  - Atrial fibrillation

IMAGING STUDIES

- Chest x-ray may show:
  - Evidence of COPD (e.g., flattened diaphragm, barrel chest, dilated pulmonary arteries, increased retrosternal air space)
  - Enlarged right atrium
  - Enlarged right ventricle
- Echocardiography will:
  - Detect TR
  - Estimate the severity of TR
  - Estimate the pulmonary artery pressure
  - Exclude vegetation, mass or prolapse
  - Assess left and right ventricular function
- Right-sided cardiac catheterization shows:
  - Elevated right atrial and right ventricular end-diastolic pressures
  - Large V waves

TREATMENT

- Functional TR caused by left-sided heart failure is treated in the standard manner with preload reduction, afterload reduction, or inotropic therapy (see "Heart Failure").

- Structural TR treatment depends on the underlying cause (e.g., antibiotics for infective endocarditis).
- Tricuspid valve surgery is considered in patients with severe TR from rheumatic heart disease, structural valve damage from carcinoid, congenital anomalies, or infective endocarditis.
- Surgical procedures may include:
  1. Total valve replacement
  2. Annuloplasty
  3. Converting the tricuspid valve from three leaflets to two leaflets

H. SURGERY FOR VALVULAR HEART DISEASE

- Valve replacement: artificial valves can be mechanical or biologic
- Mechanical prosthetic valves: preferred valve substitutes in adult patients who are already taking anticoagulants (e.g. for atrial fibrillation). The most important risk linked to these valves is valvular thrombosis requiring life-long anticoagulation.
  1. Ball-cage prosthesis: constructed as a ball in a metallic cage (e.g., Starr-Edwards valve; Fig. 107–16). The ball prosthesis partially obstructs blood flow, and flow through the prosthesis is turbulent. Benefit is low cost. Disadvantages are that trauma to red blood cells can result in hemolytic anemia, and the prosthesis is also very bulky.
  2. Tilting disk prosthesis: the mobile element of these valves is a tilting disc held in place by two welded struts. Older models consisted of the Bjork-Shiley valve; a newer model is the Medtronic-Hall omnicarbon prosthesis (Fig. 107–17).
  3. Bioleaflet prostheses: made of two semicircular pivoting discs constructed from pyrolytic carbon, a material considered to be less thrombogenic. Introduced in 1977, the prototype is the St. Jude valve, the most commonly implanted prosthetic valve. Newer models include the Carbomedics prosthesis (Fig. 107–18).
- Biologic valves: these valves are divided into three groups based on the origin of the biologic material—heterografts (animal origin), homografts (human donor), and autografts (tissues originating from the patient).
  1. Bioprostheses (heterografts): porcine bioprosthetic valves such as the Carpentier-Perimount (Fig. 107–19) are derived from pig aortic leaflets mounted on metal-coated stents. A major concern in these valves is degradation over time, usually manifesting as a valvular leak caused by a torn and prolapsed cusp or by commissural detachment. As a rule, most patients older than 75 years are offered a bioprosthesis.
  2. Homograft valves: valves harvested from human donors (Fig. 107–20). They have an excellent hemodynamic profile and are particularly useful in the management of infectious endocarditis because of the absence of prosthetic material.
  3. Autograft valves: the main use of autograft valves is the transfer of the pulmonary valve to the aortic position (Ross procedure), with the subsequent implantation of a pulmonary homograft into the prior position of the pulmonary valve.

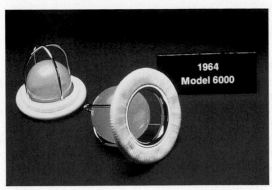

Fig 107–16
Ball-cage prosthesis. Shown is the Starr-Edwards prosthesis.
(From Crawford, MH, DiMarco JP, Paulus WJ [eds]: Cardiology, 2nd ed.
St. Louis, Mosby, 2004.)

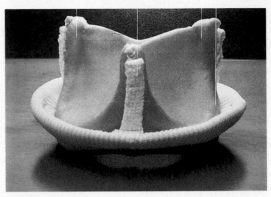

Fig 107–19
Pericardial Carpentier Perimount bioprosthesis.
(From Crawford, MH, DiMarco JP, Paulus WJ [eds]: Cardiology, 2nd ed.
St. Louis, Mosby, 2004.)

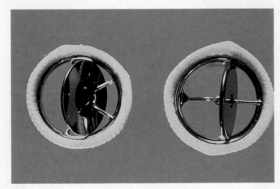

Fig 107–17
Tilting disc prostheses**. Left,** Bjork-Shiley prosthesis. **Right,**
Medtronic-Hall prosthesis.
(From Crawford, MH, DiMarco JP, Paulus WJ [eds]: Cardiology, 2nd ed.
St. Louis, Mosby, 2004.)

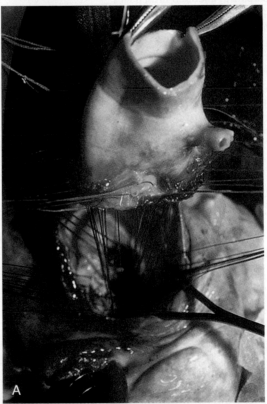

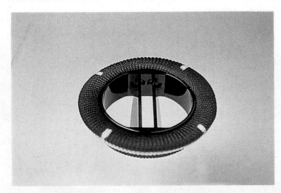

Fig 107–18
Carbomedics prosthesis.
(From Crawford, MH, DiMarco JP, Paulus WJ [eds]: Cardiology, 2nd ed.
St. Louis, Mosby, 2004.)

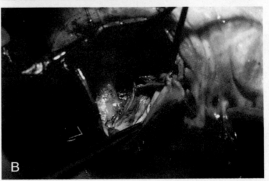

Fig 107–20
Placement of homograft in aortic position. **A,** Aortic root replacement
with homograft. **B,** Freehand aortic homograft.
(From Crawford, MH, DiMarco JP, Paulus WJ [eds]: Cardiology, 2nd ed.
St. Louis, Mosby, 2004.)

Chapter 108 / Infective endocarditis

DEFINITION
Infective endocarditis is an infection of the endocardial surface of the heart or mural endocardium.

Acute endocarditis
- Usually caused by *Staphylococcus aureus, Streptococcus pyogenes*, pneumococcus, and *Neisseria* organisms; classic clinical presentation of fever, positive blood cultures, vascular and immunologic phenomenon

Subacute endocarditis
- Usually caused by viridans streptococci in the presence of valvular pathology; less toxic, often indolent presentation, with lower fevers, night sweats, fatigue

Endocarditis in injection drug users
  Often involving *S. aureus* or *Pseudomonas aeruginosa* with variations that may be geographically influenced; tricuspid (Fig. 108–1) or multiple valvular involvement; high mortality rate, 50% to 60%

Prosthetic valve endocarditis (early)
- Usually caused by *S. epidermidis* within 2 months of valve replacement; other organisms include *S. aureus*, gram-negative bacilli, diphtheroids, *Candida* organisms

Prosthetic valve endocarditis (late)
- Typically develops more than 60 days after valvular replacement; involved organisms similar to early prosthetic valve endocarditis, including viridans streptococci, enterococci, and group D streptococci

Nosocomial endocarditis
- Secondary to intravenous catheters, total parenteral nutrition (TPN) lines, pacemakers; coagulase-negative staphylococci, *S. aureus*, and streptococci most common

PHYSICAL FINDINGS AND CLINICAL PRESENTATION
- Fever may be variable in presentation; may be high or absent
- Fever, chills, fatigue, and rigors occur in 25% to 80% of patients.
- Heart murmur may be absent in right-sided endocarditis.
- Embolic phenomenon with peripheral manifestations is found in 50% of patients (Figs. 108–2 and 108–3).
- Skin manifestations include petechiae, Osler nodes (Fig. 108–4), splinter hemorrhages (Fig. 108–5), Janeway lesions (Fig. 108–6).
- Splenomegaly is more common with subacute course.

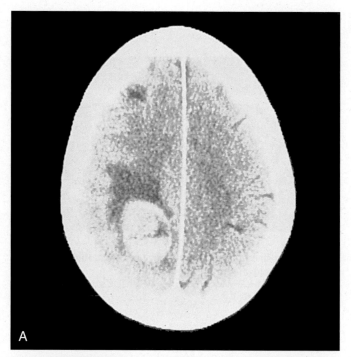

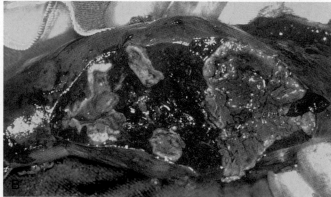

Fig 108–1
Tricuspid valve endocarditis.
There are large vegetations on the leaflets and the chordae tendineae.
(From Crawford, MH, DiMarco JP, Paulus WJ [eds]: Cardiology, 2nd ed. St. Louis, Mosby, 2004.)

Fig 108–2
A, CT scan of cerebral abscess. **B,** Multiple abscesses and ischemic necroses of the spleen. These were the result of peripheral emboli in acute endocarditis caused by *Staphylococcus aureus*. They developed after admission of this patient to the hospital.
(From Cohen J, Powderly WG: Infectious Diseases, 2nd ed. St. Louis, Mosby, 2004.)

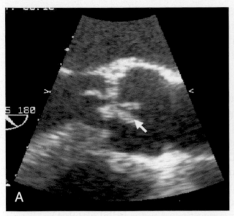 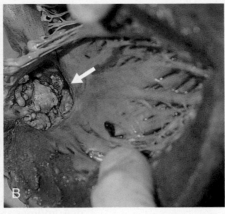 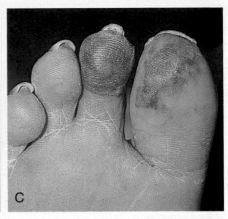

Fig 108-3
Infective endocarditis in end-stage renal disease. **A,** Transesophageal echocardiogram showing vegetation on the aortic valve *(arrow)*.
B, Vegetation on the aortic valve found at biopsy *(arrow)*. **C,** Septic embolization of the toes.
(From Johnson RJ, Feehally J: Comprehensive Clinical Nephrology, 2nd ed. St. Louis, Mosby, 2000.)

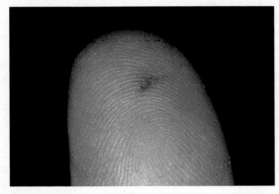

Fig 108-4
Osler node on the thumb during subacute endocarditis. This
was a rounded, tender, inflamed mass about 5 mm in diameter.
(From Cohen J, Powderly WG: Infectious Diseases, 2nd ed. St. Louis,
Mosby, 2004.)

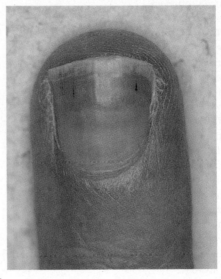

Fig 108-5
Splinter hemorrhages.
(From Swartz MH: Textbook of Physical Diagnosis, 5th ed. Philadelphia,
WB Saunders, 2006.)

CAUSE

Streptococcal and staphylococcal infections are the most
common causes of infective endocarditis. Variation in incidence may occur as a result of the patient's risk for developing
infection.

Acute endocarditis
- *S. aureus*
- *Streptococcus pneumoniae*
- Streptococcal species, groups A through G
- *Haemophilus influenzae*

Subacute endocarditis
- Viridans streptococci (alpha-hemolytic)
- *Streptococcus bovis*
- Enterococci
- *S. aureus*

Endocarditis in injection drug users
- *S. aureus*
- *P. aeruginosa*
- *Candida* species
- Enterococci

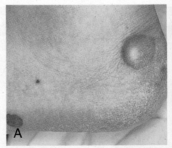 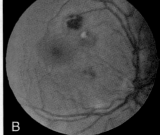

Fig 108-6
A, Skin lesions (Janeway spots) on the foot, **B,** Septic emboli of the
retina. These were the results of peripheral emboli in acute endocarditis caused by *Staphylococcus aureus* and were present in this patient
on admission to the hospital.
(From Cohen J, Powderly WG: Infectious Diseases, 2nd ed. St. Louis,
Mosby, 2004.)

Prosthetic valve endocarditis (early)
- *S. epidermidis*
- *S. aureus*
- Gram-negative bacilli
- Group D streptococci

Prosthetic valve endocarditis (late)
- *S. epidermidis*
- Viridans streptococci
- *S. aureus*
- Enterococci and group D streptococci

Nosocomial endocarditis
- Coagulase-negative *Staphylococcus*
- *S. aureus*
- Streptococci: viridans, group B, enterococcus

Hacek organisms
- Fastidious gram-negative bacilli
- *Haemophilus parainfluenzae*
- *Haemophilus aphrophilus*
- *Actinobacillus actinomycetemcomitans*
- *Cardiobacterium hominis*
- *Eikenella corrodens*
- *Kingella kingae*

RISK FACTORS
- Poor dental hygiene
- Long-term hemodialysis
- Diabetes mellitus
- HIV infection
- Mitral valve prolapse

DIFFERENTIAL DIAGNOSIS
- Brain abscess
- Fever of unknown origin (FUO)
- Pericarditis
- Meningitis
- Rheumatic fever
- Osteomyelitis
- Salmonella
- Tuberculosis (TB)
- Bacteremia
- Pericarditis
- Glomerulonephritis

LABORATORY TESTS
- Blood cultures: three sets in first 24 hours
- More culturing if patient has received prior antibiotic
- Complete blood count (CBC; anemia possibly present, subacute)
- White blood cell count (WBC; leukocytosis is higher in acute endocarditis)
- Erythrocyte sedimentation rate (ESR) and C-reactive protein (elevated)
- Positive rheumatoid factor (subacute endocarditis)
- False-positive VDRL
- Proteinuria, hematuria, red blood cell (RBC) casts
- Electrocardiogram: look for cardiac conduction abnormalities, injury pattern, or evidence for pericarditis; any such new findings are suggestive of myocardial abscess.

IMAGING STUDIES
- Echocardiography: two-dimensional
- Transesophageal echocardiography (Fig. 108–7): more sensitive in detecting vegetations if two-dimensional echocardiography is negative; especially helpful with prosthetic valves or in detecting perivalvular disease

TREATMENT
Initial IV antibiotic therapy (before culture results) is aimed at the most likely organism:
- In patients with prosthetic valves or patients with native valves who are allergic to penicillin: vancomycin plus rifampin, 600 mg PO daily, and gentamicin
- In IV drug users: nafcillin or oxacillin plus gentamicin; if methicillin-resistant *S. aureus* (MRSA), vancomycin plus gentamicin
- In native valve endocarditis with a penicillin-susceptible streptococcal isolate: combination of penicillin and gentamicin, assuming normal renal function; a penicillase-resistant penicillin plus gentamicin can be used if acute bacterial endocarditis is present or if *S. aureus* is suspected as one of the possible causative organisms; for Hacek organisms, treat with third-generation cephalosporin.
- Ceftriaxone and an aminoglycoside can be used in viridans streptococci endocarditis.
- Antibiotic therapy after identification of the organism should be guided by susceptibility testing, preferably by formal testing by MIC (minimal inhibitory concentration).

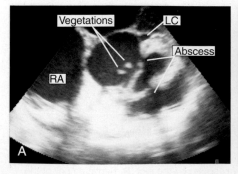
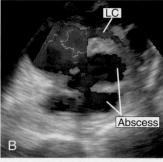

Fig 108–7
Transesophageal short-axis views through the aortic bulb in a patient with an infected aortic valve. **A,** Vegetations in the aorta can be seen, as can abscesses between the aorta and right ventricular outflow tract. **B,** The scan is positioned at the level of the main stem of the left coronary artery (LC), where flow is demonstrated. RA, right atrium. (From Crawford, MH, DiMarco JP, Paulus WJ [eds]: Cardiology, 2nd ed. St. Louis, Mosby, 2004.)

Chapter 109 **Congestive heart failure**

DEFINITION

Congestive heart failure is a pathophysiologic state characterized by congestion in the pulmonary or systemic circulation. It is caused by the heart's inability to pump sufficient oxygenated blood to meet the metabolic needs of the tissues (Fig. 109-1).

CLASSIFICATION:

The American College of Cardiology and the American Heart Association have described the following four stages of heart failure:

A. At high risk for heart failure, but without structural heart disease or symptoms of heart failure (e.g., CAD, hypertension)

B. Structural heart disease but without symptoms of heart failure

C. Structural heart disease with prior or current symptoms of heart failure

D. Refractory heart failure requiring specialized interventions

The New York Heart Association (NYHA) has defined the following functional classes:

I. Asymptomatic

II. Symptomatic with moderate exertion

III. Symptomatic with minimal exertion

IV. Symptomatic at rest

PHYSICAL FINDINGS AND CLINICAL PRESENTATION

The findings on physical examination in patients with CHF vary depending on the severity and whether the failure is right-sided or left-sided.

- Common clinical manifestations are:

1. Dyspnea on exertion initially, then with progressively less strenuous activity, and eventually manifesting when patient is at rest; caused by increasing pulmonary congestion

2. Orthopnea caused by increased venous return in the recumbent position

3. Paroxysmal nocturnal dyspnea (PND) resulting from multiple factors (increased venous return in the recumbent position, decreased PaO_2, decreased adrenergic stimulation of myocardial function)

4. Nocturnal angina resulting from increased cardiac work (secondary to increased venous return)

5. *Cheyne-Stokes respiration:* alternating phases of apnea and hyperventilation caused by prolonged circulation time from lungs to brain

6. Fatigue, lethargy resulting from low cardiac output

- Patients with failure of the left side of the heart will have the following abnormalities on physical examination: pulmonary rales, tachypnea, S_3 gallop, cardiac murmurs (AS, AR, MR), paradoxical splitting of S_2.

- Patients with failure of right side of the heart manifest with jugular venous distention (Fig. 109-2), peripheral edema, perioral and peripheral cyanosis, congestive hepatomegaly, ascites, hepatojugular reflux.

- In patients with heart failure, elevated jugular venous pressure and a third heart sound are each independently associated with adverse outcomes.

- Acute precipitants of CHF exacerbations are noncompliance with salt restriction, pulmonary infections, arrhythmias, medications (e.g., calcium channel blockers, antiarrhythmic agents), and inappropriate reductions in CHF therapy.

CAUSE

Left ventricular failure

- Systemic hypertension
- Valvular heart disease (AS, aortic regurgitation [AR], MR)
- Cardiomyopathy, myocarditis
- Bacterial endocarditis
- Myocardial infarction
- HOCM

Left ventricular failure is further differentiated according to systolic dysfunction (low ejection fraction) and diastolic dysfunction (normal or high ejection fraction), or stiff ventricle. It is important to make this distinction because treatment is significantly different (see "Treatment"). Patients with heart failure and a normal ejection fraction have significant abnormalities in active relaxation and passive stiffness. In these patients, the pathophysiologic cause of elevated diastolic pressures and heart failure is abnormal diastolic function.

- Common causes of systolic dysfunction are post-MI, cardiomyopathy, and myocarditis.
- Causes of diastolic dysfunction are hypertensive cardiovascular disease, valvular heart disease (AS, AR, MR, IHSS), and restrictive cardiomyopathy.

Right ventricular failure

- Valvular heart disease (mitral stenosis)
- Pulmonary hypertension
- Bacterial endocarditis (right-sided)
- Right ventricular infarction

Biventricular failure:

- Left ventricular failure
- Cardiomyopathy
- Myocarditis
- Arrhythmias
- Anemia
- Thyrotoxicosis
- Arteriovenous fistula
- Paget's disease
- Beriberi

DIFFERENTIAL DIAGNOSIS

- Cirrhosis
- Nephrotic syndrome
- Venous occlusive disease
- COPD, asthma
- Pulmonary embolism
- Acute respiratory disease syndrome (ARDS)
- Heroin overdose
- Pneumonia

LABORATORY TESTS

- CBC (to rule out anemia, infections), blood urea nitrogen (BUN), creatinine, electrolytes, liver enzymes, thyroid-stimulating hormone (TSH)
- BNP is a cardiac neurohormone specifically secreted from the ventricles in response to volume expansion and pressure overload. Elevated levels are indicative of left ventricular

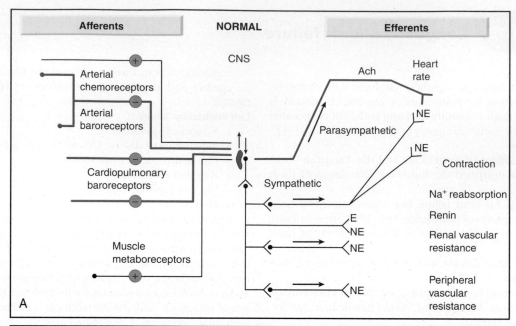

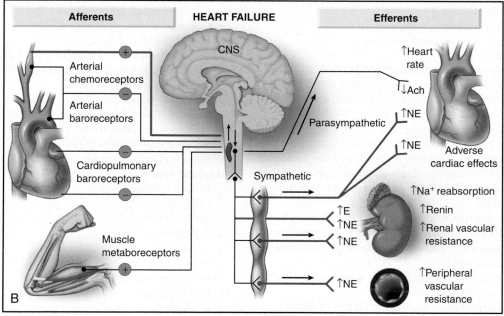

Fig 109–1

Mechanisms for generalized sympathetic activation and parasympathetic withdrawal in heart failure. **A,** Under normal conditions, inhibitory (−) inputs from arterial and cardiopulmonary baroreceptor afferent nerves are the principal influence on sympathetic outflow. Parasympathetic control of heart rate is also under potent arterial baroreflex control. Efferent sympathetic traffic and arterial catecholamines are low, and heart rate variability is high. **B,** As heart failure progresses, inhibitory input from arterial and cardiopulmonary receptors decreases and excitatory (+) input increases. The net response to this altered balance includes a generalized increase in sympathetic nerve traffic, blunted parasympathetic and sympathetic control of heart rate, and impairment of the reflex sympathetic regulation of vascular resistance. Anterior wall ischemia has additional excitatory effects on efferent sympathetic nerve traffic. See text for details. Ach, acetylcholine; CNS, central nervous system; E, epinephrine; Na+, sodium; NE, norepinephrine.

(From Floras JS: Alterations in the sympathetic and parasympathetic nervous system in heart failure. In Mann DL [ed]; Heart Failure: A Companion to Braunwald's Heart Disease. Philadelphia, Elsevier, 2004, pp 247-278.)

dysfunction. Bedside measurement of BNP is useful in establishing or excluding the diagnosis of CHF in patients with acute dyspnea. Elevated BNP levels are also strong predictors of survival in patients with heart failure, and possibly even in asymptomatic patients.

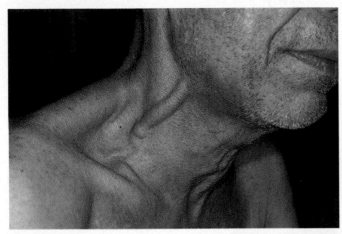

Fig 109-2
Neck vein distention.
(From Swartz MH: Textbook of Physical Diagnosis, 5th ed. Philadelphia, WB Saunders, 2006.)

IMAGING STUDIES
- Standard 12-lead ECG is useful to diagnose ischemic heart disease and obtain information about rhythm abnormalities. Over 25% of patients with CHF have some form of intraventricular conduction abnormality manifested as an increased QRS duration on ECG. The most common pattern is LBBB.
- Chest x-ray (Fig. 109–3)
  1. Pulmonary venous congestion
  2. Cardiomegaly with dilation of the involved heart chamber
  3. Pleural effusions
- Two-dimensional echocardiography is useful to assess global and regional left ventricular function and estimate the ejection fraction.
- Exercise stress testing may be useful for evaluating concomitant coronary disease and assess degree of disability. The decision to perform exercise stress testing should be individualized.
- Cardiac catheterization remains an excellent method to evaluate ventricular diastolic properties, significant coronary artery disease, or valvular heart disease; however, it is invasive. The decision to perform cardiac catheterization should be individualized.

TREATMENT
- Determine if CHF is secondary to systolic or diastolic dysfunction and treat accordingly.

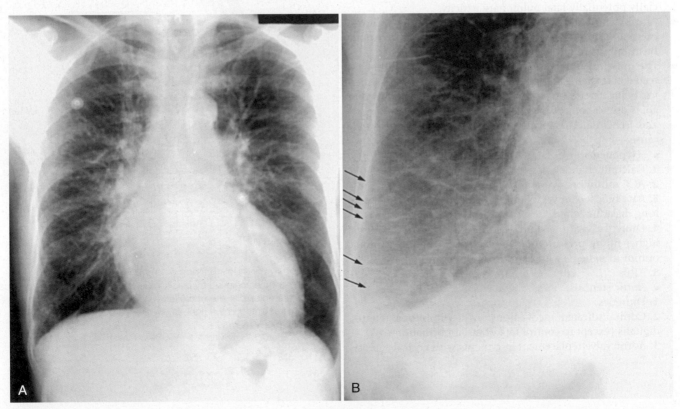

Fig 109-3
Early findings of congestive heart failure. **A,** The major signs on the upright PA chest radiograph are cardiomegaly and redistribution of the pulmonary vascularity. Normally, the vessels in the lower lobes are more prominent than those in the upper lobes; however, here they appear at least equally prominent. **B,** On a close-up view in another patient, small horizontal lines can be seen at the very periphery of the lung *(arrows)*. These are known as *Kerley B lines* and represent fluid in the interlobular septa.
(From Mettler FA, Guibertau MJ, Voss CM, Urbina CE: Primary Care Radiology. Philadelphia, Elsevier, 2000.)

- Identify and correct precipitating factors (e.g., anemia, thyrotoxicosis, infections, increased sodium load, medical noncompliance).
- Decrease cardiac workload in patients with systolic dysfunction: restrict patients' activity only during periods of acute decompensation; the risk of thromboembolism during this period can be minimized by using SC or low-molecular-weight heparin (LMWH). In patients with mild to moderate symptoms, aerobic training may improve symptoms and exercise capacity.
- Restrict sodium intake to less than 2 g/day.
- Restricting fluid intake to 2 liters or less may be useful in patients with hyponatremia.
- ACE inhibitors, diuretics, and beta blockers are effective treatments for CHF secondary to systolic dysfunction. Other useful agents are angiotensin II receptor blockers (ARBs) and direct vasodilating drugs (hydralazine, isosorbide). Nesiritide should be reserved for patients who present to the hospital with acutely decompensated heart failure and dyspnea at rest for whom standard combination therapy with diuretics and nitroglycerin has been inadequate.
- Surgical revascularization should be considered in patients with both heart failure and severe limiting angina.
- Antiarrhythmic therapy with amiodarone has a modest effect in reducing mortality in patients with CHF; however, it is not recommended for general use in CHF. Its benefits must be weighed against the risk for adverse effects, especially potentially fatal pulmonary toxicity.
- Atriobiventricular pacing (Fig. 109–4) significantly improves exercise tolerance and quality of life in patients with chronic heart failure and intraventricular conduction delay.
- The initial treatment of diastolic heart failure should be directed at reducing the congestive state with the use of diuretics, being careful not to avoid excessive diuresis. Long-term goals are to control hypertension, tachycardia, congestion, and ischemia. Therapeutic options are determined by the cause.
  - Hypertension
  1. Calcium channel blockers (verapamil)
  2. ACE inhibitors
  3. Beta blockers or verapamil to control heart rate and prolong diastolic filling
  4. Diuretics: vigorous diuresis should be avoided, because a higher filling pressure may be needed to maintain cardiac output in patients with diastolic dysfunction.
  5. ARBs
  - Aortic stenosis
  1. Diuretics
  2. Contraindicated medications: ACE inhibitors, nitrates, digitalis (except to control rate of atrial fibrillation)
  3. Aortic valve replacement in patients with critical stenosis

- Aortic insufficiency and mitral regurgitation
1. ACE inhibitors increase cardiac output and decrease pulmonary wedge pressure. They are the agents of choice, along with diuretics.
2. Hydralazine combined with nitrates can be used if ACE inhibitors are not tolerated.
3. Surgery
- IHSS
1. Beta blockers or verapamil
2. Contraindicated medications (they increase outlet obstruction by decreasing the size of the left ventricle in end systole): diuretics, digitalis, ACE inhibitors, hydralazine
3. Restoration of intravascular volume with IV saline solution if necessary in acute pulmonary edema
4. Dual-chamber (DDD) pacing is useful in select patients.

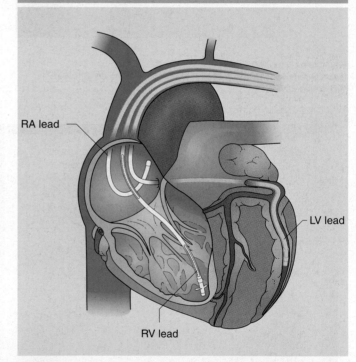

CARDIAC RESYNCHRONIZATION THERAPY

RA lead

LV lead

RV lead

Fig 109–4

Cardiac resynchronization therapy. Atrioventricular synchronous biventricular pacing is achieved by placing a lead through the coronary sinus to pace the epicardial site of the left ventricular (LV) wall (LV lead). More leads are implanted in the right atrium (RA lead) and in the right ventricular apex (RV lead).
(From Crawford, MH, DiMarco JP, Paulus WJ [eds]: Cardiology, 2nd ed. St. Louis, Mosby, 2004.)

Chapter 110 Cardiogenic pulmonary edema

DEFINITION
Cardiogenic pulmonary edema is a life-threatening condition caused by severe left ventricular decompensation.

PHYSICAL FINDINGS AND CLINICAL PRESENTATION
- Dyspnea with rapid, shallow breathing
- Diaphoresis, perioral and peripheral cyanosis
- Pink, frothy sputum
- Moist, bilateral pulmonary rales
- Increased pulmonary second sound, S_3 gallop (in association with tachycardia)
- Bulging neck veins

CAUSE
Increased pulmonary capillary pressure secondary to:
- Acute myocardial infarction
- Exacerbation of CHF
- Valvular regurgitation (e.g., mitral regurgitation)
- Ventricular septal defect
- Severe myocardial ischemia
- Mitral stenosis
- Other: cardiac tamponade, endocarditis, myocarditis, arrhythmias, cardiomyopathy, hypertensive crisis

DIFFERENTIAL DIAGNOSIS
- Noncardiogenic pulmonary edema
- Pulmonary embolism
- Exacerbation of asthma
- Exacerbation of COPD
- Sarcoidosis
- Pulmonary fibrosis
- Viral pneumonitis and other pulmonary infections

LABORATORY TESTS
- Arterial blood gases (ABGs): respiratory and metabolic acidosis, decreased Pao_2, increased Pco_2, low pH

Note: The patient may initially show respiratory alkalosis secondary to hyperventilation in attempts to maintain Pao_2.

IMAGING STUDIES
- Chest x-ray examination (Fig. 110–1)
  1. Pulmonary congestion with Kerley B lines; fluffy perihilar infiltrates in the early stages; bilateral interstitial alveolar infiltrates
  2. Pleural effusions
- Echocardiography
  1. Useful to evaluate valvular abnormalities, diastolic versus systolic dysfunction

2. Can aid in differentiation of cardiogenic versus noncardiogenic pulmonary edema

3. Can also estimate pulmonary capillary wedge pressure and rule out presence of myxoma or atrial thrombus
- Right heart catheterization (select patients): cardiac pressures in cardiogenic pulmonary edema reveal increased pulmonary artery diastolic pressure and PCWP 25 mm Hg or higher.

TREATMENT
All the following steps can be performed concomitantly:
- 100% oxygen by face mask
- IV furosemide
- Vasodilator therapy with nitrates, and nitroprusside
- Morphine: 2 to 4 mg, IV, SC, IM; may repeat every 15 minutes as needed.
- Afterload reduction with ACE inhibitors
- Dobutamine: parenteral inotropic agent of choice in severe cases of cardiogenic pulmonary edema.

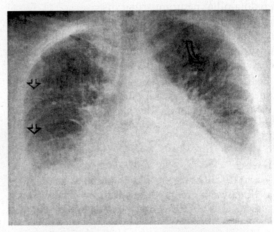

Fig 110–1
Severe cardiogenic interstitial edema. The axial interstitium is thickened (bronchovascular or Kerley A, *curved arrow*). Prominent septal lines (Kerley B) are seen in the periphery of the right lung *(arrows)*. (From Grainger RG, Allison DJ, Adam A, Dixon AK [eds]: Grainger & Allison's Diagnostic Radiology, 4th ed. London, Harcourt, 2001.)

Chapter 111   Cardiomyopathies

A. DILATED (CONGESTIVE) CARDIOMYOPATHY

DEFINITION

Cardiomyopathies are a group of diseases primarily involving the myocardium and characterized by myocardial dysfunction that is not the result of hypertension, coronary atherosclerosis, valvular dysfunction, or pericardial abnormalities. In dilated cardiomyopathy, the heart is enlarged, and both ventricles are dilated.

PHYSICAL FINDINGS AND CLINICAL PRESENTATION

- Increased jugular venous pressure
- Small pulse pressure
- Pulmonary rales, hepatomegaly, peripheral edema
- S_3, S_4
- Mitral regurgitation, tricuspid regurgitation (less common)

CAUSE

- Idiopathic
- Alcoholism (15% to 40% of all cases in Western countries)
- Collagen-vascular disease (SLE, rheumatoid arthritis [RA], polyarteritis, dermatomyositis)
- Postmyocarditis
- Peripartum (last trimester of pregnancy or 6 mo postpartum)
- Heredofamilial neuromuscular disease
- Toxins (cobalt, lead, phosphorus, carbon monoxide, mercury, doxorubicin (Fig. 111–1), daunorubicin)
- Nutritional (beriberi, selenium deficiency, carnitine deficiency, thiamine deficiency)
- Cocaine, heroin, organic solvents ("glue sniffer's heart")
- Irradiation
- Acromegaly, osteogenesis imperfecta, myxedema, thyrotoxicosis, diabetes
- Hypocalcemia
- Antiretroviral agents (zidovudine, didanosine, zalcitabine)
- Phenothiazines
- Infections (viral [HIV], rickettsial, mycobacterial, toxoplasmosis, trichinosis, Chagas' disease [Fig. 111–2])
- Hematologic (e.g., sickle cell anemia)

DIFFERENTIAL DIAGNOSIS

- Frank pulmonary disease
- Valvular dysfunction
- Pericardial abnormalities
- Coronary atherosclerosis
- Psychogenic dyspnea

IMAGING STUDIES

Chest x-ray

- Massive cardiac enlargement
- Interstitial pulmonary edema

ECG

- Left ventricular hypertrophy with ST-T wave changes
- RBBB or LBBB
- Arrhythmias (atrial fibrillation, PVC, premature atrial contraction [PAC], ventricular tachycardia)

Echocardiography (Fig. 111–3)

- Low ejection fraction with global akinesia

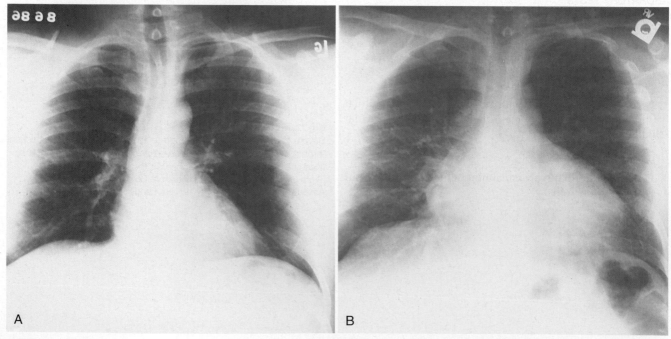

A   B

Fig 111–1

Cardiomyopathy. In this case, cardiomyopathy is caused by cancer chemotherapy with doxorubicin. **A,** An initial chest x-ray examination demonstrates a normal-sized heart. **B,** After several therapeutic courses of doxorubicin, there has been marked enlargement in the cardiac silhouette because of multichamber dilation.

(From Mettler FA, Guibertau MJ, Voss CM, Urbina CE: Primary Care Radiology. Philadelphia, Elsevier, 2000.)

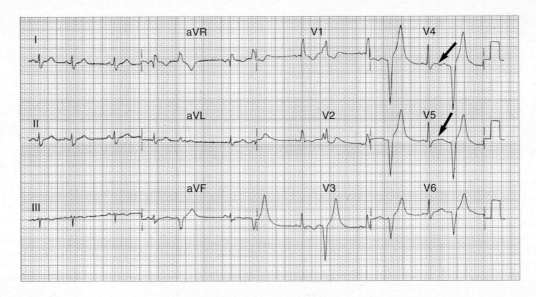

Fig 111–2

ECG in Chagas' disease. Note right bundle branch block, ventricular bigeminy, and convex upward ST-T-segment elevation in leads V_3 to V_5 (arrows), suggestive of a left ventricular aneurysm.

(From Crawford, MH, DiMarco JP, Paulus WJ [eds]: Cardiology, 2nd ed. St. Louis, Mosby, 2004.)

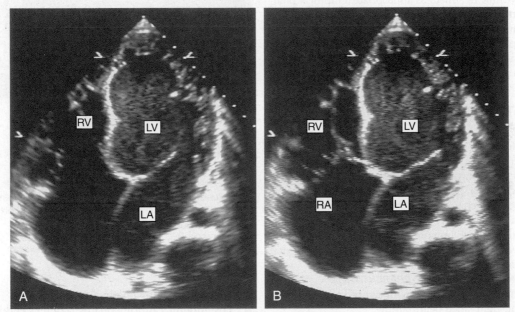

Fig 111–3

Dilated cardiomyopathy. Diastolic **(A)** and systolic **(B)** echocardiographic images demonstrating dilated cardiomyopathy with severe biventricular systolic dysfunction. Spontaneous contrast is noted in the left ventricle, consistent with stagnant flow. LA, left atrium; LV, left ventricle; RA, right atrium; RV, right ventricle.

(From Crawford, MH, DiMarco JP, Paulus WJ [eds]: Cardiology, 2nd ed. St. Louis, Mosby, 2004.)

TREATMENT

- Treatment of underlying disease (SLE, alcoholism)
- Treat CHF (cause of death in 70% of patients) with sodium restriction, diuretics, ACE inhibitors,beta blockers, spironolactone, and digitalis (Fig. 111–4).
- Vasodilators (combined with nitrates and ACE inhibitors) are effective agents in all symptomatic patients with left ventricular dysfunction.

- Prevent thromboembolism with oral anticoagulants in all patients with atrial fibrillation and in patients with moderate or severe failure.
- Low-dose beta blockade with carvedilol or other beta blockers may improve ventricular function by interrupting the cycle of reflex sympathetic activity and controlling tachycardia.

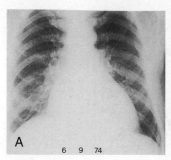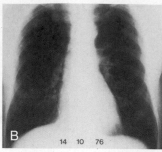

Fig 111–4
Congestive cardiomyopathy. **A,** Before full treatment, the heart is large, with some prominence of the left ventricle, although all chambers are enlarged. There is a small right pleural effusion, redistribution of blood to the upper zones, and slight pulmonary edema. **B,** After full treatment, the heart has reverted to normal size and the lungs are clear. (From Grainger RG, Allison DJ, Adam A, Dixon AK [eds]: Grainger & Allison's Diagnostic Radiology, 4th ed. London, Harcourt, 2001.)

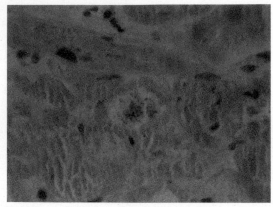

Fig 111–5
Endomyocardial biopsy in a patient with hemochromatosis. This photomicrograph shows intracellular iron deposits (blue) in a myocardial biopsy stained with Pearl's iron stain.
(Courtesy of Dr. H. Thomas Aretz, MGH Department of Pathology.)

- Diltiazem and ACE inhibitors have also been reported to have a long-term beneficial effect in idiopathic dilated cardiomyopathy.
- Use antiarrhythmic treatment as appropriate. Empirical pharmacologic suppression of asymptomatic ventricular ectopy does not reduce risk of sudden death or improve long-term survival. In patients with severe left ventricular dysfunction and/or symptomatic and sustained ventricular tachycardia, the use of an automatic ICD should be considered.

B. RESTRICTIVE CARDIOMYOPATHY

DEFINITION
Cardiomyopathies are a group of diseases primarily involving the myocardium and characterized by myocardial dysfunction that is not the result of hypertension, coronary atherosclerosis, valvular dysfunction, or pericardial abnormalities. Restrictive cardiomyopathies are characterized by decreased ventricular compliance, usually secondary to infiltration of the myocardium. These patients have impaired ventricular filling and reduced diastolic volume, normal systolic function, and normal or near-normal myocardial thickness.

PHYSICAL FINDINGS AND CLINICAL PRESENTATION
Restrictive cardiomyopathy presents with symptoms of progressive left-sided and right-sided heart failure:
- Edema, ascites, hepatomegaly, distended neck veins
- Fatigue, weakness (secondary to low output)
- Kussmaul's sign: may be present
- Regurgitant murmurs
- Possible prominent apical impulse

CAUSE
- Infiltrative and storage disorders (glycogen storage disease, amyloidosis, sarcoidosis, hemochromatosis [Fig. 111–5])
- Scleroderma
- Radiation
- Endocardial fibroelastosis (Fig. 111–6)
- Endomyocardial fibrosis
- Idiopathic
- Toxic effects of anthracycline
- Carcinoid heart disease, metastatic cancers

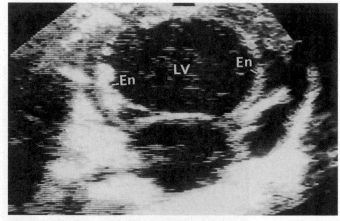

Fig 111–6
Cross-sectional echocardiogram, apical two-chamber view of endocardial fibroelastosis. Note the enlargement of the left ventricular (LV) cavity size. The cavity is abnormally round, and the amplitude of endocardial (En) and subendocardial echoes is increased.
(From Grainger RG, Allison DJ, Adam A, Dixon AK [eds]: Grainger & Allison's Diagnostic Radiology, 4th ed. London, Harcourt, 2001.)

- Diabetic cardiomyopathy
- Eosinophilic cardiomyopathy (Löffler's endocarditis)

DIFFERENTIAL DIAGNOSIS
- Coronary atherosclerosis
- Valvular dysfunction
- Pericardial abnormalities
- Chronic lung disease
- Psychogenic dyspnea

IMAGING STUDIES
- Chest x-ray
  1. Moderate cardiomegaly
  2. Possible evidence of CHF (pulmonary vascular congestion, pleural effusion)
- ECG
  1. Low voltage with ST-T wave changes
  2. Possible frequent arrhythmias, left axis deviation, and atrial fibrillation

- Echocardiogram: increased wall thickness and thickened cardiac valves (especially in patients with amyloidosis)
- Cardiac catheterization to distinguish restrictive cardiomyopathy from constrictive pericarditis
- MRI may also be useful to distinguish restrictive cardiomyopathy from constrictive pericarditis (thickness of the pericardium more than 5 mm in the latter).

TREATMENT
- Control CHF by restricting salt.
- Cardiomyopathy caused by hemochromatosis may respond to repeated phlebotomies to decrease iron deposition in the heart.
- Sarcoidosis may respond to corticosteroid therapy.
- Corticosteroid and cytotoxic drugs may improve survival in patients with eosinophilic cardiomyopathy.
- There is no effective therapy for other causes of restrictive cardiomyopathy.

C. HYPERTROPHIC CARDIOMYOPATHY

DEFINITION
Cardiomyopathies are a group of diseases primarily involving the myocardium (Fig. 111–7) and characterized by myocardial dysfunction that is not the result of hypertension, coronary atherosclerosis, valvular dysfunction, or pericardial abnormalities. In hypertrophic cardiomyopathy (HCM), there is marked hypertrophy of the myocardium and disproportionally greater thickening of the intraventricular septum (Fig. 111–8) than that of the free wall of the left ventricle (asymmetrical septal hypertrophy [ASH]).

PHYSICAL FINDINGS AND CLINICAL PRESENTATION
- Hypertrophic cardiomyopathy may be suspected on the basis of abnormalities found on physical examination. Classic findings include:
  1. Harsh, systolic, diamond-shaped murmur at the left sternal border or apex that increases with Valsalva maneuver and decreases with squatting
  2. Paradoxical splitting of S_2 (if left ventricular obstruction is present)

  3. S_4
  4. Double or triple apical impulse
- Increased obstruction can occur with:
  1. Drugs: digitalis, beta-adrenergic stimulators (isoproterenol, dopamine, epinephrine), nitroglycerin, vasodilators, diuretics, alcohol
  2. Hypovolemia
  3. Tachycardia
  4. Valsalva maneuver
  5. Standing position
- Decreased obstruction is seen with:
  1. Drugs: beta-adrenergic blockers, calcium channel blockers, disopyramide, α-adrenergic stimulators
  2. Volume expansion
  3. Bradycardia
  4. Hand grip exercise
  5. Squatting position
- Clinical manifestations are as follows:
  1. Dyspnea
  2. Syncope (usually seen with exercise)
  3. Angina (decreased angina in recumbent position)
  4. Palpitations

CAUSE
- Autosomal dominant trait with variable penetrance caused by mutations in any of 1 to 10 genes, each encoding proteins of cardiac sarcomere
- Sporadic occurrence

DIFFERENTIAL DIAGNOSIS
- Coronary atherosclerosis
- Valvular dysfunction
- Pericardial abnormalities
- Chronic pulmonary disease
- Psychogenic dyspnea

IMAGING STUDIES
- Chest x-ray: may be normal or may show cardiomegaly (Fig. 111–9).
- Two-dimensional echocardiography (Fig. 111–10) is used to establish the diagnosis. Findings include ventricular hypertrophy, ratio of septum thickness to left ventricular

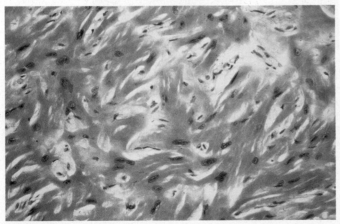

Fig 111–7
Myocyte disarray—myocardial section demonstrating myocyte disarray. Individual myocytes vary in length and diameter and contain abnormal nuclei. There are abnormal intercellular connections, and cells form circles around areas of increased connective tissue (H&E).
(Courtesy of Professor M. Davies, St. George's Hospital School, London.)

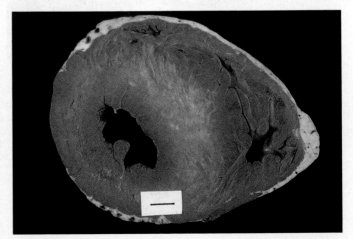

Fig 111–8
Severe asymmetrical hypertrophy of the interventricular septum and a disordered pattern of large muscle bundles in hypertrophic cardiomyopathy.
(Courtesy of Professor M. Davies, St. George's Hospital School, London.)

wall thickness higher than 1.3:1, and increased ejection fraction.
- CT or MRI (Fig. 111–11) may be of diagnostic value when echocardiographic studies are technically inadequate. MRI is also useful in identifying segmental LVH undetectable by echocardiography.

- ECG is abnormal in 75% to 95% of patients: left ventricular hypertrophy, abnormal Q waves in anterolateral and inferior leads (Fig. 111–12)
- 24-hour Holter monitor to screen for potential lethal arrhythmias (principal cause of syncope or sudden death in obstructive cardiomyopathy) should be performed initially and annually.

TREATMENT
- Advise avoidance of alcohol, dehydration, and strenuous exertion.
- Propranolol
- Verapamil also decreases left ventricular outflow obstruction by improving filling and probably reducing myocardial ischemia.
- IV saline infusion in addition to propranolol or verapamil is indicated in patients with CHF.
- Disopyramide is a useful antiarrhythmic because it is also a negative inotrope, resulting in further decrease in outflow gradient.
- Avoid use of digitalis, diuretics, nitrates, and vasodilators.
- Encouraging results have been reported on the use of DDD pacing for hemodynamic and symptomatic benefit in patients with drug-resistant hypertrophic obstructive cardiomyopathy.
- Implantable defibrillators are a safe and effective therapy in HCM patients prone to ventricular arrhythmias.

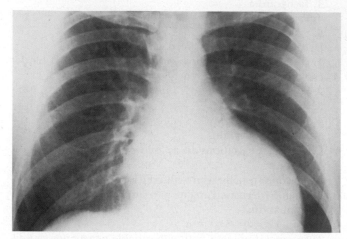

Fig 111–9
Hypertrophic cardiomyopathy: extreme left ventricular hypertrophy. (From Grainger RG, Allison DJ, Adam A, Dixon AK [eds]: Grainger & Allison's Diagnostic Radiology, 4th ed. London, Harcourt, 2001.)

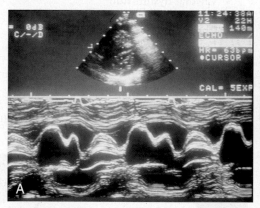 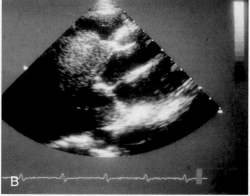

Fig 111–10
Left ventricular outflow tract obstruction. **A,** M-mode echocardiogram in a patient with asymmetrical septal hypertrophy and left ventricular outflow tract obstruction demonstrating asymmetrical septal hypertrophy and systolic anterior motion (SAM) of the mitral valve. The timing and duration of contact caused by SAM between the mitral valve and the septum can be used to estimate the severity of the outflow gradient. **B,** Two-dimensional echocardiogram in a patient with left ventricular outflow tract obstruction demonstrating the characteristic SAM of the anterior mitral valve leaflet. As the distal portion of the leaflet bends toward the septum, it makes contact with the septum and causes obstruction. (From Crawford, MH, DiMarco JP, Paulus WJ [eds]: Cardiology, 2nd ed. St. Louis, Mosby, 2004.)

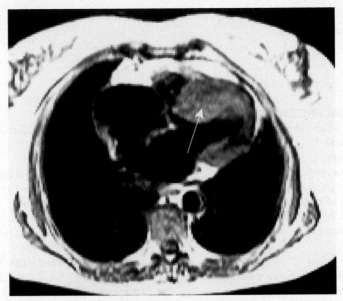

Fig 111–11
A spin-echo MR image in a transverse plane of a patient with hypertrophic cardiomyopathy. Note the asymmetrical thickening of the interventricular septum *(arrow).*
(From Grainger RG, Allison DJ, Adam A, Dixon AK [eds]: Grainger & Allison's Diagnostic Radiology, 4th ed. London, Harcourt, 2001.)

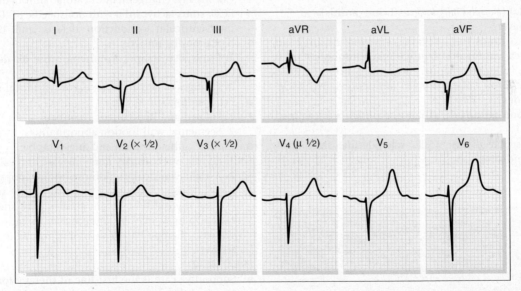

Fig 111–12
Hypertrophic cardiomyopathy simulating inferolateral infarction. This 11-year-old girl had a family history of hypertrophic cardiomyopathy. Note the W-shaped QS waves and the QRS complexes in the inferior and lateral precordial leads.
(From Goldberger AL: Myocardial Infarction: Electrocardiographic Differential Diagnosis, 4th ed. St. Louis, Mosby-Year Book, 1991.)

Chapter 112 Myocarditis

DEFINITION
Myocarditis is an inflammatory condition of the myocardium (Fig. 112–1).

PHYSICAL FINDINGS AND CLINICAL PRESENTATION
- Persistent tachycardia out of proportion to fever
- Faint S_1, S_4 sound on auscultation
- Murmur of mitral regurgitation
- Pericardial friction rub if associated with pericarditis
- Signs of biventricular failure (hypotension, hepatomegaly, peripheral edema, distention of neck veins, S_3)
- Patients may present with a history of recent flulike syndrome (fever, arthralgias, malaise).

CAUSE
- Infection
  1. Viral (coxsackie B virus, CMV, echovirus, polio virus, adenovirus, mumps, HIV, Epstein-Barr virus [EBV])
  2. Bacterial (*Staphylococcus aureus*, *Clostridium perfringens*, diphtheria, and any severe bacterial infection)
  3. Mycoplasma
  4. Mycotic (*Candida*, *Mucor*, *Aspergillus*)
  5. Parasitic (*Trypanosoma cruzi*, *Trichinella*, *Echinococcus*, amoeba, *Toxoplasma*)
  6. *Rickettsia rickettsii*
  7. Spirochetal (*Borrelia burgdorferi*—Lyme carditis)
- Rheumatic fever
- Secondary to drugs (e.g., cocaine, emetine, doxorubicin, sulfonamides, isoniazid, methyldopa, amphotericin B, tetracycline, phenylbutazone, lithium, 5-FU, phenothiazines, interferon alfa, tricyclic antidepressants, cyclophosphamides)
- Toxins (carbon monoxide, ethanol, diphtheria toxin, lead, arsenicals)
- Collagen-vascular disease (SLE, scleroderma, sarcoidosis, Kawasaki syndrome)
- Sarcoidosis

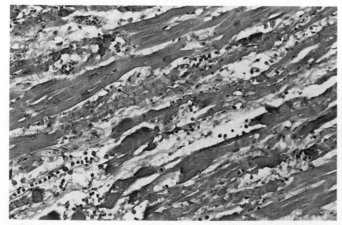

Fig 112–1
Acute viral myocarditis, with a characteristic mononuclear infiltrate. (From Cohen J, Powderly WG: Infectious Diseases, 2nd ed. St. Louis, Mosby, 2004.)

- Radiation
- Postpartum

DIFFERENTIAL DIAGNOSIS
- Cardiomyopathy
- Acute myocardial infarction
- Valvulopathies

LABORATORY TESTS
- Elevated cardiac TnT is suggestive of myocarditis in patients with clinically suspected myocarditis. A normal level does not rule out the diagnosis.
- Increased CK (with elevated MB fraction, lactate dehydrogenase [LDH]), and aspartate transaminase (AST) secondary to myocardial necrosis
- Increased ESR (nonspecific but may be of value in following the progress of the disease and the response to therapy)
- Increased WBC (increased eosinophils if parasitic infection)
- Viral titers (acute and convalescent)
- Cold agglutinin titer, ASLO titer, blood cultures
- Lyme disease antibody titer

IMAGING STUDIES
See Figure 112–2.
- Chest x-ray: enlargement of cardiac silhouette
- ECG: sinus tachycardia with nonspecific ST-T wave changes; interventricular conduction defects and bundle branch block may be present.
  1. Lyme disease and diphtheria cause all degrees of heart block.
  2. Changes of acute MI can occur with focal necrosis.
- Echocardiogram
  1. Dilated and hypokinetic chambers
  2. Segmental wall motion abnormalities
- Cardiac catheterization and angiography:
  1. To rule out coronary artery disease and valvular disease
  2. A right ventricular endomyocardial biopsy can confirm the diagnosis, although a negative biopsy result does not exclude myocarditis. Recent studies have shown that myocardial biopsy may be unnecessary, because immunosuppression therapy based on biopsy results is generally ineffective.

TREATMENT
- Supportive care is the first line of therapy for patients with myocarditis.
- Restrict physical activity (to decrease cardiac work). Bed rest is advisable during viremia.
- Treat underlying cause (e.g., use specific antibiotics for bacterial infection).
- Treat CHF with diuretics, ACE inhibitors, and salt restriction. A beta blocker may be added once clinical stability has been achieved. Digoxin should be used with caution and only at low doses.
- If ventricular arrhythmias are present, treat with quinidine or procainamide.
- Provide anticoagulation to prevent thromboembolism.
- Use preload and afterload reducing agents for treating cardiac decompensation.

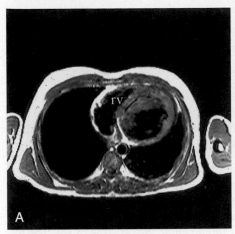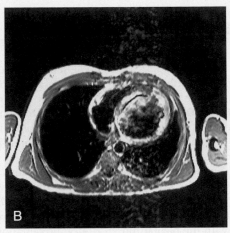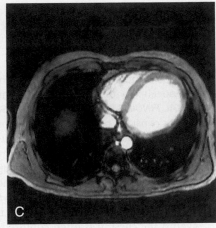

Fig 112–2

Spin-echo images acquired before **(A)** and after **(B)** intravenous Gd-DTPA injection in a patient with acute myocarditis. Note the dilated left ventricle (LV) and diffuse enhancement of left ventricular myocardial signal intensity following the intravenous administration of Gd-DTPA. **C,** Corresponding gradient-echo image.

(From Grainger RG, Allison DJ, Adam A, Dixon AK [eds]: Grainger & Allison's Diagnostic Radiology, 4th ed. London, Harcourt, 2001.)

- Corticosteroid use is contraindicated in early infectious myocarditis; it may be justified in only select patients with intractable CHF, severe systemic toxicity, and severe life-threatening arrhythmias.

- Immunosuppressive drugs (prednisone with cyclosporine or azathioprine) do not have any significant effect on the prognosis of myocarditis and should not be used in the routine treatment of patients with myocarditis. Immunosuppression may have a role in the treatment of myocarditis from systemic autoimmune disease (e.g., SLE, scleroderma) and in patients with idiopathic giant cell myocarditis.

Chapter 113 Pericarditis

DEFINITION

Pericarditis is the inflammation (or infiltration) of the pericardium associated with a wide variety of causes (see "Cause").

PHYSICAL FINDINGS AND CLINICAL PRESENTATION

- Severe constant pain that localizes over the anterior chest and may radiate to arms and back; it can be differentiated from myocardial ischemia, because the pain intensifies with inspiration and is relieved by sitting up and leaning forward (the pain of myocardial ischemia is not pleuritic).
- Pericardial friction rub is best heard with the patient upright and leaning forward and by pressing the stethoscope firmly against the chest. It is often confused with the pleural rub. The pericardial friction rub corresponds temporally to movement of the heart within the pericardial sac. Typically, the rub is a high-pitched scratchy or squeaky sound heard best at the left sternal border at end expiration. It typically consists of three short scratchy sounds:
  1. Systolic component
  2. Diastolic component
  3. Late diastolic component (associated with atrial contraction)

  However, in reality, the rub is reported to be triphasic in about half the patients, biphasic in a third, and monophasic in the remainder.
- Cardiac tamponade may be occurring if the following are observed:
  1. Tachycardia
  2. Low blood pressure and pulse pressure
  3. Distended neck veins
  4. Paradoxical pulse (pulsus paradoxus)

CAUSE

- Idiopathic (possibly postviral). In 9 of 10 patients with acute pericarditis, the cause is either viral or unknown (idiopathic).
- Infectious (viral, bacterial [1% to 2%], tuberculous [4%], fungal, amebic, toxoplasmosis)
- Collagen-vascular disease (SLE, rheumatoid arthritis, scleroderma, vasculitis, dermatomyositis): 3% to 5 % of cases
- Drug-induced lupus syndrome (procainamide, hydralazine, phenytoin, isoniazid, rifampin, doxorubicin, mesalamine)
- Acute MI (transmural myocardial infarction)
- Trauma or post-traumatic
- After MI (Dressler's syndrome)
- After pericardiotomy
- After mediastinal radiation (e.g., patients with Hodgkin's disease)
- Uremia
- Sarcoidosis
- Neoplasm (primary or metastatic): 7% of cases
- Leakage of aortic aneurysm in pericardial sac
- Familial Mediterranean fever
- Rheumatic fever
- Leukemic infiltration
- Other: anticoagulants, amyloidosis, immune thrombocytopenic purpura (ITP)

DIFFERENTIAL DIAGNOSIS

- Angina pectoris
- Pulmonary infarction
- Dissecting aneurysm
- GI abnormalities (e.g., hiatal hernia, esophageal rupture)
- Pneumothorax
- Hepatitis
- Cholecystitis
- Pneumonia with pleurisy

LABORATORY TESTS

Generally, laboratory tests are not clinically helpful and the clinical presentation should guide the ordering of any. The following tests may be useful in the absence of an obvious cause:

- CBC with differential
- Viral titers (acute and convalescent)
- ESR (not specific but may be of value in following the course of the disease and the response to therapy)
- Antinuclear antibody (ANA), rheumatoid factor
- Purified protein derivative (PPD), ASLO titers
- BUN, creatinine
- Blood cultures
- Cardiac isoenzymes (usually normal, but mild elevations of CK-MB may occur because of associated epicarditis). Plasma troponins are elevated in 35% to 50% of patients with pericarditis.
- Pericardiocentesis is indicated in patients with pericardial tamponade and in those with known or suspected purulent or neoplastic pericarditis. The fluid should be analyzed for RBC and WBC counts, cytology, glucose, LDH, protein, pH, triglyceride level and cultured. Polymerase chain reaction (PCR) assays or elevated levels of adenosine deaminase activity (more than 30 U/liter) are useful when suspecting tuberculous pericarditis.
- Pericardial biopsy may be helpful in recurrent tamponade.

IMAGING STUDIES

- Echocardiogram to detect and determine amount of pericardial effusion (Fig. 113–1); absence of effusion does not rule out the diagnosis of pericarditis. Divergence of right and left ventricular systolic pressures is present in cardiac tamponade and constrictive pericarditis.
- ECG: varies with the evolutionary stage of pericarditis (Fig. 113–2))
1. Acute phase: PR segment depression and diffuse ST segment elevations (particularly evident in the precordial leads), which can be distinguished from acute MI by:
   a. Absence of reciprocal ST segment depression in oppositely oriented leads (reciprocal ST segment depression may be seen in aV_R and VI)
   b. Elevated ST segments concave upward
   c. Absence of Q waves
2. Intermediate phase: return of ST segment to baseline, and T wave inversion in leads previously showing ST segment elevation

3. Late phase: resolution of the T wave changes
- Chest radiography: done primarily to rule out abnormalities of the mediastinum or lung fields that may be responsible for the pericarditis
1. Cardiac silhouette appears enlarged if more than 250 mL of fluid has accumulated (Fig. 113–3).
2. Calcifications around the heart may be seen with constrictive pericarditis.

TREATMENT

- Limitation of activity until the pain abates
- Anti-inflammatory therapy (NSAIDs, aspirin preferred in patients with recent MI)
- Colchicine may be used as an alternative in patients intolerant to NSAIDs and corticosteroids or can be used in combination with NSAIDs.
- Prednisone for up to 4 weeks may be added for patients with severe forms of acute pericarditis and suspected connective tissue disease.
- Consider ventricular rate control with verapamil or diltiazem because of the propensity for atrial fibrillation in these patients.
- Close observation of patients for signs of cardiac tamponade
- Avoidance of anticoagulants (increased risk of hemopericardium)

Treatment of underlying cause

1. Bacterial pericarditis: systemic antibiotics and surgical drainage of pericardium
2. Collagen vascular disease and idiopathic: NSAIDs, prednisone
3. Uremic: dialysis

POTENTIAL COMPLICATIONS FROM PERICARDITIS

1. Pericardial effusion: the time required for pericardial effusion to develop is of critical importance. If the rate of accumulation is slow, the pericardium can gradually stretch and accommodate a large effusion (up to 1000 mL), whereas rapid accumulation can cause tamponade with as little as 200 mL of fluid.

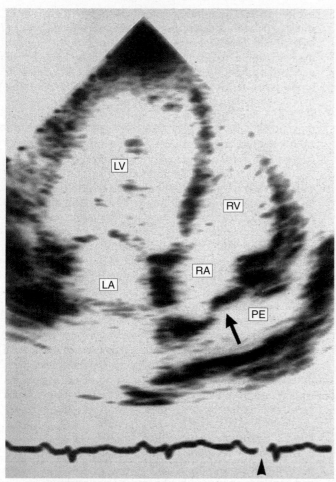

Fig 113–1
Echocardiograph of a patient with a large circumferential pericardial effusion. LA, left atrium; LV, left ventricle; PE, pericardial effusion; RA, right atrium; RV, right ventricle.
(From Crawford, MH, DiMarco JP, Paulus WJ [eds]: Cardiology, 2nd ed. St. Louis, Mosby, 2004.)

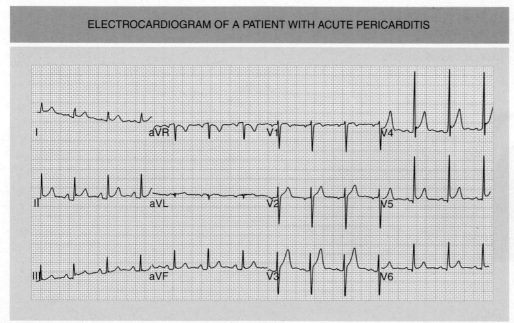

ELECTROCARDIOGRAM OF A PATIENT WITH ACUTE PERICARDITIS

Fig 113–2
Electrocardiogram of a patient with acute pericarditis. Note the diffuse ST elevation and PR depression.
(From Crawford, MH, DiMarco JP, Paulus WJ [eds]: Cardiology, 2nd ed. St. Louis, Mosby, 2004.)

2. Chronic constrictive pericarditis
   a. Physical examination reveals jugular venous distention, *Kussmaul's sign* (increase in jugular venous distention during inspiration as a result of increased venous pulse), pericardial knock (early diastolic filling sound heard 0.06 to 0.1 second after S$_2$), clear lungs, tender hepatomegaly, pedal edema, ascites.
   b. Chest x-ray: clear lung fields, normal or slightly enlarged heart, pericardial calcification
   c. ECG: low-voltage QRS complex
   d. Echocardiography: may show pericardial thickening or may be normal. CT or MRI may also aid diagnosis.
   e. Cardiac catheterization
   f. Therapy: surgical stripping or removal of both layers of the constricting pericardium
3. Cardiac tamponade: occurs in 15% of patients with idiopathic pericarditis but in almost 60% of those with neoplastic, tuberculous, or purulent pericarditis
   a. Signs and symptoms: dyspnea, orthopnea, interscapular pain

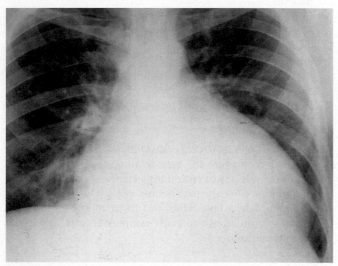

Fig 113–3
Cardiomegaly in a patient who has periocarditis. The presence of a water bottle heart on this plain film suggests a large pericardial effusion.
(From Cohen J, Powderly WG: Infectious Diseases, 2nd ed. St. Louis, Mosby, 2004.)

b. Physical examination: distended neck veins, distant heart sounds, decreased apical impulse, diaphoresis, tachypnea, tachycardia, *Ewart's sign* (an area of dullness at the angle of the left scapula caused by compression of the lungs by the pericardial effusion), pulsus paradoxus (decrease in systolic blood pressure more than 10 mm Hg during inspiration), hypotension, narrowed pulse pressure
c. Chest x-ray: cardiomegaly (water bottle configuration of the cardiac silhouette may be seen) with clear lungs; the chest x-ray film may be normal when acute tamponade occurs rapidly in the absence of prior pericardial effusion.
d. ECG reveals decreased amplitude of the QRS complex, variation of the R wave amplitude from beat to beat *(electrical alternans)*. This results from the heart's oscillating in the pericardial sac from beat to beat and frequently occurs with neoplastic effusions.
e. Echocardiography: detects effusions as small as 30 mL; a paradoxical wall motion may also be seen.
f. Cardiac catheterization: equalization of pressures within chambers of the heart, elevation of right atrial pressure, with a prominent x but no significant y descent.
g. MRI or CT can also be used to diagnose pericardial effusions (Fig. 113–4).
h. Therapy for pericardial tamponade consists of immediate pericardiocentesis, preferably by needle paracentesis with the use of echocardiography, fluoroscopy, or CT; in patients with recurrent effusions (e.g., neoplasms), placement of a percutaneous drainage catheter or pericardial window draining in the pleural cavity may be necessary.
4. Effusive-constrictive pericarditis
   a. Uncommon pericardial syndrome characterized by concomitant tamponade as a result of tense pericardial effusion and constriction caused by the visceral pericardium.
   b. Extensive epicardiectomy is the procedure of choice in patients requiring surgery

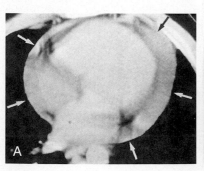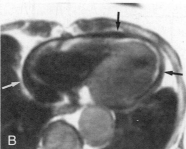

Fig 113–4
Pericardial effusion. **A,** Contrast-enhanced CT scan shows a band of fluid attenuation *(arrows)* surrounding the heart. **B,** Axial spin-echo MR image. The pericardial effusion is seen as a homogeneous signal void *(arrows)* surrounding the heart, subjacent to the pericardial fat.
(From Grainger RG, Allison DJ, Adam A, Dixon AK [eds]: Grainger & Allison's Diagnostic Radiology, 4th ed. London, Harcourt, 2001.)

Chapter 114: Cor pulmonale

114

Chapter 114 | Cor pulmonale

DEFINITION
Cor pulmonale is an alteration in the structure and function of the right ventricle caused by pulmonary hypertension caused by diseases of the lungs or pulmonary vasculature.

EPIDEMIOLOGY AND DEMOGRAPHICS
- Cor pulmonale is the third most common cardiac disorder after the age of 50.
- More common in men than in women

PHYSICAL FINDINGS AND CLINICAL PRESENTATION
- Dyspnea, fatigue, chest pain, or syncope with exertion
- Rarely, cough and hemoptysis
- Right upper quadrant abdominal pain and anorexia
- Hoarseness
- Jugular venous distention, peripheral edema, hepatic congestion, and a right ventricular third heart sound
- Tricuspid regurgitation, V wave on jugular venous pulse, and pulsatile hepatomegaly if severe
- Increased intensity of the pulmonic component of S_2

CAUSE
- 80% to 90% of cases of cor pulmonale are caused by COPD.
- Mechanisms leading to pulmonary hypertension include:
  1. Pulmonary vasoconstriction resulting from any condition causing alveolar hypoxia or acidosis
  2. Anatomic reduction of the pulmonary vascular bed (e.g., emphysema, interstitial lung disease, pulmonary emboli)
  3. Increased blood viscosity (e.g., polycythemia vera, Waldenström's macroglobulinemia)
  4. Increased pulmonary blood flow (e.g., left-to-right shunts)

DIAGNOSIS
- Evidence of pulmonary hypertension and findings of right-sided heart failure not caused by left-sided heart failure or congenital heart disease.

DIFFERENTIAL DIAGNOSIS
- Left heart failure
- Pulmonary veno-occlusive disease
- Neuromuscular diseases causing hypoventilation (e.g., amyotrophic lateral sclerosis [ALS])
- Disorders of ventilatory control (e.g., sleep apnea syndromes, primary central hypoventilation)

LABORATORY TESTS
- CBC may show erythrocytosis secondary to chronic hypoxia.
- ABGs confirming hypoxemia and acidosis or hypercapnia
- Pulmonary function tests

IMAGING STUDIES
- Chest x-ray (Fig. 114–1)
- Electrocardiogram
- Echocardiogram
- Radionuclide ventriculography
- Cardiac MRI
- Right heart catheterization
- Chest CT

TREATMENT
The treatment of cor pulmonale is directed at the underlying cause while at the same time reversing hypoxemia, improving RV contractility, decreasing pulmonary artery vascular resistance, and improving pulmonary hypertension.
- Continuous positive airway pressure (CPAP) is used in patients with obstructive sleep apnea.

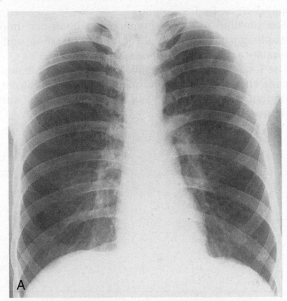
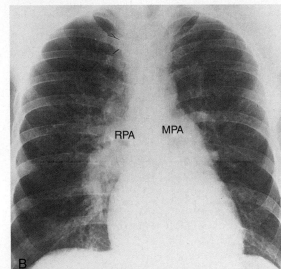

Fig 114–1
Progressive pulmonary arterial hypertension. **A,** This patient initially presented with a relatively normal chest radiograph. **B,** However, several years later, there are increasing heart size as well as marked dilation of the main pulmonary artery (MPA) and right pulmonary artery (RPA). Rapid tapering of the arteries as they proceed peripherally is suggestive of pulmonary hypertension and is sometimes referred to as pruning. (From Mettler FA, Guibertau MJ, Voss CM, Urbina CE: Primary Care Radiology, Philadelphia, Elsevier, 2000.)

- Phlebotomy is reserved as adjunctive therapy in polycythemia patients (hematocrit, 55%) who have acute decompensation of cor pulmonale or remain polycythemic despite long-term oxygen therapy.
- Pulmonary embolism is the most common cause of acute cor pulmonale.
- Acute pulmonary exacerbating conditions should be treated.
- Long-term oxygen supplementation has improved survival in hypoxemic patients with COPD.
- RV volume overload should be treated with diuretics (e.g., furosemide); however, overdiuresis can reduce RV filling and decrease cardiac output.
- Theophylline and sympathomimetic amines may improve diaphragmatic excursion, myocardial contraction, and pulmonary artery vasodilation.
- The long-term use of vasodilators, including nitrates, calcium channel blockers, and angiotensin-converting enzyme inhibitors, at present, do not result in significant survival improvement.

Chapter 115   Arrhythmias

A. PAROXYSMAL ATRIAL TACHYCARDIA

DEFINITION
Paroxysmal atrial tachycardia (PAT) is a group of arrhythmias that generally originate as re-entrant rhythm from the AV node and are characterized by sudden onset and abrupt termination.

PHYSICAL FINDINGS AND CLINICAL PRESENTATION
- Patient is usually asymptomatic.
- Patient may be aware of "fast" heartbeat.
- Persistent tachycardia may precipitate CHF or hypotension during acute MI.

CAUSE
- Preexcitation syndromes (Wolff-Parkinson-White [WPW] syndrome)
- Atrial septal defect
- Acute MI

IMAGING STUDIES
ECG (Fig. 115–1)
- Absolutely regular rhythm at rate of 150 to 220 beats/min is present.
- P waves may or may not be seen (the presence of P waves depends on the relationship of atrial to ventricular depolarization).

TREATMENT
- Valsalva maneuver in the supine position is the most effective way to terminate supraventricular tachycardia (SVT); carotid sinus massage (after excluding occlusive carotid disease) is also commonly used to elicit vagal efferent impulses.

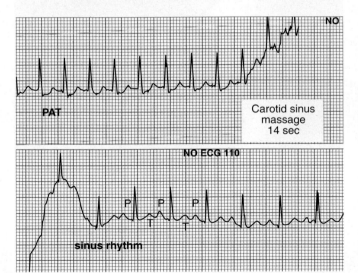

Fig 115–1
Supraventricular tachycardia (PAT). The upper and lower rows are part of one continuous strip. In the upper row, no definite P waves are visible. The diagnosis of this electrocardiogram is therefore supraventricular tachyarrhythmia. The ventricular rate is approximately 185 beats/min. In the lower strip, taken at the end of the carotid sinus massage, sinus rhythm has appeared. However, the heart rate is still rapid (approximately 135 beats/min).
(From Goldberger E: Treatment of Cardiac Emergencies, 5th ed. St. Louis, Mosby, 1990.)

- Synchronized DC shock is used if patient shows signs of cardiogenic shock, angina, or HF.
- Adenosine is considered by many the first choice of therapy for treatment of almost all episodes of SVT unresponsive to vagal maneuvers.
- IV verapamil and IV metoprolol are also effective.

B. MULTIFOCAL ATRIAL TACHYCARDIA

DEFINITION
Multifocal atrial tachycardia is a supraventricular, moderately rapid arrhythmia (rate, 100 to 140 beats/min) with P waves having at least three or more different morphologies.

PHYSICAL FINDINGS AND CLINICAL PRESENTATION
- Palpitation
- Lightheadedness
- Syncope
- Symptoms of the underlying pulmonary disease
- Physical findings associated with the underlying pulmonary disease

CAUSE
- Exact mechanism unknown
- Associated abnormalities include hypoxia, hypercarbia, acidosis, electrolyte disturbances, and digitalis toxicity.

DIFFERENTIAL DIAGNOSIS
- Atrial fibrillation (see Fig. 115–4)
- Atrial flutter (see Fig. 115–6)
- Sinus tachycardia
- Paroxysmal atrial tachycardia (see Fig. 115–1)
- Extrasystoles

WORKUP
- ECG (Fig. 115–2)
- Electrolytes
- Arterial blood gases, pulmonary function tests in COPD patients
- Digoxin level in patients on digoxin

TREATMENT
- Improve the pulmonary or metabolic dysfunction if possible.
- Calcium blockers
- Beta blockers if not contraindicated by obstructive lung disease
- If the arrhythmia is asymptomatic, it can be left untreated.

C. ATRIAL FIBRILLATION

DEFINITION
Atrial fibrillation is totally chaotic atrial activity caused by simultaneous discharge of multiple atrial foci.

PHYSICAL FINDINGS AND CLINICAL PRESENTATION
Clinical presentation is variable:
- Most common complaint: palpitations
- Fatigue, dizziness, lightheadedness in some patients
- A few completely asymptomatic patients
- Cardiac auscultation revealing irregularly irregular rhythm.
- Cardiac thrombi (Fig. 115–3) and subsequent stroke can develop in patients with atrial fibrillation and no anticoagulation.

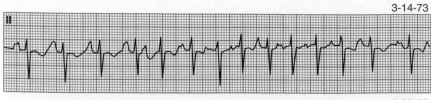

3-14-73

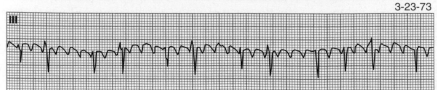

3-23-73

A   5502   56M

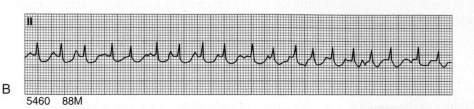

B   5460   88M

Fig 115–2

Multifocal atrial tachycardia. **A,** The patient has chronic obstructive pulmonary disease. The tracing on 3-14-73 shows multifocal atrial tachycardia. The rhythm changes to atrial flutter with varying atrioventricular conduction on 3-23-73. **B,** Tracing obtained from an 88-year-old man with mitral insufficiency. The multifocal atrial tachycardia closely resembles atrial fibrillation with rapid ventricular response. (From Chou TC: Electrocardiography in Clinical Practice, 4th ed. Philadelphia, WB Saunders, 1996.).

CAUSE
- Coronary artery disease
- MS, MR, AS, AR
- Thyrotoxicosis
- Pulmonary embolism, COPD
- Pericarditis
- Myocarditis, cardiomyopathy
- Tachycardia-bradycardia syndrome
- Alcohol abuse
- MI
- WPW syndrome
- Obesity: the excess risk of AF associated with obesity appears to be mediated by left atrial dilation.
- Other causes: left atrial myxoma, atrial septal defect, carbon monoxide poisoning, pheochromocytoma, idiopathic, hypoxia, hypokalemia, sepsis, pneumonia

DIFFERENTIAL DIAGNOSIS
- Multifocal atrial tachycardia
- Atrial flutter
- Frequent atrial premature beats

LABORATORY TESTS
- Thyroid-stimulating hormone (TSH), free thyroxine (T_4)
- Serum electrolytes

IMAGING STUDIES
- ECG (Fig. 115–4)
  1. Irregular, nonperiodic wave forms (best seen in V_1) reflecting continuous atrial re-entry
  2. Absence of P waves
  3. Conducted QRS complexes showing no periodicity
- Echocardiography to evaluate left atrial size and detect valvular disorders
- Holter monitor: useful only in select patients to evaluate paroxysmal atrial fibrillation

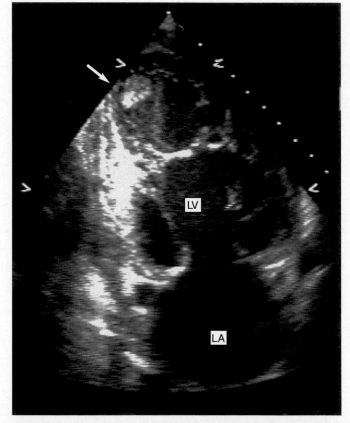

Fig 115–3

Apical thrombus. Two-dimensional echocardiographic image demonstrating left ventricular apical thrombus *(arrow)* in a patient with severe left ventricular dysfunction. LA, left atrium; LV, left ventricle. (From Crawford, MH, DiMarco JP, Paulus WJ [eds]: Cardiology, 2nd ed. St. Louis, Mosby, 2004.)

TREATMENT

New-onset atrial fibrillation

- If the patient is hemodynamically unstable, perform synchronized cardioversion.
- If the patient is hemodynamically stable, treatment options include diltiazem, verapamil, esmolol, or digoxin.
- IV heparin or SC LMWH followed by warfarin
- The *maze procedure* with its recent modifications creating electrical barriers to the macroreentrant circuits that are thought to underlie atrial fibrillation is being performed

with good results in several medical centers (preservation of sinus rhythm in >95% of patients without the use of long-term antiarrhythmic medication). Clear indications for its use remain undefined. Generally, surgery is reserved for patients with rapid heart rate refractory to pharmacologic therapy or who cannot tolerate pharmacologic therapy.

- Catheter-based radiofrequency ablation procedures (Fig. 115–5) designed to eliminate atrial fibrillation represent newer approaches to atrial fibrillation. Restoration and maintenance of sinus rhythm by catheter ablation without

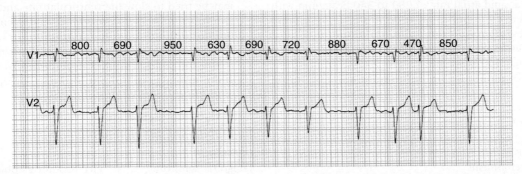

Fig 115–4
Atrial fibrillation. Chest leads V₁ and V₂ are shown. Notice the irregularly irregular RR intervals and the oscillations on the baseline caused by the rapid, chaotic, atrial electrical activity.
(From Crawford, MH, DiMarco JP, Paulus WJ [eds]: Cardiology, 2nd ed. St. Louis, Mosby, 2004.)

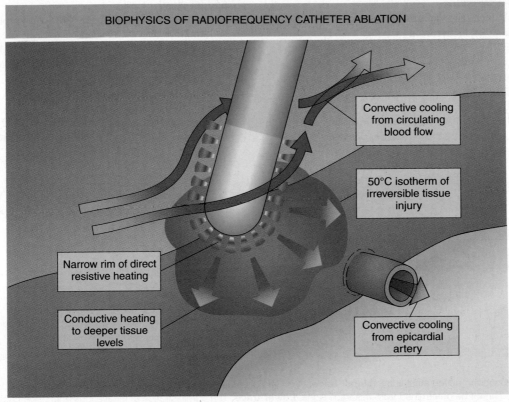

Fig 115–5
Radiofrequency catheter ablation from the tip of an electrode catheter to the endocardial surface. The cut-away view shows the narrow rim of direct resistive heating and heat conduction to deeper tissue layers to create the pathologic lesion. Convective cooling on the endocardial surface by circulating blood flow cools the electrode and decreases the lesion diameter on the endocardium. The convective cooling from epicardial arterial blood flow protects these vessels from excessive heating.
(From Crawford, MH, DiMarco JP, Paulus WJ [eds]: Cardiology, 2nd ed. St. Louis, Mosby, 2004.)

the use of drugs in patients with congestive heart failure and atrial fibrillation significantly improve cardiac function, symptoms, exercise capacity, and quality of life.

- Implantable pacemakers and defibrillators that combine pacing and cardioversion therapies to prevent and treat atrial defibrillation are likely to have an increasing role in the future management of atrial fibrillation.

D. ATRIAL FLUTTER

DEFINITION
Atrial flutter is a rapid atrial rate of 280 to 340 beats/min with varying degrees of intraventricular block. It is a macroreentrant tachycardia, most often involving right atrial tissue.

PHYSICAL FINDINGS AND CLINICAL PRESENTATION
- Approximately 150 beats/min
- Symptoms of cardiac failure, lightheadedness, and angina pectoris

CAUSE
- Atherosclerotic heart disease
- MI
- Thyrotoxicosis
- Pulmonary embolism
- Mitral valve disease
- Cardiac surgery
- COPD
- Atrial flutter can also occur spontaneously or as a result of organization of atrial fibrillation from antiarrhythmic therapy.

DIFFERENTIAL DIAGNOSIS
- Atrial fibrillation (see Fig. 115–4)
- Paroxysmal atrial tachycardia (see Fig. 115–1)

LABORATORY TESTS
- Thyroid function studies
- Serum electrolytes

IMAGING STUDIES
ECG (Fig. 115–6)
- Regular, sawtooth, or F wave pattern, best seen in leads II, III, and aVF and secondary to atrial depolarization
- AV conduction block (2:1, 3:1, or varying)

TREATMENT
- Valsalva maneuver or carotid sinus massage usually slows the ventricular rate (increases grade of AV block) and may make flutter waves more evident.
- DC cardioversion is the treatment of choice for acute management of atrial flutter.
- Overdrive pacing in the atrium may also terminate atrial flutter. This method is especially useful in patients who have recently undergone cardiac surgery and still have temporary atrial pacing wires.
- In absence of cardioversion, IV diltiazem or digitalization may be tried to slow the ventricular rate and convert flutter to fibrillation. Esmolol, verapamil, and adenosine may also be effective.
- Radiofrequency ablation to interrupt the atrial flutter is effective for patients with chronic or recurring atrial flutter and is generally considered first-line therapy in those with recurrent episodes of atrial flutter.

E. LONG-QT SYNDROME

DEFINITION
Long-QT syndrome is an electrocardiographic abnormality characterized by a corrected QT interval longer than 0.44 second and associated with an increased risk of developing life-threatening ventricular arrhythmias.

PHYSICAL FINDINGS AND CLINICAL PRESENTATION
- Syncope caused by ventricular tachycardia
- Sudden death
- Abnormal ECG (prolonged QT) in asymptomatic relatives of known case.

  The calculated QTc should be less than 440 milliseconds. If the patient has atrial fibrillation, take the average of the longest and shortest QTc intervals.
- Routine (baseline) ECG finding.

CAUSE
- Cardiac repolarization abnormality (Fig. 115–7)
- Congenital cause (chromosome 3 or 7 abnormality)

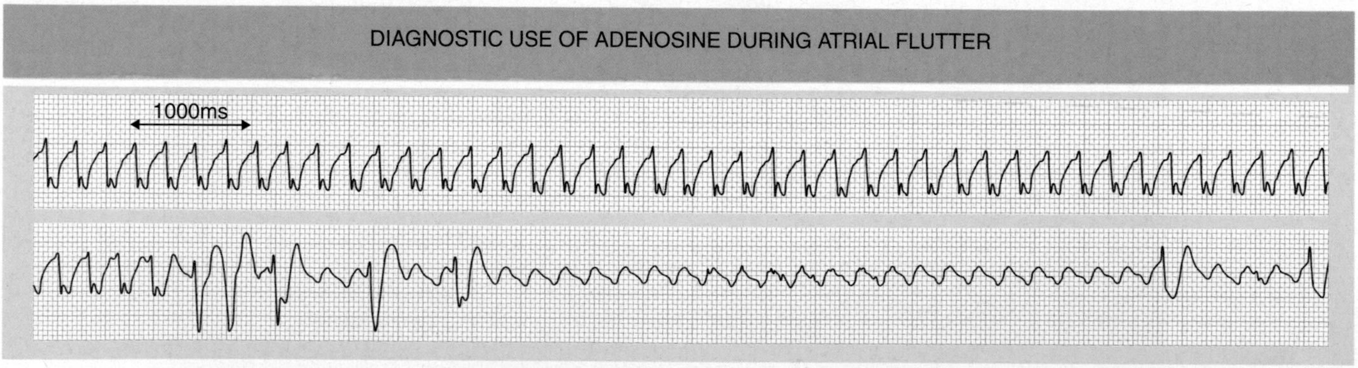

DIAGNOSTIC USE OF ADENOSINE DURING ATRIAL FLUTTER

Fig 115–6
Diagnostic use of adenosine during atrial flutter. **Upper trace,** Wide QRS complex tachycardia with cycle length of 250 milliseconds. The mechanism of tachycardia cannot be determined from this trace alone. **Lower trace,** The administration of intravenous adenosine causes transient atrioventricular block and reveals the underlying atrial flutter.
(From Crawford, MH, DiMarco JP, Paulus WJ [eds]: Cardiology, 2nd ed. St. Louis, Mosby, 2004.)

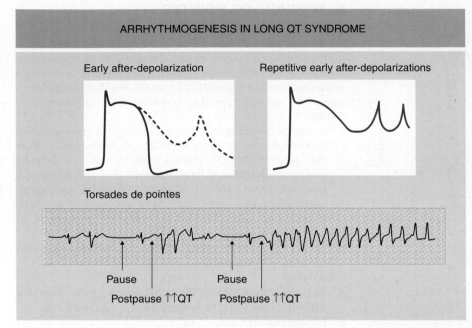

ARRHYTHMOGENESIS IN LONG QT SYNDROME

Early after-depolarization

Repetitive early after-depolarizations

Torsades de pointes

Pause   Pause
Postpause ↑↑QT   Postpause ↑↑QT

Fig 115–7
Electrophysiologic basis of arrhythmogenesis in the long-QT syndrome. On prolongation of the action potential, particularly at slow stimulation rates and in the presence of a lowered extracellular bath potassium concentration, depolarization can occur during phase 3 of the action potential before full repolarization; this is known as an early afterdepolarization (dotted line). Repetitive early afterdepolarization (right) can occur under certain conditions, which may lead to multiple abnormal depolarizations. In the polymorphic ventricular tachycardia torsades de pointes, premature ventricular beats lead to a pause that results in marked, postpause QT prolongation, which ultimately leads to the sustained arrhythmia. (From Crawford, MH, DiMarco JP, Paulus WJ [eds]: Cardiology, 2nd ed. St. Louis, Mosby, 2004.)

- Acquired causes:
  - Drugs (dofetilide, ibutilide, bepridil, quinidine, procainamide, sotalol, amiodarone, disopyramide, phenothiazines, and antiemetic agents [droperidrol, domperidone], tricyclic antidepressants, quinolones, astemizole, or cisapride given with ketoconazole or erythromycin, clarithromycin, and antimalarials), particularly in patients with asthma or those using potassium-lowering medications
  - Hypokalemia, hypomagnesemia
  - Liquid protein diet
  - Central nervous system (CNS) lesions
  - Mitral valve prolapse

DIAGNOSIS
Diagnostic criteria for the congenital long-QT syndrome can be calculated using a point system.
- ECG criteria
  Corrected QT > 480 milliseconds: 3 points
  Corrected QT = 460 to 480 milliseconds: 2 points
  Corrected QT = 450 to 460 milliseconds: 1 point (males)
  Torsades de pointes: 2 points
  T wave alternans: 1 point
  Notched T wave in three leads: 1 point
  Bradycardia: 0.5 point
- History
  Syncope with stress: 2 points
  Syncope without stress: 1 point
  Congenital deafness: 0.5 points
  Definite family history: 1 point if long-QT (LQT) syndrome
  Unexplained cardiac death in first-degree relative: 0.5 point under age 30
- Total score ≥ 4: definite long-QT syndrome
- Total score = 2 to 3: intermediate probability
- Total score ≤ 1: low probability

TREATMENT
- Asymptomatic sporadic forms with no complex ventricular arrhythmias: no treatment

- Risk stratification
  - High risk (less than 50% of cardiac events): QTc > 500 milliseconds and LQT1 and LQT2, or male with LQT3
  - Moderate risk (30% to 50%): QTc > 500 milliseconds in female with LQT3 or LQTc < 500 milliseconds in male with LQT3 or in female with LQT2 or LQT 3
  - Low risk (<30%): QTc < 500 milliseconds and LQT1 and/or male with LQT2
- General recommendations
  - Avoid competitive sports
  - Beta blocker at maximum tolerated dose
  - Cardiology referral is recommended for all cases. Pacemaker and ICD may be advised.

F. VENTRICULAR TACHYCARDIA

DEFINITION
Ventricular tachycardia is defined as three or more consecutive beats of ventricular origin (wide QRS) at a rate between 100 and 200 beats/min (Fig. 115–8). When the QRS complexes of the ventricular tachycardia (VT) are of the same shape and amplitude, the rhythm is termed *monomorphic VT*; when the QRS complexes vary in shape and amplitude, the rhythm is termed *polymorphic VT*. Polymorphic VT can be further subclassified based on its association with a normal or prolonged QT interval. Polymorphic VT occurring in the presence of a long-QT is termed *torsades de pointes* (see below). Cardiomyopathies are often associated with ventricular tachycardia. Arrhythmogenic right ventricular dysplasia (Fig. 115–9) can cause ventricular arrhythmias in children and young adults.

TREATMENT
- Antiarrhythmics: Procainamide, amiodarone, lidocaine
- Electrophysiologic mapping followed by surgical treatment can be performed for recurrent tachycardia, generally in combination with CABG. Currently, the use of transvenous ICDs is the most common nonpharmacologic intervention in patients with life-threatening arrhythmias.

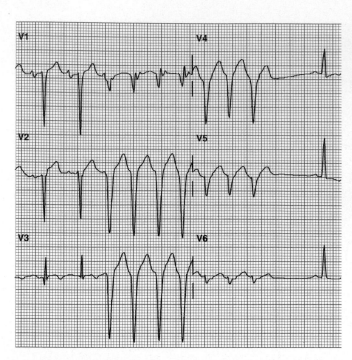

Fig 115–8
Short run of nonsustained ventricular tachycardia.
(From Khan MG: Rapid ECG Interpretation, 4th ed. Philadelphia, WB Saunders, 2003.)

G. TORSADE DE POINTES

DEFINITION

Torsades de pointes (Fig. 115–10) is a form of ventricular tachycardia manifested by episodes of alternating electrical polarity, with the amplitude of the QRS complex twisting around an isoelectric baseline resembling a spindle. Rhythm usually starts with a PVC and is preceded by widening of the QT interval.

CAUSE

- It may be caused by electrolyte disturbances (hypokalemia, hypomagnesemia, hypocalcemia), antiarrhythmic drugs that prolong the QT interval (procainamide, quinidine, disopyramide), *N*-acetylprocainamide, droperidol, amiodarone, phenothiazines, haloperidol, tricyclic antidepressants, terfenadine, astemizole, ketoconazole, erythromycin, trimethoprim-sulfamethoxazole, high-dose methadone, or cocaine.
- Torsades de pointes is also associated with hereditary long-QT interval syndromes.

TREATMENT

- Electrical termination of the tachycardia with cardioversion when the ventricular tachyarrhythmia is sustained
- Intravenous infusion of isoproterenol to decrease the QT interval and prevent recurrences
- Elimination of contributing factors (correction of electrolyte abnormalities, discontinuation of suspected drugs); early diagnosis of hereditary long-QT syndromes and treatment

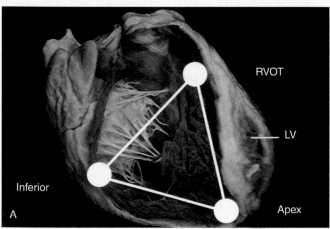

Fig 115–9
Arrhythmogenic right ventricular dysplasia. **A,** An autopsy specimen shows the triangle of Marcus, with typical areas of fibrofatty degeneration in the inferior, apical, and right ventricular outflow tract regions. **B,** Ventricular tachycardia with a left bundle pattern and superior axis from a patient with this condition. LV, left ventricle; RVOT, right ventricular outflow tract.
(From Crawford, MH, DiMarco JP, Paulus WJ [eds]: Cardiology, 2nd ed. St. Louis, Mosby, 2004.)

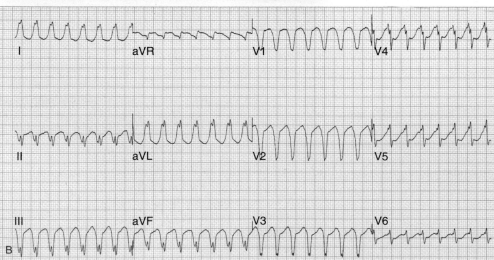

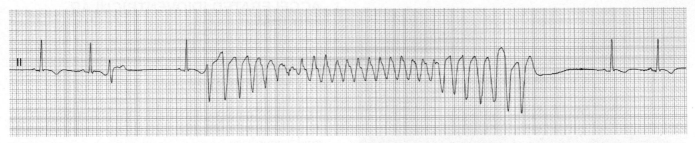

Fig 115–10
Torsades de pointes after conversion of atrial fibrillation. This patient had received intravenous ibutilide and converted to sinus rhythm. Shortly afterward, this episode of polymorphic ventricular tachycardia was recorded.
(From Crawford, MH, DiMarco JP, Paulus WJ [eds]: Cardiology, 2nd ed. St. Louis, Mosby, 2004.)

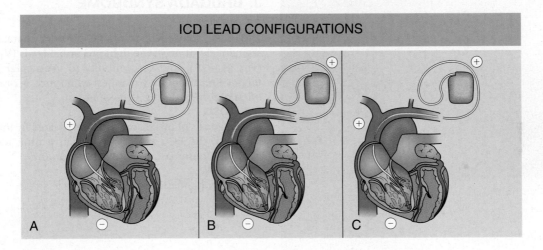

ICD LEAD CONFIGURATIONS

A   B   C

Fig 115–11
Endocardial defibrillation electrode configurations. **A,** Dual-coil configuration with the cathode in the distal coil at the right ventricle and the anode in the proximal coil at the superior vena cava–right atrium. **B,** Single-lead unipolar defibrillation system with the cathode in the right ventricle and the anode in the ICD can. **C,** Triad configuration with the cathode in the right ventricle and the anode in the proximal coil and the ICD can. ICD, implantable cardioverter-defibrillator.
(From Crawford, MH, DiMarco JP, Paulus WJ [eds]: Cardiology, 2nd ed. St. Louis, Mosby, 2004.)

with alpha$_1$-adrenergic receptor blocking agents. Surgical sympathectomy and use of ICDs (Figs. 115–11 and 115–12) should also be considered in high-risk patients with hereditary long-QT syndrome.

● Intravenous magnesium sulfate may be helpful, even if magnesium levels are normal.
● Sequential overdrive pacing if the episodes of torsades de pointes are sustained and appear to be precipitated by bradycardia

H. VENTRICULAR FIBRILLATION

DEFINITION
Ventricular fibrillation (VF) is characterized by a chaotic ventricular rhythm with disorganized spread of impulses throughout the ventricles (Fig. 115–13). VF with low-amplitude waves (less than 3 mm) is termed *fine VF*. Waves that are more easily visible are described as coarse. VF is the most common cause of out of hospital cardiac arrest. Fatality rate is more than 95%.

TREATMENT
The current guidelines recommend considering the use of amiodarone or lidocaine for shock-resistant VF. Recent trials (ALIVE trial) have indicated that the survival rate is considerably higher with the use of amiodarone instead of lidocaine.

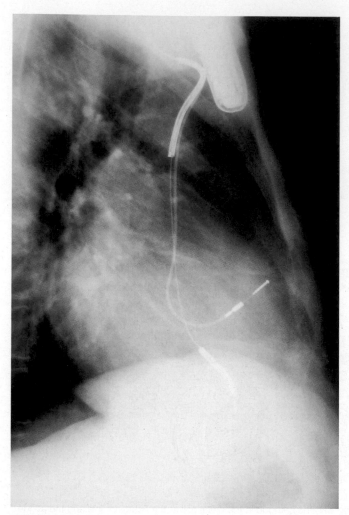

Fig 115–12
Lateral chest X-ray showing a dual-chamber implantable cardioverter-defibrillator.
(From Crawford, MH, DiMarco JP, Paulus WJ [eds]: Cardiology, 2nd ed. St. Louis, Mosby, 2004.)

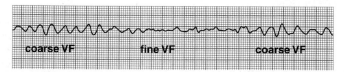

Fig 115–13
Ventricular fibrillation (VF). Coarse and fine fibrillatory waves are shown.
(From Goldberger E: Treatment of Cardiac Emergencies, 5th ed. St. Louis, Mosby, 1990.)

I. ACCELERATED IDIOVENTRICULAR RHYTHM

- Ventricular rate of 60 to 100 beats/min, at times interspersed with brief runs of sinus rhythm (Fig. 115–14). QRS > 0.12 second, T wave frequently in opposite direction of QRS complex, P waves usually absent.
- Usually seen in acute MI during the first 12 hours and also particularly common following successful reperfusion therapy. It can also be seen with digitalis toxicity and subarachnoid hemorrhage.
- Generally benign and transient, not requiring any therapy
- Atrioventricular sequential pacing may be necessary if the dissociation between atria and ventricles impairs ventricular filling and decreases cardiac output.

J. BRUGADA SYNDROME

DEFINITION
This is an autosomal dominant disorder characterized by ST segment elevation in the right precordial leads (V_1 to V_3), RBBB (Fig. 115–15), and susceptibility to ventricular tachyarrhythmias. Clinically, it may manifest with syncope or cardiac arrest, often occurring during sleep or at rest.

DIAGNOSIS
The diagnosis of this disorder is complicated by the intermittent nature of the ECG pattern. Provocative drug testing may be necessary to unmask the Brugada syndrome.

TREATMENT
- ICD implantation to prevent cardiac arrest

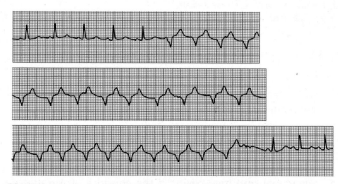

Fig 115–14
Accelerated isochronic (isorhythmic) ventricular rhythm.
(From Cerra FB: Manual of Critical Care. St. Louis, Mosby, 1987.)

RESTING ECG IN BRUGADA SYNDROME

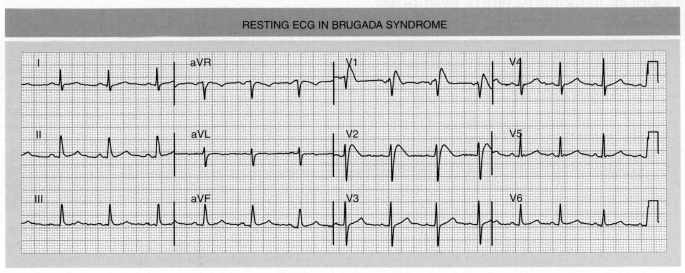

Fig 115–15
Resting ECG of a patient with Brugada syndrome. Note right bundle branch block–like pattern and ST segment elevation in leads V_1 and V_2.
(From Crawford, MH, DiMarco JP, Paulus WJ [eds]: Cardiology, 2nd ed. St. Louis, Mosby, 2004.)

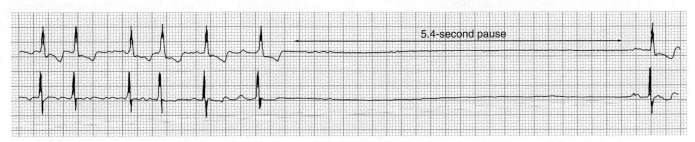

Fig 115–16
Bradycardia-tachycardia syndrome. This ambulatory ECG recording was obtained in a 79-year-old man with near-syncope. The beginning of the tracing shows atrial fibrillation. When the atrial fibrillation terminates, a 5.4-second pause occurs until the sinus note recovers.
(From Crawford, MH, DiMarco JP, Paulus WJ [eds]: Cardiology, 2nd ed. St. Louis, Mosby, 2004.)

K. SICK SINUS SYNDROME

DEFINITION
Sick sinus syndrome (tachycardia-bradycardia syndrome) is a group of cardiac rhythm disturbances characterized by abnormalities of the sinus node including (1) sinus bradycardia, (2) sinus arrest or exit block, (3) combinations of sinoatrial or atrioventricular conduction defects, and (4) supraventricular tachyarrhythmias. These abnormalities may coexist in a single patient so that a patient may have episodes of bradycardia and episodes of tachycardia.

PHYSICAL FINDINGS AND CLINICAL PRESENTATION
- Lightheadedness, dizziness, syncope, palpitations
- Arterial embolization (e.g., stroke) associated with atrial fibrillation
- Physical examination may be normal or reveal abnormalities (e.g., heart murmurs or gallop sounds) associated with the underlying heart disease.

CAUSE
- Fibrosis or fatty infiltration involving the sinus node, atrioventricular node, the His bundle, or its branches
- In addition, inflammatory or degenerative changes of the nerves and ganglia surrounding the sinus nodes and other sclerodegenerative changes may be found.

DIFFERENTIAL DIAGNOSIS
- Bradycardia: atrioventricular block
- Tachycardia: atrial fibrillation
- Atrial flutter
- Paroxysmal atrial tachycardia
- Sinus tachycardia

WORKUP
- ECG (Fig. 115–16)
- Ambulatory cardiac rhythm monitoring
- 24-hour ambulatory ECG (Holter)
- Event recorder
- Electrophysiologic testing, including sinus nodal recovery time and sinoatrial conduction time

TREATMENT
- Permanent pacemaker placement if symptoms are present
- The drug treatment of the tachycardia (e.g., with digitalis or calcium channel blockers) may worsen or bring out the bradycardia and become the reason for pacemaker requirement.

L. WOLFF-PARKINSON-WHITE SYNDROME

DEFINITION

Wolff-Parkinson-White syndrome is an electrocardiographic abnormality associated with earlier than normal ventricular depolarization following the atrial impulse and predisposing the affected person to tachyarrhythmias.

PHYSICAL FINDINGS AND CLINICAL PRESENTATION

Paroxysmal tachycardias

- 10% of WPW patients age 20 to 40 years
- 35% of WPW patients older than 60 years

The type of tachycardia is:

- Reciprocating tachycardia at 150 to 250 beats/min (80%)
- Atrial fibrillation (15%)
- Atrial flutter (5%)

WPW Preexcitation

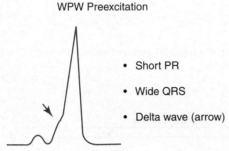

- Short PR
- Wide QRS
- Delta wave (arrow)

Fig 115–17
Preexcitation via the bypass tract in Wolff-Parkinson-White (WPW) syndrome is associated with the triad of findings shown here.
(From Goldberger AL, Goldberger E: Clinical Electrocardiography: A Simplified Approach, 5th ed. St. Louis, Mosby, 1994.)

- Ventricular tachycardia: rare
- Sudden death: rare (less than 1 in 1000 cases)

CAUSE AND PATHOGENESIS

- Existence of accessory pathways (Kent bundles)
- If the accessory pathway is capable of anterograde conduction, two parallel routes of AV conduction are possible, one subject to delay through the AV mode, the other without delay through the accessory pathway. The resulting QRS complex is a fusion beat, with the delta wave representing ventricular activation through the accessory pathway.
- Tachycardias occur when, because of different refractory periods, conduction is anterograde in one pathway (usually the normal AV pathway) and retrograde in the other (usually the accessory pathway). Some patients (5% to 10%) with WPW syndrome have multiple accessory pathways.
- In patients with WPW, development of atrial fibrillation may be associated with very rapid ventricular rates caused by atrial ventricular conduction over the anomalous AV pathway.

DIAGNOSIS

Three basic features characterize the ECG abnormalities in WPW syndrome (Fig. 115–17):

- PR interval < 120 milliseconds
- QRS complex > 120 milliseconds with a slurred, slowly rising onset of QRS in some leads (delta wave)
- ST-T wave changes (Fig. 115–18)

Variants

- Lown-Ganong-Levine syndrome: atriohisian pathway with short PR interval and normal QRS complex on ECG (no delta wave)
- Atriofascicular accessory pathways: duplication of the AV node, with normal baseline ECG

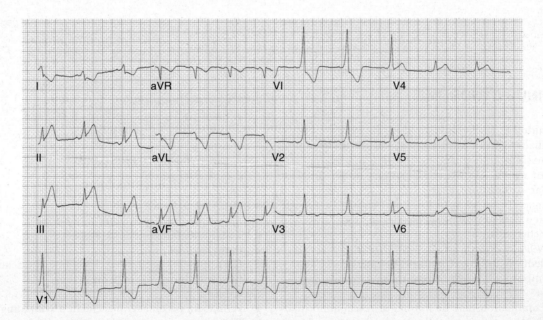

Fig 115–18
ECG in a 57-year-old man with Wolff-Parkinson-White syndrome and acute inferior transmural ischemia. Preexcitation and delta waves are evident, but ST segment elevation in leads II, III, aVF, V$_5$ and V$_6$, with reciprocal ST segment depression in leads I and aVL, remain as markers for the ischemia.
(From Crawford, MH, DiMarco JP, Paulus WJ [eds]: Cardiology, 2nd ed. St. Louis, Mosby, 2004.)

TREATMENT
- No treatment in the absence of tachyarrhythmias
- Symptomatic tachyarrhythmias
  - Acute episode: adenosine, verapamil, or diltiazem can be used to terminate an episode of reciprocal tachycardia.
  - Digitalis should not be used because it can reduce refractoriness in the accessory pathway and accelerate the tachycardia. Cardioversion should be used in the presence of hemodynamic impairment.
  - Treatment of atrial fibrillation: procainamide
  - Electrical or surgical ablation of the accessory pathway

M. ATRIOVENTRICULAR CONDUCTION DEFECTS

(1) First-degree atrioventricular block
DEFINITION
This is prolongation of the PR interval of more than 0.2 second (at a rate of 70 beats/min), which remains constant from beat to beat (Fig. 115–19).

CAUSE
- Vagal stimulation: first-degree AV block may be a normal finding in individuals with no history of cardiac disease, especially in athletes.
- Degenerative changes in the AV conduction system
- Ischemia at the AV nodes (seen particularly in cases of inferior wall MI)
- Drugs (digitalis, quinidine, procainamide, adenosine, calcium channel blockers, beta blockers, digitalis, amiodarone)
- Cardiomyopathies
- Aortic regurgitation
- Lyme carditis
- Hyperkalemia
- Complication of bacterial endocarditis

TREATMENT
- None necessary

(2) Second-degree atrioventricular block
DEFINITION
This is blockage of some (but not all) impulses from the atria to the ventricles.

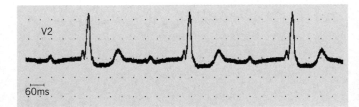

Fig 115–19
First-degree atrioventricular (AV) block. The PR interval is particularly prolonged, to 320 milliseconds. Major prolongation of the PR interval is almost always caused by a delay within the AV node. In this case, associated right bundle branch block is observed.
(From Crawford, MH, DiMarco JP, Paulus WJ [eds]: Cardiology, 2nd ed. St. Louis, Mosby, 2004.)

Mobitz type I (Wenckebach)
DEFINITION
- Progressive prolongation of the PR interval before an impulse is completely blocked; the cycle repeats periodically.
- Cycle with dropped beat is less than two times the previous cycle.
- Site of block: usually AV nodal (proximal to the bundle of His)

CAUSE
- Same as for first-degree AV block

DIAGNOSIS
ECG (Fig. 115–20)
- Gradual prolongation of PR interval leading to a blocked beat
- Shortened PR interval after the dropped beat

TREATMENT
- Usually transient; no treatment is necessary.
- If symptomatic (e.g., dizziness), atropine, 1 mg (may repeat once after 5 minutes) can be tried to increase AV conduction; if no response, insert temporary pacemaker.
- If block is secondary to drug (e.g., digitalis), discontinue the drug.
- If associated with anterior wall MI and wide QRS escape rhythm, consider insertion of a temporary pacemaker.
- Significant AV block post-MI may be caused by adenosine produced by the ischemic myocardium. These arrhythmias, which may be resistant to conventional therapy, such as atropine, may respond to theophylline (an adenosine antagonist).

Mobitz type II
DEFINITION
This is a sudden interruption of AV conduction without prior prolongation of the PR interval; the site of the block is infranodal.

CAUSE
- Degenerative changes in His-Purkinje system and any cause of first-degree AV block
- Acute anterior wall MI more commonly, but any MI can cause the block
- Calcific aortic stenosis
- Complication of bacterial endocarditis
- Lyme carditis

DIAGNOSIS
ECG (Fig. 115–21)
- Fixed duration of PR interval
- Sudden appearance of blocked beats

TREATMENT
- Pacemaker insertion, because this type of block is usually permanent and often progresses to complete AV block

(3) Third-degree atrioventricular block (complete atrioventricular block)
DEFINITION
All AV conduction is completely blocked, and the atria and ventricles have separate independent rhythms.

CAUSE
- Same as for Mobitz II; incidence is 5.8% in early MI (greater in inferior-posterior infarctions)
- Cardiomyopathy

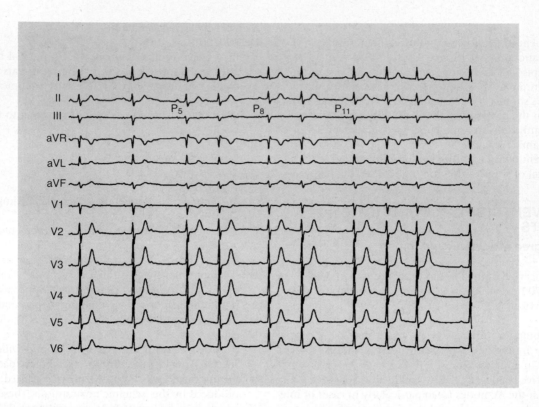

Fig 115–20
Second-degree type 1 atrioventricular (AV) block and 2:1 AV block. Three periods of Wenckebach-type AV block are shown starting with P waves 5, 8, and 11. In the first two periods of block, only one PR is prolonged before the dropped beat, described as 3:2 Wenckebach periods. In the third period of block, after a major PR prolongation following the second P wave of the period, the subsequent PR prolongation is less marked. This is described as a 4:3 Wenckebach block. Note that the P-P interval is constant. In the right part of the tracing, there is an intermittent 2:1 PR relation. Alternating 2:1 AV block with 3:2 and 4:3 Wenckebach sequences suggests that the lesion responsible for this pattern of AV block is located within the AV node.
(From Crawford, MH, DiMarco JP, Paulus WJ [eds]: Cardiology, 2nd ed. St. Louis, Mosby, 2004.)

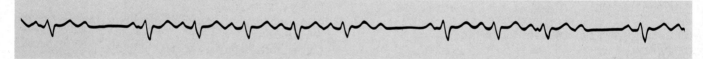

Fig 115–21
Mobitz type 2 second-degree atrioventricular block. Shown is the ECG lead II in a patient with intermittent sudden unexpected blockade of a singe P wave, without discernible increase in the preceding PR interval.
(From Crawford, MH, DiMarco JP, Paulus WJ [eds]: Cardiology, 2nd ed. St. Louis, Mosby, 2004.)

- Trauma
- Cardiovascular surgery
- Congenital
- Any cause of first-degree AV block and Mobitz I

DIAGNOSIS

ECG:

- There is no relationship between the P waves and the QRS complexes. P waves constantly change their relationship to the QRS complexes (Fig. 115–22).
- Ventricular rate usually < 50 beats/min (may be higher in congenital forms)
- Ventricular rate generally lower than the atrial rate
- QRS wide

Symptoms

- Dizziness, palpitations
- Stokes-Adams syncopal attacks
- CHF
- Angina

TREATMENT

- Immediate pacemaker insertion unless the patient has congenital third-degree AV block and is completely asymptomatic. A temporary pacer could be used until a a permanent pacer is used.

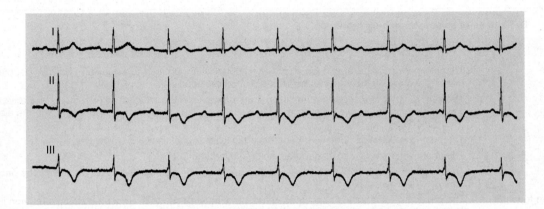

Fig 115–22

Complete atrioventricular (AV) block with narrow QRS escape and complete AV dissociation. The atrial rate is slightly more than twice as fast as the ventricular escape rate. None of the sinus P waves is able to penetrate the escape focus and depolarize it. The normal shape of the QRS complex suggests that the escape focus originates in the AV node. The AV dissociation here is the direct result of AV block.
(From Crawford, MH, DiMarco JP, Paulus WJ [eds]: Cardiology, 2nd ed. St. Louis, Mosby, 2004.)

Cardiac pacemakers

- Table 116–1 describes select pacemaker features
- Figure 116–1 illustrates placement of a dual-chamber pacemaker.
- Pacing artifacts on ECG are shown in Figure 116–2.
- The indications for temporary pacemaker in an acute MI setting are as follows:
  - Complete heart block with anterior wall MI
  - Alternating bundle branch block
- Bifascicular block (new RBBB with left anterior hemiblock or left posterior hemiblock)
- Mobitz II
- Mobitz I with anterior or inferior wall MI, with wide QRS escape rhythm
- Symptomatic sinus bradycardia unresponsive to atropine or isoproterenol
- New RBBB with anterior wall MI
- New LBBB with anterior wall MI

TABLE 116–1	Definitions of select pacemaker features
Feature	**Explanation**
Threshold	The minimum stimulus amplitude at any given pulse width required to achieve myocardial depolarization (= capture) consistently outside the heart's refractory period
Impedance	The sum of all forces opposing the flow of current in an electrical circuit. In pacemaker systems, the impedance is determined by the resistance of the leads, the tissue between the electrodes, and the electrode-tissue interfaces.
Sensing	The peak-to-peak amplitude (in mV) of the intracardiac signal (P wave or R wave)
Slew rate	The change in intracardiac electrogram voltage over time (dV/dt)
Sensitivity	The level in millivolts (mV) that an intracardiac electrogram must exceed to be sensed by the pacemaker; acts as a filter for noise
Rate-adaptive function	The pacemaker is able to change paced heart rate in response to a sensor indicating alteration in activity. This is indicated for patients with chronotropic incompetence.
Mode switch	Automatic change of the pacing mode from DDD or VDD to a nonatrial tracking mode: WI, VDI, or DDI in case of atrial fibrillation, atrial flutter, or other supraventricular tachyarrhythmia
Rate hysteresis	Delaying onset of ventricular pacing to preserve normal physiologic activation and contraction—for example, starting ventricular pacing with a rate of 110 beats/min in case of decrease in heart rate below 50 beats/min in patients with recurrent vasovagal syncope
Rate-adaptive AV delay	Automatically shortening of the AV delay in case of increasing heart rate
AV hysteresis	Automatic search scan for spontaneous ventricular events during a prolonged AV interval. In case of spontaneous ventricular events, the AV interval remains extended to preserve intrinsic AV conduction.

AV, atrioventricular.
From Crawford, MH, DiMarco JP, Paulus WJ (eds): Cardiology, 2nd ed. St. Louis, Mosby, 2004.

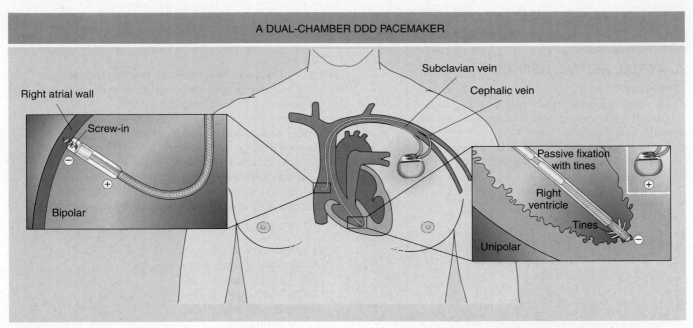

A DUAL-CHAMBER DDD PACEMAKER

Fig 116–1
Dual-chamber pacemaker (DDD). It is implanted in the left pectoral region, with the atrial bipolar lead implanted via the left cephalic vein and actively fixated in the right atrium, and the ventricular unipolar lead implanted via the left subclavian vein and passively fixated with tines captured in the right ventricular myocardial trabeculae.
(From Crawford, MH, DiMarco JP, Paulus WJ [eds]: Cardiology, 2nd ed. St. Louis, Mosby, 2004.)

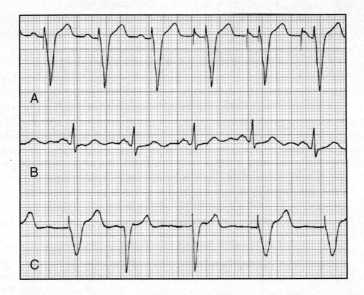

Fig 116–2
ECG during pacing. **A,** DDD pacing. To the left are spontaneous P waves followed by ventricular pacing, and to the right is pacing in the atrium and ventricle. **B,** Bipolar AAI pacing. **C,** Unipolar WI pacing. Note the small pacing artifacts caused by bipolar pacing **(B),** in contrast to the large pacing artifacts caused by unipolar pacing **(A, C)**.
(From Crawford, MH, DiMarco JP, Paulus WJ [eds]: Cardiology, 2nd ed. St. Louis, Mosby, 2004.)

Chapter 117   Congenital heart disease

A. ATRIAL SEPTAL DEFECT

DEFINITION
Atrial septal defect (ASD) is an abnormal opening in the atrial septum that allows for blood flow between the atria. There are several forms (Fig. 117–1):
- Ostium primum: defect low in the septum
- Ostium secundum: occurs mainly in the region of the fossa ovalis
- Sinus venous defect: less common form, involves the upper part of the septum

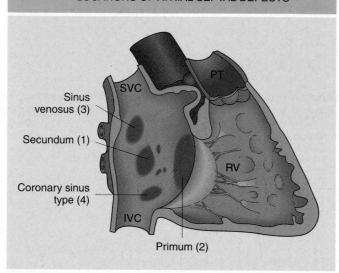

LOCATIONS OF ATRIAL SEPTAL DEFECTS

Fig 117–1
Locations of atrial septal defects. 1-4, Order of frequency of occurrence, with 1 being the most frequent. IVC, inferior vena cava; PT, pulmonary trunk; RV, right ventricle; SVC, superior vena cava. (From Crawford, MH, DiMarco JP, Paulus WJ [eds]: Cardiology, 2nd ed. St. Louis, Mosby, 2004.)

PHYSICAL FINDINGS AND CLINICAL PRESENTATION
- Pansystolic murmur best heard at apex secondary to mitral regurgitation (ostium primum defect)
- Widely split S_2
- Visible and palpable pulmonary artery pulsations
- Ejection systolic flow murmur
- Prominent right ventricular impulse
- Cyanosis and clubbing (severe cases)
- Exertional dyspnea
- Patients with small defects: generally asymptomatic

CAUSE
- Unknown

DIFFERENTIAL DIAGNOSIS
- Primary pulmonary hypertension
- Pulmonary stenosis
- Rheumatic heart disease
- Mitral valve prolapse
- Cor pulmonale

IMAGING STUDIES
- ECG (Fig. 117–2)
  1. Ostium primum defect: left axis deviation, RBBB, prolongation of PR interval
  2. Sinus venous defect: leftward deviation of P axis
  3. Ostium secundum defect: right axis deviation, right bundle-branch block
- Chest x-ray (Fig. 117–3): cardiomegaly, enlargement of right atrium and ventricle, increased pulmonary vascularity, small aortic knob
- Echocardiography (Fig. 117–4) with saline bubble contrast and Doppler flow studies (Fig. 117–5): may demonstrate the defect and presence of shunting. Transesophageal echocardiography is much more sensitive than transthoracic echocardiography in identifying sinus venous defects and is preferred by some for the initial diagnostic evaluation.
- Cardiac catheterization: confirms the diagnosis in patients who are candidates for surgery. It is useful if the patient has

ELECTROCARDIOGRAPHIC FINDINGS IN SECUNDUM ARTIAL SEPTAL DEFECT

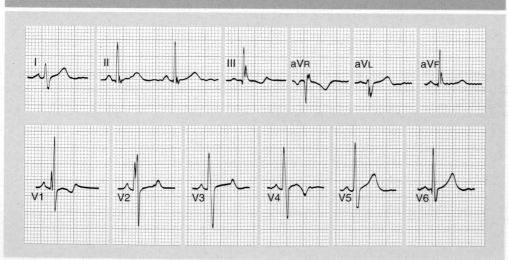

Fig 117–2
Electrocardiographic findings in secundum atrial septal defect from a 9-year-old patient. The patient is in normal sinus rhythm. There is right deviation of the frontal plane QRS axis, and right ventricular volume overload is manifested by rsR in lead V_1 and terminal widening of the S wave in lead V_6. (From Crawford, MH, DiMarco JP, Paulus WJ [eds]: Cardiology, 2nd ed. St. Louis, Mosby, 2004.)

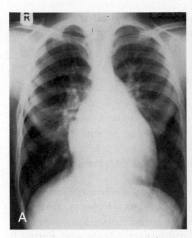
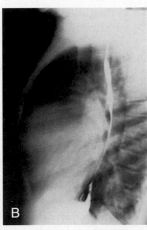

Fig 117–3
Atrial septal defect. **A,** Frontal view. The heart shadow is bulky and triangular in shape with its axis extending downward. There is a slight bulge on the left cardiac border and an increased curvature of the right heart border. The main pulmonary artery is large and the lung vessels are enlarged, indicating a left-to-right shunt. **B,** Lateral view. The entire large heart is in contact with the sternum, even though the sternum is slightly bulged forward. There is no evidence of left atrial enlargement.
(From Grainger RG, Allison DJ, Adam A, Dixon AK [eds]: Grainger & Allison's Diagnostic Radiology, 4th ed. London, Harcourt, 2001.)

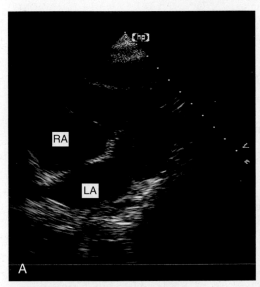
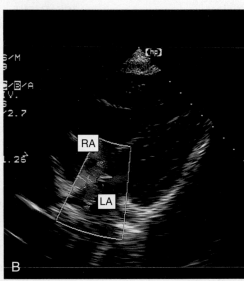

Fig 117–4
Subcostal two-dimensional echocardiographic examination. **A,** Two-dimensional echocardiography. The defect is located in the middle portion of the atrial septum. **B,** Color flow mapping. The left-to-right shunt at atrial levels is characterized as a velocity volume moving across the plane of the atrial septum and is displayed as an orange-red signal moving toward the transducer. LA, left atrium; RA, right atrium.
(From Crawford, MH, DiMarco JP, Paulus WJ [eds]: Cardiology, 2nd ed. St. Louis, Mosby, 2004.)

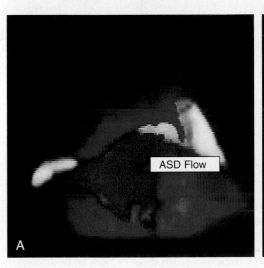
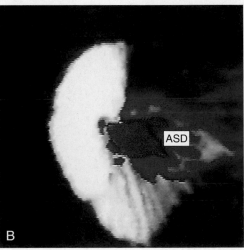

Fig 117–5
Three-dimensional volume-rendered color flow images. These images can be used to visualize three-dimensional intracardiac flow phenomena (i.e., the flow convergence region and vena contracta). **A,** View of the ASD perpendicular to the atrial septum. **B,** View of the ASD from the right atrium. ASD, atrial septal defect.
(From Crawford, MH, DiMarco JP, Paulus WJ [eds]: Cardiology, 2nd ed. St. Louis, Mosby, 2004.)

some anatomic finding on echocardiography that is not completely clear or has significant elevation of pulmonary artery pressures.

TREATMENT
- Children and infants: closure of ASD before age 10 years is indicated if pulmonary-to-systemic flow ratio is more than 1.5:1.
- Adults: closure is indicated in symptomatic patients with shunts more than 2:1.
- Surgery should be avoided in patients with pulmonary hypertension with reversed shunting (Eisenmenger's syndrome) because of increased risk of right heart failure.
- Transcatheter closure is advocated in children when feasible.
- Prophylactic beta blocker therapy to prevent atrial arrhythmias should be considered in adults with ASD.
- Surgical closure is indicated in all patients with ostium primum defect and significant shunting unless patient has significant pulmonary vascular disease.

B. ANOMALOUS PULMONARY ARTERY VENOUS CONNECTION

DEFINITION
This is a group of abnormalities in which one or more pulmonary veins connect to the systemic venous circulation. This group of defects can be divided into two major categories:
- Partial anomalous pulmonary venous connection (PAPVC): one or more of the pulmonary veins, but not all of them, connect abnormally (Fig. 117–6).

- Total anomalous pulmonary venous connection (TAPVC): all pulmonary veins connect abnormally to the systemic venous circulation.

DIAGNOSIS
- Echocardiography (Fig. 117–7)
- Cardiac catheterization

CLINICAL PRESENTATION
- PAPVC: many patients are asymptomatic in early life.
  - The presenting complaint in many patients is an abnormal chest x-ray or a cardiac murmur.
  - When symptoms occur, the most common complaint is exercise intolerance.
- TAPVC: cyanosis and respiratory distress are the presenting complaints. The chest radiograph shows abnormal pulmonary venous markings with diffuse, linear reticular pattern and often overt pulmonary edema and Kerley B lines (Fig. 117–8).

TREATMENT
Surgical correction is indicated for TAPVC and for PAPVC with significant increased pulmonary blood flow.

C. VENTRICULAR SEPTAL DEFECT

DEFINITION
- Ventricular septal defect (VSD) refers to an abnormal communication in the septum separating the right and left ventricles.
- VSDs may be large or small, single or multiple.

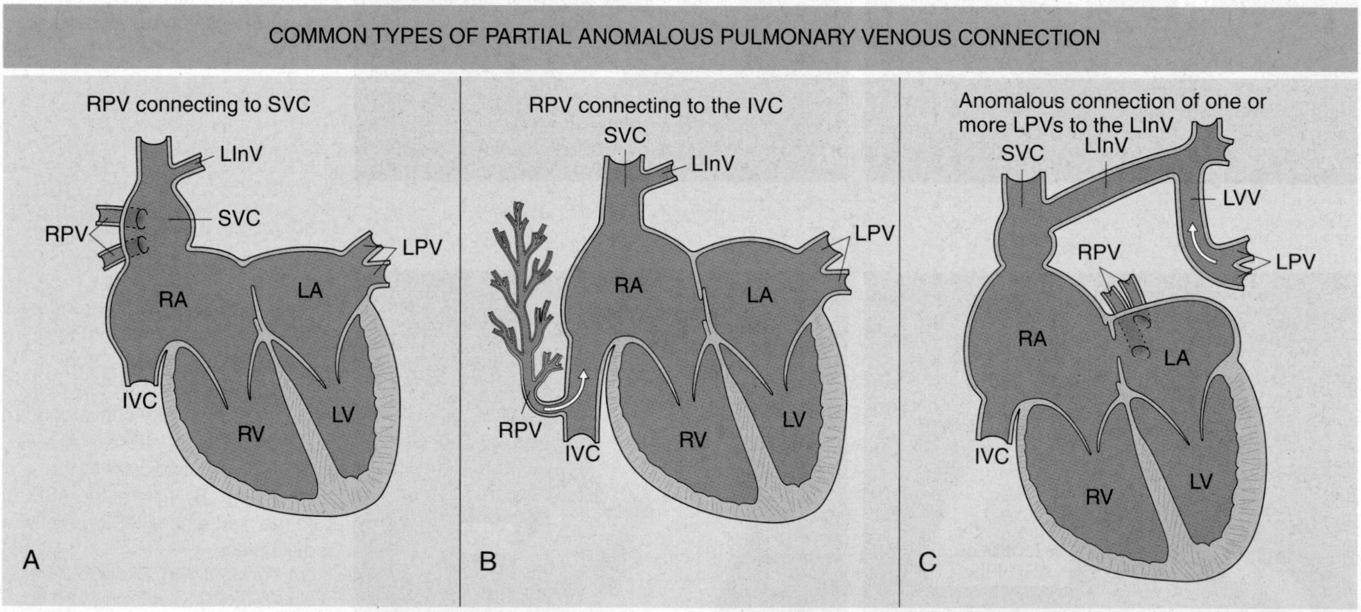

COMMON TYPES OF PARTIAL ANOMALOUS PULMONARY VENOUS CONNECTION

Fig 117–6
Common types of partial anomalous pulmonary venous connection (PAPVC). **A,** Right pulmonary veins (RPV) connecting to superior vena cava (SVC). Usually, right upper and middle lobe veins connect separately to the SVC between the azygous vein and SVC–right atrium (RA) junction. Often, a sinus venosus type of atrial septal defect is present. **B,** RPV connecting to the inferior vena cava (IVC). Usually, most or all of the RPVs form a confluence that enters the IVC as a singe trunk. The trunk forms in the right hilum, passes inferiorly and to the left, and enters the IVC just above or below the diaphragm. This type of PAPVC is found in the scimitar syndrome. **C,** Anomalous connection of one or more left pulmonary veins (LPVs) to the left innominate vein (LInV) by way of a left vertical vein (LW), also called a persistent left SVC. LA, left atrium; LV, left ventricle; RV, right ventricle.
(From Crawford, MH, DiMarco JP, Paulus WJ [eds]: Cardiology, 2nd ed. St. Louis, Mosby, 2004.)

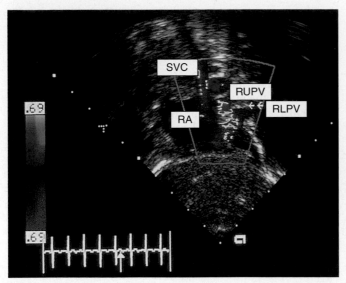

Fig 117-7
Color Doppler examination in partial anomalous pulmonary venous connection. The subcostal sagittal view shows anomalous drainage of the right upper pulmonary vein (RUPV) and right lower pulmonary vein (RLPV) to the back wall of the right atrium (RA). The left pulmonary veins in SVC, superior vena cava.
(From Crawford, MH, DiMarco JP, Paulus WJ [eds]: Cardiology, 2nd ed. St. Louis, Mosby, 2004.)

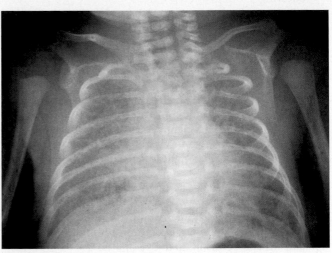

Fig 117-8
Chest radiograph in infracardiac total anomalous pulmonary venous connection with severe pulmonary venous obstruction. The heart size is normal but the pulmonary vascular markings are abnormal. Diffuse, stippled densities form a linear reticular pattern that fans out from the hilar regions. The cardiac borders are obscured. Kerley B lines are present.
(From Crawford, MH, DiMarco JP, Paulus WJ [eds]: Cardiology, 2nd ed. St. Louis, Mosby, 2004.)

- VSDs are located at various anatomic regions of the septum (Fig. 117-9) and classified as the following:
  1. Membranous (75% to 80%): most common defect that can extend into the vascular septum.
  2. Canal or inlet defects (8%): commonly lie beneath the septal leaflet of the tricuspid valve and often seen in patients with Down syndrome.
  3. Muscular or trabecular defects (5% to 20%): can be single or multiple, small or large.
  4. Subarterial defect (5% to 7%): least common; also called outlet, infundibular, or supracristal defect; commonly found beneath the aortic valve, leading to aortic valve prolapse and regurgitation

PHYSICAL FINDINGS AND CLINICAL PRESENTATION
- Clinical presentation is dictated by the size of the defect and direction and volume of the VSD shunt, along with the ratio of the pulmonary-to-systemic vascular resistance.
- Infants at birth may be asymptomatic because of elevated pulmonary artery pressure and resistance. Over the next few weeks, pulmonary arterial resistance decreases, allowing more blood shunting through the VSD into the right ventricle, with subsequent increased flow into the lungs, left atrium, and left ventricle, causing LV volume overload. Tachypnea, failure to thrive, and congestive heart failure ensue.
- In adults with VSD, the shunt is left to right in the absence of pulmonary stenosis and pulmonary hypertension, and patients typically manifest with symptoms of heart failure (e.g., shortness of breath, orthopnea, and dyspnea on exertion).

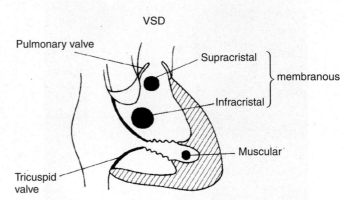

Fig 117-9
Anatomic varieties of ventricular septal defect (VSD) as seen from the right ventricular (RV) side. Membranous ventricular septal defect is the most frequent type of VSD. The most frequent variety of membranous VSD is the infracristal variety, situated below the right and noncoronary aortic cusps (on the left ventricular side) and exiting below the crista supraventricularis on the RV side. The supracristal (also known as infundibular) variety is much less frequent and exits immediately below the pulmonary valve, above the crista. A muscular ventricular septal defect Is usually small, often multiple, and occurs in the muscular septum.
(From Grainger RG, Allison DJ, Adam A, Dixon AK [eds]: Grainger & Allison's Diagnostic Radiology, 4th ed. London, Harcourt, 2001.)

- A spectrum of physical findings may be seen, including the following:
  1. Holosystolic murmur heard best along the left sternal border
  2. Systolic thrill
  3. Mid-diastolic rumble heard at the apex
  4. S_3
  5. Rales
- With the development of pulmonary hypertension:
  1. Augmented pulmonic component of S_2
  2. Cyanosis, clubbing, right ventricular heave, and signs of right heart failure (seen in Eisenmenger's complex, with reversal of the shunt in a right-to-left direction)

CAUSE
- Usually congenital (focus of this review), but may occur post-MI
- After acute myocardial infarction (MI): rupture of the intraventricular septum typically occurs within 3 to 5 days after acute MI and occurs in up to 2% of MIs.

DIFFERENTIAL DIAGNOSIS
Based on physical examination, the diagnosis of VSD may be confused with other causes of systolic murmurs such as mitral regurgitation, aortic stenosis, asymmetrical septal hypertrophy, and pulmonary stenosis.

LABORATORY TESTS
- Laboratory tests are not specific, but may offer insight into the severity of the disease.

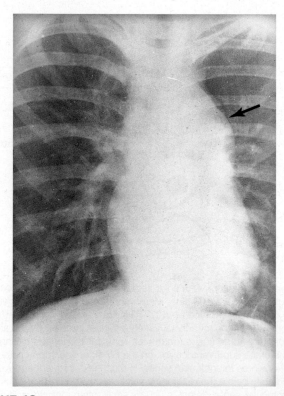

Fig 117–10
Typical chest radiogram in a septal defect with elevated pulmonary resistance. The image was taken in a 17-year-old patient with an unrepaired ventricular septal defect. The cardiac size is normal. The main pulmonary artery is enlarged *(arrow)*. The peripheral pulmonary vessels are small.
(From Crawford, MH, DiMarco JP, Paulus WJ [eds]: Cardiology, 2nd ed. St. Louis, Mosby, 2004.)

- CBC may show polycythemia, especially in patients with Eisenmenger's complex.
- Arterial blood gases may show hypoxemia.

IMAGING STUDIES
- Chest x-ray findings (Fig. 117–10) in patients with VSD:
  1. Cardiomegaly resulting from volume overload directly related to the magnitude of the shunt
  2. Enlargement of the proximal pulmonary arteries, along with redistribution and pruning of the distal pulmonary vessels resulting from sustained pulmonary hypertension
- ECG findings vary according to the size of the VSD and whether pulmonary hypertension is present. In large VSDs with pulmonary hypertension, right axis deviation is seen along with evidence of right ventricular hypertrophy.
- Echocardiography (Fig. 117–11) is the imaging modality of choice in the diagnosis of VSD.
  1. Two-dimensional echo and color Doppler display the size and location of the VSD.
  2. Continuous-wave Doppler not only approximates the gradient between the left and right ventricles, but also estimates the pulmonary artery pressure.
  3. Magnitude of shunt can be determined by calculation of the pulmonary-to-systemic flow ratio on echocardiography.
- Cardiac catheterization (Fig. 117–12) measures right heart pressures as well as detects and estimates the size of the shunt by calculation of the pulmonary-to-systemic flow ratio.
- Ventriculography also locates the VSD.

TREATMENT
The decision to treat a VSD depends on its type, size, shunt severity, pulmonary vascular resistance, functional capacity, and associated valvular abnormalities.
- In young children, small asymptomatic VSDs with a pulmonary-to-systemic blood flow ratio ≤1.5:1 and no evidence of pulmonary hypertension observed.
- Oxygen and low-salt diet are recommended in patients with congestive heart failure.
- Surgery is indicated for the following:
  1. Infants with congestive heart failure
  2. Children between the ages of 1 to 6 years with persistent VSD and a pulmonary-to-systemic blood flow ratio >2:1.
  3. Adults with VSD and flow ratios >1.5:1

D. TETRALOGY OF FALLOT

DEFINITION
Tetralogy of Fallot (TOF) is a congenital heart deformity (Fig. 117–13) consisting of the following four features:
- VSD
- Infundibular stenosis leading to obstruction to the RV outflow tract
- Overriding aorta
- Right ventricular hypertrophy (RVH)

PHYSICAL FINDINGS AND CLINICAL PRESENTATION
- Of the four major features of TOF, infundibular stenosis leading to right ventricular outflow tract obstruction and VSD are the primary defects leading to
  1. Right-to-left shunting and hypoxemia
  2. Altered RV hemodynamics
  3. Decreased pulmonary blood flow
- These pathophysiologic concepts subsequently result in common manifestations of TOF, including the following:

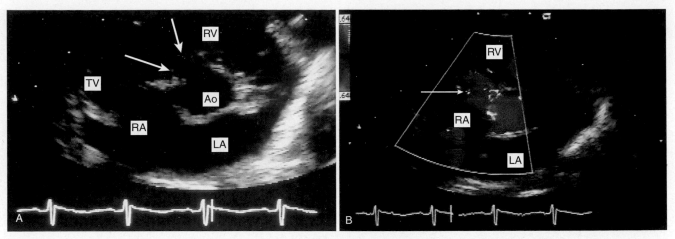

Fig 117–11

Parasternal short-axis echocardiographic scan of a membranous ventricular septal defect (VSD) in. **A,** This two-dimensional image was obtained in an infant with a membranous VSD. The defect *(between arrows)* is located beneath the tricuspid valve (TV), between 9 and 11 o'clock around the aortic annulus (Ao). The VSD measures approximately 6 mm. **B,** The same image with color flow Doppler color added. The Doppler color-flow jet is red-orange *(arrow)* because the direction of the flow is from the left ventricle into the right ventricle (RV), or toward the transducer. LA, left atrium; RA, right atrium.

(From Crawford, MH, DiMarco JP, Paulus WJ [eds]: Cardiology, 2nd ed. St. Louis, Mosby, 2004.)

1. Cyanosis secondary to increased RV pressure from infundibular stenosis, resulting in the shunting of deoxygenated blood from the RV through the VSD into the left ventricle, thus bypassing the lungs
2. Dyspnea on exertion
3. Clubbing
4. Child assuming a squatting position after exercise, increasing systemic vascular resistance, thereby decreasing right-to-left shunting
5. Low birth weight and growth rate
6. Palpable RV impulse
7. Systolic thrill along the left sternal border
8. Single second heart sound, inaudible P_2 component
9. Systolic ejection murmur resulting from RV outflow tract obstruction

CAUSE
- Unknown

DIFFERENTIAL DIAGNOSIS
- Asthma
- Isolated VSD
- Pulmonary atresia
- Patent ductus arteriosus
- Aortic stenosis
- Pneumothorax

LABORATORY TESTS
- CBC with polycythemia resulting from long-standing cyanosis
- ABGs with hypoxemia, normal pH, and P_{CO_2}
- Pulse oximetry
- ECG commonly demonstrating RVH, defined as right axis deviation > 90 degrees with an R wave greater than S wave in lead V_1; right atrial enlargement with peaked p wave amplitude > 2.5 mm in the inferior leads or initial portion of the p wave > 1.5 mm in lead V_1

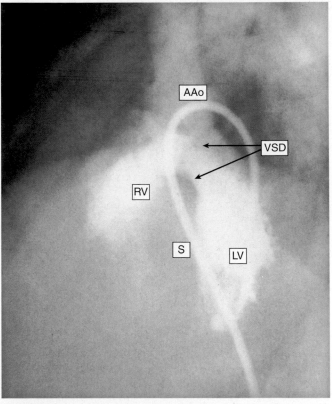

Fig 117–12

Left ventriculogram in patient with membranous ventricular septal defect (VSD). A long axial projection is shown. The catheter course is from the inferior vena cava to the right atrium, left atrium, and left ventricle. The interventricular septum (S) is well outlined. There is a high membranous defect *(between arrows)* illustrated by the presence of contrast crossing from the left to the right ventricle. AAo, ascending aorta; RV, right ventricle; LV, left ventricle.

(From Crawford, MH, DiMarco JP, Paulus WJ [eds]: Cardiology, 2nd ed. St. Louis, Mosby, 2004.)

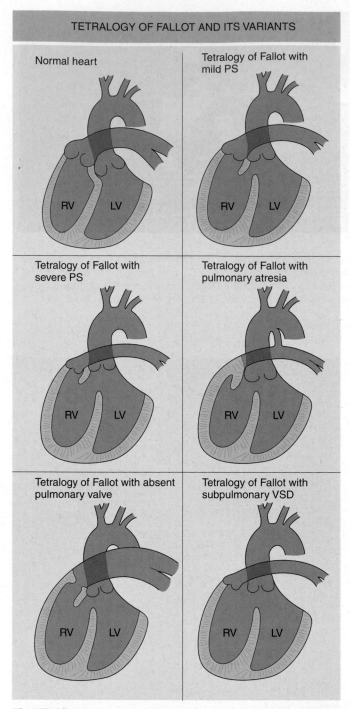

TETRALOGY OF FALLOT AND ITS VARIANTS

Normal heart

Tetralogy of Fallot with mild PS

Tetralogy of Fallot with severe PS

Tetralogy of Fallot with pulmonary atresia

Tetralogy of Fallot with absent pulmonary valve

Tetralogy of Fallot with subpulmonary VSD

Fig 117–13
Tetralogy of Fallot and its variants. LV, left ventricle; PS, pulmonary stenosis; RV, right ventricle; VSD, ventricular septal defect.
(From Crawford, MH, DiMarco JP, Paulus WJ [eds]: Cardiology, 2nd ed. St. Louis, Mosby, 2004.)

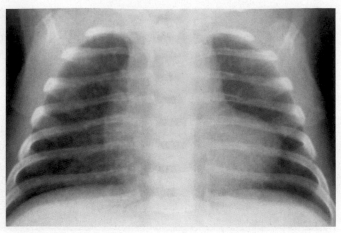

Fig 117–14
Tetralogy of Fallot showing boot-shaped heart.
(From Grainger RG, Allison DJ, Adam A, Dixon AK [eds]: Grainger & Allison's Diagnostic Radiology, 4th ed. London, Harcourt, 2001.)

IMAGING STUDIES
- Chest x-ray (Fig. 117–14) revealing boot-shaped heart, commonly described as "coeur en sabot"; prominent RV with decreased pulmonary vascularity
- ECG (Fig. 117–15): right axis deviation, right ventricular hypertrophy
- Echocardiography (Fig. 117–16) demonstrating VSD with a stenotic RV outflow tract and an overriding aorta
- Cardiac catheterization and angiography (Fig. 117–17) aid in the determination of the severity of right-to-left shunting, localization of the VSD, and anatomic assessment of the RV outflow tract, pulmonary artery, and coronary artery anatomy.

TREATMENT
- Oxygen.
- Knee-chest position in hypoxemic spells helps reduce venous return and increase systemic vascular resistance, thus decreasing right-to-left shunting.
- Acute treatment of any infant or child with TOF who is cyanotic with respiratory distress is aimed at increasing systemic vascular resistance and decreasing right-to-left shunting. Intravenous beta blockers are used to decrease RV outflow tract contractility and subcutaneous morphine can be used to decrease venous return.
- Palliative repair includes procedures increasing pulmonary blood flow, thus reducing right-to-left shunting. Examples of palliative procedures include the Blalock-Taussig shunt, whereby a shunt is made between the subclavian artery and pulmonary artery, the Waterston shunt, attaching the ascending aorta to right pulmonary artery, and the Potts shunt attaching the descending aorta to left pulmonary artery.
- Complete surgical repair has good success and involves closing the VSD with a Dacron patch and relieving the RV outflow tract obstruction. It is recommended for almost every patient with TOF.

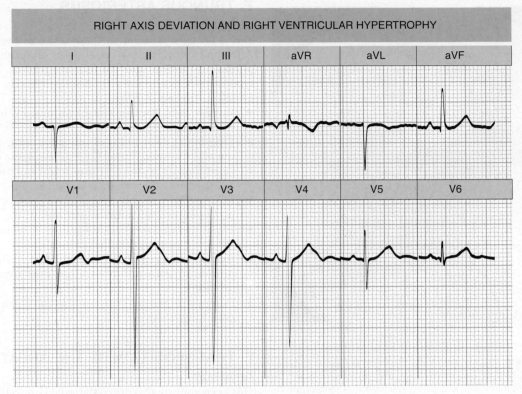

RIGHT AXIS DEVIATION AND RIGHT VENTRICULAR HYPERTROPHY

| I | II | III | aVR | aVL | aVF |

| V1 | V2 | V3 | V4 | V5 | V6 |

Fig 117-15
Right axis deviation and right ventricular hypertrophy in tetralogy of Fallot. This ECG is from a 5-year-old boy.
(From Crawford, MH, DiMarco JP, Paulus WJ [eds]: Cardiology, 2nd ed. St. Louis, Mosby, 2004.)

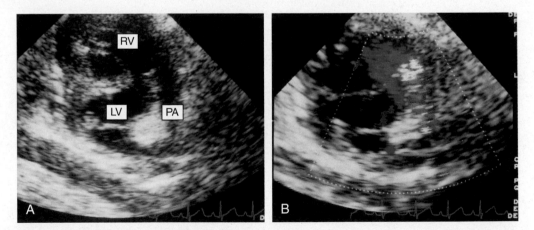

Fig 117-16
Right ventricular outflow in tetralogy of Fallot. **A,** Echocardiogram showing infundibular stenosis. **B,** Echocardiogram showing accelerated flow in yellow and red, with a mosaic pattern. LV, left ventricle; PA, pulmonary artery; RV, right ventricle.
(From Crawford, MH, DiMarco JP, Paulus WJ [eds]: Cardiology, 2nd ed. St. Louis, Mosby, 2004.)

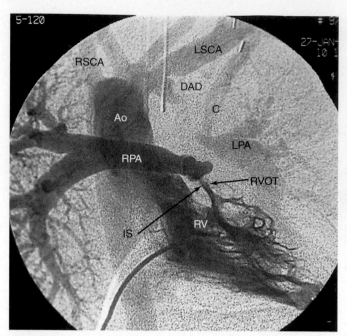

Fig 117–17

Tetralogy of Fallot. This right ventricular (RV) angiogram, shallow right anterior oblique view, shows a long stenosis of the right ventricular outflow tract (RVOT), filling of a right aortic arch (Ao), and displacement of the infundibular septum (IS). There is also interruption of the left pulmonary artery (LPA), which is filled faintly by collaterals (C). DAD, ductus arteriosus diverticulum; LSCA, left subclavian artery; RPA, right pulmonary artery; RSCA, right subclavian artery.

(From Grainger RG, Allison DJ, Adam A, Dixon AK [eds]: Grainger & Allison's Diagnostic Radiology, 4th ed. London, Harcourt, 2001.)

E. TRUNCUS ARTERIOSUS

DEFINITION

This is a congenital anomaly that consists of a ventricular septal defect and a single arterial vessel giving off coronary arteries, the pulmonary arteries and the ascending aorta. The four main types of truncus arteriosus are described in (Fig. 117–18).

CLINICAL PRESENTATION

- Variable with the amount of pulmonary blood flow and truncal valve regurgitation
- Tachycardia, tachypnea, excessive sweating, and poor feeding may be noted during the first few weeks of life.
- Chest x-ray (Fig. 117–19) may reveal cardiomegaly and increased pulmonary vascular markings.
- ECG generally reveals normal sinus rhythm, ventricular hypertrophy, and left atrial hyperthrophy.
- Two-dimensional echocardiography is essential in the non-invasive diagnosis of truncus arteriosus.
- Cardiac catheterization and angiography (Fig. 117–20) will provide accurate morphologic and hemodynamic data.

TREATMENT

- Diuretics to control CHF, intracardiac repair. Surgical mortality ranges between 5% and 10%.

F. TRANSPOSITION OF THE GREAT ARTERIES

DEFINITION

This is an abnormal ventriculoarterial connection of the great arteries. The aorta arises from the morphologic right ventricle and the pulmonary artery arises from the morphologic left ventricle.

THE FOUR MAIN TYPES OF TRUNCUS ARTERIOSUS AND THEIR FREQUENCIES			
Van Praagh type A1	Van Praagh type A2	Van Praagh type A3	Van Praagh type A4
Collett–Edwards I	Collett–Edwards II or III		
50% of cases	30% of cases	5% of cases	15% of cases
Pulmonary trunk arises from truncus	Two PAs arise from truncus	One PA arises from truncus, PDA or MAPCA	With interrupted aortic arch

Fig 117–18

The four main types of truncus arteriosus and their frequencies. Van Praagh type A1 is the most common, in which the pulmonary trunk originates from the truncus. Van Praagh type A2 is the second most common, in which the right pulmonary artery (PA) and the left PA originate separately from the truncus. Van Praagh type A3 is rare, in which only one PA originates from the truncus and the ductus arteriosus or aortopulmonary collateral arteries connect to the PA in the affected lung. Van Praagh type A4, characterized by association of an interrupted aortic arch, is the third most common. MAPCA, major aortopulmonary collateral artery; PDA, patent ductus arteriosus.

(From Crawford, MH, DiMarco JP, Paulus WJ [eds]: Cardiology, 2nd ed. St. Louis, Mosby, 2004.)

CLINICAL PRESENTATION

- Cyanosis is the most prominent symptom and, in the absence of a VSD, is almost always apparent within the first day of life.
- Murmur, cardiomegaly, and respiratory distress are inconsistent findings.
- Heart failure is evident only if there is an associated large VSD

DIAGNOSIS:

- Chest x-ray: egg-shaped heart (Fig. 117–21)
- Echocardiography (Fig. 117–22)
- Arteriography (Fig. 117–23)

TREATMENT

- Prostaglandin E
- Balloon atrial septostomy
- Atrial switch operation (Mustard technique)
- Arterial switch operations (Fig.117–24)

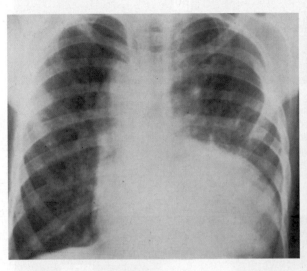

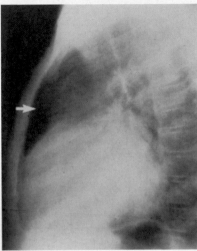

Fig 117–19

Truncus arteriosus. The classic silhouette has a blunt, rounded, cardiac apex, deeply concave pulmonary bay, and right-sided aortic arch. Note the small central pulmonary arteries on both front and lateral radiographs. Note the characteristic gap (arrow), which would have been occupied by a normal right ventricular outflow.
(From Grainger RG, Allison DJ, Adam A, Dixon AK [eds]: Grainger & Allison's Diagnostic Radiology, 4th ed. London, Harcourt, 2001.)

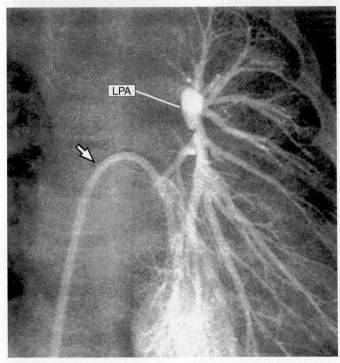

Fig 117–20

Pulmonary venous wedge injection in a patient with truncus arteriosus type A3 of Van Praagh and absent left pulmonary artery from aortic origin of the left pulmonary artery (LPA) from the descending aorta. The arrow is pointing to the catheter.
(From Crawford, MH, DiMarco JP, Paulus WJ [eds]: Cardiology, 2nd ed. St. Louis, Mosby, 2004.)

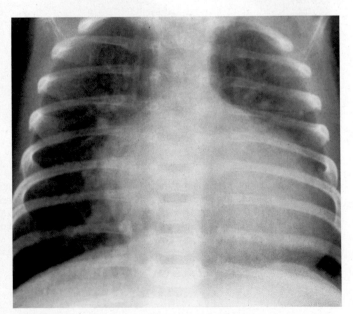

Fig 117–21

Transposition of great arteries—ventriculoarterial discordance. Note the egg-shaped heart, narrow superior mediastinum (pedicel) on frontal film, and pulmonary plethora.
(From Grainger RG, Allison DJ, Adam A, Dixon AK [eds]: Grainger & Allison's Diagnostic Radiology, 4th ed. London, Harcourt, 2001.)

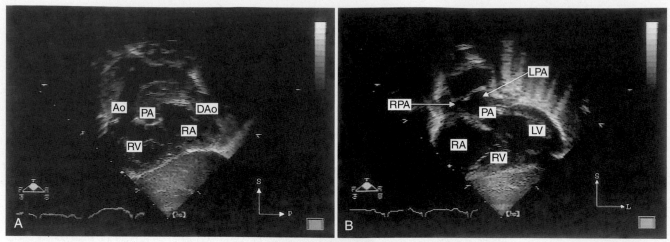

Fig 117–22
Echocardiography in transposition of the great vessels. The diagnosis of transposition of the great vessels is currently established using echocardiography. The definitive views are obtained from the subcostal window. **A,** The aorta (Ao) can be seen to arise from the right ventricle (RV) in a subcostal sagittal plane. **B,** The main pulmonary artery, branching into right and left pulmonary arteries, can be seen arising from the left ventricle in a subcostal coronal plane. DAo, descending aorta; PA, pulmonary artery; RA, right atrium.
(From Crawford, MH, DiMarco JP, Paulus WJ [eds]: Cardiology, 2nd ed. St. Louis, Mosby, 2004.)

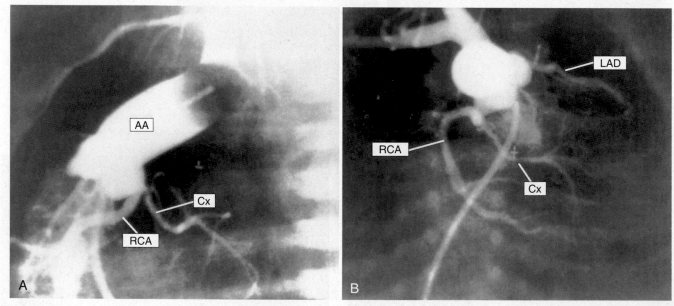

Fig 117–23
Load-back aortogram in a patient with {S,D,D} transposition of the great arteries and circumflex coronary artery arising from the right coronary artery (RCA). **A,** Lateral projection. **B,** Anteroposterior projection. AA, ascending aorta; Cx, circumflex coronary artery; LAD, left anterior descending coronary artery; {S,D,D}, visceroatrial situs solitus (S), D-ventricular loop (D), and D-transposition (D).
(From Crawford, MH, DiMarco JP, Paulus WJ [eds]: Cardiology, 2nd ed. St. Louis, Mosby, 2004.)

ARTERIAL SWITCH OPERATIONS

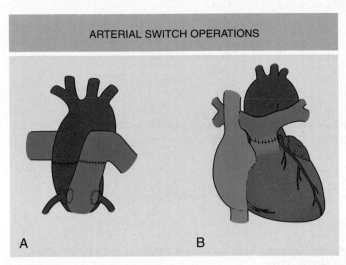

A   B

Fig 117–24

Arterial switch operations for transposition of the great vessels. **A,** Currently, patients undergo the arterial switch operation, which consists of transecting the great vessels and suturing them to the opposite valve annulus, in addition to performing a coronary artery transfer. **B,** Because this operation stretches the right pulmonary artery, the Lecompte maneuver is usually performed as part of the arterial switch operation.
(From Crawford, MH, DiMarco JP, Paulus WJ [eds]: Cardiology, 2nd ed. St. Louis, Mosby, 2004.)

EBSTEIN'S ANOMALY OF THE TRICUSPID VALVE

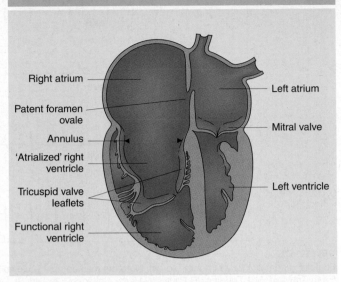

Right atrium
Patent foramen ovale
Annulus
'Atrialized' right ventricle
Tricuspid valve leaflets
Functional right ventricle
Left atrium
Mitral valve
Left ventricle

Fig 117–25

Ebstein's anomaly of the tricuspid valve. Note the enlarged right atrium, the atrialized portion of the right ventricle between the tricuspid valve annulus and the valve leaflets, and the diminutive functional right ventricle.
(From Crawford, MH, DiMarco JP, Paulus WJ [eds]: Cardiology, 2nd ed. St. Louis, Mosby, 2004.)

G. EBSTEIN'S ANOMALY

DEFINITION

This is a congenital cardiac malformation characterized by varying degrees of downward displacement of the posterior and septal leaflets of the tricuspid valve into the right ventricle (Fig. 117–25). Most cases are accompanied by an atrial level communication (patent foramen ovale or true atrial septal defect)

CLINICAL PRESENTATION

The physiology of the lesion varies with the degree of valvular deformity. Consequently, presentation can vary from a decompensated fetus at 18 weeks' gestation to an incidental finding at autopsy in an older person.

- ECG usally reveals normal sinus rhythm and right atrial enlargement (Fig. 117–26).
- Arrhythmias, especially supraventricular tachycardia secondary to Wolff-Parkinson-White syndrome, are common in patients who have Ebstein's anomaly (20%).
- Chest x-ray usually reveals marked cardiomegaly.
- Echocardiography demonstrates a large right atrium and severe tricuspid regurgitation (Fig. 117–27).

TREATMENT

This can be medical (endocarditis prophylaxis, prostaglandin E, inhaled nitric oxide to decrease pulmonary vascular resistance) or surgical and is individualized on the basis of the age of the patient and the predominant findings.

H. PATENT DUCTUS ARTERIOSUS

DEFINITION

Patent ductus ateriosus (PDA) is persistent patency of the fetal ductus arteriosus after birth. It causes a left-to-right shunt distal to the tricuspid valve. There are six distinct types of PDA (Fig. 117–28).

CLINICAL PRESENTATION

- Most patients with PDA do not have any symptoms.
- PDA is usually detected during routine auscultation in which the typical "machinery murmur" is heard.
- Some patients may have signs of decreased exercise tolerance.
- In infancy, poor feeding and slow weight gain herald cardiac failure resulting from large left-to-right shunt across the ductus.
- Systolic blood pressure may be elevated as a result of increased stroke volume.

DIAGNOSIS

- Doppler echocardiography (Fig. 117–29)
- Heart catheterization shows an oxygen step-up in the pulmonary artery compared with the oxygen saturation in the right ventricle, which is highest at the pulmonary bifurcation.

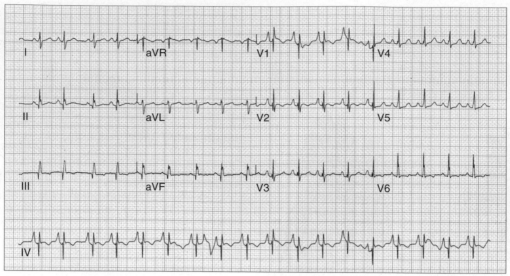

Fig 117–26
Ebstein's anomaly in a 21-month-old girl. Note the marked right atrial enlargement, as indicated by tall P waves in lead V₁ and the rsR′ pattern. (From Crawford, MH, DiMarco JP, Paulus WJ [eds]: Cardiology, 2nd ed. St. Louis, Mosby, 2004.)

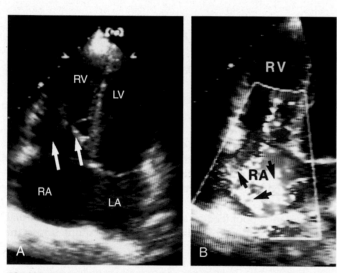

Fig 117–27
Ebstein's anomaly producing a large right atrium. **A,** Apical four-chamber view shows displacement of the attachments of the tricuspid valve leaflets *(arrows)* toward the right ventricular apex. **B,** Apical four-chamber view using color flow Doppler shows severe tricuspid regurgitation *(arrows show direction of flow)*. LA, left atrium; LV, left ventricle; RA, right atrium; RV, right ventricle.
(From Grainger RG, Allison DJ, Adam A, Dixon AK [eds]: Grainger & Allison's Diagnostic Radiology, 4th ed. London, Harcourt, 2001.)

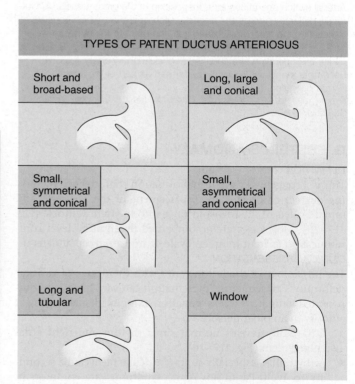

TYPES OF PATENT DUCTUS ARTERIOSUS

Short and broad-based	Long, large and conical
Small, symmetrical and conical	Small, asymmetrical and conical
Long and tubular	Window

Fig 117–28
Types of patent ductus arteriosus (PDA). There are six distinct types of PDA. This classification is important for choosing the appropriate closure device in terms of type and dimensions.
(From Crawford, MH, DiMarco JP, Paulus WJ [eds]: Cardiology, 2nd ed. St. Louis, Mosby, 2004.)

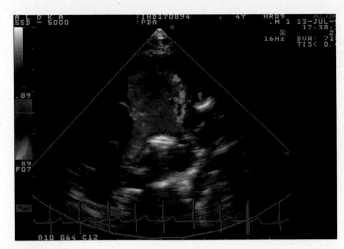

Fig 117–29
Color flow mapping of patent ductus arteriosus. In the two-dimensional image, the diastolic backflow into the main pulmonary artery (MPA) can be seen (red-yellow).
(From Crawford, MH, DiMarco JP, Paulus WJ [eds]: Cardiology, 2nd ed. St. Louis, Mosby, 2004.)

TREATMENT

● Closure of the PDA. This is now commonly accomplished by transcatheter implantation of a closure device (preferably a coil) after measurement of the PDA.

COARCTATION OF THE AORTA

DEFINITION

This is localized, discrete narrowing of the thoracic aorta .It is a relatively common abnormality, occurring in approximately 8% of patients with congenital heart disease.

CLINICAL PRESENTATION

This is variable, depending on the nature of associated cardiac lesions and severity of narrowing. In isolated coarctation, most patients are asymptomatic. Systolic hypertension and heart murmur are the most common symptoms in children and adolescents

DIAGNOSIS

● Chest x-ray: the heart may be mildly enlarged. Typically, there may be a visible indentation at the site of coarctation, especially on the frontal film, producing rib notching (Fig. 117–30). Radial angiography (Fig. 117–31) is useful for assessing the anatomy of the aortic arch before surgical repair.

TREATMENT

● Balloon dilation angioplasty (Fig. 117–32)

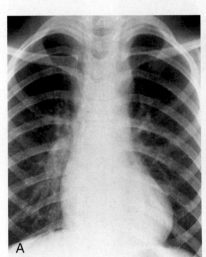 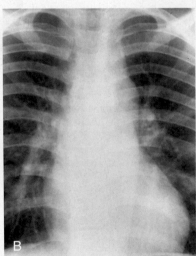 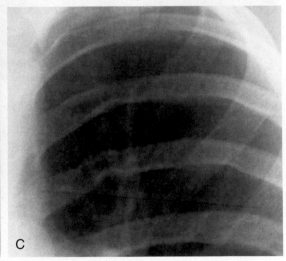

Fig 117–30
Coarctation. These two patients show abnormalities of aortic contour. **A,** Flat aortic knuckle with a bulge from the enlarged subclavian artery above it. **B,** There is prominence of the aorta below the level of the coarctation. **C,** Rib notching.
(From Grainger RG, Allison DJ, Adam A, Dixon AK [eds]: Grainger & Allison's Diagnostic Radiology, 4th ed. London, Harcourt, 2001.)

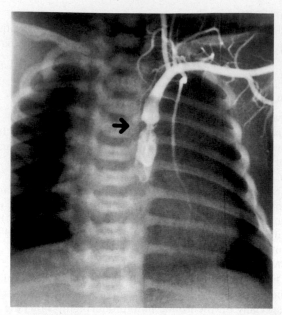

Fig 117–31
Frontal view obtained by using left radial angiography. The *arrow* shows the discrete-type coarctation of the aorta.
(From Crawford, MH, DiMarco JP, Paulus WJ [eds]: Cardiology, 2nd ed. St. Louis, Mosby, 2004.)

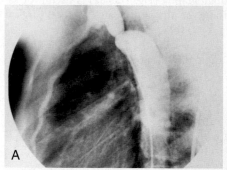
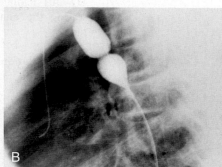
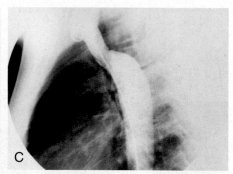

Fig 117–32
Balloon angioplasty for native coarctation of the aorta. Shown are typical aortograms in the lateral view before **(A)**, during **(B)**, and after **(C)** balloon angioplasty.
(From Crawford, MH, DiMarco JP, Paulus WJ [eds]: Cardiology, 2nd ed. St. Louis, Mosby, 2004.)

Chapter 118 Atrial myxoma

DEFINITION
Atrial myxoma (Fig. 118–1) is a benign neoplasm of mesenchymal origin, and is the most common primary tumor of the heart (50% of all primary tumors of the heart). Figure 118–2 reveals the characteristic appearance of the four most common benign tumors of the heart.

PHYSICAL FINDINGS AND CLINICAL PRESENTATION
Patients with atrial myxomas characteristically present in one of three ways:

- Atrioventricular valve obstruction (e.g., mitral or tricuspid valve)
  1. Dyspnea on exertion
  2. Orthopnea
  3. Paroxysmal nocturnal dyspnea
  4. Edema
  5. Dizziness, lightheadedness, or syncope
  6. Elevated jugular venous pressure
  7. Loud S_1, increased intensity of the P_2 component of S_2 secondary to pulmonary hypertension
  8. Systolic murmurs of mitral regurgitation or tricuspid regurgitation and diastolic murmurs of mitral stenosis or tricuspid stenosis, depending on from which chamber the myxoma arises
  9. Third heart sound, called a tumor plop
  10. Atrial fibrillation, with an irregularly irregular pulse
- Systemic embolization may occur in up to 30% of cases, leading to:
  1. Cerebrovascular accidents
  2. Pulmonary embolism
  3. Paradoxical embolism
- Constitutional symptoms
  1. Fever
  2. Weight loss
  3. Arthralgias
  4. Raynaud's phenomenon

CAUSE
- Most cases (90%) of atrial myxomas are sporadic with no known cause.
- In the remaining 10% of cases, a familial pattern occurs having an autosomal dominant transmission.
- Some patients with familial cardiac myxomas have Carney's syndrome, which consists of myxomas in other locations, skin pigmentation, and tumors of endocrine origin.

DIFFERENTIAL DIAGNOSIS
- Primary valvular diseases: mitral stenosis, mitral regurgitaiton, tricuspid stenosis, tricuspid regurgitation
- Endocarditis
- Atrial thrombus
- Pulmonary embolism
- Carcinoid heart disease
- Ebstein's anomaly

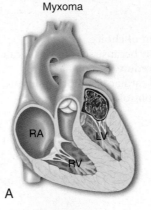
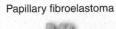
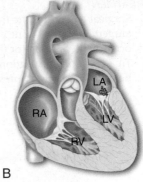
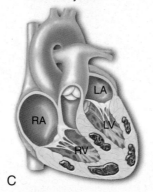
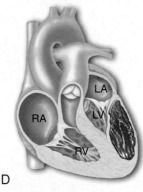

Myxoma Papillary fibroelastoma

Rhabdomyomas Fibroma

Fig 118–2
Characteristic appearance of the four most common benign primary cardiac tumors. **A,** Myxomas are typically a 5- to 6-cm globular mass, attached to the fossa ovalis in the left atrium, and can prolapse through the mitral valve. **B,** Papillary fibroelastomas are small (<1 cm) frond-like masses attached to the mitral or aortic valve. **C,** Rhabdomyomas usually present as multiple, rounded, small (<2 cm) masses throughout the left and right ventricular myocardium. **D,** Fibromas are large, singular, 3-to 10-cm dense masses, typically found in the anterior free wall of the left ventricle (LV). LA, left atrium; RA, right atrium; RV, right ventricle.
(From Zipes DP, Libby P, Bonow RO, Braunwald E [eds]: Braunwald's Heart Disease, 7th ed. Philadelphia, Elsevier, 2005.)

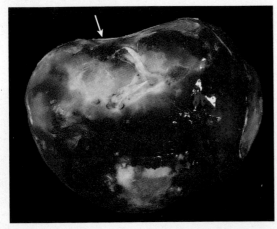

Fig 118–1
Large spheric left atrial myxoma. It has a smooth shiny surface with thrombosed red areas. There is a broad attachment base *(arrow)*.
(From Crawford, MH, DiMarco JP, Paulus WJ [eds]: Cardiology, 2nd ed. St. Louis, Mosby, 2004.)

LABORATORY TESTS

Although not very specific, the following laboratory values may be abnormal in patients with atrial myxomas:

- CBC: anemia, polycythemia, thrombocytopenia may occur.
- Erythrocyte sedimentation rate, C-reactive protein, and serum immunoglobulins are commonly elevated.
- ECG: patients with atrial myxomas may have findings of left atrial enlargement, right atrial enlargement, atrial fibrillation, atrial flutter, premature ventricular contractions, or ventricular tachycardia.

IMAGING STUDIES

- Echocardiography (Fig. 118–3): initial test of choice in suspected cases of atrial myxoma
- Chest x-ray: altered cardiac contour and chamber enlargement
- Transesophageal echocardiography: may visualize and better define cardiac masses not noticeable by transthoracic echocardiography
- MRI: delineates size, shape, and tumor characterizations
- Cardiac catheterization: may be required to rule out concomitant coronary artery disease in anticipation of surgical excision of the tumor.

TREATMENT

- Surgical excision is the treatment of choice.
- Surgery should be done promptly because sudden death can occur while waiting for the procedure.
- Treatment of constitutional and cardiac symptoms: diuresis, heart rate and blood pressure control, fever control

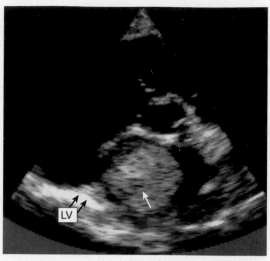

Fig 118–3

Large left atrial myxoma. This two-dimensional echocardiogram (short-axis view) shows a large left atrial myxoma *(white arrow)* prolapsing into the left ventricle (LV; *black arrows*) during diastole. (Courtesy of Dr. J.G. Pickering.)

Chapter 119 | Peripheral arterial disease

DEFINITION

Peripheral arterial disease (PAD) usually refers to atherosclerotic obstruction of the arteries to the lower extremity.

PHYSICAL FINDINGS AND CLINICAL PRESENTATION

- Almost 50% of the patients with PAD experience no symptoms, making PAD an underdiagnosed and undertreated condition.
- Approximately one third of patients with PAD present with intermittent claudication described as an aching or cramping leg pain brought on by exertion and relieved with rest that can progress with time; however, relying on the classic history of claudication alone will miss 85% to 90% of patients with PAD.
- Pain at rest, occurring commonly at night when the patient is supine
- Diminished pulses
- Bruits heard over the distal aorta, iliac, or femoral arteries
- Rubor with prolonged capillary refill on dependency (Fig. 119–1)
- Cool skin temperature
- Trophic changes of hair loss and muscle atrophy
- Nonhealing ulcers, necrotic tissue (Fig. 119–2), and gangrene possible

CAUSE

The primary cause of peripheral arterial disease is atherosclerosis. Atherosclerotic lesions of the arteries to the lower extremities subsequently lead to stenosis of peripheral vessels and inability to supply oxygenated blood to working limb muscles to meet the demand.

DIFFERENTIAL DIAGNOSIS

- Spinal stenosis
- Degenerative joint disease of the lumbar spine and hips
- Muscle cramps
- Compartment syndrome
- Varicose veins (Fig. 119–3)

WORKUP

- The initial workup in any patient suspected of having PAD includes measuring the ankle-brachial index (ABI). The ABI is calculated by dividing the highest ankle systolic pressure using the dorsalis pedis or posterior tibial artery by the highest systolic pressure from either arm.
- A diagnosis of PAD is based on the presence of limb symptoms or an ABI.
- The severity of PAD is based on the ABI at rest and during treadmill exercise (1 to 2 miles/hr, 5 minutes, or symptom-limited) and is classified as follows:
  1. Mild: ABI at rest 0.71 to 0.90 or ABI during exercise > 0.50
  2. Moderate: ABI at rest 0.41 to 0.70 or ABI during exercise > 0.20
  3. Severe: ABI at rest <0.40 or ABI during exercise <0.20

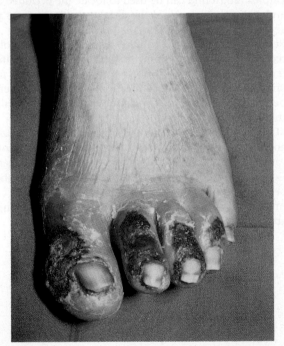

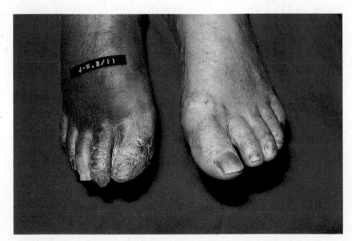

Fig 119–1
Red and warm ischemic foot in dependent position. In patients who have severe, chronic, critical leg ischemia, the skin color is often red and the temperature is increased in the sitting or standing position. The skin temperature of this patient was 5.4°F (3°C) higher at the dorsum of the ischemic right foot than at the same area of the left nonischemic foot.
(From Crawford, MH, DiMarco JP, Paulus WJ [eds]: Cardiology, 2nd ed. St. Louis, Mosby, 2004.)

Fig 119–2
Ischemic skin ulcer induced by trauma from shoes. This patient with peripheral arterial occlusive disease suffered severe superficial skin necrosis of several toes because of shoes that were too tight.
(From Crawford, MH, DiMarco JP, Paulus WJ [eds]: Cardiology, 2nd ed. St. Louis, Mosby, 2004.)

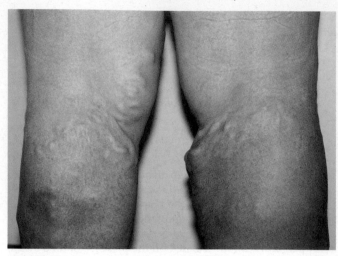

Fig 119–3
Marked varicosities of the politeal fossa.
(From Swartz MH: Textbook of Physical Diagnosis, 5th ed. Philadelphia, WB Saunders, 2006.)

LABORATORY TESTS
- Lipid profile
- Blood glucose
- HgbA$_{1c}$ levels in diabetic patients

IMAGING STUDIES
- Duplex ultrasound can be used to locate the occluded areas and assess the patency of the distal arterial system or prior vein grafts.
- Rest or exercise pulse volume recordings. Pulse volume recording measures volume of limb flow per pulse in different segments of the limb (e.g., thigh, calf, ankle, metatarsals, and toes). It helps localize the site of the stenosis because the contour of the pulse wave changes distally to the occlusion.
- MRA can be used as a noninvasive approach to visualize the aorta and peripheral lower extremity arteries. A major advantage of MRA is that it does not require contrast agents.
- Contrast CT may be used, but alternative modalities should be used in patients with renal failure.
- Angiography remains the gold standard for visualizing the arterial anatomy before revascularization.

TREATMENT
- PAD patients with no prior history of a cardiac event are to be considered as a cardiovascular "equivalent," with risks of future cardiovascular events similar to patients with prior MIs.
- Diet counseling (e.g., salt restriction in hypertension, American Diabetes Association [ADA] caloric diets for diabetics)
- Foot care should be stressed (wearing properly fitting shoes, daily cleaning, meticulous wound care)
- Exercise training, walking 30 to 60 min/day at about 2 miles/hr to near-maximal pain every day for 6 months, improves exercise capacity, walking distance, and quality of life.
- Aggressive management of risk factors for PAD:
  1. Tobacco counseling and smoke cessation programs are indispensable in decreasing the progression of disease as well as reducing the mortality rate from cardiovascular events in patients with PAD.
  2. Management of hypertension.
  3. Tight glycemic control (A$_1$Cs <6.5%) in diabetic patients with PAD results in prevention of microvascular complications.
  4. Control of dyslipidemia reduces severity of claudication symptoms.
- Aspirin daily is recommended for secondary disease prevention in patients with cardiovascular disease.
- Clopidogrel also provides protection from cardiovascular and cerebrovascular events associated with PAD.
- Pentoxyphylline may provide a small benefit in walking distance when compared with placebo.
- Cilostazol has been shown to increase the distance that symptomatic patients with infrainguinal PAD can walk significantly, but should not be given to patients with congestive heart failure and an ejection fraction <40.
- Surgical revascularization is indicated in patients with refractory rest pain, limb ischemia, nonhealing ulcers, or gangrene, and in a select group of patients with functional disability. Common surgical procedures:
  1. Aortoiliofemoral reconstruction
  2. Infrainguinal bypass (e.g., femoropopliteal, femorotibial)
  3. Extra-anatomic bypass (e.g., axillofemoral or femorofemoral bypass)
- Angioplasty is used for short discrete stenotic lesions in the iliac or femoropopliteal artery.

Chapter 120 | Venous ulcers and stasis dermatitis

DEFINITION

Venous ulcers are shallow wounds with irregular borders that usually occur on the lower extremities above or over the malleoli. These ulcerations develop because of high venous pressures caused by incompetent valves or obstructed veins. Stasis dermatitis refers to an inflammatory skin disease of the lower extremities, commonly seen in patients with chronic venous insufficiency.

PHYSICAL FINDINGS AND CLINICAL PRESENTATION

- Patients with venous stasis often have chronic skin changes on their lower limbs, including hyperpigmentation, hyperkeratosis, and dependent edema (Fig. 120–1). Skin color changes are caused by the extravasation of red blood cells and the resultant deposition of hemosiderin.
- Venous dermatitis or stasis dermatitis is common in these patients and is characterized by pruritic, red, and scaly eczematous changes.
- Smooth white plaques of atrophic sclerosis are known as atrophie blanche and can be a clue that the patient has venous disease.
- Venous ulcers are shallow full-thickness ulcers, with irregular borders and areas of granulation tissue. Necrosis is extremely rare.
- Patients often report a long history of dependent lower extremity edema and aching pain in the legs that are often worse after standing for long periods.

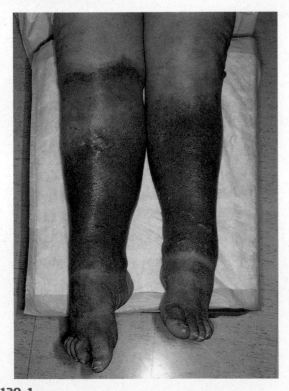

Fig 120–1
Chronic venous stasis.
(From Swartz MH: Textbook of Physical Diagnosis, 5th ed. Philadelphia, WB Saunders, 2006.)

CAUSE

- Venous stasis develops from valvular incompetence or obstruction, resulting in venous hypertension. Some have proposed that venous hypertension leads to malformation of capillaries, causing leakage of fluid and reduced blood flow to the skin. The resultant hypoxic tissue is prone to ulceration after minor trauma. The underlying vascular deficiency also impedes wound healing.

DIFFERENTIAL DIAGNOSIS

- Peripheral arterial disease (with ischemia and necrosis) (see Fig. 119–2)
- Diabetic ulceration (often secondary to neuropathy) (see Fig. 285–7)
- Decubitus ulceration (caused by pressure over a bony prominence) (see Fig. 30–1)
- Vasculitis (with erythema and bullae) (see Fig. 16–18)
- Necrotic ulceration from infection (see Fig. 28–1)
- Basal cell carcinoma or squamous cell carcinoma (see Fig. 22–16)
- Nerobiosis lipoidica (see Fig. 285–9)

WORKUP

- The majority of patients can be diagnosed clinically from the physical examination; however, up to 25% of patients have concomitant arterial disease. In these patients an ankle-brachial index should be determined. Arterial insufficiency is suggested by an ABI < 1.0.
- Patients with lower extremity ulcers should also be evaluated for diabetes.
- If vasculitis is suspected, a biopsy of the edge of the ulcer can confirm the diagnosis.
- Any wound that is present for more than 3 months should be biopsied to rule out malignancy.

IMAGING STUDIES

- If the ulcer appears infected, consider MRI of underlying bones to evaluate for osteomyelitis.

TREATMENT

- The goal of therapy is to improve venous return to the heart, thus decreasing edema, inflammation, and tissue ischemia.
- First-line treatment includes compression bandages and elevation of the leg above the heart for at least 30 minutes three to four times daily. Multilayer compression bandages, composed of an absorbent layer, elastic wrap, and an outer adherent layer, have been shown to accelerate healing over single-layer treatments. Bandages should be used until the ulcers heal.
- Smaller ulcers can be treated using compression stockings. Knee-high stockings with graded pressure providing at least 35 to 40 mm Hg of pressure at the ankle and 20 to 25 mm Hg at the knee are most effective.
- Compression with either bandages or stockings is to be used only after arterial disease has been excluded because it can cause limb ischemia.
- Surgical intervention is not routine; however, options include sclerotherapy, replacement of venous valves, ligation, and stripping of veins. Skin grafts are also an option for nonhealing wounds.

- Moist occlusive dressings and certain topical agents can aid in the healing of venous ulcers.
- Dressings can be nonadherent (Telfa), occlusive (Tegaderm, DuoDerm), or medicated, such as the Unna boot. Occlusive bandages have the advantage of reducing pain and can be changed by the patient every 5 to 7 days. Additionally, these bandages do not increase the rate of wound infection if used appropriately.
- Daily aspirin is recommended to accelerate healing.
- Underlying systemic hypertension and diabetes should be aggressively treated.

- Pentoxifylline may improve healing through its antithrombotic effects as well as fibrinolytic properties. The antiplatelet/vasodilator cilostazol also has been shown to be an effective adjuvant to compression therapy.
- Antiseptics such as iodine cause cellular toxicity and should not be used on ulcers. In addition, silver sulfadiazine (Silvadene), neomycin, and bacitracin are common causes of contact dermatitis and skin irritation and are not recommended.
- Systemic antibiotics are not indicated unless there are obvious signs of infection. including erythema, heat, purulent drainage, and pain.

Chapter 121 Lymphedema

DEFINITION

Lymphedema refers to excessive accumulation of interstitial protein-rich fluid, typically resulting from impaired regional lymphatic drainage.

PHYSICAL FINDINGS AND CLINICAL PRESENTATION

Edema

- Painless and progressive
1. Initially, the edema is pitting and smooth; however, with advanced cases, the edema becomes nonpitting (this depends on the extent of fibrosis that has occurred).
2. Elevation of the extremity resolves the swelling in the early stages but not in the advanced stages.
- More often unilateral (Fig. 121–1) but, depending on the cause, can be bilateral
- Not always restricted to the lower extremities but may involve the genitals, face, or upper extremities (e.g., arm swelling after mastectomy)
- *Stemmer's sign* (squaring of the toes caused by edema in the digits)
- Buffalo hump appearance of the dorsum of the foot
- Loss of the ankle contour, giving a tree trunk appearance to the leg (Fig. 121–2)

Skin

- Hard, thick, leathery skin secondary to fibrosis induced by chronic stasis
- Occasional drainage of lymph
- Infections (cellulitis, lymphangitis, onychomycosis)

CAUSE

Lymphedema is caused by a reduction in lymphatic transport and is classified into primary and secondary forms.

Primary idiopathic lymphedema is thought to result from developmental abnormalities such as lymphatic hypoplasia and functional insufficiency or absence of lymphatic valves. Subclasses of this type of lymphedema include the following:

- Congenital lymphedema
1. Detected at birth or recognized within the first 2 years of life
2. Involving one or both extremities, usually the entire leg
3. May be familial (Milroy's disease)
- Lymphedema praecox
1. Onset in teenage years
2. Usually unilateral
3. Most common form of primary lymphedema (up to 94% of cases)

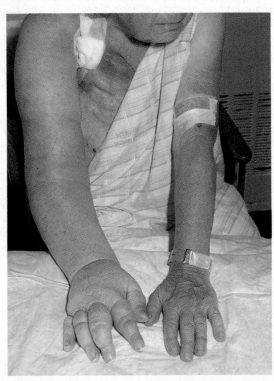

Fig 121–1
Lymphedema.
(From Swartz MH: Textbook of Physical Diagnosis, 5th ed. Philadelphia, WB Saunders, 2006.)

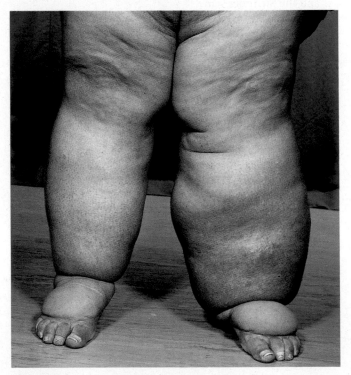

Fig 121–2
In lymphedema, loss of the ankle contour gives a tree trunk appearance to the leg.
(From Lebwohl MG, Heymann WR, Berth-Jones J, Coulson I [eds]: Treatment of Skin Disease. St. Louis, Mosby, 2002.)

4. More common in females (10:1), suggesting that estrogen plays a role in pathogenesis

5. May be familial (Meige's disease)

- Lymphedema tarda

1. Usually occurs after the age of 30 years

2. Uncommon, accounting for less than 10% of cases of primary lymphedema

Secondary lymphedema develops after disruption or obstruction of the lymphatic system as a consequence of the following:

- Surgery for malignant tumors (e.g., breast, prostate, lymphoma)
- Edema of the arm after axillary lymph node dissection is the most common cause of lymphedema in the United States.
- Incidence of lymphedema is approximately 14% in post mastectomy patients with adjuvant radiation.

TREATMENT

- Inflammation (streptococci, filariasis)
- Filariasis is most common cause of lymphedema worldwide
- Trauma
- Radiation with lymph node removal

DIFFERENTIAL DIAGNOSIS

- Lymphedema is primarily a clinical diagnosis made on the basis of physical features that distinguish it from other causes of chronic edema of the extremities, such as the presence of cutaneous and subcutaneous fibrosis (peau d'orange) and the Stemmer sign.
- When physical examination is inconclusive, other available imaging tests can help make the diagnosis: isotopic lymphoscintigraphy, indirect and direct lymphography, lymphatic capillaroscopy, MRI, CT, ultrasound
- Isoptopic lymphoscintigraphy is currently considered the gold standard for diagnosis of lymphedema.
- Exclude other causes of edema (e.g., cirrhosis, nephrosis, CHF, myxedema, hypoalbuminemia, chronic venous stasis, reflex sympathetic dystrophy, obstruction from abdominal or pelvic malignancy).

LABORATORY TESTS

- BUN, creatinine (Cr), liver function tests, albumin, urine analysis, thyroid function tests (TFTs) are obtained to exclude possible systemic causes of edema.
- Noninvasive venous studies help exclude venous insufficiency.
- Genetic testing may be practical in defining a specific hereditary syndrome with a discrete gene mutation, such as lymphedema-distichiasis (*FOXC2*) and some forms of Milroy disease (vascular endothelial growth factor receptor 3 [VEGFR-3]).

IMAGING STUDIES

- Lymphoscintigraphy:

1. Diagnostic image of choice

2. Sensitivity and specificity of 100% in diagnosing lymphedema

- CT scan: to exclude malignancy leading to obstruction
- Duplex ultrasound to rule out venous obstruction as a cause for edema
- Lymphangiography:

1. Available but rarely used

2. May be requested by surgeons considering repair or excision of tissue for lymphedema

3. Difficult to perform; most information can be obtained from the nuclear lymphoscintigram

TREATMENT

Complex decongestive therapy (CDT) is backed by long-standing experience as the primary treatment of choice for lymphedema in children and adults. It involves a two-stage treatment program:

1. Reduce leg swelling and size:
   - Leg elevation
   - Limb massage
   - Pneumatic leg compression

2. Maintain edema-free state:
   - Elastic support stockings that are properly fitted according to compression pressure and length are essential to prevent edema from returning.
   - Compression pressures are graduated; most of the pressure is distal, with less and less pressure from the stockings moving proximally.
   - Compression pressures range from 20 to 30 mm Hg, 30 to 40 mm Hg, 40 to 50 mm Hg, and 50 to 60 mm Hg. Most prefer 40 to 50 mm Hg for lymphedema.
   - The length should cover the edematous site. Choices include below-knee, thigh-high, and pantyhose lengths.
   - No drugs have been shown to be beneficial. Diuretics, in particular, should not be used because they may promote the development of volume depletion.
   - Treat infections, such as lymphangitis (usually caused by group A streptococcus), with antibiotics. Clotrimazole 1% cream should be applied daily to dried fissured areas between the toes to prevent fungal infections.
   - In secondary lymphedema, treating the underlying cause is indicated (e.g., prostate cancer, breast cancer). If the cause is filariasis caused by the parasites *Wuchereria bancrofti* or *Brugia malayi,* treatment is diethylcarbamazine citrate.
   - Surgery for chronic lymphedema should act as an adjunct to CDT or as an alternative if CDT has proved unsuccessful.

- Operative treatment is considered for the following:
   - Continued increase in leg size, despite medical treatment
   - Impaired leg function
   - Recurrent infections
   - Emotional lability secondary to the cosmetic appearance

Chapter 122   Deep vein thrombosis

DEFINITION

Deep vein thrombosis (DVT) is the development of thrombi (Fig. 122–1) in the deep veins of the extremities or pelvis.

PHYSICAL FINDINGS AND CLINICAL PRESENTATION

- Pain and swelling of the affected extremity (Fig. 122–2)
- In lower extremity DVT, leg pain on dorsiflexion of the foot (Homans' sign)
- Physical examination may be unremarkable

CAUSE

The cause is often multifactorial (prolonged stasis, coagulation abnormalities, vessel wall trauma). The following are risk factors for DVT:

- Prolonged immobilization (3 days or more)
- Postoperative state
- Trauma to pelvis and lower extremities
- Birth control pills, high-dose estrogen therapy; conjugated equine estrogen but not esterified estrogen is associated with increased risk of DVT; estrogen plus progestin is associated with doubling the risk of venous thrombosis.
- Visceral cancer (lung, pancreas, alimentary tract, GU tract)
- Age older than 60 years
- History of thromboembolic disease
- Hematologic disorders (e.g., antithrombin III deficiency, protein C deficiency, protein S deficiency, heparin cofactor II deficiency, sticky platelet syndrome, G20210A prothrombin mutation, lupus anticoagulant, dysfibrinogenemias, anticardiolipin antibody, hyperhomocystinemia, concurrent homocystinuria, high levels of factors VIII, XI, and factor V Leiden mutation)
- Pregnancy and early puerperium
- Obesity, CHF
- Surgery, fracture, or injury involving lower leg or pelvis
- Surgery requiring more than 30 minutes of anesthesia
- Gynecologic surgery (particularly gynecologic cancer surgery)
- Recent travel (within 2 weeks, lasting more than 4 hours)
- Smoking and abdominal obesity
- Central venous catheter or pacemaker insertion
- Superficial vein thrombosis, varicose veins

DIFFERENTIAL DIAGNOSIS

- Superficial thrombophlebitis
- Ruptured Baker's cyst
- Cellulitis (see Fig. 28–1)
- Lymphangitis (see Fig. 28–2)
- Achilles tendinitis
- Hematoma
- Muscle or soft tissue injury, stress fracture
- Varicose veins, lymphedema
- Arterial insufficiency (see Fig. 285–7)
- Abscess
- Claudication
- Venous stasis (see Fig. 120–1)

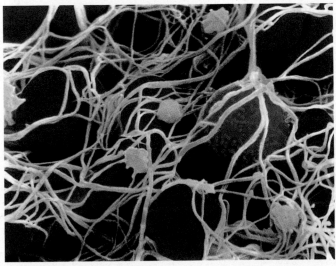

Fig 122–1
A colored scanning electron micrograph of a blood clot or thrombus. Red blood cells (erythrocytes) are seen trapped in a web of insoluble fibrin polymer (white). Platelets (green) and a white blood cell (yellow) have become enmeshed in the clot.
(Courtesy of the Science Photo Gallery.)

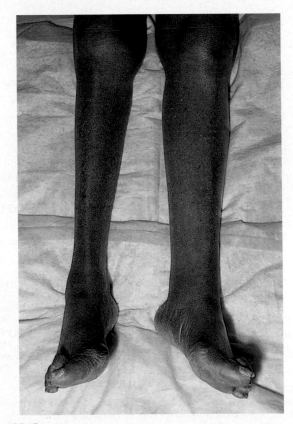

Fig 122–2
Deep vein thrombosis.
(From Swartz MH: Textbook of Physical Diagnosis, 5th ed. Philadelphia, WB Saunders, 2006.)

LABORATORY TESTS

- Laboratory tests are not specific for DVT. Baseline prothrombin time (PT), international normalized ratio (INR), partial thromboplastin time (PTT), and platelet count should be determined for all patients before starting anticoagulation.
- Use of D-dimer assay by enzyme-linked immunosorbent assay (ELISA) may be useful in the management of suspected DVT. The combination of a normal D-dimer study on presentation, together with a normal compression venous ultrasound, is useful to exclude DVT and generally eliminates the need to repeat ultrasound at 5 to 7 days. DVT can be ruled out in patients who are clinically unlikely to have DVT and who have a negative D-dimer test. Compressive ultrasonography can be safely omitted in such patients. Figure 122–3 depicts a clinical algorithm for DVT.
- Laboratory evaluation of young patients with DVT, patients with recurrent thrombosis without obvious causes, and those with a family history of thrombosis should include determination of protein S, protein C, fibrinogen, antithrombin III level, lupus anticoagulant, anticardiolipin antibodies, factor V Leiden, factor VIII, factor IX, and plasma homocysteine levels.

IMAGING STUDIES

- Compression ultrasonography (Fig. 122–4) is generally preferred as the initial study because it is noninvasive and can be repeated serially (useful to monitor suspected acute DVT). It offers good sensitivity for detecting proximal vein thrombosis (in the popliteal or femoral vein). Its disadvantages are poor visualization of deep iliac and pelvic veins and poor sensitivity in isolated or nonocclusive calf vein thrombi.
- Contrast venography (Fig. 122–5) is the gold standard for evaluation of DVT of the lower extremity. It is, however, invasive and painful. Additional disadvantages are the increased risk of phlebitis, new thrombosis, renal failure, and hypersensitivity reaction to contrast media; it also gives poor visualization of the deep femoral vein in the thigh and internal iliac vein and its tributaries.

TREATMENT

- Anticoagulation: heparin followed by warfarin
- Insertion of an inferior vena cava filter (Fig. 122–6) to prevent pulmonary embolism is recommended in patients with contraindications to anticoagulation.
- Thrombolytic therapy (streptokinase) can be used in rare cases (unless contraindicated) in patients with extensive iliofemoral venous thrombosis and a low risk of bleeding.

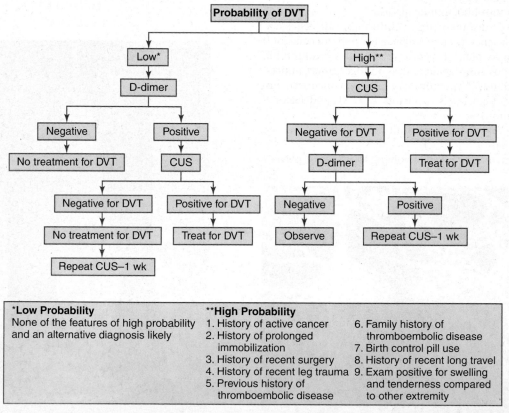

Fig 122–3

Clinical algorithm for deep venous thrombosis (DVT). CUS, compression ultrasonography.
(From Ferri F: Practical Guide to the Care of the Medical Patient, 7th ed. St. Louis, Mosby, 2007.)

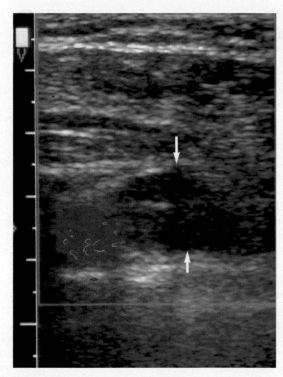

Fig 122–4
Doppler ultrasound appearance of deep vein thrombosis. The superficial femoral vein is filled with echogenic material representing thrombus and no flow can be identified in the vein on Doppler evaluation. Flow can be identified in the adjacent artery on color Doppler evaluation (arrows).
(From Crawford, MH, DiMarco JP, Paulus WJ [eds]: Cardiology, 2nd ed. St. Louis, Mosby, 2004.)

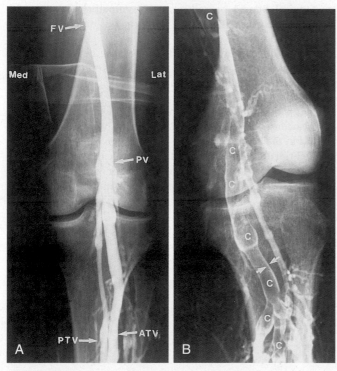

Fig 122–5
Venous thrombosis about the knee. **A,** A normal contrast venogram near the knee shows the contrast material coming up the anterior (ATV) and posterior (PTV) tibial veins into the popliteal vein (PV) and then into the femoral vein (FV). **B,** A venogram in a different patient with leg swelling demonstrates that the veins are filled with clot (C). A small amount of contrast agent is able to pass by and outline the clot in some veins *(arrows)*.
(From Mettler FA, Guibertau MJ, Voss CM, Urbina CE: Primary Care Radiology. Philadelphia, Elsevier, 2000.)

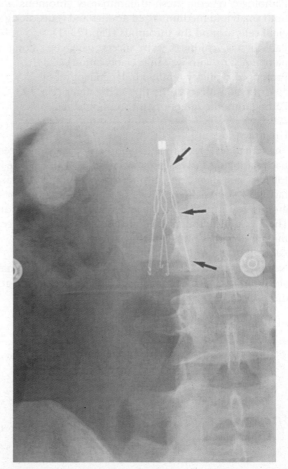

Fig 122–6
Inferior vena cava filter. An expandable wire mesh basket *(arrows)* has been placed in the inferior vena cava. This can be done by pushing the device out of a catheter and allowing it to expand in place. This keeps the large clots from traveling from the lower extremities and pelvis, up the inferior vena cava, and into the lung.
(From Mettler FA, Guibertau MJ, Voss CM, Urbina CE: Primary Care Radiology. Philadelphia, Elsevier, 2000.)

Chapter 123 Thromboangiitis obliterans (Buerger's disease)

DEFINITION

Thromboangiitis obliterans (Buerger's disease) is an occlusive inflammatory disease of the small to medium-sized arteries of the upper and lower extremities The disease typically occurs before the age of 50 years and is found predominantly in men who smoke.

PHYSICAL FINDINGS AND CLINICAL PRESENTATION

- Peripheral vascular disease occurring predominantly in men before the age of 50 years
- Typically, affects the arms and the legs and not just the lower extremities as does arteriosclerosis
- Found solely in tobacco smokers, with improvement in those who abstain
- Associated with migratory thrombophlebitis
- No other atherosclerotic risk factors (e.g., diabetes, cholesterol, or hypertension)
- Angiographic criteria (see "Imaging Studies")
- Pathologic criteria: fresh inflammatory thrombus within both small and medium-sized arteries and veins, along with giant cells around the thrombus (Fig. 123–1).
- Paresthesias, coldness, skin ulcers, gangrene, along with pain at rest or with walking (claudication)
- Prolonged capillary refill with dependent rubor
- Necrotic skin ulcers at the tips of the digits (Fig. 123–2)
- Pathognomonic migratory thrombophlebitis

CAUSE

- Unknown
- The remarkable feature is the close association between tobacco smoking and disease exacerbation. If abstinence from tobacco is adhered to, thromboangiitis obliterans takes a favorable course. If smoking is continued, the disease progresses, leading to gangrene and small-digit amputations.
- There is some thought of a genetic predisposition because the prevalence is higher in the Far East.

IMAGING STUDIES

- Noninvasive vascular studies help differentiate proximal occlusive disease characteristic of arteriosclerosis from the distal disease typical of thromboangiitis obliterans.

- Angiography findings in thromboangiitis obliterans include the following:
  1. Involvement of distal small and medium-sized vessels
  2. Occlusions are segmental, multiple, smooth, and tapered (Fig. 123–3)
  3. Collateral circulation gives a tree root or spider leg appearance.
  4. Both upper and lower extremities are involved.

TREATMENT

- Abstaining from smoking is the only way to stop the progression of the disease. Medical and surgical treatments will prove to be futile if the patient continues to smoke. Exacerbation of ischemic ulcers is directly related to tobacco use.
- The goal of medical treatment is to provide relief of ischemic pain and healing of ischemic ulcers. If the patient does not completely abstain from tobacco, medical measures will not be helpful.
- Prostaglandin vasodilator therapy given IV or intra-arterially provides some relief of pain but does not change the course of the disease.
- Epidural anesthesia and hyperbaric oxygen have a vasodilator effect and have been shown to help relieve pain from ischemic ulcers.
- Surgical bypass procedures and sympathectomy, as with medical treatment, will not be efficacious unless the patient stops smoking.
- Surgical bypass may be difficult because the occlusions of thromboangiitis obliterans are distal. Nevertheless, if successfully done, this can lead to rapid healing of ischemic ulcers.
- Sympathectomy leads to increased flow by decreasing the vasoconstriction of distal vessels and also has been shown to aid in the healing and relief of pain from ischemic ulcers.
- Débridement must be done on necrotic ulcers, if needed.
- Amputation is frequently required for gangrenous digits; however, below-knee or above-knee amputations are rarely necessary.

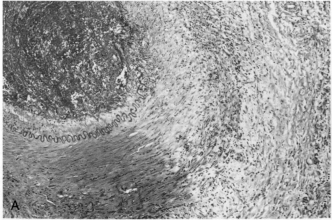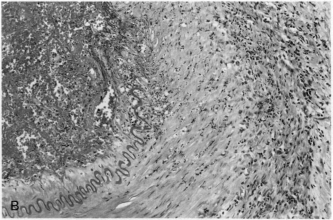

Fig 123–1

A, B, Buerger's disease. This acute lesion shows panmural inflammation, with abscess formation and thrombosis.
(From McKee PH, Calonje E, Granter SR [eds]: Pathology of the Skin With Clinical Correlation, 3rd ed. St. Louis, Mosby, 2005.)

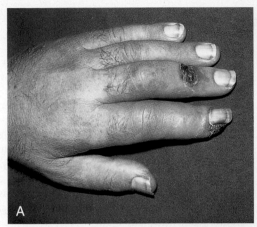
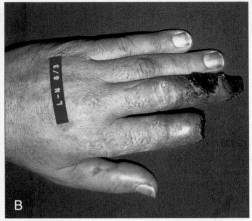
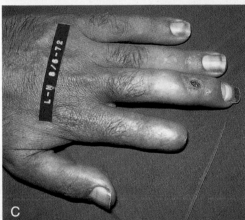

Fig 123-2

Buerger's disease. This 42-year-old man has typical criteria for Buerger's disease. Two toes on the left foot were amputated 5 years ago, after which the patient stopped smoking. **A, B,** Three weeks before these photographs were taken, he started smoking again and developed severe ischemia in several fingers. **C,** Four weeks after cessation of smoking, healing of the ulcers was complete.

(From Crawford, MH, DiMarco JP, Paulus WJ [eds]: Cardiology, 2nd ed. St. Louis, Mosby, 2004.)

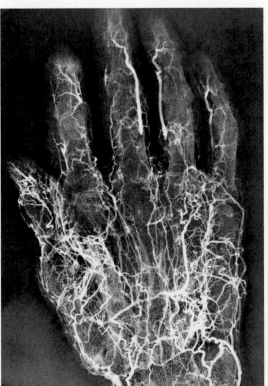

Fig 123-3

Angiographic findings in the hand of a patient with Buerger's disease. Several of the digital arteries are occluded, with acral skin necrosis as a result.

(Courtesy of Professor Bollinger, Zürich.)

Chapter 124   Abdominal aortic aneurysm

DEFINITION

An abdominal aortic aneurysm (AAA) is a permanent localized dilation of the abdominal aortic artery to at least 50% when compared with the normal diameter. The normal diameter in men is 2.3 cm, and in women it is 1.9 cm.

PHYSICAL FINDINGS AND CLINICAL PRESENTATION

- The physical examination, although not very sensitive for AAA <5 cm in size, has a sensitivity of 82% for detecting AAA >5 cm.
- Pulsatile epigastric mass that may or may not be tender (Fig. 124–1)
- Abdominal pain radiating to the back, flank, and groin
- Early satiety, nausea, and vomiting caused by compression of adjacent bowel
- Venous thrombosis from iliocaval venous compression
- Discoloration and pain of the feet with distal embolization of the thrombus within the aneurysm
- Flank and groin pain from ureteral obstruction and hydronephrosis
- Rupture presents as shock, hypoperfusion, and abdominal distention.
- Rare presentations include hematemesis or melena with abdominal and back pain in patients with aortoenteric fistulas. Aortocaval fistula produces loud abdominal bruits.

CAUSE

- Atherosclerotic (degenerative or nonspecific; Fig. 124–2)
- Genetic (e.g., Ehlers-Danlos syndrome)
- Trauma
- Cystic medial necrosis (Marfan syndrome)
- Arteritis, inflammatory
- Mycotic, infected (syphilis)
- Tobacco smoking significantly increases the risk of aneurysm

DIFFERENTIAL DIAGNOSIS

Almost 75% of AAAs are asymptomatic and are discovered on routine examination or serendipitously when ordering studies for other complaints. This must be considered in the differential:

- Abdominal pain
- Back pain

IMAGING STUDIES

- Abdominal ultrasound (Fig. 124–3) is almost 100% accurate in identifying an aneurysm and estimating the size to within 0.3 to 0.4 cm. It is not very good for estimating the proximal extension to the renal arteries or involvement of the iliac arteries.
- CT (Fig. 124–4) is recommended for preoperative aneurysm imaging and estimating the size to within 0.3 mm. There are no false-negatives, and the CT scan can localize the proximal extent, detect the integrity of the wall, and rule out rupture.
- Angiography gives detailed arterial anatomy, localizing the aneurysm relative to the renal and visceral arteries. This is the definitive preoperative study for surgeons.
- MRI can also be used, but it is more expensive and not always readily available.

TREATMENT

- AAA rupture is an emergency. Surgery is the only chance for survival.
- On diagnosing an AAA, surveillance ultrasound for sizing with recommendations for prophylactic surgery for AAA >5.5 cm remains safe, with very low rates of AAA rupture (less than 1%).

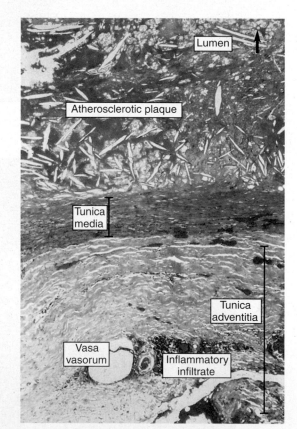

Fig 124–2
Histologic section through the wall of a typical abdominal aortic aneurysm. There is an atherosclerotic plaque on the luminal surface. The tunica media, which in a normal aorta is comprised of a thick layer of smooth muscle and elastin, is thin and exhibits marked loss of smooth muscle cells. The tunica adventitia is thick, disorganized, and inflamed. The inflammatory infiltrate is particularly prominent around the vasa vasorum.
(From Crawford, MH, DiMarco JP, Paulus WJ [eds]: Cardiology, 2nd ed. St. Louis, Mosby, 2004.)

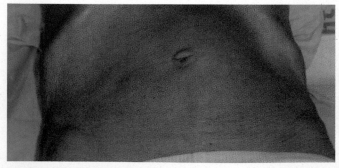

Fig 124–1
In thin individuals, an aortic aneurysm may be seen as a pulsating swelling in the upper abdomen.
(Courtesy of S. Ray.)

- The most commonly used predictor of rupture is the maximum diameter of the AAA. For AAA with baseline diameters >3.5 cm, 4.0 cm, 4.5 cm, and 5 cm, the recommended screening intervals are 36, 24, 12, and 3 months, respectively.
- For AAAs 5.5 cm or larger, surgery is recommended, provided there is no contraindication (e.g., MI within 6 months, refractory CHF, life expectancy less than 2 years, severe residual from cerebrovascular accident [CVA]). Figure 124–5 presents techniques of endovascular aortic aneurysm repair.
- Mortality after rupture is more than 90% because most patients do not reach the hospital on time. Of those patients who reach the hospital, the mortality rate is still 50%, compared with the 4% mortality rate for elective repair of a nonruptured aorta.

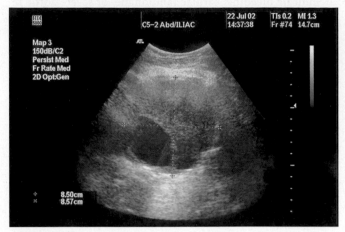

Fig 124–3
Ultrasound appearance of an abdominal aortic aneurysm, seen in cross section. Sonography is highly accurate in diagnosing and measuring infrarenal aortic aneurysms.
(Courtesy of M. Ellis.)

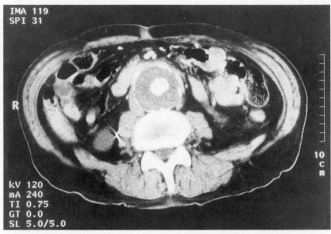

Fig 124–4
CT scan of an abdominal aortic aneurysm. Contrast in the lumen of the vessel, a thick layer of mural thrombus, and calcification in the aneurysm wall are shown.
(From Crawford, MH, DiMarco JP, Paulus WJ [eds]: Cardiology, 2nd ed. St. Louis, Mosby, 2004.)

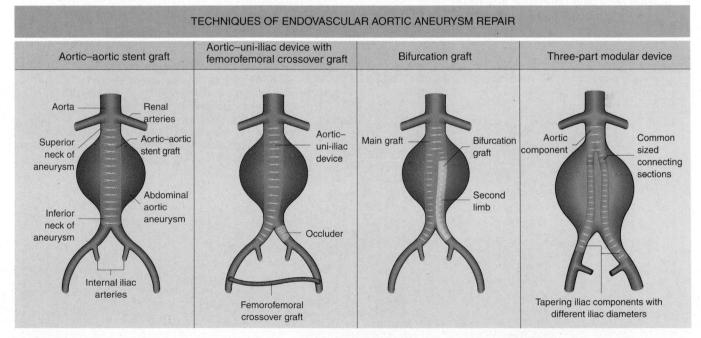

Fig 124–5
Techniques of endovascular aortic aneurysm repair. The aortic-aortic stent graft was the configuration of the early aneurysm stent graft systems. In practice, the inferior aneurysm neck is not usually of adequate length to achieve a seal, and aortic-aortic tube grafts are now rarely used. The aortic–uni-iliac device with a femorofemoral crossover graft appears inelegant at first glance, but these types of grafts, particularly the custom-made devices, permit great flexibility in anatomic dimensions and thus enable patients whose aneurysms are not suitable for other graft configurations to receive endovascular treatment. The bifurcation graft is the configuration of choice for most patients. Most bifurcation grafts are modular devices, in which the main graft resembles a pair of long trousers with one leg cut short. This is deployed in the aneurysm, with the upper neck placed below the renal arteries and the long limb secured in the common iliac artery. The second trouser leg is then deployed via the contralateral groin to join the short limb of the main graft to the opposite common iliac artery. The early endovascular bifurcation grafts were complicated to use and required thick delivery systems; improvements in technology have simplified use and slimmed down delivery catheters to allow percutaneous deployment in some cases.
(From Crawford, MH, DiMarco JP, Paulus WJ [eds]: Cardiology, 2nd ed. St. Louis, Mosby, 2004.)

Chapter 125 · Aortic dissection

DEFINITION
Aortic dissection occurs when an intimal tear allows blood to dissect between medial layers of the aorta.

RISK FACTORS
- Hypertension
- Atherosclerosis
- Family history of aortic aneurysms
- Vasculitis
- Disorders of collagen
- Bicuspid aortic valve
- Aortic coarctation
- Turner's syndrome
- Crack cocaine
- Trauma

CLASSIFICATION
The majority of aortic dissections originate in the ascending or descending aorta; there are three major classifications:
- DeBakey type I ascending and descending aorta, type II ascending aorta, type III descending aorta
- Stanford type A ascending aorta (proximal), type B descending aorta (distal; Fig. 125–1)

PHYSICAL FINDINGS AND CLINICAL PRESENTATION
- Sudden onset of very severe chest pain, at its peak at onset
- Little radiation to neck, shoulder, arm
- Sharp, tearing, or ripping pain
- Anterior chest pain (ascending dissection)
- Back pain (descending dissection)
- Syncope, abdominal pain, CHF, malperfusion may occur
- Most with severe hypertension, 25% with hypotension (systolic blood pressure [SBP] <100 mm Hg), which can indicate bleeding, cardiac tamponade, or severe aortic regurgitation
- Pulse and blood pressure differentials common (38%) caused by partial compression of subclavian arteries
- Aortic regurgitation in 18% to 50% of cases of proximal dissection
- Myocardial ischemia caused by coronary artery compression
- Stroke in 5% to 10% of patients

CAUSE
- Unknown, risk factors known. Chronic hypertension (HTN) affects arterial wall composition.
- Medial degeneration of aorta appears to be responsible.
- Aortic dissection reflects systemic illness of the vasculature.
- Major inherited connective tissue disorders affect arterial wall—Marfan syndrome, Ehlers-Danlos syndrome, and familial forms of thoracic aneurysm and dissection.

DIFFERENTIAL DIAGNOSIS
- Acute MI, angina
- Pulmonary embolism
- Aortic stenosis
- Pericarditis
- Cholecystitis
- Aortic insufficiency

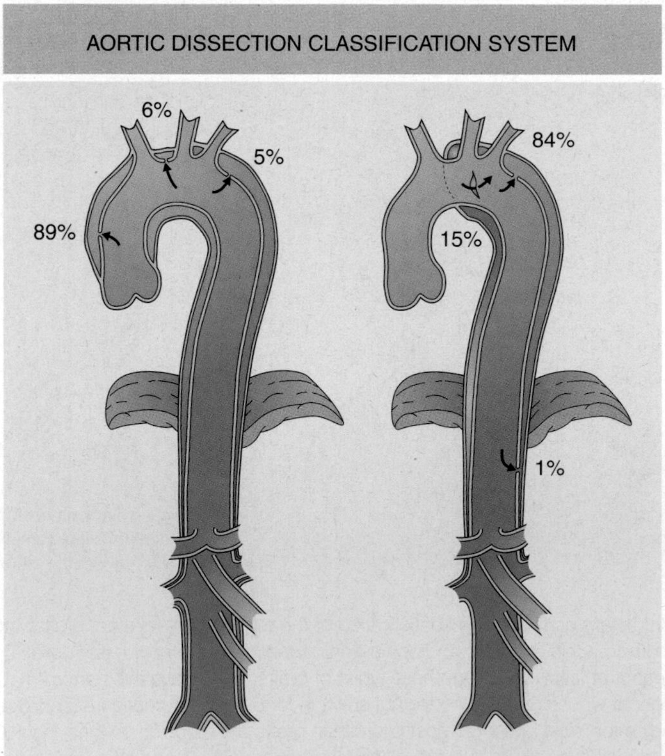

AORTIC DISSECTION CLASSIFICATION SYSTEM

6%
5%
84%
89%
15%
1%

Fig 125–1
Aortic dissection classification system. Type A is defined by the involvement of the ascending aorta, irrespective of the location of the tear. In type B, the dissection does not extend into the ascending aorta. Note the distribution of the location of the entry point for each type.
(From Crawford, MH, DiMarco JP, Paulus WJ [eds]: Cardiology, 2nd ed. St. Louis, Mosby, 2004.)

LABORATORY TESTS
- ECG, cardiac troponins : helpful to rule out MI
- Highly elevated D-dimer

IMAGING STUDIES
- Greatest value in proximal lesions with sensitivity, 90.9%, specificity, 98%
- Chest x-ray (Fig. 125–2) may show widened mediastinum (62%) and displacement of aortic intimal calcium.
- Transesophageal echocardiography (Fig. 125–3), sensitivity, 97% to 100%, is the study of choice in unstable patients, but operator-dependent.
- MRI (Fig. 125–4): sensitivity, 90% to 100%, is gold standard, but not suitable for stable intubated patients
- CT (Fig. 125–5): sensitivity, 83% to 100%

- Test of choice depends on clinical circumstances and availability. Accuracy of tests is almost equal in skilled hands.
- With medium or high pretest probability, a second diagnostic test should be done if the first is negative.

TREATMENT
- IV propanolol, metoprolol, or labetolol, followed by nitroprusside, with target SBP 100 to 120 mm Hg.
- IV calcium channel blockers with negative inotropy may be used.
- Multiple medications may be needed.
- Proximal dissections require emergent surgery to prevent rupture or pericardial effusion. Distal embolization may occur during surgery (Fig. 125–6).
- Distal dissections are treated medically unless distal organ involvement or impending rupture occurs.
- Endovascular stent placement is a new treatment, especially for older high-risk surgical patients.

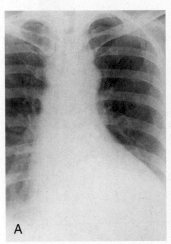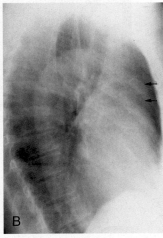

Fig 125–2
Large intrapericardial dissecting aortic aneurysm (frontal and lateral chest films). **A,** In the frontal view, the aorta looks normal. **B,** In the lateral view, the large aortic root can be seen above the cardiac shadow, bulging forward *(arrow)* and almost meeting the sternum.
(From Grainger RG, Allison DJ, Adam A, Dixon AK [eds]: Grainger & Allison's Diagnostic Radiology, 4th ed. London, Harcourt, 2001.)

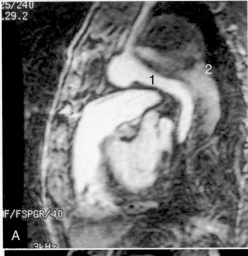
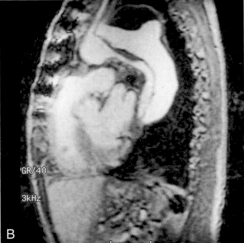

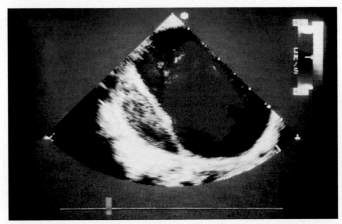

Fig 125–3
Transesophageal echocardiogram showing dissecting aortic aneurysm.
(From Crawford, MH, DiMarco JP, Paulus WJ [eds]: Cardiology, 2nd ed. St. Louis, Mosby, 2004.)

Fig 125–4
Longitudinal MRI in a chronic type B dissection extending into the arch. **A,** Early phase showing (1) the entry point and (2) a faint visualization of the outline of the aneurysm. **B,** Late phase demonstrating partial opacification of the aneurysm and extension of the dissection along the subclavian artery.
(Courtesy of Dr. Loren Ketai, University of New Mexico, Albuquerque, NM.)

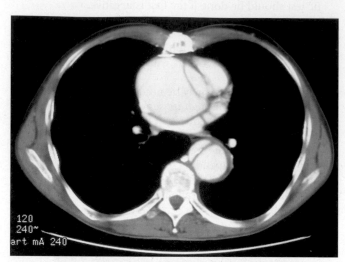

Fig 125-5
Spiral CT in acute type A dissection extending into the descending aorta. The ascending aorta is dilated. The intimal flap is clearly seen in both the ascending and descending aorta.
(Courtesy of Dr. Loren Ketai, University of New Mexico, Albuquerque, NM.)

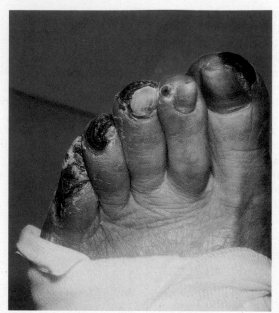

Fig 125-6
Distal embolization during aortic aneurysm surgery.
(From Crawford, MH, DiMarco JP, Paulus WJ [eds]: Cardiology, 2nd ed. St. Louis, Mosby, 2004.)

Chapter 126   Syncope

DEFINITION

Syncope is the transient loss of consciousness that results from an acute global reduction in cerebral blood flow. Syncope should be distinguished from other causes of transient loss of consciousness.

PHYSICAL FINDINGS AND CLINICAL PRESENTATION

- Blood pressure: if low, consider orthostatic hypotension; if unequal in both arms (difference >20 mm Hg), consider subclavian steal or dissecting aneurysm. (*Note*: Blood pressure and heart rate should be recorded in the supine and standing positions.) If there is a drop in BP but no change in HR, the patient may be on a beta blocker or may have an autonomic neuropathy.
- Pulse: if patient has tachycardia, bradycardia, or irregular rhythm, consider arrhythmia.
- Heart: if there are murmurs present suggestive of aortic stenosis (AS) or HOCM, consider syncope secondary to left ventricular outflow obstruction; if there are JVD and distal heart sounds, consider cardiac tamponade.
- Carotid sinus pressure: can be diagnostic if it reproduces symptoms and other causes are excluded; a pause of more than 3 seconds or a systolic BP drop of more than 50 mm Hg without symptoms or less than 30 mm Hg with symptoms when sinus pressure is applied separately on each side for less than 5 seconds is considered abnormal. This test should be avoided in patients with carotid bruits or cerebrovascular disease; ECG monitoring, IV access, and bedside atropine should be available when carotid sinus pressure is applied.

CAUSE

- Neurally mediated syncope
  1. Psychophysiologic (emotional upset, panic disorders, hysteria)
  2. Visceral reflex (micturition, defecation, food ingestion, coughing, ventricular contraction; glossopharyngeal neuralgia)
  3. Carotid sinus pressure
  4. Reduction of venous return caused by Valsalva maneuver
- Orthostatic hypotension
  1. Hypovolemia
  2. Vasodilator medications
  3. Autonomic neuropathy (diabetes, amyloid, Parkinson's disease, multisystem atrophy)
  4. Pheochromocytoma
  5. Carcinoid syndrome
- Cardiac
  1. Reduced cardiac output
     a. Left ventricular outflow obstruction (aortic stenosis, hypertrophic cardiomyopathy)
     b. Obstruction to pulmonary flow (pulmonary embolism, pulmonic stenosis, primary pulmonary hypertension)
     c. MI with pump failure
     d. Cardiac tamponade
     e. Mitral stenosis
     f. Reduction of venous return (atrial myxoma, valve thrombus)
     g. Beta blockers

  2. Arrhythmias or asystole
     a. Extreme tachycardia (>160 to 180 beats/min)
     b. Severe bradycardia (<30 to 40 beats/min)
     c. Sick sinus syndrome
     d. AV block (second- or third-degree)
     e. Ventricular tachycardia or fibrillation
     f. Long-QT syndrome
     g. Pacemaker malfunction
     h. Psychotropic medications and beta blockers

DIFFERENTIAL DIAGNOSIS

- Seizure
- Vertebrobasilar transient ischemic attack (TIA) usually manifests as diplopia, vertigo, ataxia, but not loss of consciousness. Isolated episodes of transient loss of consciousness (TLOC) without accompanying neurologic symptoms are unlikely to be a TIA.
- Recreational drugs, alcohol
- Functional causes, such as stress and somatoform disorders
- Sleep disorders, such as sleep attacks and narcolepsy, are also in the differential for TLOC.
- Head trauma

WORKUP

The history is crucial to diagnosing the cause of syncope and may suggest a diagnosis that can be evaluated with directed testing. History is also important to determine other causes for TLOC, such as seizure.

- Sudden loss of consciousness: consider cardiac arrhythmias.
- Gradual loss of consciousness: consider orthostatic hypotension, vasodepressor syncope, hypoglycemia.
- History of aura before loss of consciousness (LOC) or prolonged confusion (more than 1 minute), amnesia, or lethargy after LOC suggests seizure rather than syncope.
- Patient's activity at the time of syncope:
  1. Micturition, coughing, defecation: consider syncope secondary to decreased venous return.
  2. Turning head or while shaving: consider carotid sinus syndrome.
  3. Physical exertion in a patient with murmur: consider aortic stenosis.
  4. Arm exercise: consider subclavian steal syndrome.
  5. Assuming an upright position: consider orthostatic hypotension.
- Associated events:
  1. Chest pain: consider MI, pulmonary embolism.
  2. Palpitations: consider arrhythmias.
  3. Incontinence (urine or fecal) and tongue biting are associated with seizure or syncope.
  4. Brief, transient shaking after LOC may represent myoclonus from global cerebral hypoperfusion and not seizures. However, sustained tonic-clonic muscle action is more suggestive of seizure.
  5. Focal neurologic symptoms or signs point to a neurologic event, such as a seizure with residual deficits (e.g. Todd's paralysis) or cerebral ischemic injury.

6. Psychological stress: syncope may be vasovagal.
- Review current medications, particularly antihypertensive and psychotropic drugs.

LABORATORY TESTS
- Routine blood tests rarely yield diagnostically useful information and should be done only if they are specifically suggested by the results of the history and physical examination. The following are commonly ordered tests:
  - Pregnancy test should be considered in women of childbearing age
  - CBC to rule out anemia, infection
  - Electrolytes, BUN, creatinine, magnesium, calcium to rule out electrolyte abnormalities and evaluate fluid status
  - Serum glucose level
  - Cardiac isoenzymes should be obtained if the patient gives a history of chest pain before the syncopal episode.
  - ABGs to rule out pulmonary embolus, hyperventilation (when suspected)
  - Evaluate drug and alcohol levels when suspecting toxicity.

IMAGING STUDIES
- Echocardiography is useful in patients with a heart murmur to rule out AS, HOCM, or atrial myxoma.
- If seizure is suspected, CT and/or MRI of the head and electroencephalography may be useful.
- If head trauma or neurologic signs are noted on examination, CT or MRI may be helpful.
- If pulmonary embolism is suspected, spiral chest CT or ventilation-perfusion scan should be done.
- If arrhythmias are suspected, a 24-hour Holter monitor and admission to a telemetry unit is appropriate. Generally, Holter monitoring is rarely useful, revealing a cause for syncope in less than 3% of cases. Loop recorders (Fig. 126–1)

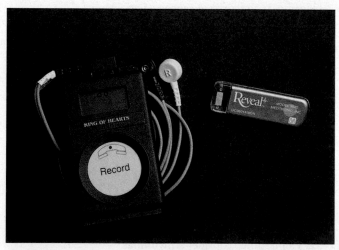

Fig 126–1
External loop recorder (left) and implantable loop recorder (right). The external loop recorder uses two skin electrodes with wires attached to a pager-style device. The implantable loop recorder has sensing electrodes on the external shell. It is inserted into the left chest region, permitting prolonged monitoring.
(From Crawford, MH, DiMarco JP, Paulus WJ [eds]: Cardiology, 2nd ed. St. Louis, Mosby, 2004.)

that can be activated after a syncopal episode to retrieve information about the cardiac rhythm during the preceding 4 minutes add considerable diagnostic yield in patients with unexplained syncope.
- Implantable cardiac monitors that function as permanent loop recorders (Fig. 126–2) or ICDs, which are placed subcutaneously in the pectoral region with the patient under local anesthesia, are useful in patients with cardiac syncope.
- Electrophysiologic studies may be indicated in patients with structural heart disease and/or recurrent syncope.
- ECG to rule out arrhythmias; may be diagnostic in 5% to 10% of patients

TILT-TABLE TESTING
- Useful to support a diagnosis of neurally mediated syncope. Patients older than age 50 should have stress testing before tilt-table testing. Positive results would preclude tilt-table testing.
- Indicated in patients with recurrent episodes of unexplained syncope, as well as for patients in high-risk occupations (e.g., pilots, bus drivers). The test is also useful for identifying patients with a prominent bradycardic response who may benefit from implantation of a permanent pacemaker.
- It is performed by keeping the patient in an upright posture on a tilt table with footboard support. The angle of the tilt table varies from 60 to 80 degrees. The duration of upright posture during tilt-table testing varies from 25 to 45 minutes (Fig. 126–3).
- The hallmark of neurally mediated syncope is severe hypotension associated with a paradoxical bradycardia triggered by a specific stimulus. The diagnosis of neurally mediated syncope is likely if upright tilt testing reproduces these hemodynamic changes in less than 15 minutes and causes presyncope or syncope.

PSYCHIATRIC EVALUATION
- May be indicated in young patients without heart disease who have frequently recurring transient loss of consciousness and other somatic symptoms
- Generalized anxiety disorder, pain disorder, and major depression predispose patients to neurally mediated reactions and may result in syncope.

TREATMENT
- Varies with the underlying cause of syncope (e.g., pacemaker in patients with syncope secondary to complete heart block)
- Ensure proper hydration; consider thromboembolic disease stockings (TEDS) and salt tablets.
- Eliminate medications that may induce hypotension.
- Syncope caused by orthostatic hypotension is treated with volume replacement in patients with intravascular volume depletion. Also consider midodrine to promote venous return via adrenergic-mediated vasoconstriction and fludrocortisone (Florinef) for its mineralocorticoid effects to increase intravascular volume

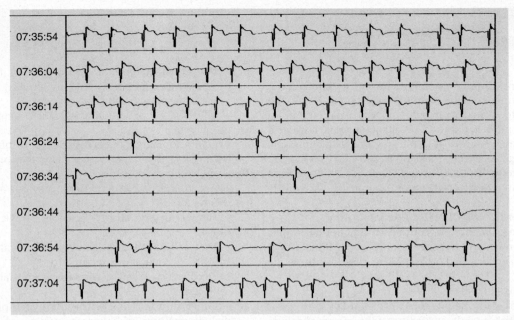

Fig 126–2
Rhythm strip obtained with an implantable loop recorder in a 69-year-old man who had experienced two syncopal episodes in the previous 18 months. Each line represents 10 seconds of a single-lead rhythm strip. Note marked bradycardia, with a 14-second pause. Syncope resolved after implantation of a permanent pacemaker.
(From Crawford, MH, DiMarco JP, Paulus WJ [eds]: Cardiology, 2nd ed. St. Louis, Mosby, 2004.)

DISPOSITION

Prognosis varies with the age of the patient and the cause of the syncope. Generally, the following apply:

• Benign prognosis (very low 1-year morbidity) in patients:
1. Age younger than 30 years and having noncardiac syncope
2. Age older than 70 years and having vasovagal-psychogenic syncope or syncope of unknown cause
• Poor prognosis (high mortality and morbidity) in patients with cardiac syncope
• Patients with the following risk factors have a higher 1-year mortality: abnormal ECG, history of ventricular arrhythmia, history of CHF

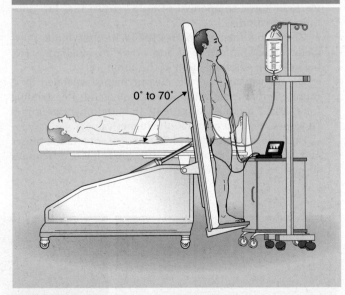

70° TILT TEST USING MOTORIZED TABLE WITH A FOOTPLATE

0° to 70°

Fig 126-3
A 70-degree tilt test using a motorized table with a footplate. Not illustrated are ECG leads for monitoring, and a cuff or continuous blood pressure monitor.
(From Crawford, MH, DiMarco JP, Paulus WJ [eds]: Cardiology, 2nd ed. St. Louis, Mosby, 2004.)

Chapter 127 Hypertension

DEFINITION

The Joint National Committee on Prevention, Detection, Evaluation, and Treatment of High Blood Pressure (JNC 7) has classified normal blood pressure in adults as less than 120 mm Hg systolic and 80 mm Hg diastolic. "Prehypertension" is defined as systolic pressure of 120 to 139 mm Hg or diastolic pressure 80 to 89 mm Hg. Stage 1 hypertension is systolic BP 140 to 159 mm Hg or diastolic BP 90 to 99 mm HG. Stage 2 hypertension is systolic BP 160 mm Hg or higher or diastolic BP 100 mm Hg or higher.

PHYSICAL FINDINGS AND CLINICAL PRESENTATION

Physical examination may be entirely within normal limits, except for the presence of hypertension. A proper initial physical examination on a hypertensive patient should include the following:

- Measure height and weight.
- Evaluate skin for the presence of café-au-lait spots (neurofibromatosis), uremic appearance (chronic renal failure [CRF]), striae (Cushing's syndrome).
- Perform careful funduscopic examination to evaluate for hypertensive retinopathy (Fig. 127–1): check for papilledema, retinal exudates, hemorrhages, arterial narrowing, AV compression.
- Examine the neck for carotid bruits, distended neck veins, or enlarged thyroid gland.
- Perform extensive cardiopulmonary examination: check for loud aortic component of S_2, S_4, ventricular lift, murmurs, arrhythmias.
- Check abdomen for masses (pheochromocytoma, polycystic kidneys), presence of bruits over the renal artery (renal artery stenosis), dilation of the aorta.
- Obtain two or more BP measurements separated by 2 minutes with the patient supine or seated and after standing for at least 2 minutes. Measure BP in both upper extremities (if values are discrepant, use the higher value).
- Examine arterial pulses (dilated or absent femoral pulses and BP higher in upper extremities than lower extremities suggest aortic coarctation).
- Note the presence of truncal obesity (Cushing's syndrome) and pedal edema (CHF, nephrosis).
- Perform full neurologic assessment.
- The clinical evaluation should help determine whether the patient has primary or secondary (possibly reversible) hypertension, target organ disease is present, and cardiovascular risk factors in addition to hypertension are noted.

Pertinent history

- Age at onset of hypertension, previous antihypertensive therapy
- Family history of hypertension, stroke, cardiovascular disease
- Diet, salt intake, alcohol, drugs (e.g., oral contraceptives, NSAIDs, decongestants, steroids)
- Occupation, lifestyle, socioeconomic status, psychological factors
- Other cardiovascular risk factors: hyperlipidemia, obesity, diabetes mellitus, carbohydrate intolerance
- Symptoms of secondary hypertension:
1. Headache, palpitations, excessive perspiration (possible pheochromocytoma)
2. Weakness, polyuria (consider hyperaldosteronism)
3. Claudication of lower extremities (seen with coarctation of aorta)

CAUSE

- Essential (primary) hypertension (85%)
- Drug-induced or drug-related (5%)
- Renal hypertension (5%)
1. Renal parenchymal disease (3%)
2. Renovascular hypertension (<2%)
- Endocrine (4% to 5%)
1. Oral contraceptives (4%)
2. Primary aldosteronism (0.5%)
3. Pheochromocytoma (0.2%)
4. Cushing's syndrome and chronic steroid therapy (0.2%)
5. Hyperparathyroidism or thyroid disease (0.2%)
- Coarctation of the aorta (0.2%)
- Figure 127–2 presents some factors involved in the regulation of blood pressure.

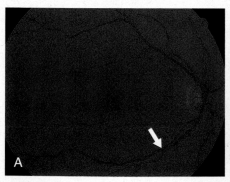
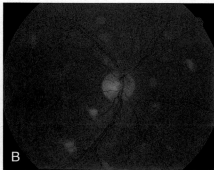
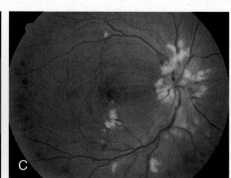

Fig 127–1
Different grades of hypertensive retinopathy. **A,** Mild hypertensive retinopathy, with arteriolar narrowing and arteriovenous nicking. **B,** Moderate hypertensive retinopathy, with cotton wool spots (nerve fiber layer infarcts) and arteriovenous nicking. **C,** Malignant hypertension with papilledema, cotton wool spots, macular yellow exudates (star formation pattern), and retinal hemorrhages.
(Courtesy of J. Kinyoun.)

LABORATORY TESTS

- Urinalysis: for evidence of renal disease
- BUN, creatinine: to rule out renal disease. High-serum creatinine is a predictor of cardiovascular risk in essential hypertension.
- Serum electrolyte levels: low potassium is suggestive of primary aldosteronism, diuretic use.
- Screening for coexisting diseases that may adversely affect prognosis:
  1. Fasting serum glucose
  2. Serum lipid panel, uric acid, calcium
  3. If pheochromocytoma is suspected: plasma metanephrine level, 24-hour urine for vanillylmandelic acid (VMA) and metanephrines

IMAGING STUDIES

- ECG: check for presence of left ventricular hypertrophy (LVH) with strain pattern. If found on ECG, an echocardiogram (Fig. 127–3) can be used to assess left ventriculat hypertrophy further.
- MRA of the renal arteries: in suspected renovascular hypertension (renal artery stenosis)

TREATMENT

Lifestyle modifications:

- Lose weight if overweight.
- Limit alcohol intake to 1 oz of ethanol or less/day in men or 0.5 oz or less/day in women.
- Exercise (aerobic) regularly (at least 30 minutes/day, most days).
- Reduce sodium intake to less than 100 mmol/day (less than 2.3 g of sodium).
- Maintain adequate dietary potassium (more than 3500 mg/day) intake.
- Stop smoking and reduce dietary saturated fat and cholesterol intake for overall cardiovascular health. Consume a diet rich in fruits and vegetables.
- For patients with prehypertension and diabetes or chronic kidney disease, aggressive pharmacologic treatment should be undertaken to reduce blood pressure to less than 130/80 mm Hg.

Antihypertensive drug therapy should be initiated in patients with stage 1 hypertension. The choice of antihypertensive agent should be individualized and based on coexisting disorders:

- CHF: ACE inhibitors, ARBs, beta blockers, diuretics, aldosterone antagonists
- Post-MI: beta blockers, ACE inhibitors, aldosterone antagonists
- High cardiovascular risk: beta blockers, ACE inhibitors, calcium channel blockers, diuretics
- Diabetes: ACE inhibitors, ARBs, calcium channel blockers, beta blockers, diuretics
- Chronic kidney disease: ACE inhibitors, ARBs
- Recurrent stroke prevention: ACE inhibitors, diuretics
- Two-drug combination is necessary for most patients with stage 2 hypertension. Combination of a diuretic with another agent is preferred unless there are compelling indications to use other agents.
- When selecting drugs, also consider the cost of the medication, metabolic and subjective side effects, and drug-drug interactions.

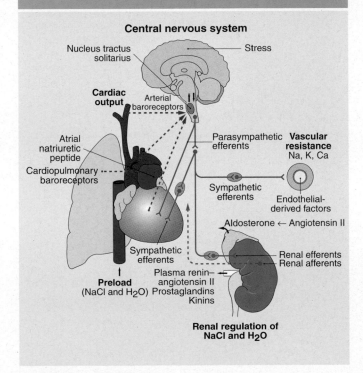

Fig 127–2
Some factors involved in the regulation of blood pressure.
(From Johnson RJ, Feehally J: Comprehensive Clinical Nephrology, 2nd ed. St. Louis, Mosby, 2000.)

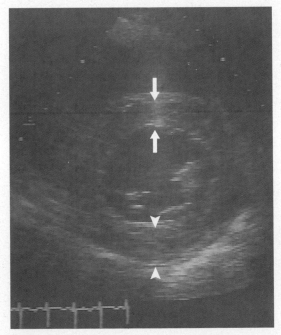

Fig 127–3
Echocardiogram showing concentric left ventricular hypertrophy. Septal thickness *(between large arrows)* and posterior wall thickness *(between arrowheads)* are increased to 16 mm in a patient with essential hypertension (normal is 11 mm or less).
(Courtesy of A. Pearlman.)

REFERENCES

Crawford MH, DiMarco JP, Paulus WJ: Cardiology, ed 2, St. Louis, 2004, Mosby

Ferri, F: Practical Guide to the Care of the Medical Patient, ed 7, St. Louis, 2007 Mosby

Ferri, F: Ferri's Clinical Advisor, 2007, St. Louis, 2007, Mosby

Souhami RL, Moxham J: Textbook of Medicine, ed 4, London, 2002, Churchill Livingstone

Zipes DB, Libby P, Bonow RO, Braunwald E: Braunwald's Heart disease, ed 7, Philadelphia, 2005, Elsevier

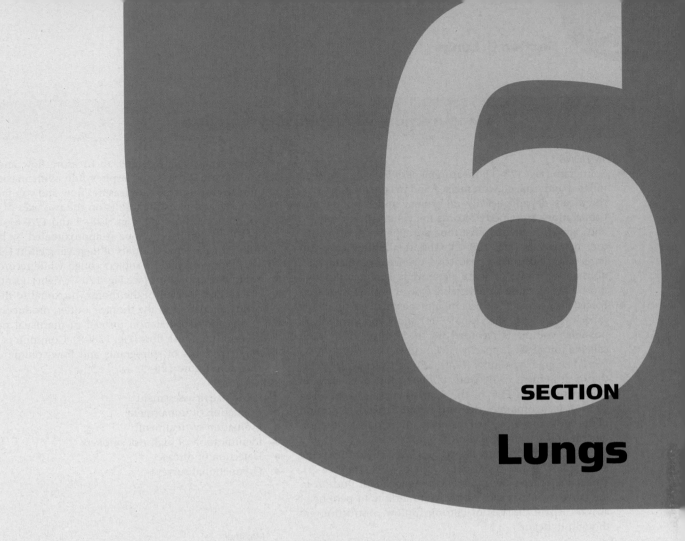

SECTION
Lungs

Chapter 128: Measurement of respiratory function
Chapter 129: Asthma
Chapter 130: Chronic obstructive pulmonary disease
Chapter 131: Alpha$_1$-antitrypsin deficiency
Chapter 132: Lung neoplasms
Chapter 133: Diseases of the pleura
Chapter 134: Occupational lung disease
Chapter 135: Interstitial lung disease

Chapter 136: Idiopathic pulmonary fibrosis
Chapter 137: Pulmonary infiltrations
Chapter 138: Atelectasis
Chapter 139: Respiratory infections
Chapter 140: Acute respiratory distress syndrome
Chapter 141: Pulmonary hypertension
Chapter 142: Altitude sickness
Chapter 143: Pulmonary embolism

Chapter 128   **Measurement of respiratory function**

DEFINITIONS

- Spirogram (Fig. 128–1): measurement of the volumes of air inhaled and exhaled with relaxed and maximal effort. Measurements depend heavily on patient understanding and cooperation. Spirometry records the volume of air inhaled and exhaled plotted against time during a series of ventilatory maneuvers (Fig. 128–2). Abnormal spirometric patterns reflect obstructive, restrictive, or mixed ventilatory abnormalities; none of these patterns is specific, although most diseases cause a predictable type of ventilatory defect.
- Forced vital capacity: subject inhales maximally to total lung capacity (TLC) and then exhales as rapidly and forcefully as possible. Volume is recorded on the abscissa of a graph called a forced vital capacity (FVC) curve.
- Forced expiratory volume (FEV): FEV at 1 second (FEV_1) is the measurement of dynamic volume most often used in conjunction with FVC in the analysis of spirometry (Fig. 128–3). It incorporates the early, effort-dependent portion of the curve, but enough of the midportion to make it reproducible and sensitive for clinical purposes.
- Average forced expiratory flow (FEF): FEF 25% to 75% is the average flow between 25% and 75% of FVC (Fig. 128–4). This value reflects the most effort-independent portion of the curve, which is most sensitive to airflow in peripheral airways where diseases of chronic airflow obstruction are thought to begin.

- Flow-volume relationships: to measure flow and volume, the subject inspires and expires fully with maximal effort into an instrument that measures flow and volume simultaneously, and plots the results on the two axes of an x-y recorder or oscilloscope (Figs. 128–5 and 128–6). The maximal flow-volume envelope is approximated by having the subject make repeated trials of increasing effort (Fig. 128–7, left), or by having the subject cough while recording flow-volume relationships (see Fig. 128–7, right). Central airway obstruction located in the thorax, proximal to the tracheal carina and distal to the thoracic outlet, produces a plateau during forced exhalation instead of the usual rise to and descent from peak flow (Fig. 128–8). Common pathophysiologic patterns of spirograms and flow-volume curves are shown in Figure 128–9.

INDICATIONS

- Preoperative assessment
- Evaluation of impairment
- Evaluation of treatment
- Identification of high-risk smokers
- Detection of disease
- Occupational surveys

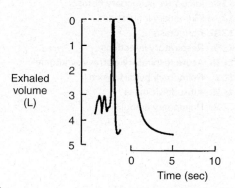

Fig 128–1

Spirogram obtained in a normal subject. The subject breathes quietly (slow recording speed) then takes a maximal inspiration followed by a maximal expiration without concern for time (VC). The subject then takes a maximal inspiration (rapid recording speed) exhales completely forcefully and as rapidly as possible (FVC).
(From Murray JF, Nadel JA [eds]: Textbook of Respiratory Medicine, 3rd ed. Philadelphia, WB Saunders, 2000, p 785.)

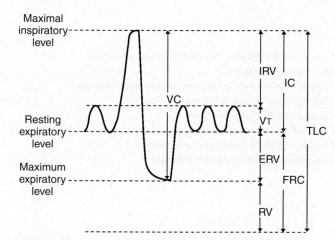

Fig 128–2

Volumes—there are four volumes, which do not overlap: (1) tidal volume (V_T) is the volume of gas inhaled or exhaled during each respiratory cycle; (2) inspiratory reserve volume (IRV) is the maximal volume of gas inspired from end-inspiration; (3) expiratory reserve volume (ERV) is the maximal volume of gas exhaled from end-expiration; and (4) residual volume (RV) is the volume of gas remaining in the lungs following a maximal exhalation. Capacities—there are four capacities, each of which contains two or more primary volumes: (1) total lung capacity (TLC) is the amount of gas contained in the lung at maximal inspiration; (2) vital capacity (VC) is the maximum volume of gas that can be expelled from the lungs by a forceful effort following maximal inspiration, without regard for the time involved; (3) inspiratory capacity (IC) is the maximal volume of gas that can be inspired from the resting expiratory level; and (4) functional residual capacity (FRC) is the volume of gas in the lungs at resting end-expiration.
(From Murray JF, Nadel JA [eds]: Textbook of Respiratory Medicine, 3rd ed. Philadelphia, WB Saunders, 2000, p 783.)

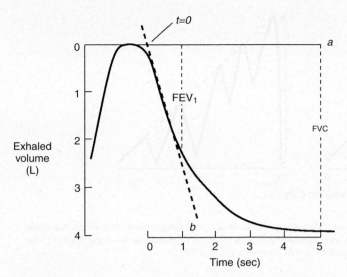

Fig 128–3

Back-extrapolation to define time zero. This diagram illustrates the measurement of forced expiratory volume (FEV_1) using the back-extrapolation method to define time zero, or the point during the forced vital capacity (FVC) maneuver when the subject began to blow as hard and fast as possible. A solid horizontal line (a) indicates the level of maximal inhalation. A heavy dashed line (b) passes through the steepest portion of volume-time tracing. The intersection point of these two lines becomes time zero, as indicated, from which timing is initiated; 1 second after time zero, the vertical dashed line is drawn, indicating FEV_1, and 5 seconds later, another vertical dashed line is drawn, indicating FVC.
(From Murray JF, Nadel JA [eds]: Textbook of Respiratory Medicine, 3rd ed. Philadelphia, WB Saunders, 2000, p 786.)

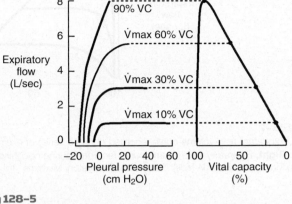

Fig 128–5

From a series of isovolume pressure-flow (IVPF) curves at varying vital capacities (left), it is possible to construct a maximal flow-volume curve (right). $\dot{V}$max = maximal expiratory flow. A similar flow-volume curve can be obtained by simply plotting expired flow against volume using an x-y recorder during a single forced expiratory vital capacity maneuver.
(From Murray JF, Nadel JA [eds]: Textbook of Respiratory Medicine, 3rd ed. Philadelphia, WB Saunders, 2000, p 787.)

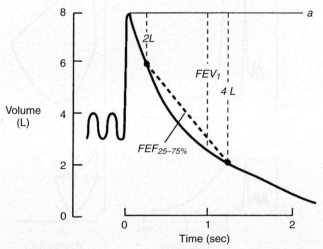

Fig 128–4

Determination of forced expiratory flow ($FEF_{25-75\%}$). A heavy dashed line connects two points on the volume-time curve of the forced vital capacity (FVC) maneuver. One point is marked when 25% of the FVC (2 L) has been exhaled; the other point is marked when 75% of the FVC (4 L) has been exhaled from the level of maximal inhalation indicated by the solid line (a). The elapsed time between these two points is 1 second; thus, the $FEF_{25-75\%}$ = 2 L/sec.
(From Murray JF, Nadel JA [eds]: Textbook of Respiratory Medicine, 3rd ed. Philadelphia, WB Saunders, 2000, p 786.)

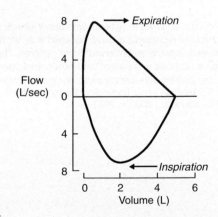

Fig 128–6

Flow-volume curve recorded during inspiration and expiration in a normal subject.
(From Murray JF, Nadel JA [eds]: Textbook of Respiratory Medicine, 3rd ed. Philadelphia, WB Saunders, 2000, p 788)

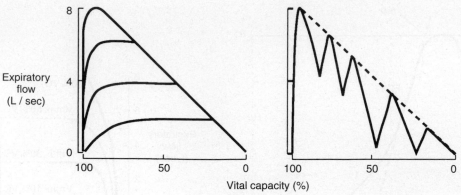

Fig 128-7
Left, Expiratory flow-volume curve recorded during a series of expirations with increasing efforts, finally producing a maximal flow-volume envelope. **Right,** Expiratory flow-volume curve recorded during coughing (solid line), approximating the maximal flow-volume envelope (dashed line). (From Murray JF, Nadel JA [eds]: Textbook of Respiratory Medicine, 3rd ed. Philadelphia, WB Saunders, 2000, p 789.)

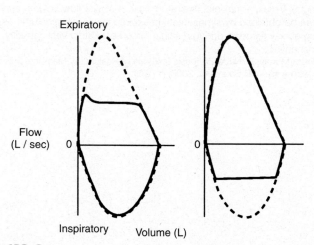

Fig 128-8
Flow-volume curves obtained in patients with upper airway obstruction. The dashed line represents a curve obtained in a normal subject with the same vital capacity as observed in the patients. The solid line indicates a curve obtained in a patient with intrathoracic obstruction *(left)* and another patient with extrathoracic obstruction *(right)*. (From Murray JF, Nadel JA [eds]: Textbook of Respiratory Medicine, 3rd ed. Philadelphia, WB Saunders, 2000, p 790.)

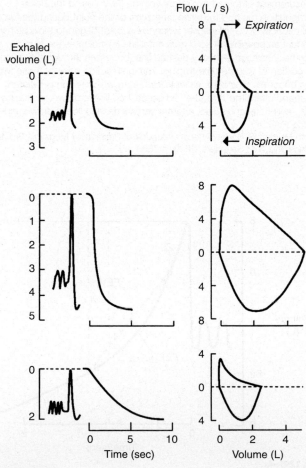

Fig 128-9
Spirogram and flow-volume curves obtained in a patient with a restrictive ventilatory defect *(top),* a normal subject *(middle),* and a patient with an obstructive ventilatory defect *(bottom).* (From Murray JF, Nadel JA [eds]: Textbook of Respiratory Medicine, 3rd ed. Philadelphia, WB Saunders, 2000, p 805.)

DEFINITION

The American Thoracic Society defines asthma as a "disease characterized by an increased responsiveness of the trachea and bronchi to various stimuli and manifested by a widespread narrowing of the airways that changes in severity either spontaneously or as a result of treatment." *Status asthmaticus* can be defined as a severe continuous bronchospasm.

PHYSICAL FINDINGS AND CLINICAL PRESENTATION

Physical examination varies with the stage and severity of asthma and may reveal only increased inspiratory and expiratory phases of respiration.

CAUSE

- Intrinsic asthma: occurs in patients who have no history of allergies; may be triggered by upper respiratory infections or psychological stress
- Extrinsic asthma (allergic asthma): brought on by exposure to allergens (e.g., dust mites, cat allergen, industrial chemicals)
- Exercise-induced asthma: seen most frequently in adolescents; manifests with bronchospasm following initiation of exercise and improves with discontinuation of exercise
- Drug-induced asthma: often associated with use of nonsteroidal anti-inflammatory drugs (NSAIDs), beta blockers, sulfites, and certain foods and beverages
- There is a strong association of the *ADAM 33* gene with asthma and bronchial hyperresponsiveness.

DIFFERENTIAL DIAGNOSIS

- Congestive heart failure (CHF)
- Chronic obstructive pulmonary disease (COPD)
- Pulmonary embolism (in adult and older patients)
- Foreign body aspiration (most frequent in younger patients)
- Pneumonia and other upper respiratory infections
- Rhinitis with postnasal drip
- Tuberculosis (TB)
- Hypersensitivity pneumonitis
- Anxiety disorder
- Wegener's granulomatosis
- Diffuse interstitial lung disease

WORKUP

- For symptomatic adults and children older than 5 years who can perform spirometry, asthma can be diagnosed after a medical history and physical examination documenting an episodic pattern of respiratory symptoms and from spirometry that indicates partially reversible airflow obstruction (>12% increase and 200 mL in FEV_1 after inhaling a short bronchodilator or receiving a short [2- to 3-week] course of oral corticosteroids). For children younger than 5 years, spirometry is generally not feasible. Young children with asthma symptoms should be treated as having suspected asthma once alternative diagnoses are ruled out.
- Following diagnosis, it is necessary to classify the severity of asthma and monitor at every visit. The following questions are important in assessing patients with asthma:
- In the past 2 weeks, how many times have you:
  - Had problems with coughing, wheezing, shortness of breath, or chest tightness during the day?
  - Awakened at night from sleep because of coughing or other asthma symptoms?
  - Awakened in the morning with asthma symptoms?
  - Had asthma symptoms that did not improve within 15 minutes of inhaling a short-acting $beta_2$ agonist?
  - Missed days from school or work?
  - Had symptoms while exercising or playing?
- What are your highest and lowest peak flow rates (Fig. 129–1) since your last visit?
- Has your peak flow dropped below ___ L/min (80% of personal best) since your last visit?

LABORATORY AND PULMONARY FUNCTION TESTS

Laboratory tests are usually not necessary and can be normal if performed during a stable period. The following laboratory and PFT abnormalities may be present during an acute bronchospasm:

- Arterial blood gases (ABGs) can be used in staging the severity of an asthmatic attack:
  - Mild: decreased Pao_2 and $Paco_2$, increased pH
  - Moderate: decreased Pao_2, normal $Paco_2$, normal pH
  - Severe: marked decreased Pao_2, increased $Paco_2$, and decreased pH
- Complete blood count (CBC), leukocytosis with left shift may indicate the existence of bacterial infection.
- Spirometry is recommended at the initial assessment and at least every 1 to 2 years after treatment is initiated and when the symptoms and peak expiratory flow have stabilized. Spirometry as a monitoring measure may be performed more frequently, if indicated, based on severity of symptoms and the disease's lack of response to treatment.
- Pulmonary function studies: during acute severe bronchospasm, FEV_1 is <1 L and peak expiratory flow rate (PEFR) is <80 L/min.

IMAGING STUDIES

- Chest x-ray: usually normal, may show evidence of thoracic hyperinflation (e.g., flattening of the diaphragm, increased volume over the retrosternal air space) (Fig. 129–2).
- Electrocardiography: tachycardia, nonspecific ST-T wave changes are common during an asthmatic attack; may also show cor pulmonale, right bundle branch block, right axial deviation, counterclockwise rotation.

STAGES OF ASTHMA AND TREATMENT

1. Mild intermittent asthma
   a. Symptoms less than two times weekly
   b. Asymptomatic or normal peak expiratory flows between exacerbations
   c. Exacerbations are brief (hours to days).
   d. No daily medications are needed. Use short-acting inhaled $beta_2$ agonists as needed (e.g., albuterol, terbutaline) as needed.
2. Mild persistent asthma
   a. Symptoms more often than two times weekly, but less than once daily
   b. Exacerbations may affect activity.
   c. Treat with daily low-dose inhaled corticosteroids and short-acting beta agonist as needed (consider mast cell degranulation inhibitors—e.g., cromolyn and nedocromil).

d. Although guidelines recommend daily treatment in patients with mild persistent asthma recent trials have shown that it may be possible to treat mild persistent asthma with short, intermittent courses of inhaled or oral corticosteroids when symptoms worsen, thus maintaining control with the least amount of medication without adverse effects on the clinical outcome.

3. Moderate persistent asthma

a. Daily symptoms or daily use of short-acting inhaled beta agonist

b. Exacerbations more than two times weekly, affecting daily activity and possibly lasting for days

c. Treat with moderate-dose inhaled corticosteroids and long-acting beta agonist (consider leukotriene receptor antagonist). Continue use of short-acting beta agonist.

4. Severe persistent asthma

a. Continual symptoms

b. Limited physical activity, frequent exacerbations

c. Treat with high-dose inhaled corticosteroids and long-acting beta agonist (may require oral steroids). Continue use of short-acting beta agonist.

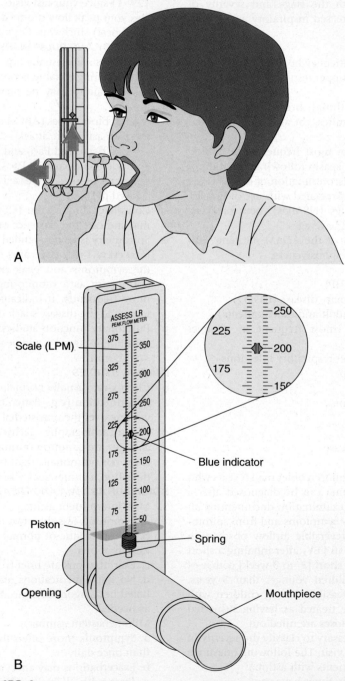

Fig 129–1

A, Patient using a peak flowmeter. **B,** Typical peak flowmeter used to monitor asthma severity.
(From Fireman P: Atlas of Allergies and Immunology, 3rd ed. St. Louis, Mosby, 2006.)

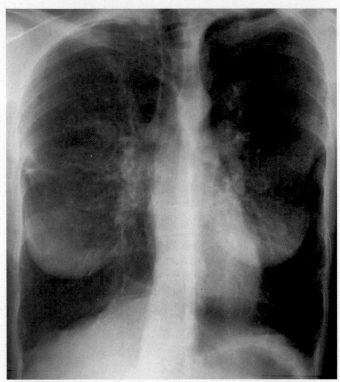

Fig 129–2

Posterioanterior chest radiograph in a patient with chronic and severe
asthma. The chest is overinflated. Bronchial wall thickening is also
present, mainly in the upper lobes.

(From Grainger RG, Allison DJ, Adam A, Dixon AK [eds]: Grainger &
Allison's Diagnostic Radiology, 4th ed. London, Harcourt, 2001.)

Chapter 130 Chronic obstructive pulmonary disease

DEFINITION

COPD is a disorder characterized by the presence of airflow limitation that is not fully reversible. COPD encompasses emphysema, characterized by loss of lung elasticity and destruction of lung parenchyma with enlargement of air spaces, and chronic bronchitis, characterized by obstruction of small airways (Fig. 130–1) and productive cough longer than 3 months'

duration for more than 2 successive years. Patients with COPD are classically subdivided into two major groups based on their appearance:

1. "Blue bloaters" are patients with chronic bronchitis; the name is derived from the bluish tinge of the skin (secondary to chronic hypoxemia and hypercapnia) and from the frequent presence of peripheral edema (secondary to cor pulmonale); chronic cough with production of large amounts of sputum is characteristic.

2. "Pink puffers" are patients with emphysema; they have a cachectic appearance but pink skin color (adequate oxygen saturation); shortness of breath is manifested by pursed-lip breathing and use of accessory muscles of respiration.

PHYSICAL FINDINGS AND CLINICAL PRESENTATION

- Blue bloaters (chronic bronchitis): peripheral cyanosis, productive cough, hemoptysis (Fig. 130–2) tachypnea, tachycardia
- Pink puffers (emphysema): dyspnea, pursed-lip breathing with use of accessory muscles for respiration, decreased breath sounds

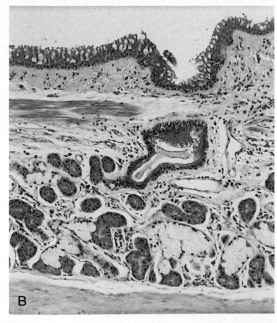

Fig 130–1
Bronchial wall in normal patient. **A,** Normal pseudostratified columnar epithelium with few goblet cells overlies smooth muscle and a submucosal gland. Cartilage is at the bottom of the figure (H&E, ×100). **B,** Bronchial wall from a patient with chronic bronchitis. Hyperplastic epithelium with mucous cell metaplasia overlies a hypertrophied submucosal gland (H&E, ×100).
(From Cohen J, Powderly WG: Infectious Diseases, 2nd ed. St. Louis, Mosby, 2004.)

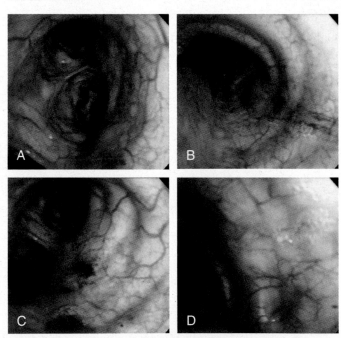

Fig 130–2
Chronic bronchitis is responsible for almost 25% of all cases of nonmassive hemoptysis. Bronchoscopy in this figure shows significantly hypertrophied and prominent submucosal capillaries in many lobar and segmental bronchi (**A-D**) in a patient with chronic bronchitis and frequent streaky hemoptysis. The capillaries tend to bleed on hard coughing and instrumentation with the bronchoscope. The capillaries are branches of the bronchial arterial system. Similar prominent mucosal capillary hypertrophy can be seen in bronchiectasis, mitral stenosis, and severe congestive cardiac failure. Early (within 48 hours of onset) bronchoscopy is more likely to provide the diagnosis than when it is delayed.
(From Gold WM, Murray JF, Nadel JA: Atlas of Procedures in Respiratory Medicine. Philadelphia, WB Saunders, 2002.)

- Possible wheezing in patients with chronic bronchitis and emphysema
- Features of chronic bronchitis and emphysema in many patients with COPD
- Acute exacerbation of COPD is mainly a clinical diagnosis and generally manifests with worsening dyspnea, increase in sputum purulence, and increase in sputum volume.

CAUSE
- Tobacco exposure
- Occupational exposure to pulmonary toxins (e.g., cadmium)
- Atmospheric pollution
- Alpha$_1$ antitrypsin deficiency (rare; <1% of COPD patients) (see Chapter 131)

DIFFERENTIAL DIAGNOSIS
- CHF (see Fig. 109–3)
- Asthma (see Fig. 129–2)
- Respiratory infections (see Fig. 139–2)
- Bronchiectasis (see Fig. 139–38)
- Cystic fibrosis (see Fig. 139–31)
- Neoplasm (see Fig. 132–5)
- Pulmonary embolism (see Fig. 143–3)
- Sleep apnea, obstructive
- Hypothyroidism

LABORATORY TESTS
- CBC may reveal leukocytosis with shift to the left during acute exacerbation.
- Sputum may be purulent with bacterial respiratory tract infections (Fig. 130–3). Sputum staining and cultures are usually reserved for cases refractory to antibiotic therapy.
- ABGs: normocapnia, mild to moderate hypoxemia may be present.
- Pulmonary function testing (PFT): the primary physiologic abnormality in COPD is an accelerated decline in FEV$_1$ from the normal rate in adults older than 30 years of approximately 30 mL/yr to almost 60 mL/yr. PFT results in COPD reveal abnormal diffusing capacity, increased total lung ca-

pacity and/or residual volume, fixed reduction in FEV$_1$ in patients with emphysema; normal diffusing capacity, reduced FEV$_1$ in patients with chronic bronchitis. Patients with COPD can generally be distinguished from asthmatics by their incomplete response to albuterol (change in FEV$_1$ <200 mL and 12%) and absence of an abnormal bronchoconstrictor response to methacholine or other stimuli. However, almost 40% of patients with COPD respond to bronchodilators.

IMAGING STUDIES
Chest x-ray (Fig. 130–4):
- Hyperinflation with flattened diaphragm, tending of the diaphragm at the rib, and increased retrosternal chest space
- Decreased vascular markings and bullae in patients with emphysema
- Thickened bronchial markings and enlarged right side of the heart in patients with chronic bronchitis

TREATMENT
- Weight loss in patients with chronic bronchitis
- Avoidance of tobacco use and elimination of air pollutants
- Supplemental oxygen, through nasal O$_2$ or a face mask to ensure oxygen saturation >90% measured by pulse oximetry
- Pulmonary toilet: careful nasotracheal suction is indicated only in patients with excessive secretions and inability to expectorate. Mechanical percussion of the chest as applied by a physical or respiratory therapist is often performed but generally ineffective with acute exacerbations of COPD.
- Pharmacologic treatment should be administered in a stepwise approach according to the severity of disease and patient's tolerance for specific drugs.
  1. Bronchodilators improve symptoms, quality of life, and exercise tolerance and decrease incidence of exacerbations.
  2. Short-acting beta$_2$ agonists (e.g., albuterol, metered-dose inhaler [MDI], one or two puffs every 4 to 6 hours PRN) are acceptable in patients with mild, variable symptoms. Long-acting inhaled agents (e.g., salmeterol or formoterol, one or two puffs twice daily are preferred in patients with mild to moderate or continuous symptoms.
  3. Anticholinergics (e.g., ipratropium [Atrovent] inhaler, two puffs four times daily) are also effective and are available in combination with albuterol (Combivent). Tiotropium (Spiriva HandiHaler) is a newer long-acting bronchodilator. It is effective for the long-term, once-daily maintenance treatment of bronchospasm.
  4. Addition of inhaled steroids is helpful. Phosphodiesterase inhibitors (theophylline) are reserved for patients unresponsive to the above measures.
- Acute exacerbation of COPD can be treated with:
  1. Aerosolized beta$_2$ agonists
  2. Anticholinergic agents, which have equivalent efficacy to inhaled beta-adrenergic agonists
  3. Short courses of systemic corticosteroids have been shown to improve spirometric and clinical outcomes.
  4. Use of noninvasive positive pressure ventilation (NIPPV) decreases the risk of endotracheal intubation and decreases intensive care unit (ICU) admission rates.
  5. The role of inhaled corticosteroids in COPD is controversial. Although some trials have demonstrated mild improvement in patients' symptoms and decreased frequency of exacerbations, most pulmonologists believe that these drugs are ineffective in most patients with COPD but should be

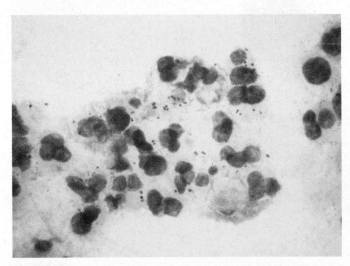

Fig 130–3
Gram-stained smear of sputum containing *Moraxella catarrhalis*. Sample from a patient suffering from an acute exacerbation of chronic bronchitis showing Gram-negative diplococci and leukocytes (*M. catarrhalis*). (From Cohen J, Powderly WG: Infectious Diseases, 2nd ed. St. Louis, Mosby, 2004.)

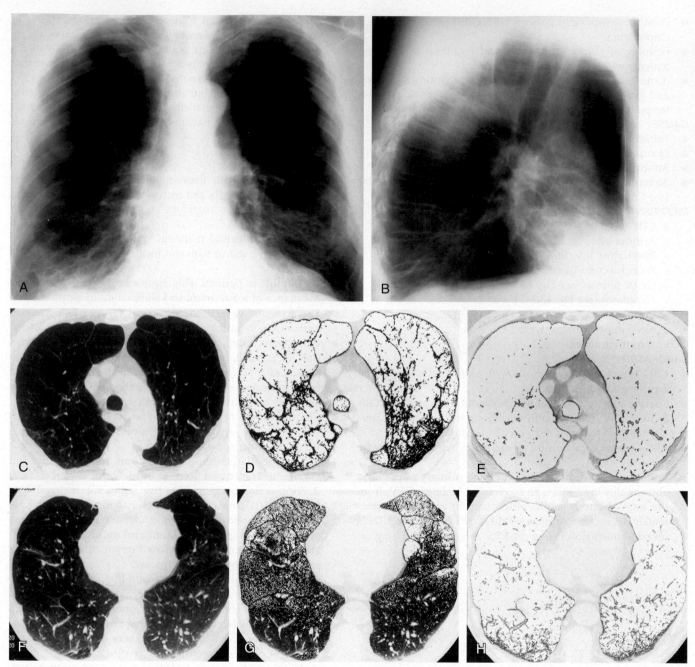

Fig 130–4

A 68-year-old man with severe upper lobe predominant emphysema. Posteroanterior **(A)** and **(B)** lateral chest radiographs demonstrate pulmonary hyperinflation with flat hemidiaphragms, a large retrosternal clear space, an enlarged anteroposterior chest dimension (barrel-shaped chest), hyperlucent upper lobes with a paucity of upper lobe vessels, and crowding of lower lobe vessels just above the diaphragm. **C,** Axial high-resolution CT scan with density-mask technique applied at attenuation thresholds of −900 HU **(D)** and −700 HU **(E)** and below. Similar images have been taken of the lower lobes **(F, G, H)**. The images demonstrate extensive low-attenuation regions without definable walls and sparse pulmonary vessels, more severe in the upper lobes than the lower lungs. Density mask technique images at −900 HU demonstrate the emphysema in white, whereas density-mask technique images at −700 HU and below outline the entire lung volume.

(From Grainger RG, Allison DJ, Adam A, Dixon AK [eds]: Grainger & Allison's Diagnostic Radiology, 4th ed. London, Harcourt, 2001.)

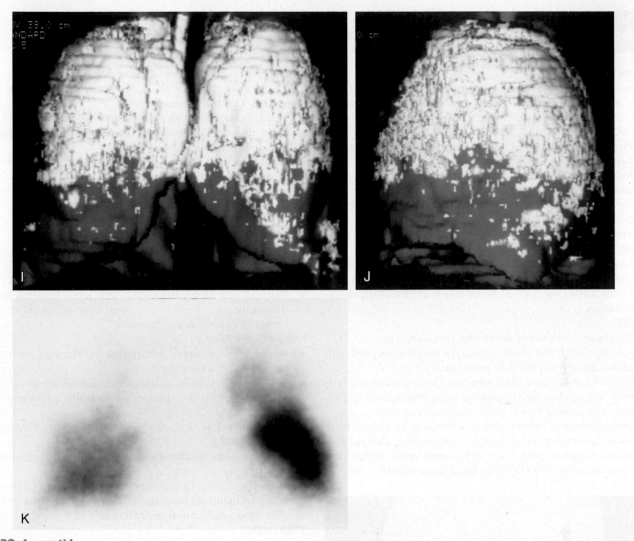

Fig 130–4—cont'd
A 68-year-old man with severe upper lobe predominant emphysema, continued. Anterior **(I)** and lateral three-dimensional **(J)** shaded surface display reconstructions of the lungs demonstrate the emphysema in white (all pixels less than −900 HU) superimposed on the gray-shaded total lung volume (all pixels less than −700 HU). Note the upper lobe distribution of emphysema; 66% of the upper halves of the lungs and 26% of the lower lung represents emphysema, for a CT ratio of 2.6. **K,** An anterior image from a planar ^{99m}Tc-macroaggregated albumin perfusion scan demonstrates focal absence of radiotracer in the upper portions of both lungs, corresponding to the CT areas of most severe emphysema.
(From Grainger RG, Allison DJ, Adam A, Dixon AK [eds]: Grainger & Allison's Diagnostic Radiology, 4th ed. London, Harcourt, 2001.)

considered for patients with moderate to severe airflow limitation who have persistent symptoms despite optimal bronchodilator therapy.
- Antibiotics are indicated in suspected respiratory infection (e.g., increased purulence and volume of phlegm).
  1. *Haemophilus influenzae, Streptococcus pneumoniae* are frequent causes of acute bronchitis.
  2. Oral antibiotics of choice are azithromycin, levofloxacin, amoxicillin-clavulanate, and cefuroxime.
  3. The use of antibiotics is beneficial in exacerbations of COPD presenting with increased dyspnea and sputum purulence (especially if the patient is febrile).
- Guaifenesin may improve cough symptoms and mucus clearance; however, mucolytic medications are generally ineffective. Their benefits may be greatest in patients with more advanced disease.

Chapter 131   Alpha₁-antitrypsin deficiency

DEFINITION
Alpha₁-antitrypsin deficiency is a genetic deficiency of the protease inhibitor, alpha₁-antitrypsin, that results in a predisposition to pulmonary emphysema and hepatic cirrhosis.

PHYSICAL FINDINGS AND CLINICAL PRESENTATION
- Physical findings and clinical presentation are varied and dependent on phenotype (see "Cause")
- Most often affects the lungs but can also involve the liver and skin
- Typically associated with early-onset, severe, lower lobe–predominant emphysema; bronchiectasis may also be seen
- Symptoms are similar to typical COPD presentation (dyspnea, cough, sputum production).
- Liver involvement includes neonatal cholestasis, cirrhosis in children and adults, and primary carcinoma of the liver.
- Panniculitis (Fig. 131–1) is the major dermatologic manifestation.

CAUSE
- Degree of deficiency is dependent on phenotype.
- MM represents the normal genotype and is associated with alpha₁-antitrypsin levels in the normal range.
- Mutation most commonly associated with emphysema is Z, with homozygote (ZZ) resulting in an approximately 85% deficit in plasma alpha₁-antitrypsin concentrations.
- Development of emphysema is believed to be a result from an imbalance between the proteolytic enzyme, elastase, produced by neutrophils, and alpha₁-antitrypsin, which normally protects lung elastin by inhibiting elastase.

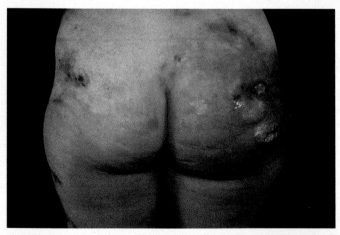

Fig 131–1
Alpha₁-antitrypsin deficiency–associated panniculitis. Note the extensive involvement of the buttocks in this young woman.
(Courtesy of Dr. M. R. Pittelkow, Mayo Clinic, Rochester, Minn.)

- Deficiency of alpha₁-antitrypsin increases risk of early-onset emphysema, but not all alpha₁-antitrypsin–deficient individuals will develop lung disease.
- Smoking increases risk and accelerates onset of COPD.
- Liver disease is caused by pathologic accumulation of alpha₁-antitrypsin in hepatocytes.
- Similar to lung disease, skin involvement is thought to be secondary to unopposed proteolysis in skin.

DIFFERENTIAL DIAGNOSIS
- See COPD (see Chapter 130)
- See cirrhosis (see Chapter 176)

WORKUP
- Suspicion for alpha₁-antitrypsin deficiency usually results from emphysema developing at an early age and with basilar predominance of disease.
- Suspicion for alpha₁-antitrypsin deficiency resulting in liver disease or skin involvement may arise when other more common etiologies are excluded.

LABORATORY TESTS
- Serum level of alpha₁-antitrypsin is decreased or not detected in severe lung disease.
- Investigate possibility of abnormal alleles with genotyping.
- Pulmonary function testing is generally consistent with typical COPD.
- Liver biopsy (Fig. 131–2) will identify liver involvement

IMAGING STUDIES
- Chest x-ray shows characteristic emphysematous changes at lung bases.
- High-resolution chest computed tomography (CT) usually confirms the lower lobe–predominant emphysema and may also show significant bronchiectasis.

TREATMENT
- Avoidance of smoking is paramount.
- Avoidance of other environmental and occupational exposures that may increase risk of COPD
- Acute exacerbations of COPD secondary to alpha₁-antitrypsin deficiency are treated in a similar fashion to typical COPD exacerbations.
- The goal of treatment in alpha₁-antitrypsin deficiency is to increase serum alpha₁-antitrypsin levels above a minimum protective threshold.
- Although there are several therapeutic options under investigation, IV administration of pooled human alpha₁-antitrypsin is currently the only approved method to raise serum alpha₁-antitrypsin levels.
- Organ transplantation for patients with end-stage lung or liver disease is also an option.

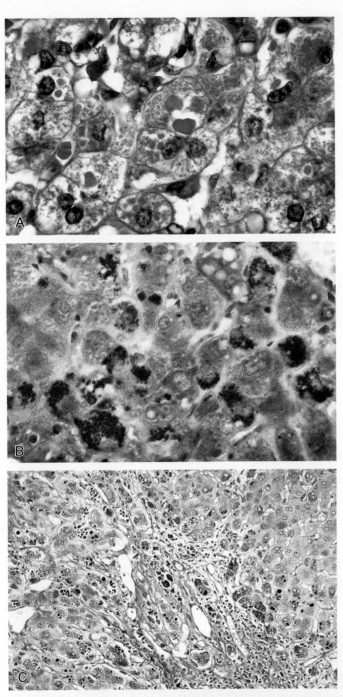

Fig 131–2
Alpha₁-antitrypsin deficiency. **A,** Variably sized eosinophilic globules are present in periportal hepatocytes. **B,** Immunostaining for alpha₁-antitrypsin confirms the nature of the globules. Larger globules tend to stain only around the periphery. **C,** Alpha₁-antitrypsin globules (demonstrated with periodic acid–Schiff stain after diastase digestion) tend to be concentrated in the periportal areas in noncirrhotic liver.
(From Silverberg SG, Frable WJ, Wick MR, et al [eds]: Principles and Practice of Surgical Pathology and Cytopathology, 4th ed. Philadelphia, Elsevier, 2006.)

Chapter 132   Lung neoplasms

DEFINITION

A primary lung neoplasm is a malignancy arising from lung tissue. The World Health Organization distinguishes 12 types of pulmonary neoplasms. The major types are squamous cell carcinoma, adenocarcinoma, small cell carcinoma, and large cell carcinoma. However, the crucial difference in the diagnosis of lung cancer is between small cell and non–small cell types, because the prognosis and therapeutic approach are different. Selective characteristics of lung carcinomas are as follows:

- Adenocarcinoma: represents 35% of lung carcinomas; frequently located in the midlung and periphery; initial metastases are to lymphatics, frequently associated with peripheral scars
- Squamous cell (epidermoid): 20% to 30% of lung cancers; central location; metastasis by local invasion; frequent cavitation and obstructive phenomena
- Small cell (oat cell): 20% of lung carcinomas; central location; metastasis through lymphatics; associated with lesion of the short arm of chromosome 3; high cavitation rate
- Large cell: 15% to 20% of lung carcinomas; frequently located in the periphery; metastasis to central nervous system (CNS) and mediastinum; rapid growth rate with early metastasis
- Bronchoalveolar: 5% of lung carcinomas; frequently located in the periphery; may be bilateral; initial metastasis through lymphatic, hematogenous, and local invasion; no correlation with cigarette smoking; cavitation rare

PHYSICAL FINDINGS AND CLINICAL PRESENTATION

- Weight loss, fatigue, fever, anorexia, dysphagia
- Cough, hemoptysis, dyspnea, wheezing
- Chest, shoulder, and bone pain
- Paraneoplastic syndromes
  1. Eaton-Lambert syndrome: myopathy involving proximal muscle groups
  2. Endocrine manifestations: hypercalcemia, ectopic ACTH, SIADH

3. Neurologic: subacute cerebellar degeneration, peripheral neuropathy, cortical degeneration
4. Musculoskeletal: polymyositis, clubbing (Fig. 132–1), hypertrophic pulmonary osteoarthropathy
5. Hematologic or vascular: migratory thrombophlebitis, marantic thrombosis, anemia, thrombocytosis, or thrombocytopenia
6. Cutaneous: acanthosis nigricans, dermatomyositis
- Pleural effusion (10% of patients), recurrent pneumonias (secondary to obstruction), localized wheezing
- Superior vena cava syndrome (see Chapter 103)
  1. Obstruction of venous return of the superior vena cava is most commonly caused by bronchogenic carcinoma or metastasis to paratracheal nodes.
  2. The patient usually complains of headache, nausea, dizziness, visual changes, syncope, and respiratory distress.
  3. Physical examination reveals distention of thoracic and neck veins, edema of face and upper extremities, facial plethora, and cyanosis.
- *Horner's syndrome:* constricted pupil, ptosis, facial anhidrosis caused by spinal cord damage between C8 and T1 secondary to a superior sulcus tumor (bronchogenic carcinoma of the extreme lung apex); a superior sulcus tumor associated with ipsilateral Horner's syndrome and shoulder pain is known as a *Pancoast tumor* (Fig. 132–2).

CAUSE

- Tobacco abuse
- Environmental agents (e.g., radon) and industrial agents (e.g., ionizing radiation, asbestos, nickel, uranium, vinyl chloride, chromium, arsenic, coal dust)

DIFFERENTIAL DIAGNOSIS

- Pneumonia (see Fig. 139–4)
- TB (see Fig. 139–36)
- Metastatic carcinoma to the lung
- Lung abscess (see Fig. 139–13)
- Granulomatous disease (see Fig. 137–14)

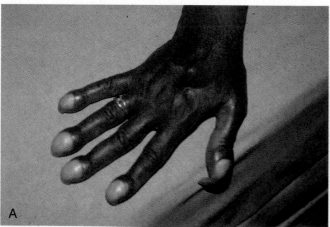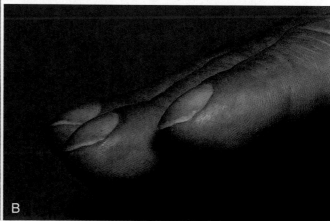

Fig 132–1

Clubbing. **A,** Hereditary clubbing without skin changes of pachydermoperiostitis. **B,** Acquired clubbing showing loss of the angle at the base of the nail.

(From Hochberg MC, Silman AJ, Smolen JS, et al [eds]: Rheumatology, 3rd ed, St. Louis, Mosby, 2003.)

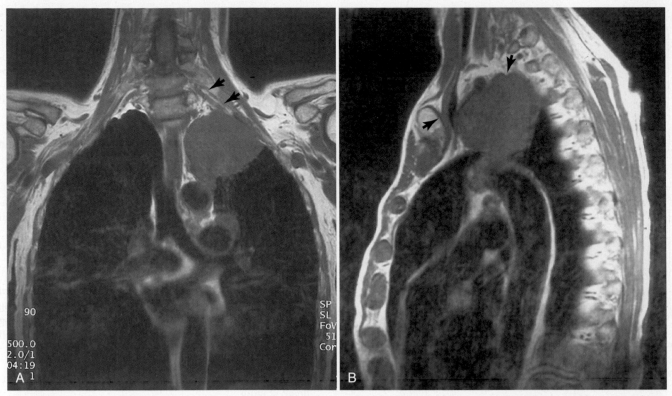

Fig 132–2
MRI scan of a Pancoast tumor. **A,** Coronal image. **B,** Sagittal image. A large tumor in the left upper lobe has invaded the soft tissues, displacing the vascular structures anteriorly *(arrows).* The brachial plexus has also been invaded *(arrowheads).*
(From Grainger RG, Allison DJ, Adam A, Dixon AK [eds]: Grainger & Allison's Diagnostic Radiology, 4th ed. London, Harcourt, 2001.)

- Carcinoid tumor
- Mycobacterial and fungal diseases (see Fig. 139–25)
- Sarcoidosis (see Fig. 137–6)
- Viral pneumonitis (see Fig. 139–16)
- Benign lesions that simulate thoracic malignancy:

1. Lobar atelectasis: pneumonia, TB, chronic inflammatory disease, allergic bronchopulmonary aspergillosis

2. Multiple pulmonary nodules: septic emboli, Wegener's granulomatosis, sarcoidosis, rheumatoid nodules, fungal disease, multiple pulmonary arteriovenous fistulas

3. Mediastinal adenopathy: sarcoidosis, lymphoma, primary TB, fungal disease, silicosis, pneumoconiosis, drug-induced (e.g., phenytoin, trimethadione)

4. Pleural effusion: CHF, pneumonia with parapneumonic effusion, TB, viral pneumonitis, ascites, pancreatitis, collagen-vascular disease

LABORATORY TESTS
Obtain a tissue diagnosis (Fig. 132–3). Various modalities are available:

- Biopsy of any suspicious lymph nodes (e.g., supraclavicular node)
- Flexible fiberoptic bronchoscopy (Fig. 132–4): brush and biopsy specimens are obtained from any visualized endobronchial lesions.

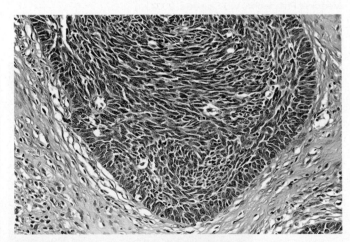

Fig 132–3
Squamous cell carcinoma, basaloid variant. Invasive tumor shows whorled, poorly differentiated, nonkeratinizing squamous cells with palisading around the edge in a manner reminiscent of cutaneous basal cell carcinoma.
(From Silverberg SG, Frable WJ, Wick MR, et al [eds]: Principles and Practice of Surgical Pathology and Cytopathology, 4th ed. Philadelphia, Elsevier, 2006.)

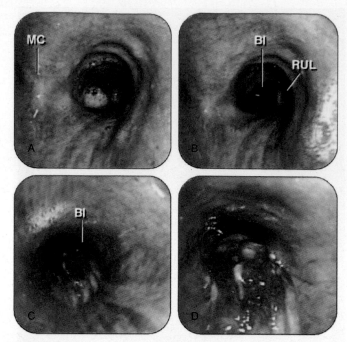

Fig 132-4
Bronchogenic carcinoma. Bronchoscopy is commonly used to diagnose respiratory neoplasms. **A,** View from the distal trachea reveals collection of mucus in the right bronchus intermedius (BI). **B,** Following suctioning of the mucus, an obstructing lesion can be seen in the BI. **C,** Close-up reveals partial obstruction of BI. **D,** Further close-up indicates distal extension of the tumor. It is important to clear the mucus and necrotic tissue before attempting brush or biopsy. Biopsy in this patient revealed squamous cell carcinoma. MC = main carina; RUL = right upper lobe.
(From Gold WM, Murray JF, Nadel JA: Atlas of Procedures in Respiratory Medicine. Philadelphia, WB Saunders, 2002.)

- Transbronchial needle aspiration: done via a special needle passed through the bronchoscope; this technique is useful to sample mediastinal masses or paratracheal lymph nodes.
- Transthoracic fine-needle aspiration biopsy with fluoroscopic or CT scan guidance to evaluate peripheral pulmonary nodules
- Mediastinoscopy and anteromedial sternotomy in suspected tumor involvement of the mediastinum
- Pleural biopsy in patients with pleural effusion
- Thoracentesis of pleural effusion and cytologic evaluation of the obtained fluid: may confirm diagnosis

IMAGING STUDIES

- Chest x-ray (Fig. 132-5): the radiographic presentation often varies with the cell type. Pleural effusion, lobar atelectasis, and mediastinal adenopathy can accompany any cell types.
- CT scan of chest (Fig. 132-6): to evaluate mediastinal and pleural extension of suspected lung neoplasms.
- Positron emission tomography (PET; Fig. 132-7), with ^{18}F-fluorodeoxyglucose (^{18}FDG-PET), a metabolic marker of malignant tissue, is superior to CT scanning in detecting mediastinal and distant metastases in non–small cell lung cancer. It is useful for preoperative staging of non–small cell lung cancer.

STAGING

- Following confirmation of diagnosis, patients should undergo staging.
1. The international staging system is the most widely accepted staging system for non–small cell lung cancer. In this system, stage 1 (N0, no lymph node involvement) and stage 2 (N1, spread to ipsilateral bronchopulmonary or hilar lymph nodes) include localized tumors for which surgical resection is the preferred treatment. Stage 3 is subdivided into 3A

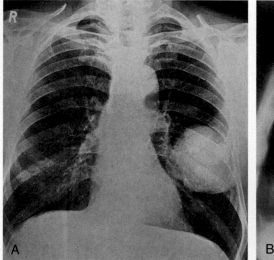

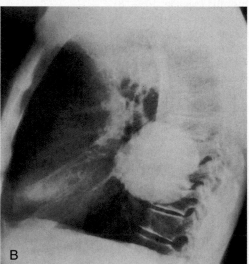

Fig 132-5
Bronchial carcinoma in left lower lobe showing typical rounded, slightly lobular configuration. The mass shows a notch posteriorly. **A,** posterior anterior view. **B,** lateral view.
(From Grainger RG, Allison DJ, Adam A, Dixon AK [eds]: Grainger & Allison's Diagnostic Radiology, 4th ed. London, Harcourt, 2001.)

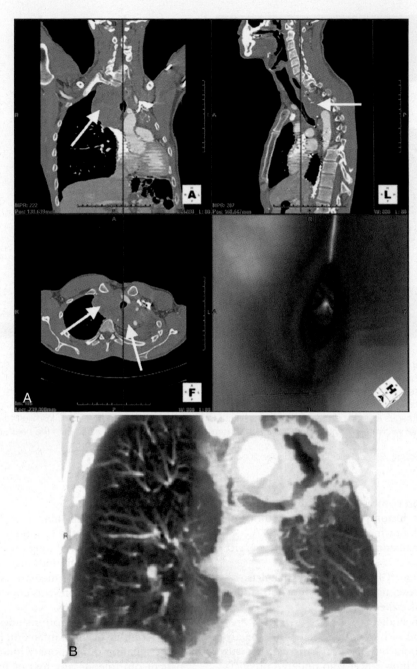

Fig 132–6
Lung cancer. **A,** Axial CT scans (lower left) shows a mediastinal mass *(arrows)* narrowing the airway. Coronal (top left) and sagittal (top right) reconstructed images show narrowing of the airway by mass *(arrows)*. Virtual bronchoscopy image (lower right) shows an endoluminal view of the narrowed airway. **B,** Coronal reconstruction of CT data in a different patient shows a cavitating mass in the left upper lobe.
(Courtesy of Dr. Leo Lawler, Johns Hopkins University School of Medicine, Baltimore.)

(potentially resectable) and 3B. The surgical management of stage IIIA disease (N2, involvement of ipsilateral mediastinal nodes) is controversial. Only 20% of N2 disease is considered minimal disease (involvement of only one node) and technically resectable. Stage 4 indicates metastatic disease. The pathologic staging system uses a tumor–nodal involvement–metastasis (TNM) system.

2. In patients with small cell lung cancer, a more practical accepted staging system is the one developed by the Veterans Administration Lung Cancer Study Group (VALG). This system contains two stages:
a. Limited stage: disease confined to the regional lymph nodes and to one hemithorax (excluding pleural surfaces)
b. Extensive stage: disease spread beyond the confines of limited stage disease

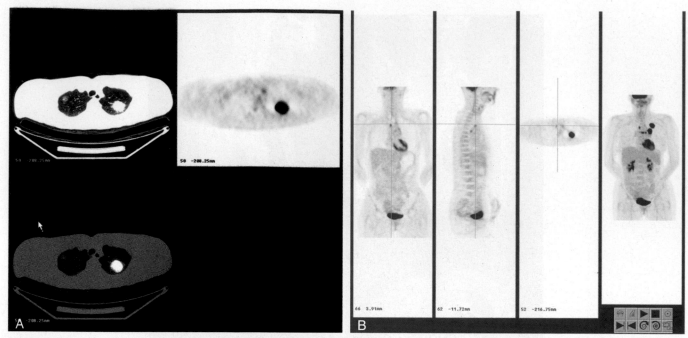

Fig 132–7

A, PET and CT scans. The upper left image is CT, the upper right image is PET, and the lower image is PET and CT data fused. The CT scan shows a smaller right apical nodule and a large left upper lung nodule. The PET scan shows increased uptake of ^{18}F-fluorodeoxyglucose (FDG) in the left apical nodule, consistent with cancer, whereas only minimal uptake is seen in the right apical lesion, consistent with benign disease. Fused PET and CT scans confirm the location of increased apical FDG uptake, as in the left lung nodule. **B,** Whole-body images from PET scans of the patient shown in **A**. The images include coronal, sagittal, transverse, and projection whole-body views, from left to right. They show cancer in the left upper lung, mediastinal involvement, and a right paratracheal tumor focus. Normal uptake is seen in the heart, brain, and excretory system (bladder).

(From Abeloff MD: Clinical Oncology, 3rd ed. Philadelphia, Elsevier, 2004.)

3. Pretreatment staging procedures for lung cancer patients, in addition to complete history and physical examination, generally include the following tests:
   a. Chest x-ray (posteroanterior [PA] and lateral views), electrocardiography
   b. Laboratory evaluation: CBC, electrolytes, platelets, calcium, phosphate, glucose, renal and liver function studies, ABGs; PPD in high-risk patient
   c. Pulmonary function studies
   d. CT scan of chest and PET scan: there is a >50% relative reduction in futile thoracotomies for patients with suspected non–small cell lung cancer who undergo preoperative assessment with ^{18}FDG-PET in addition to conventional workup
   e. Mediastinoscopy or anterior mediastinotomy in patients being considered for possible curative lung resection
   f. Biopsy of any accessible suspect lesions
   g. CT scans of liver and brain; radionuclide scans of bone in all patients with small cell carcinoma of the lung and patients with non–small cell lung neoplasms suspected of involving these organs
   h. Bone marrow aspiration and biopsy only in select patients with small cell carcinoma of the lung. In the absence of an increased lactate dehydrogenase (LDH) or cytopenia, routine bone marrow examination is generally not recommended.

TREATMENT
Non–small cell lung carcinoma
- Surgical resection is the best hope for cure in patients with operable non–small cell lung cancer.
   1. Surgical resection is indicated in patients with limited disease (not involving mediastinal nodes, ribs, pleura, or distant sites). This represents approximately 15% to 30% of cases at initial diagnosis.
   2. Preoperative evaluation includes review of cardiac status (e.g., recent myocardial infarction [MI], major arrhythmias) and evaluation of pulmonary function (to determine if the patient can tolerate any loss of lung tissue). Pneumonectomy is possible if the patient has a preoperative $FEV_1 \geq 2$ L or if the maximal ventilatory volume (MVV) is >50% of predicted capacity. Individuals with $FEV_1 >1.5$ L are suitable for lobectomy without further evaluation unless there is evidence of interstitial lung disease or undue dyspnea on exertion. In that case, the diffusing capacity of the lung for carbon monoxide (DL_{CO}) should be measured. If the DL_{CO} is <80% predicted normal, the individual is generally not operable.
   3. Preoperative chemotherapy should be considered in patients with more advanced disease (stage IIIA) who are being considered for surgery, because it increases the median survival time in patients with non–small cell lung cancer compared with the use of surgery alone.

4. Postoperative adjuvant chemotherapy (chemotherapy given after surgical resection of an apparently localized tumor to eradicate occult metastases) significantly increases 5-year survival in patients with completely resected stage IB or stage II non–small cell lung cancer and good performance status.

- Treatment of unresectable non–small cell carcinoma of the lung:

1. Radiotherapy can be used alone or in combination with chemotherapy; it is used primarily for treatment of CNS and skeletal metastases, superior vena cava syndrome, and obstructive atelectasis. Although thoracic radiotherapy is generally considered standard therapy for stage 3 disease, it has limited effect on survival. Palliative radiotherapy should be delayed until symptoms occur, because immediate therapy offers no advantage over delayed therapy and results in more adverse events from the radiotherapy.

2. Chemotherapy: various combination regimens are available. Current drugs of choice are paclitaxel plus carboplatin or cisplatin; cisplatin plus vinorelbine; gemcitabine plus cisplatin; carboplatin or cisplatin plus docetaxel. The overall results are disappointing, and none of the standard regimens for non–small cell lung cancer is clearly superior to the others. Gefitinib and erlotinib are oral inhibitors of epidermal growth factor receptor (EGFR) tyrosine kinase. Both agents are approved only for patients who have failed at least one prior chemotherapy regimen. Sensitivity of lung neoplasms to these agents is seen primarily in tumors with somatic mutations in the tyrosine kinase domain (more common in adenocarcinomas found in patients who have never smoked and in Asian patients).

3. The addition of chemotherapy to radiotherapy improves survival in patients with locally advanced, unresectable non–small cell lung cancer. The absolute benefit is relatively small, however, and should be balanced against the increased toxicity associated with the addition of chemotherapy.

Small cell lung cancer

- Limited stage disease: standard treatments include thoracic radiotherapy and chemotherapy (cisplatin and etoposide).
- Extensive stage disease: standard treatments include combination chemotherapy (cisplatin or carboplatin plus etoposide or combination of irinotecan and cisplatin)/
- Prophylactic cranial irradiation for patients in complete remission to decrease the risk of CNS metastasis

DISPOSITION

- The 5-year survival rate of patients with non–small cell carcinoma when the disease is resectable is approximately 30%.
- Median survival time in patients with limited stage disease and small cell lung cancer is 15 months; in patients with extensive stage disease, it is 9 months.

Chapter 133   Diseases of the pleura

A. PLEURAL EFFUSION

LOCALIZATION OF PLEURAL EFFUSION

1. Physical examination: dullness to percussion, loss of tactile fremitus
2. Chest x-ray (Fig. 133–1): posteroanterior view is usually sufficient in identifying the fluid collection, but in cases of equivocal effusions, a lateral decubitus chest x-ray can demonstrate layering out of the pleural fluid. Effusions larger than 1 cm on a lateral decubitus film are usually sufficiently large to remove at the bedside without additional imaging.

3. Fluoroscopy, ultrasonography, or CT guidance in performing thoracentesis if the fluid collection has the following qualities:
   a. Less than 10 mm thick
   b. Not freely movable on the lateral decubitus x-ray view

DIAGNOSTIC THORACENTESIS

1. Position patient in a sitting position with arms and head supported on a bedside adjustable table (Fig. 133–2).
2. Identify the area of effusion by gentle percussion.

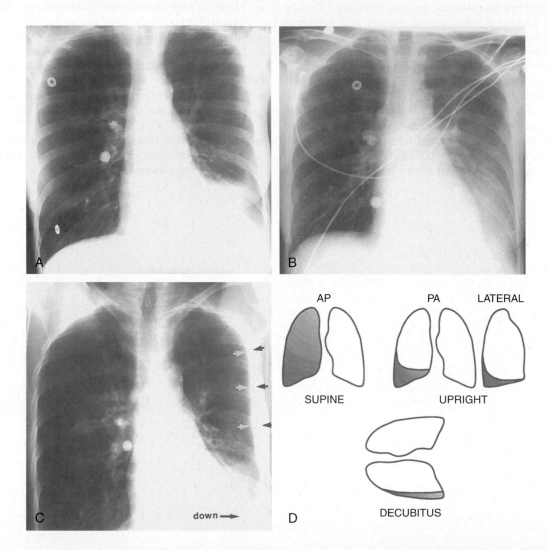

Fig 133–1

The appearance of pleural effusions depending on patient position. **A,** On an upright PA chest radiograph, a large left pleural effusion obscures the left hemidiaphragm, the left costophrenic angle, and the left cardiac border. **B,** On a supine AP view, the fluid runs posteriorly, causing a diffuse opacity over the lower two thirds of the left lung; the left hemidiaphragm remains obscured. This can easily mimic left lower lobe infiltrate or left lower lobe atelectasis. **C,** With a left lateral decubitus view, the left side of the patient is dependent, and the pleural effusion can be seen to be free-moving and layering *(arrows)* along the lateral chest wall. **D,** These findings are shown diagrammatically as well for a right pleural effusion. (From Mettler FA, Guibertau MJ, Voss CM, Urbina CE: Primary Care Radiology. Philadelphia, Elsevier, 2000.)

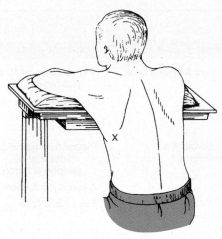

Fig 133–2
Patient position for thoracentesis.
(From Suratt PM, Gibson RS [eds]: Manual of Medical Procedures. St. Louis, Mosby, 1982.)

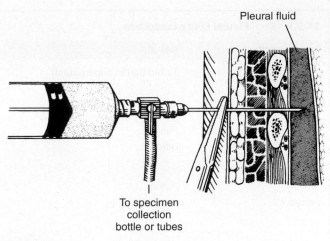

Pleural fluid

To specimen collection bottle or tubes

Fig 133–3
Fluid removal through thoracentesis needle and a three-way stopcock.
(From Suratt PM, Gibson RS [eds]: Manual of Medical Procedures. St. Louis, Mosby, 1982.)

3. Clean the area with povidone-iodine solution and maintain strict aseptic technique.
4. Insert the needle in the posterior chest (approximately 5 to 10 cm lateral to the spine, in the midpoint between the spine and the posterior axillary line) in one or two interspaces below the point of dullness to percussion.
5. Anesthetize the skin and subcutaneous tissues with 1% to 2% lidocaine using a 25-gauge needle.
6. Make sure that the needle is positioned and advanced above the superior margin of the rib (the intercostal nerve and the blood supply are located near the inferior margin). Walk the needle over the superior margin of the rib and deeper into the interspace, anesthetizing the intercostal muscle layers.
7. Apply negative pressure as the needle is advanced. In thin patients, this needle is often long enough to reach the pleural space. If pleural fluid is withdrawn, anesthetize the pleura adequately and note the depth at which it was reached. If it is not reached, use a longer 20- or 22-gauge syringe with 1% to 2% lidocaine, advance it slowly with negative pressure along the same track as the prior needle, anesthetize the pleura adequately, and advance the needle into the pleural space. If the purpose of the thoracentesis is for diagnosis only, a 30- to 50-mL syringe may then be attached and pleural fluid withdrawn for diagnostic studies.

If the purpose of the thoracentesis is for fluid removal, proceed further, as below. Place a clamp on the needle at skin level to mark the depth, remove the needle, and note the depth of insertion needed for the thoracentesis needle.
8. In the previous puncture site, insert a 17-gauge needle (flat bevel) attached to a 30-mL syringe via a three-way stopcock connected to a drainage tube (Fig. 133–3).
9. Slowly advance the needle (above the superior margin of the rib) and gently aspirate while advancing.
10. Keep a clamp or hemostat on the needle at the level previously marked to prevent it from inadvertently advancing forward. Many thoracentesis kits will have a catheter that can be advanced over the needle to remove the risk of having a sharp needle within the pleural space.
11. Remove the necessary amount of pleural fluid (usually 100 mL for diagnostic studies), but do not remove more than 1000 mL of fluid at any one time because of increased risk of pulmonary edema or hypotension (pneumothorax from needle laceration of the visceral pleura is also much more likely to occur if an effusion is completely drained).

PLEURAL FLUID EXAMINATION
Table 133–1 describes common tests performed on pleural fluid.

TABLE 133-1 Pleural fluid examination

Investigation	Result	Possible causes	Comment
Visual inspection	Turbid (turbid supernatant)	Chylothorax, pseudochylothorax	Triglycerides >110 mg/dL (1.2 mmol/L)
			Cholesterol >200 mg/dL (5.2 mmol/L)
	Pus	Empyema	
	Blood	Malignancy, tuberculosis, trauma, embolism	Pleural fluid hematocrit >50% that of peripheral blood
Smell	Putrid	Empyema	Anaerobic infection
Protein	<3g/dl (30 g/L)	Transudate (but also seen in malignancy, parapneumonic effusions)	See Light's criteria
	>3g/dl (30 g/L)	Exudate, effusion in diuretic treated cardiac failure	See Light's criteria
Lactate dehydrogenase	Pleural fluid to serum ratio >0.6	Exudate	Indicates pleural inflammation
	Pleural fluid level >two thirds upper limit normal serum level		
Amylase	Raised salivary amylase	Esophageal rupture, malignancy	
	Raised pancreatic amylase	Acute or chronic pancreatitis	
Glucose	<60 mg/dL (3.3 mmol/L)	Malignancy, tuberculosis, rheumatoid arthritis, parapneumonic effusion	
pH	In parapneumonic effusions:	Uncomplicated parapneumonic effusion	
	≥7.3		
	>7.2 and <7.3	May progress to empyema	Requires close observation; expert advice recommended
	≤7.2	Empyema	Tube drainage recommended
Ultrasound	Loculations	Empyema	Consider tube drainage

B. MESOTHELIOMA

DEFINITION
Malignant mesothelioma is a rare neoplastic lesion associated with asbestos exposure. There are three major histologic subtypes: epithelial (most common), sarcomatous, and mixed (epithelial, sarcomatous).

PHYSICAL FINDINGS AND CLINICAL PRESENTATION
- Dyspnea
- Nonpleuritic chest pain
- Fever, weight loss, sweats, fatigue, loss of appetite
- Dysphagia, superior vena cava syndrome, Horner's syndrome in advanced stages
- Auscultation may reveal unilateral loss of breath sounds.
- Dullness on percussion may be present.

CAUSE
- Asbestos exposure
- Other reported potentially causal factors include prior radiation therapy and extravasated Thorotrast, zeolite, and erionite fibers.

DIFFERENTIAL DIAGNOSIS
- Metastatic adenocarcinomas (from the lung, breast, ovary, kidney, stomach, or prostate)

LABORATORY TESTS
- Pleural biopsy (Fig. 133–4) for tissue diagnosis (Fig. 133–5). Diagnostic thoracentesis is generally insufficient for diagnosis, because pleural effusions may only reveal atypical mesothelial cells.
- Immunohistochemistry is useful to distinguish adenocarcinoma from epithelial malignant mesothelioma (mesotheliomas are generally carcinoembryonic antigen (CEA)–negative and cytokeratin-positive)
- Thrombocytosis and anemia may be found on initial laboratory evaluation.

IMAGING STUDIES
- Chest x-ray (Fig. 133–6) may reveal pleural plaques, pleural thickening, or calcifications in the diaphragm.
- CT scan (Fig. 133–7) of the chest and abdomen and bone scan are used to assess the extent of disease.

TREATMENT
- Operable patient (epithelial type, no positive nodes, confined to pleura, adequate PFT results): the two surgical techniques for therapeutic intervention are decortication (pleurectomy) and extrapleural pneumonectomy. Postoperative chemotherapy with cisplatin, doxorubicin, and cyclophos-

phamide and subsequent external beam radiation are used in some centers with limited success.

- Inoperable patient (disease too extensive, sarcomatous or mixed histology type, poor PFT results): supportive care plus or minus radiation therapy for symptoms or supportive care plus chemotherapy. Combined modality therapies (surgery, radiation therapy, chemotherapy, and biologics) have also been used to reduce both local and distant recurrences. The

combination of pemetrexed (an antimetabolite that inhibits enzymes involved in folate metabolism) and cisplatin is often used for chemotherapy of unresectable malignant pleural mesothelioma.

- Intrapleural instillation of cisplatin or biologics (e.g., interferons, interleukin-2) is generally limited to very early disease because it can only penetrate a limited depth of the tumor and there is a propensity of the pleural space to become progressively obliterated with advancing disease.
- The role of radiation therapy in the treatment of mesotheliomas remains uncertain. It is often used for palliation of local pain despite lack of trials to prove its usefulness.
- Obliteration of the pleural space (pleurodesis) with instillation of tetracycline, bleomycin, or biologic substances such as *Cryptosporidium parvum* into the pleural cavity is often tried when attempting to treat recurrent symptomatic pleural effusions.

C. PNEUMOTHORAX

DEFINITION

A spontaneous pneumothorax (SP) is defined as the accumulation of air into the pleural space, collapsing the lung. This can be primary SP (i.e., without any obvious underlying lung disease) or secondary SP (i.e., with underlying lung disease).

PHYSICAL FINDINGS AND CLINICAL PRESENTATION

- Sudden onset of pleuritic chest pain (90%)
- Dyspnea (80%)
- Tachycardia
- Diminished breath sounds
- Decreased tactile fremitus
- Hyperresonance

CAUSE

- In primary SP, rupture of small blebs usually located near the apex of the upper lobes is a common cause. Although rare, loud music has recently been documented as a contributing cause of primary SP.

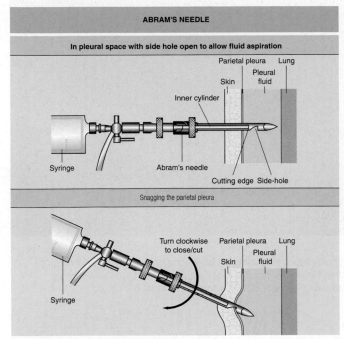

Fig 133–4
Abram's needle. The curved arrow shows clockwise rotation of the inner cylinder to close the side hole.
(From Cohen J, Powderly WG: Infectious Diseases, 2nd ed. St. Louis, Mosby, 2004.)

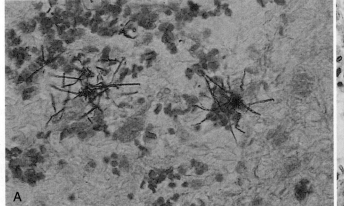 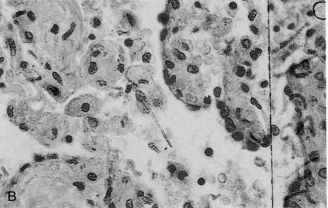

Fig 133–5
Mesothelioma. Asbestos bodies can be counted in properly prepared specimens and are generally expressed as the number of fibers per gram of wet weight lung. Although urban dwellers commonly have 500 fibers/g, some workers with significant induscial exposure have counts in the millions. Microscopic sections shown here exhibit asbestos fibers within lung tissue **(A)** and within a mesothelioma **(B)**, an extremely rare finding. A ferruginous body (not shown) is an iron-coated asbestos fiber.
(Courtesy of Brigham and Women's Hospital, Pathology Department, Boston.)

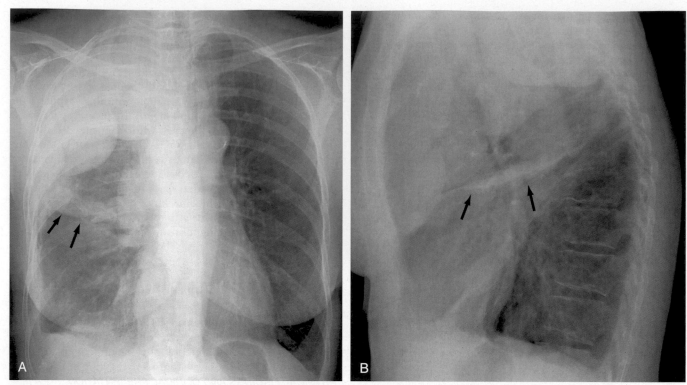

Fig 133–6
Malignant pleural thickening, PA **(A)** and lateral **(B)** chest radiographs. Malignant pleural thickening is characteristically lobulated and nodular. The extensive right-sided disease in this patient was caused by mesothelioma. Notice the extension of the tumors into the fissure *(arrows)*. (From Grainger RG, Allison DJ, Adam A, Dixon AK [eds]: Grainger & Allison's Diagnostic Radiology, 4th ed. London, Harcourt, 2001.)

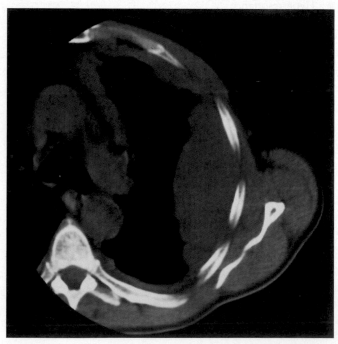

Fig 133–7
Malignant mesothelioma. Typical appearance of a lobulated, soft-tissue mass encasing the lung, with reduction in volume of the affected hemithorax. The overlying ribs are intact.
(From Grainger RG, Allison DJ, Adam A, Dixon AK [eds]: Grainger & Allison's Diagnostic Radiology, 4th ed. London, Harcourt, 2001.)

- In secondary SP, COPD is the most common cause but can also be associated with pneumonia, bronchogenic carcinoma, mesothelioma, sarcoidosis, tuberculosis, cystic fibrosis, and many other lung diseases.

DIFFERENTIAL DIAGNOSIS
- Pleurisy (see Fig. 143–3)
- Pulmonary embolism
- Myocardial infarction
- Pericarditis (see Fig. 113–3)
- Asthma (see Fig. 129–2)
- Pneumonia (see Fig. 139–4)

WORKUP
- Includes pulse oxymetry or ABGs, chest x-ray and, in some cases, CT scan of the chest

LABORATORY TESTS
- ABGs may show hypoxemia and hypocapnia secondary to hyperventilation.

IMAGING STUDIES
- Spontaneous pneumothorax is usually confirmed by chest x-ray (Fig. 133–8). X-ray findings reveal pleural line with absence of vessel markings peripheral to this line.
  1. Expiratory films are better at demarcating the pneumothorax pleural line.
  2. Films should be done with patient standing, not supine.
- CT scan can be done in suspected but difficult to visualize pneumothoraces.

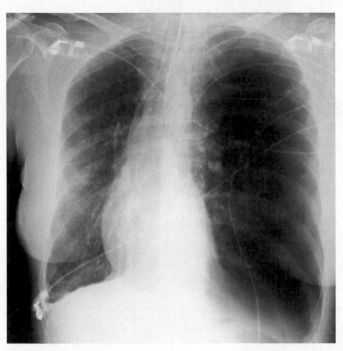

Fig 133–8

Pneumothorax. This AP recumbent chest radiograph of a 48-year-old woman 17 months after right lung transplantation for chronic obstructive pulmonary disease shows a large left tension pneumothorax, causing shift of the mediastinum to the right. The patient underwent a left upper lobectomy and a left lower lobe lobectomy for the treatment of recurrent left pneumothorax.

(From Grainger RG, Allison DJ, Adam A, Dixon AK [eds]: Grainger & Allison's Diagnostic Radiology, 4th ed. London, Harcourt, 2001.)

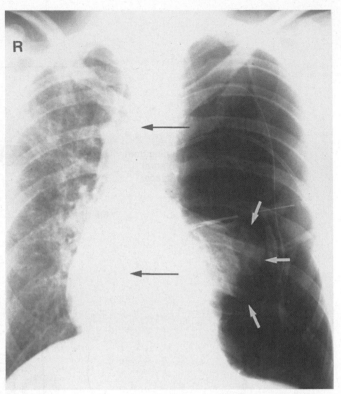

Fig 133–9

Tension pneumothorax. On this PA chest radiograph, the left hemithorax is very dark or lucent because the left lung has collapsed completely *(white arrows)*. The tension pneumothorax can be identified by the fact that the mediastinal contents, including the heart, are shifted toward the right *(black arrows)*, and the left hemidiaphragm is flattened and depressed.

(From Mettler FA, Guibertau MJ, Voss CM, Urbina CE: Primary Care Radiology. Philadelphia, Elsevier, 2000.)

TREATMENT

- Supplemental oxygen increases the rate of pneumothorax absorption.
- Cautious observation in the asymptomatic patient with <15% pneumothorax can be done but requires close daily outpatient monitoring.
- Aspiration using a small IV catheter in the second intercostal space midclavicular line attached to a three-way stopcock and a large syringe. Air is aspirated until resistance, excess cough by the patient, or <2.5 L of fluid is taken out. Repeat films are done immediately after aspiration and again in 24 hours.

- Chest tube insertion has been recommended for patients with primary SP who failed observation and simple aspiration and for all patients with secondary SP.
- There is no firm consensus on the optimal treatment (simple aspiration versus chest tube insertion) for a first episode of primary SP.
- In tension pneumothorax (Fig. 133–9), the mediastinal contents, including the heart, are shifted to one side. Treatment consists of emergent needle decompression (Fig. 133–10).

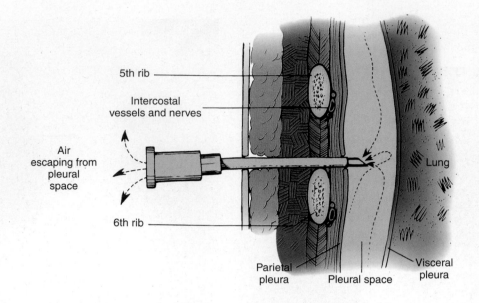

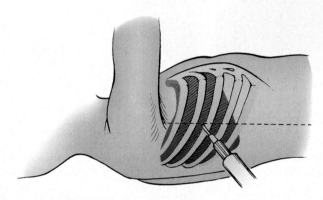

Fig 133–10
Needle decompression of tension pneumothorax. This procedure is performed only for tension pneumothorax in patients with hemodynamic instability.
(From Auerbach P: Wilderness Medicine, 5th ed. St. Louis, Mosby, 2006.)

Chapter 134 | Occupational lung disease

A. ASBESTOSIS

DEFINITION

Asbestosis is a slowly progressive diffuse interstitial fibrosis resulting from dose-related inhalation exposure to fibers of asbestos.

PHYSICAL FINDINGS AND CLINICAL PRESENTATION

- Insidious onset of shortness of breath with exertion is usually the first sign of asbestosis.
- Dyspnea becomes more severe as the disease advances; with time, progressively less exertion is tolerated.
- Cough is frequent and usually paroxysmal, dry, and nonproductive.
- Scant mucoid sputum may accompany the cough in the later stages of the disease.
- Fine end-respiratory crackles (rales, crepitions) are heard more predominantly in the lung bases.
- Digital clubbing, edema, and jugular venous distention are present.

CAUSE

- Inhalation of asbestos fibers (Fig. 134–1)

DIFFERENTIAL DIAGNOSIS

- Silicosis (see Fig. 134–4)
- Siderosis, other pneumoconioses (see Fig. 134–5)
- Lung cancer (see Fig. 132–5)
- Atelectasis (see Fig. 138–1)

LABORATORY AND PULMONARY FUNCTION TESTS

- Pulmonary function testing: decreased vital capacity, decreased total lung capacity, decreased carbon monoxide gas transfer
- ABGs: hypoxemia, hypercarbia in advanced stages

IMAGING STUDIES

- Chest x-ray
  - Small irregular shadows in lower lung zones
  - Thickened pleural, calcified plaques (present under diaphragms and lateral chest wall; Fig. 134–2)

TREATMENT

- Smoking cessation, proper nutrition, exercise program to maximize available lung function
- Home oxygen therapy PRN
- Removal of patient from further asbestos fiber exposure
- Prompt identification and treatment of respiratory infections
- Supplemental oxygen on a PRN basis
- Annual influenza vaccination, pneumococcal vaccination

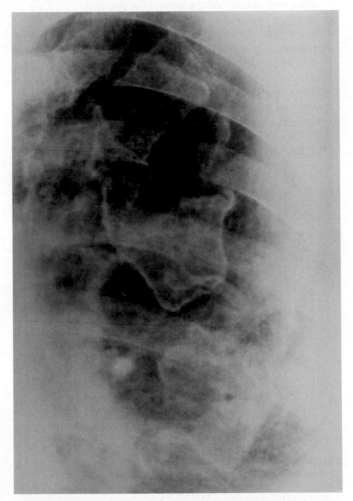

Fig 134–2
Pleural plaques. The margins of the lesions are well-defined and angulated.
(From Grainger RG, Allison DJ, Adam A, Dixon AK [eds]: Grainger & Allison's Diagnostic Radiology, 4th ed. London, Harcourt, 2001.)

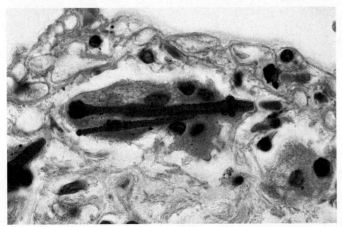

Fig 134–1
Asbestosis. Asbestos bodies have knobs at each end and a central body that appears beaded along a central thread-like fiber.
(From Silverberg SG, Frable WJ, Wick MR, et al [eds]: Principles and Practice of Surgical Pathology and Cytopathology, 4th ed. Philadelphia, Elsevier, 2006.)

B. SILICOSIS

DEFINITION
Silicosis is a lung disease attributable to the inhalation of silica (silicon dioxide) in crystalline form (quartz) or in cristobalite or tridymite forms.

PHYSICAL FINDINGS AND CLINICAL PRESENTATION
- Dyspnea
- Cough
- Wheezing
- Abnormal chest x-ray in an asymptomatic person

CAUSE
- Silica particles are ingested by alveolar macrophages, which in turn release oxidants causing cell injury and cell death, attract fibroblasts, and activate lymphocytes, increasing immunoglobulins in the alveolar space.
- Hyperplasia of alveolar epithelial cells occurs.
- Collagen accumulates in the interstitium.
- Neutrophils also accumulate and secrete proteolytic enzymes, which leads to tissue destruction and emphysema.
- Silica dust may be carcinogenic (not proved).
- Exposure to silicosis predisposes to tuberculosis.
- Some patients develop rheumatoid silicotic pulmonary nodules (Fig. 134–3) and may have arthritic symptoms of rheumatoid arthritis (Caplan's syndrome). Scleroderma has also been associated with silicosis.

DIFFERENTIAL DIAGNOSIS
- Other pneumoconioses, berylliosis, hard metal disease, asbestosis (see Fig. 134–2)
- Sarcoidosis (see Fig. 137–6)
- Tuberculosis (see Fig. 139–36)
- Interstitial lung disease (see Fig. 135–1)
- Hypersensitivity pneumonitis
- Lung cancer (see Fig. 132–5)
- Langerhans' cell granulomatosis (histiocytosis X) (see Fig. 328–2)
- Granulomatous pulmonary vasculitis (see Fig. 137–14)

DIAGNOSTIC IMAGING
- Chest x-ray (Fig. 134–4)

Chronic silicosis
- Characteristic finding: small, rounded lung parenchymal opacities
- Hilar lymphadenopathy with eggshell calcifications
- Pleural plaques (uncommon)

Accelerated silicosis (progressive massive fibrosis)
- Large parenchymal lesions resulting from coalesced small nodules

Acute silicosis
- Ground-glass appearance of the lung fields
- Chest CT scan
- Pulmonary function tests
- Combination of obstructive and restrictive changes with or without reduction in diffusing capacity
- Bronchoscopy with lung biopsy in uncertain cases

TREATMENT
- Prevention (industrial hygiene)
- Treatment of associated tuberculosis if present
- Supportive measures (oxygen, bronchodilators)
- Lung transplantation

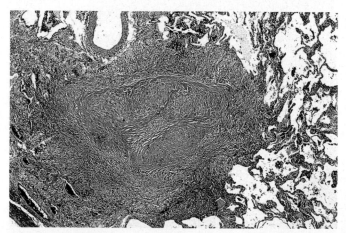

Fig 134–3
Silicosis. The diagnostic lesion of silicosis is the silicotic nodule, which is comprised of a central whorled mass of acellular hyalinized collagen, surrounded by layers of macrophages and plasma cells.
(From Silverberg SG, Frable WJ, Wick MR, et al [eds]: Principles and Practice of Surgical Pathology and Cytopathology, 4th ed. Philadelphia, Elsevier, 2006.)

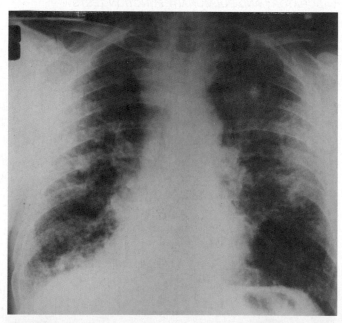

Fig 134–4
Silicosis. The nodules are coarser than those seen in coal worker's pneumoconiosis, with a linear component caused by fibrosis. There is eggshell calcification of the hilar lymph nodes.
(From Grainger RG, Allison DJ, Adam A, Dixon AK [eds]: Grainger & Allison's Diagnostic Radiology, 4th ed. London, Harcourt, 2001.)

C. PNEUMOCONIOSIS

DEFINITION
This is a parenchymal lung disease caused by chronic inhalation of coal mine dust and characterized pathologically by an inflammatory lesion composed of coal mine dust–filled macrophages surrounding respiratory bronchioles and accompanied by fibrosis.

PHYSICAL FINDINGS AND CLINICAL PRESENTATION
- Dyspnea
- Cough
- Wheezing
- Sputum production

DIFFERENTIAL DIAGNOSIS
- Other pneumoconioses, berylliosis, hard metal disease, asbestosis (see Fig. 134–2), silicosis (see Fig. 134–4)
- Sarcoidosis (see Fig. 137–6)
- Tuberculosis (see Fig. 139–36)
- Interstitial lung disease (see Fig. 135–1)
- Hypersensitivity pneumonitis
- Lung cancer (see Fig. 132–5)
- Langerhans' cell granulomatosis (histiocytosis X) (see Fig. 328–2)
- Granulomatous pulmonary vasculitis (see Fig. 137–14)

DIAGNOSTIC IMAGING
- Chest x-ray (Fig. 134–5)
- Chest CT scan
- Pulmonary function tests; reduced FEV_1 and FEV_1/FVC ratio
- Bronchoscopy with lung biopsy in uncertain cases

TREATMENT
- Prevention (industrial hygiene)
- Supportive measures (oxygen, bronchodilators)
- Lung transplantation

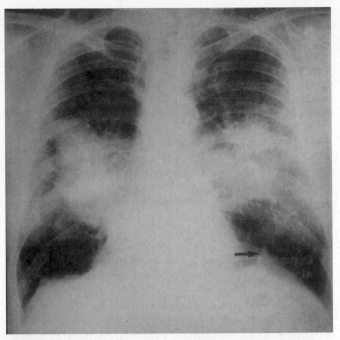

Fig 134–5
Coal worker's pneumoconiosis with progressive, massive fibrosis. Large, bilateral, soft tissue masses are present, which have caused shrinkage of the lungs. Note the angulation of the left hemidiaphragm *(arrow)* caused by traction on the inferior pulmonary ligament. (From Grainger RG, Allison DJ, Adam A, Dixon AK [eds]: Grainger & Allison's Diagnostic Radiology, 4th ed. London, Harcourt, 2001.)

Chapter 135 Interstitial lung disease

DEFINITION

Diffuse interstitial lung disease is a group of blood disorders involving the lung interstitium and characterized by inflammation of the alveolar structures and progressive parenchymal fibrosis.

PHYSICAL FINDINGS AND CLINICAL PRESENTATION

- The patient generally presents with progressive dyspnea and nonproductive cough; other clinical manifestations vary with the underlying disease process.
- Physical examination typically shows end-respiratory dry rales (Velcro rales), cyanosis, clubbing, and right-sided heart failure.

CAUSE

- Occupational and environmental exposures: pneumoconiosis, asbestosis, organic dust, gases, fumes, berylliosis, silicosis
- Granulomatous lung disease: sarcoidosis, infections (e.g., fungal, mycoba cterial)
- Drug-induced: bleomycin, busulfan, methotrexate, chlorambucil, cyclophosphamide, carmustine (BCNU), gold salts, tetrazolium chloride, amiodarone, tocainide, penicillin, zidovudine, sulfonamide
- Radiation pneumonitis
- Connective tissue diseases: systemic lupus erythematosus (SLE), rheumatoid arthritis, dermatomyositis
- Idiopathic pulmonary fibrosis: bronchiolitis obliterans, interstitial pneumonitis, desquamative interstitial pneumonia (DIP)
- Infections: viral pneumonia, *Pneumocystis* pneumonia
- Others: Wegener's granulomatosis, Goodpasture's syndrome, eosinophilic granuloma, lymphangitic carcinomatosis, chronic uremia, chronic gastric aspiration, hypersensitivity pneumonitis, lipoid pneumonia, lymphoma, lymphoid granulomatosis

DIFFERENTIAL DIAGNOSIS

- CHF (see Fig. 109-3)
- Chronic renal failure (see Fig. 203-6)
- Lymphangitic carcinomatosis
- Sarcoidosis (see Fig. 137-6)
- Allergic alveolitis (hypersensitivity pneumonitis)

LABORATORY TESTS

- ABGs provide only limited information; initially, ABGs may be normal but with progression of the disease, hypoxemia may be present.
- Anti–neutrophil cytoplasmic antibody (c-ANCA) is frequently positive in Wegener's granulomatosis.
- Anti–glomerular basement membrane (anti-GBM) and antipulmonary basement membrane antibody are often present in Goodpasture's syndrome.
- Pulmonary function testing: findings are generally consistent with restrictive disease (decreased vital capacity [VC], TLC, and diffusing capacity).
- Bronchoscopy with bronchioloalveolar lavage is useful to characterize the pulmonary inflammatory response. The effector cell population in patients with interstitial lung disease consists of two major cell types:
    1. Lymphocytes (e.g., sarcoidosis, berylliosis, silicosis, hypersensitive pneumonitis)
    2. Neutrophils (e.g., asbestosis, collagen-vascular disease, idiopathic pulmonary fibrosis)

IMAGING STUDIES

- Chest x-ray may be normal in 10% of patients.
- Ground-glass appearance is often an early finding (Fig. 135-1).
- A coarse reticular pattern is usually a late finding (Fig. 135-2).
- CHF causing interstitial changes on chest x-ray must always be ruled out.

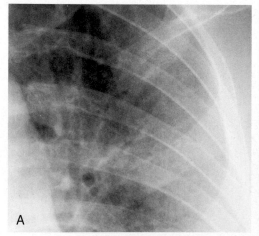 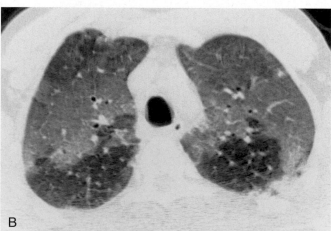

Fig 135–1

Ground-glass pattern. **A,** Ground-glass opacification in the left upper zone of a patient with *Pneumocystis* pneumonia. There is obscuration of some of the pulmonary vasculature, but this pattern is easily overlooked. **B,** The patchy distribution of the ground-glass opacification on CT scan makes this abnormality more easily recognizable.

(From Grainger RG, Allison DJ, Adam A, Dixon AK [eds]: Grainger & Allison's Diagnostic Radiology, 4th ed. London, Harcourt, 2001.)

- Differential diagnosis of interstitial patterns include the following: pulmonary fibrosis, pulmonary edema, *Pneumocystis carinii* pneumonia (PCP), TB, sarcoidosis, eosinophilic granuloma, pneumoconiosis, and lymphangitic spread of carcinoma.
- Gallium-67 scanning plays a limited role in the evaluation of interstitial lung disease because it is not specific and a negative result does not exclude the disease (e.g., patients with end-stage fibrosis may have a negative scan).

TREATMENT

- Treatment of infectious process with appropriate antibiotic therapy
- Supplemental oxygen in patients with significant hypoxemia
- Corticosteroids in symptomatic patients with sarcoidosis
- Immunosuppressive therapy in select cases (e.g., cyclophosphamide in patients with Wegener's granulomatosis)
- Treatment of any complications (e.g., pneumothorax, pulmonary embolism)

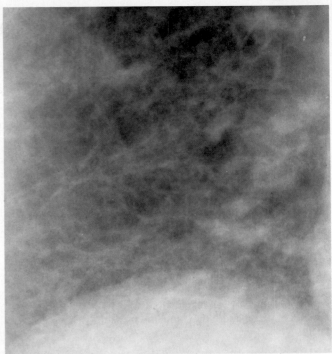

Fig 135–2
Interstitial lung disease reticular pattern. Magnified view of the right lower lung showing a
reticular pattern consisting of numerous intersecting lines creating a network in a patient with fibrosing alveolitis.
(From Grainger RG, Allison DJ, Adam A, Dixon AK [eds]: Grainger & Allison's Diagnostic Radiology, 4th ed. London, Harcourt, 2001.)

| Chapter 136 | **Idiopathic pulmonary fibrosis** |

DEFINITION

Idiopathic pulmonary fibrosis (IPF) is a specific form of chronic fibrosing interstitial pneumonia with histopathology characteristic of usual interstitial pneumonia (UIP).

PHYSICAL FINDINGS AND CLINICAL PRESENTATION

- Initial presentation is consistent and insidious exertional dyspnea and nonproductive cough. Over many months, dyspnea is the most prominent symptom
- Associated symptoms (fever, myalgia) may be present but are not common and suggest another diagnosis.
- Tachypnea to compensate for stiff noncompliant lung
- Fine bibasilar inspiratory crackles in >80% of patients, with progression upward as the disease advances
- Clubbing in 25% to 50% of patients
- Cyanosis, cor pumonale, right ventricular heave, peripheral edema may occur.
- Extrapulmonary involvement does not occur, but weight loss, malaise, and fatigue may be present.

CAUSE

- Unknown
- Numerous hypotheses, including environmental insults, such as metal and wood dust, infectious causes, chronic aspiration, or exposure to certain drugs (antidepressants)
- New research suggests little role for inflammation; fibrosis may be the major issue.

DIFFERENTIAL DIAGNOSIS

- Sarcoidosis (see Fig. 137–6)
- Drug-induced lung diseases
- Connective tissue disease with similar clinical and pathologic presentations
- Other idiopathic interstitial pneumonias:
  Desquamative interstitial pneumonia
  Respiratory bronchitis interstitial lung disease
  Acute interstitial pneumonia
  Nonspecific interstitial pneumonia
  Cryptogenic organizing pneumonia
  Bronchiolitis obliterans organizing pneumonia
  Occupational exposure (e.g., asbestos, silica) may cause pneumoconiosis that mimics IPF.
  - It is important to differentiate these from IPF pathologically because IPF responds better to treatment.

WORKUP

- Almost all patients have an abnormal chest x-ray at presentation, with bilateral reticular opacities most prominent in the periphery and lower lobes. Peripheral honeycombing may be seen (Fig. 136–1).
- High-resolution CT scan shows patchy peripheral reticular abnormalities with intralobular linear opacities, irregular septal thickening, subpleural honeycombing, and ground-glass appearance.
- Pulmonary function tests show restrictive impairment with reduced vital capacity and total lung capacity: obstructive picture only seen in smokers with IPF; reduced DL_{CO}

- Laboratory abnormalities: mild anemia; increases in erythrocyte sedimentation rate (ESR), LDH, C-reactive protein (CRP); low titers in ANA and rheumatoid factor (RF) are seen in up to 30% of patients.
- Limited role for bronchioalveolar lavage in diagnosis or monitoring IPF. A lone increase in lymphocytes is uncommon; if found, another diagnosis should be excluded.
- Gold standard for diagnosis is lung biopsy (open thoracotomy or video-assisted thorascopy) Hallmark features: heterogeneous distribution of parenchymal fibrosis against background of mild inflammation (UIP)
- Transbronchial lung biopsies generally do not provide a large enough sample to make the diagnosis.
- Among experienced clinicians, a combination of clinical and radiographic features is often enough to establish the diagnosis.

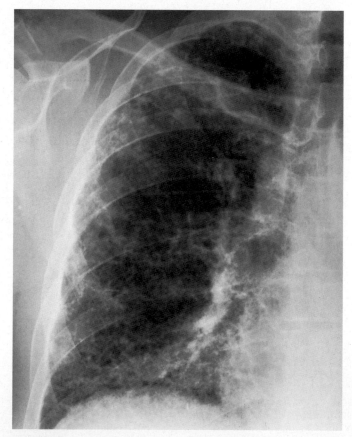

Fig 136–1
Honeycombing in classic idiopathic pulmonary fibrosis is predominantly peripheral and basilar.
(From Grainger RG, Allison DJ, Adam A, Dixon AK [eds]: Grainger & Allison's Diagnostic Radiology, 4th ed. London, Harcourt, 2001.)

- Lung biopsies are often not done because of other medical problems, especially severe COPD; however, they are critical to evaluate for the potential of a more treatable disease, especially in patients with any atypical features.
- The diagnosis will be missed in one third of new-onset IPF cases.

TREATMENT

- No proved treatment for IPF
- Much focus has been on anti-inflammatory medications, especially corticosteroids. Current thinking suggests that fibrosis, not inflammation, is a major issue.
- Many studies that have evaluated treatment responses have grouped together several forms of idiopathic interstitial pneumonia under the IPF label.

- A trial of corticosteroids at 0.5 mg/kg for 4 weeks, 0.25 mg/kg for 8 weeks, and then tapered down, combined with azathioprine or cyclophosphamide for 3 to 6 months is reasonable; 10% to 30% of patients may respond.
- Treatment is continued for up to 18 months if the patient improves or is stable. Long-term treatment is recommended only with objective evidence of continued improvement or stabilization.
- Single lung transplantation should be considered, especially in younger healthier patients.
- Treatment options include cytotoxic agents and antifibrotic agents (colchicine, pirfenidone, interferon gamma-1b), alone or in combination with corticosteroids.

Chapter 137   Pulmonary infiltrations

A. SARCOIDOSIS

DEFINITION

Sarcoidosis is a chronic systemic granulomatous disease characterized histologically by the presence of nonspecific, noncaseating granulomas (Fig. 137–1).

PHYSICAL FINDINGS AND CLINICAL PRESENTATION

- Clinical manifestations often vary with the stage of the disease and degree of organ involvement; patients may be asymptomatic, but a chest x-ray may demonstrate findings consistent with sarcoidosis . Almost 50% of patients with sarcoidosis are diagnosed by incidental findings on chest x-ray.

- Frequent manifestations:
  1. Pulmonary manifestations: dry, nonproductive cough, dyspnea, chest discomfort
  2. Constitutional symptoms: fatigue, weight loss, anorexia, malaise
  3. Visual disturbances: blurred vision, ocular discomfort, conjunctivitis, iritis, uveitis, retinitis (Fig. 137–2)
  4. Dermatologic manifestations: erythema nodosum (Fig. 137–3), macules, papules, subcutaneous nodules, erythematous plaques (Fig. 137–4) hyperpigmentation, lupus pernio
  5. Myocardial disturbances: arrhythmias, cardiomyopathy (Fig. 137–5)
  6. Splenomegaly, hepatomegaly
  7. Rheumatologic manifestations: arthralgias have been reported in up to 40% of patients.
  8. Neurologic and other manifestations: cranial nerve palsies, diabetes insipidus, meningeal involvement, parotid enlargement, hypothalamic and pituitary lesions, peripheral adenopathy

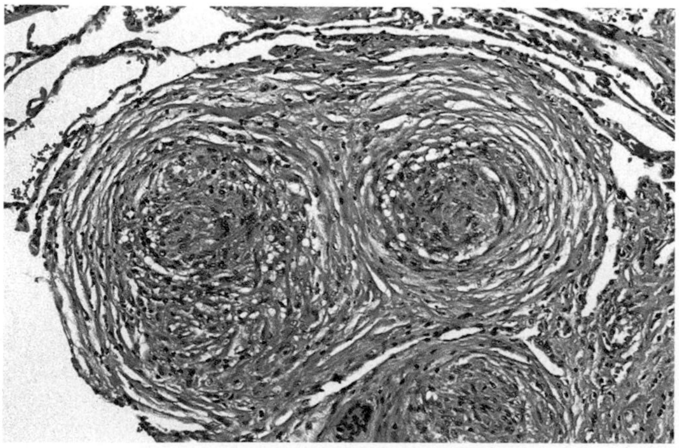

CAUSE

- Unknown. Multiple lines of evidence suggest that sarcoidosis may result from the interaction of multiple genes with environmental exposures or infection.

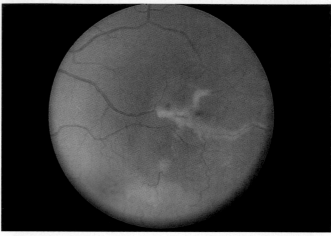

Fig 137–2
Retinal inflammatory vascular sheathing (vasculitis). This case occurred secondary to sarcoidosis.
(From Cohen J, Powderly WG: Infectious Diseases, 2nd ed. St. Louis, Mosby, 2004.)

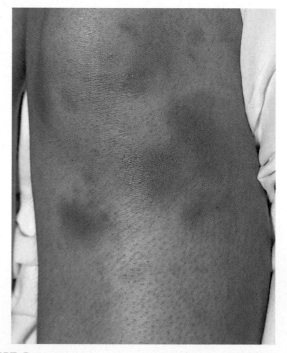

Fig 137–3
Erythema nodosum secondary to acute sarcoidosis.
(From Hochberg MC, Silman AJ, Smolen JS, et al [eds]: Rheumatology, 3rd ed. St. Louis, Mosby, 2003.)

Fig 137–1
Sarcoidosis. The hallmark of sarcoidosis is the presence of well-formed, tuberculoid granulomas without central necrosis.
(From Silverberg SG, Frable WJ, Wick MR, et al [eds]: Principles and Practice of Surgical Pathology and Cytopathology, 4th ed. Philadelphia, Elsevier, 2006.)

DIFFERENTIAL DIAGNOSIS

- TB (see Figs. 102–9 and 139–6)
- Lymphoma (see Figs. 102–7 and 316–3)
- Hodgkin's disease (see Fig. 315–3)
- Metastases
- Pneumoconioses (see Fig. 134–5)
- Enlarged pulmonary arteries
- Infectious mononucleosis
- Lymphangitic carcinomatosis
- Idiopathic hemosiderosis
- Alveolar cell carcinoma
- Pulmonary eosinophilia
- Hypersensitivity pneumonitis
- Fibrosing alveolitis
- Collagen disorders
- Parasitic infection

LABORATORY TESTS

Laboratory abnormalities:

- Hypergammaglobulinemia, anemia, leukopenia
- Liver function test (LFT) abnormalities
- Hypercalcemia, hypercalciuria (secondary to increased GI absorption, abnormal vitamin D metabolism, and increased calcitriol production by sarcoid granuloma)
- Cutaneous anergy to *Trichophyton, Candida,* mumps, and tuberculin
- Angiotensin-converting enzyme (ACE): elevated in approximately 60% of patients with sarcoidosis; nonspecific and generally not useful in following the course of the disease
- Biopsy should be done on accessible tissues suspected of sarcoid involvement (conjunctiva, skin, lymph nodes); bronchoscopy with transbronchial biopsy is the procedure of choice in patients without any readily accessible site.

IMAGING STUDIES

- Chest x-ray (Fig. 137–6) and CT scan (Fig. 137–7): adenopathy of the hilar and paratracheal nodes is a frequent finding; parenchymal changes may also be present, depending on the stage of the disease (stage 0, normal x-ray; stage I, bilateral hilar adenopathy; stage II, stage I plus pulmonary infiltrate; stage III, pulmonary infiltrate without adenopathy); stage IV, advanced fibrosis with evidence of honeycombing, hilar retraction, bullae, cysts, and emphysema).
- PFT results (spirometry and diffusing capacity of the lung for carbon dioxide): may be normal or may reveal a restrictive and/or obstructive pattern
- Gallium-67 scan (Fig. 137–8): will localize in areas of granulomatous infiltrates; however, it is not specific. The panda sign (localization in the lacrimal and salivary glands, giving a panda appearance to the face) is suggestive of sarcoidosis.

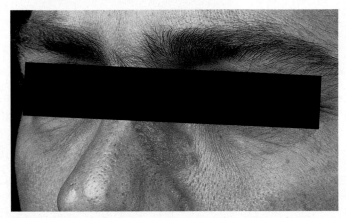

Fig 137–4
Sarcoidosis—erythematous plaque on the nose.
(Courtesy of the Institute of Dermatology, London.)

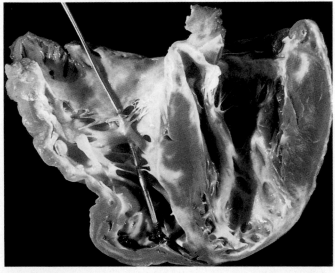

Fig 137–5
Explanted heart specimen showing gross pathologic features of sarcoidosis. A pacing wire traverses the tricuspid valve with its tip near the right ventricular apex. There is dense fibrous tissue replacing significant portions of the myocardium.
(From Hochberg MC, Silman AJ, Smolen JS, et al [eds]: Rheumatology, 3rd ed, St. Louis, Mosby, 2003.)

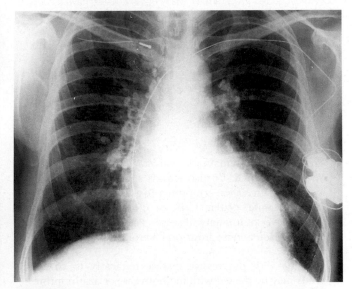

Fig 137–6
Eggshell calcification in sarcoidosis. There is extensive calcification of the hilar and mediastinal lymph nodes; the calcification has a peripheral (eggshell) configuration, particularly in lymph nodes at the right hilum. Cardiac involvement necessitated pacemaker implantation.
(From Grainger RG, Allison DJ, Adam A, Dixon AK [eds]: Grainger & Allison's Diagnostic Radiology, 4th ed. London, Harcourt, 2001.)

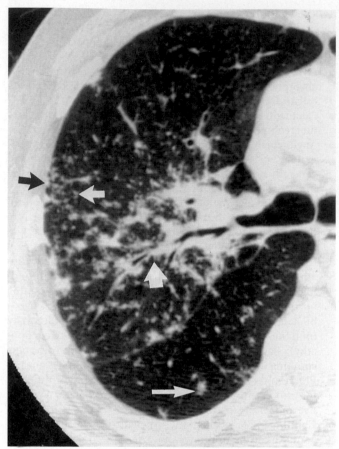

Fig 137-7
Pulmonary sarcoidosis on high-resolution CT. There are nodules of varying sizes: small interstitial nodules 1 to 2 mm in diameter *(intermediate white arrow),* irregular and larger nodules *(thin white arrow),* and subpleural nodules *(black arrow).* Many of the nodules have a subpleural distribution (particularly along the oblique fissure) as well as a bronchocentric distribution giving an irregular bronchovascular-lung interface *(broad white arrow).*
(Courtesy of Dr. F. Gleeson, Oxford, England.)

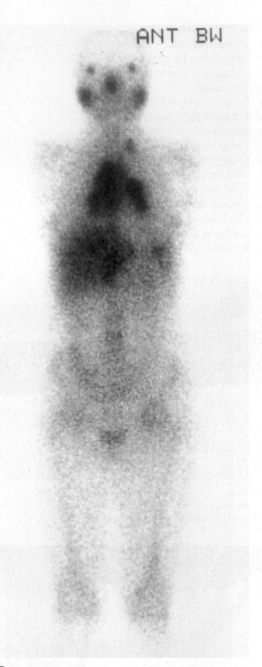

Fig 137-8
Abnormal gallium scan in sarcoidosis. The scan shows uptake in the lacrimal, parotid, and salivary glands (panda sign) as well as mediastinal lymph nodes (lambda sign) and lungs.
(From Hochberg MC, Silman AJ, Smolen JS, et al [eds]: Rheumatology, 3rd ed, St. Louis, Mosby, 2003.)

TREATMENT

- Corticosteroids remain the mainstay of therapy when treatment is required. Corticosteroids should be considered in patients with severe symptoms (e.g., dyspnea, chest pain), hypercalcemia, ocular, CNS, or cardiac involvement, and progressive pulmonary disease. Patients with interstitial lung disease benefit from oral steroid therapy for 6 to 24 months.
- Patients with progressive disease refractory to corticosteroids may be treated with methotrexate or azathioprine.
- Hydroxychloroquine is effective for chronic disfiguring skin lesions.
- NSAIDs are useful for musculoskeletal symptoms and erythema nodosum.
- Pulmonary rehabilitation in patients with significant respiratory insufficiency

B. WEGENER'S GRANULOMATOSIS

DEFINITION

Wegener's granulomatosis is a multisystem disease generally consisting of a classic triad:

1. Necrotizing granulomatous lesions in the upper or lower respiratory tract
2. Generalized focal necrotizing vasculitis involving both arteries and veins
3. Focal glomerulonephritis of the kidneys

Limited forms of the disease can also occur and may evolve into the classic triad. Wegener's granulomatosis can be classified using the ELK classification, which identifies the three major sites of involvement: *E*, ears, nose, and throat or respiratory tract; *L*, lungs; *K*, kidneys.

PHYSICAL FINDINGS AND CLINICAL PRESENTATION

- Clinical manifestations often vary with the stage of the disease and degree of organ involvement; 90% of patients present with symptoms involving the upper or lower airways or both.
- Frequent manifestations include the following:
  1. Upper respiratory tract: chronic sinusitis, chronic otitis media, mastoiditis, nasal crusting, obstruction and epistaxis, nasal septal perforation, nasal lacrimal duct stenosis, saddle nose deformities (resulting from cartilage destruction; Fig. 137–9)
  2. Lung: hemoptysis, multiple nodules, diffuse alveolar pattern, consolidation, abscesses (Fig. 137–10)
  3. Kidney: renal insufficiency, glomerulonephritis (Fig. 137–11)

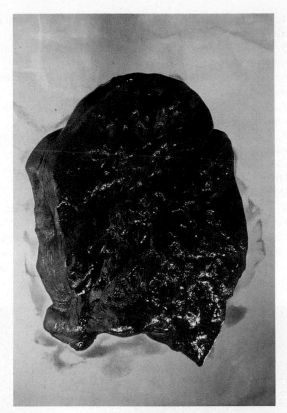

Fig 137–10
Wegener's granulomatosis. This postmortem lung specimen shows consolidation and numerous abscesses.
(Courtesy of Dr. B. Corrin, Brompton Hospital, London.)

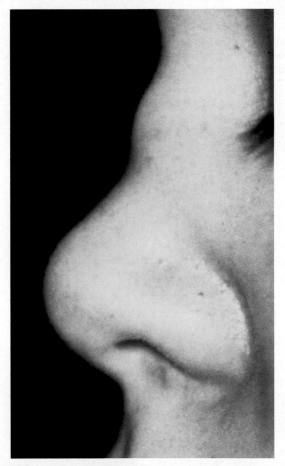

Fig 137–9
Saddle nose deformity resulting from collapse of the nasal cartilage in Wegener's granulomatosis.
(From Hochberg MC, Silman AJ, Smolen JS, et al [eds]: Rheumatology, 3rd ed, St. Louis, Mosby, 2003.)

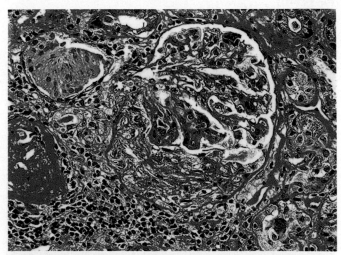

Fig 137–11
Segmental necrotizing glomerulonephritis with crescent formation, the classic renal histopathology in Wegener's granulomatosis. Immunofluorescence studies in this disease show a paucity of immunoglobulin and complement deposition.
(From Hochberg MC, Silman AJ, Smolen JS, et al [eds]: Rheumatology, 3rd ed, St. Louis, Mosby, 2003.)

4. Skin: necrotizing skin lesions, purpuric macules and papules (Fig. 137–12)

5. Nervous system: mononeuritis multiplex, cranial nerve involvement

6. Joints: monarthritis or polyarthritis (nondeforming), usually affecting large joints

7. Mouth: chronic ulcerative lesions of the oral mucosa, mulberry gingivitis

8. Eye: proptosis, uveitis, episcleritis, retinal and optic nerve vasculitis

CAUSE

● Unknown

DIFFERENTIAL DIAGNOSIS

● Other granulomatous lung diseases (e.g., sarcoidosis, [see Fig. 137–6] lymphomatoid granulomatosis [see Fig. 137–20], Churg-Strauss syndrome [see Fig. 137–16], necrotizing sarcoid granulomatosis, bronchocentric granulomatosis)

● Neoplasms (see Fig. 132–5) (especially lymphoproliferative disease)

● Goodpasture's syndrome
● Bacterial or fungal sinusitis
● Midline granuloma
● Viral infections (see Fig. 139–16)
● Other causes of glomerulonephritis (e.g., poststreptococcal nephritis)

LABORATORY TESTS

● Positive test for cytoplasmic pattern of ANCA (c-ANCA; Fig. 137–13)

● Anemia, leukocytosis

● Urinalysis: may reveal hematuria, red blood cell (RBC) casts, and proteinuria

● Elevated serum creatinine, decreased creatinine clearance

● Increased ESR, positive rheumatoid factor, and elevated CRP may be found.

IMAGING STUDIES

● Chest x-ray and CT (Fig. 137–14): may reveal bilateral multiple nodules, cavitated mass lesions, pleural effusion (20%). Up to one third of patients without pulmonary signs or symptoms have an abnormal chest x-ray.

● PFTs: useful in detecting stenosis of the airways

● Biopsy of one or more affected organs should be attempted; the most reliable source for tissue diagnosis is the lung (Fig. 137–15). Lesions in the nasopharynx (if present) can be easily biopsied but biopsy is positive in only 20%. Biopsy of radiographically abnormal pulmonary parenchyma provides the highest yield (>90%).

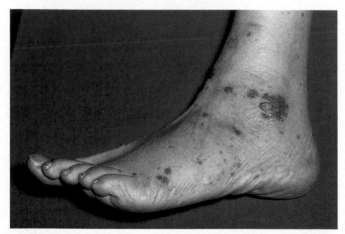

Fig 137–12
Wegener's granulomatosis—multiple purpuric macules and papules. (Courtesy of Dr. D. McGibbon, St. Thomas' Hospital, London.)

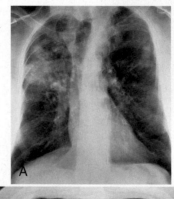

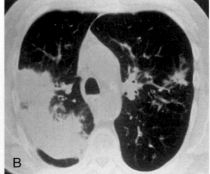

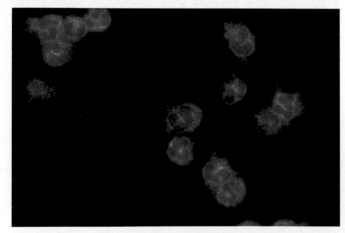

Fig 137–13
Wegener's granulomatosis—anti–neutrophil cytoplasmic antibodies. (Courtesy of Dr. G. Swana, St. Thomas' Hospital, London.)

Fig 137–14
Wegener's granulomatosis. **A,** Chest radiograph showing bilateral patchy air space opacities. There is no evidence of cavitation. **B,** CT through the upper zones with multifocal regions of dense parenchymal opacification.
(From Grainger RG, Allison DJ, Adam A, Dixon AK [eds]: Grainger & Allison's Diagnostic Radiology, 4th ed. London, Harcourt, 2001.)

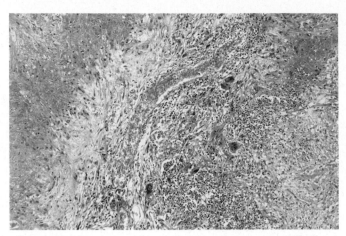

Fig 137–15
Wegener's granulomatosis. This lung section shows extensive necrosis associated with a granulomatous infiltrate containing Langhans' giant cells. These appearances resemble pulmonary tuberculosis.
(From McKee PH, Calonje E, Granter SR [eds]: Pathology of the Skin With Clinical Correlation, 3rd. St. Louis, Mosby, 2005.)

TREATMENT
- Prednisone and cyclophosphamide are generally effective and are used to control clinical manifestations; once the disease is controlled, prednisone is tapered and cyclophosphamide is continued. Other potentially useful agents in patients intolerant to cyclophosphamide are methotrexate, azathioprine, and mycophenolate mofetil.
- Trimethoprim-sulfamethoxazole (TMP-SMX) therapy may represent a useful alternative in patients with lesions limited to the upper or lower respiratory tracts in the absence of vasculitis or nephritis. Treatment with TMP-SMX also reduces the incidence of relapses in patients with Wegener's granulomatosis in remission. It is also useful in preventing *Pneumocystis carinii* pneumonia, which occurs in 10% of patients receiving induction therapy.
- Methotrexate represents an alternative to cyclophosphamide in patients who do not have immediately life-threatening disease.

C. CHURG-STRAUSS SYNDROME (ALLERGIC GRANULOMATOSIS)

DEFINITION
Churg-Strauss syndrome (CSS) refers to a systemic vasculitis accompanied by severe asthma, hypereosinophilia, and necrotizing vasculitis with extravascular eosinophil granulomas.

PHYSICAL FINDINGS AND CLINICAL PRESENTATION
The clinical picture of CSS typically consists of three partially overlapping phases:
1. The prodromal phase or allergic phase characterized by severe adult-onset asthma, with or without allergic rhinitis (70%), sinusitis, headache, cough, and wheezing. This phase can last several years.
2. The eosinophilic phase characterized by peripheral eosinophilia and eosinophilic infiltration of the lungs and GI tract, producing signs and symptoms of cough, fever, anorexia, weight loss, sweats, malaise, nausea, vomiting, abdominal pain, and diarrhea.

3. The vasculitic phase, which may involve any organ, including the heart (most frequent), lungs, peripheral nerves, kidneys, lymph nodes, muscle, CNS, and skin, and manifesting in chest pain, dyspnea, hemoptysis, migratory polyarthralgia, myalgias, peripheral neuropathy (mononeuritis multiplex), joint swelling, skin rash, and signs of CHF.

CAUSE
- The cause of Churg-Strauss syndrome is unknown. A hypersensitivity allergic response to an unknown allergen has been proposed, with eosinophils and IgE playing a direct role in pathogenesis.
- The National Institutes of Health (NIH) has investigated the observed relation between asthma therapy and the development of CSS and found that symptoms of CSS typically appear as oral corticosteroids are being decreased or discontinued. Development of the vasculitis appeared to be unmasked by the tapering of corticosteroids and not triggered by leukotriene receptor-1 antagonists, as previously reported.
- Reports of CSS developing in severe asthmatics after vaccination or desensitization therapy have led some to conclude that massive or nonspecific immunologic stimulation should be used with caution in patients with unstable asthma.
- Although similar and at times grouped with patients with polyarteritis nodosa (PAN) or Wegener's granulomatosis (WG), Churg-Strauss syndrome differs in the following ways:
  1. Churg-Strauss syndrome vasculitis involves not only small arteries but also veins and venules.
  2. Churg-Strauss syndrome, unlike PAN, predominantly involves the lungs. Other organs affected include the heart, GI, CNS, kidneys, and skin.
  3. Kidney involvement is much less common in CSS than in WG. Pulmonary lesions in WG usually involve the upper respiratory tract versus peripheral lung parenchyma in CSS.
  4. Churg-Strauss biopsy shows necrotizing vasculitis along with a granulomatous extravascular reaction infiltrated by eosinophils.

DIAGNOSIS
The American College of Rheumatology (ACR) has established criteria for the diagnosis of Churg-Strauss syndrome. At least four of the following six criteria must be met to make the diagnosis:
- Asthma
- Eosinophilia >10% on WBC count
- Mononeuropathy or polyneuropathy
- Migratory pulmonary infiltrates
- Paranasal sinus abnormalities
- Extravascular eosinophils on biopsy

The presence of any four or more of the six criteria yields a sensitivity of 85% and a specificity of 99.7%. The combination of asthma and eosinophilia in patients with vasculitis was found by the ACR to be 90% sensitive and 99% specific for CSS.

DIFFERENTIAL DIAGNOSIS
- Polyarteritis nodosa (see Fig. 300–4)
- Wegener's granulomatosis (see Fig. 137–14)
- Sarcoidosis (see Fig. 137–6)
- Löffler's syndrome

- Henoch-Schönlein purpura
- Allergic bronchopulmonary aspergillosis (see Fig. 336–11)
- Rheumatoid arthritis (see Fig. 291–7)
- Leukocytoclastic vasculitis

LABORATORY TESTS

- CBC with differential may reveal one diagnostic criterion—eosinophilia with counts ranging from 5,000 to 10,000 eosinophils/mm³.
- ESR is usually elevated as a marker of inflammation.
- Blood urea nitrogen (BUN) and creatinine may be elevated, suggesting renal involvement.
- Urinalysis may show hematuria and proteinuria.
- 24-hour urine for protein if higher than than 1 g/day is a poor prognostic factor.
- ANCAs, although not diagnostic of Churg-Strauss syndrome, are found in up to 70% of patients, usually with a perinuclear staining pattern.
- Stools may be occult blood positive because of enteric involvement during eosinophilic phase.
- Aspartate transaminase (AST), alanine aminotransferase (ALT), and creatine phosphokinase (CPK) may indicate liver or muscle (skeletal or cardiac) involvement.
- RA and ANA may be positive.
- Biopsy substantiates the diagnosis. Surgical lung biopsy is the gold standard. Transbronchial biopsy is rarely helpful. Necrotizing vasculitis and extravascular necrotizing granulomas, usually with eosinophilic infiltrates, are suggestive of CSS. The presence of eosinophils in extravascular tissues is most specific for CSS.

IMAGING STUDIES

- Chest x-ray is abnormal in 37% to 77% of cases and can show asymmetrical, patchy, migratory infiltrates, interstitial lung disease, or nodular infiltrates. Small pleural effusions are found in 29% of cases. CT (Fig. 137–16) may reveal nodules and ground-glass attenuation.
- Lung lesions in CSS are noncavitating, as opposed to those characteristic of Wegener's granulomatosis.
- Paranasal sinus films may reveal sinus opacification.
- Angiography is sometimes done in patients with mesenteric ischemia or renal involvement.

TREATMENT

- Corticosteroids are the treatment of choice.
- A drop in the eosinophil count and ESR documents a response. ANCAs do not reliably correspond with disease activity.
- Cyclophosphamide plus corticosteroids are used in patients with multiorgan involvement and poor prognostic factors. Azathioprine or high-dose IV immunoglobulin (IVIg) have shown benefit in patients with severe disease and in patients unresponsive to corticosteroids. Corticosteroids in combination with interferon-alfa have also been used in refractory cases.
- Many patients with persistent symptoms of asthma will require long-term corticosteroids, even if vasculitis is no longer present.

D. GOODPASTURE'S SYNDROME

DEFINITION

Goodpasture's syndrome is characterized by the idiopathic recurrence of alveolar hemorrhage (Fig. 137–17) and rapidly progressive glomerulonephritis. It can also be defined by the triad of glomerulonephritis, pulmonary hemorrhage, and antibody to basement membrane antigens.

PHYSICAL FINDINGS AND CLINICAL PRESENTATION

- Dyspnea, cough, hemoptysis

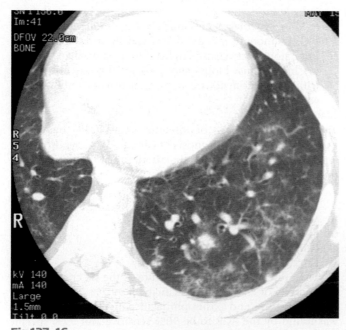

Fig 137–16
Sixteen-year-old woman with Churg-Strauss vasculitis. High-resolution CT scan shows patchy ground-glass attenuation and several nodules. The largest nodule is surrounded by a halo of ground-glass attenuation, suggestive of pulmonary hemorrhage.
(From Grainger RG, Allison DJ, Adam A, Dixon AK [eds]: Grainger & Allison's Diagnostic Radiology, 4th ed. London, Harcourt, 2001.)

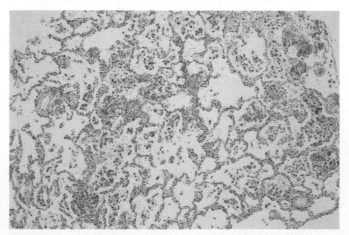

Fig 137–17
Alveolar hemorrhage in a patient with Goodpasture's syndrome; open lung biopsy.
(Courtesy of Dr. E. Mary Thompson.)

- Skin pallor, fever, arthralgias (may be mild or absent at the time of initial presentation)

CAUSE
- Presence of glomerular basement membrane (GBM) antibody deposition in kidneys and lungs with subsequent pulmonary hemorrhage and glomerulonephritis (Fig. 137–18)

DIFFERENTIAL DIAGNOSIS
- Wegener's granulomatosis (see Fig. 137–14)
- SLE (see Fig. 293–5)
- Systemic necrotizing vasculitis
- Idiopathic rapidly progressive glomerulonephritis
- Drug-induced renal pulmonary disease (e.g., penicillamine)

LABORATORY TESTS
- Presence of circulating serum anti-GBM antibodies
- Absence of circulating immunocomplexes, antineutrophils, cytoplasmic antibodies, and cryoglobulins

- Urinalysis revealing microscopic hematuria and proteinuria
- Elevated BUN and creatinine from rapidly progressive glomerulonephritis
- Immunofluorescence studies of renal biopsy material: linear deposits of anti-GBM antibody, often accompanied by C3 deposition
- Anemia from iron deficiency (secondary to blood loss and iron sequestration in the lungs)

IMAGING STUDIES
- Chest x-ray: fluffy alveolar infiltrates, evidence of pulmonary hemorrhage (Fig. 137–19)

TREATMENT
- Plasma exchange therapy
- Immunosuppressive therapy with prednisone and cyclophosphamide
- Dialysis support in patients with renal failure

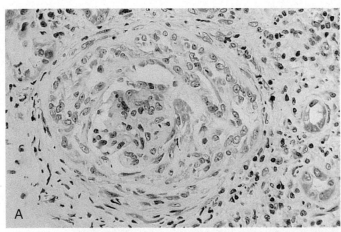 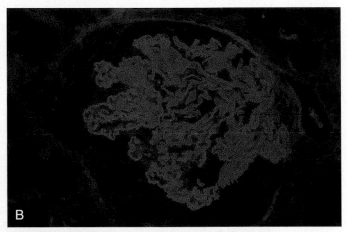

Fig 137–18
Renal biopsy in Goodpasture's syndrome. **A,** Glomerulus from a patient with Goodpasture's syndrome, showing a recent, mostly cellular crescent. **B,** Direct immunofluorescence study showing ribbon-like linear deposition of IgG along the glomerular basement membrane (GBM). The glomerular tuft is slightly compressed by cellular proliferation, forming a crescent.
(Courtesy of Dr. Richard Herriot)

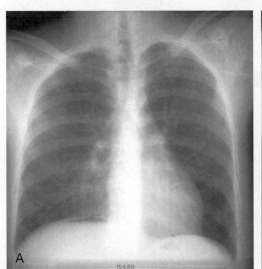 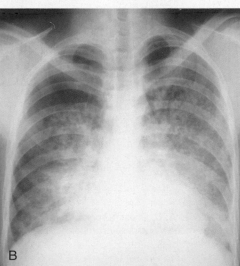

Fig 137–19
A, Chest radiograph of patient with lung hemorrhage. **B,** Radiograph taken 4 days later shows the evolution of alveolar shadowing caused by lung hemorrhage.
(From Johnson RJ, Feehally J: Comprehensive Clinical Nephrology, 2nd ed. St. Louis, Mosby, 2000.)

E. LYMPHOMATOID GRANULOMATOSIS

DEFINITION

- Lymphomatoid granulomatosis (LG) is an angiocentric and angiodestructive lymphoproliferative disorder associated with the transformation of B lymphocytes by Epstein-Barr virus (EBV).
- Although the lesions are characterized by angioinvasion of both reactive and atypical lymphocytes, the disorder is not an inflammatory vasculitis in the classic sense. Rather, it comprises part of a disease continuum, one end of which mimics systemic vasculitis clinically. At the other end of this continuum, the pathologic process merges with an aggressive form of diffuse, large B-cell lymphoma.
- Because of its propensity to cause constitutional symptoms, lung nodules, renal dysfunction, and a polymorphic inflammatory infiltrate associated with necrosis, this disorder may mimic Wegener's granulomatosis

CLINICAL PRESENTATION

- Most patients with LG have pulmonary involvement manifesting with cough, pleuritic chest pain, and dyspnea.
- Pulmonary nodules are a classic manifestation (Fig. 137–20).
- Skin lesions usually consist of subcutaneous nodules that are painful, erythematous and tender, ranging from 1 to 4 cm. These lesions may resemble eythema nodosum.
- The nodules sometimes erode through the skin, causing ulcers (Fig. 137–21).

DIAGNOSIS

Biopsy reveals an angiocentric and angiodestructive infiltrate comprised of atypical lymphoreticular cells (Fig. 137–22). At the malignant end of the disease continuum, the disease is essentially a B-cell lymphoma rich in T cells.

TREATMENT

- Corticosteroids
- Chemotherapy

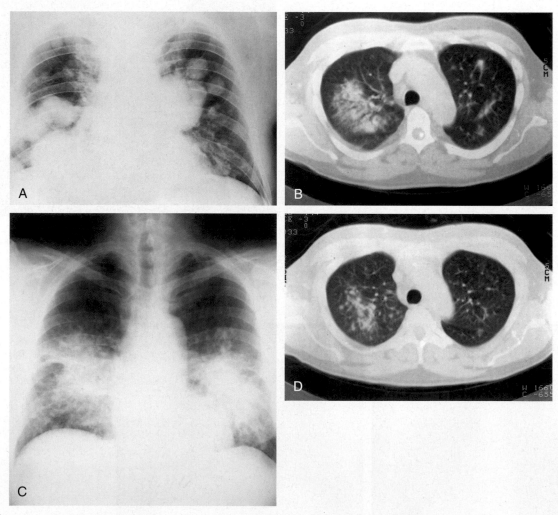

Fig 137–20
Radiologic studies in lymphomatoid granulomatosis. **A, C,** Chest radiographs showing bilateral pulmonary nodules of varying sizes.
B, D, Cuts from a CT study showing bilateral pulmonary nodules accompanied by interstitial changes.
(Courtesy of Fredric B. Askin and Stanley S, Siegelman.)

F. INTERSTITIAL PNEUMONIA

Interstitial pneumonia, which is a histologic and not a clinical or radiographic diagnosis, can be secondary to infections such as cytomegalovirus pneumonia and is also being recognized with increasing frequency among the pulmonary complications of HIV infection. Lymphocytic interstitial pneumonia (LIP) is characterized by a histologic pattern of diffuse infiltration of the alveolar walls and peribronchial areas by non-neoplastic mature lymphocytes, plasma cells with Russell bodies, plasmacytoid lymphocytes, and immunoblasts, as well as by nodular aggregates of lymphoid cells, with or without germinal centers. On chest x-ray (Fig. 137–23), diffuse bilateral reticulonodular infiltrates are commonly demonstrated, often with associated hilar adenopathy, and occasionally a predominantly nodular pattern is observed.

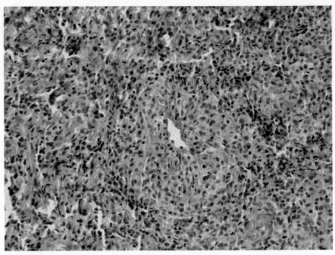

Fig 137–22
Lymphomatoid granulomatosis. A mixture of small lymphocytes, macrophages, and immunoblast-like cells infiltrates a vessel at the center of the photomicrograph.
(From Silverberg SG, Frable WJ, Wick MR, et al [eds]: Principles and Practice of Surgical Pathology and Cytopathology, 4th ed. Philadelphia, Elsevier, 2006.)

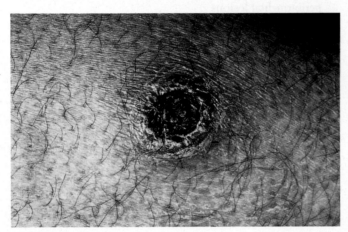

Fig 137–21
Cutaneous ulcer in a patient with lymphomatoid granulomatosis.
(From Hochberg MC, Silman AJ, Smolen JS, et al [eds]: Rheumatology, 3rd ed, St. Louis, Mosby, 2003.)

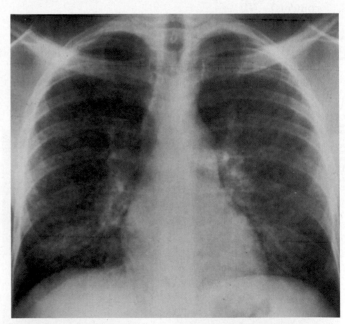

Fig 137–23
Lymphocytic interstitial pneumonia (LIP). A PA chest film demonstrates reticulonodular densities throughout both lungs and bilateral hilar lymphadenopathy. This combination of abnormalities is characteristic of LIP, but is also found in fungal or mycobacterial disease.
(From Grainger RG, Allison DJ, Adam A, Dixon AK [eds]: Grainger & Allison's Diagnostic Radiology, 4th ed. London, Harcourt, 2001.)

Chapter 138   Atelectasis

DEFINITION
Atelectasis is the collapse of lung volume.

PHYSICAL FINDINGS AND CLINICAL PRESENTATION
- Decreased or absent breath sounds
- Abnormal chest percussion
- Cough, dyspnea, decreased vocal fremitus and vocal resonance
- Diminished chest expansion, tachypnea, tachycardia

CAUSE
- Mechanical ventilation with higher FiO_2
- Chronic bronchitis
- Cystic fibrosis
- Endobronchial neoplasms
- Foreign bodies
- Infections (e.g., TB, histoplasmosis)
- Extrinsic bronchial compression from neoplasms, aneurysms of ascending aorta, enlarged left atrium
- Sarcoidosis
- Silicosis
- Anterior chest wall injury, pneumothorax
- Alveolar injury (e.g., toxic fumes, aspiration of gastric contents)
- Pleural effusion, expanding bullae
- Chest wall deformity (e.g., scoliosis)
- Muscular weaknesses or abnormalities (e.g., neuromuscular disease)
- Mucus plugs from asthma, allergic bronchopulmonary aspergillosis, postoperative state

DIFFERENTIAL DIAGNOSIS
- Neoplasm (see Fig. 132–5)
- Pneumonia (see Fig. 139–4)
- Encapsulated pleural effusion (see Fig. 133–1)
- Abnormalities of the brachiocephalic vein and left pulmonary ligament

IMAGING STUDIES
- Chest x-ray will confirm the diagnosis (Fig. 138–1A).
- CT scan (see Fig. 138–1B) indicated with suspected endobronchial neoplasm or extrinsic bronchial compression
- Fiberoptic bronchoscopy (select patients) is useful for removal of foreign body or evaluation of endobronchial and peribronchial lesions.

TREATMENT
- Deep breathing, mobilization of the patient
- Incentive spirometry
- Tracheal suctioning
- Humidification
- Chest physiotherapy with percussion and postural drainage
- Positive-pressure breathing (continuous positive airway pressure [CPAP] by face mask, positive end-expiratory pressure [PEEP] for patients on mechanical ventilation)
- Use of mucolytic agents (e.g., acetylcysteine)
- Recombinant human DNase in patients with cystic fibrosis
- Bronchodilator therapy in select patients

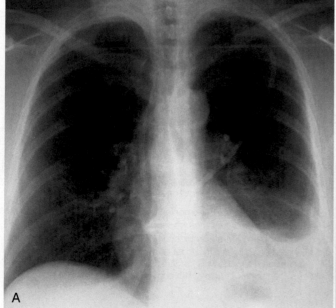
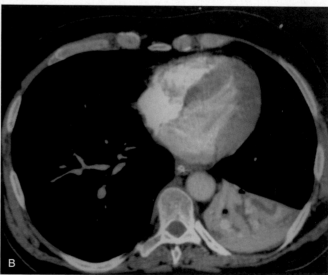

Fig 138–1
Retrocardiac atelectasis. **A,** PA radiograph shows left lower-lobe atelectasis, 2½ days after upper abdominal surgery. **B,** In a different patient, CT scan shows left lower lobe atelectasis. Some of the bronchi are open (air-filled), whereas others are plugged (mucus-filled).
(From Grainger RG, Allison DJ, Adam A, Dixon AK [eds]: Grainger & Allison's Diagnostic Radiology, 4th ed. London, Harcourt, 2001.)

Chapter 139 | **Respiratory infections**

A. BACTERIAL PNEUMONIA

DEFINITION

Bacterial pneumonia is an infection involving the lung parenchyma.

PHYSICAL FINDINGS AND CLINICAL PRESENTATION

- Fever, tachypnea, chills, tachycardia, cough
- Presentation varies with the cause of pneumonia, the patient's age, and the clinical situation:

  1. Patients with streptococcal pneumonia usually present with high fever, shaking chills, pleuritic chest pain, cough, and copious production of purulent sputum.

  2. *Mycoplasma pneumoniae*: insidious onset; headache; dry, paroxysmal cough, worse at night; myalgias; malaise; sore throat; extrapulmonary manifestations (e.g., erythema multiforme, aseptic meningitis, urticaria, erythema nodosum) may be present.

  3. *Chlamydia pneumoniae*: persistent, nonproductive cough; low-grade fever; headache; sore throat

  4. *Legionella pneumophila*: fever, mild cough, mental status change, myalgias, diarrhea, respiratory failure

  5. Older or immunocompromised hosts with pneumonia may initially present with only minimal symptoms (e.g., low-grade fever, confusion); respiratory and nonrespiratory symptoms are less commonly reported by older patients with pneumonia.

  6. Generally, auscultation of patients with pneumonia reveals crackles and diminished breath sounds.

  7. Percussion dullness is present if the patient has pleural effusion.

CAUSE

- *Streptococcus pneumoniae* (Fig. 139–1)
- *Haemophilus influenzae*
- *Legionella pneumophila* (1% to 5% of adult pneumonias)

- *Klebsiella, Pseudomonas, Escherichia coli*
- *Staphylococcus aureus*
- Atypical organisms such as *Mycoplasma pneumoniae* (Fig. 139–2), and *Legionella pneumophila* are implicated in up to 40% of cases of community-acquired pneumonias.
- Pneumococcal infection is responsible for 50% to 75% of community-acquired pneumonias, whereas gram-negative organisms cause more than 80% of nosocomial pneumonias
- Predisposing factors include the following:

  1. COPD: *H. influenzae, S. pneumoniae, L. pneumophila*

  2. Seizures: aspiration pneumonia

  3. Compromised hosts: *L. pneumophila* (Fig. 139–3), gram-negative organisms (Fig. 139–4)

  4. Alcoholism: *Klebsiella, S. pneumoniae, H. influenzae*

  5. HIV: *S. pneumoniae* (Fig. 139–5)

  6. IV drug addicts with right-sided bacterial endocarditis: *S. aureus* (Fig. 139–6)

  7. Older patients with comorbid diseases: *Chlamydia pneumoniae* (Fig. 139–7)

DIFFERENTIAL DIAGNOSIS

- Exacerbation of chronic bronchitis
- Pulmonary embolism or infarction (see Fig. 143–3)
- Lung neoplasm (see Fig. 132–5)
- Bronchiolitis
- Sarcoidosis (see Fig. 137–6)

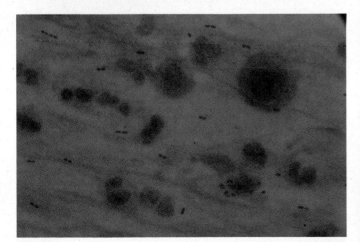

Fig 139–1
Streptococcus pneumoniae is a gram-positive diplococcus, 0.5 to 2.0 μm in diameter. It may be spheric, lanceolate, or elongated in pairs or short chains. It may lose its gram-positive nature in aged culture and on exposure to beta-lactam antibiotics and leukocyte lysozyme.
(From Gold WM, Murray JF, Nadel JA: Atlas of Procedures in Respiratory Medicine. Philadelphia, WB Saunders, 2002.)

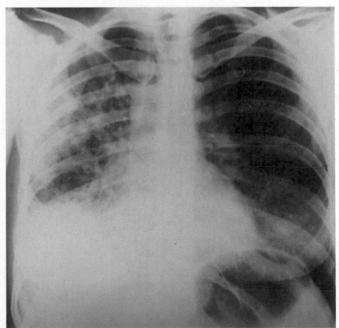

Fig 139–2
Mycoplasma pneumoniae pneumonia. Consolidation is unilateral and shows two patterns common with this infection. In the lower zone, consolidation is homogeneous, whereas in the mid and upper zones, it is heterogeneous and nodular.
(From Grainger RG, Allison DJ, Adam A, Dixon AK [eds]: Grainger & Allison's Diagnostic Radiology, 4th ed. London, Harcourt, 2001.)

- Hypersensitivity pneumonitis
- Pulmonary edema (see Fig. 110–1)
- Drug-induced lung injury
- Viral pneumonias (see Fig. 139–16)
- Fungal pneumonias (see Fig. 132–21)

- Parasitic pneumonias
- Atypical pneumonia (see Fig. 139–2)
- Tuberculosis (see Fig. 139–36)

LABORATORY TESTS

- CBC with differential. WBC count is elevated, usually with left shift.

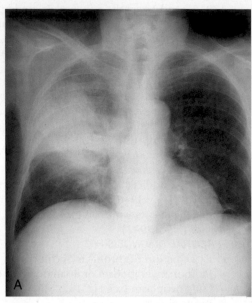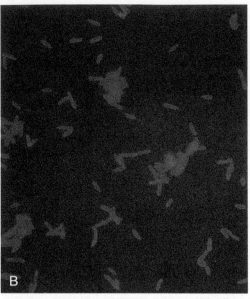

Fig 139–3
Legionnaire disease in a renal transplant recipient. **A,** Chest radiograph showing a right lower lobe pneumonia. **B,** Culture of sputum showing *Legionella pneumophila*, as identified by immunofluorescent staining with a specific antibody.
(Courtesy of R. Johnson.)

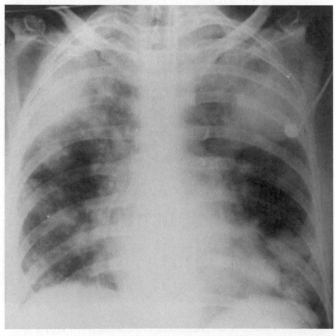

Fig 139–4
Pseudomonas aeruginosa pneumonia. Multifocal disseminated nodular consolidations in a patient on a respirator are seen.
(From Grainger RG, Allison DJ, Adam A, Dixon AK [eds]: Grainger & Allison's Diagnostic Radiology, 4th ed. London, Harcourt, 2001.)

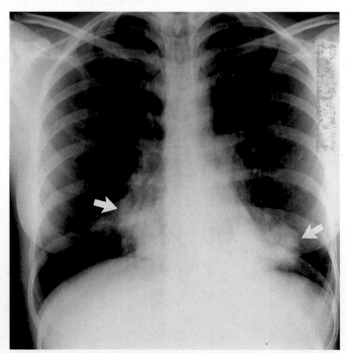

Fig 139–5
Streptococcus pneumoniae pneumonia, bilateral lower zone consolidation (*arrows*). Although pneumococcal pneumonia is typically unifocal, multifocal involvement is not uncommon.
(From Grainger RG, Allison DJ, Adam A, Dixon AK [eds]: Grainger & Allison's Diagnostic Radiology, 4th ed. London, Harcourt, 2001.)

- Blood cultures (hospitalized patients only): positive in approximately 20% of cases of pneumococcal pneumonia
- Pulse oximetry or ABGs: hypoxemia with partial pressure of oxygen <60 mm Hg while the patient is breathing room air is a standard criterion for hospital admission.
- Direct immunofluorescent examination of sputum when suspecting *L. pneumophila* (e.g., direct fluorescent antibody [DFA] stain is a highly specific and rapid test for detecting legionellae in clinical specimens).
- Serologic testing for HIV in select patients

IMAGING STUDIES

- Chest x-ray: findings vary with the stage and type of pneumonia and the hydration of the patient. Usually, pneumococcal pneumonia presents with a segmental lobe infiltrate (Fig. 139-8).
- Diffuse infiltrates on chest x-ray can be seen with *L. pneumophila*, *M. pneumoniae*, viral pneumonias, *P. carinii*, miliary TB, aspiration, aspergillosis.

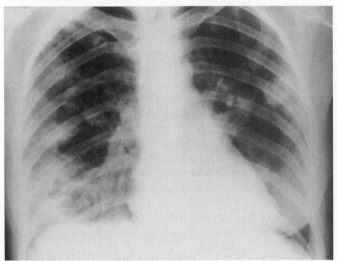

Fig 139–6
Staphylococcus aureus infection in a drug abuser. Multiple disseminated nodular consolidations are confluent in the right lower zone; several have cavitated. The appearance is typical of hematogenous dissemination.
(From Grainger RG, Allison DJ, Adam A, Dixon AK [eds]: Grainger & Allison's Diagnostic Radiology, 4th ed. London, Harcourt, 2001.)

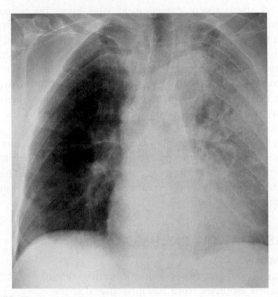

Fig 139–7
Chlamydia pneumoniae reinfection pneumonia in a 63-year-old man.
(From Cohen J, Powderly WG: Infectious Diseases, 2nd ed. St. Louis, Mosby, 2004.)

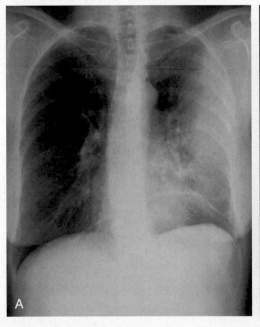

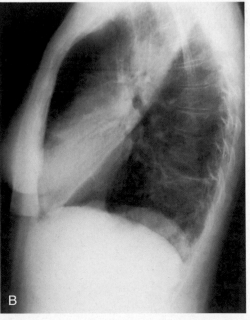

Fig 139–8
A, Large pneumonia obscures the left heart border, producing the silhouette sign. **B,** Lateral view confirms the presence of pneumonia in left upper lobe.
(From Grainger RG, Allison DJ, Adam A, Dixon AK [eds]: Grainger & Allison's Diagnostic Radiology, 4th ed. London, Harcourt, 2001.)

- An initial chest x-ray is also useful to rule out the presence of any complications (pneumothorax, empyema, abscesses).

TREATMENT

- Initial antibiotic therapy should be based on clinical, radiographic, and laboratory evaluations.
- Macrolides (azithromycin or clarithromycin) or levofloxacin are effective for empirical outpatient treatment of community-acquired pneumonia; cefotaxime or a beta-lactam or beta-lactamase inhibitor can be added in patients with more severe presentation who insist on outpatient therapy. Duration of treatment ranges from 7 to 14 days.
- In the hospital setting, patients admitted to the general ward can be treated empirically with a second- or third-generation cephalosporin (ceftriaxone, ceftizoxime, cefotaxime, or cefuroxime) plus a macrolide (azithromycin or clarithromycin) or doxycycline. An antipseudomonal quinolone (levofloxacin, moxifloxacin) may be substituted in place of the macrolide or doxycycline.
- In hospitalized patients at risk for *P. aeruginosa* infection, empirical treatment may consist of an antipseudomonal beta-lactam (cefepime or piperacillin-tazobactam) *plus* an aminoglycoside *plus* an antipseudomonal quinolone or macrolide.

B. ASPIRATION PNEUMONIA

DEFINITION

Aspiration pneumonia is a lung infection caused by bacterial organisms aspirated from nasopharyngeal space.

PHYSICAL FINDINGS AND CLINICAL PRESENTATION

- Shortness of breath, tachypnea, cough, sputum, fever after vomiting, or difficulty swallowing
- Rales, rhonchi, often diffusely throughout lung

CAUSE

- Complex interaction of causes, ranging from chemical (often acid) pneumonitis following aspiration of sterile gastric contents (generally not requiring antibiotic treatment) to bacterial aspiration

Community-acquired aspiration pneumonia

- Generally results from predominantly anaerobic mouth bacteria (anaerobic and microaerophilic streptococci, fusobacteria, gram-positive anaerobic non–spore-forming rods), *Bacteroides* spp. *(melaninogenicus, intermedius, oralis, ureolyticus), Haemophilus influenzae,* and *Streptococcus pneumoniae*
- Rarely caused by *Bacteroides fragilis* or *Eikenella corrodens*
- High-risk groups: older individuals, alcoholics, IV drug users, patients who are obtunded, those with esophageal disorders, seizures (Fig. 139–9), poor dentition, stroke victims, or recent dental manipulations

Hospital-acquired aspiration pneumonia

- Often occurs among older patients and others with diminished gag reflex, those with nasogastric tubes, intestinal obstruction, or ventilator support, and especially those exposed to contaminated nebulizers or unsterile suctioning (Fig. 139–10)
- High-risk groups: seriously ill hospitalized patients (especially patients with coma, acidosis, alcoholism, uremia, diabetes mellitus, nasogastric intubation, or recent antimicrobial therapy, who are frequently colonized with aerobic gram-negative rods); patients undergoing anesthesia; those with strokes, dementia, swallowing disorders; older individuals; and those receiving antacids or H_2 blockers (but not sucralfate)
- Hypoxic patients receiving concentrated O_2 have diminished ciliary activity, encouraging aspiration
- Causative organisms:

1. Anaerobes listed earlier, although in many studies gram-negative aerobes (60%) and gram-positive aerobes (20%) predominate

2. *E. coli, P. aeruginosa, S. aureus, Klebsiella, Enterobacter, Serratia,* and *Proteus* spp., *H. influenzae, S. pneumoniae, Legionella,* and *Acinetobacter* spp. (sporadic pneumonias) in two thirds of cases

3. Fungi, including *Candida albicans,* in fewer than 1%

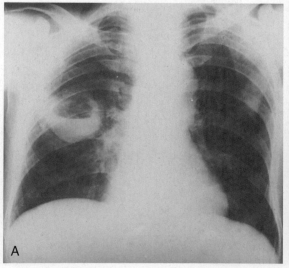
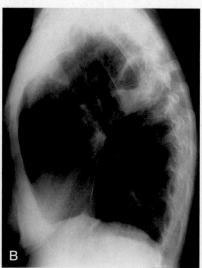

Fig 139–9
Mixed anaerobic infection in an epileptic. **A,** PA view. **B,** Lateral view. There is little in the way of consolidation; the main finding is a thick-walled cavity containing an air-fluid level. The site, the superior segment of the lower lobe, is typical.
(From Grainger RG, Allison DJ, Adam A, Dixon AK [eds]: Grainger & Allison's Diagnostic Radiology, 4th ed. London, Harcourt, 2001.)

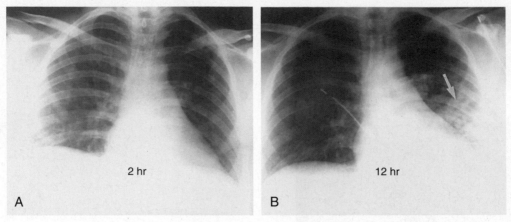

Fig 139–10
Aspiration pneumonia. **A,** A chest radiograph obtained immediately after aspiration may be normal. **B,** The chemical pneumonia takes 6 or 12 hours to cause an alveolar infiltrate *(arrow)*.
(From Mettler FA, Guibertau MJ, Voss CM, Urbina CE: Primary Care Radiology. Philadelphia, Elsevier, 2000.)

DIFFERENTIAL DIAGNOSIS
- Other necrotizing or cavitary pneumonias (especially tuberculosis, gram-negative pneumonias)
- Pulmonary tuberculosis

LABORATORY TESTS
- CBC: leukocytosis often present
- Sputum Gram stain
  1. Often useful when carefully prepared immediately after obtaining suctioned or expectorated specimen, examined by experienced observer
  2. Only specimens with multiple WBCs and rare or absent epithelial cells should be examined.
  3. Unlike nonaspiration pneumonias (e.g., pneumococcal), multiple organisms may be present.
  4. Long slender rods suggest anaerobes.
  5. Sputum from pneumonia caused by acid aspiration may be devoid of organisms.
  6. Cultures should be interpreted in light of morphology of visualized organisms.

IMAGING STUDIES
- Chest x-ray often reveals bilateral, diffuse, patchy infiltrates, posterior segment upper lobes.
- Aspiration pneumonias of several days' or longer duration may reveal necrosis (especially community-acquired anaerobic pneumonias) and even cavitation with air-fluid levels, indicating lung abscess.

TREATMENT
- Airway management to prevent repeated aspiration
- Acute aspiration of acidic gastric contents without bacteria may not require antibiotic therapy; consult infectious diseases or pulmonary expert.
- Community acquired: levofloxacin or ceftriaxone
- Nursing-home acquired: levofloxacin or piperacillin-tazobactam, or ceftazidime
- Hospital acquired: piperacillin-tazobactam, or clindamycin or cefoxitin
- Knowledge of resident flora in the microenvironment of the aspiration in the hospital is crucial to intelligent antibiotic selection; consult infection control nurse or hospital epidemiologist.

- Confirmed *Pseudomonas* pneumonia should be treated with antipseudomonal beta-lactam agent plus an aminoglycoside until antimicrobial sensitivities confirm that less toxic agents may replace aminoglycoside.

C. LUNG ABSCESS

DEFINITION
A lung abscess is an infection of the lung parenchyma resulting in a necrotic cavity containing pus (Fig. 139–11).

PHYSICAL FINDINGS AND CLINICAL PRESENTATION
- Symptoms are generally insidious and prolonged, occurring for weeks to months
- Fever, chills, and sweats
- Cough
- Sputum production (purulent with foul odor)
- Pleuritic chest pain
- Hemoptysis
- Dyspnea
- Malaise, fatigue, and weakness
- Tachycardia and tachypnea
- Dullness to percussion, whispered pectoriloquy, and bronchophony
- Amphoric breath sounds (low-pitched sound of air moving across a large open cavity)

CAUSE
- The most important factor predisposing to lung abscess is aspiration.
- Following aspiration as a major predisposing factor is periodontal disease.
- Lung abscess is rare in an edentulous person.
- Approximately 90% of lung abscesses are caused by anaerobic microorganisms (*Bacteroides fragilis, Fusobacterium nucleatum, Peptostreptococcus,* microaerophilic *Streptococcus*). Pulmonary actinomycosis will also generate lung abscess.
- In most cases, anaerobic infection is mixed with aerobic or facultative anaerobic organisms (*S. aureus, E. coli, K. pneumoniae, P. aeruginosa*).
- Parasitic organisms, including *Paragonimus westermani* and *Entamoeba histolytica*

529

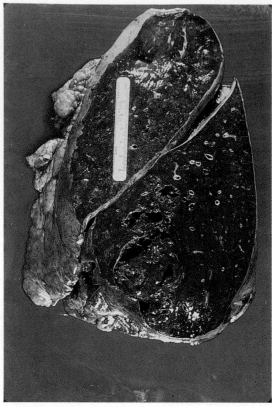

Fig 139–11
Cross section of a lung abscess.
(From Cohen J, Powderly WG: Infectious Diseases, 2nd ed. St. Louis, Mosby, 2004.)

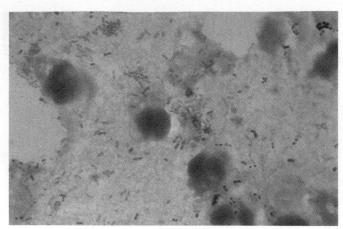

Fig 139–12
Gram stain of lower respiratory tract secretions. The patient had a lung abscess caused by oropharyngeal streptococci and anaerobes.
(From Cohen J, Powderly WG: Infectious Diseases, 2nd ed. St. Louis, Mosby, 2004.)

- Fungi, including *Aspergillus, Cryptococcus, Histoplasma, Blastomyces,* and *Coccidioides*
- Immunocompromised hosts may become infected with *Aspergillus,* mycobacteria, *Nocardia, Legionella micdadei,* and *Rhodococcus equi.*

DIAGNOSIS

Lung abscess may be primary or secondary.
- Primary lung abscess refers to infection from normal host organisms within the lung (e.g., aspiration, pneumonia).
- Secondary lung abscess results from other preexisting conditions (e.g., endocarditis, underlying lung cancer, pulmonary emboli).

Lung abscess may be acute or chronic.
- Acute lung abscess is present if symptoms are less than 4 to 6 weeks.
- Chronic lung abscess is present if symptoms are longer than 6 weeks.

DIFFERENTIAL DIAGNOSIS

The differential diagnosis is similar to that for cavitary lung lesions:
- Bacterial (anaerobic, aerobic, infected bulla, empyema, actinomycosis, tuberculosis)
- Fungal (histoplasmosis, coccidioidomycosis, blastomycosis, aspergillosis, cryptococcosis)
- Parasitic (amebiasis, echinococcosis)
- Malignancy (primary lung carcinoma, metastatic lung disease, lymphoma, Hodgkin's disease)

- Wegener's granulomatosis, sarcoidosis, endocarditis, septic pulmonary emboli

LABORATORY TESTS

- CBC with leukocytosis
- Bacteriologic studies
  1. Sputum Gram stain and culture (commonly contaminated by oral flora)
  2. Percutaneous transtracheal aspiration
  3. Percutaneous transthoracic aspiration
  4. Fiberoptic bronchoscopy using bronchial brushings or bronchoalveolar lavage is the most widely used intervention when trying to obtain diagnostic bacteriologic cultures (Fig. 139–12).
- Blood cultures on some occasions may be positive
- If an empyema is present, obtaining empyema fluid via thoracentesis may isolate the organism.

IMAGING STUDIES

- Chest x-ray reveals cavitary lesion with an air fluid level (Fig. 139–13).
- Lung abscesses are most commonly found in the posterior segment of the right upper lobe.
- Chest CT scan (Fig. 139–14) can localize and size the lesion and assist in differentiating lung abscesses from other pathologic processes (e.g., tumor, empyema, infected bulla, etc.)

TREATMENT

- Penicillin, 1 to 2 million U IV, every 4 hours until improvement (e.g., afebrile, decrease in sputum production) followed by penicillin VK 500 mg PO daily for the next 2 to 3 weeks but usually requiring longer 6- to 8-week courses
- Metronidazole is given with penicillin at doses of 7.5 mg/kg IV every 6 hours, followed by metronidazole PO, 500 mg twice to four times daily.
- Clindamycin is an alternative choice if concerned about penicillin-resistant organisms. The dose is 600 mg IV every 8 hours until improvement, followed by 300 mg PO every 6 hours.

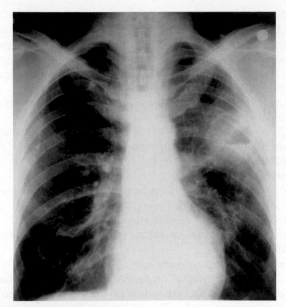

Fig 139–13
A lung abscess showing an air-fluid level.
(From Cohen J, Powderly WG: Infectious Diseases, 2nd ed. St. Louis, Mosby, 2004.)

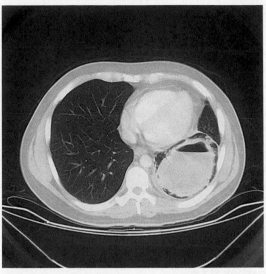

Fig 139–14
CT scan of a lung abscess showing an air-fluid level.
(From Cohen J, Powderly WG: Infectious Diseases, 2nd ed. St. Louis, Mosby, 2004.)

Chronic therapy
- Bronchoscopy to assist with drainage and/or diagnosis is indicated in patients who fail to respond to antibiotics or if there is suspected underlying malignancy.
- Surgery is indicated on rare occasions (<10%) in patients with complications of lung abscess

D. VIRAL PNEUMONIA

DEFINITION
Viral pneumonia is infection of the pulmonary parenchyma caused by a viral agent. The most important viruses are discussed in the following sections.

PHYSICAL FINDINGS AND CLINICAL PRESENTATION
Influenza
- Fever
- Uncomfortable or lethargic appearance
- Prominent dry cough (rarely hemoptysis)
- Flushed integument and erythematous mucous membranes
- Rales or rhonchi

Respiratory syncytial virus
- Fever
- Tachypnea
- Prolonged expiration
- Wheezes and rales

Adenoviruses
- Hoarseness
- Pharyngitis
- Tachypnea
- Cervical adenitis

Measles
- Conjunctivitis
- Rhinorrhea
- Koplik's spots

- Exanthem
- Pneumonitis
  1. May occur as a complication in 3% to 4% of adolescents and young adults
  2. Coincident with rash
  3. May also develop following apparent recovery from measles
- Fever
- Dry cough

Varicella
- Fever
- Maculopapular or vesicular rash
  1. Becomes encrusted
  2. Pneumonia typically 1 to 6 days after rash appears
  3. Pneumonia accompanied by cough, and occasionally hemoptysis
- Few auscultatory abnormalities noted on examination of the lungs

Cytomegalovirus
- Fever
- Paroxysmal cough
- Occasional hemoptysis
- Diffuse adenopathy when pneumonia occurs after transfusion

CAUSE
Viral infection can lead to pneumonia in immunocompetent and immunocompromised hosts.

DIFFERENTIAL DIAGNOSIS
- Bacterial pneumonia, which frequently complicates (i.e., can follow or be simultaneous with) viral (especially influenza) pneumonia
- Other causes of atypical pneumonia:
  1. *Mycoplasma*
  2. *Chlamydia*
  3. *Coxiella*

4. Legionnaires' disease
- Acute repiratory distress syndrome (ARDS)

WORKUP

- Information about the prevalent strain of influenza virus can be obtained from local health departments or from the Centers for Disease Control and Prevention.
- Viral diagnostic tests are usually not necessary once an outbreak has been defined.
- Influenza and other viruses can be cultured from respiratory secretions during the initial few days of the illness (special media and techniques necessary).
- Paired sera antibody titers are also useful.
- Monoclonal antibody tests are available for influenza and other respiratory viruses.
- Measles and adenovirus pneumonia are usually diagnosed clinically.
- Polymerase chain reaction (PCR) assay may be able to rapidly detect and identify viral nucleic acid.
- Open lung biopsy is required for definite diagnosis of cytomegalovirus (CMV) pneumonia (Fig. 139–15).

LABORATORY TESTS

- Sputum Gram stain (usually produced in scanty amounts) typically shows few polymorphonuclear leukocytes and few bacteria.
- WBC count may vary from leukopenic to modest elevation, usually without a leftward shift.
- Disseminated intravascular coagulation has occasionally complicated adenovirus type 7 pneumonia.
- Multinucleated giant cells on Tzanck preparation of an unroofed vesicular lesion are useful in diagnosing varicella in a patient with an infiltrate (also found in herpes simplex).
- Severe immunosuppression is associated with symptomatic CMV pneumonia (usually reactivation of latent infection, or in previously seronegative recipients from the donor).
- Hypoxemia may be profound.
- Cultures may be helpful in identifying superinfecting bacterial pathogens.
- When they occur, parapneumonic pleural effusions are exudative.

IMAGING STUDIES

- Chest x-ray examination may demonstrate a spectrum of findings from ill-defined, patchy, or generalized interstitial infiltrates (Fig. 139–16).
- A localized dense alveolar infiltrate suggests a superimposed bacterial pneumonia.
- Small calcified nodules may develop as a radiographic residual of varicella pneumonia.
- CT of chest (Fig. 139–17) is indicated when diagnosis is uncertain or complications are suspected.

TREATMENT

General

- Measures to diminish person-to-person transmission
- Modified bed rest
- Maintenance of adequate hydration
- Possible ventilatory support for severe pneumonia or ARDS

Influenza

- Yearly prophylactic strain-specific influenza vaccination (only subvirion vaccine should be used in children younger than 13 years) can be given to prevent infection.
- Amantadine and rimantadine (not commercially available) for influenza A. Early use can speed recovery from small airways dysfunction, but whether it influences the development or course of pneumonia is uncertain.
- Amantadine is also effective prophylactically while it is administered.
- Aerosolized ribavirin and amantadine may have a role in severe influenza pneumonia but have not been approved for this indication.

Respiratory syncytial virus

- Isolation techniques are important in limiting the spread of respiratory syncytial virus (RSV) infections.
- Immunoglobulins with a high RSV-neutralizing antibody titer are beneficial in treatment.
- Ribavirin aerosol is effective for severe RSV pneumonia.

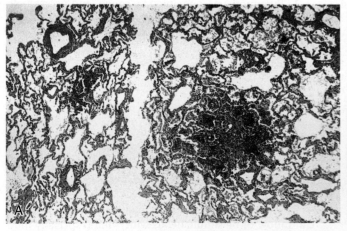
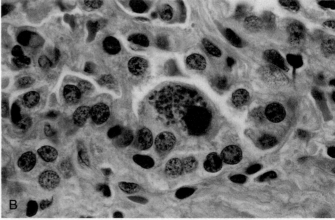

Fig 139–15
Cytomegalovirus (CMV) pneumonia. **A,** Hemorrhagic nodules are accompanied by varying degrees of diffuse alveolar damage. **B,** The intranuclear inclusion of CMV is distinctive.
(From Silverberg SG, Frable WJ, Wick MR, et al [eds]: Principles and Practice of Surgical Pathology and Cytopathology, 4th ed. Philadelphia, Elsevier, 2006.)

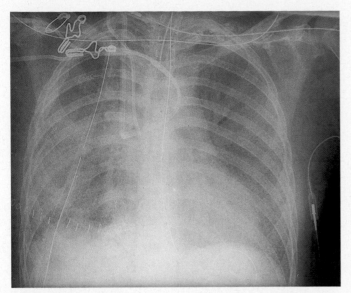

Fig 139–16
Cytomegalovirus pneumonia in an allogeneic stem cell transplant recipient with diffuse bilateral interstitial lung infiltrates on chest radiography. (From Cohen J, Powderly WG: Infectious Diseases, 2nd ed. St. Louis, Mosby, 2004.)

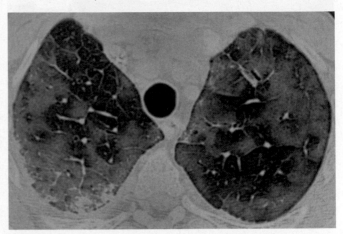

Fig 139–17
Cytomegalovirus (CMV) pneumonia. This high-resolution CT of a 32-year-old man 29 months after bilateral lung transplantation for cystic fibrosis shows bilateral multifocal areas of ground-glass attenuation. Bronchoscopic biopsy showed numerous CMV inclusion bodies. (From Grainger RG, Allison DJ, Adam A, Dixon AK [eds]: Grainger & Allison's Diagnostic Radiology, 4th ed. London, Harcourt, 2001.)

Adenoviruses
- No effective antiadenovirus agent.
- Intestinal inoculation of respiratory adenoviruses has been used to immunize military recruits successfully.
- Although they produce no disease in recipients, the viruses may be shed chronically and may infect others at a later date.
- These vaccines are not available for civilian populations.

Varicella
- Varicella pneumonia can be treated with IV acyclovir.
- Adults who develop chickenpox should be considered for acyclovir treatment, which may prevent the development of pneumonia.
- Live attenuated varicella vaccine has been successfully used in clinical trials.
- Varicella-zoster immune globulin should be administered within 4 days of exposure to prevent or modify the disease in susceptible persons.
- Nonimmunized persons exposed to varicella are potentially infectious between 10 and 21 days after exposure.

Measles
- No effective antimeasles agent
- Effective measles vaccine is available:
  1. The vaccine should be administered at 15 months.
  2. A second dose should be administered when starting school.
- Live attenuated vaccine or gamma globulin can prevent measles in unvaccinated persons if administered early following exposure.
- Vitamin A given PO for 2 days reduces morbidity and mortality from measles in exposed children.
- Severe acute respiratory syndrome (SARS)–associated coronaviruses
  1. No vaccine currently available.
  2. Combination therapy with lopinavir-ritonavir and ribavirin may reduce viral load.

E. ANTHRAX

DEFINITION
Anthrax is an acute infectious disease caused by the spore-forming bacterium *Bacillus anthracis*.

PHYSICAL FINDINGS AND CLINICAL PRESENTATION
Symptoms of disease vary depending on how the disease was contracted, but usually occur within 7 days after exposure.
The serious forms of human anthrax are inhalation anthrax, cutaneous anthrax, and intestinal anthrax.
- Inhalation anthrax begins with a brief prodrome resembling a viral respiratory illness, followed by development of hypoxia and dyspnea, with radiographic evidence of mediastinal widening. Host factors, dose of exposure, and chemoprophylaxis may affect the duration of the incubation period. Initial symptoms include mild fever, muscle aches, and malaise and may progress to respiratory failure and shock; meningitis often develops.
- Cutaneous anthrax is characterized by a skin lesion evolving from a papule, through a vesicular stage (Fig. 139–18) to a depressed black eschar (Fig. 139–19). The incubation period ranges from 1 to 12 days. The lesion is usually painless, but patients also may have fever, malaise, headache, and regional lymphadenopathy. The eschar dries and falls off in 1 to 2 weeks, with little scarring.
- Gastrointestinal anthrax is characterized by severe abdominal pain followed by fever and signs of septicemia. Bloody diarrhea and signs of acute abdomen may occur. This form of anthrax usually follows after eating raw or undercooked contaminated meat and can have an incubation period of 1 to 7 days. Gastric ulcers may occur and may be associated with hematemesis. Oropharyngeal and abdominal forms of the disease have been described. Involvement

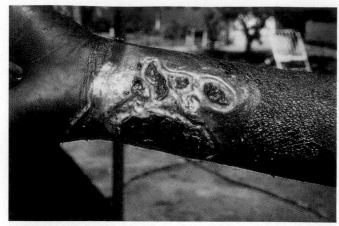

Fig 139–18
Anthrax—multiple lesions on the forearm.
(Courtesy of Dr. J. Frean and the late Dr. M. Isaäcson, MD, University of Witwatersrand, Johannesburg, South Africa.)

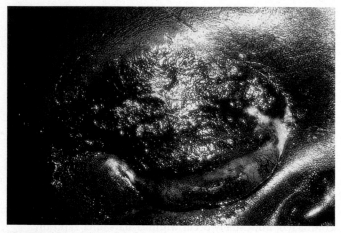

Fig 139–19
Anthrax—cutaneous disease is the most common manifestation in humans. This black crusted lesion is typical.
(Courtesy of Dr. J. Frean and the late Dr. M. Isaäcson, MD, University of Witwatersrand, Johannesburg, South Africa.)

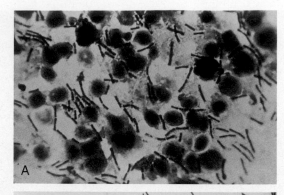

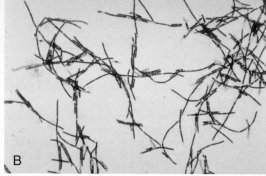

Fig 139–20
Bacillus anthracis. **A,** *Bacillus anthracis* appearing as gram-positive bacilli. **B,** The typical jointed bamboo rod appearance of the organism from blood cultures.
(Courtesy of the Centers for Disease Control and Prevention and Dr. William A. Clark.)

of the pharynx is usually characterized by lesions at the base of the tongue, dysphagia, fever, and regional lymphadenopathy. Lower bowel inflammation typically causes nausea, loss of appetite, and fever followed by abdominal pain, hematemesis, and bloody diarrhea.

CAUSE
The disease is caused by *Bacillus anthracis,* a gram-positive, spore-forming bacillus. It is aerobic, nonmotile, nonhemolytic on sheep's blood agar, and grows readily at 37° C, forming large colonies with irregularly tapered outgrowths (a Medusa's head appearance or joint bamboo rod; Fig. 139–20). In the host, it appears as single organisms or chains of two or three bacilli.

DIFFERENTIAL DIAGNOSIS
- Inhalation anthrax must be distinguished from influenza-like illness (ILI) and tularemia. Most cases of ILI are associated with nasal congestion and rhinorrhea, which are unusual in inhalation anthrax. Additional distinguishing factors are the usual absence of an abnormal chest x-ray in ILI (see later).

- Cutaneous anthrax should be distinguished from staphylococcal disease, ecthyma, ecthyma gangrenosum, plague, brown recluse spider bite, and tularemia.
- The differential diagnosis of gastrointestinal anthrax includes viral gastroenteritis, shigellosis, and yersiniosis.

LABORATORY TESTS
- Presumptive identification is based on Gram stain of material from skin lesion, cerebrospinal fluid (CSF), or blood showing encapsulated gram-positive bacilli.
- Confirmatory tests are performed at specialized labs. Virulent strains grow on nutrient agar in the presence of 5% CO_2. Susceptibility to lysis by gamma phage or direct fluorescent antibody (DFA) staining of cell wall polysaccharide antigen are also useful confirmatory tests.
- Serologic testing by enzyme-linked immunosorbent assay (ELISA) can confirm the diagnosis.
- A skin test (anthracin test) that detects anthrax cell-mediated immunity is also available in specialized laboratories.

IMAGING STUDIES
Chest x-ray usually reveals mediastinal widening (Fig. 139–21). Additional findings include infiltrates and pleural effusion.

TREATMENT
- Most naturally occurring *B. anthracis* strains are sensitive to penicillin. The FDA has approved penicillin, doxycycline, and ciprofloxacin for the treatment of inhalational anthrax infection.

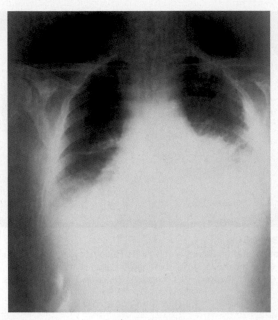

Fig 139–21
Imaging abnormalities associated with anthrax. This chest radiograph demonstrates a widened mediastinum caused by inhalational anthrax. (Courtesy of the Centers for Disease Control and Prevention and Dr. P. S. Brachman.)

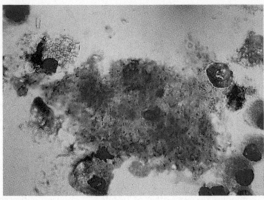

Fig 139–22
Wright-Giemsa stained specimen of an induced sputum specimen showing clusters of *Pneumocystis jiroveci* organisms. (From Cohen J, Powderly WG: Infectious Diseases, 2nd ed. St. Louis, Mosby, 2004.)

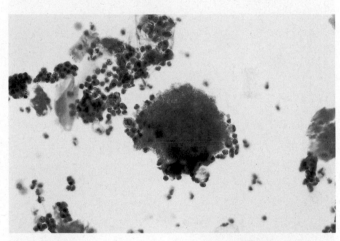

Fig 139–23
Pneumocystis in bronchial washing. Clusters of organisms enmeshed in fibrin and surrounded by a few inflammatory cells. There is a vague outline of small cysts, but trophozoites are not seen with the Papanicolaou stain (×1000). (From Silverberg SG, Frable WJ, Wick MR, et al [eds]: Principles and Practice of Surgical Pathology and Cytopathology, 4th ed. Philadelphia, Elsevier, 2006.)

F. *PNEUMOCYSTIS* PNEUMONIA

DEFINITION
Pneumocystis pneumonia (PCP is a serious respiratory infection caused by the organism *Pneumocystis jiroveci* (formerly known as *P. carinii*).

PHYSICAL FINDINGS AND CLINICAL PRESENTATION
- Fever, cough, shortness of breath present in almost all cases
- Lungs frequently clear to auscultation, although rales occasionally present
- Cyanosis and pronounced tachypnea in severe cases
- Hemoptysis unusual
- Spontaneous pneumothorax
- Extrapulmonary involvement rare

CAUSE
- *Pneumocystis jiroveci* (formerly *P. carinii*) recently reclassified as a fungal organism
- Reactivation of dormant infection

DIFFERENTIAL DIAGNOSIS
- Other opportunistic respiratory infections:
    1. Tuberculosis (see Fig. 139–36)
    2. Histoplasmosis (see Fig. 336–20)
    3. Cryptococcosis (see Fig. 336–25)
- Nonopportunistic infections:
    1. Bacterial pneumonia (see Fig. 139–4)
    2. Viral pneumonia (see Fig. 139–16)
    3. Mycoplasmal pneumonia (see Fig. 139–2)
    4. Legionellosis (see Fig. 139–3)
- Occurs almost exclusively in the setting of profound depression of cellular immunity

LABORATORY TESTS
- ABG or pulse oximetry monitoring
- Elevated LDH in the majority of cases
- HIV antibody test if cause of underlying immune deficiency state is unclear
- Sputum examination for cysts of PCP; (Fig. 139–22) and to exclude other pathogens
- Bronchoscopy with bronchoalveolar lavage (Fig. 139–23) or lung biopsy (Fig. 139–24) for diagnosis if sputum examination is negative or equivocal

IMAGING STUDIES
- Chest x-ray (Fig. 139–25)
- CT scan (Fig. 139–26)
- Diffuse uptake on gallium scanning of the lungs is suggestive but not diagnostic.

TREATMENT
- Trimethoprim-sulfamethoxazole
- Pentamidine
- Either regimen with prednisone

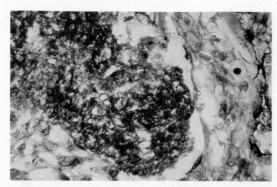

Fig 139–24
Gomori methenamine silver stain of lung tissue showing characteristic *P. jiroveci* cysts.
(From Cohen J, Powderly WG: Infectious Diseases, 2nd ed. St. Louis, Mosby, 2004.)

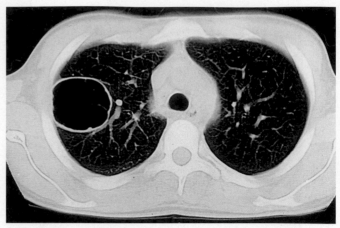

Fig 139–26
Six weeks after treatment of moderate *Pnuemocystis* pneumonia. The chest CT scan shows large, thin-walled bullae of the right lung.
(From Cohen J, Powderly WG: Infectious Diseases, 2nd ed. St. Louis, Mosby, 2004.)

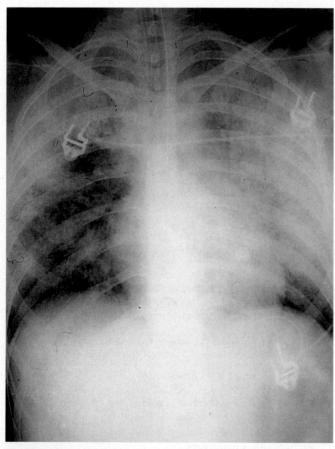

Fig 139–25
Severe *Pneumocystis* pneumonia. This shows an extensive alveolar interstitial infiltrate, with consolidation of the left lung and upper right lobe.
(Courtesy of A. Cabié.)

G. EMPYEMA

DEFINITION
This is an accumulation of pus in the pleural space, most often caused by bacterial infection.

PHYSICAL FINDINGS AND CLINICAL PRESENTATION
- May be abrupt and dramatic or chronic and insidious depending on the causative agent and host factors
- Typically presents as progressive pleuritic chest pain, persistent fever, and other sustained signs and symptoms of infection
- In anaerobic empyema, particularly that caused by actinomycetes, the clinical picture may be dominated by systemic symptoms and signs, such as weight loss, malaise, and low-grade fever.
- A slowly enlarging chest wall mass
- As a complication of thoracic trauma or surgery, empyema typically results from superinfection of blood or other material in the pleural space several days following the event.
- The physical findings of empyema are those of pleural effusion. Decreased breath sounds and dullness to percussion over the involved part of the thorax are typical. Systemic signs of infection include fever, tachycardia, leukocytosis and, occasionally, warmth and erythema over the involved area.

CAUSE
Infection of the lung parenchyma spreading to pleural space is caused by the following:
- *Streptococcus pneumoniae*
- *Haemophilus influenzae*
- *Staphylococcus aureus*
- *Legionella* spp.
- *Mycobacterium tuberculosis*
- Actinomyces spp.
- A variety of oral anaerobic bacteria

DIFFERENTIAL DIAGNOSIS
- Uninfected parapneumonic effusion (see Fig. 133–1)
- Congestive heart failure (see Fig. 109–3)
- Malignancy involving the pleura (see Fig. 133–6)
- Tuberculous pleurisy (see Fig. 139–36)
- Collagen vascular disease (particularly rheumatoid lung [see Fig. 291–7] and SLE [see Fig. 293–5])

LABORATORY TESTS
- Complete blood count; ABGs
- Blood cultures.

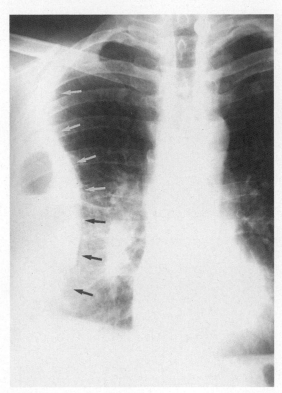

Fig 139–27
Empyema. On an upright chest radiograph, a lenticular density is seen along the lateral chest wall. An air-fluid level is also seen within this. (From Mettler FA, Guibertau MJ, Voss CM, Urbina CE: Primary Care Radiology. Philadelphia, Elsevier, 2000.)

- Pleural fluid analysis, including cell count and differential, LDH and protein levels, pH, Gram stain and culture. Empyema fluid is expected to have the characteristics of pleural exudates with a ratio of pleural fluid protein to serum protein of 0.5 or higher or a ratio of pleural fluid LDH to serum LDH of 0.6 or higher. In addition, the presence of gross pus, visible organisms on Gram stain of the pleural fluid, pleural fluid glucose less than 50 mg/dL or pleural fluid pH below 7 are characteristic of empyema. Any of these latter findings justifies immediate drainage by chest tube or surgery because of the high risk of loculation and progressive systemic infection.

IMAGING STUDIES
- Chest x-ray (Fig. 139–27)
- Lateral decubitus view to establish the presence of free fluid in the pleural space
- CT to establish the presence of fluid loculation, underlying mass lesions, and other intrathoracic pathology

TREATMENT
- Prompt drainage by thoracostomy (chest tube) or open thoracotomy
- Antibiotics directed at suspected or proved bacterial or fungal pathogens
- Thoracoscopy or instillation of thrombolytic agents (streptokinase or urokinase) may be considered in refractory loculated empyema.

H. BRONCHIECTASIS
DEFINITION
Bronchiectasis is the abnormal dilation and destruction of bronchial walls, which may be congenital or acquired.
PHYSICAL FINDINGS AND CLINICAL PRESENTATION
- Moist crackles at lung bases
- Cough with expectoration of large amount of purulent sputum
- Fever, night sweats, generalized malaise, weight loss
- Hemoptysis
- Halitosis, skin pallor
- Clubbing (infrequent)

CAUSE
- Cystic fibrosis
- Lung infections (pneumonia, lung abscess, TB, fungal infections, viral infections)
- Abnormal host defense (panhypogammaglobulinemia, Kartagener's syndrome, AIDS, chemotherapy)
- Localized airway obstruction (congenital structural defects, foreign bodies, neoplasms)
- Inflammation (inflammatory pneumonitis, granulomatous lung disease, allergic aspergillosis)

DIFFERENTIAL DIAGNOSIS
- TB (see Fig. 139–36)
- Asthma (see Fig. 129–2)
- Chronic bronchitis or chronic sinusitis
- Interstitial fibrosis (see Fig. 136–1)
- Chronic lung abscess (see Fig. 139–13)
- Foreign body aspiration (see Fig. 139–10)
- Cystic fibrosis (see Fig. 139–31)
- Lung carcinoma (see Fig. 132–5)

LABORATORY TESTS
- Sputum for Gram stain, C&S, and acid-fast bacteria (AFB)
- CBC with differential (leukocytosis with left shift, anemia)
- Serum protein electrophoresis to evaluate for hypogammaglobulinemia
- Antibody test for aspergillosis
- Sweat test in patients with suspected cystic fibrosis

IMAGING STUDIES
- Chest x-ray (Fig. 139–28): hyperinflation, crowded lung markings, small cystic spaces at the bases of the lungs.
- High-resolution CT scanning of the chest has become the best tool to detect cystic lesions and exclude underlying obstruction from neoplasm.
- Bronchoscopy may be helpful to evaluate hemoptysis, rule out obstructive lesions, and remove mucus plugs.

TREATMENT
- Postural drainage (reclining prone on a bed with the head down on the side) and chest percussion with the use of inflatable vests or mechanical vibrators applied to the chest may enhance removal of respiratory secretions.
- Adequate hydration
- Supplemental oxygen for hypoxemia
- Antibiotic therapy is based on the results of sputum, Gram stain, and C&S; in patients with inadequate or inconclusive results, empirical therapy with amoxicillin-clavulanate, doxycycline, or cefuroxime is recommended.
- Bronchodilators are useful in patients with demonstrable airflow obstruction.

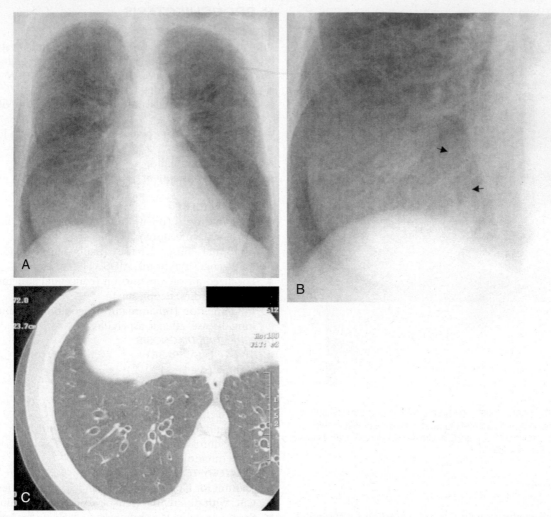

Fig 139–28
Cylindrical bronchiectasis in a 55-year-old woman with long-standing rheumatoid arthritis. **A, B,** Chest radiograph shows diffuse airway wall thickening with multiple dilated bronchi, most evident in the right lower lobe *(arrows).* **C,** High-resolution CT confirms marked cylindrical right lower lobe bronchiectasis.
(From Grainger RG, Allison DJ, Adam A, Dixon AK [eds]: Grainger & Allison's Diagnostic Radiology, 4th ed. London, Harcourt, 2001.)

I. CYSTIC FIBROSIS

DEFINITION
Cystic fibrosis (CF) is an autosomal recessive disorder characterized by dysfunction of exocrine glands (Fig. 139–29).

PHYSICAL FINDINGS AND CLINICAL PRESENTATION
- Failure to thrive in children
- Increased anterior-posterior chest diameter
- Basilar crackles and hyperresonance to percussion
- Digital clubbing
- Chronic cough
- Abdominal distention
- Greasy, smelly feces

CAUSE
- Chromosome 7 gene mutation (*CFTR* gene) resulting in abnormalities in chloride transport and water flux across the surface of epithelial cells; the abnormal secretions cause obstruction of glands and ducts in various organs and subsequent damage to exocrine tissue (recurrent pneumonia, atelectasis, bronchiectasis, diabetes mellitus, biliary cirrhosis, cholelithiasis, intestinal obstruction, increased risk of GI malignancies).

DIFFERENTIAL DIAGNOSIS
- Immunodeficiency states
- Celiac disease
- Asthma
- Recurrent pneumonia

LABORATORY TESTS
- Pilocarpine iontophoresis (sweat test): diagnostic of CF in children if sweat chloride is more than 60 mmol/L (more than 80 mmol/L in adults) on two separate tests on consecutive days. Repeat testing may be necessary, because not all infants have sufficient quantities of sweat for reliable testing
- DNA testing may be useful for confirming the diagnosis and providing genetic information for family members.

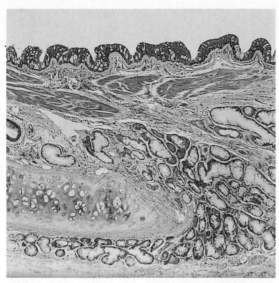

Fig 139–29
A cystic fibrosis submucosal gland demonstrates marked hypertrophy and dilated gland ducts with mucoid secretions. The surface epithelium has marked goblet cell metaplasia (H&E, ×100).
(From Cohen J, Powderly WG: Infectious Diseases, 2nd ed. St. Louis, Mosby, 2004.)

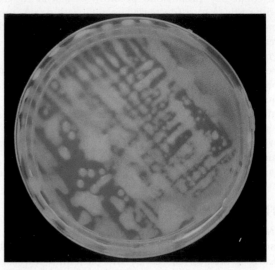

Fig 139–30
Mucoid colonies of a strain of *Pseudomonas aeruginosa* isolated from a patient with cystic fibrosis.
(Courtesy of Professor E. Bingen.)

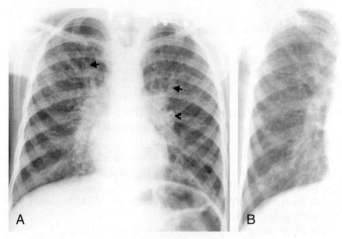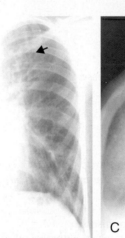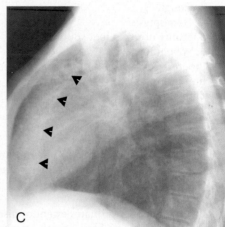

Fig 139–31
Evolution of cystic fibrosis in a young male. **A,** Chest radiograph at age 7 shows extensive bilateral bronchial wall thickening, manifested by ring shadows of end-on bronchi *(arrowhead),* and train track' for bronchi seen in profile *(arrows).* **B, C,** Frontal and lateral chest radiographs obtained 12 years later show progression of airway disease, with extensive cystic bronchiectasis *(arrow)* in the left upper lobe. The obscuration of the left heart border and the hazy density over the left hemithorax on the frontal view are caused by left upper lobe atelectasis. *Arrowheads* on the lateral view indicate the anteriorly displaced major fissure.
(From Grainger RG, Allison DJ, Adam A, Dixon AK [eds]: Grainger & Allison's Diagnostic Radiology, 4th ed. London, Harcourt, 2001.)

- Sputum C&S (Fig. 139–30) and Gram stain (frequent bacterial infections with *Staphylococcus aureus, Pseudomonas aeruginosa* [most common virulent respiratory pathogen], *Haemophilus influenzae*)
- Low albumin level, increased 72-hour fecal fat excretion
- Pulse oximetry or ABGs: hypoxemia
- Pulmonary function studies: decreased TLC, forced vital capacity, pulmonary diffusing capacity

IMAGING STUDIES

- Chest x-ray (Fig. 139–31): may reveal focal atelectasis, peribronchial cuffing, bronchiectasis, increased interstitial markings, hyperinflation

- High-resolution chest CT scan: bronchial wall thickening, cystic lesions, ring shadows (bronchiectasis)

TREATMENT

- Postural drainage and chest percussion
- Encouragement of regular exercise and proper nutrition
- Psychosocial evaluation and counseling of patient and family members
- Antibiotic therapy based on results of Gram stain and C&S of sputum
- Bronchodilators for patients with airflow obstruction
- Chronic pancreatic enzyme replacement

- Alternate-day prednisone possibly beneficial in children with cystic fibrosis (decreased hospitalization rate, improved pulmonary function); routine use of corticosteroids not recommended in adults
- Proper nutrition and vitamin supplementation
- Recombinant human deoxyribonuclease is useful to improve mucociliary clearance by liquefying difficult to clear pulmonary secretions
- Intermittent administration of inhaled tobramycin has been reported beneficial in CF.
- Treatment of impaired glucose tolerance and diabetes mellitus
- Pneumococcal vaccination, yearly influenza vaccination

J. TUBERCULOSIS

DEFINITION

Pulmonary TB is an infection of the lung and, occasionally, surrounding structures, caused by the bacterium *Mycobacterium tuberculosis.*

PHYSICAL FINDINGS AND CLINICAL PRESENTATION

- Primary pulmonary TB infection generally asymptomatic
- Reactivation pulmonary TB
  1. Fever
  2. Night sweats
  3. Cough
  4. Hemoptysis
  5. Scanty nonpurulent sputum
  6. Weight loss
- Progressive primary pulmonary TB disease: same as reactivation pulmonary TB
- TB pleurisy
  1. Pleuritic chest pain
  2. Fever
  3. Shortness of breath
- Rare massive, suffocating, fatal hemoptysis secondary to erosion of pulmonary artery in a cavity *(Rasmussen aneurysm)*
- Chest examination
  1. Not specific
  2. Usually underestimates extent of disease
  3. Rales accentuated following a cough (posttussive rales)

CAUSE

Mycobacterium tuberculosis (Mtb), is a slow-growing, aerobic, non–spore-forming, nonmotile bacillus, with a lipid-rich cell wall.

1. Lacks pigment
2. Produces niacin
3. Reduces nitrate
4. Produces heat-labile catalase
5. Mtb staining, acid-fast and acid-alcohol fast by Ziehl-Neelsen method, appearing as red, slightly bent, beaded rods 2 to 4 microns long (acid-fast bacilli [AFB]), against a blue background (Fig. 139–32)
6. PCR to detect less than 10 organisms/mL in sputum (compared with the requisite 10,000 organisms/mL for AFB smear detection)
7. Culture
   a. Growth on solid media (Lowenstein-Jensen, Middlebrook 7H11 agar) in 2 to 6 weeks (Fig. 139–33)

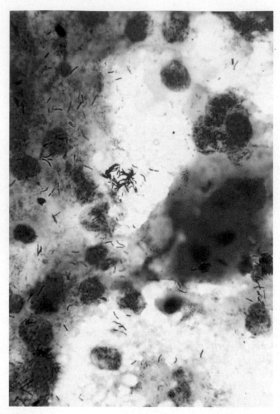

Fig 139–32
Ziehl-Neelsen acid-fast stain of sputum containing 4+ tubercle bacilli. (Courtesy of S. Froman and A. Gaytan.)

   b. Growth in liquid media (BACTEC, using a radioactive carbon source for early growth detection) often in 9 to 16 days
   c. Enhanced in a 5% to 10% carbon dioxide atmosphere
8. DNA fingerprinting (based on restriction fragment length polymorphism [RFLP])
   a. Facilitates immediate identification of Mtb strains in early-growing cultures
   b. False-negatives possible if growth suboptimal
9. Humans are the only reservoir for Mtb
10. Transmission
    a. Facilitated by close exposure to high-velocity cough (unprotected by proper mask or respirators) from patient with AFB-positive sputum and cavitary lesions, producing aerosolized droplets containing AFB, which are inhaled directly into alveoli
    b. Occurs in prisons, nursing homes, and hospitals

Pathogenesis

1. AFB (Mtb) is ingested by macrophages in alveoli, then transported to regional lymph nodes where spread is contained.
2. Some AFB may reach the bloodstream and disseminate widely.
3. Primary TB (asymptomatic, minimal pneumonitis in lower or midlung fields, with hilar lymph adenopathy) essentially an intracellular infection, with multiplication of organisms continuing for 2 to 12 weeks after primary exposure, until cell-mediated hypersensitivity (detected by positive skin test

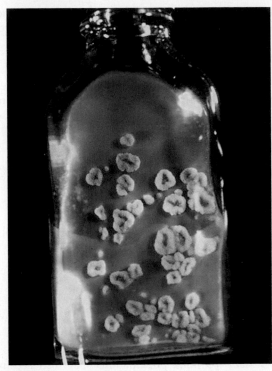

Fig 139–33
Primary isolate of *Mycobacterium tuberculosis* grown from sputum on Lowenstein-Jensen medium displaying cauliflower or verrucose colonies. These are also characteristic of other mycobacteria. (Courtesy of S. Froman and A. Gaytan.)

reaction to tuberculin purified protein derivative [PPD]) matures, with subsequent containment of infection

4. Local and disseminated AFB therefore contained by T-cell–mediated immune responses
   a. Recruitment of monocytes
   b. Transformation of lymphocytes with secretion of lymphokines
   c. Activation of macrophages and histiocytes
   d. Organization into granulomas, where organisms may survive in macrophages (Langhans' giant cells), but within which multiplication essentially ceases (95%) and from which spread is prohibited
5. Progressive primary pulmonary disease
   a. May immediately follow the asymptomatic phase
   b. Necrotizing pulmonary infiltrates
   c. Tuberculous bronchopneumonia
   d. Endobronchial TB
   e. Interstitial TB
   f. Widespread miliary lung lesions
6. Postprimary TB pleurisy with pleural effusion
   a. Develops after early primary infection, although often before conversion to positive PPD
   b. Results from pleural seeding from a peripheral lung lesion or rupture of lymph node into pleural space
   c. May produce a large (sometimes hemorrhagic) exudative effusion (with polymorphonuclear cells early, rapidly replaced by lymphocytes), frequently without pulmonary infiltrates

d. Generally resolves without treatment
   e. Portends a high risk of subsequent clinical disease, and therefore must be diagnosed and treated early (pleural biopsy and culture) to prevent future catastrophic TB illness
   f. May result in disseminated extrapulmonary infection
7. Reactivation pulmonary TB
   a. Occurs months to years following primary TB
   b. Preferentially involves the apical posterior segments of the upper lobes and superior segments of the lower lobes
   c. Associated with necrosis and cavitation of involved lung, hemoptysis, chronic fever, night sweats, weight loss
   d. Spread within lung occurs via cough and inhalation
8. Reinfection TB
   a. May mimic reactivation TB
   b. Ruptured caseous foci and cavities, which may produce endobronchial spread
9. Mtb in both progressive primary and reactivation pulmonary TB
   a. Intracellular (macrophage) lesions (undergoing slow multiplication)
   b. Closed caseous lesions (undergoing slow multiplication)
   c. Extracellular, open cavities (undergoing rapid multiplication)
   d. Isoniazid (INH) and rifampin are effective in all three sites
   e. Pyrazinamide (PZA) especially active within acidic macrophage environment
   f. Extrapulmonary reactivation disease also possible
10. Rapid local progression and dissemination in infants with devastating illness before PPD conversion occurs
11. Most symptoms (fever, weight loss, anorexia) and tissue destruction (caseous necrosis) from cytokines and cell-mediated immune responses
12. Mtb has no important endotoxins or exotoxins
13. Granuloma formation related to tumor necrosis factor (TNF) secreted by activated macrophages

DIFFERENTIAL DIAGNOSIS
- Necrotizing pneumonia (anaerobic, gram-negative) (see Fig. 139–4)
- Histoplasmosis (see Fig. 336–20)
- Coccidioidomycosis (see Fig. 336–25)
- Melioidosis
- Interstitial lung diseases (rarely) (see Fig. 135–2)
- Cancer (see Fig. 135–5)
- Sarcoidosis (see Fig. 137–6)
- Silicosis (see Fig. 134–4)
- Paragonimiasis
- Rare pneumonias
  1. *Rhodococcus equi* (cavitation)
  2. *Bacillus cereus* (50% hemoptysis)
  3. *Eikenella corrodens* (cavitation)

WORKUP
- Sputum for AFB stains
- Chest x-ray
- PPD
1. Recent conversion from negative to positive within 3 months of exposure is highly suggestive of recent infection.
2. Single positive PPD is not helpful diagnostically.
3. Negative PPD never rules out acute TB.

4. Be sure that positive PPD does not reflect booster phenomenon (prior positive PPD may become negative after several years and return to positive only after second repeated PPD; repeat second PPD within 1 week), which thus may mimic skin test conversion.

5. Positive PPD reaction is determined as follows:
   a. Induration after 72 hours of intradermal injection of 0.1 mL of tuberculin skin test (5 TU-PPD)
   b. 5-mm induration if HIV-positive (or other severe immunosuppressed state affecting cellular immune function), close contact of active TB, fibrotic chest lesions
   c. 10-mm induration if in high-medical risk group (immunosuppressive disease or therapy, renal failure, gastrectomy, silicosis, diabetes), foreign-born high-risk group (Southeast Asia, Latin America, Africa, India), low socioeconomic group, IV drug addict, prisoner, health care worker
   d. 15-mm induration if low risk

6. Anergy antigen testing (using mumps, *Candida*, tetanus toxoid) may identify patients truly anergic to PPD and these antigens, but results often confusing; not recommended

7. Patients with TB may be selectively anergic only to PPD.

8. Positive PPD indicates prior infection but does not itself confirm active disease.

● A new diagnostic test for latent tuberculosis infection, known as the QuantiFERON TB gold test (QFT-G), is now available. This is a blood test that measures interferon response to specific *M. tuberculosis* antigens. The test is FDA-approved and is available in some large TB centers and state health departments. It may assist in distinguishing true positive reactions from individuals with latent tuberculosis from PPD reactions related to nontuberculous mycobacteria, prior BCG vaccination, or difficult to interpret skin test results from those with dermatologic conditions or immediate allergic reactions to PPD. The diagnostic usefulness of the test as a replacement or supplement to the standard PPD is not yet fully determined.

LABORATORY TESTS

● Sputum for AFB stains and culture
   1. Induced sputum if patient not coughing productively
● Sputum from bronchoscopy (Fig. 139–34) if high suspicion of TB with negative expectorated induced sputum for AFB
   1. Positive AFB smear is essential before or shortly after treatment to ensure subsequent growth for definitive diagnosis and sensitivity testing
   2. Consider lung biopsy (Fig. 139–35) if sputum negative, especially if infiltrates are predominantly interstitial

IMAGING STUDIES

● Chest x-ray (Fig. 139–36)
   1. Primary infection reflected by calcified peripheral lung nodule with calcified hilar lymph node
   2. Reactivation pulmonary TB
      a. Necrosis
      b. Cavitation (especially on apical lordotic views)
      c. Fibrosis and hilar retraction
      d. Bronchopneumonia
      e. Interstitial infiltrates
      f. Miliary pattern
      g. Many previous presentations may also accompany progressive primary TB.
   3. TB pleurisy
      a. Pleural effusion, often rapidly accumulating and massive
   4. TB activity not established by single chest x-ray.
   5. Serial chest x-rays are excellent indicators of progression or regression.

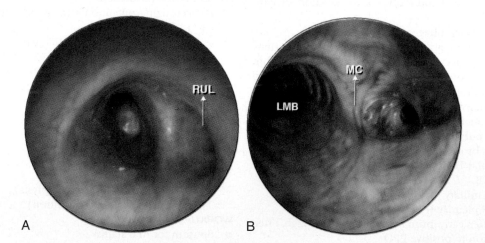

A   B

Fig 139–34
A, Endobronchial tuberculosis with endobronchial granuloma distal to right upper lobe bronchus (RUL). **B,** Tuberculous stricture of right main stem bronchus. Main carina (MC) and left main stem bronchus (LMB) are normal. Postinfectious strictures usually follow endobronchial tuberculosis. Tuberculosis can lead to mucosal and submucosal granulomas, mucosal ulcerations, endobronchial polyps, and bronchial stenosis. Erosion into a bronchus by a mediastinal lymph node may mimic a neoplasm. The diagnostic rate from bronchoscopy in tuberculosis is about 72%, and bronchoscopy is the only procedure to provide the diagnosis in 20% to 45% of patients with active tuberculosis. However, routine culture of bronchoscopic specimens has a diagnostic yield of only 6%. In military tuberculosis, bronchoscopic brushings, washings, and bronchoscopic lung biopsy (BLB) are diagnostic in up to 80% of patients.
(From Gold WM, Murray JF, Nadel JA: Atlas of Procedures in Respiratory Medicine. Philadelphia, WB Saunders, 2002.)

TREATMENT

- Compliance (rigid adherence to treatment regimen) chief determinant of success.
  1. Supervised, directly observed therapy (DOT) recommended for all patients and mandatory for unreliable patients
- Preferred adult regimen: DOT
  1. Isoniazid (INH), 15 mg/kg (maximum, 900 mg) + rifampin, 600 mg + ethambutol (EMB), 30 mg/kg (maximum, 2500 mg) + pyrazinamide (PZA; 2 g [<50 kg]; 2.5 g [51 to 74 kg]; 3 g [>75 kg]) three times weekly for 6 months
  2. Alternative, more complicated DOT regimens
- Rifapentine, a rifampin derivative with a much longer serum half-life, was shown to be as effective when administered weekly (with weekly isoniazid) as conventional regimens for drug-sensitive pulmonary tuberculosis in non–HIV-infected patients.
- Short-course daily therapy: adult
  1. HIV-negative patient: 6 months total therapy (2 months INH, 300 mg + rifampin, 600 mg + EMB, 15 mg/kg [maximum, 2500 mg]) + PZA (1.5 g [<50 kg]; 2 g [51 to 74 kg]; 2.5 g [>75 kg]) daily and until smear negative and sensitivity confirmed; then INH + rifampin daily × 4 months
  2. HIV-positive patient: 9 months total therapy (2 months INH + rifampin + EMB + PZA daily until smear negative and sensitivity confirmed; then INH + rifampin daily × 7 months)
  3. Continue treatment at least 3 months following conversion to negative cultures.
- Drug resistance (often multiple drug resistance to TB [MDRTB]) increased by the following:
  1. Prior treatment
  2. Acquisition of TB in developing countries
  3. Homelessness

  4. AIDS
  5. Prisoners
  6. IV drug addicts
  7. Known contact with MDRTB
- Never add single drug to failing regimen.
- Never treat TB with fewer than two to three drugs or two to three new additional drugs.
- Monitor for clinical toxicity (especially hepatitis).
  1. Patient and physician awareness that anorexia, nausea, right upper quadrant pain, and unexplained malaise require immediate cessation of treatment.
  2. Evaluation of LFT results
     a. Minimal aspartate aminotransferase (AST). Alanine aminotransferase (ALT) elevations without symptoms generally transient and not clinically significant
- Preventive treatment for PPD conversion only (infection without disease).
  1. Must be certain that chest x-ray is negative and patient has no symptoms of TB
  2. INH, 300 mg daily for 6 to 12 months; at least 12 months if HIV-positive
  3. Most important groups:
     a. HIV-positive
     b. Close contact of active TB
     c. Recent converter
     d. Old TB on chest x-ray
     e. IV drug addict
     f. Medical risk factor
     g. High-risk foreign country
     h. Homeless

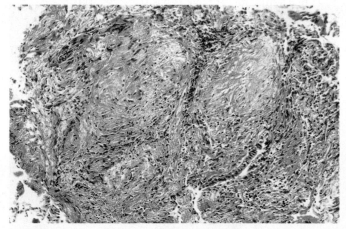

Fig 139–35

Mycobacterium tuberculosis—noncaseating granulomas with multinucleated giant cells in the submucosa of a bronchus; transbronchial biopsy (H&E, ×100; *M. tuberculosis* isolated in cultures).
(From Silverberg SG, Frable WJ, Wick MR, et al [eds]: Principles and Practice of Surgical Pathology and Cytopathology, 4th ed. Philadelphia, Elsevier, 2006.)

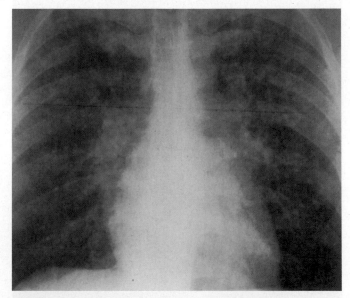

Fig 139–36

Tuberculosis. A PA chest film demonstrates a diffuse, bilateral, coarse nodular interstitial pattern associated with right hilar adenopathy. This combination of findings should suggest the presence of fungal or mycobacterial disease.
(From Grainger RG, Allison DJ, Adam A, Dixon AK [eds]: Grainger & Allison's Diagnostic Radiology, 4th ed. London, Harcourt, 2001.)

K. MILIARY TUBERCULOSIS

DEFINITION

Miliary tuberculosis (TB) is an infection of disseminated hematogenous disease, caused by the bacterium *Mycobacterium tuberculosis*. It is often characterized as resembling millet seeds on examination. Extrapulmonary disease may occur in almost every organ site.

PHYSICAL FINDINGS AND CLINICAL PRESENTATION

- See also "Cause"
- Common symptoms
  1. High intermittent fever
  2. Night sweats
  3. Weight loss
- Symptoms referable to individual organ systems may predominate.
  1. Meninges
  2. Pericardium
  3. Liver
  4. Kidneys, bladder (Fig. 139–37)
  5. Bone
  6. GI tract (Fig. 139–38)
  7. Lymph nodes

  8. Serous spaces
     a. Pleural (Fig. 139–39)
     b. Pericardial
     c. Peritoneal
     d. Joint
  9. Skin
  10. Lung: cough, shortness of breath
- Adrenal insufficiency possible caused by infection of adrenal gland
- TB hepatitis
  1. Tender liver
  2. Obstructive enzymes (alkaline phosphatase) elevated out of proportion to minimal hepatocellular enzymes (ALT, AST) and bilirubin
- TB meningitis
  1. Gradual-onset headache
  2. Minimal meningeal signs
  3. Malaise
  4. Low-grade fever (may be absent)
  5. Sudden stupor or coma
  6. Cranial nerve VI palsy
- TB pericarditis
  1. Effusions resembling TB pleurisy
  2. Cardiac tamponade
- Skeletal TB
  1. Large joint arthritis (with effusions resembling TB pericarditis)
  2. Bone lesions (especially ribs)
  3. Pott's disease
     a. TB spondylitis, especially of lower thoracic spine
     b. Paraspinous TB abscess
     c. Possible psoas abscess
     d. Frequent cord compression (often relieved by steroids)
- Genitourinary TB
  1. Renal TB (Fig. 139–40)
     a. Papillary necrosis
     b. Destruction of renal pelvis (Fig. 139–41)
     c. Strictures of upper third of ureters

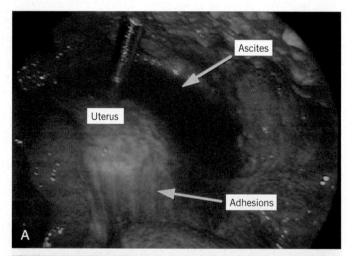

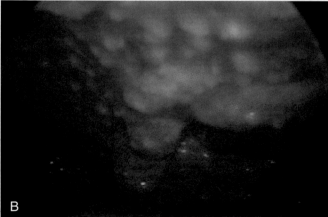

Fig 139–37
Laparoscopic views in genitourinary tuberculosis. **A,** Free and loculated ascites and fine fibrous adhesions. **B,** Miliary nodular exudate in the anteiror wall.
(From Cohen J, Powderly WG: Infectious Diseases, 2nd ed. St. Louis, Mosby, 2004.)

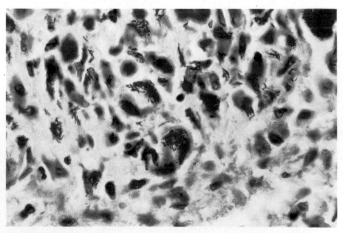

Fig 139–38
Acid-fast stain of tissue in miliary tuberculosis. The cells are packed with mycobacteria (×1000).
(From Silverberg SG, Frable WJ, Wick MR, et al [eds]: Principles and Practice of Surgical Pathology and Cytopathology, 4th ed. Philadelphia, Elsevier, 2006.)

        d. Hematuria
        e. Pyuria with misleading bacte rial cultures
        f. Preserved renal function
- Gastrointestinal TB
    1. Diarrhea
    2. Pain
    3. Obstruction
    4. Bleeding
    5. Especially common with AIDS

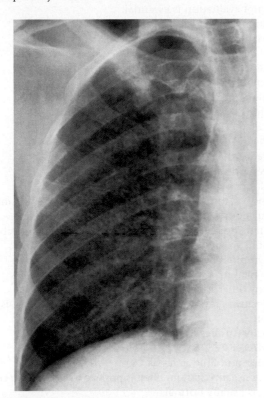

Fig 139–39
Miliary pattern in tuberculosis consists of numerous nodules of uniform size.
(From Grainger RG, Allison DJ, Adam A, Dixon AK [eds]: Grainger & Allison's Diagnostic Radiology, 4th ed. London, Harcourt, 2001.)

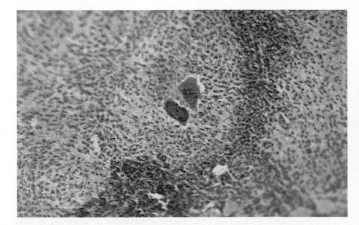

Fig 139–40
Tuberculosis granuloma. The granuloma is comprised of Langhans' giant cells (two large cells in the center), surrounding epithelioid cells, and a rim of lymphocytes.
(Courtesy of Dr. Sathi Bai Panikker Kottayam.)

6. Bowel lesions
    a. Circumferential ulcers
    b. Short strictures
    c. Calcified granulomas
    d. TB mesenteric caseous adenitis
    e. Abscess, but rare fistula formation
    f. Often difficult to distinguish from granulomatous bowel disease (Crohn's disease)
- TB peritonitis
    1. Fluid resembles TB pleurisy
    2. PPD often negative
    3. Tender abdomen
    4. Doughy peritoneal consistency, often with ascites
    5. Peritoneal biopsy indicated for diagnosis
- TB lymphadenitis (*scrofula*; Fig. 139–42)
    1. May involve all node groups
    2. Common adenopathies
        a. Cervical
        b. Supraclavicular
        c. Axillary
        d. Retroperitoneal
    3. Biopsy generally needed for diagnosis
    4. Surgical resection of nodes may be necessary
    5. Especially common with AIDS

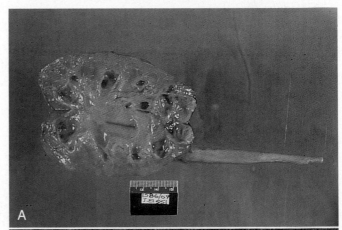

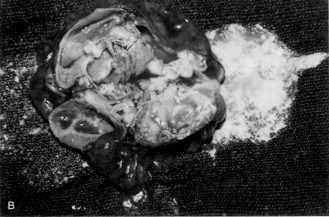

Fig 139–41
Ulcerocavernous lesions. **A,** Cut section of kidney showing areas of destruction in medulla and renal cortex. **B,** Cut section of kidney showing areas of cavitation and caseation necrosis (whitish chalky material).
(Courtesy of Professor K. Sasidhara.)

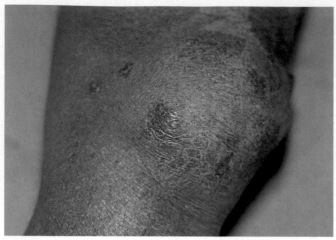

Fig 139–42
Scrofuloderma in a 60-year-old patient. A biopsy confirmed tuberculoid granulation tissue and the patient responded well to antituberculous therapy.
(From Cohen J, Powderly WG: Infectious Diseases, 2nd ed. St. Louis, Mosby, 2004.)

- Cutaneous TB
  1. Skin infection from autoinoculation or dissemination
  2. Nodules or abscesses
  3. Tuberculids (possibly allergic reactions)
  4. Erythema nodosum
- Miscellaneous presentations
  1. TB laryngitis
  2. TB otitis
  3. Ocular TB
     a. Choroidal tubercles
     b. Iritis
     c. Uveitis
     d. Episcleritis
  4. Adrenal TB
  5. Breast TB

CAUSE
- *Mycobacterium tuberculosis* (Mtb), a slow growing, aerobic, non–spore-forming, nonmotile bacillus
- Humans are the only reservoir for Mtb.
- Pathogenesis
  1. AFB (Mtb) are ingested by macrophages in alveoli, and then transported to regional lymph nodes, where spread is contained.
  2. Some AFB reach the bloodstream and disseminate widely.
  3. Immediate active disseminated disease may ensue or a latent period may develop.
  4. During latent period, T-cell immune mechanisms contain infection in granulomas until later reactivation occurs as a result of immunosuppression or other undefined factors in conjunction with reactivated pulmonary TB or alone.
- Miliary TB may occur as a consequence of the following:
  1. Primary infection: inability to contain primary infection leads to a hematogenous spread and progressive disseminated disease.
  2. In late chronic TB and in those with advanced age or poor immunity, a continuous seeding of the blood may develop and lead to disseminated disease.

DIFFERENTIAL DIAGNOSIS
- Widespread sites of possible dissemination associated with myriad differential diagnostic possibilities
- Lymphoma
- Typhoid fever
- Brucellosis
- Other tumors
- Collagen-vascular disease

WORKUP
- Prompt evaluation is essential.
- Sputum for AFB stain and culture
- Chest x-ray
- PPD
- Fluid analysis and culture wherever available
  1. Sputum
  2. Blood: particularly helpful in patients with AIDS
  3. Urine
  4. CSF
  5. Pleural
  6. Pericardial
  7. Peritoneal
  8. Gastric aspirates
- Biopsy of any involved tissue is advisable to make immediate diagnosis.
  1. Transbronchial biopsy preferred and easily accessible
  2. Bone marrow
  3. Lymph node
  4. Scrotal mass if present
  5. Any other involved site
  6. Positive granuloma or AFB on biopsy specimen is diagnostic.
- Imaging studies as needed

LABORATORY TESTS
- Culture and fluid analysis
- Smear-negative sputum often is positive weeks later on culture.
- CBC is usually normal.
- ESR is usually elevated.

IMAGING STUDIES
- Chest x-ray examination (may or may not be positive)
- CT scan or MRI of brain
  1. Tuberculoma
  2. Basilar arachnoiditis
- Endoscopic evaluation or barium studies of bowel

TREATMENT
- Therapy should be initiated immediately. Do not wait for definitive diagnosis.
- More rapid response to chemotherapy by disseminated TB foci than cavitary pulmonary TB.
- Treatment for 6 months with INH plus rifampin plus PZA.
  1. Treatment for 12 months often required for bone and renal TB
  2. Prolonged treatment often required for CNS and pericardial involvement
  3. Prolonged treatment often required for all disseminated TB in infants.
- Compliance (rigid adherence to treatment regimen) is the chief determinant of success.
  1. Supervised DOT is recommended for all patients.
  2. Supervised DOT is mandatory for unreliable patients.
- Steroids are often helpful additions in fulminant miliary disease with hypoxemia and DIC.

| Chapter 140 | **Acute respiratory distress syndrome** |

DEFINITION

Acute respiratory distress syndrome (ARDS) is a form of noncardiogenic pulmonary edema that results from acute damage to the alveoli. It is characterized by acute diffuse infiltrative lung lesions with resulting interstitial and alveolar edema, severe hypoxemia, and respiratory failure. The definition of ARDS includes the following three components:

1. Ratio of PaO_2 to FiO_2 ≤200 regardless of the level of PEEP
2. Detection of bilateral pulmonary infiltrates on frontal chest x-ray (Fig. 140–1)
3. Pulmonary artery wedge pressure (PAWP) ≤18 mm Hg or no clinical evidence of elevated left atrial pressure on the basis of chest radiograph or other clinical data

The cardinal feature of ARDS, refractory hypoxemia, is caused by the formation of protein-rich alveolar edema after damage to the integrity of the lung's alveolar capillary barrier.

PHYSICAL FINDINGS AND CLINICAL PRESENTATION

Signs and symptoms

1. Dyspnea
2. Chest discomfort
3. Cough
4. Anxiety

Physical examination

1. Tachypnea
2. Tachycardia
3. Hypertension
4. Coarse crepitations of both lungs
5. Fever may be present if infection is the underlying cause.

CAUSE

- Sepsis (>40% of cases)
- Aspiration: near-drowning, aspiration of gastric contents (>30% of cases)
- Trauma (>20% of cases)
- Multiple transfusions, blood products
- Drugs (e.g., overdose of morphine, methadone, heroin; reaction to nitrofurantoin)
- Noxious inhalation (e.g., chlorine gas, high O_2 concentration)
- Postresuscitation
- Cardiopulmonary bypass
- Pneumonia
- Burns
- Pancreatitis
- A history of chronic alcohol abuse significantly increases the risk of developing ARDS in critically ill patients.

DIFFERENTIAL DIAGNOSIS

- Cardiogenic pulmonary edema (see Fig. 110–1)
- Viral pneumonitis (see Fig. 139–16)
- Lymphangitic carcinomatosis

LABORATORY TESTS

- ABGs
  1. Initially: varying degrees of hypoxemia, generally resistant to supplemental oxygen
  2. Respiratory alkalosis, decreased PCO_2
  3. Widened alveolar-arterial gradient
  4. Hypercapnia as the disease progresses

- Bronchoalveolar lavage
  1. The most prominent finding is an increased number of polymorphonucleocytes.
  2. The presence of eosinophilia has therapeutic implications, because these patients respond to corticosteroids.
- Blood and urine cultures

IMAGING STUDIES

- Chest x-ray (see Fig. 140–1A)
  - The initial chest radiogram might be normal in the initial hours after the precipitating event.
  - Bilateral interstitial infiltrates are usually seen within 24 hours; they often are more prominent in the bases and periphery.
  - White out of both lung fields can be seen in advanced stages.
- CT scan of chest (see Fig. 140–1B): diffuse consolidation with air bronchograms, bullae, pleural effusions. Pneumomediastinum and pneumothoraces may also be present.

TREATMENT

- Ventilatory support
  - Blood and urine cultures and trial of antibiotics in presumed sepsis (routine administration of antibiotics in all cases of ARDS is not recommended).
  - Fluid management
  - Positioning the patient: changes in position can improve oxygenation by improving the distribution of perfusion to ventilated lung regions; repositioning (lateral decubitus positioning) should be attempted in patients with hypoxemia that is not responsive to other medical interventions. Placing patients with acute respiratory failure in a prone position improves their oxygenation but does not improve their survival.
- Nutritional support: nutritional support, preferably administered by the enteral route, is necessary to maintain adequate colloid oncotic pressure and intravascular volume. The inclusion of eicosapentaenoic acid from fish oil may be beneficial in improving ventilation requirements and length of stay in patients with ARDS.
- Tracheostomy: tracheostomy is warranted in patients requiring more than 2 weeks of mechanical ventilation.
- Stress ulcer prophylaxis with sucralfate suspension (via nasogastric tube), IV proton pump inhibitors (PPIs), or IV H_2 blockers.

DISPOSITION

- Prognosis for ARDS varies with the underlying cause. Prognosis is worse in patients with chronic liver disease, nonpulmonary organ dysfunction, sepsis, and advanced age.
- Elevated values of dead space fraction [($PaCO_2$ − $PeCO_2$)/$PaCO_2$] (normal is <0.3) is associated with an increased risk of death.
- Overall mortality rate varies between 32% and 45%. Most deaths are attributable to sepsis or multiorgan dysfunction rather than primary respiratory causes.

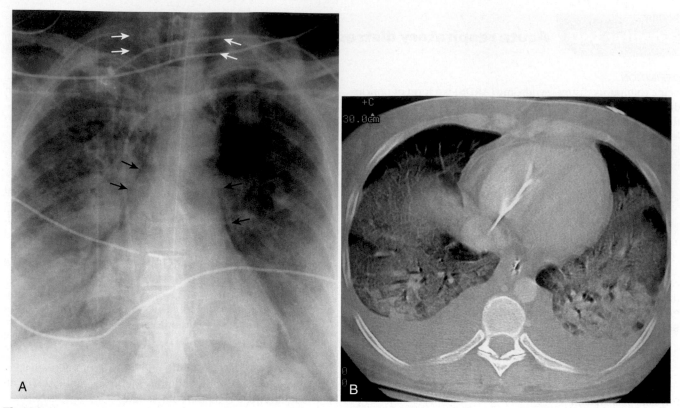

Fig 140-1
Acute respiratory distress syndrome (ARDS) caused by extrapulmonary disease. **A,** Chest radiograph 2¹/₂ days after postoperative hemorrhage. There is diffuse ground-glass opacification, slightly greater on the right than the left. For unknown reasons, the left apex is spared. Incidentally noted are signs of barotrauma pneumomediastinum *(black arrows),* and subcutaneous air in the neck *(white arrows).* **B,** CT scan taken a few hours earlier shows almost symmetrical bilateral ground-glass opacification throughout the lower lobes. There are bilateral effusions, which are commonly seen in ARDS on CT, but missed on the supine portable radiograph.
(From Grainger RG, Allison DJ, Adam A, Dixon AK [eds]: Grainger & Allison's Diagnostic Radiology, 4th ed. London, Harcourt, 2001.)

DEFINITION

Pulmonary hypertension (PH) is abnormally elevated pressure in the arterial side of the pulmonary circulation, usually defined as mean pulmonary pressure >25 mm Hg at rest or greater than 30 mm Hg with exercise. Sustained elevation in pulmonary arterial pressure caused by increased pulmonary venous pressure, hypoxic pulmonary vasoconstriction, or increased flow is often referred to as secondary pulmonary hypertension.

PHYSICAL FINDINGS AND CLINICAL PRESENTATION

Primary pulmonary hypertension
- PPH is insidious and may go undetected for years.
- Exertional dyspnea is the most common presenting symptom (60%).
- Fatigue and weakness
- Syncope
- Chest pain
- Loud P_2 component of the second heart sound
- Right-sided S_4
- Jugular venous distention
- Abdominal distention, ascites
- Prominent parasternal (RV) impulse
- Holosystolic tricuspid regurgitation murmur heard best along the left fourth parasternal line that increases in intensity with inspiration
- Peripheral edema

Secondary pulmonary hypertension
- Similar to PPH but depends on the underlying cause (e.g., left-sided CHF, mitral stenosis, COPD)

CAUSE
- The cause of PPH is unknown. Most cases are sporadic, but there is a 6% to 12% familial incidence.
- PPH is associated with several known risk factors: portal hypertension and liver cirrhosis, appetite-suppressant drugs (fenfluramine), and HIV disease.
- Several genetic abnormalities have been associated with the familial form of PPH, many of which are mutations in the genes that code for members of the transforming growth factor β (TGF-β) family of receptors (BMPR-II, ALK-1) on chromosome 2q33.
- Familial PPH is an autosomal-dominant disease with variable penetrance, affecting only about 10% to 20% of carriers.
- Several factors have been identified that play roles in the pathogenesis of PPH, including a genetic predisposition, endothelial cell dysfunction, abnormalities in vasomotor control, thrombotic obliteration of the vascular lumen, and vascular remodeling through cell proliferation and matrix production (Fig. 141–1). An emerging theory involves abnormal membrane potassium channels modulating calcium kinetics.
- Secondary pulmonary hypertension is primarily caused by underlying pulmonary and cardiac conditions, including the following:
  1. Pulmonary thromboembolic disease
  2. Chronic obstructive pulmonary disease (COPD)
  3. Interstitial lung disease
  4. Obstructive sleep disorder
  5. Neuromuscular diseases causing hypoventilation (e.g., amyotrophic lateral sclerosis [ALS])
  6. Collagen-vascular disease (e.g., SLE, CREST syndrome, systemic sclerosis)
  7. Pulmonary venous disease
  8. Left ventricular failure resulting from hypertension, coronary artery disease, aortic stenosis, and cardiomyopathy
  9. Valvular heart disease (e.g., mitral stenosis, mitral regurgitation)
  10. Congenital heart disease with left-to-right shunting (e.g., atrial septal defect [ASD])

DIAGNOSIS
- The normal pulmonary arterial systolic pressure ranges from 18 to 30 mm Hg and the diastolic pressure ranges from 4 to 12 mm Hg.
- PH is a hemodynamic diagnosis involving two stages: detection of elevated pressure in the pulmonary arteries, and characterization of this abnormality to determine its cause by ruling out secondary causes.
- Right-heart catheterization must be performed in all patients suspected of having PH to establish the diagnosis and document pulmonary hemodynamics.
- Primary pulmonary hypertension is a diagnosis of exclusion; all secondary causes as mentioned earlier must be excluded.

DIFFERENTIAL DIAGNOSIS
See "Cause"

WORKUP
- Screening for the presence of PH using Doppler echocardiography is warranted in individuals with a known predisposing genetic mutation or first-degree relative with idiopathic PPH, scleroderma, congenital heart disease with left-to-right shunt, or portal hypertension undergoing evaluation for orthotopic liver transplantation.

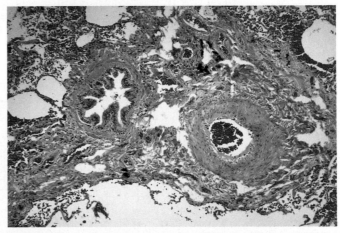

Fig 141–1
Pulmonary hypertension, grade I. There is muscular hypertrophy, muscular arteries have thickened walls. Luminal narrowing is typically present and may be prominent.
(From Silverberg SG, Frable WJ, Wick MR, et al [eds]: Principles and Practice of Surgical Pathology and Cytopathology, 4th ed. Philadelphia, Elsevier, 2006.)

- The workup of a patient suspected of having PPH includes a detailed evaluation of the heart and lungs. Blood tests, chest x-ray, pulmonary function tests, CT scan of the chest, radionuclide studies of the heart and lungs, echocardiography, electrocardiography, pulmonary angiography, and right and left heart catheterization are all useful to exclude secondary causes of pulmonary hypertension.
- Once the diagnosis has been made, functional assessment should be undergone to determine disease prognosis and potential treatment options.
- The degree of functional impairment as assessed by the World Health Organization (WHO) classification system and the 6-minute walk test are useful ways to monitor disease progression and assess response to treatment.

LABORATORY TESTS

- CBC is usually normal in PPH but may show secondary polycythemia.
- ABGs show low P_{O_2} and oxygen saturation.
- PFT is done to exclude obstructive or restrictive lung disease.
- Overnight oximetry and sleep study to rule out sleep apnea/hypopnea
- ECG (Fig. 141–2) may show evidence of right atrial enlargement (tall P wave >2.5 mV in leads II, III, aVF) and right ventricular enlargement (right axis deviation >100 and R wave > S wave in lead V_1).
- Other blood tests: ANA titer to screen for underlying connective tissue disease, HIV serology, LFT, and antiphospholipid antibodies.
- Assessment of exercise capacity is a key part of the evaluation of PH in characterizing the disease and determining prognosis and treatment options. The 6-minute walk test and cardiopulmonary exercise testing with gas exchange measurements are the most commonly used methods of assessment.

IMAGING STUDIES

- Chest x-ray (Fig. 141–3) shows enlargement of the main and hilar pulmonary arteries with rapid tapering of the distal vessels. Right ventricular enlargement may be evident on lateral films.
- Spiral CT scan of chest or lung perfusion scan (V/Q scan) are useful in excluding chronic pulmonary embolism.
- Transthoracic Doppler echocardiography, including M-mode, two-dimensional, pulse, continuous, and color Doppler, assesses ventricular function, excludes significant valvular pathology, and visualizes abnormal shunting of blood between heart chambers if present. It also provides an estimate of pulmonary artery systolic pressure that has been shown by most studies to correlate well with pressures measured by right-heart catheterization.
- MRI (Fig. 141–4)
- Pulmonary angiogram is done in patients with suspicious V/Q scans.
- Cardiac catheterization is performed to measure pulmonary artery pressures directly and to detect any shunting of blood.

TREATMENT

- Oxygen therapy to improve alveolar oxygen flow in primary and secondary pulmonary hypertension
- Avoidance of vigorous exercise
- Chest physiotherapy
- PPH
  1. Diuretics improve dyspnea and peripheral edema.
  2. Vasodilator treatment is usually done with hemodynamic monitoring and includes IV adenosine, epoprostenol (prostacyclin) nitric oxide, or oral sildenafil.
- Secondary pulmonary hypertension treatment is aimed at the underlying cause.
- Chronic anticoagulation with warfarin is recommended to prevent thromboses and has been shown to prolong life in patients with PPH.

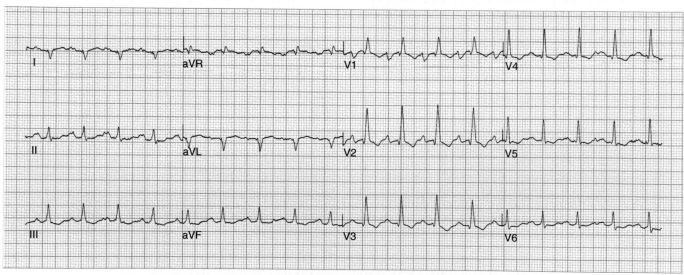

Fig 141–2

ECG from a patient with advanced pulmonary hypertension demonstrating right axis deviation, right ventricular hypertrophy, and right atrial enlargement.
(From Crawford MH, DiMarco JP, Paulus WJ [eds]: Cardiology, 2nd ed. St. Louis, Mosby, 2004.)

- Calcium channel blockers may alleviate pulmonary vaso-constriction and prolong life in about 20% of patients with PPH. Nifedipine and diltiazem are the agents of choice.
- Epoprostenol
- Iloprost
- Bosentan
- Sildenafil
- Lung transplantation and heart-lung transplantation are other options in end-stage class IV patients. Atrial septostomy may be performed as a bridge to transplantation. The defect can be closed at the time of transplantation.

- Atrial septostomy is recommended for individuals with a room air SaO_2 >90% who suffer from severe right heart failure (with refractory ascites), despite maximal diuretic therapy or who have signs of impaired systemic blood flow (such as syncope) caused by reduced left heart filling.
- Lung transplant recipients with PPH had survival rates of 73% at 1 year, 55% at 3 years, and 45% at 5 years.

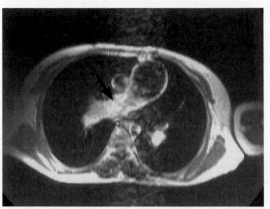

Fig 141–4
MRI scan of pulmonary hypertension. The MR spin-echo image (echo time, 40 msec) through the right pulmonary artery of a patient with pulmonary hypertension caused by ventricular septal defect. The high signal in the right pulmonary artery *(arrow)* is caused by sluggish blood flow rather than a pulmonary embolus.
(From Grainger RG, Allison DJ, Adam A, Dixon AK [eds]: Grainger & Allison's Diagnostic Radiology, 4th ed. London, Harcourt, 2001.)

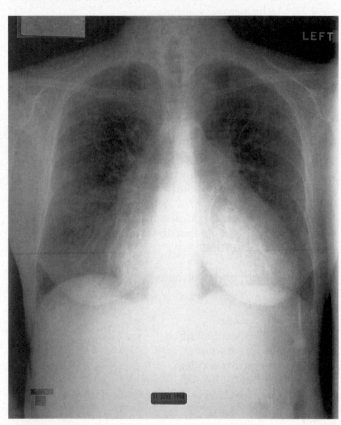

Fig 141–3
Chest radiograph in a patient with severe intrinsic pulmonary vascular disease demonstrating enlargement of the main pulmonary artery, right ventricle, and right atrium.
(From Crawford MH, DiMarco JP, Paulus WJ [eds]: Cardiology, 2nd ed. St. Louis, Mosby, 2004.)

Chapter 142 — Altitude sickness

DEFINITION

Altitude sickness refers to a spectrum of illnesses related to hypoxia occurring in people rapidly ascending to high altitudes. Common acute syndromes occurring at high altitudes include acute mountain sickness, high-altitude pulmonary edema, and high-altitude cerebral edema.

PHYSICAL FINDINGS AND CLINICAL PRESENTATION

Acute mountain sickness (AMS)

- Occurs within hours to a few days after rapid ascent over 8000 feet (2500 m)
- Headache is the most common symptom
- Dizziness and lightheadedness
- Nausea, vomiting, loss of appetite
- Fatigue, nail changes (Fig. 142–1)
- Sleep disturbance
- AMS can evolve into high-altitude pulmonary edema (HAPE) and high-altitude cerebral edema (HACE)

Pulmonary edema

- Occurs usually during the second night after rapid ascent over 8000 feet (2500 m)

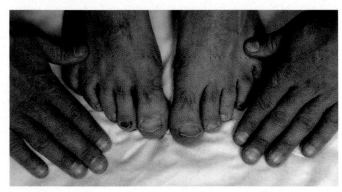

Fig 142–1
Everest nails that developed in a 40-year-old man who climbed Cho/Oyu [8254m (27,063 feet)], in the Mount Everest region. White bands are seen on all nail beds; their width and distance from the base plate are proportional to the time spent at high altitude, and proportional to the time since exposure to high altitude.
(From Crawford MH, DiMarco JP, Paulus WJ [eds]: Cardiology, 2nd ed. St. Louis, Mosby, 2004.)

- Dyspnea at rest
- Dry cough
- Chest tightness
- Tachycardia, tachypnea, rales, cyanosis, with pink-tinged frothy sputum

High-altitude cerebral edema

- Usually presents several days after AMS
- Confusion, irritability, drowsiness, stupor, hallucinations
- Headache, nausea, vomiting
- Ataxia, paralysis, seizures
- Coma and death may develop within hours of the first symptoms.

CAUSE

- As one ascends to altitudes above sea level, the atmospheric pressure decreases. Although the percentage of oxygen in the air remains the same, the partial pressure of oxygen decreases with altitude.
- Thus, the cause of altitude sickness is primarily hypoxia resulting from low partial pressures of oxygen.
- The body responds to low oxygen partial pressures through a process of acclimatization.

DIAGNOSIS

The diagnosis of altitude sickness is made by clinical presentation and physical findings described earlier.

DIFFERENTIAL DIAGNOSIS

- Dehydration
- Carbon monoxide poisoning
- Hypothermia
- Infection
- Substance abuse
- Congestive heart failure
- Pulmonary embolism
- Cerebrovascular accident

LABORATORY TESTS

- Laboratory tests are not very useful in diagnosing altitude sickness.

IMAGING STUDIES

- Chest x-ray (Fig. 142–2) may show prominent pulmonary arteries, Kerley B lines, and patchy edema.
- CT scan of the head showing diffuse or patchy edema

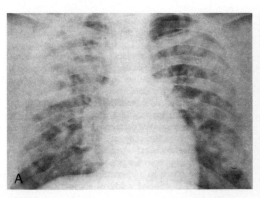
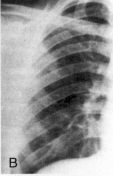
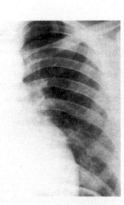

Fig 142–2
Chest radiographs of a young male with high-altitude pulmonary embolism. **A,** The patchy supradiaphragmatic distribution, normal-sized heart, and prominent pulmonary arteries are typical. **B,** Near-complete resolution after 48 hours of supplemental oxygen is typical.
(From Crawford MH, DiMarco JP, Paulus WJ [eds]: Cardiology, 2nd ed. St. Louis, Mosby, 2004.)

TREATMENT

- Stop the ascent to allow acclimatization or start to descend until symptoms have resolved.
- Oxygen, 4 to 6 L/min, is used for severe AMS, HAPE, and HACE.
- Portable hyperbaric bags are useful if available at the site.
- Avoid dehydration.
- Aspirin, 325 mg PO every 6 hours, can be used for headaches in AMS.

- Acetazolamide, 125-250 mg PO twice daily, has been shown to alleviate symptoms of AMS and HAPE.
- Nifedipine, 10 mg sublingual, followed by long-acting nifedipine, 30 mg twice daily, used for patients with HAPE who cannot descend immediately.
- Dexamethasone, 4 mg PO every 6 hours, is used in patients with severe AMS, HAPE, and HACE.

Chapter 143 | Pulmonary embolism

DEFINITION
Pulmonary embolism (PE) refers to the lodging of a thrombus or other embolic material from a distant site in the pulmonary circulation.

PHYSICAL FINDINGS AND CLINICAL PRESENTATION
- Most common symptom: dyspnea
- Chest pain: may be nonpleuritic or pleuritic (infarction)
- Syncope (massive PE)
- Fever, diaphoresis, apprehension
- Hemoptysis, cough
- Evidence of deep venous thrombosis (DVT) may be present (e.g., swelling and tenderness of extremities)
- Cardiac examination: may reveal tachycardia, increased pulmonic component of S_2, murmur of tricuspid insufficiency, right ventricular heave, right-sided S_3
- Pulmonary examination: may demonstrate rales, localized wheezing, friction rub
- Most common physical finding: tachypnea

CAUSE
- Thrombus, fat, or other foreign material
- Risk factors for PE
  1. Prolonged immobilization
  2. Postoperative state
  3. Trauma to lower extremities
  4. Estrogen-containing birth control pills
  5. Prior history of DVT or PE
  6. CHF
  7. Pregnancy and early puerperium
  8. Visceral cancer (lung, pancreas, alimentary and genitourinary tracts)
  9. Trauma, burns
  10. Advanced age
  11. Obesity
  12. Hematologic disease (e.g., antithrombin III deficiency, protein C deficiency, protein S deficiency, lupus anticoagulant, polycythemia vera, dysfibrinogenemia, paroxysmal nocturnal hemoglobinuria, factor V Leiden mutation, G20210A prothrombin mutation)
  13. COPD, diabetes mellitus
  14. Prolonged air travel

DIFFERENTIAL DIAGNOSIS
- Myocardial infarction
- Pericarditis
- Pneumonia
- Pneumothorax
- Chest wall pain
- GI abnormalities (e.g., peptic ulcer, esophageal rupture, gastritis)
- CHF
- Pleuritis
- Anxiety disorder with hyperventilation
- Pericardial tamponade
- Dissection of aorta
- Asthma

LABORATORY TESTS
- ABGs generally reveal decreased Pao_2 and $Paco_2$ and increased pH; normal results do not rule out PE.
- Alveolar-arteriolar (A-a) oxygen gradient, a measure of the difference in oxygen concentration between alveoli and arterial blood, is a more sensitive indicator of the alteration in oxygenation than Pao_2; it can easily be calculated using the information from ABGs. A normal A-a gradient among patients without history of PE or DVT makes the diagnosis of PE unlikely.
- Plasma D-dimer measurement: D-dimer assays by ELISA detect the presence of plasmin-mediated degradation products of fibrin that contain cross-linked D fragments in the whole blood or plasma. A normal plasma D-dimer level is useful to exclude pulmonary embolism in patients with a nondiagnostic lung scan and a low pretest probability of PE. However, it cannot be used to rule in the diagnosis because it increases with many other disorders (e.g., metastatic cancer, trauma, sepsis, postoperative state).
- ECG (Fig. 143–1) is abnormal in 85% of patients with acute PE. Frequent abnormalities include sinus tachycardia; nonspecific ST-segment or T wave changes; S-I, Q-III, T-III pat-

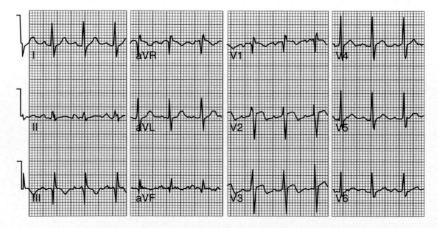

Fig 143–1
Acute massive pulmonary embolus with the characteristic S_1Q_3 pattern and more common but nonspecific changes, including incomplete right bundle branch block and ST segment elevation in leads V_1 through V_3, with terminal T wave inversion.
(From Braunwald E: Heart Disease: A Textbook of Cardiovascular Medicine, 5th ed. Philadelphia, WB Saunders, 1997.)

tern (10% of patients); S-I, S-II, S-III pattern; T wave inversion in V_1 to V_6; acute right bundle branch block (RBBB); new-onset atrial fibrillation; ST segment depression in lead II; and right ventricular strain.

IMAGING STUDIES

- A diagnostic algorithm for suspected pulmonary embolism is shown in Figure 143–2.
- Chest x-ray may be normal; suggestive findings include elevated diaphragm, pleural effusion, dilation of pulmonary artery (Fig. 143–3), infiltrate or consolidation, abrupt vessel cutoff, and atelectasis. A wedge-shaped consolidation in the middle and lower lobes is suggestive of a pulmonary infarction and is known as *Hampton's hump.*
- Spiral CT (Fig. 143–4) is an excellent modality for diagnosing PE. It may be used instead of a lung scan and is favored

in patients with baseline lung abnormalities on initial chest x-ray. It has the added advantage of detecting other pulmonary pathology that can mimic pulmonary embolism. Newer generation CT scanners (e.g., four-slice multidetector row CT) are highly accurate in diagnosing PE and, when coupled with D-dimer testing, may eliminate the need for additional testing.

- Lung scan (Fig. 143–5) in patients with normal chest x-ray examination:

1. A normal lung scan rules out PE.

2. A ventilation-perfusion mismatch is suggestive of PE, and a lung scan interpretation of high probability is confirmatory.

- Angiography (Fig. 143–6): pulmonary angiography is the gold standard; however, it is invasive, expensive, and not

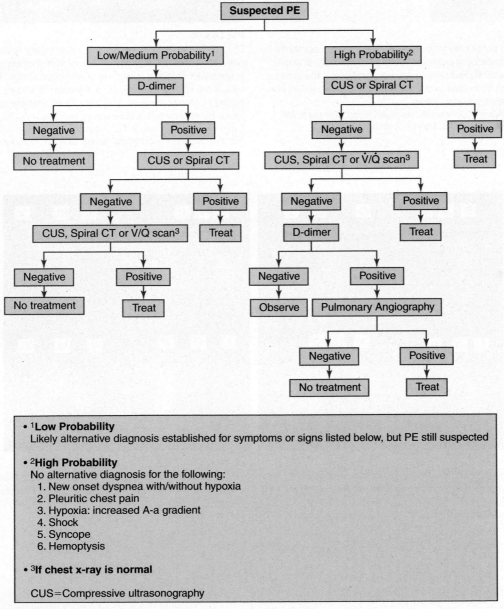

Fig 143–2
Clinical algorithm for pulmonary embolism (PE).
(From Ferri F: Practical Guide to the Care of the Medical Patient, 7th ed. St. Louis, Mosby, 2007.)

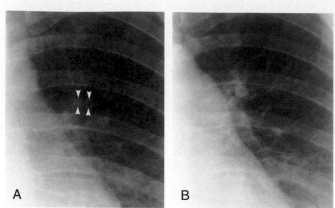

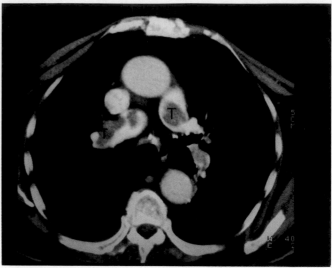

Fig 143–3

Plain radiography in pulmonary embolism. **A,** The anterior segmental bronchus and accompanying pulmonary artery are normally of similar diameter *(arrowheads).* **B,** Following pulmonary embolism, the anterior segmental artery has increased in caliber. Note also the increased convex bulge of the main pulmonary artery.
(From Grainger RG, Allison DJ, Adam A, Dixon AK [eds]: Grainger & Allison's Diagnostic Radiology, 4th ed. London, Harcourt, 2001.)

Fig 143–4

Spiral CT scan from a patient with a pulmonary embolus. A ventilation-perfusion radionuclide study gave a high probability result. A series of images was obtained with 5-mm collimation and a pitch of 1 (5 mm/sec) at the end of an intravenous injection of 100 mL of dilute (150 mg/mL) contrast medium. The thrombotic material appears as soft tissue filling defects in both main pulmonary arteries.
(From Grainger RG, Allison DJ, Adam A, Dixon AK [eds]: Grainger & Allison's Diagnostic Radiology, 4th ed. London, Harcourt, 2001.)

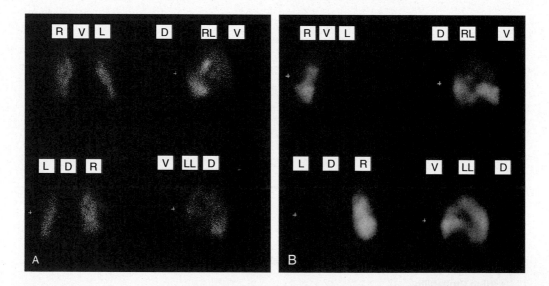

Fig 143–5

Ventilation-perfusion lung scan in massive pulmonary embolism. **A,** Normal pattern on the ventilation scan. **B,** The complete disappearance of the entire left lung from the perfusion scan indicates proximal occlusion of the left pulmonary artery. D, dorsal; L, left; LL, left lobe; R, right; RL, right lobe; V, ventral.
(From Crawford MH, DiMarco JP, Paulus WJ [eds]: Cardiology, 2nd ed. St. Louis, Mosby, 2004.)

readily available in some clinical settings. Gadolinium-enhanced magnetic resonance angiography (MRA) of the pulmonary arteries has a moderate sensitivity and high specificity for the diagnosis of PE. MRA is best reserved for select patients when CT and/or lung scans are inconclusive and the risk of pulmonary angiography is high.

TREATMENT

- Heparin by continuous infusion for at least 5 days. Many experts recommend a larger initial IV heparin bolus (15,000 to 20,000 U) to block platelet aggregation and thrombi and subsequent release of vasoconstrictive substances.

- Thrombolytic agents (urokinase, tissue plasminogen activator [tPA], streptokinase): provide rapid resolution of clots; thrombolytic agents are the treatment of choice in patients with massive PE who are hemodynamically unstable and with no contraindication to their use..

- Long-term treatment is generally carried out with warfarin therapy started on day 1 or 2 and given in a dose to maintain the internation normalized ratio (INR) at 2 to 3.

- If thrombolytics and anticoagulants are contraindicated (e.g., GI bleeding, recent CNS surgery, recent trauma) or if the patient continues to have recurrent PE despite anticoagulation therapy, vena caval interruption is indicated by transvenous placement of a Greenfield vena caval filter.

- Acute pulmonary artery embolectomy may be indicated in a patient with massive pulmonary emboli and refractory hypotension.

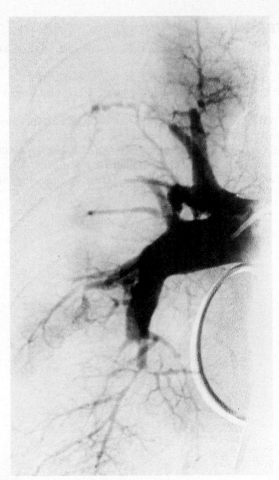

Fig 143–6
Digital subtraction pulmonary arteriogram of the right lung of a patient with recurrent pulmonary emboli. Note the complete occlusion of several of the large pulmonary arteries and abrupt changes in arterial caliber.
(From Grainger RG, Allison DJ, Adam A, Dixon AK [eds]: Grainger & Allison's Diagnostic Radiology, 4th ed. London, Harcourt, 2001.)

REFERENCES

Cohen J, Powderly WG: Infectious Diseases, 2nd ed 2, St. Louis, Mosby, 2004.

Ferri F: Ferri's Clinical Advisor 2007. St. Louis, Mosby, 2007.

Ferri F: Practical Guide to the Care of the Medical Patient, 7th ed. St. Louis, Mosby, 2007.

Gold WM, Murray JF, Nadel JA: Atlas of Procedures in Respiratory Care Medicine, Philadelphia, WB Saunders, 2002.

Grainger RG, Allison DJ, Adam A, Dixon AK (eds): Grainger & Allison's Diagnostic Radiology, 4th ed. London, Harcourt, 2001.

Hochberg MC, Silman AJ, Smolen JS, et al (eds): Rheumatology, 3rd ed. St. Louis, Mosby, 2003.

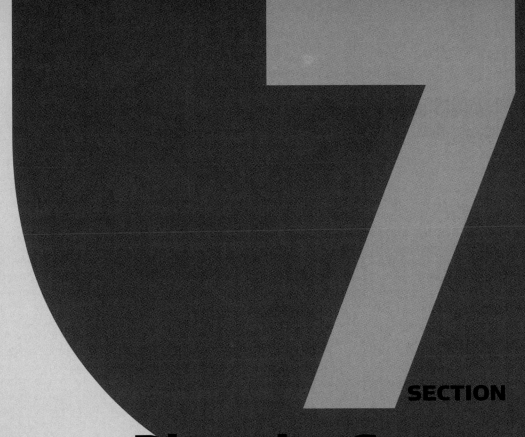

SECTION

Digestive System

Esophagus
Chapter 144: Zenker's diverticulum
Chapter 145: Gastroesophageal reflux
Chapter 146: Hiatal hernia
Chapter 147: Mallory-Weiss tear
Chapter 148: Barrett's esophagus
Chapter 149: Esophageal carcinoma
Chapter 150: Rings and webs
Chapter 151: Achalasia
Chapter 152: Esophageal spasm
Chapter 153: Esophageal varices

Stomach and duodenum
Chapter 154: Gastritis
Chapter 155: Peptic ulcer
Chapter 156: Gastric carcinoma
Chapter 157: Intestinal obstruction

Small intestine
Chapter 158: Celiac disease
Chapter 159: Meckel's diverticulum
Chapter 160: Inguinal and femoral hernias
Chapter 161: Appendicitis
Chapter 162: Crohn's colitis

Colon
Chapter 163: Ulcerative colitis
Chapter 164: Diverticular disease
Chapter 165: Familial polyposis syndrome
Chapter 166: Peutz-Jeghers syndrome
Chapter 167: Gardner's syndrome
Chapter 168: Colorectal cancer

Disorders of the anus, anal canal, and perianal region
Chapter 169: Hemorrhoids
Chapter 170: Anal fissure
Chapter 171: Perirectal abscess
Chapter 172: Fistula

Pancreas
Chapter 173: Acute pancreatitis
Chapter 174: Chronic pancreatitis
Chapter 175: Carcinoma of the pancreas

Liver
Chapter 176: Cirrhosis
Chapter 177: Ascites
Chapter 178: Hepatorenal syndrome
Chapter 179: Primary biliary cirrhosis
Chapter 180: Hemochromatosis
Chapter 181: Nonalcoholic steatohepatitis
Chapter 182: Hepatocellular carcinoma
Chapter 183: Hepatic infections
Chapter 184: Autoimmune hepatitis

Gallbladder and bile ducts
Chapter 185: Cholelithiasis
Chapter 186: Cholecystitis
Chapter 187: Cholangiocarcinoma

Gastrointestinal Infections
Chapter 188: Viral gastroenteritis
Chapter 189: Salmonellosis
Chapter 190: Cholera
Chapter 191: Whipple's disease
Chapter 192: Mesenteric adenitis
Chapter 193: Pseudomembranous colitis

Vascular
Chapter 194: Mesenteric ischemia
Chapter 195: Portal vein thrombosis
Chapter 196: Budd-Chiari syndrome

Endocrine gastrointestinal disorders
Chapter 197: Carcinoid
Chapter 198: Gastrinoma (Zollinger-Ellison syndrome)
Chapter 199: Glucagonoma

ESOPHAGUS

Chapter 144   Zenker's diverticulum

DEFINITION

Zenker's (hypopharyngeal, pharynoesophageal) diverticulum refers to the acquired physiologic obstruction of the esophageal introitus that results from mucosal herniation (false diverticulum) posteriorly between the cricopharyngeus muscle and the inferior pharyngeal constrictor muscle (Fig. 144–1).

PHYSICAL FINDINGS AND CLINICAL PRESENTATION

Small Zenker's diverticulum may be asymptomatic. As they become larger, symptoms include:
- Dysphagia to solids and liquids
- Regurgitation of undigested food
- Sensation of globus or fullness in the neck
- Cough
- Halitosis
- Aspiration pneumonia
- Weight loss
- Voice changes

CAUSE

The specific cause of Zenker's diverticulum is not known; however, the leading hypothesis suggests the following:
- During swallowing, there is raised intraluminal pressure secondary to the incomplete opening of the cricopharyngeus muscle (improperly timed relaxation) before the bolus of food can be driven forward into the stomach.
- Discordination of the swallowing mechanism leads to increased pressure on the mucosa of the hypopharynx resulting in the slow progressive distention of the mucosa in the weakest area of the esophagus, namely the posterior wall. The end result being the formation of a false diverticulum where food elements and secretions may be lodged, causing the symptoms listed previously.

DIFFERENTIAL DIAGNOSIS

The differential diagnosis is similar to anyone presenting with dysphagia:
- Achalasia (see Fig. 151–1)
- Esophageal spasm (see Fig. 152–1)
- Esophageal carcinoma (see Fig. 169–2)
- Esophageal webs
- Peptic stricture (see Fig. 155–2)
- Lower esophageal (Schatzkis) ring (see Fig. 150–2)
- Foreign bodies
- Central nervous system (CNS) disorders (stroke, Parkinson's disease, ALS, multiple sclerosis, myasthenia gravis, muscular dystrophies)
- Dermatomyositis
- Infection

IMAGING STUDIES

- Barium swallow is the diagnostic procedure of choice. Radiographically, Zenker's diverticulum is easily demonstrated with a barium contrast study.
- Endoscopy to rule out neoplasia is indicated if barium studies show mucosal irregularities.
- Oropharyngeal-esophageal scintigraphy is also an effective, sensitive, and simple diagnostic study for both qualitative and quantitative analyses.
- Barium swallow characteristically demonstrates a herniated sac with a narrow diverticular neck that typically originates just proximal to the cricopharyngeus at the level of C5-C6.
- A chest x-ray is performed in cases of suspected aspiration pneumonia.

TREATMENT

- Soft mechanical diet can be tried in patients with symptoms of dysphagia. Avoid seeds, skins, and nuts.
- Endoscopic techniques (esophagodiverticulostomy) have largely replaced conventional treatment by open surgery; these include:
  1. Endoscopic stapler diverticulotomy (some recommend it as the initial treatment of choice)
  2. Microendoscopic carbon dioxide laser surgical diverticulotomy
- Surgery is the recommended treatment for symptomatic patients with Zenker's diverticulum.
  - Surgical treatment relieves symptoms (dysphagia, cough, aspiration) in nearly all patients with Zenker's diverticulum.
  - Surgical procedures include:
    1. Cervical diverticulectomy with cricopharyngeal myotomy (most common approach)
    2. Diverticulopexy or diverticular inversion with cricopharyngeal myotomy
    3. Diverticulectomy alone
    4. Cricopharyngeal myotomy alone
  - Surgical mortality >1.5%

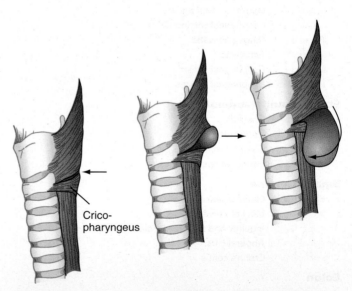

Fig 144–1
Formation of pharyngoesophageal (Zenker's) diverticulum. *Left,* Herniation of the pharyngeal mucosa and submucosa occurs at the point of transition (*arrow*) between the oblique fibers of the thyropharyngeus muscle and the more horizontal fibers of the cricopharyngeus muscle. *Center and right,* As the diverticulum enlarges, it dissects toward the left side and downward into the superior mediastinum in the prevertebral space.
(From Townsend CM, Beauchamp RD, Evers BM, Mattox KL [eds]: Sabiston Textbook of Surgery, 17th ed. Philadelphia, WB Saunders, 2004.)

Chapter 145   Gastroesophageal reflux

DEFINITION
Gastroesophageal reflux disease (GERD) is a motility disorder characterized primarily by heartburn and caused by the reflux of gastric contents into the esophagus.

PHYSICAL FINDINGS AND CLINICAL PRESENTATION
- Physical examination: generally unremarkable
- Clinical signs and symptoms: heartburn, dysphagia, sour taste, regurgitation of gastric contents into the mouth
- Chronic cough and bronchospasm
- Chest pain, laryngitis, early satiety, abdominal fullness, and bloating with belching
- Dental erosions in children

CAUSE
- Incompetent lower esophageal sphincter (LES)
- Medications that lower LES pressure (e.g., calcium channel blockers, beta-adrenergic blockers, theophylline, anticholinergics)
- Foods that lower LES pressure (e.g., chocolate, yellow onions, peppermint)
- Tobacco abuse, alcohol, coffee
- Pregnancy
- Gastric acid hypersecretion
- Hiatal hernia (controversial) present in >70% of patients with GERD; however, most patients with hiatal hernia are asymptomatic
- Obesity is associated with a statistically significant increase in the risk for GERD symptoms, erosive esophagitis, and esophageal carcinoma

DIFFERENTIAL DIAGNOSIS
- Peptic ulcer disease (see Fig. 155–1)
- Unstable angina
- Esophagitis (from infections such as herpes, *Candida*), medication induced (doxycycline, potassium chloride)
- Esophageal spasm (nutcracker esophagus)(see Fig. 152–1)
- Cancer of esophagus (see Fig. 149–2)

WORKUP
Endoscopy will identify abnormalities associated with reflux esophagitis (Fig. 145–1) and will rule out carcinoma

LABORATORY TESTS
- The 24-hour esophageal pH monitoring and Bernstein test are sensitive diagnostic tests; however, they are not very practical and generally not done. They are useful in patients with atypical manifestations of GERD, such as chest pain or chronic cough.
- Esophageal manometry is indicated in patients with refractory reflux in whom surgical therapy is planned.

IMAGING STUDIES
Upper gastrointestinal (GI) series can identify ulcerations and strictures; however, it may miss mucosal abnormalities. It may be useful in patients unwilling to have endoscopy or with medical contraindications to the procedure. Only one third of patients with GERD have radiographic signs of esophagitis on upper GI (UGI) series.

TREATMENT
- Lifestyle modifications with avoidance of foods (e.g., citrus- and tomato-based products) and drugs that exacerbate reflux (e.g., caffeine, beta blockers, calcium channel blockers, alpha-adrenergic agonists, theophylline). Lifestyle modification must be followed lifelong, because this is generally an irreversible condition.
- Avoidance of tobacco and alcohol use
- Elevation of head of bed (4 to 8 inches) using blocks
- Avoidance of lying down directly after late or large evening meals
- Weight reduction, decreased fat intake
- Proton pump inhibitors (PPIs) are safe, tolerated, and very effective in most patients.
- For refractory cases: surgery with Nissen fundoplication.

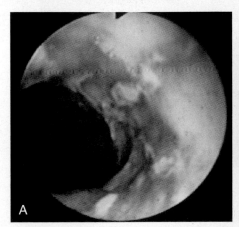 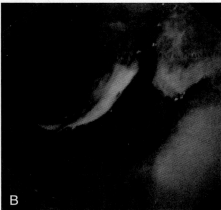 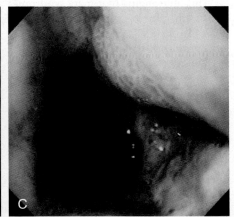

Fig 145–1
Endoscopic images of the lower esophagus in cases of reflux esophagitis, showing (**A**) linear ulceration, (**B**) extensive circumferential ulceration, and (**C**) deep ulceration.
(From Grainger RG, Allison DJ, Adam A, Dixon AK [eds]: *Grainger and Allison's Diagnostic Radiology*, 4th ed. Philadelphia, Churchill Livingstone, 2001.)

Chapter 146 / Hiatal hernia

DEFINITION
A hiatal hernia is the herniation of a portion of the stomach into the thoracic cavity through the diaphragmatic esophageal hiatus.

PHYSICAL FINDINGS AND CLINICAL PRESENTATION
Most patients with hiatal hernias are asymptomatic. Symptomatic patients present similarly to patients with GERD.
- Heartburn
- Dysphagia
- Regurgitation
- Chest pain
- Postprandial fullness
- GI bleed
- Dyspnea
- Hoarseness
- Wheezing with bowel sounds heard over the left lung base

CAUSE
- Hiatal hernias are classified as:
  1. Type I: Sliding, axial, or concentric hiatal hernia (most common type, 99%). The GE junction protrudes through the hiatus into the thoracic cavity
  2. Type II: Paraesophageal hernia (1%). The GE junction stays at the level of the diaphragm, but part of the stomach bulges into the thoracic cavity and stays there at all times, not being affected by swallowing
  3. Type III: Mixed (rare), a combination of types I and II
  4. Type IV: Large defect in hiatus that allows other intra-abdominal organs to enter the hernia sac
- Hiatal hernias are thought to develop from an imbalance between normal pulling forces of the esophagus through the diaphragmatic hiatus during swallowing and the supporting structures maintaining normal esophagogastric junction positioning in association with repetitive stretching that results in rupture of the phrenoesophageal membrane.

DIFFERENTIAL DIAGNOSIS
- Peptic ulcer disease (see Fig. 155–1)
- Unstable angina (coronary syndrome)
- Esophagitis (e.g., *Candida*, herpes, NSAIDs, etc.) (see Fig. 145–1)
- Esophageal spasm (see Fig. 152–1)
- Barrett's esophagus (see Fig. 148–1)
- Schatzki's ring (see Fig. 150–2)
- Achalasia (see Fig. 151–1)
- Zenker's diverticulum (see Fig. 144–1)
- Esophageal cancer (see Fig. 149–2)

IMAGING STUDIES
- Barium contrast UGI series best defines the anatomic abnormality (Fig. 146–1). A hiatal hernia is considered to be present if the gastric cardia is herniated 2 cm above the hiatus. UGI may reveal a tortuous esophagus.
- Upper GI endoscopy is useful to document the presence of a hiatal hernia and also to exclude common associated findings of esophagitis and Barrett's esophagus. A hiatal hernia

can be found incidentally and is diagnosed if >2 cm of gastric rugal fold is seen above the margins of the diaphragmatic crura.

TREATMENT
- Lifestyle modifications with avoidance of foods and drugs that decrease lower esophageal pressure (e.g. caffeine, chocolate, mint, calcium channel blockers, and anticholinergics). Weight loss
- Avoid large quantities of food with meals
- Sleep with the head of the bed elevated 4 to 6 inches with blocks placed at base of the bed
- Antacids, H_2 antagonists, PPIs may be useful to relieve symptoms.
- When indicated, surgery (laparoscopic or open) can be done in patients with refractory symptoms impairing quality of life and causing both intestinal (e.g., recurrent GI bleeds) and extraintestinal complications (e.g., aspiration pneumonia, asthma, and ENT complications).
- Prophylactic surgery is a consideration in all patients with paraesophageal hiatal hernias because they have a higher incidence of strangulation.

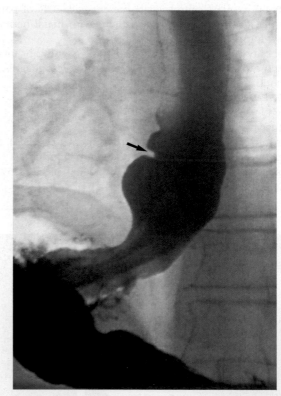

Fig 146–1
A sliding hiatal hernia confirmed by the presence of an incisural notch (*arrow*) on the greater curve aspect.
(From Grainger RG, Allison DJ, Adam A, Dixon AK [eds]: Grainger and Allison's Diagnostic Radiology, 4th ed. Philadelphia, Churchill Livingstone, 2001.)

Chapter 147   Mallory-Weiss tear

DEFINITION
A Mallory-Weiss tear (MWT) is a longitudinal mucosal laceration in the region of the gastroesophageal junction.

PHYSICAL FINDINGS AND CLINICAL PRESENTATION
- Vomiting, retching, or vigorous coughing will often, but not always, precede hematemesis.
- Patients may be clinically stable or present with tachycardia, hypotension, melena, or hematochezia.
- Bleeding may be self-limited or severe.
- Tears may be seen in association with other upper GI tract lesions, including hiatal hernia (present in as many as 90% of patients), ulcers and erosions (fig. 147–1), and esophageal varices, particularly in alcoholics.

CAUSE
- An acute increase in intra-abdominal pressure is transmitted to the esophagus, resulting in mucosal laceration.
- Vomiting may be associated with alcohol use, ketoacidosis, ulcer disease, uremia, pancreatitis, cholecystitis, pregnancy, or myocardial infarction.
- Tears may be iatrogenic, related to endoscopy (EGD), especially in struggling or retching patients, esophageal dilation, lower esophageal pneumatic disruption therapy for achalasia, transesophageal echocardiography, or in association with polyethylene glycol electrolyte colonic lavage preparation.

DIFFERENTIAL DIAGNOSIS
- Esophageal or gastric varices (see Fig. 153–1)
- Esophagitis/esophageal ulcers (peptic or pill-induced) (see Fig. 145–1)
- Gastric erosions (see Fig. 154–1)
- Gastric or duodenal ulcer (see Fig. 155–1)
- Arteriovenous malformations
- Neoplasms (usually gastric) (see Fig. 156–3)

WORKUP
- EGD (see Fig. 147–1) is the diagnostic method of choice to identify lacerations and/or erosions.

TREATMENT
- Supportive care
- Aspirin, NSAIDs, and anticoagulants should be held
- Patients with active bleeding or hemodynamic instability require large-bore IVs, fluid resuscitation, and transfusion of blood products as appropriate
- NG decompression and antiemetics may be considered
- Endoscopic therapy for patients with active or ongoing hemorrhage.
- Arterial embolization in patients with active bleeding who are poor surgical candidates
- Laparotomy, with gastrotomy and oversewing of the tear, is required in a small percentage of patients with uncontrolled bleeding

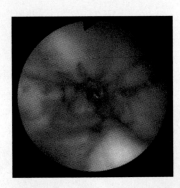
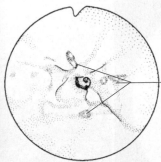

Multiple discrete erosions in mild esophagitis

Fig 147–1
Endoscopic view of grade A esophagitis with solitary erosions.
(From Forbes A, Misiewicz J, Compton C, et al: Atlas of Clinical Gastroenterology, 3rd ed. Edinburgh, Elsevier Mosby, 2005.)

Chapter 148 Barrett's esophagus

DEFINITION

Barrett's esophagus occurs when the squamous lining of the lower esophagus is replaced by metaplastic, intestinalized columnar epithelium (Fig. 148–1). The condition is associated with an increased risk of adenocarcinoma of the esophagus.

CLINICAL PRESENTATION

Symptoms

- Typically, chronic (>5 years) heartburn
- Dysphagia for solid food
- May be an incidental finding on EGD
- Less frequent: chest pain, hematemesis, or melena

Physical findings

- Nonspecific; can be completely normal
- Epigastric tenderness on palpation

CAUSE

- Metaplasia is thought to result from re-epithelialization of esophageal tissue injured secondary to chronic GERD.
- Patients with Barrett's esophagus tend to have more severe esophageal motility disturbances (decreased lower esophageal sphincter pressure, ineffective peristalsis) and greater esophageal acid exposure on 24-hour pH monitoring.
- Intresophageal bile reflux may also play a role in the pathogenesis.
- Familial clustering of GERD and Barrett's esophagus suggests a genetic predisposition, but no gene has yet been identified.
- Progression from metaplasia to carcinoma is associated with changes in gene structure and expression.

DIFFERENTIAL DIAGNOSIS

- GERD, uncomplicated (see Fig. 145–1)
- Erosive esophagitis (see Fig. 147–1)
- Gastritis (see Fig. 154–1)
- Peptic ulcer disease (see Fig. 155–1)
- Angina (coronary syndrome)
- Malignancy (see Fig. 149–2)
- Stricture or Schatzki's ring (see Fig. 150–2)

WORKUP

- EGD with biopsy for diagnosis.
- Diagnosis requires the presence of intestinal metaplasia in columnar epithelium proximal to the gastroesophageal junction. Longer segment Barrett's esophagus is more readily diagnosed.

TREATMENT

- Lifestyle modifications, elevating head of bed, avoiding chocolate, tobacco, caffeine, mints, and certain drugs (see Gastroesophageal Reflux Disease).
- Chronic acid suppression is often necessary to control symptoms and promote healing.
- PPIs are most effective.
- Antireflux surgery may be considered for management of GERD and associated sequelae.
- Patients should have EGD surveillance of their Barrett's esophagus.

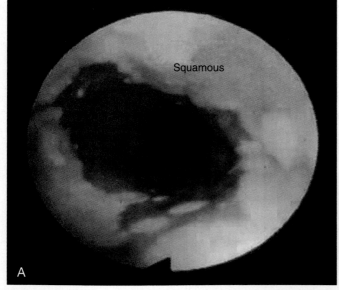
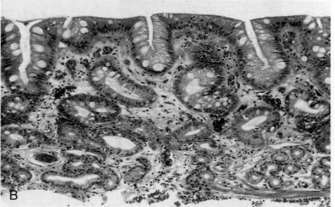

Fig 148–1

Barrett's esophagus is defined by both endoscopic and histologic components, Endoscopically, there must be visible pink columnar epithelium within the tubular esophagus (**A**) that histologically has intestinalized metaplastic columnar epithelium defined by the presence of true goblet cells (**B**) on this HANDE stain. Barrett's esophagus should not be diagnosed without both components.
(From Silverberg SG: Principles and Practice of Surgical Pathology and Cytopathology, 4th ed. Philadelphia, Churchill Livingstone, 2006.)

Chapter 149   **Esophageal carcinoma**

DEFINITION

Esophageal tumors are defined as benign and malignant tumors arising from the esophagus. Approximately 15% of esophageal cancers arise in the cervical esophagus, 50% in the middle third of the esophagus, and 35% in the lower third. Eighty-five percent of esophageal tumors are squamous cell carcinoma (arising from squamous epithelium) (Fig. 149–1). Adenocarcinomas arise from columnar epithelium in the distal esophagus, which have become dysplastic secondary to chronic gastric reflux.

CLINICAL PRESENTATION

Symptoms and signs

- Dysphagia: initially occurs with solid foods and gradually progresses to include semisolids and liquids; later signs usually indicate incurable disease with tumor involving more than 60% of the esophageal circumference, and occur in 74% of patients.
- Weight loss: many patients present with weight loss usually of short duration. Weight loss >10% of body mass is an independent predictor of poor prognosis.
- Hoarseness: suggests recurrent laryngeal nerve involvement.
- Odynophagia: an unusual symptom.
- Cervical adenopathy: usually involving supraclavicular lymph nodes.
- Dry cough: suggests tracheal involvement.

- Aspiration pneumonia: caused by development of a fistula between the esophagus and trachea.
- Massive hemoptysis or hematemesis: results from the invasion of vascular structures.
- Advanced disease spreads to liver, lungs, and pleura.
- Hypercalcemia: usually associated with squamous cell carcinoma because of the secretion of a tumor peptide similar to the parathyroid hormone.

CAUSE

Pathogenesis of esophageal cancers is due to chronic recurrent oxidative damage from any of the following etiologic agents, which cause inflammation, esophagitis, increased cell turnover, and ultimately, initiation of the carcinogenic process.

ETIOLOGIC AGENTS

- Excess alcohol consumption: accounts for 80% to 90% of esophageal cancer in the United States; whiskey is associated with a higher incidence than wine or beer.
- Tobacco and alcohol use combined increases risk substantially.
- Other ingested carcinogens:
  - Nitrates (converted to nitrites): South Asia, China
  - Smoked opiates: northern Iran
  - Fungal toxins in pickled vegetables
- Mucosal damage:
  - Long-term exposure to extremely hot tea
  - Lye ingestion
  - Radiation-induced strictures
  - Chronic achalasia: incidence is 7 times.
- Host susceptibility secondary to precancerous lesions:
- Plummer-Vinson syndrome (Paterson-Kelly): glossitis with iron deficiency
- Chronic GERD leading to Barrett's esophagus and adenocarcinoma (whites are affected more than blacks).

DIFFERENTIAL DIAGNOSIS

- Achalasia of the esophagus (see Fig. 151–1)
- Scleroderma of the esophagus
- Diffuse esophageal spasm (see Fig. 152–1)
- Esophageal rings and webs (see Fig. 150–2)
- Barrett's esophagus (see Fig. 148–1)

IMAGING STUDIES

- Esophagogram can identify large esophageal lesions (Fig. 149–2).
- In contrast to benign esophageal leiomyomata, which cause narrowing with preservation of normal mucosal pattern, esophageal carcinomas cause ragged ulcerating mucosal changes in association with deeper infiltration.
- Esophagoscopy is the diagnostic procedure of choice. It is performed to visualize tumor (Fig. 149–2) and obtain histopathologic confirmation. In conjunction, an endoscopic sonogram may be performed to determine the depth of tumor invasion.
- Endoscopic biopsies fail to recover malignant tissue one third of the time, thus cytologic examination of tumor brushings should be routinely performed.
- Examination of the fundus of the stomach via retroflexion of the endoscope is also imperative.

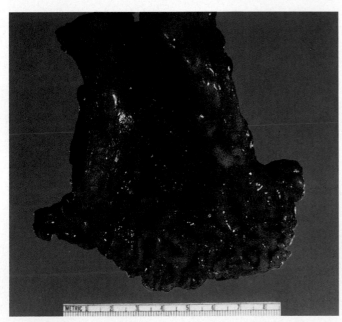

Fig 149–1

The distal-most part of the esophageal mucosa is replaced by squamous cell carcinoma, which has a nodular and erosive appearance. The wall is infiltrated by tumor.

(From Silverberg SG: Principles and Practice of Surgical Pathology and Cytopathology, 4th ed. Philadelphia, Churchill Livingstone, 2006.)

- Chest and abdominal CT scans should be performed to determine the extent of tumor spread to mediastinum, para-aortic lymph nodes, and liver.

TREATMENT

SURGICAL RESECTION

- Surgical resection of squamous cell and adenocarcinoma of the lower third of the esophagus is indicated if there is no widespread metastasis. Usually stomach or colon is used for esophageal replacement.

RADIATION THERAPY:

- Squamous cell carcinomas are more radiosensitive than adenocarcinoma. Radiation achieves good local control and is an excellent palliative modality for obstructive symptoms. Most effective for upper esophageal tumors.

COMBINATION CHEMOTHERAPY, RADIATION Rx, AND SURGICAL Rx:

- Single-agent chemotherapy results in significant tumor regression in 15% to 25% of patients.
- Combination chemotherapy including cisplatin achieves significant tumor reduction in 30% to 60% of patients.

Fig 149–2
Radiologic (**A**) and endoscopic (**B**) images of bulky squamous carcinomas in the mid esophagus.
(From Grainger RG, Allison DJ, Adam A, Dixon AK [eds]: Grainger and Allison's Diagnostic Radiology, 4th ed. Philadelphia, Churchill Livingstone, 2001.)

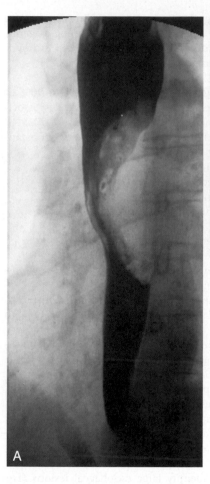

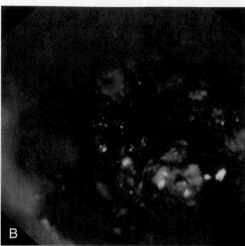

Chapter 150 Rings and webs

- Esophageal webs can be diagnosed by endoscopy (Fig. 150-1) or esophagogram (Fig. 150-2).
- Cervical esophageal webs may cause dysphagia.
- Patients wirh Plummer-Vinson syndrome have a cervical esophageal web, chronic iron deficiency anemia, atrophic oral mucosa, glossitis, and spoon-shaped nails (koilonychias).
- Treatment consists of esophageal dilation and correction of nutritional deficiencies.

- Lower esophageal webs *(Schatzki's ring)* occur at the squamocolumnar junction and appear as annular structures on esophagogram (see Fig. 150-2).
- Intermittent dysphagia may occur, although most patients are asymptomatic.
- Treatment in symptomatic patients consists of periodic dilatations and antireflux medical therapy

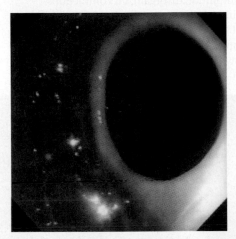

Fig 150-1
Typical endoscopic view of a fibrotic Schatski's ring that will require dilation.
(From Grainger RG, Allison DJ, Adam A, Dixon AK [eds]: Grainger and Allison's Diagnostic Radiology, 4th ed. Philadelphia, Churchill Livingstone, 2001.)

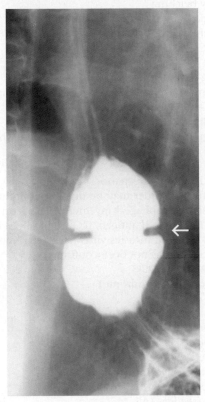

Fig 150-2
Esophagogram shows a distal esophageal (Schatzki's) ring (*arrow*).
(Courtesy of Ronelle A. Dubrow, MD, M. D. Anderson Cancer Center, Houston, TX.)

Chapter 151 | **Achalasia**

DEFINITION
Achalasia is a motility disorder of the esophagus characterized by inadequate relaxation of the LES and ineffective peristalsis of esophageal smooth muscle. The result is functional obstruction of the esophagus.

PHYSICAL FINDINGS AND CLINICAL PRESENTATION
Symptoms
- Difficulty belching
- Dysphagia to both solids and liquids
- Chest pain and/or heartburn
- Globus
- Frequent hiccups
- Vomiting of undigested food
- Symptoms of aspiration such as nocturnal cough; possible dyspnea and pneumonia

Physical findings
- Focal lung examination abnormalities and wheezing also possible

CAUSE
- Etiology is poorly understood.
- This motility disorder may be due to autoimmune degeneration of the esophageal myenteric plexus. An association with the HLA class II antigen, DQw1, has been noted.
- Herpes zoster and measles virus have been implicated, but the association has not been confirmed.

DIFFERENTIAL DIAGNOSIS
- Angina (coronary syndrome)
- Bulimia
- Anorexia nervosa
- Gastric bezoar
- Gastritis (see Fig. 154–1)
- Peptic ulcer disease (see Fig. 155–1)
- Postvagotomy dysmotility
- Esophageal disease:
  - GERD (see Fig. 145–1)
  - Sarcoidosis
  - Amyloidosis
  - Esophageal stricture
  - Esophageal webs and rings (see Fig. 150–2)
  - Scleroderma
  - Barrett's esophagus (see Fig. 148–1)
  - Chagas' disease (see Fig. 332–24)
  - Esophagitis
  - Diffuse esophageal spasm (see Fig. 152–1)
- Malignancy:
  - Esophageal cancer (see Fig. 149–2)
  - Infiltrating gastric cancer (see Fig. 156–3)
  - Lung cancer
  - Lymphoma

IMAGING STUDIES
Barium swallow with fluoroscopy may demonstrate:
- Uncoordinated or absent esophageal contractions
- An acutely tapered contrast column ("bird's beak") (Fig. 151–1)
- Dilation of the distal (smooth muscle portion) esophagus
- Esophageal air fluid level
Manometry may be indicated if barium swallow is inconclusive. Characteristic abnormalities are as follows:
- Low-amplitude disorganized contractions
- High intresophageal resting pressure
- High LES pressure
- Inadequate LES relaxation after swallow
Direct visualization by endoscopy can rule out other causes of dysphagia.

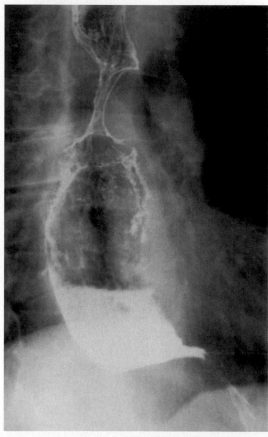

Fig 151–1
An example of achalasia as demonstrated by the typical bird's beak appearance of the distal esophagus together with a stricture carcinoma at the level of the carina. The patient had a 20-year history of untreated dysphagia, which had recently become more severe. (From Grainger RG, Allison DJ, Adam A, Dixon AK [eds]: Grainger and Allison's Diagnostic Radiology, 4th ed. Philadelphia, Churchill Livingstone, 2001.)

TREATMENT

All nonpharmacologic therapies including surgical procedures.

● Mechanical dilation may benefit up to 90% of patients.

● Surgical: Open and thoracoscopic esophagomyotomy is available and effective (90%).

● Medications may be useful when the only goal is short-term symptom relief. Lower esophageal sphincter pressure may be lowered by 50% through sublingual use of long-acting nitrates (e.g., isosorbide dinitrate 5 to 20 mg) or calcium channel blockers (e.g., nifedipine 10 to 30 mg). However, side effects are common and duration of relief tends to be short.

● Botulinum toxin injection will benefit up to 85% of patients, but up to half of these patients will require repeat injections.

Chapter 152 Esophageal spasm

DEFINITION

- Diffuse esophageal spasm (DES) is an esophageal motility disorder manifesting clinically with chest pain and/or dysphagia
- The character of the chest pain may mimic myocardial ischemia and is responsible for innumerable hospital admission to rule out myocardial infarction.
- The origin of DES is unknown. Emotional stress, peptic ulcer disease, pancreatitis, and gallstones may trigger esophageal spasm in susceptible patients.

DIAGNOSIS

- Diagnosis: Barium swallow may reveal the classic "corkscrew" appearance (Fig. 152–1). Manometry may reveal repetitive contractions. However, both studies may be normal if the patient is not experiencing spasms at the time of the test.

TREATMENT

- Treatment: avoidance of trigger factors, calcium channel blockers, nitrates. Thoracic esophagomyotomy in resistant case; however, results have been disappointing.

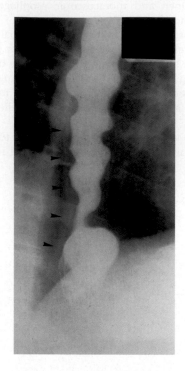

Fig 152–1
An example of diffuse esophageal spasm with marked irregular contractions. Some thickening of the esophageal wall can also be seen (*arrowheads*). A corkscrew esophagus.
(From Grainger RG, Allison DJ, Adam A, Dixon AK [eds]: Grainger and Allison's Diagnostic Radiology, 4th ed. Philadelphia, Churchill Livingstone, 2001.)

Chapter 153   Esophageal varices

DEFINITION

- Esophageal varices are dilated sumucosal veins that communicate with the portocollateral circulation and the systemic venous system. They are a common complication of cirrhosis.

DIAGNOSIS

- Diagnosis is best made with endoscopy (Fig. 153–1). UGI series (Fig. 153–2) will also identify varices.
- Patients with cirrhosis should undergo an upper endoscopy examination once a year to evaluate for varices.

TREATMENT

- Esophageal bleeding is a major cause of death in patients with cirrhosis and hypertension.
- The risk factors for variceal hemorrhage include continued alcohol use, poor liver function, portal venous pressure gradient greater than 2 mm Hg, and large varices. Nonselective beta blockers (propranolol or nadolol given in a dose to reduce resting heart rate <25%) are recommended as primary prophylaxis to prevent esophageal variceal bleeding in patients with medium-large esophageal varices. Endoscopic variceal ligation (EVL) can be used in patients who are intolerant to beta-blocker therapy.
- The acute management of bleeding varices includes the following:

  a. Resuscitation (intravenous fluids and blood transfusion) and correction of any coagulation abnormalities (fresh frozen plasma).

  b. Octreotide, terlipressin, somatostatin

  c. Emergency endoscopic sclerotherapy or variceal band ligation

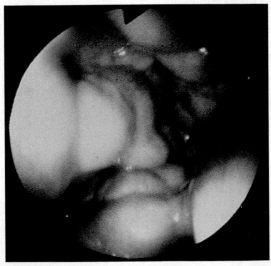

Fig 153–1
Endoscopic view of esophageal varices.
(From Cohen J, Powderly WG: Infectious Diseases, 2nd ed. St Louis, Mosby, 2004.)

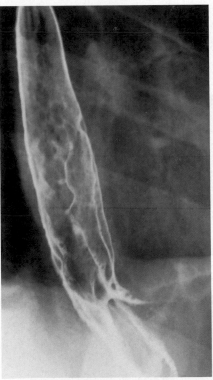

Fig 153–2
Uphill varices demonstrated in the lower esophagus as serpiginous filling defects. These are unusually prominent on this erect image.
(From Grainger RG, Allison DJ, Adam A, Dixon AK [eds]: Grainger and Allison's Diagnostic Radiology, 4th ed. Philadelphia, Churchill Livingstone, 2001.)

STOMACH AND DUODENUM

Chapter 154 **Gastritis**

DEFINITION
Histologically, gastritis refers to inflammation in the stomach. Endoscopically, gastritis refers to a number of abnormal features such as erythema, erosions, and subepithelial hemorrhages (Fig. 154–1). Gastritis can also be subdivided into erosive, nonerosive, and specific types of gastritis with distinctive features both endoscopically and histologically.

PHYSICAL FINDINGS AND CLINICAL PRESENTATION
- Patients with gastritis generally present with nonspecific clinical signs and symptoms (e.g., epigastric pain, abdominal tenderness, bloating, anorexia, and nausea [with or without vomiting]). Symptoms may be aggravated by eating.
- Epigastric tenderness in acute alcoholic gastritis (may be absent in chronic gastritis).
- Foul-smelling breath.
- Hematemesis ("coffee-ground" emesis).

CAUSE
- Alcohol, NSAIDs (Fig. 154–2), stress (critically ill patients usually on mechanical respiration), hepatic or renal failure, multiorgan failure
- *Helicobacter pylori* infection (Fig. 154–3)
- Bile reflux, pancreatic enzyme reflux
- Gastric mucosal atrophy, portal hypertension gastropathy
- Irradiation

DIFFERENTIAL DIAGNOSIS
- Peptic ulcer disease (see Fig. 155–1)
- GERD (see Fig. 145–1)
- Nonulcer dyspepsia
- Gastric lymphoma or carcinoma (see Fig. 156–3)
- Pancreatitis (see Fig. 173–4)
- Gastroparesis

LABORATORY TESTS
- *H. pylori* testing via endoscopic biopsy, urea breath test, stool antigen test (*H. pylori* stool antigen), or specific antibody test is recommended:
- Vitamin B_{12} level in patients with atrophic gastritis.
- Hct (low if significant bleeding has occurred).

TREATMENT
- Avoidance of mucosal irritants such as alcohol and NSAIDs
- Lifestyle modifications with avoidance of tobacco and foods that trigger symptoms
- Eradication of *H. pylori*, when present, can be accomplished with various regimens:
  1. PPI bid *plus* amoxicillin 500 mg bid *plus* metronidazole 500 mg for 10 days.
  2. PPI bid *plus* clarithromycin 500 mg bid *and* metronidazole 500 mg bid for 10 days. This regimen is useful in those with penicillin allergy.

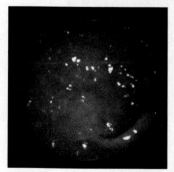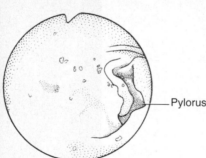

Pylorus

Fig 154–1
Endoscopic appearance of antral gastritis associated with Helcobacter pylori.
(From Forbes A, Misiewicz J, Compton C, et al: Atlas of Clinical Gastroenterology, 3rd ed. Edinburgh, Elsevier Mosby, 2005.)

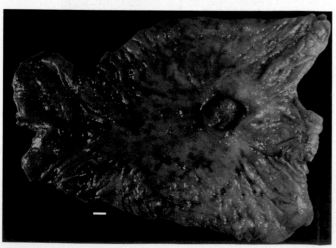

Fig 154–2
Nonsteroidal anti-inflammatory drug-induced acute hemorrhagic gastritis. Numerous punctate erosions pepper the mucosa of the gastric body. An acute ulcer is located high on the lesser curve of the body (bar = 1 cm). (From Silverberg SG: Principles and Practice of Surgical Pathology and Cytopathology, 4th ed. Philadelphia, Churchill Livingstone, 2006.)

- Prophylaxis and treatment of stress gastritis with sucralfate suspension 1 g orally q4-6h, H$_2$-receptor antagonists, or PPIs in patients on ventilator support
- Misoprostol or PPIs in patients on chronic NSAID therapy

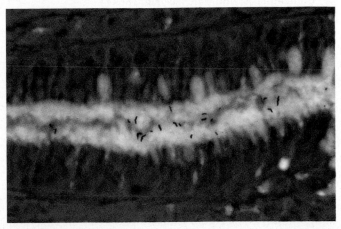

Fig 154–3
Helicobacter pylori. Curvilinear bacilli are most easily detected in the mucus of the gastric pits after staining with various silver impregnation methods (Steiner).
(From Silverberg SG: Principles and Practice of Surgical Pathology and Cytopathology, 4th ed. Philadelphia, Churchill Livingstone, 2006.)

Chapter 155 | Peptic ulcer

DEFINITION

Peptic ulcer disease (PUD) is an ulceration in the stomach or duodenum resulting from an imbalance between mucosal protective factors and various mucosal damaging mechanisms (see "Cause").

PHYSICAL FINDINGS AND CLINICAL PRESENTATION

- Physical examination is often unremarkable.
- Patient may have epigastric tenderness, tachycardia, pallor, hypotension (from acute or chronic blood loss), nausea and vomiting (if pyloric channel is obstructed), boardlike abdomen and rebound tenderness (if perforated), and hematemesis or melena (with a bleeding ulcer).

CAUSE

Often multifactorial; the following are common mucosal damaging factors:

- *Helicobacter pylori* infection. *H. pylori* is the major cause of peptic ulcer disease. It is found in more than 70% of patients with duodenal ulcers and gastric ulcers in the United States. Rates are much higher (>90%) in other parts of the world. Eradication of *H. pylori* markedly reduces peptic ulcer recurrence.
- Medications (NSAIDs, glucocorticoids)
- Incompetent pylorus or LES
- Bile acids
- Impaired proximal duodenal bicarbonate secretion
- Decreased blood flow to gastric mucosa
- Acid secreted by parietal cells and pepsin secreted as pepsinogen by chief cells
- Cigarette smoking
- Alcohol

DIFFERENTIAL DIAGNOSIS

- GERD (see Fig. 145–1)
- Cholelithiasis syndrome (see Fig. 186–1)
- Pancreatitis (see Fig. 173–5)
- Gastritis (see Fig. 154–1)
- Nonulcer dyspepsia
- Neoplasm (gastric carcinoma [see Fig. 156–3], lymphoma, pancreatic carcinoma [see Fig. 175–4])
- Angina pectoris, MI, pericarditis
- Dissecting aneurysm
- Other: high small bowel obstruction, pneumonia, subphrenic abscess, early appendicitis (see Fig. 161–1)

WORKUP

- Diagnostic modalities include endoscopy or UGI series. Endoscopy is preferred (Fig. 155–1)

LABORATORY TESTS

H. pylori testing via endoscopic biopsy, urea breath test, stool antigen test (*H. pylori* stool antigen), or specific antibody test. Additional laboratory evaluation is indicated only in specific cases (e.g., CBC when suspecting GI bleeding amylase level in suspected pancreatitis, serum gastrin level in suspected Zollinger-Ellison [Z-E] syndrome).

IMAGING STUDIES

Conventional UGI barium studies identify approximately 70% to 80% of PUD (Fig. 155–2); accuracy can be increased to approximately 90% by using double contrast.

TREATMENT

- Lifestyle changes: stop smoking, avoid NSAIDs and alcohol
- Eradication of *H. pylori*, when present
- PUD patients testing negative for *H. pylori* should be treated with antisecretory agents: Histamine-2 receptor antagonists (H₂RAs), Proton pump inhibitors (PPIs)

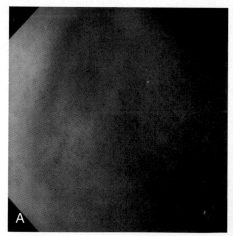 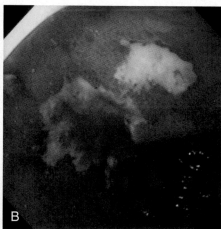 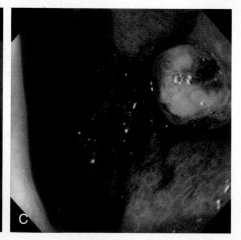

Fig 155–1
Endoscopic pictures of the stomach and duodenum. (**A**) Erythema of the gastric antrum. This appearance correlates poorly with histologic gastritis and may be a normal finding. (**B**) Duodenal ulceration. (**C**) Gastric ulcer. Note the clot in the base indicating recent bleeding and high risk of rebleed and the endoscope entering the stomach through the cardia.
(From Cohen J, Powderly WG: Infectious Diseases, 2nd ed. St Louis, Mosby, 2004.)

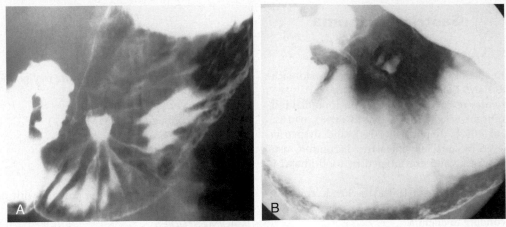

Fig 155–2
En face appearance of benign gastric ulcer. (**A**) Posterior wall ulcer is nearly filled with barium in this RPO projection. Thin regular radiating folds (best seen around inferior border of the ulcer) are seen converging to the ulcer. (**B**) Unfilled benign ulcer crater is outlined by a "ring" shadow. This ulcer is surrounded by a prominent ring of edema, the lucent area around the crater.
(From Grainger RG, Allison DJ, Adam A, Dixon AK [eds]: Grainger and Allison's Diagnostic Radiology, 4th ed. Philadelphia, Churchill Livingstone, 2001.)

Chapter 156 Gastric carcinoma

DEFINITION
Gastric cancer is an adenocarcinoma arising from the stomach.

PHYSICAL FINDINGS AND CLINICAL PRESENTATION
- Medical history may reveal complaints of postprandial fullness with significant weight loss (70% to 80%), nausea/emesis (20% to 40%), dysphagia (20%), and dyspepsia, usually unrelieved by antacids; epigastric discomfort, usually lessened by fasting and exacerbated by food intake, is also common.
- Epigastric or abdominal mass (30% to 50%), epigastric pain.
- Skin pallor secondary to anemia.
- Hard, nodular liver: generally indicates metastatic disease to the liver.
- Hemoccult-positive stools.
- Ascites, lymphadenopathy, or pleural effusions: may indicate metastasis. Metastatic adenocarcinoma of the stomach to an area near the umbilicus is known as "*Sister Mary Joseph's nodule*" (Fig. 156–1). Gastric cancer metastatic to the ovary is known as a "*Krukenberg tumor*"(Fig. 156–2)

CAUSE
Risk factors
- Chronic *H. pylori* gastritis.
- Tobacco abuse, alcohol consumption
- Food additives (nitrosamines), smoked foods, occupational exposure to heavy metals, rubber, asbestos
- Chronic atrophic gastritis with intestinal metaplasia, hypertrophic gastritis, and pernicious anemia

DIAGNOSIS
Diagnosis is best accomplished by endoscopy (Fig. 156–3) and biopsy. UGI series will also demonstrate abnormalities (Fig. 156–4)

DIFFERENTIAL DIAGNOSIS
- Gastric lymphoma (5% of gastric malignancies)
- Hypertrophic gastritis
- Peptic ulcer (see Fig. 155–1)
- Reflux esophagitis (see Fig. 145–1)

LABORATORY TESTS
- Microcytic anemia
- Hemoccult-positive stools
- Hypoalbuminemia
- Abnormal liver enzymes in patients with metastasis to the liver

IMAGING STUDIES
- Abdominal CT (Fig. 156–4) scan to evaluate for metastasis (70% accurate for regional node metastases)

TREATMENT
- Gastrectomy with regional lymphadenectomy is performed in patients with curative potential (<30% of patients at time of diagnosis). Postoperative adjuvant chemoradiotherapy using 5-fluorouracil (5-FU) and leucovorin is now the standard of care for resected patients able to tolerate such treatment.
- When surgical cure is not possible, palliative resection may prolong duration and quality of life.
- Chemotherapy (FAM: 5-FU, Adriamycin, and mitomycin C) may provide some palliation; however, it generally does not prolong survival. Chemotherapy with docetaxel, cisplatin, and 5-FU can be used for chemotherapy-naive patients with metastatic or locally recurrent gastric cancer.

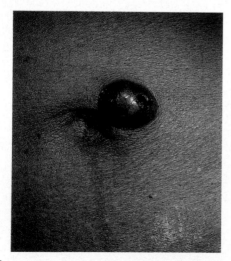

Fig 156–1
Sister Mary Joseph's nodule. Metastatic adenocarcinoma of the stomach to an area near the umbilicus.
(From Callen JP, Jorizzo JL, Bolognia JL, et al: Dermatological Signs of Internal Disease, 3rd ed. Philadelphia, WB Saunders, 2003.)

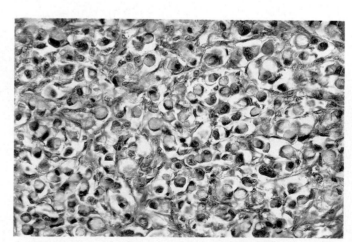

Fig 156–2
Krukenberg tumor. The ovarian stroma is diffusely infiltrated by malignant signet-ring cells in this example of gastric cancer metastatic to the ovary.
(From Silverberg SG: Principles and Practice of Surgical Pathology and Cytopathology, 4th ed. Philadelphia, Churchill Livingstone, 2006.)

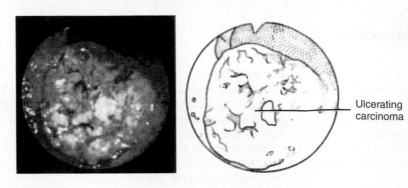

Fig 156–3
Endoscopic appearance of an obvious, ulcerating carcinoma.
(From Forbes A, Misiewicz J, Compton C, et al: Atlas of Clinical Gastroenterology, 3rd ed. Edinburgh, Elsevier Mosby, 2005.)

Ulcerating carcinoma

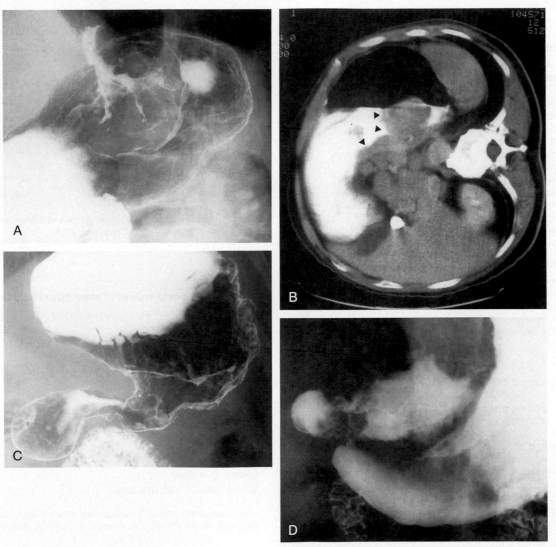

Fig 156–4
Advanced gastric cancer. (**A**) Large polypoid mass of the cardia. Tumors in this region are becoming more common for unknown reasons.
(**B**) Polypoid mass of the cardia shown on CT (*arrowheads*). Patient was imaged in right lateral decubitus position. (**C**) Large circumferential mass in the body of the stomach with a shelf at the proximal stomach. (**D**) Large ulcerated mass in the antrum. This is often referred to as a *"Carman"* ulcer.
(From Grainger RG, Allison DJ, Adam A, Dixon AK [eds]: Grainger and Allison's Diagnostic Radiology, 4th ed. Philadelphia, Churchill Livingstone, 2001.)

Chapter 157 | Intestinal obstruction

- Dilation of the bowel occurs in mechanical intestinal obstruction, paralytic ileus, and air swallowing. The radiologic differences of these different causes depend mainly on the size and distribution of the loops of the bowel. Box 157–1 describes the various causes of abdominal distention.
- The normal bowel gas pattern is shown in Fig. 157–1
- Table 157–1 describes the radiographic distinction between small bowel and large bowel dilation
- Common causes of small bowel fluid levels are described in Table 157–2.

Diagnostic imaging
- Small bowel obstruction: plain film (Fig. 157–2), CT scan (Fig. 157–3). Small bowel primary lymphoma (Fig. 157–4) may initially manifest with symptoms of bowel obstruction.
- Paralytic ileus (Fig. 157–5)
- Gallstone ileus (Fig. 157–6)
- Large bowel obstruction (Fig. 157–7)
- Toxic megacolon (Fig. 157–8)

Box 157–1 Abdominal distention

Nonmechanical Obstruction

Excessive intraluminal gas
Intra-abdominal infection
Trauma
Retroperitoneal irritation (renal colic, neoplasms, infections, hemorrhage, ruptured abdominal aortic aneurysm [AAA])
Vascular insufficiency (thrombosis, embolism)
Mechanical ventilation
Extra-abdominal infection (sepsis, pneumonia, empyema, osteomyelitis of spine)
Metabolic/toxic abnormalities (hypokalemia, uremia, lead poisoning)
Chemical irritation (perforated ulcer, bile, pancreatitis)
Peritoneal inflammation
Severe pain, pain medications
Pseudo-obstruction in the elderly (Ogilvie's syndrome)

Mechanical Obstruction

Neoplasm (intraluminal, extraluminal)
Adhesions, endometriosis
Infection (intra-abdominal abscess, diverticulitis)
Gallstones
Foreign body, bezoars
Pregnancy
Hernias
Volvulus
Stenosis at surgical anastomosis, radiation stenosis
Fecaliths
Inflammatory bowel disease
Gastric outlet obstruction
Hematoma
Other: parasites, superior mesenteric artery syndrome, pneumatosis intestinalis, annular pancreas, Hirschsprung's disease, intussusception, meconium

From Ferri F: Practical Guide to the Care of the Medical Patient, 7th ed. St Louis, Mosby, 2007.

TABLE 157–1 The distinction between small bowel and large bowel dilation

	Small bowel	Large bowel
Haustra	Absent	Present
Valvula conniventes	Present in jejunum	Absent
Number of loops	Many	Few
Distribution of loops	Central	Peripheral
Radius of curvature of loop	Small	Large
Diameter of loop	30-50 mm	50 mm+
Solid feces	Absent	May be present

From Grainger RG, Allison D: Grainger and Allison's Diagnostic Radiology, 4th ed. Philadelphia, Churchill Livingstone, 2001.

TABLE 157–2 Some causes of small bowel fluid levels

Small bowel obstruction
Large bowel obstruction
Paralytic ileus
Gastroenteritis
Hypokalemia
Uraemia
Jejunal diverticulosis
Mesenteric thrombosis
Saline cathartics
Peritoneal metastases (usually <25 mm long)
Cleansing enemas
Normal (always <25 mm long)

From Grainger RG, Allison D: Grainger and Allison's Diagnostic Radiology, 4th ed. Philadelphia, Churchill Livingstone, 2001.

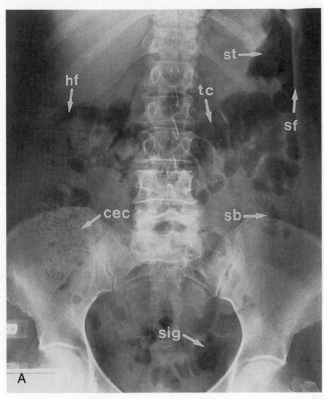

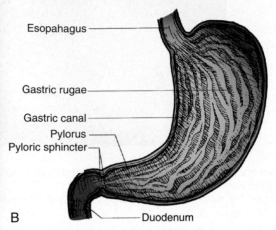

- Esopahagus
- Gastric rugae
- Gastric canal
- Pylorus
- Pyloric sphincter
- Duodenum

B

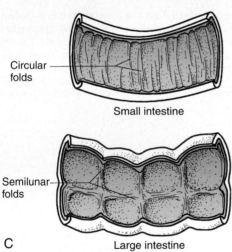

- Circular folds

Small intestine

- Semilunar folds

C

Large intestine

Fig 157–1

A to C, Normal bowel gas pattern. Gas is normally swallowed and can be seen in the stomach (st). Small amounts of air normally can be seen in the small bowel (sb), and this is usually in the left mid-abdomen or central portion of the abdomen. In this patient, gas can be seen throughout the entire colon, including the cecum (cec). In the area where the air is mixed with feces, there is a mottled pattern. Cloverleaf-shaped collections of air are seen in the hepatic flexure (hf), transverse colon (tc), splenic flexure (sf), and sigmoid (sig).

(From Mettler FA, Guibertau MJ, Voss CM, Urbina CE: Primary Care Radiology. Philadelphia, Elsevier, 2000.)

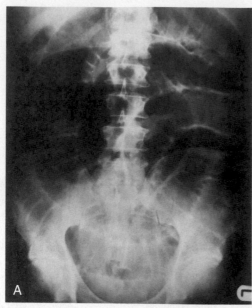
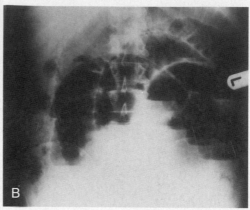

Fig 157–2

Small bowel obstruction: (**A**) supine, (**B**) erect. Very distended small bowel identified by its central position, multiple loops, and valvula conniventes. Nondistended ascending colon can be identified.

(From Grainger RG, Allison DJ, Adam A, Dixon AK [eds]: Grainger and Allison's Diagnostic Radiology, 4th ed. Philadelphia, Churchill Livingstone, 2001.)

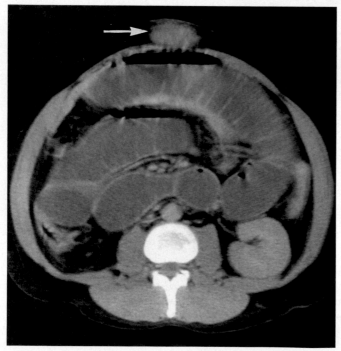

Fig 157–3

Small intestine obstruction. A section through the mid abdomen shows dilated, mainly fluid-filled, small-intestine loops. The stretched valvula conniventes can clearly be identified in some segments. The obstruction was due to an incarcerated paraumbilical hernia, the edge of which can be identified (*arrow*).

(From Grainger RG, Allison DJ, Adam A, Dixon AK [eds]: Grainger and Allison's Diagnostic Radiology, 4th ed. Philadelphia, Churchill Livingstone, 2001.)

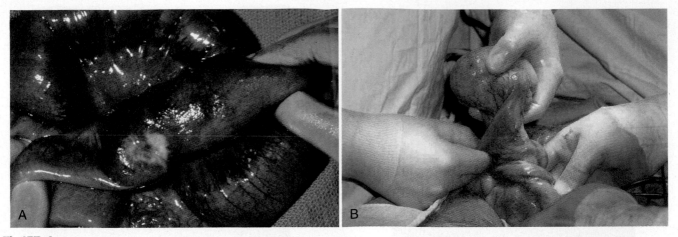

Fig 157–4
A, Small bowel primary lymphoma, diagnosed at laparotomy for bowel obstruction, Bowel proximal to obstruction is dilated, whereas distal bowel is decompressed. Treatment was surgical resection and primary anastomosis. **B,** Small bowel primary lymphoma, diagnosed at laparotomy for symptoms of bowel obstruction. Treatment was resection of segment of bowel with tumor and primary anastomosis.
(From Young NS, Gerson SL, High KA [eds]: Clinical Hematology, St Louis, Mosby, 2006.)

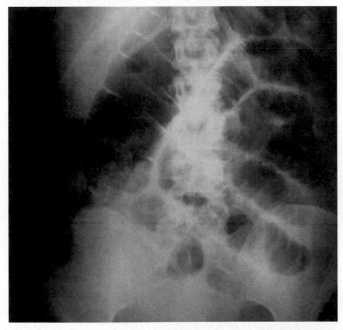

Fig 157–5
Paralytic ileus: supine. There is considerable gaseous distention of both the small and large bowels. This 34-year-old woman had 3 days earlier undergone a hysterectomy; with conservative treatment, she settled within 2 days.
(From Grainger RG, Allison DJ, Adam A, Dixon AK [eds]: Grainger and Allison's Diagnostic Radiology, 4th ed. Philadelphia, Churchill Livingstone, 2001.)

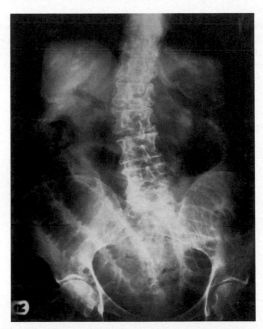

Fig 157–6
Gallstone ileus. Supine radiograph showing evidence of small bowel obstruction. In addition, gas can be identified within the right and left hepatic ducts and the common bile duct. The 79-year-old woman presented with a 5-day history of abdominal pain and vomiting.
(From Grainger RG, Allison DJ, Adam A, Dixon AK [eds]: Grainger and Allison's Diagnostic Radiology, 4th ed. Philadelphia, Churchill Livingstone, 2001.)

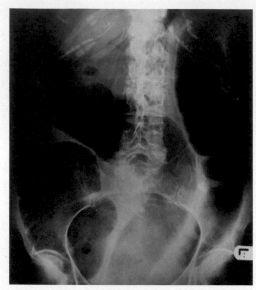

Fig 157–7
Large bowel obstruction: supine. Gas-filled, distended large bowel and cecum. Competent ileocecal valve has resulted in no dilation of small bowel. An 84-year-old woman with carcinoma of the sigmoid. (From Grainger RG, Allison DJ, Adam A, Dixon AK [eds]: Grainger and Allison's Diagnostic Radiology, 4th ed. Philadelphia, Churchill Livingstone, 2001.)

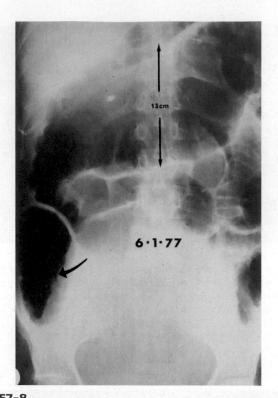

Fig 157–8
Toxic megacolon. The colon is grossly dilated (13 cm), and some mucosal islands are seen in the cecum (curved arrow). There is loss of haustration and marked small-bowel distention. (From Grainger RG, Allison DJ, Adam A, Dixon AK [eds]: Grainger and Allison's Diagnostic Radiology, 4th ed. Philadelphia, Churchill Livingstone, 2001.)

SMALL INTESTINE

Chapter 158 | Celiac disease

DEFINITION

Celiac disease is a chronic disease characterized by malabsorption and diarrhea precipitated by ingestion of food products containing gluten.

PHYSICAL FINDINGS AND CLINICAL PRESENTATION

- Physical examination may be entirely within normal limits.
- Weight loss, dyspepsia, short stature, and failure to thrive (Fig. 158–1) may be noted in children and infants.
- Weight loss, fatigue, and diarrhea are common in adults.
- Abdominal pain, nausea, and vomiting are unusual.
- Pallor as a result of iron deficiency anemia is common.
- Atypical forms of the disease are being increasingly recognized and include osteoporosis, short stature, anemia, infertility, and neurologic problems. Manifestations of calcium deficiency, such as tetany and seizures, are rare and can be exacerbated by coexistent magnesium deficiency.
- Angular cheilitis, aphthous ulcers, atopic dermatitis, and dermatitis herpetiformis are frequently associated with celiac disease.

CAUSE

- Celiac sprue is considered an autoimmune-type disease with tissue transglutaminase (tTG) suggested as a major autoantigen. It results from an inappropriate T-cell–mediated immune response against ingested gluten in genetically predisposed individuals who carry either *HLA-DQ2* or *HLA-DQ8* genes. There is sensitivity to gliadin, a protein fraction of gluten found in wheat, rye, and barley.
- Timing of introduction of gluten into the infant diet is associated with the appearance of celiac disease in children at risk. Children initially exposed to gluten in the first 3 months of life have a fivefold increased risk.

DIFFERENTIAL DIAGNOSIS

- Inflammatory bowel disease (IBD) (see Figs. 163–2, 162–4)
- Laxative abuse
- Intestinal parasitic infestations
- Other: irritable bowel syndrome, tropical sprue, chronic pancreatitis, Zollinger-Ellison syndrome, cystic fibrosis (children), lymphoma (see Fig. 157–4), eosinophilic gastroenteritis, short bowel syndrome, Whipple's disease (see Fig. 191–1)

LABORATORY TESTS

- Iron deficiency anemia (microcytic anemia, low ferritin level)
- Folic acid deficiency
- Vitamin B_{12} deficiency, hypomagnesemia, hypocalcemia
- IgA endomysial antibodies are a good screening test for celiac disease, except in the case of patients with IgA deficiency. IgA tissue transglutaminase (TTG) antibody by ELISA is a newer and very accurate serologic test for celiac sprue.
- Biopsy of the small bowel is helpful in confirming a suspected diagnosis when positive, but a negative result does not rule out the diagnosis. It may be reasonable in children with significant elevations of TTG levels (>100 U) to first try a gluten-free diet and consider biopsy in those who do not improve with diet.
- Human leukocyte antigen DQ2DQ8 testing is highly sensitive (90% to 95%) for celiac disease but not very specific. Its greatest diagnostic value is in its negative predictive value, making it useful when negative in ruling out the disease.

IMAGING STUDIES

- An endoscopic view of the duodenum in celiac disease is shown in (Fig. 158–2). Capsule endoscopy can be used to evaluate the small-intestinal mucosa, especially if future innovations will allow adequate mucosal biopsy.

TREATMENT

- Patients should be instructed on a gluten-free diet (avoidance of wheat, rye, and barley). Oats do not damage the mucosa in celiac disease.
- Correct nutritional deficiencies with iron, folic acid, calcium, vitamin B_{12}, as needed.
- Prednisone 20 to 60 mg qd gradually tapered is useful in refractory cases.
- Lifelong gluten-free diet is necessary.

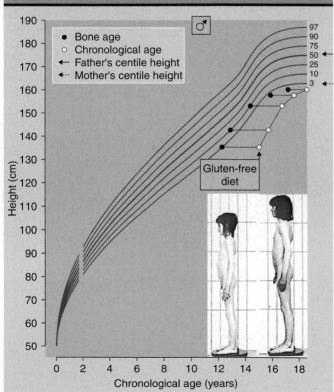

A Child with Occult Celiac Disease with Short Stature, Before and After Treatment

- ● Bone age
- ○ Chronological age
- ← Father's centile height
- ←- - Mother's centile height

Gluten-free diet

Height (cm) / Chronological age (years)

Fig 158–1

A child with occult celiac disease with short stature, before and after treatment. The effect on growth of introducing a gluten-free diet is shown. Note the delayed bone age at the start of treatment.
(From Besser CM, Thorner MO: Comprehensive Clinical Endocrinology, 3rd ed. St Louis, Mosby, 2002.)

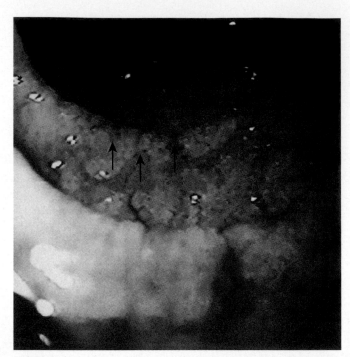

Fig 158-2
Endoscopic view of scalloped duodenal folds (*arrows*) in a patient with celiac disease.
(From Silverberg SG: Principles and Practice of Surgical Pathology and Cytopathology, 4th ed. Philadelphia, Churchill Livingstone, 2006.)

Chapter 159 | Meckel's diverticulum

DEFINITION
Meckel's diverticulum is an ileal diverticulum located 100 cm proximal to the cecum. It results from failure of the omphalomesenteric duct to obliterate completely (as it should by the eighth week of gestation).

PHYSICAL FINDINGS AND CLINICAL PRESENTATION
- Painless lower GI bleeding (4%)
- Intestinal obstruction secondary to intussusception, volvulus, herniation, or entrapment of a loop of bowel through a defect in the diverticular mesentery (6%)
- Meckel's diverticulitis mimics acute appendicitis (5%)
- Rare primary tumor arising from diverticulum (carcinoid, sarcoma, leiomyoma, adenocarcinoma)
- Asymptomatic (80% to 95%)

CAUSE AND PATHOGENESIS
- As a remnant of the omphalomesenteric duct, Meckel's diverticulum contains all layers of the intestinal wall and has its own mesentery and blood supply (branch of the superior mesenteric artery) (Fig. 159–1).
- The majority of complicated cases of Meckel's diverticulum contain ectopic mucosa (75% gastric, 15% pancreatic). It causes ulceration and bleeding of ileal mucosa adjacent to the acidic ectopic gastric secretions. Alkaline secretions of ectopic pancreatic tissue can also cause ulcerations.

DIFFERENTIAL DIAGNOSIS
- Appendicitis (see Fig. 161–1)
- Crohn's disease (see Fig. 162–8)
- All causes of lower GI bleeding (polyp, colon cancer, AV malformation, diverticulosis, hemorrhoids)

WORKUP
- Diagnosis is often made intraoperatively when the preoperative diagnosis is appendicitis.
- Preoperative detection of symptomatic Meckel's diverticulum requires a high index of suspicion.
- In the case of GI bleeding of unknown sources, a technetium scan (Fig. 159–2) will identify Meckel's diverticulum (sensitivity: 85% in children, 62% in adults; specificity: 95% in children, 9% in adults)
- In patients with suspected small bowel obstruction, intussusception, or diverticulitis, a CT scan of the abdomen/pelvis is helpful.

TREATMENT
- Surgical resection in symptomatic patients.
- There is controversy regarding the need to remove an incidentally found diverticulum, with most surgeons arguing in favor of resection.

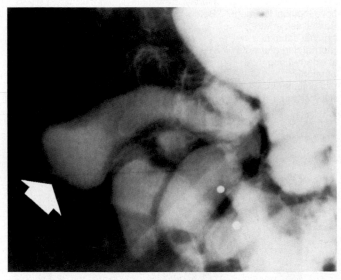

Fig 159–1
Meckel's diverticulum. A blind-ending sac is shown arising from the antimesentric border of the distal ileum (*arrow*).
(From Grainger RG, Allison DJ, Adam A, Dixon AK [eds]: Grainger and Allison's Diagnostic Radiology, 4th ed. Philadelphia, Churchill Livingstone, 2001.)

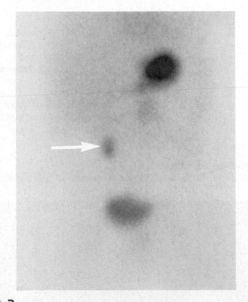

Fig 159–2
Radionuclide image of Meckel's diverticulum. Increased radionuclide uptake by ectopic gastric mucosa (*arrow*) in the Meckel's diverticulum. The patient was an 11-month-old boy who presented with acute bleeding.
(Courtesy of Dr. Kieran McHugh and reproduced with permission from Nolan DJ: Schweiz Med Wochenschr 128:109-114, 1998.)

Chapter 160 | **Hernias**

- Figure 160–1 describes the differential diagnosis of inguinal and femoral hernias

- Figure 160–2 shows a right direct inguinal hernia
- A left indirect inguinal hernia is shown in Figure 160–3.
- Treatment is surgical in symptomatic patients.

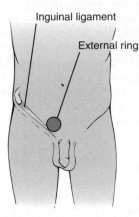
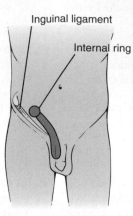
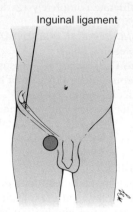

DIRECT INGUINAL HERNIA

INDIRECT INGUINAL HERNIA

FEMORAL HERNIA

Feature	Direct Inguinal*	Indirect Inguinal*	Femoral
Occurrence	Middle-aged and elderly men	All ages	Least common: More frequently found in women
Bilaterality	55%	30%	Rarely
Origin of swelling	Above inguinal ligament. Directly behind and through external ring.	Above inguinal ligament. Hernial sac enters inguinal canal at internal ring and exits at external ring.	Below inguinal ligament
Scrotal involvement	Rarely	Commonly	Never
	At side of finger in inguinal canal	At tip of finger in inguinal canal	Not felt by finger in inguinal canal; mass below canal

Fig 160–1
Differential diagnosis of hernias.
(From Swartz MH: Textbook of Physical Diagnosis, ed 5, Philadelphia, WB Saunders, 2006.)

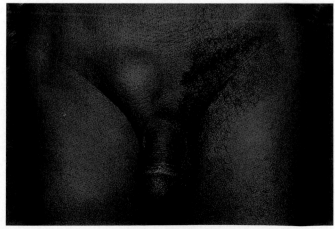

Fig 160–2
Right direct inguinal hernia.
(From Swartz MH: Textbook of Physical Diagnosis, ed 5, Philadelphia, WB Saunders, 2006.)

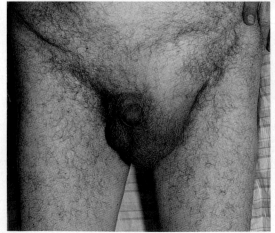

Fig 160–3
Left indirect inguinal hernia.
(From Swartz MH: Textbook of Physical Diagnosis, ed 5, Philadelphia, WB Saunders, 2006.)

Chapter 161 | Appendicitis

DEFINITION
Appendicitis is the acute inflammation of the appendix.

PHYSICAL FINDINGS AND CLINICAL PRESENTATION
- Abdominal pain: initially the pain may be epigastric or peri-umbilical in nearly 50% of patients; it subsequently localizes to the RLQ within 12 to 18 hours. Pain can be found in the back or right flank if appendix is retrocecal or in other abdominal locations if there is malrotation of the appendix.
- Pain with right thigh extension (psoas sign), low-grade fever: temperature may be >38° C if there is appendiceal perforation.
- Pain with internal rotation of the flexed right thigh *(obturator sign)* is present.
- RLQ pain on palpation of the LLQ *(Rovsing's sign):* physical examination may reveal right-sided tenderness in patients with pelvic appendix.
- Point of maximum tenderness is in the RLQ *(McBurney's point)*.
- Nausea, vomiting, tachycardia, cutaneous hyperesthesias at the level of T12 can be present.

CAUSE
Obstruction of the appendiceal lumen with subsequent vascular congestion, inflammation, and edema; common causes of obstruction are:
- Fecaliths: 30% to 35% of cases (most common in adults)
- Foreign body: 4% (fruit seeds, pinworms, tapeworms, roundworms, calculi)
- Inflammation: 50% to 60% of cases (submucosal lymphoid hyperplasia [most common etiology in children, teens])
- Neoplasms: 1% (carcinoids, metastatic disease, carcinoma)

DIFFERENTIAL DIAGNOSIS
- Intestinal: regional cecal enteritis (see Fig. 162–5), incarcerated hernia, cecal diverticulitis (see Fig. 164–3), intestinal obstruction, perforated ulcer, perforated cecum, Meckel's diverticulitis (see Fig. 159–1)
- Reproductive: ectopic pregnancy (see Fig. 258–2), ovarian cyst, torsion of ovarian cyst, salpingitis, tubo-ovarian abscess, Mittelschmerz endometriosis, seminal vesiculitis
- Renal: renal and ureteral calculi (see Fig. 216–6), neoplasms, pyelonephritis
- Vascular: leaking aortic aneurysm
- Psoas abscess
- Trauma
- Cholecystitis (see Fig. 186–1)
- Mesenteric adenitis (see Fig. 192–1)

LABORATORY TESTS
- CBC with differential reveals leukocytosis with a left shift in 90% of patients with appendicitis. Total WBC count is generally lower than 20,000/mm³. Higher counts may be indicative of perforation. Less than 4% have a normal WBC and differential. A low Hgb and Hct in an older patient should raise suspicion for GI tract carcinoma.
- Microscopic hematuria and pyuria may occur in <20% of patients.

IMAGING STUDIES
- CT of the right lower quadrant of the abdomen (Fig. 161–1) has a sensitivity of >90% and an accuracy >94% for acute appendicitis. A distended appendix, periappendiceal inflammation, and a thickened appendiceal wall are indicative of appendicitis.
- Ultrasonography (see Fig. 161–1) has a sensitivity of 75% to 90% for the diagnosis of acute appendicitis, although it is highly operator dependent and difficult in patients with large body habitus. Ultrasound is useful, especially in younger women when diagnosis is unclear. Normal ultrasonographic findings should not deter surgery if the history and physical examination are indicative of appendicitis.

TREATMENT
- Urgent appendectomy (laparoscopic or open), correction of fluid and electrolyte imbalance with vigorous IV hydration and electrolyte replacement
- IV antibiotic prophylaxis to cover gram-negative bacilli and anerobes

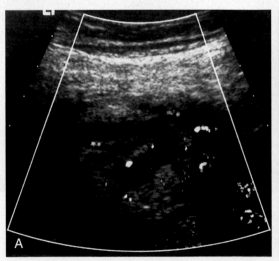
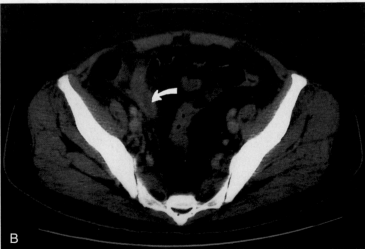

Fig 161–1
Appendicitis. (**A**) Ultrasound shows a thickened hypoechoic tubular blind-ended structure in the right iliac fossa. The surrounding fat is hyperechoic. (**B**) CT shows the thickened inflamed appendix (*arrow*). (Courtesy of Dr. A. McLean, St Bartholomew's Hospital, London.)

Chapter 162   Crohn's colitis

DEFINITION
Crohn's disease is an inflammatory disease of the bowel most commonly involving the terminal ileum and manifesting primarily with diarrhea, abdominal pain, fatigue, and weight loss.

PHYSICAL FINDINGS AND CLINICAL PRESENTATION
- Abdominal tenderness, mass, or distention
- Chronic or nocturnal diarrhea
- Weight loss, fever, night sweats
- Hyperactive bowel sounds in patients with partial obstruction, bloody diarrhea
- Delayed growth and failure of normal development in children
- Perianal and rectal abscesses, mouth and lip ulcers (Fig. 162–1), and atrophic glossitis
- Extraintestinal manifestations: joint swelling, tenderness and erosion (Fig. 162–2) hepatosplenomegaly, erythema nodosum, cutaneous polyarteritis (Fig. 162–3), clubbing, tenderness to palpation of the sacroiliac joints
- Symptoms may be intermittent with varying periods of remission

CAUSE
Unknown. Pathophysiologically, Crohn's disease involves an immune system dysfunction.

DIFFERENTIAL DIAGNOSIS
- Ulcerative colitis (see Fig. 163–2)
- Infectious diseases (TB, *Yersinia, Salmonella* [see Fig. 189–2], *Shigella, Campylobacter*)
- Parasitic infections (amebic infection [see Fig. 332–10])
- Pseudomembranous colitis (see Fig. 183–2)
- Ischemic colitis in elderly patients (see Fig. 184–2)
- Lymphoma (see Fig. 157–4)
- Colon carcinoma (see Fig. 168–1)
- Diverticulitis (see Fig. 164–3)
- Radiation enteritis
- Collagenous colitis
- Fungal infections (*Histoplasma, Actinomyces*)
- Gay bowel syndrome (in homosexual patient)
- Carcinoid tumors (see Fig. 197–6)
- Celiac sprue (see Fig. 158–2)
- Mesenteric adenitis (see Fig. 192–1)

LABORATORY TESTS
- Decreased Hgb and Hct from chronic blood loss, effect of inflammation on bone marrow, and malabsorption of vitamin B_{12}

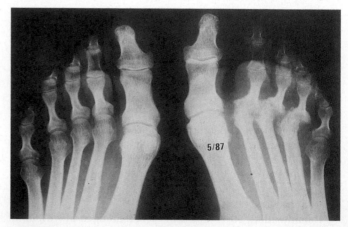

Fig 162–2
Erosive metatarsophalangeal joint lesions in a patient with Crohn's disease (asymmetrical joint involvement).
(From Hochberg MC, Silman AJ, Smolen JS, et al [eds]: Rheumatology, 3rd ed. St Louis, Mosby, 2003.)

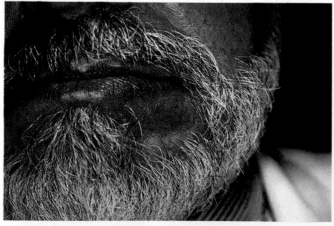

Fig 162–1
Oral Crohn's disease: there is swelling of the lips and a reddened, indurated area of skin adjacent to the lower vermilion, typical for skin involvement by Crohn's disease.
(From McKee PH, Calonje E, Granter SR [eds]: Pathology of the Skin With Clinical Correlations, 3rd ed. St Louis, Mosby, 2005.)

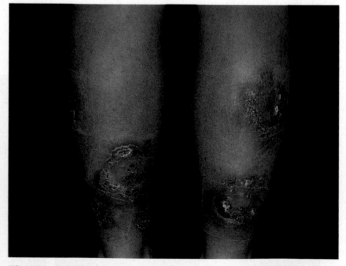

Fig 162–3
This patient with Crohn's disease also has cutaneous polyarteritis.
(From Hochberg MC, Silman AJ, Smolen JS, et al [eds]: Rheumatology, 3rd ed. St Louis, Mosby, 2003.)

- Hypokalemia, hypomagnesemia, hypocalcemia, and low albumin in patients with chronic diarrhea
- Vitamin B_{12} and folate deficiency
- Elevated ESR

ENDOSCOPIC EVALUATION

Endoscopic features of Crohn's disease include asymmetrical and discontinued disease, deep longitudinal fissures, cobblestone appearance (Fig. 162–4), presence of strictures. Thickening of the bowel wall (Fig 162–5), crypt distortion and inflammation are also present. Granulomas (Fig. 162–6) may be present.

IMAGING STUDIES

- Barium imaging studies (when performed) reveal deep ulcerations (often longitudinal and transverse) and segmental lesions (skip lesions, strictures, fistulas, cobblestone appearance of mucosa [Fig. 162–7] caused by submucosal inflammation); "thumbprinting" is common, "string sign" in terminal ileum may be noted. Although the diagnosis may be suggested by radiographic studies, it should be confirmed by endoscopy and biopsy when possible.
- CT of abdomen (Fig. 162–8) is helpful in identifying abscesses and other complications.
- In 5% to 10% of patients with IBD, a clear distinction between ulcerative colitis and Crohn's disease cannot be made. Generally, Crohn's disease can be distinguished from ulcerative colitis by presence of transmural involvement and the frequent presence of noncaseating granulomas and lymphoid aggregates on biopsy.

TREATMENT

- Oral salicylates, mesalamine (Asacol, Rowasa)
- Corticosteroids for moderate to severe active Crohn's disease.
- Immunosuppressants can be used for severe, progressive disease.
- Metronidazole may be useful for colonic fistulas and for treatment of mild to moderate active Crohn's disease.

- Infliximab, a chimeric monoclonal antibody targeting tumor necrosis factor-α, is effective in the treatment of enterocutaneous fistulas.
- Natalizumab, a selective adhesion-molecule inhibitor, has been reported effective in increasing the rate of remission and response in patients with active Crohn's disease.

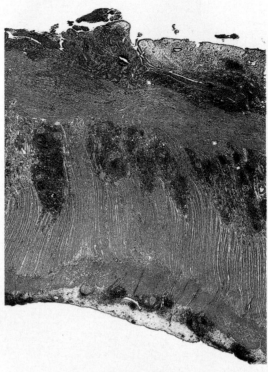

Fig 162–5
Crohn's colitis. Note the marked thickening of the wall due to the presence of submucosal fibrosis and hypertrophy of the muscularis propria. (From Silverberg SG: Principles and Practice of Surgical Pathology and Cytopathology, 4th ed. Philadelphia, Churchill Livingstone, 2006.)

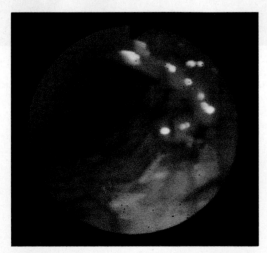

Fig 162–4
Endoscopy revealing cobblestone formation in a patient with Crohn's disease.
(From Hochberg MC, Silman AJ, Smolen JS, et al [eds]: Rheumatology, 3rd ed. St Louis, Mosby, 2003.)

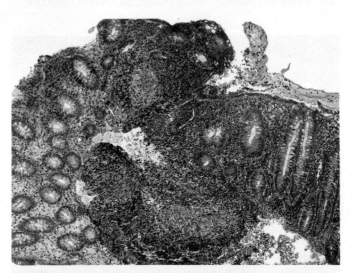

Fig 162–6
Small granuloma in a colonic biopsy from a patient with active Crohn's disease.
(From Silverberg SG: Principles and Practice of Surgical Pathology and Cytopathology, 4th ed. Philadelphia, Churchill Livingstone, 2006.)

- Hydrocortisone enema bid or tid is useful for proctitis.
- Most patients who have anemia associated with Crohn's disease respond to iron supplementation. Erythropoietin is useful in patients with anemia refractory to treatment with iron and vitamins.

- Surgical referral for segmental resection (Fig. 162–9) is needed for complications such as abscess formation, obstruction, strictures (Fig. 162–10), fistulas, toxic megacolon, refractory disease, or severe hemorrhage. A conservative surgical approach is necessary, because surgery is not curative. Multiple surgeries may also result in short bowel syndrome.

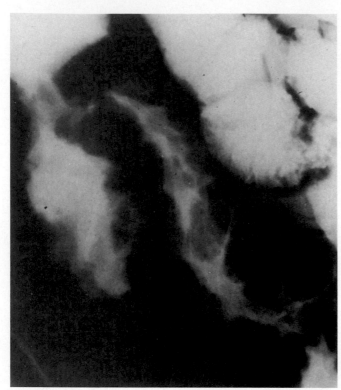

Fig 162–7
Cobblestoning of the terminal ileum, thickening of the wall of the terminal ileum, and an enlarged ileocecal valve in Crohn's disease.
(From Grainger RG, Allison DJ, Adam A, Dixon AK [eds]: Grainger and Allison's Diagnostic Radiology, 4th ed. Philadelphia, Churchill Livingstone, 2001.)

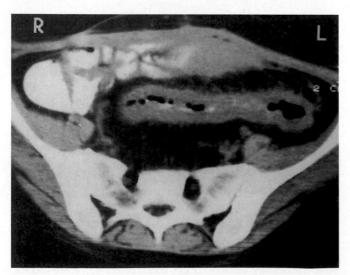

Fig 162–8
Computed tomography scan in Crohn's disease. Thickening of the intestinal wall with some asymmetry is shown in a long segment of ileum. Mesenteric thickening and infiltration are also seen.
(Courtesy of Dr. L. Engelholm.)

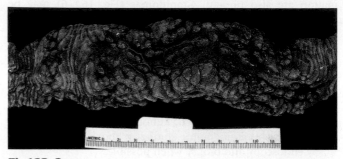

Fig 162–9
Segmental resection of small bowel showing cobblestoning ulceration in Crohn's disease.
(From Silverberg SG: Principles and Practice of Surgical Pathology and Cytopathology, 4th ed. Philadelphia, Churchill Livingstone, 2006.)

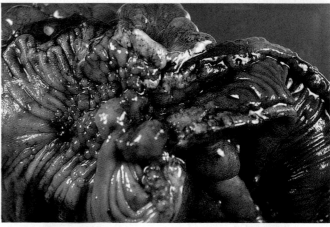

Fig 162–10
Crohn's ileitis with formation of a short stricture.
(From Silverberg SG: Principles and Practice of Surgical Pathology and Cytopathology, 4th ed. Philadelphia, Churchill Livingstone, 2006.)

COLON

Chapter 163 | **Ulcerative colitis**

DEFINITION
Ulcerative colitis is a chronic inflammatory bowel disease of undetermined etiology.

PHYSICAL FINDINGS AND CLINICAL PRESENTATION
- Patients with ulcerative colitis often present with bloody diarrhea accompanied by tenesmus, fever, dehydration, weight loss, anorexia, nausea, and abdominal pain.
- Abdominal distention and tenderness.
- Bloody diarrhea.
- Fever, evidence of dehydration.
- Evidence of extraintestinal manifestations may be present: liver disease, sclerosing cholangitis, iritis, uveitis, episcleritis, arthritis, sacroiliitis (Fig. 163–1), erythema nodosum, pyoderma gangrenosum, aphthous stomatitis.

DIFFERENTIAL DIAGNOSIS
- Crohn's disease (see Fig. 162–4)
- Bacterial infections
  1. Acute: *Campylobacter, Yersinia, Salmonella,* (see Fig. 189–2) *Shigella, Chlamydia, Escherichia coli, Clostridium difficile,* gonococcal proctitis
  2. Chronic: Whipple's disease (see Fig. 191–1), TB enterocolitis
- Irritable bowel syndrome
- Protozoal and parasitic infections (amebiasis [see Fig. 332–10], giardiasis, cryptosporidiosis)
- Neoplasm (intestinal lymphoma (see Fig. 157–4), carcinoma of colon (see Fig. 168–1))
- Ischemic bowel disease (see Fig. 194–2)
- Diverticulitis (see Fig. 164–3)
- Celiac sprue (see Fig. 158–2), collagenous colitis, radiation enteritis, endometriosis, gay bowel syndrome

LABORATORY TESTS
- Anemia, high sedimentation rate (in severe colitis) are common.
- Potassium, magnesium, calcium, albumin may be decreased.

- Antineutrophil cytoplasmic antibodies (ANCA) with a perinuclear staining pattern (pANCA) can be found in >45% of patients; there is an increased frequency in treatment-resistant left-sided colitis, suggesting a possible association between these antibodies and a relative resistance to medical therapy in patients with ulcerative colitis.
- Colonoscopy to establish the presence of mucosal inflammation: typical endoscopic findings in ulcerative colitis are friable mucosa, diffuse, uniform erythema replacing the usual mucosal vascular pattern, and pseudopolyps (Fig. 163–2); rectal involvement is invariably present if the disease is active

IMAGING STUDIES
Image studies are generally not indicated. Air-contrast barium enema, when used, may reveal continuous involvement (including the rectum), pseudo polyps, decreased mucosal pattern, and fine superficial ulcerations.

TREATMENT
The therapeutic options vary with the degree of disease (mild, severe, fulminant) and areas of involvement (distal, extensive):
- Mild or moderate disease can be treated with mesalamine. It can be administered as an enema or suppository for patients with distal colonic disease. Oral forms can deliver therapeutic concentrations to the more proximal small bowel or distal ileum.
- Olsalazine is often useful for maintenance of remission of ulcerative colitis in patients intolerant to sulfasalazine. Usual dose is 500 mg bid taken with food.
- Balsalazide is useful for mild to moderately active ulcerative colitis.
- Severe disease usually responds to oral corticosteroids. Corticosteroid suppositories or enemas are also useful for distal colitis.
- Fulminant disease generally requires hospital admission and parenteral corticosteroids. IV cyclosporine can also be used in severe refractory cases; renal toxicity is a potential complication.

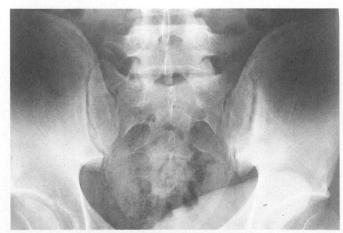

Fig 163–1
Asymmetrical sacroiliitis in a patient with inflammatory bowel disease. (From Hochberg MC, Silman AJ, Smolen JS, et al [eds]: Rheumatology, 3rd ed. St Louis, Mosby, 2003.)

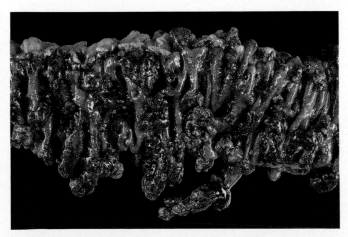

Fig 163–2
Ulcerative colitis with numerous large inflammatory polyps.

- Surgery is indicated in patients who fail to respond to intensive medical therapy. Colectomy is usually curative in these patients and also eliminates the high risk of developing adenocarcinoma of the colon (10% to 20% of patients develop it after 10 years with the disease); newer surgical techniques allow for the preservation of the sphincter.
- Correct nutritional deficiencies; TPN with bowel rest may be necessary in severe cases; folate supplementation may reduce the incidence of dysplasia and cancer in chronic ulcerative colitis.
- Avoid oral feedings during acute exacerbation to decrease colonic activity; a low-roughage diet may be helpful in *early* relapse.

- Psychotherapy is useful in most patients. Referral to self-help groups is also important because of the chronicity of the disease and the young age of most patients.
- Colonoscopic surveillance and multiple biopsies should be instituted approximately 10 years after diagnosis because of the increased risk of colon carcinoma.
- Erythropoietin is useful in patients with anemia refractory to treatment with iron and vitamins.
- The clinical course is variable; 15% to 20% of patients will eventually require colectomy; >75% of patients treated medically will experience relapse.

Chapter 164   Diverticular disease

DEFINITIONS

- Colonic diverticula are herniations of mucosa and submucosa through the muscularis (Fig. 164–1). They are generally found along the colon's mesenteric border at the site where the vasa recta penetrates the muscle wall (anatomic weak point).
- *Diverticulosis* is the asymptomatic presence of multiple colonic diverticula.
- *Diverticulitis* is an inflammatory process or localized perforation of diverticulum.

PHYSICAL FINDINGS AND CLINICAL PRESENTATION

- Physical examination in patients with diverticulosis is generally normal.
- Painful diverticular disease can present with LLQ pain, often relieved by defecation; location of pain may be anywhere in the lower abdomen because of the redundancy of the sigmoid colon.
- Diverticulitis can cause muscle spasm, guarding, and rebound tenderness predominantly affecting the LLQ.

CAUSE

- Diverticular disease is believed to be secondary to low intake of dietary fiber.

DIFFERENTIAL DIAGNOSIS

- Irritable bowel syndrome
- IBD (see Fig. 163–2)
- Carcinoma of colon (see Fig. 168–1)
- Endometriosis (see Fig. 232–2)
- Ischemic colitis (see Fig. 194–2)
- Infections (pseudomembranous colitis [see Fig. 193–2], appendicitis [see Fig. 161–1], pyelonephritis [see Fig. 213–2], PID [see Fig. 250–1])
- Lactose intolerance
- Celiac disease (see Fig. 158–2)

LABORATORY TESTS

- WBC count in diverticulitis reveals leukocytosis with left shift.
- Microcytic anemia can be present in patients with chronic bleeding from diverticular disease. MCV may be elevated in acute bleeding secondary to reticulocytosis.

IMAGING STUDIES

- Barium enema should only be considered in patients unwilling to undergo colonoscopy or with contraindications to the procedure. When performed, barium enema will demonstrate multiple diverticula (Fig. 164–2) and muscle spasm ("sawtooth" appearance of the lumen) in patients with painful diverticular disease. Barium enema can be hazardous and should not be performed in the acute stage of diverticulitis because it may produce free perforation.
- A CT scan of the abdomen (Fig. 164–3) can be used to diagnose acute diverticulitis; typical findings are thickening of the bowel wall, fistulas, or abscess formation.

TREATMENT

- Increases in dietary fiber intake and regular exercise to improve bowel function
- NPO and IV hydration in severe diverticulitis; NG suction if ileus or small bowel obstruction is present

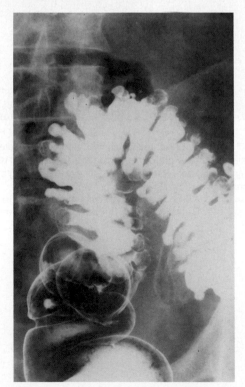

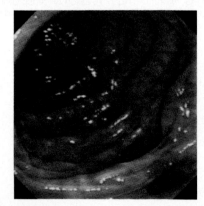

Fig 164–1
Colonoscopic appearance of diverticular disease affecting the sigmoid colon.
(From Forbes A, Misiewicz J, Compton C, et al: Atlas of Clinical Gastroenterology, 3rd ed. Edinburgh, Elsevier Mosby, 2005.)

Fig 164–2
Diverticular disease showing typical muscle changes in the sigmoid and diverticula arising from the apices of the clefts between interdigitating muscle folds.
(From Grainger RG, Allison DJ, Adam A, Dixon AK [eds]: Grainger and Allison's Diagnostic Radiology, 4th ed. Philadelphia, Churchill Livingstone, 2001.)

A. TREATMENT OF DIVERTICULITIS
- Broad-spectrum antibiotics
- Surgical treatment consisting of resection of involved areas and re-anastomosis (if feasible); otherwise a diverting colostomy with re-anastomosis can be performed when infection has been controlled

B. DIVERTICULAR HEMORRHAGE:
1. Bleeding is painless and stops spontaneously in the majority of patients (60%); it is usually caused by erosion of a blood vessel by a fecalith present within the diverticular sac. Angiography may be necessary to exclude the sources of lower GI bleeding such as colonic adenocarcinoma (Fig. 164–4) or angiodysplasia (Fig. 164–5).
2. Medical therapy consists of blood replacement and correction of volume and any clotting abnormalities.

3. Colonoscopic treatment with epinephrine injections, bipolar coagulation, or both may prevent recurrent bleeding and decrease the need for surgery.
4. Surgical resection is necessary if bleeding does not stop spontaneously after administration of 4 to 5 U of PRBCs or recurs with severity within a few days; if attempts at localization are unsuccessful, total abdominal colectomy with ileoproctostomy may be indicated (high incidence of rebleeding if segmental resection is performed without adequate localization).

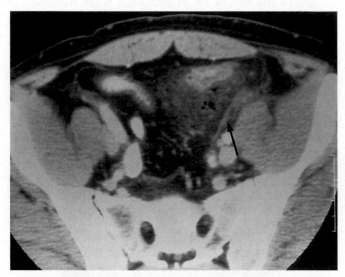

Fig 164–3
Sigmoid diverticulitis. Enhanced CT shows haziness associated with extraluminal air in the sigmoid mesocolon due to perforated diverticulitis, also manifested as a thickened sigmoid wall. Thickening at the root of the sigmoid mesocolon is also present (*arrow*).
(From Grainger RG, Allison DJ, Adam A, Dixon AK [eds]: Grainger and Allison's Diagnostic Radiology, 4th ed. Philadelphia, Churchill Livingstone, 2001.)

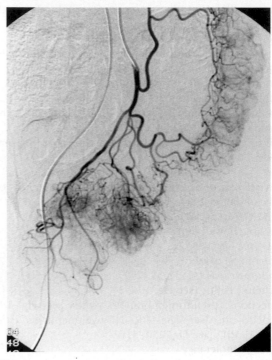

Fig 164–4
A selective inferior mesenteric artery angiogram shows an area of focal hypovascularity in the proximal sigmoid colon with occlusion of the vasa recta in a patient with a colonic adenocarcinoma.
(From Grainger RG, Allison DJ, Adam A, Dixon AK [eds]: Grainger and Allison's Diagnostic Radiology, 4th ed. Philadelphia, Churchill Livingstone, 2001.)

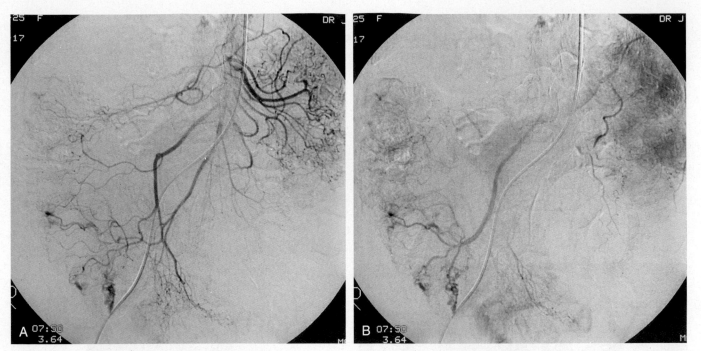

Fig 164–5
(**A**) Arterial phase of superior mesenteric artery angiogram demonstrates the classic findings of angiodysplasia with enlargement of the vessels supplying the antimesenteric border of the cecum and several vascular lakes. (**B**) Early venous phase of the same study, although there is still some peripheral arterial branch filling in the ileum, shows the early filling, prominent draining veins from three focal areas cecal angiodysplasia. (From Grainger RG, Allison DJ, Adam A, Dixon AK [eds]: Grainger and Allison's Diagnostic Radiology, 4th ed. Philadelphia, Churchill Livingstone, 2001.)

Chapter 165   Familial polyposis syndrome

- Familial adenomatous polyposis (FAP) is an autosomal dominant inherited disorder caused by a mutation of the APC gene on the long arm of chromosome 5 and manifested by the development of numerous (>100) adenomas by the late teens (Fig. 165–1). Thirty percent of cases of FAP are de novo germline mutations, and thus patients present without a family history of the disease.
- Clinically patients may present with bleeding, diarrhea, and mucous discharge.

- Diagnosis is made by colonoscopy. Barium enema if performed will show numerous sessile polyps (Fig. 165–2).
- All patients will develop colon cancer if left untreated. Treatment consists of proctocolectomy with restorative ileostomy once the diagnosis is made.
- Screening of family members is mandatory.

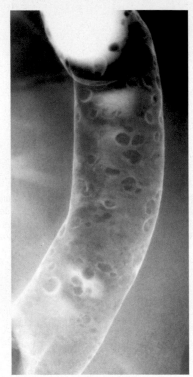

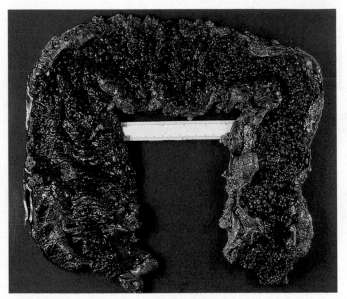

Fig 165–1
In familial polyposis, the luminal surface of the bowel is carpeted with hundreds of adenomas of varying sizes. The intervening flat mucosa often contains adenomatous epithelium.
(From Silverberg SG: Principles and Practice of Surgical Pathology and Cytopathology, 4th ed. Philadelphia, Churchill Livingstone, 2006.)

Fig 165–2
Familial adenomatous polyposis with numerous sessile polyps.
(From Grainger RG, Allison DJ, Adam A, Dixon AK [eds]: Grainger and Allison's Diagnostic Radiology, 4th ed. Philadelphia, Churchill Livingstone, 2001.)

Chapter 166	**Peutz-Jeghers syndrome**

PHYSICAL FINDINGS AND CLINICAL PRESENTATION

- Transmission: autosomal dominant with incomplete penetrance
- Disease expression
  1. Stomach, small and large intestinal hamartomas (Fig. 166–1) with bands of smooth muscle in the lamina propria
  2. Pigmented lesions around mouth (lips and buccal mucosa) (Fig. 166–2), nose, hands, feet (Fig. 166–3), genital, and perineal areas
  3. Ovarian tumors
  4. Sertoli cell testicular tumors
  5. Airway polyps
  6. Pancreatic cancer
  7. Breast cancer
  8. Urinary tract polyps
- Cumulative lifetime cancer risk
  1. Colon cancer: 39%
  2. Stomach cancer: 29%
  3. Small intestine cancer: 13%
  4. Pancreatic cancer: 36%
  5. Breast cancer: 54%
  6. Ovarian cancer: 10%
  7. Sertoli cell tumor: 9%
  8. Overall cancer risk: 93%
- Clinical manifestation
  1. Gastrointestinal, small bowel obstruction, intussusception, GI bleeding

TREATMENT

- Colonoscopies with polypectomies
- Screening for breast cancer, testicular cancer, possibly ovarian cancer

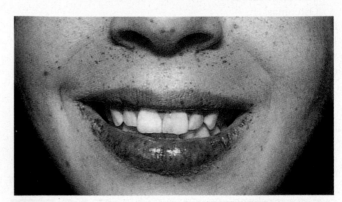

Fig 166–2
Peutz-Jeghers syndrome. Note the pigmentary changes.
(From Swartz MH: Textbook of Physical Diagnosis, 5th ed. Philadelphia, WB Saunders, 2006.)

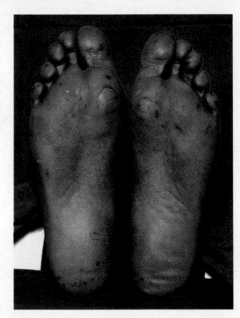

Fig 166–3
Peutz-Jeghers syndrome: multiple darkly pigmented larger macular lesions on the soles. (Courtesy of the Institute of Dermatology, London.)

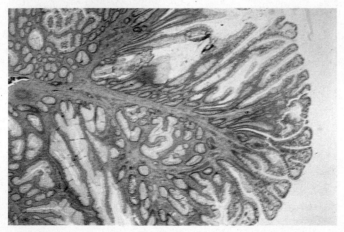

Fig 166–1
Peutz-Jeghers hamartoma. Treelike network of muscularis radiates up into the lamina propria and supports epithelium without cytologic atypia.
(From Silverberg SG: Principles and Practice of Surgical Pathology and Cytopathology, 4th ed. Philadelphia, Churchill Livingstone, 2006.)

Chapter 167   Gardner's syndrome

DEFINITION

Gardner's syndrome is a variant of familial adenomatous polyposis (FAP), with prominent extraintestinal manifestations. It is an autosomal dominant condition characterized by:

- Adenomatous intestinal polyps (Fig. 167–1)
- Soft tissue tumors
- Osteomas

PHYSICAL FINDINGS AND CLINICAL PRESENTATION

Phenotypic variability seen in individuals and families with the same mutation. Soft tissue and bone abnormalities may precede intestinal disease.

- Congenital hypertrophy of the retinal pigment epithelium (often the first sign)
- Dental abnormalities: supernumerary or unerupted teeth
- Soft tissue lesions: epidermoid (Fig. 167–2) or sebaceous cysts, fibromas, lipomas, desmoid tumors
- Skull, mandible, long bone osteomas (Fig. 167–3)
- Abdominal mass, occult blood in stool

CAUSE

- Caused by mutations of the adenomatous polyposis coli (APC) gene on chromosome 5q21; over 300 mutations have been identified. The site of the mutation may explain the prominent extraintestinal lesions that differentiate Gardner's syndrome from other variants of FAP.
- Spontaneous mutations are responsible for 20% to 30% of cases.

DIAGNOSIS

In individuals with a family history, diagnosis is confirmed by >100 adenomatous polyps in the colon, >3 pigmented ocular lesions on funduscopic examination, or genetic testing.

DIFFERENTIAL DIAGNOSIS

- FAP (see Fig. 165–1)
- Turcot's syndrome
- Attenuated adenomatous polyposis coli
- Peutz-Jeghers syndrome (see Figs. 166–1, 166–2)
- Juvenile polyposis
- MYH polyposis

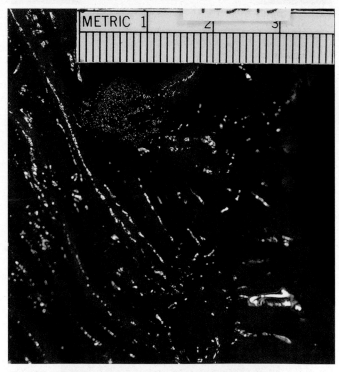

Fig 167–1
This segment of bowel contains an adenoma on a lengthy stalk. When small, adenomas may be grossly indistinguishable from hyperplastic polyps. Adenomas larger than 5 mm, such as this one, have a granular red surface and usually appear lobulated and raspberry-like. The tan stalk is covered with normal mucosa.
(From Silverberg SG: Principles and Practice of Surgical Pathology and Cytopathology, 4th ed. Philadelphia, Churchill Livingstone, 2006.)

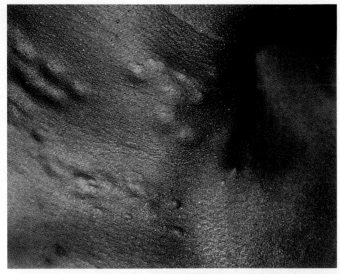

Fig 167–2
Gardner's syndrome. Multiple epidermoid cysts are present in this patient with adenomatous colonic polyps.
(From Callen JP, Jorizzo JL, Bolognia JL, et al: Dermatological Signs of Internal Disease, 3rd ed. Philadelphia, WB Saunders, 2003.)

DIAGNOSTIC SCREENING OPTIONS

Screening should be offered to first-degree relatives of affected individuals >10 years of age and individuals with >100 colorectal adenomas.

Protein Truncation Testing

- Genetic test; serum in vitro synthesized protein assay.
- Able to identify a mutation in 80% of families with FAP. To ensure that the family has a detectable mutation, test an affected family member first.
- If positive in the affected individual, the test can differentiate with 100% accuracy affected and unaffected family members. If negative in the affected individual, screening family members will not be useful in determining disease status.
- If there is no known family history, screening the individual in question is reasonable. A positive test rules in FAP, but a negative test does not rule it out.
- Other genetic tests (sequencing, linkage, single-strand conformation polymorphism testing) can be considered if protein truncation testing is not informative.

Note: Genetic counseling should be performed and written informed consent obtained before genetic testing.

Colonoscopy

- Pedigrees with an identified APC mutation:
- Positive genetic tests: annual colonoscopy beginning at age 12 years
- Negative genetic test: colonoscopy at age 25 years
- Pedigrees with an unidentified APC mutation: family members should have annual colonoscopy starting at age 12 years; every 2 years starting at age 25 years; every 3 years starting at age 35 years; and then per age-appropriate guidelines starting at age 50.

Congenital Hypertrophy of the Retinal Pigment Epithelium (HRPE):

- Lesions occur in some families and are a reliable indicator of affected status in these families.

TREATMENT

- Colectomy is recommended once polyps are seen on sigmoidoscopy.
- Screening of remaining GI tract and screening for extraintestinal manifestations must continue after colectomy.
- Annual physical examination: history, examination, and blood tests.
- Upper endoscopy (must include the ampulla of vater): screening for gastric and duodenal polyps should begin once colonic polyps are detected and continue every 3-5 years. Screening frequency increases if polyps are present in the UGI tract.
- Other possible cancer sites should be imaged if symptoms occur or if these cancers have occurred in relatives.
- Consider celocoxib therapy to reduce polyposis
- Treat soft tissue lesions and osteomas for symptoms or cosmetic concerns
- Treat desmoid tumors if they pose a risk to adjacent structures

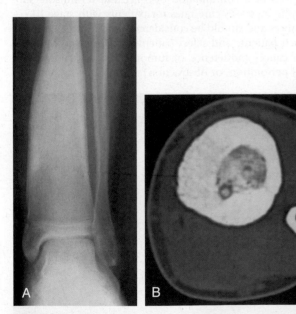

Fig 167–3
Osteoid osteoma of the tibia. (**A**) AP radiograph demonstrates dense sclerosis and expansion of the distal tibial cortex with no evidence of a nidus. (**B**) CT shows the classic appearances of the nidus, a focal lytic lesion less than 10 mm in size with central mineralization. Medullary sclerosis is also evident.
(From Grainger RG, Allison DJ, Adam A, Dixon AK [eds]: Grainger and Allison's Diagnostic Radiology, 4th ed. Philadelphia, Churchill Livingstone, 2001.)

Chapter 168 Colorectal cancer

DEFINITION

Colorectal cancer is a neoplasm arising from the luminal surface of the large bowel: descending colon (40% to 42%), rectosigmoid and rectum (30% to 33%), cecum and ascending colon (25% to 30%), transverse colon (10% to 13%).

PHYSICAL FINDINGS AND CLINICAL PRESENTATION

- Physical examination may be completely unremarkable.
- The clinical presentation of colorectal malignancies is initially vague and nonspecific (weight loss, anorexia, malaise). It is useful to divide colon cancer symptoms into those usually associated with the right side of the colon and those commonly associated with the left side of the colon, because the clinical presentation varies with the location of the carcinoma.
  1. Right side of colon
     a. Anemia (iron deficiency secondary to chronic blood loss).
     b. Dull, vague, and uncharacteristic abdominal pain may be present or patient may be completely asymptomatic.
     c. Rectal bleeding is often missed because blood is mixed with feces.
     d. Obstruction and constipation are unusual because of large lumen and more liquid stools.
  2. Left side of colon
     a. Change in bowel habits (constipation, diarrhea, tenesmus, pencil-thin stools).
     b. Rectal bleeding (bright red blood coating the surface of the stool).
     c. Intestinal obstruction is frequent because of small lumen.
- Digital rectal examination can detect approximately 50% of rectal cancers.
- Palpable abdominal masses may indicate metastasis or complications of colorectal carcinoma (abscess, intussusception, volvulus).
- Abdominal distention and tenderness are suggestive of colonic obstruction.
- Hepatomegaly may be indicative of hepatic metastasis.

CAUSE

Colorectal cancer can arise through two mutational pathways: microsatellite instability or chromosomal instability. Germline genetic mutations are the basis of inherited colon cancer syndromes; an accumulation of somatic mutations in a cell is the basis of sporadic colon cancer.

DIFFERENTIAL DIAGNOSIS

- Diverticular disease (see Fig. 164–3)
- Strictures
- IBD (see Fig. 162–4, Fig. 163–2)
- Infectious or inflammatory lesions (see Fig. 189–2)
- Adhesions
- Arteriovenous malformations
- Metastatic carcinoma (prostate, sarcoma)
- Extrinsic masses (cysts, abscesses)

IMAGING STUDIES

- Colonoscopy with biopsy (primary assessment tool) (Fig. 168–1).

- Virtual colonoscopy (VC) uses helical (spiral) CT scan to generate a two- or three-dimensional virtual colorectal image. VC does not require sedation, but like optical colonoscopy, it requires some bowel preparation (either bowel cathartics or ingestion of iodinated contrast medium with meals during the 48 hours before CT) and air insufflation. It also involves substantial exposure to radiation. In addition, patients with lesions detected by VC will require traditional colonoscopy.
- CT scan (Fig. 168–2) of abdomen/pelvis/chest to assist in preoperative staging. PET scan (Fig. 168–2) is also used for staging.

TREATMENT

- Surgical resection (Fig. 168–3): 70% of colorectal cancers are resectable for cure at presentation; 45% of patients are cured by primary resection.
- Radiation therapy is a useful adjunct to chemotherapy with fluorouracil and levamisole therapy for stage II or III rectal cancers.
- The backbone of treatment of colorectal cancer is fluorouracil (FL). Leucovorin (folinic acid) enhances the effect of fluorouracil and is given together with it. Adjuvant chemotherapy with a combination of 5-FU and levamisole substantially increases cure rates for patients with stage III colon cancer and should be considered standard treatment for all such patients and select patients with high-risk stage II colon cancer (adherence of tumor to an adjacent organ, bowel perforation, or obstruction).

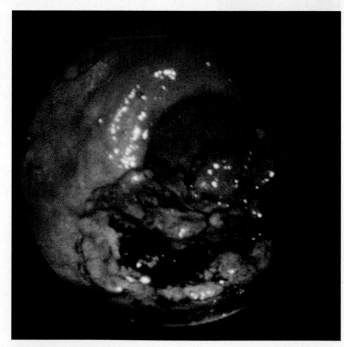

Fig 168–1

Colonoscopic appearance of hemorrhagic carcinoma in ascending colon.

(From Forbes A, Misiewicz J, Compton C, et al: Atlas of Clinical Gastroenterology, 3rd ed. Edinburgh, Elsevier Mosby, 2005.)

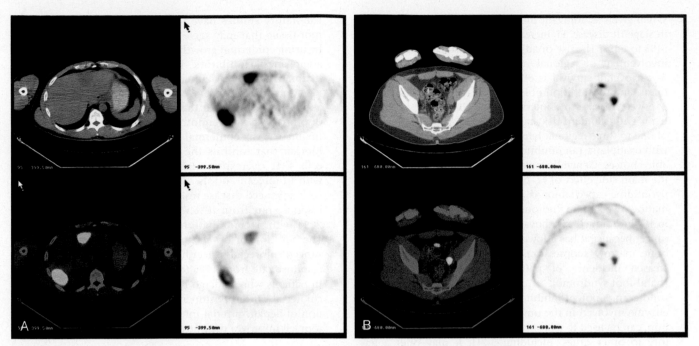

Fig 168–2
Colon cancer. **A,** Positron emission tomography (PET) and computed tomography (CT) scans display of a patient with two ^{18}fluorodeoxyglucose (FDG)-avid lesions in the liver. These are seen on the CT (*upper left*) scan, attenuation-corrected PET (*upper right*) scan, non–attenuation-corrected PET (*lower right*) scan, and fused images (*lower left*). **B,** PET and CT scans of the pelvis, oriented as in (**A**), show increased FDG uptake in a left external iliac lymph node metastasis.
(From Abeloff MD: Clinical Oncology, 3rd ed. Philadelphia, Elsevier, 2004.)

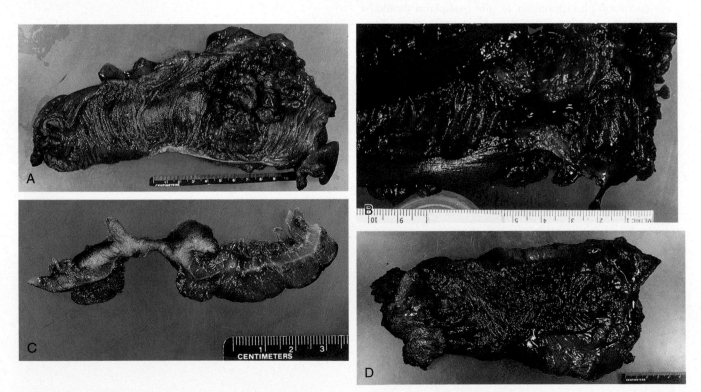

Fig 168–3
Common gross appearances of colonic carcinoma. (**A**) Exophytic carcinoma of the cecum. (**B**) Circumferential, napkin ringlike pattern of carcinoma narrowing the lumen of descending colon. (**C**) Cross-section of (**B**) showing interruption of muscularis propria by carcinoma invading full thickness of the bowel wall. (**D**) Ulcerating carcinoma in rectum, with raised edges and a necrotic center.
(From Silverberg SG: Principles and Practice of Surgical Pathology and Cytopathology, 4th ed. Philadelphia, Churchill Livingstone, 2006.)

- When given as adjuvant therapy after a complete resection in stage III disease, FL increases overall 5-year survival from 51% to 64%. The use of adjuvant FL in stage II disease (no involvement of regional nodes) is controversial because 5-year overall survival is 80% for treated or untreated patients, and the addition of FL only increases the probability of 5-year disease-free interval from 72% to 76%. For patients with standard-risk stage III tumors (e.g., involvement of one to three regional lymph nodes), both FL alone or FL with oxaliplatin (an inhibitor of DNA synthesis) are reasonable choices. Generally, reversible peripheral neuropathy is the main side effect of FL plus oxaliplatin. The oral fluoropyrimidine capecitabine is a prodrug that undergoes enzymatic conversion to fluorouracil. It is an effective alternative to IV fluorouracil as adjuvant treatment for stage III colon cancer because it has a lower incidence of mouth sores and bone marrow suppression. It does however have an increased incidence of palmar-plantar erythrodysesthesia (hand-foot syndrome).

- Irinotecan, a potent inhibitor of topoisomerase I, a nuclear enzyme involved in the unwinding of DNA during replication, can be used to treat metastatic colorectal cancer refractory to other drugs, including 5-FU; it may offer a few months of palliation but is expensive and associated with significant toxicity.

- Oxaliplatin, a third-generation platinum derivative, can be used in combination with fluorouracil and leucovorin (FL) for patients with metastatic colorectal cancer whose disease has recurred or progressed despite treatment with fluorouracil/leucovorin plus irinotecan. FL plus oxaliplatin should be considered for high-risk patients with stage III cancers (e.g., >3 involved regional nodes [N2] or tumor invasion beyond the serosa [T4 lesion]).

- Laboratory studies have identified molecular sites in tumor tissue that may serve as specific targets for treatment by using epidermal growth factor receptor antagonists and angiogenesis inhibitors. The monoclonal antibodies cetuximab and bevacizumab have been approved by the FDA for advanced colorectal cancer. Bevacizumab is an angiogenesis inhibitor that binds and inhibits the activity of human vascular endothelial growth factor (VEGF). Cetuximab is an epidermal growth factor receptor [EGFR] blocker that inhibits the growth and survival of tumor cells that overexpress EGFR. Cetuximab has synergism with irinotecan and its addition to irinotecan in patients with advanced disease resistant to irinotecan increases the response rate from 10% when cetuximab is used alone to 22% with a combination of cetuximab and irinotecan. The addition of bevacizumab to FL in patients with advanced colorectal cancer has been reported to increase the response rate from 17% to 40%.

- In patients who undergo resection of liver metastases from colorectal cancer, postoperative treatment with a combination of hepatic arterial infusion of floxuridine and IV fluorouracil improves the outcome at 2 years.

DISORDERS OF THE ANUS, ANAL CANAL, AND PERIANAL REGION

Chapter 169 | Hemorrhoids

DEFINITION
A hemorrhoid is a varicose dilation of a vein of the superior or inferior hemorrhoidal plexus, resulting from a persistent increase in venous pressure. External hemorrhoids are below the pectinate line (inferior plexus). Internal hemorrhoids (Fig. 169–1) are above the pectinate line (superior plexus)

PHYSICAL FINDINGS AND CLINICAL PRESENTATION
- Bleeding with defecation; bleeding is bright red and staining on toilet paper
- Perianal irritation
- Mucofecal staining of underclothes
- Acute external hemorrhoids: painful, swollen, and often thrombosed
- Pain on sitting, standing, or defecating (thrombosed hemorrhoid)
- Prolapse
- Constipation

CAUSE
- Low-fiber, high-fat diet
- Chronic constipation and straining with defecation
- High resting anal sphincter pressures
- Pregnancy
- Rectal surgery (i.e., episiotomy)
- Prolonged sitting
- Anal intercourse

DIFFERENTIAL DIAGNOSIS
- Fissure (see Fig. 170–1)
- Abscess (see Fig. 171–1)
- Anal fistula (see Fig. 171–2)
- Condylomata acuminata (see Fig. 27–18)
- Hypertrophied anal papille
- Rectal prolapse (see Fig. 231–12)
- Rectal polyp
- Neoplasm

WORKUP
- Inspection
- Digital rectal examination
- Anoscopy
- Sigmoidoscopy

TREATMENT
- Avoidance of constipation and straining with defecation
- Avoidance of prolonged sitting on toilet
- High-fiber diet (20 to 30 g/day). Fiber supplements to provide bulk (psyllium extracts or mucilloids)
- Increased fluid intake (six to eight glasses of water per day)
- Cleaning with mild soap and water after defecation
- Warm soaks or ice to soothe
- Sitz baths
- Medicated compresses with witch hazel
- Topical hydrocortisone (1% to 3% cream or ointment)
- Topical anesthetic spray
- Glycerin suppositories
- Stool softeners
- Surgical removal of clot from thrombosed hemorrhoid (Fig. 169–2)

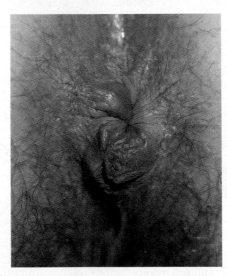

Fig 169–1
Prolapsed internal hemorrhoids.
(From Swartz MH: Textbook of Physical Diagnosis, ed 5, Philadelphia, WB Saunders, 2006.)

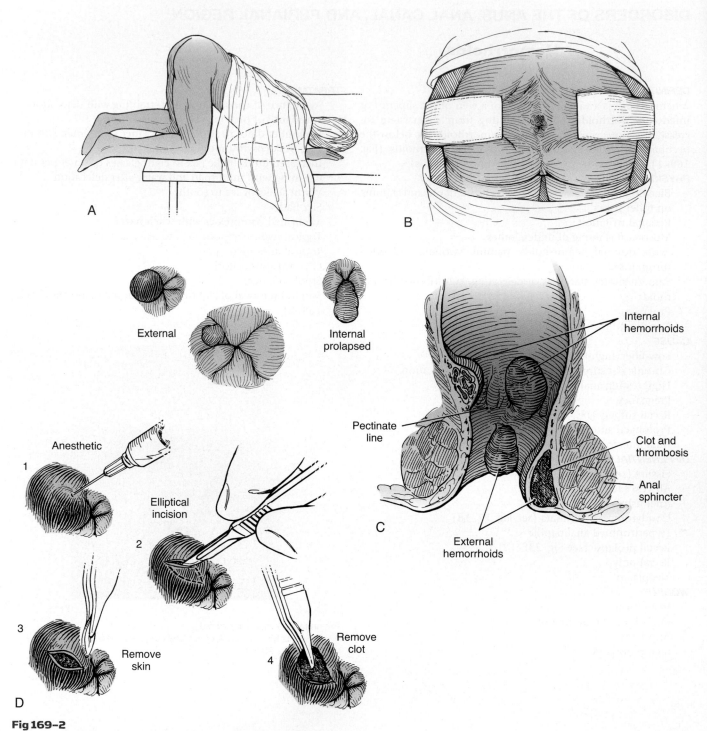

Labels within figure:

A

B

External

Internal prolapsed

Pectinate line

Internal hemorrhoids

Clot and thrombosis

Anal sphincter

External hemorrhoids

C

Anesthetic

1

Elliptical incision

2

3 Remove skin

4 Remove clot

D

Fig 169–2
Surgical removal of clot from thrombosed hemorrhoid.
(From Rosen P, Chan TC, Vilke GM, Sternbach G: Atlas of Emergency Procedures. St Louis, Mosby, 2001.)

Chapter 170 Anal fissure

DEFINITION
A fissure is a tear in the epithelial lining of the anal canal (i.e., from the dentate line to the anal verge) (Fig. 170–1).

PHYSICAL FINDINGS AND CLINICAL PRESENTATION
With separation of the buttocks a tear in the posterior midline or, less frequently, in the anterior midline will be visible

- Acute anal fissure:
  1. Sharp burning or tearing pain exacerbated by bowel movements
  2. Bright-red blood on toilet paper, a streak of blood on the stool or in the water
- Chronic anal fissure:
  1. Pruritus ani
  2. Pain seldom present
  3. Intermittent bleeding
  4. Sentinel tag at the caudal aspect of the fissure (Fig. 170–1), hypertrophied anal papilla at the proximal end

CAUSE
- Most are initiated after passage of a large, hard stool
- May result from frequent defecation and diarrhea
- Bacterial infections: TB, syphilis, gonorrhea, chancroid, lymphogranuloma venereum
- Viral infections: herpes simplex virus, cytomegalovirus, human immunodeficiency virus
- Inflammatory bowel disease (IBD): Crohn's disease, ulcerative colitis
- Trauma: surgery (hemorrhoidectomy), foreign bodies, anal intercourse
- Malignancy: carcinoma, lymphoma, Kaposi's sarcoma

TREATMENT
- Sitz baths
- High-fiber diet
- Increased oral fluid intake
- Local anesthetic jelly (may exacerbate pruritus ani)
- Nitroglycerin ointment
- Suppositories *not* recommended
- Surgery

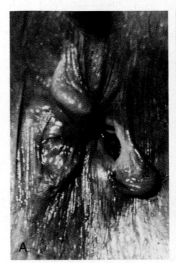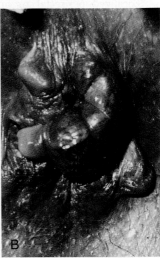

Fig 170–1
An anterior fissure-in-ano associated with a large sentinel skin tag **(A)** and the large fibrovascular anal polyp in the same patient **(B)**. (From Forbes A, Misiewicz JJ, Compton CC, et al [eds]: Atlas of Clinical Gastroenterology, 3rd ed. Edinburgh, Elsevier Mosby, 2005.)

Chapter 171   Perirectal abscess

DEFINITION

A perirectal abscess is a localized inflammatory process that can be associated with infections of soft tissue and anal glands based on anatomic location. Perianal and perirectal abscesses may be simple or complex, causing suppuration. Infections in these spaces may be classified as superficial perianal or perirectal with involvement in the following anatomic spaces: ischiorectal, intersphincteric, perianal, and supralevator

PHYSICAL FINDINGS AND CLINICAL PRESENTATION

- Localized perirectal or anal pain—often worsened with movement or straining
- Perirectal erythema or cellulitis
- Perirectal mass by inspection or palpation (Fig. 171–1)
- Fever and signs of sepsis with deep abscess
- Urinary retention

CAUSE

- Polymicrobial aerobic and anerobic bacteria involving one of the anatomic spaces (see Definition), often associated with localized trauma
- Microbiology: most bacteria are polymicrobial, mixed enteric and skin flora
- Predominant anerobic bacteria: *Bacteroides fragilis*, *Peptostreptococcus spp.*, *Prevotella spp.*
- Predominant agrobic bacteria: *Staphylococcus aureus*, *Streptococcus spp.*, *Escherichia coli*

DIAGNOSIS

- Many patients will have predisposing underlying conditions including:
  - Malignancy or leukemia
  - Immune deficiency
  - Diabetes mellitus
  - Recent surgery
  - Steroid therapy

DIFFERENTIAL DIAGNOSIS

- Crohn's disease (inflammatory bowel disease) (Fig. 171–2)
- Pilonidal disease
- Hidradenitis suppurativa (see Fig. 15–11)
- Hemorrhoids (see Fig. 169–1)
- Cancerous lesions
- Anal fissure (see Fig. 170–1)
- Fistula (Fig. 171–2)
- Proctitis—often STD-associated, including: syphilis, gonococcal, chlamydia, chancroid, condylomata acuminata, HSV (see Fig. 226–26)
- AIDS-associated: Kaposi's sarcoma, lymphoma, CMV

WORKUP

- Examination of rectal, perirectal/perineal areas
- Rule out necrotic process and crepitance suggesting deep tissue involvement
- Local aerobic and anaerobic cultures
- Blood cultures if toxic, febrile, or compromised
- Possible sigmoidoscopy

TREATMENT

- Incision and drainage of abscess
- Débridement of necrotic tissue
- Rule out need for fistulectomy
- Local wound care-packing
- Sitz baths
- Antibiotic treatment: Directed toward coverage for mixed skins and enteric flora
- Outpatient-oral: Amoxicillin/clavulanic acid, ciprofloxacin plus metronidazole or clindamycin
- Inpatient-intravenous: Ampicillin/sulbactam, cefotetan, piperacillin/tazobactam, imipenem

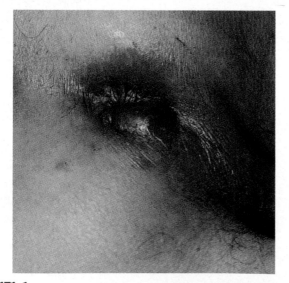

Fig 171–1
A perianal abscess.
(From Forbes A, Misiewicz JJ, Compton CC, et al [eds]: Atlas of Clinical Gastroenterology, 3rd ed. Edinburgh, Elsevier Mosby, 2005.)

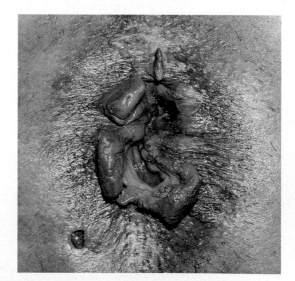

Fig 171–2
Crohn's disease: edematous skins tags, bluish discoloration, ulceration, and sepsis are manifest—there is also a fistula.
(From Forbes A, Misiewicz JJ, Compton CC, et al [eds]: Atlas of Clinical Gastroenterology, 3rd ed. Edinburgh, Elsevier Mosby, 2005.)

Chapter 172 Fistula

DEFINITION
A fistula is an inflammatory tract with a secondary (external) opening in the perianal skin and a primary (internal) opening in the anal canal at the dentate line. It originates in an abscess in the intersphincteric space of the anal canal. Fistulas can be classified as follows:
1. Intersphincteric: fistula track passes within the intersphincteric plane to the perianal skin; most common
2. Trans-sphincteric: fistula track passes from the internal opening, through the internal and external sphincter, and into the ischiorectal fossa to the perianal skin; frequent
3. Suprasphincteric: after passing through the internal sphincter, fistula tract passes above the puborectalis and then tracts downward, lateral to the external sphincter, into the ischiorectal space to the perianal skin; uncommon; if abscess cavity extends cephalad, a supralevator abscess possibly palpable on rectal examination
4. Extrasphincteric: fistula tract passes from the rectum, above the levators, through the levator muscles to the ischiorectal space and perianal skin; rare

With a horseshoe fistula, the tract passes from one ischiorectal fossa to the other behind the rectum.

PHYSICAL FINDINGS AND CLINICAL PRESENTATION
- Acute stage: perianal swelling, pain, and fever
- Chronic stage: history of rectal drainage or bleeding; previous abscess with drainage
- Tender external fistulous opening (see Fig. 171–2), with 2 to 3 cm of the anal verge, with purulent or serosanguineous drainage on compression; the greater the distance from the anal margin, the greater the probability of a complicated upward extension

CAUSE
- Most common: nonspecific cryptoglandular infection (skin or intestinal flora)
- Fistulas more common when intestinal microorganisms are cultured from the anorectal abscess
- Tuberculosis
- Lymphogranuloma venereum
- Actinomycosis
- Inflammatory bowel disease (IBD): Crohn's disease, ulcerative colitis
- Trauma: surgery (episiotomy, prostatectomy), foreign bodies, anal intercourse
- Malignancy: carcinoma, leukemia, lymphoma
- Treatment of malignancy: surgery, radiation

DIFFERENTIAL DIAGNOSIS
- Hidradenitis suppurativa (see Fig. 15–11)
- Pilonidal sinus
- Bartholin's gland abscess (see Fig. 231–10) or sinus
- Infected perianal sebaceous cysts (see Fig. 171–1)

WORKUP
- Digital rectal examination:
- Gentle probing of external orifice to avoid creating a false tract; 50% do not have clinically detectable opening
- Anoscopy
- Proctosigmoidoscopy to exclude inflammatory or neoplastic disease

LABORATORY TESTS
- Rectal biopsy if diagnosis of IBD or malignancy suspected; biopsy of external orifice is useless

IMAGING STUDIES
- Colonoscopy if:
  1. Diagnosis of IBD or malignancy is suspected
  2. History of recurrent or multiple fistulas
  3. Patient <25 years of age
- Small bowel series: occasionally obtained for reasons similar to above
- Fistulography: unreliable; but may be helpful in complicated fistulas

TREATMENT
- Treatment of choice: surgery
- Broad-spectrum antibiotic given if:
  1. Cellulitis present
  2. Patient is immunocompromised
  3. Valvular heart disease present
  4. Prosthetic devices present
- Stool softener/laxative

PANCREAS

Chapter 173 Acute pancreatitis

DEFINITION
- Acute pancreatitis is an inflammatory process of the pancreas with intrapancreatic activation of enzymes that may also involve peripancreatic tissue and/or remote organ systems.

PHYSICAL FINDINGS AND CLINICAL PRESENTATION
- Epigastric tenderness and guarding; pain usually developing suddenly, reaching peak intensity within 10 to 30 minutes, severe and lasting several hours without relief
- Hypoactive bowel sounds (secondary to ileus)
- Tachycardia, shock (secondary to decreased intravascular volume)
- Confusion (secondary to metabolic disturbances)
- Fever
- Tachycardia, decreased breath sounds (atelectasis, pleural effusions, ARDS)
- Jaundice (secondary to obstruction or compression of biliary tract)
- Ascites (secondary to tear in pancreatic duct, leaking pseudocyst)
- Palpable abdominal mass (pseudocyst, phlegmon, abscess, carcinoma)
- Evidence of hypocalcemia *(Chvostek's sign* [see Fig. 269–3A], *Trousseau's sign* [see Fig. 269–3B])
- Evidence of intra-abdominal bleeding (hemorrhagic pancreatitis):
  1. Gray-bluish discoloration around the umbilicus *(Cullen's sign)* (Fig. 173–1)
  2. Bluish discoloration involving the flanks *(Grey Turner's sign)* (Fig. 173–2)
- Tender subcutaneous nodules (caused by subcutaneous fat necrosis) (Fig. 173–3)

CAUSE
- In >90% of cases: biliary tract disease (calculi or sludge) or alcohol
- Drugs (e.g., thiazides, furosemide, corticosteroids, tetracycline, estrogens, valproic acid, metronidazole, azathioprine, methyldopa, pentamidine, ethacrynic acid, procainamide, sulindac, nitrofurantoin, ACE inhibitors, danazol, cimetidine, piroxicam, gold, ranitidine, sulfasalazine, isoniazid, acetaminophen, cisplatin, opiates, erythromycin)
- Abdominal trauma
- Surgery
- ERCP
- Infections (predominantly viral infections)
- Peptic ulcer (penetrating duodenal ulcer) (see Fig. 155–1)
- Pancreas divisum (congenital failure to fuse of dorsal or ventral pancreas)
- Idiopathic
- Pregnancy
- Vascular (vasculitis, ischemic) (see Fig. 194–4)
- Hypolipoproteinemia (types I, IV, and V)
- Hypercalcemia
- Pancreatic carcinoma (primary or metastatic) (see Fig. 175–4)
- Renal failure
- Hereditary pancreatitis
- Occupational exposure to chemicals: methanol, cobalt, zinc, mercuric chloride, creosol, lead, organophosphates, chlorinated naphthalenes
- Others: scorpion bite, obstruction at ampulla region (neoplasm, duodenal diverticula, Crohn's disease), hypotensive shock

DIFFERENTIAL DIAGNOSIS
- Peptic ulcer disease (PUD) (see Fig. 155–1)
- Acute cholangitis, biliary colic (see Fig. 186–1)
- High intestinal obstruction (See Fig. 157–2)
- Early acute appendicitis (See Fig. 161–1)
- Mesenteric vascular obstruction (see Fig. 194–4)
- Diabetic ketoacidosis
- Pneumonia (basilar)

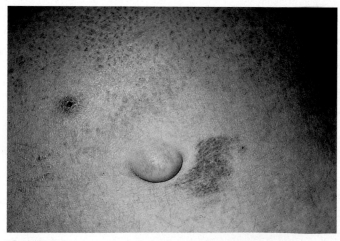

Fig 173–1
Periumbilical purpura (Cullen's sign) associated with acute hemorrhagic pancreatitis.
(From Callen JP, Jorizzo JL, Bolognia JL, et al: Dermatological Signs of Internal Disease, 3rd ed. Philadelphia, WB Saunders, 2003.)

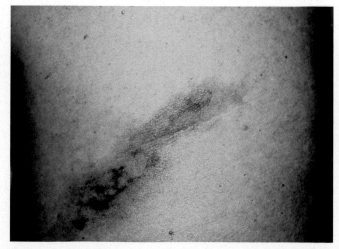

Fig 173–2
Purpura of the left flank (Grey Turner's sign) in a patient with acute hemorrhagic pancreatitis.
(From Callen JP, Jorizzo JL, Bolognia JL, et al: Dermatological Signs of Internal Disease, 3rd ed. Philadelphia, WB Saunders, 2003.)

- Myocardial infarction (inferior wall)
- Renal colic
- Ruptured or dissecting aortic aneurysm
- Mesenteric ischemia (see Fig. 194–3)

LABORATORY TESTS

Pancreatic enzymes

- Amylase is increased, usually elevated in the initial 3 to 5 days of acute pancreatitis.
- Serum lipase levels are elevated in acute pancreatitis; the elevation is less transient than serum amylase; concomitant evaluation of serum amylase and lipase increases diagnostic accuracy of acute pancreatitis. An elevated lipase/amylase ratio is suggestive of alcoholic pancreatitis.
- Elevated serum trypsin levels are diagnostic of pancreatitis (in absence of renal failure); measurement is made by radioimmunoassay. Although not routinely available, the serum trypsin level is the most accurate laboratory indicator for pancreatitis.
- Rapid measurement of urinary trypsinogen-2 (if available) is useful in the ER as a screening test for acute pancreatitis in patients with abdominal pain; a negative dipstick test for urinary trypsinogen-2 generally rules out acute pancreatitis with a high degree of probability, whereas a positive test indicates need for further evaluation.

Additional tests

- CBC: reveals leukocytosis; Hct may be initially increased secondary to hemoconcentration; decreased Hct may indicate hemorrhage or hemolysis.
- BUN is increased secondary to dehydration.
- Elevation of serum glucose in previously normal patient correlates with the degree of pancreatic malfunction and may be related to increased release of glycogen, catecholamines, and glucocorticoid release and decreased insulin release.
- Serum chemistry: AST and LDH are increased secondary to tissue necrosis; bilirubin and alkaline phosphatase may be increased secondary to common bile duct obstruction. A threefold or greater rise in serum ALT concentrations is an excellent indicator (95% probability) of biliary pancreatitis.

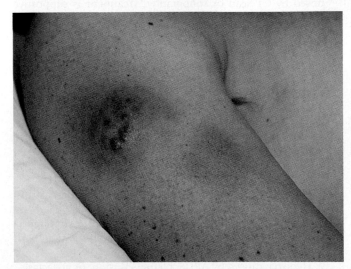

Fig 173–3
Painful nodules and plaques as a result of subcutaneous fat necrosis. (From Callen JP, Jorizzo JL, Bolognia JL, et al: Dermatological Signs of Internal Disease, 3rd ed. Philadelphia, WB Saunders, 2003.)

- Serum calcium is decreased secondary to saponification, precipitation, and decreased PTH response.
- ABGs: Pao_2 may be decreased secondary to ARDS, pleural effusion(s); pH may be decreased secondary to lactic acidosis, respiratory acidosis, and renal insufficiency.
- Serum electrolytes: potassium may be increased secondary to acidosis or renal insufficiency, sodium may be increased secondary to dehydration.

IMAGING STUDIES

- Abdominal plain film is useful initially to distinguish other conditions that may mimic pancreatitis (perforated viscus); it may reveal localized ileus (sentinel loop), pancreatic calcifications (chronic pancreatitis) (Fig. 173–4), blurring of left psoas shadow, dilation of transverse colon, calcified gallstones.
- Chest x-ray may reveal elevation of one or both diaphragms, pleural effusions, basilar infiltrates, platelike atelectasis.
- Abdominal ultrasonography is useful in detecting gallstones (sensitivity of 60% to 70% for detecting stones associated with pancreatitis). It is also useful for detecting pancreatic pseudocysts (see Fig. 173–8); its major limitation is the presence of distended bowel loops overlying the pancreas.
- CT scan (Fig. 173–5) is superior to ultrasonography in identifying pancreatitis and defining its extent, and it also plays a role in diagnosing pseudocysts (they appear as a well-defined area surrounded by a high-density capsule); GI fistulation or infection of a pseudocyst can also be identified by the presence of gas within the pseudocyst.
- Magnetic resonance cholangiopancreatography (MRCP) is also a useful diagnostic modality if a surgical procedure is not anticipated.
- ERCP (Fig. 173–6) should not be performed during the acute stage of disease unless it is necessary to remove an impacted stone in the ampulla of Vater; patients with severe or worsening pancreatitis but without obstructive jaundice (biliary obstruction) do not benefit from early ERCP and papillotomy.

TREATMENT

- Bowel rest with avoidance of PO liquids or solids during the acute illness
- Avoidance of alcohol and any drugs associated with pancreatitis

General measures

- Maintain adequate intravascular volume with vigorous IV hydration.
- Patient should remain NPO until clinically improved, stable, and hungry. Enteral feedings are preferred over total parenteral nutrition (TPN). Parenteral nutrition may be necessary in patients who do not tolerate enteral feeding or in whom an adequate infusion rate cannot be reached within 2 to 4 days.
- Nasogastric suction is useful only in severe pancreatitis to decompress the abdomen in patients with ileus.
- Control pain: IV morphine or fentanyl
- Correct metabolic abnormalities (e.g., replace calcium and magnesium as necessary).

Specific measures

- Pancreatic or peripancreatic infection develops in 40% to 70% of patients with pancreatic necrosis (Fig. 173–7). However, IV antibiotics should not be used prophylactically for all cases of pancreatitis; their use is justified if the patient

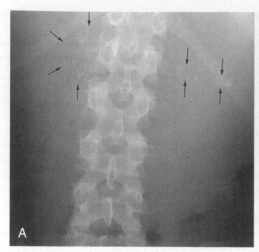 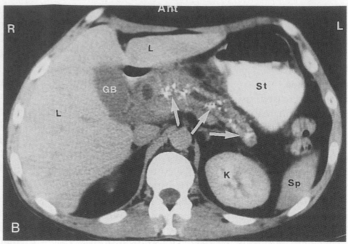

Fig 173–4

Calcification in chronic pancreatitis. Rarely on a plain film of the abdomen (**A**), a horizontal band of calcification can be seen extending across the upper midabdomen (*arrows*). Calcification within the pancreas is much easier to see on a transverse computed tomography scan of the upper abdomen (**B**). Calcification is seen as white speckled areas within the pancreas (*arrows*). The darker areas within the pancreas represent dilated common and pancreatic ducts. L = liver; GB = gallbladder; St = stomach; K = kidney; Sp = spleen.
(From Mettler FA, Guibertau MJ, Voss CM, Urbina CE: Primary Care Radiology. Philadelphia, Elsevier, 2000.)

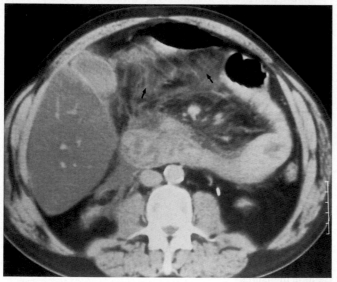

Fig 173–5

Spread of acute pancreatitis. Enhanced CT demonstrates the inflammatory changes of acute pancreatitis spreading along the transverse mesocolon (*arrows*) toward the transverse colon. Phlegmonous extension through the small bowel mesentery is also present.
(From Grainger RG, Allison DJ, Adam A, Dixon AK [eds]: Grainger and Allison's Diagnostic Radiology, 4th ed. Philadelphia, Churchill Livingstone, 2001)

has evidence of septicemia, pancreatic abscess, or pancreatitis secondary to biliary calculi. Their use should generally be limited to 5 to 7 days to prevent development of fungal superinfection. Appropriate empirical antibiotic therapy should cover: *B. fragilis* and other anaerobes, *Enterococcus*
● Surgical therapy has a limited role in acute pancreatitis; it is indicated in the following:
  1. Gallstone-induced pancreatitis: cholecystectomy when acute pancreatitis subsides
  2. Perforated peptic ulcer

3. Excision or drainage of necrotic or infected foci.
● Identification and treatment of complications:
  1. Pseudocyst: round or spheroid collection of fluid, tissue, pancreatic enzymes, and blood.
    a. Diagnosed by CT scan (Fig. 173–8) or sonography
    b. Treatment: CT scan or ultrasound-guided percutaneous drainage (with a pigtail catheter left in place for continuous drainage) can be used, but the recurrence rate is high; the conservative approach is to re-evaluate the pseudocyst (with CT scan or sonography) after 6 to 7 weeks and surgically drain it if the pseudocyst has not decreased in size. Generally, pseudocysts >5 cm in diameter are reabsorbed without intervention, whereas those >5 cm require surgical intervention after the wall has matured.
  2. Phlegmon: represents pancreatic edema. It can be diagnosed by CT scan or sonography. Treatment is supportive measures because it usually resolves spontaneously.
  3. Pancreatic abscess: diagnosed by CT scan (presence of bubbles in the retroperitoneum) (Fig. 173–9); Gram staining and cultures of fluid obtained from guided percutaneous aspiration (GPA) usually identify bacterial organism. Therapy is surgical (or catheter) drainage and IV antibiotics
  4. Pancreatic ascites: usually caused by leaking of pseudocyst or tear in pancreatic duct. Paracentesis reveals very high amylase and lipase levels in the pancreatic fluid; ERCP may demonstrate the lesion. Treatment is surgical correction if exudative ascites from severe pancreatitis does not resolve spontaneously.
  5. GI bleeding: caused by concomitant alcoholic gastritis, bleeding varices, stress ulceration, or DIC.
  6. Renal failure: caused by hypovolemia resulting in oliguria or anuria, cortical or tubular necrosis (shock, DIC), or thrombosis of renal artery or vein.
  7. Hypoxia: caused by ARDS, pleural effusion, or atelectasis.

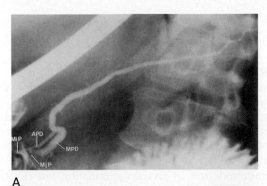

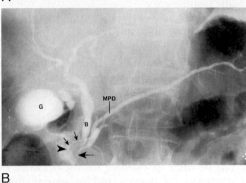

Fig 173–6
Normal pancreatic duct. (**A**) Normal ERCP shows the accessory pancreatic duct (APD) draining separately into the minor papillary (MiP), and the major pancreatic duct (MPD) draining into the major papilla (MjP). (**B**) ERCP shows filling of the main pancreatic duct (MPD), common bile duct (B) and gallbladder (G). The MPD and CBD drain into the major papillary (*large arrow*). The small accessory pancreatic duct (*small arrows*) drains separately into the minor papilla (*arrowhead*).
(From Grainger RG, Allison DJ, Adam A, Dixon AK [eds]: Grainger and Allison's Diagnostic Radiology, 4th ed. Philadelphia, Churchill Livingstone, 2001.)

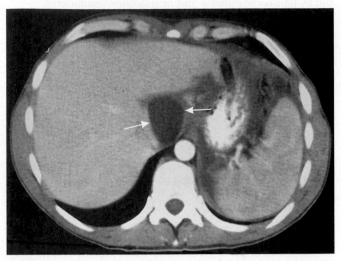

Fig 173–8
Pancreatic pseudocyst. A well-defined fluid collection with a thick wall (*arrows*) lies superior to the pancreas.
(From Grainger RG, Allison DJ, Adam A, Dixon AK [eds]: Grainger and Allison's Diagnostic Radiology, 4th ed. Philadelphia, Churchill Livingstone, 2001.)

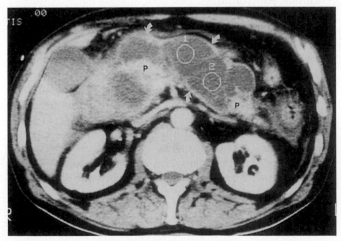

Fig 173–7
Acute necrotizing pancreatitis. Dynamic CT shows enlargement of the pancreas, a thin rim of contrast-enhancement (*arrows*), and lack of enhancement of the pancreatic parenchyma indicating almost complete gland necrosis (cursors 1 and 2 measure soft tissue density: 25 to 30 Hounsfield units). Small islands of normally enhancing parenchyma are seen (P). Patient died despite surgery.
(From Grainger RG, Allison DJ, Adam A, Dixon AK [eds]: Grainger and Allison's Diagnostic Radiology, 4th ed. Philadelphia, Churchill Livingstone, 2001.)

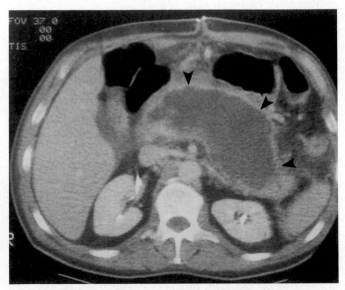

Fig 173–9
Pancreatic abscess. Dynamic CT shows a fluid collection with a contrast-enhancing capsure (*arrowheads*). Percutaneous aspiration showed the fluid to be pus. The abscess was drained successfully through percutaneous catheters.
(From Grainger RG, Allison DJ, Adam A, Dixon AK [eds]: Grainger and Allison's Diagnostic Radiology, 4th ed. Philadelphia, Churchill Livingstone, 2001.)

Chapter 174   Chronic pancreatitis

DEFINITION

Chronic pancreatitis is a recurrent or persistent inflammatory process of the pancreas (Fig. 174–1) characterized by chronic pain and by pancreatic exocrine and/or endocrine insufficiency.

PHYSICAL FINDINGS AND CLINICAL PRESENTATION

- Persistent or recurrent epigastric and LUQ pain, may radiate to the back
- Tenderness over the pancreas, muscle guarding
- Significant weight loss
- Bulky, foul-smelling stools, greasy in appearance
- Epigastric mass (10% of patients)
- Jaundice (5% to 10% of patients)

CAUSE

- Chronic alcoholism
- Obstruction (ampullary stenosis, tumor, trauma, pancreas divisum, annular pancreas)
- Hereditary pancreatitis
- Severe malnutrition
- Idiopathic
- Untreated hyperparathyroidism (hypercalcemia)
- Mutations of the cystic fibrosis transmembrane conductance regulator *(CFTR)* gene and the TF genotype
- Sclerosing pancreatitis: A form of chronic pancreatitis characterized by infrequent attacks of abdominal pain, irregular narrowing of the pancreatic duct, and swelling of the pancreatic parenchyma; these patients have high levels of serum immunoglobins (IgG4)

DIFFERENTIAL DIAGNOSIS

- Pancreatic cancer (see Fig. 175–4)
- PUD (see Fig. 155–1)
- Cholelithiasis with biliary obstruction (see Fig. 186–1)
- Malabsorption from other etiologies
- Recurrent acute pancreatitis (see Fig. 173–5)

LABORATORY TESTS

- Serum amylase and lipase may be elevated (normal amylase levels, however, do not exclude the diagnosis).
- Hyperglycemia, glycosuria, hyperbilirubinemia, and elevated serum alkaline phosphatase may also be present.
- 72-hour fecal fat determination (rarely performed) reveals excess fecal fat.
- Bentiromide test or secretin stimulation test can confirm pancreatic insufficiency.
- Elevated levels of serum IgG4 are found in sclerosing pancreatitis, but not in other disorders of the pancreas.

IMAGING STUDIES

- Plain abdominal radiographs may reveal pancreatic calcifications (95% specific for chronic pancreatitis) (Fig. 173–4).
- Ultrasound of abdomen may reveal duct dilation, pseudocyst, calcification, and presence of ascites.
- CT scan of abdomen is useful for the detection of calcifications, to evaluate for ductal dilation, and for ruling out pancreatic cancer.
- ERCP can be used to evaluate for the presence of dilated ducts, strictures, pseudocysts, and intraductal stones.
- Use of fine needle aspiration (FNA) and endoscopic ultrasound (EUS) are newer diagnostic modalities.

TREATMENT

- Avoidance of alcohol
- Frequent, small-volume, low-fat meals
- Avoidance of narcotics if possible (simple analgesics or NSAIDs can be used)
- Treatment of steatorrhea with pancreatic supplements
- Octreotide may be useful for pain secondary to idiopathic chronic pancreatitis
- Treatment of complications (e.g., type 1 DM)
- Glucocorticoid therapy in patients with sclerosing pancreatitis can induce clinical remission and significantly decrease serum concentrations of IgG4, immune complexes, and the IgG4 subclass of immune complexes
- Surgical intervention may be necessary to eliminate biliary tract disease and improve flow of bile into the duodenum by eliminating obstruction of pancreatic duct.
- ERCP with endoscopic sphincterectomy and stone extraction is useful in select patients.
- Transduodenal sphincteroplasty or pancreaticojejunostomy in select patients. Surgery should also be considered in patients with intractable pain.

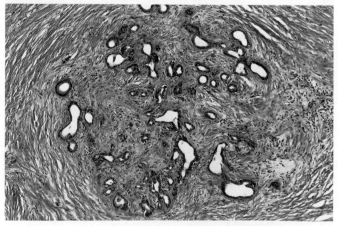

Fig 174–1

Chronic pancreatitis is characterized by fibrosis, chronic inflammation, and acinar drop-out. The lobular arrangement of the remaining ductules is retained.
(From Silverberg SG: Principles and Practice of Surgical Pathology and Cytopathology, 4th ed. Philadelphia, Churchill Livingstone, 2006.)

Chapter 175   Carcinoma of pancreas

DEFINITION
Pancreatic cancer is an adenocarcinoma derived from the epithelium of the pancreatic duct.

PHYSICAL FINDINGS AND CLINICAL PRESENTATION
Presenting symptoms
- Jaundice
- Abdominal pain
- Weight loss
- Anorexia/change in taste
- Nausea
- Uncommonly: GI bleeding, acute pancreatitis, back pain, depression

Physical findings
- Icterus
- Cachexia
- Excoriations from scratching pruritic skin, superficial migratory thrombophlebitis (Fig. 175–1)

CAUSE
Unknown, but several conditions have been associated with pancreatic cancer:
- Smoking
- Alcoholism
- Gallstones
- Diabetes mellitus
- Chronic pancreatitis

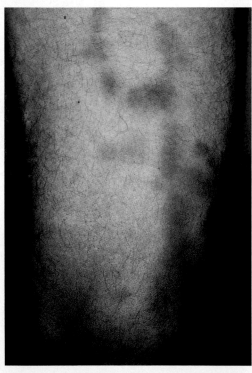

Fig 175–1
Multiple erythematous linear cords caused by superficial migratory thrombophlebitis.
(From Callen JP, Jorizzo JL, Bolognia JL, et al: Dermatological Signs of Internal Disease, 3rd ed. Philadelphia, WB Saunders, 2003.)

- Diet rich in animal fat
- Occupational exposures: oil refining, paper manufacturing, chemical industry

DIFFERENTIAL DIAGNOSIS
- Common duct cholelithiasis (see Fig. 185–3)
- Cholangiocarcinoma (see Fig. 187–1)
- Common duct stricture
- Sclerosing cholangitis (see Fig. 187–2)
- Primary biliary cirrhosis (see Fig. 179–1)
- Drug-induced cholestasis (e.g., phenothiazines)
- Chronic hepatitis (see Fig. 187–17)
- Sarcoidosis (see Fig. 137–3)
- Other pancreatic tumors (islet cell tumor, cystadenocarcinoma, epidermoid carcinoma, sarcomas, lymphomas) (see Fig. 197–4)

WORKUP

Routine laboratory test	% Abnormal
Alkaline phosphatase	80
Bilirubin	55
Total protein	15
Amylase	15
Hematocrit	60

IMAGING STUDIES
There is no evidence-based consensus on the optimal preoperative imaging assessment of patients with suspected pancreatic cancer. In patients with malignant bile duct obstruction who are surgical candidates, various combinations of PTC (Fig. 175–2), ERCP (Fig. 175–3), angiography, endoscopic ultrasound, MR plus MRCP and contrast-enhanced CT (Fig. 175–4) should be undertaken to assess the operability of the lesion.

Imaging	% Abnormal
Noninvasive	
Abdominal ultrasonography	60
Abdominal CT scan (without or with contrast [IV or oral])	90
Abdominal MR image	90
Invasive	
Endoscopic retrogradecholangio-pancreatography (ERCP)	90
CT scan or ultrasonography-guided needle aspiration cytology (Fig. 175–5)	90-95

TREATMENT
Surgery
Curative pancreatectomy (Whipple's procedure) is appropriate for only 10% to 20% of patients whose lesion is <5 cm, solitary, and without metastases. Surgical mortality is 5%. Adjuvant chemotherapy may improve postoperative survival.
- Palliative surgery (for biliary decompression/diversion)
- Palliative therapeutic endoscopic retrograde cholangio-pancreatography (ERCP) using stents

Chemotherapy
- The best combination chemotherapy using streptozotocin, mitomycin C, and 5-FU provides only a 19-week median survival.

Radiation

- External beam radiation for palliation of pain

Other

- Combined chemotherapy and radiation provides a median survival of 11 months
- Celiac plexus block by an experienced anesthesiologist provides pain relief in 80% to 90% of cases

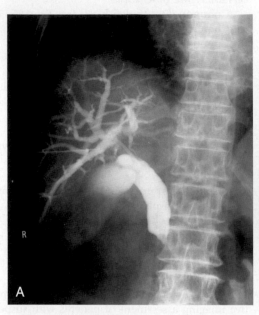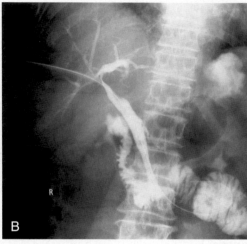

Fig 175–2

Malignant biliary obstruction due to carcinoma of the head of the pancreas. Palliation by a metallic stent. (**A**) This PTC shows obstruction of the distal bile ducts by a surgically incurable carcinoma of the head of pancreas. (**B**) A horizontal right duct was catheterized and the stricture was crossed. A 70-mm-long, 10-mm-diameter Wallstent was inserted across the stricture during the same procedure, enabling immediate internal biliary drainage. The patient was discharged home the next day.

(From Grainger RG, Allison DJ, Adam A, Dixon AK [eds]: Grainger and Allison's Diagnostic Radiology, 4th ed. Philadelphia, Churchill Livingstone, 2001.)

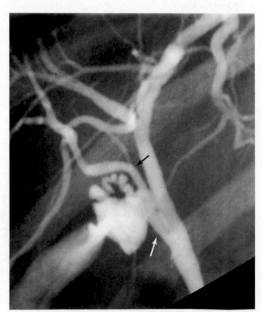

Fig 175–3

ERCP. Low insertion of a right segmental duct (*black arrow*) close to the cystic duct insertion (*white arrow*).

(From Grainger RG, Allison DJ, Adam A, Dixon AK [eds]: Grainger and Allison's Diagnostic Radiology, 4th ed. Philadelphia, Churchill Livingstone, 2001.)

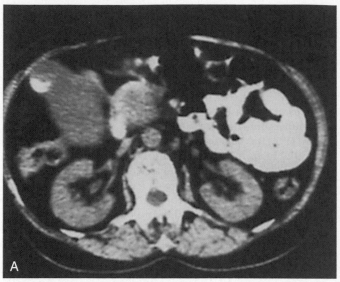
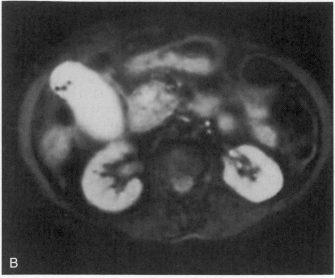

Fig 175–4
Carcinoma of the head of the pancreas with Courvoisier gallbladder and stones. CT (**A**) and IR 1500/44/100 (**B**) scans. The head of the pancreas is enlarged and has a high signal intensity in (**B**). A carcinoma 30 mm in diameter was found at surgery.
(From Grainger RG, Allison DJ, Adam A, Dixon AK [eds]: Grainger and Allison's Diagnostic Radiology, 4th ed. Philadelphia, Churchill Livingstone, 2001.)

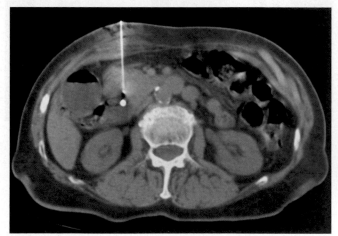

Fig 175–5
CT-guided biopsy of the pancreas. A pancreatic mass is present and there is a plastic biliary stent in situ. Using an anterior approach, a 22-gauge needle has been inserted into the mass for biopsy. Fine-needle aspirate revealed adenocarcinoma.
(From Grainger RG, Allison DJ, Adam A, Dixon AK [eds]: Grainger and Allison's Diagnostic Radiology, 4th ed. Philadelphia, Churchill Livingstone, 2001.)

LIVER

Chapter 176 Cirrhosis

DEFINITION

Cirrhosis is defined histologically as the presence of fibrosis and regenerative nodules in the liver (Fig. 176–1). It can be classified as micronodular, macronodular, and mixed; however, each form may be seen in the same patient at different stages of the disease. Cirrhosis manifests clinically with portal hypertension, hepatic encephalopathy, and variceal bleeding.

PHYSICAL FINDINGS AND CLINICAL PRESENTATION

Variable with etiology and stage of cirrhosis

SKIN: Jaundice (Fig. 176–2), palmar erythema (alcohol abuse) (Fig. 176–3), spider angiomata (Fig. 176–4), ecchymosis (thrombocytopenia or coagulation factor deficiency), dilated abdominal wall veins, xerotic eczema (Fig. 176–5), dilated superficial periumbilical vein (caput meduse) (Fig. 176–6), increased pigmentation (hemochromatosis [see Fig. 180–1]), xanthomas (primary biliary cirrhosis; see Fig. 179–1), needle tracks (viral hepatitis)

EYES: Kayser-Fleischer rings (corneal copper deposition seen in Wilson's disease [see Fig. 40–3]; best diagnosed with slit lamp examination), scleral icterus

BREATH: Fetor hepaticus (musty odor of breath and urine found in cirrhosis with hepatic failure)

CHEST: Possible gynecomastia in men

ABDOMEN: Tender hepatomegaly (congestive hepatomegaly), small, nodular liver (cirrhosis), palpable, nontender gallbladder (neoplastic extrahepatic biliary obstruction), palpable spleen (portal hypertension), venous hum auscultated over periumbilical veins (portal hypertension), ascites (portal hypertension, hypoalbuminemia) (Fig. 176–7)

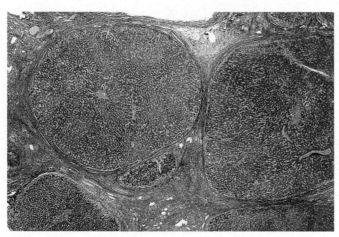

Fig 176–1
Advanced cirrhosis after longstanding chronic hepatitis C.
(From Silverberg SG: Principles and Practice of Surgical Pathology and Cytopathology, 4th ed. Philadelphia, Churchill Livingstone, 2006.)

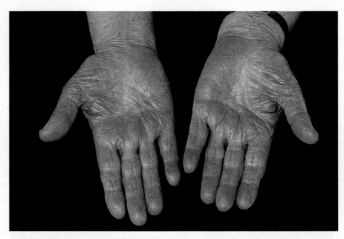

Fig 176–3
Palmar erythema (liver palms). Gross reddening of the thenar and hypothenar eminences and fingers with sparing of the center of the palm.
(From Forbes A, Misiewicz JJ, Compton CC, et al [eds]: Atlas of Clinical Gastroenterology, 3rd ed. Edinburgh, Elsevier Mosby, 2005.)

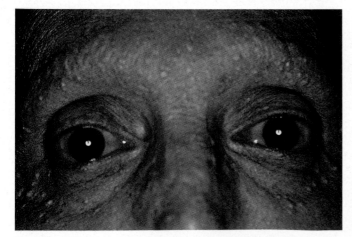

Fig 176–2
Jaundice.
(From Swartz MH: Textbook of Physical Diagnosis, 5th ed. Philadelphia, WB Saunders, 2006.)

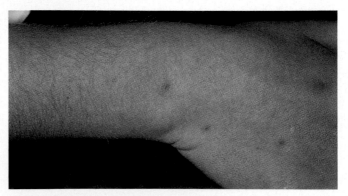

Fig 176–4
Spider angioma on the arm.
(From Callen JP, Jorizzo JL, Bolognia JL, et al: Dermatological Signs of Internal Disease, 3rd ed. Philadelphia, WB Saunders, 2003.)

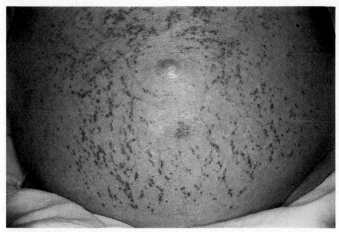

Fig 176-5
Dilated abdominal wall veins along with xerotic eczema associated with cirrhosis and portal hypertension.
(Courtesy of Neil Fenske, MD, Tampa, FL.)

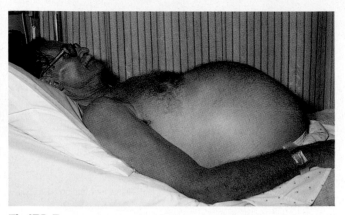

Fig 176-7
Ascites.
(From Swartz MH: Textbook of Physical Diagnosis, 5th ed. Philadelphia, WB Saunders, 2006.)

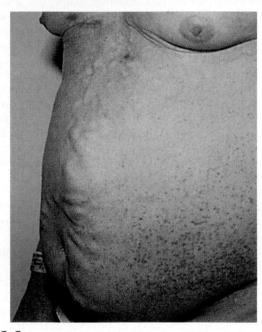

Fig 176-6
Abdominal venous patterns
(From Swartz MH: Textbook of Physical Diagnosis, 5th ed. Philadelphia, WB Saunders, 2006.)

RECTAL EXAMINATION: Hemorrhoids (see Fig. 169-1) (portal hypertension), guaiac-positive stools (alcoholic gastritis, bleeding esophageal varices, PUD, bleeding hemorrhoids)

GENITALIA: Testicular atrophy in males (chronic liver disease, hemochromatosis)

EXTREMITIES: Pedal edema (hypoalbuminemia, failure of right side of the heart), arthropathy (see Fig. 180-3) (hemochromatosis)

NEUROLOGIC: Flapping tremor, asterixis (hepatic encephalopathy), choreoathetosis, dysarthria (Wilson's disease)

CAUSE
● Alcohol abuse

● Secondary biliary cirrhosis, obstruction of the common bile duct (stone, stricture, pancreatitis, neoplasm, sclerosing cholangitis)
● Drugs (e.g., acetaminophen, isoniazid, methotrexate, methyldopa)
● Hepatic congestion (e.g., CHF, constrictive pericarditis, tricuspid insufficiency, thrombosis of the hepatic vein, obstruction of the vena cava)
● Primary biliary cirrhosis
● Hemochromatosis
● Chronic hepatitis B or C
● Wilson's disease
● Alpha-1 antitrypsin deficiency
● Infiltrative diseases (amyloidosis, glycogen storage diseases, hemochromatosis)
● Nutritional: jejunoileal bypass
● Others: parasitic infections (schistosomiasis), idiopathic portal hypertension, congenital hepatic fibrosis, systemic mastocytosis, autoimmune hepatitis, hepatic steatosis, IBD

LABORATORY TESTS
● Decreased Hgb and Hct, elevated MCV, presence of stomatocytes (Fig. 176-8), increased BUN and creatinine (the BUN may also be "normal" or low if the patient has severely diminished liver function), decreased sodium (dilutional hyponatremia), decreased potassium (as a result of secondary aldosteronism or urinary losses).
Decreased glucose in a patient with liver disease is indicative of severe liver damage
● Other laboratory abnormalities:
1. Alcoholic hepatitis and cirrhosis: there may be mild elevation of ALT and AST, usually <500 IU; AST > ALT (ratio >2:3).
2. Extrahepatic obstruction: there may be moderate elevations of ALT and AST to levels <500 IU.
3. Viral, toxic, or ischemic hepatitis: there are extreme elevations (>500 IU) of ALT and AST.
4. Transaminases may be normal despite significant liver disease in patients with jejunoileal bypass operations or hemochromatosis or after methotrexate administration.

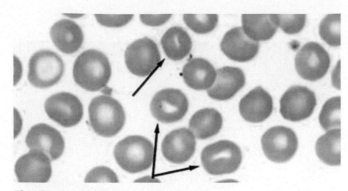

Fig 176–8
Stomatocytes in a patient with liver disease.
(From Young NS, Gerson SL, High KA [eds]: Clinical Hematology. St Louis, Mosby, 2006.)

5. Alkaline phosphatase elevation can occur with extrahepatic obstruction, primary biliary cirrhosis, and primary sclerosing cholangitis.

6. Serum LDH is significantly elevated in metastatic disease of the liver; lesser elevations are seen with hepatitis, cirrhosis, extrahepatic obstruction, and congestive hepatomegaly.

7. Serum γ-glutamyl transpeptidase (GGTP) is elevated in alcoholic liver disease and may also be elevated with cholestatic disease (primary biliary cirrhosis, primary sclerosing cholangitis).

8. Serum bilirubin may be elevated; urinary bilirubin can be present in hepatitis, hepatocellular jaundice, and biliary obstruction.

9. Serum albumin: significant liver disease results in hypoalbuminemia.

10. Prothrombin time: an elevated PT (INR) in patients with liver disease indicates severe liver damage and poor prognosis.

11. Presence of hepatitis B surface antigen implies acute or chronic hepatitis B.

12. Presence of antimitochondrial antibody suggests primary biliary cirrhosis, chronic hepatitis.

13. Elevated serum copper, decreased serum ceruloplasmin, and elevated 24-hours urine is indicative of Wilson's disease.

14. Protein immunoelectrophoresis may reveal decreased α-1 globulins (α-1 antitrypsin deficiency), increased IgA (alcoholic cirrhosis), increased IgM (primary biliary cirrhosis), increased IgG (chronic hepatitis, cryptogenic cirrhosis).

15. An elevated serum ferritin and increased transferrin saturation are suggestive of hemochromatosis.

16. An elevated blood ammonia suggests hepatocellular dysfunction; serial values, however, are generally not useful in following patients with hepatic encephalopathy, because there is poor correlation between blood ammonia level and degree of hepatic encephalopathy.

17. Serum cholesterol is elevated in cholestatic disorders.

18. Antinuclear antibodies (ANA) may be found in autoimmune hepatitis.

19. Alpha fetoprotein: levels >1000 pg/mL are highly suggestive of primary liver cell carcinoma.

20. Hepatitis C viral testing identifies patients with chronic hepatitis C infection.

21. Elevated level of serum globulin (especially γ-globulins), positive ANA test may occur with autoimmune hepatitis.

IMAGING STUDIES

- Ultrasonography is the procedure of choice for detection of gallstones and dilation of common bile ducts.
- CT scan is useful for detecting mass lesions in the liver and pancreas, assessing hepatic fat content, identifying idiopathic hemochromatosis, diagnosing of Budd-Chiari syndrome, dilation of intrahepatic bile ducts, and detection of varices and splenomegaly.
- Technetium-99m sulfur colloid scanning is infrequently used. It can be useful for diagnosing cirrhosis (there is a shift of colloid uptake to the spleen, bone marrow), identifying hepatic adenomas (cold defect is noted), diagnosing Budd-Chiari syndrome (there is increased uptake by the caudate lobe).
- ERCP is the procedure of choice for diagnosing periampullary carcinoma, common duct stones; it is also useful in diagnosing primary sclerosing cholangitis.
- Percutaneous transhepatic cholangiography (PTC) is useful when evaluating patients with cholestatic jaundice and dilated intrahepatic ducts by ultrasonography; presence of intrahepatic strictures and focal dilation is suggestive of primary sclerosing cholangitis (PSC).
- Percutaneous liver biopsy (Fig. 176–9) is useful in evaluating hepatic filling defects, diagnosing hepatocellular disease or hepatomegaly, evaluating persistently abnormal liver function tests, and diagnosing hemachromatosis, primary biliary cirrhosis, Wilson's disease, glycogen storage diseases, chronic hepatitis, autoimmune hepatitis, infiltrative diseases, alcoholic liver disease, drug-induced liver disease, and primary or secondary carcinoma.

TREATMENT

Treatment varies with etiology of cirrhosis

- Avoid any hepatotoxins (e.g., ethanol, acetaminophen); improve nutritional status.
- Remove excess body iron with phlebotomy and deferoxamine in patients with hemochromatosis.
- Remove copper deposits with D-penicillamine in patients with Wilson's disease.
- Long-term ursodiol therapy will slow the progression of primary biliary cirrhosis. It is, however, ineffective in primary sclerosing cholangitis.
- Glucocorticoids (prednisone 20 to 30 mg/day initially or combination therapy or prednisone and azathioprine) is useful in autoimmune hepatitis.
- Liver transplantation may be indicated in otherwise healthy patients (age <65 years) with sclerosing cholangitis, chronic hepatitis cirrhosis, or primary biliary cirrhosis with prognostic information suggesting <20% chance of survival without transplantation; contraindications to liver transplantation are AIDS, most metastatic malignancies, active substance abuse, uncontrolled sepsis, and uncontrolled cardiac or pulmonary disease.
- Treatment of complications of portal hypertension (ascites, esophagogastric varices, hepatic encephalopathy, and hepatorenal syndrome).

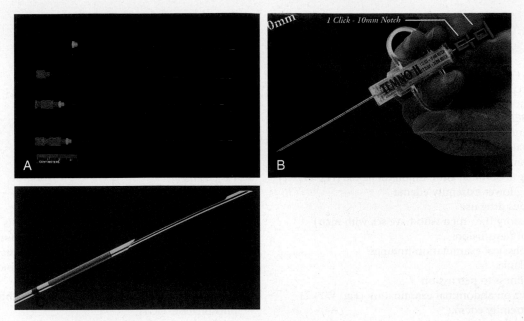

Fig 176-9
Biopsy needles. (**A**) Chiba needles for aspiration biopsy. (**B**) Automated biopsy needle (Temno, Bauer). (**C**) Close-up view of notched cutting tip of Temno needle.
(From Grainger RG, Allison DJ, Adam A, Dixon AK [eds]: Grainger and Allison's Diagnostic Radiology, 4th ed. Philadelphia, Churchill Livingstone, 2001.)

Chapter 177   Ascites

DEFINITION

Ascites is the accumulation of excess fluid in the peritoneal cavity, most commonly caused by liver cirrhosis.

CLINICAL PRESENTATION

- Important information to elicit within history:
  - Viral hepatitis
  - Alcoholism
  - Increasing abdominal girth, umbilical hernia (Fig. 177–1)
  - Increasing lower extremity edema
  - Intravenous drug use
  - Sexual history (i.e., men who have sex with men)
  - History of transfusions
- Important physical examination findings:
  - Bulging flanks
  - Flank dullness to percussion
  - Fluid wave on abdominal examination (Fig. 177–2)
  - Lower extremity edema
  - Shifting dullness "succussion splash" (see Fig. 177–2) on abdominal examination
  - Physical signs associated with liver cirrhosis: spider angiomas (see Fig. 176–4), jaundice (see Fig. 176–2), loss of body hair, Dupuytren's contracture (see Fig. 304–11), muscle wasting, bruising, palmar erythema, gynecomastia (see Fig. 284–2), testicular atrophy, hemorrhoids (see Fig. 169–1), caput meduse (see Fig. 176–6)

CAUSE

Pathophysiology of ascites: increased hepatic resistance to portal flow leads to portal hypertension. The splanchnic vessels respond by increased secretion of nitric oxide causing splanchnic artery vasodilation. Early in the disease increased plasma volume and increased cardiac output compensate for this vasodilation. However, as disease progresses the effective arterial blood volume decreases causing sodium and fluid retention through activation of the renin-angiotensin system. The change in capillary pressure causes increased permeability and retention of fluid in the abdomen.

DIFFERENTIAL DIAGNOSIS

- Chronic parenchymal liver disease, leading to portal hypertension
- Peritoneal carcinomatosis
- Congestive heart failure
- Peritoneal tuberculosis
- Nephrotic syndrome
- Pancreatitis

LABORATORY TESTS

- Initial evaluation should always include:
  - Diagnostic paracentesis. Laboratory tests on this fluid should include a CBC with differential, albumin, total protein, culture and a Gram stain. Optional tests on paracentesis fluid (depending on patient's history) include amylase, LDH, acid-fast bacilli and glucose levels
  - AST, ALT, total and direct bilirubin, albumin, alkaline phosphatase, GGTP
  - CBC, coagulation studies
  - Electrolytes, BUN, creatinine

A serum to ascites albumin gradient (SAAG) should be calculated in all patients. If the SAAG is greater than 1.1, the cause of ascites can be attributed to portal hypertension. If SAAG is less than 1.1, a nonportal hypertension etiology of ascites must be sought.

IMAGING STUDIES

- Endoscopy of the upper GI tract to evaluate for esophageal varices if ascites is secondary to portal hypertension.
- Abdominal ultrasound is the most sensitive measure for detecting ascitic fluid; a CT scan is a viable alternative (Fig. 177–3).

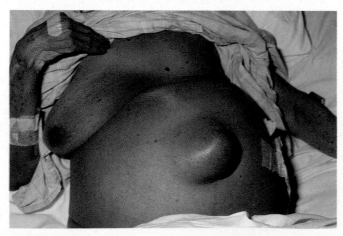

Fig 177–1

Ascites with umbilical hernia.
(From Swartz MH: Textbook of Physical Diagnosis, 5th ed. Philadelphia, WB Saunders, 2006.)

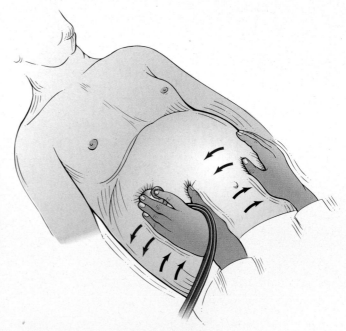

Fig 177–2

"Succussion splash" technique for assessing distention of abdominal viscera.
(From Swartz MH: Textbook of Physical Diagnosis, 5th ed. Philadelphia, WB Saunders, 2006.)

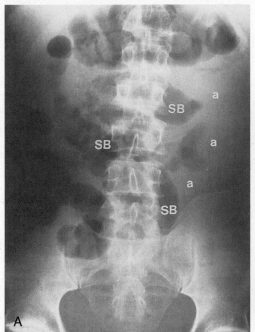
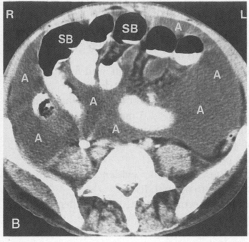

Fig 177–3

Ascites. On a plain film of the abdomen (**A**), only gross amount of ascites (a) can be identified. This is usually seen, because the ascites have caused a rather gray appearance of the abdomen and pushed the gas-containing loops of small bowel (SB) toward the most nondependent and central portion of the abdomen. A transverse computed tomography scan (**B**) shows a cross-sectional view of the same appearance with the air- and contrast-filled small bowel (SB) floating in the ascitic fluid (A).
(From Mettler FA, Guibertau MJ, Voss CM, Urbina CE: Primary Care Radiology. Philadelphia, Elsevier, 2000.)

- Liver biopsy in select patients (i.e., those with portal hypertension of uncertain etiology).

TREATMENT

- Sodium-restricted diet (maximum 60-90 milliequivalents per day).
- Fluid restriction to 1 liter per day in patients with hyponatremia.
- Patients with moderate-volume ascites causing only moderate discomfort may be treated on an outpatient basis with the following diuretic regimen: spironolactone 50-200 mg daily or amiloride 5-10 mg daily. Add furosemide 20-40 mg per day in the first several days of treatment, monitoring renal functions carefully for signs of prerenal azotemia (in patients without edema goal weight loss is 300-500 grams/day, in patients with edema 800-1000 grams/day).
- Patients with large-volume ascites causing marked discomfort or decrease in activities of daily living may also be treated as outpatients if there are no complications. There are two options for treatment in these patients: (1) large-volume paracentesis or (2) diuretic therapy until loss of fluid is noted (maximum spironolactone 400 mg daily and Lasix 160 mg daily). There is generally no difference in long-term mortality; however paracentesis is faster, more effective, and associated with fewer adverse effects.
- Five percent to 10% of patients with large-volume ascites will be refractory to high-dose diuretic treatment. Treatment strategies include repeated large-volume paracentesis with infusion of albumin every 2-4 weeks or placement of a transjugular intrahepatic portosystemic shunt (TIPS) (Fig. 177–4).

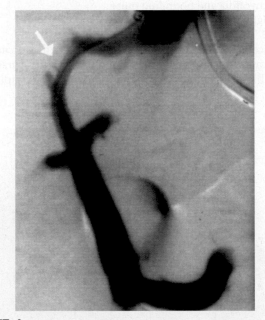

Fig 177–4

Transjugular intrahepatic portosystemic stent-shunt (TIPS). An intrahepatic tract has been created between the right hepatic vein and the right portal vein. The tract is dilated and stented, creating a shunt as demonstrated on shuntogram. (Courtesy of Dr. W. K. Tso.)

Chapter 178 Hepatorenal syndrome

DEFINITION

Hepatorenal syndrome (HRS) is a condition of intense renal vasoconstriction and kidney damage (Fig. 178–1) resulting from loss of renal autoregulation occurring as a complication of severe liver disease. Criteria for hepatorenal syndrome are:

1. Serum creatinine concentration >1.5 mg/dL or 24 hours creatinine clearance <40 mL/minutes
2. Absence of shock, ongoing infection, and fluid loss, and no current treatment with nephrotoxic drugs
3. Absence of sustained improvement in renal function (decrease in serum creatinine to <1.5 mg/dL after discontinuation of diuretics and a trial of plasma expansion)
4. Absence of proteinuria (<500 mg/day) or hematuria (<50 RBC/high power field)
5. Absence of ultrasonographic evidence of obstructive uropathy or parenchymal renal disease
6. Urinary sodium concentration <10 mmol/liter

There are two types of hepatorenal syndrome:

Type 1: progressive impairment in renal function as defined by a doubling of initial serum creatinine above 2.5 mg/dL in <2 weeks

Type 2: stable or slowly progressive impairment of renal function not meeting the above criteria

PHYSICAL FINDINGS AND CLINICAL PRESENTATION

- Evidence of cirrhosis is usually present: jaundice (see Fig. 176–2), spider angiomas (see Fig. 176–4), splenomegaly, ascites (see Fig. 177–1), fetor hepaticus, pedal edema
- Hepatic encephalopathy: flapping tremor (asterixis), coma
- Tachycardia and bounding pulse
- Oliguria

CAUSE

An exacerbation of end-stage liver disease, HRS may occur after significant reduction of effective blood volume (e.g., paracentesis, GI bleeding, diuretics) or in the absence of any precipitating factors.

DIFFERENTIAL DIAGNOSIS

- Prerenal azotemia: response to sustained plasma expansion is good (prompt diuresis with volume expansion).
- Acute tubular necrosis: urinary sodium >30, FENa >1.5%, urinary/plasma creatinine ratio <30, urine/plasma osmolality ratio = 1, urine sediment reveals casts and cellular debris, there is no significant response to sustained plasma expansion.

LABORATORY TESTS

- Obtain serum electrolytes, BUN, creatinine, osmolality, urinalysis, urinary sodium, urinary creatinine, urine osmolality.
- Calculate fractional excretion of sodium (FENa).
- In HRS: urinary sodium <10 mEq/L, FENa <1%, urinary plasma creatinine ratio >30, urine-plasma osmolality ratio >1.5, urine sediment is unremarkable.

IMAGING STUDIES

Renal ultrasound may be indicated if renal obstruction is suspected.

TREATMENT

- Volume challenge (to increase mean arterial pressure) followed by large-volume paracentesis (to increase cardiac output and decrease renal venous pressure) may be useful to distinguish HRS from prerenal azotemia in patients with FENa <1%. In patients with prerenal azotemia, the increase in renal perfusion pressure and renal blood flow will result in prompt diuresis; the volume challenge can be accomplished by giving a solution of 100 g of albumin in 500 mL of isotonic saline.
- The only effective treatment of HRS is liver transplantation; ornipressin is used in some liver units to avoid further deterioration of renal function in patients awaiting liver transplantation. Generally, dopamine and prostaglandins are ineffective in treating patients with hepatorenal syndrome.

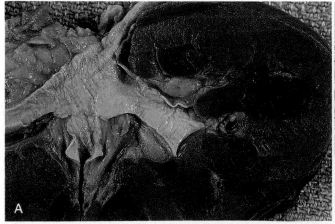
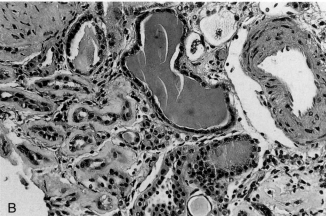

Fig 178–1

Hepatorenal syndrome. (**A**) In this gross photograph the kidney parenchyma has acquired a green color, a finding which is occasionally seen in cases with cholemic nephrosis. (**B**) Abundant bile pigmentation in tubular cells, evidence of tubular simplification and bile-containing casts (×350). (From Silverberg SG: Principles and Practice of Surgical Pathology and Cytopathology, 4th ed. Philadelphia, Churchill Livingstone, 2006.)

- Liver transplantation may be indicated in otherwise healthy patients (age preferably <65 years) with sclerosing cholangitis, chronic hepatitis with cirrhosis, or primary biliary cirrhosis; contraindications to liver transplantation are AIDS, most metastatic malignancies, active substance abuse, uncontrolled sepsis, uncontrolled cardiac or pulmonary disease.
- Vasopressin analogues may improve renal perfusion by reversing splanchnic vasodilation, which is the hallmark of HRS, however, response is erratic.
- Treatment of hepatorenal syndrome with vasoconstrictors for 5 to 15 days in attempt to reduce serum creatinine to <1.5 mg/dL is often attempted but generally ineffective.

Chapter 179 Primary biliary cirrhosis

DEFINITION

Primary biliary cirrhosis (PBC) is a chronic, variably progressive disease most often affecting women and characterized by destruction of the small intrahepatic bile ducts leading to portal inflammation, fibrosis, cirrhosis, and clinical liver failure.

CAUSE

- Although the cause of PBC is still unknown, it is felt to be due to an environmental insult (possibly bacterial or chemical) triggering an underlying genetic predisposition that results in the persistent T lymphocyte–mediated attack on intralobular bile duct epithelial cells.
- Recent studies have identified a peptide, an enzyme complex subunit (PDC-E2) in the mitochondrial membrane, as a major autoantigen in the early pathogenesis of PBC.
- In addition to the T lymphocyte–mediated direct destruction of small bile ducts, secondary damage to hepatocytes may result from the accumulation of noxious substances such as bile acids.

PHYSICAL FINDINGS AND CLINICAL PRESENTATION

Symptoms

- Forty-eight percent to 60% of patients may be asymptomatic; 40% to 100% of these patients will go on to develop symptoms.
- Fatigue (78% patients) and pruritus (20% to 70% patients) are the usual presenting symptoms.
- Pruritus is worse at night, under constricting, coarse garments; in association with dry skin; and in hot, humid weather. The cause is unknown; it is no longer felt to be due to the retention of bile acids in skin. Pruritus may first occur during pregnancy but is distinguished from pruritus of pregnancy because it persists into the postpartum period and beyond.
- Other common signs and symptoms include hepatomegaly, jaundice, unexplained RUQ pain (10%), splenomegaly, manifestations of portal hypertension, sicca symptoms, and scleroderma-like lesions.
- Musculoskeletal complaints caused by inflammatory arthropathy in 40% to 70% of patients: 5% to 10% develop chronic RA; 10% develop "arthritis of PBC."
- Steatorrhea may be seen in advanced disease.

Physical

- Variable: dependent on stage of disease at time of presentation. Early may be completely normal.
- Twenty-five percent to 50% have hypopigmentation of skin.
- Excoriations may be present.
- Hepatomegaly (70%) and splenomegaly (initially 35%) may be present in more advanced disease.
- Xanthomas and jaundice (Fig. 179–1) appear in advanced disease. Kayser-Fleischer rings are rare and result from copper retention.
- Late physical findings mirror those of cirrhosis: spider nevi, temporal and proximal limb wasting, finger clubbing (Fig. 179–2), ascites (see Fig. 177–1), and edema.
- Other associated illnesses that should be detected and treated include hyperlipidemia (without increased risk of ASHD), hypothyroidism (20% of patients and often associated with antithyroglobulin and antimicrosomal antibodies), osteoporosis, interstitial pneumonitis, celiac disease, sarcoidosis, asymptomatic renal tubular acidosis (from copper deposition in the kidneys), fat-soluble vitamin deficiencies (especially vitamin A), hemolytic anemia, autoimmune thrombocytopenia, and coexisting autoimmune disease including Sjögren's syndrome and scleroderma.

DIAGNOSIS

- Based on three criteria:
  - Positive serum antimitochondrial antibodies (AMA)
  - Increased liver function tests (especially alkaline phosphatase) for 6 months
  - Characteristic liver histology: asymmetrical destruction of the bile ducts within the portal triads (Fig. 179–3)
- Two criteria indicate a probable diagnosis and all three criteria are required for a definite diagnosis.

DIFFERENTIAL DIAGNOSIS

- Drug-induced cholestasis
- Other etiologies of chronic liver disease and cirrhosis:
  - Alcoholic cirrhosis
  - Viral hepatitis (chronic)
  - Primary sclerosing cholangitis
  - Autoimmune chronic active hepatitis

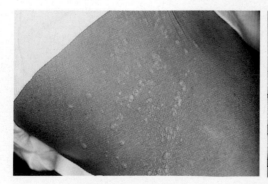 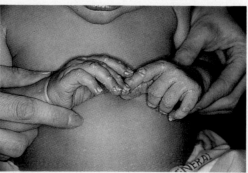

Fig 179–1
Primary biliary cirrhosis. This patient has eruptive xanthomas on a diffusely hyperpigmented background.
(Courtesy of Loren Golitz, MD, Denver, CO.)

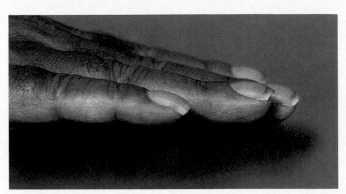

Fig 179–2
Finger clubbing associated with primary biliary cirrhosis.
(From Forbes A, Misiewicz JJ, Compton CC, et al [eds]: Atlas of Clinical Gastroenterology, 3rd ed. Edinburgh, Elsevier Mosby, 2005.)

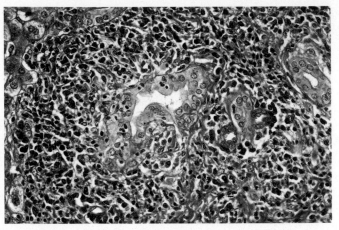

Fig 179–3
Primary biliary cirrhosis. The PAS stain after diastase digestion demonstrates the bile duct basement membrane, which has been destroyed in several places.
(From Silverberg SG: Principles and Practice of Surgical Pathology and Cytopathology, 4th ed. Philadelphia, Churchill Livingstone, 2006.)

- Chemical/toxin-induced cirrhosis
- Other hereditary or familial disorders (e.g., CF, μ-1-anti-trypsin deficiency)

LABORATORY TESTS
- Antimitochondrial antibodies (found in 95% of patients with PBC and are 98% specific).
- Antinuclear antibodies are found in approximately 50%. Nuclear-rim and nuclear-dot patterns highly specific for PBC.
- Markedly elevated alkaline phosphatase (of hepatic origin).
- Elevated GGTP.
- Elevated serum IgM levels.
- Bilirubin normal early; increases with disease progression (direct and indirect) in 60% patients. Elevated serum bilirubin is a poor prognostic sign.
- Normal or slightly elevated aminotransferases, rarely more than 5× upper limit of normal, for more than 6 months. Degree of elevation has no prognostic significance.
- Markedly elevated serum lipids in more than 50%. Total cholesterol may exceed 1000 mg/dL. No increased risk of death from atherosclerosis seen, possibly due to very high HDL levels and low serum levels of Lp(a) lipoprotein.
- Elevated ceruloplasmin.
- Percutaneous liver biopsy confirms the diagnosis, allows staging, and indicates response to therapy.

IMAGING STUDIES
If history, physical examination, blood tests, and liver biopsy are all consistent with PBC, neither imaging nor cholangiography is necessary.

TREATMENT
- Management decisions vary depending on clinical status of patient.
- No generally accepted treatment of underlying disease process.
- 20% of patients will not respond to medical therapy and proceed to liver transplantation.
- Treatment focuses on management of complications (pruritus, metabolic bone diseases, hyperlipidemia), because liver transplantation is the only definitive treatment for this disease.
- Goals of treatment: resolution of pruritus, decrease of alkaline phosphatase levels to <50% above normal, and improvement in liver biopsy histology.
- Ursodiol significantly reduces need for liver transplantation or likelihood of death after 4 years if started early. May see decreased efficacy after 10 years. Ineffective and may actually worsen disease if started in advanced stages.
- Colchicine and methotrexate yield less impressive results but are still modestly effective. Patients with PBC on methotrexate need to be monitored for the development of interstitial pneumonitis, which resolves with discontinuation of the drug.
- For the pruritus of PBC, cholestyramine resin reduces pruritus in most patients. Antihistamines at bedtime help night-time symptoms.
- Diet low in neutral triglycerides and high in medium-chain triglycerides decreases steatorrhea and improves nutritional status.
- Prompt diagnosis and treatment of acute bacterial cystitis, which occur with greater frequency in these patients.
- Treatment for osteoporosis including calcium, vitamin D should be undertaken, although only liver transplantation results in significant improvement. Bisphosphonates may be helpful.
- Vitamin A, K, and E deficiencies can be clinically important in advanced cases and respond to oral replacement.
- Esophageal variceal bleeding often happens earlier in the course of PBC than with other progressive liver diseases. These are best treated with endoscopic rubber-band ligation or TIPS shunt.
- Liver transplantation is the definitive cure and appropriate referral should be sought. Indications for transplant include unacceptable quality of life and anticipated death in 1 year, and are guided by the Mayo (MELD) scoring system.

Chapter 180 | Hemochromatosis

DEFINITION

Hemochromatosis is an autosomal recessive disorder characterized by increased accumulation of iron in various organs (adrenals, liver, pancreas, heart, testes, kidneys, pituitary) and eventual dysfunction of these organs if not treated appropriately.

PHYSICAL FINDINGS AND CLINICAL PRESENTATION

Examination may be normal; patient with advanced case may present with the following:

- Increased skin pigmentation (Fig. 180–1)
- Hepatomegaly, splenomegaly, hepatic tenderness, testicular atrophy
- Loss of body hair, peripheral edema, gynecomastia, ascites (see Fig. 177–1)
- Amenorrhea (25% of females)
- Loss of libido (50% of males)
- Arthropathy (Fig. 180–2)
- Joint pain (44%) (Fig. 180–3)
- Fatigue (45%)

CAUSE

Autosomal recessive disease linked to the region of the short arm of chromosome 6 encoding HLA-A3; the gene *HFE*, which contains two missense mutations (C 282Y and H 63D), was recently identified.

DIFFERENTIAL DIAGNOSIS

- Hereditary anemias with defect of erythropoiesis
- Cirrhosis
- Repeated blood transfusions

LABORATORY TESTS

- Transferrin saturation is the best screening test. Values >45% are an indication for further testing. When using transferring saturation to screen individuals >40 years of age, a single test may not be sufficient and sequential measurements over a period of many months to years should be considered to detect hemochromatosis before onset of fibrosis or cirrhosis. Plasma ferritin is also a good indicator of total body iron stores but may be elevated in many other conditions (inflammation, malignancy). Some authors recommend measurement of both fasting transferrin saturation and serum ferritin level as initial tests for population-based screening to detect and treat hemochromatosis before iron loading occurs.
- Elevated AST, ALT, alkaline phosphatase.
- Hyperglycemia.
- Endocrine abnormalities (decreased testosterone, LH, FSH).
- Measurement of hepatic iron index (hepatic iron concentration [HIC] divided by age) in liver biopsy specimen (Fig. 180–4) can confirm diagnosis.

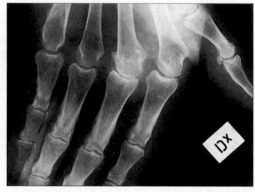

Fig 180–2
Radiograph of the hands of a 45-year-old man with hemochromatosis. There are cystic lesions of the metacarpal heads, joint space narrowing, and osteophytes at the second and third MCP joints.
(From Hochberg MC, Silman AJ, Smolen JS, et al [eds]: Rheumatology, 3rd ed. St Louis, Mosby, 2003.)

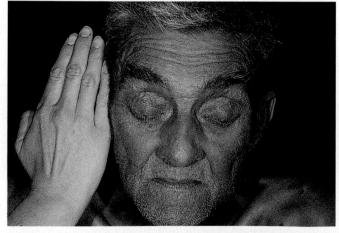

Fig 180–1
Hemochromatosis, also known as "bronze diabetes," combines diabetes mellitus, cirrhosis, and generalized hyperpigmentation. These patients have iron overload.
(From Callen JP, Greer KE, Paller AS, Swinyer LJ: Color Atlas of Dermatology, 2nd ed. Philadelphia, WB Saunders, 2000.)

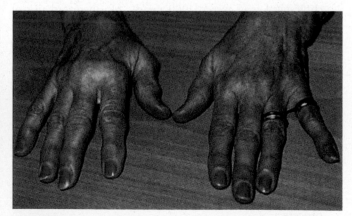

Fig 180–3
The hands of a patient with hemochromatosis. The bony swelling of the MCP joints is apparent.
(From Hochberg MC, Silman AJ, Smolen JS, et al [eds]: Rheumatology, 3rd ed. St Louis, Mosby, 2003.)

- Genetic testing (HFE genotyping for the C282Y and H63 D mutations) may be useful in select patients with liver disease and suspected iron overload (e.g., patients with transferrin saturation >40%). Genetic testing should not be performed as part of an initial routine evaluation for hereditary hemochromatosis. Once a patient has been identified, first-degree relatives of the index patient should also be screened. The *HFE* gene test is a PCR-based test usually performed on whole blood sample.

IMAGING STUDIES

CT scan or MRI of the liver (Fig. 180–5) is useful to exclude other etiologies and may in some cases show iron overload in the liver.

TREATMENT

Weekly phlebotomies of one or two units of blood (each containing approximately 250 mg of iron) should be continued until depletion of iron stores is achieved (ferritin level <50 μg/mL and transferring saturation <30%). Subsequent phlebotomies can be performed on a prn basis to maintain a transferrin saturation <50% and a ferritin level <100 μg/L.

- Deferoxamine (iron chelating agent) is generally reserved for patients with severe hemochromatosis with diffuse organ involvement (e.g., liver disease, heart disease) and when phlebotomy is not possible.

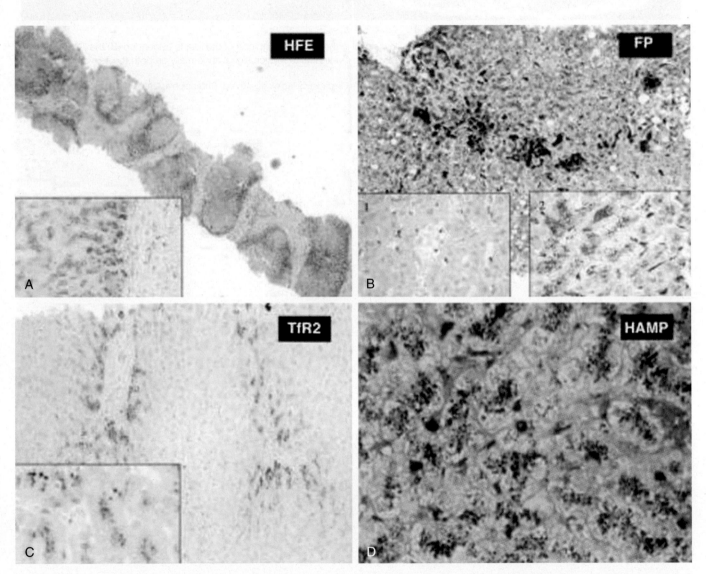

Fig 180–4

Patterns of iron deposition in primary iron-overload disorders (Perls' Prussian blue stain). **A,** Hereditary hemochromatosis, HFE-associated, with cirrhosis. Inset, iron deposits in hepatocytes. **B,** Autosomal dominant hemochromatosis, SLC40A1-associated (ferroportin disease), with advanced-stage disease. *Left inset panel,* early-stage disease with iron deposition predominantly in Kupffer cells. *Right inset panel,* late-stage disease with iron accumulation in both Kupffer cells and hepatocytes. **C,** Hereditary (TfR2-associated) hemochromatosis with periportal iron deposition. *Inset,* iron deposits in hepatocytes. **D,** Juvenile hemochromatosis, type 2B (HAMP-associated), with massive panlobular iron distribution. (From Pietrangelo A: Non-HFE hemochromatosis. Hepatology 39:21-29, 2004, with permission.)

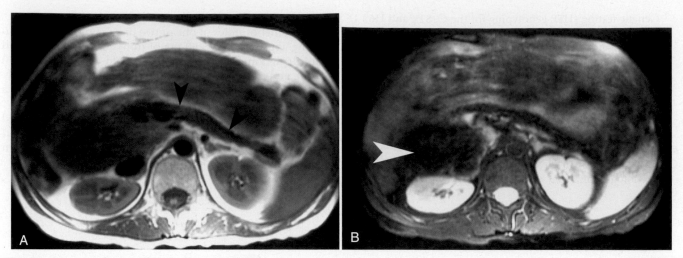

Fig 180–5

Hemochromatosis. Despite the motion artefact, the abnormally low signal in the atrophic right lobe of the liver is evident on (**B**) the T2-weighted section (*white arrowhead*). The accumulation of iron in the pancreas is so marked as to reduce signal abnormally on both the T2-weighted and T1-weighted sections (**A**, *black arrowheads*).

(From Grainger RG, Allison DJ, Adam A, Dixon AK [eds]: Grainger and Allison's Diagnostic Radiology, 4th ed. Philadelphia, Churchill Livingstone, 2001.)

Chapter 181 Nonalcoholic steatohepatitis

DEFINITION
- Nonalcoholic steatohepatitis (NASH, non-alcoholic fatty liver) represents a spectrum of diseases based on histiopathologic findings and representing a morphologic rather than a clinical diagnosis. It is liver disease occurring in patients who do not abuse alcohol and manifesting histologically by mononuclear cells and/or polymorphonuclear cells, hepatocyte ballooning, and spotty necrosis. Nonalcoholic fatty liver disease is closely associated with metabolic disorders, even in nonobese, nondiabetic subjects. It can be considered an early predictor of metabolic disorders, particularly in the normal-weight population.
- A diagnosis of nonalcoholic fatty liver disease is contingent on the following factors:
  1. Alcohol consumption in amounts less than those considered hepatotoxic
  2. Absence of serologic evidence of other hepatic diseases or disorders
  3. Liver biopsy showing predominant macrovesicular steatosis or steatohepatitis (Fig. 181-1)

PHYSICAL FINDINGS AND CLINICAL PRESENTATION
- Most patients are asymptomatic
- Patients may report a sensation of fullness or discomfort on the right side of the upper abdomen
- Nonspecific complaints of fatigue or malaise may be reported
- Hepatomegaly is generally the only positive finding on physical examination
- Acanthosis nigricans may be found in children

CAUSE
- Insulin resistance is the most reproducible factor in the development of nonalcoholic fatty liver disease
- Risk factors are obesity (especially truncal obesity), diabetes mellitus, hyperlipidemia

DIFFERENTIAL DIAGNOSIS
- Alcohol-induced liver disease (Fig. 181-2)
- Viral hepatitis (see Fig. 183-13)
- Autoimmune hepatitis (see Fig. 184-1)
- Toxin or drug-induced liver disease

WORKUP
Diagnosis is usually suspected on the basis of hepatomegaly, asymptomatic elevations of transaminases, or "fatty liver" on sonogram of abdomen in obese patients with little or no alcohol use. Liver biopsy will confirm diagnosis and provide prognostic information. It should be considered in patients with suspected advanced liver fibrosis (presence of obesity or type 2 diabetes, AST/ALT ratio 1, age >45 years).

LABORATORY TESTS
- Elevated ALT, AST: AST/ALT ratio is usually <1, but can increase as fibrosis advances
- Negative serology for infectious hepatitis; generally normal GGTP, and serum alkaline phosphatase

- Hyperlipidemia (primarily hypertriglyceridemia) may be present
- Elevated glucose levels may be present
- Prolonged prothrombin time, hypoalbuminuria, and elevated bilirubin may be present in advanced stages
- Elevated serum ferritin and increased transferrin saturation may be found in up to 10% of patients; however, hepatic iron index and hepatic iron level are normal
- Liver biopsy may show a wide spectrum of liver damage, ranging from simple steatosis to advanced fibrosis and cirrhosis

IMAGING STUDIES
- Ultrasound generally reveals diffuse increase in echogenicity as compared with that of the kidneys; CT scan reveals diffuse low-density hepatic parenchyma (Fig. 181-3).
- Occasionally patients may have focal rather than diffuse steatosis, which may be misinterpreted as a liver mass on ultrasound or CT; use of MRI in these cases will identify focal fatty infiltration.

TREATMENT
- Weight reduction of 55% to 10% in all obese patients (500 g per week in children and 1600 g per week in adults is preferred)
- No medications have been proved to directly improve liver damage from nonalcoholic fatty liver disease.
- Medications to control hyperlipidemia (e.g., fenofibrates for elevated triglycerides) and hyperglycemia (e.g., metformin) can lead to improvement in abnormal liver test results.

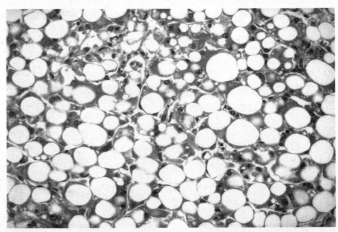

Fig 181-1
Macrovesicular steatosis in a patient with obesity and mild liver associated enzyme elevation. Most hepatocytes contain a single, large, rounded vacuole that displaces the nucleus and cytoplasm to the periphery of the cell. There is minimal inflammation.
(From Silverberg SG: Principles and Practice of Surgical Pathology and Cytopathology, 4th ed. Philadelphia, Churchill Livingstone, 2006.)

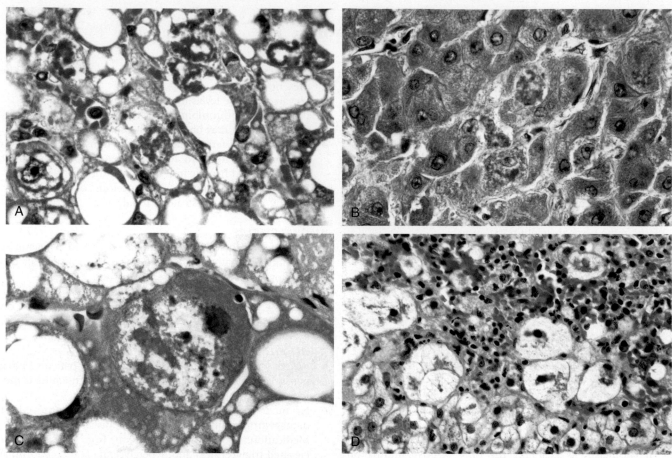

Fig 181–2
Mallory bodies. (**A**) Numerous Mallory bodies in a case of alcoholic hepatitis. Many of the hepatocytes are ballooned, making the Mallory bodies easy to detect. One large Mallory body forms a complete or open ring around the nucleus of its liver cell. (**B**) Mallory bodies in this case of alcoholic hepatitis are less easily seen because the hepatocytes are not ballooned, but heavy eosin staining brings them out. (**C**) Mallory body in a case of nonalcoholic steatohepatitis. Only a few cells contained diagnostic Mallory bodies such as these. (**D**) Mallory bodies in another case of nonalcoholic steatohepatitis. Mallory bodies are present in many cells, but most are small and thin.
(From Silverberg SG: Principles and Practice of Surgical Pathology and Cytopathology, 4th ed. Philadelphia, Churchill Livingstone, 2006.)

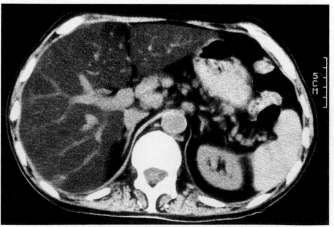

Fig 181–3
Diffuse fat infiltration. The liver parenchyma is markedly reduced in attenuation reversing the normal relationship with the spleen and blood vessels. The shape and vascular architecture of the liver are normal.
(From Grainger RG, Allison DJ, Adam A, Dixon AK [eds]: Grainger and Allison's Diagnostic Radiology, 4th ed. Philadelphia, Churchill Livingstone, 2001.)

Chapter 182 | **Hepatocellular carcinoma**

DEFINITION
Hepatocellular carcinoma (HCC) (Fig. 182–1) is a malignant tumor of the hepatocytes.

PHYSICAL FINDINGS AND CLINICAL PRESENTATION
- One third of patients are asymptomatic.
- Signs of underlying cirrhosis are often present (e.g., weight loss, ascites).
- Previously compensated cirrhosis with new ascites, encephalopathy, jaundice, or bleeding
- Paraneoplastic syndromes (hypoglycemia, erythrocytosis, hypercalcemia, severe diarrhea)

DIFFERENTIAL DIAGNOSIS
- Metastatic tumor to liver
- Benign liver tumors such as adenomas, focal nodular hyperplasia, hemangiomas
- Focal fatty infiltration

LABORATORY TESTS
- LFTs may be elevated
- Elevated alpha-fetoprotein (AFP) in 70% of patients (sensitivity 40%–65%; specificity 80%–94%)
- Paraneoplastic syndromes associated with HCC may cause hypercalcemia, hypoglycemia, and polycythemia

IMAGING STUDIES
Ultrasound, CT scan, or MRI. Ultrasound is most commonly used as a screening test for HCC in high-risk patients. CT (Fig. 182–2) and MR scans are usually performed when there is a focal lesion on US or strong clinical suspicion of HCC.

BIOPSY
Percutaneous biopsy under ultrasound or CT scan guidance usually is diagnostic. Tissue diagnosis is the gold standard (Fig. 182–3). However, HCC can be reliably diagnosed when:
- Confirmed by two imaging modalities when the nodule is >2 cm and has arterial hypervascularity or
- Single positive imaging method with AFP >400 μg/mL

SCREENING
Screening high-risk patients with US and AFP every 6 months may identify hepatocellular carcinoma at an early stage. Screening at 6- to 12-month intervals may be acceptable for healthy hepatitis B virus carriers without cirrhosis.

STAGING
According to the Barcelona-Clinic Liver Cancer (BCLC) staging classification, treatment is determined according to stage:
- Early stage: asymptomatic single tumor ≤5 cm or 3 nodules ≤3 cm
- Intermediate stage: patients with tumors that exceed early criteria but do not yet show cancer-related symptoms, vascular invasion, or metastases
- Advanced stage: patients with cancer-related symptoms
- End-stage: patients with advanced, symptomatic disease

TREATMENT
- Early stage: curative treatment (resection, liver transplantation, or percutaneous ablation). Among patients with elevated portal pressure who have <3 tumors that are <3 cm in size, surgical resection should be attempted, including transplantation or ablation.
- Intermediate stage: optimal therapeutic approach is controversial. Outcome may be improved with chemoembolization.

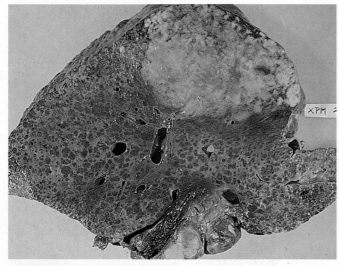

Fig 182–1
Hepatocellular carcinoma.
(From Cohen J, Powderly WG: Infectious Diseases, 2nd ed. St Louis, Mosby, 2004.)

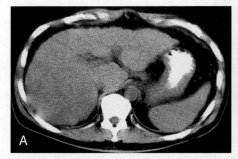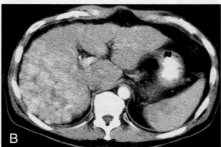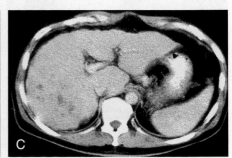

Fig 182–2
Multifocal hepatocellular carcinoma. A biphasic CT (unenhanced, **A**; arterial phase, **B**; portal phase, **C**) examination demonstrates the multifocal and extensive nature of the tumor, which is only fully apparent during the transient enhancement of the arterial phase.
(From Grainger RG, Allison DJ, Adam A, Dixon AK [eds]: Grainger and Allison's Diagnostic Radiology, 4th ed. Philadelphia, Churchill Livingstone, 2001.)

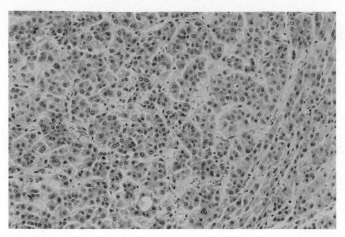

Fig 182–3

Hepatocellular carcinoma, trabecular type. Note that the cell plates are greater than three cells thick and the sinusoids are focally dilated. Nuclei are similar in size or smaller than normal but their cytoplasm is decreased for an overall increase in nuclear:cytoplasmic ratio and increase in the nuclear density greater than two times normal, the so-called small-cell change.

(From Silverberg SG: Principles and Practice of Surgical Pathology and Cytopathology, 4th ed. Philadelphia, Churchill Livingstone, 2006.)

- Advanced stage: no curative treatment. In the absence of metastatic disease or portal invasion, chemoembolization is reasonable (Fig. 182–4). Entry into clinical trials should be considered.
- End-stage: palliative care
- For patients with unresectable HCC, chemoembolization using cisplatin or doxorubicin has been shown to improve 2-year survival rates.
- Patients with advanced cirrhosis and small tumors should be considered for liver transplantation. Liver transplantation in patients with HCC has been associated with significant improvements in 5-year survival rates, which may reflect patient selection.
- For hepatitis C virus–associated HCC, postoperative treatment with interferon-alpha decreases the rate of tumor recurrence.

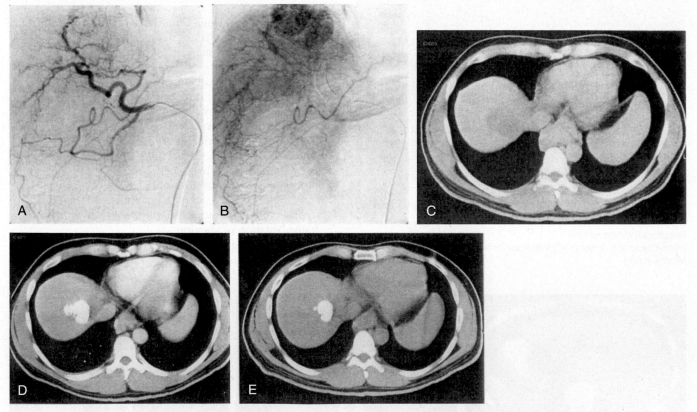

Fig 182–4

(A, B) Common hepatic artery angiogram demonstrates an area of neovascularity within the superior portion of the right lobe of the liver consistent with a hepatocellular cell carcinoma in a patient with hepatitis C–associated cirrhosis. **(C-E)** Axial CT scans performed before **(C)**, 1 month after **(D)**, and 6 months after **(E)** selective embolization using a combination of Lipiodol, *cis*-platinum, and polyvinyl alcohol, which show a gradual decrease in size of the tumor. The radiologic improvement was associated with a reduction in alpha-fetoprotien levels.

(From Grainger RG, Allison DJ, Adam A, Dixon AK [eds]: Grainger and Allison's Diagnostic Radiology, 4th ed. Philadelphia, Churchill Livingstone, 2001.)

Chapter 183 | **Hepatic infections**

A. HEPATIC ABSCESSES

DEFINITION
Liver abscess is a necrotic infection of the liver usually classified as pyogenic or amebic.

PHYSICAL FINDINGS AND CLINICAL PRESENTATION
- Fever, chills, and sweats
- Anorexia with weight loss
- Nausea, vomiting, and diarrhea
- Cough with pleuritic chest pain
- Right upper quadrant abdominal pain
- Hepatomegaly
- Splenomegaly
- Jaundice
- Pleural effusions, rales, and friction rubs may be present
- Most abscesses occur on the right lobe of the liver

CAUSE
- Pyogenic liver abscess is usually polymicrobial (E. coli [33%], *K. pneumonie* [18%], streptococcal sp [37%], *P. aeruginosa*, proteus, bacteroides [24%], fusobacterium, Actinomyces, gram-positive anerobes, and *S. aureus*).
- Pyogenic liver abscess occurs from:
  1. Biliary disease with cholangitis (accounts for approximately 21% to 30%)
  2. Gallbladder disease with contiguous spread to the liver
  3. Diverticulitis or appendicitis with spread via the portal circulation
  4. Hematogenous spread via the hepatic artery
  5. Penetrating wounds
  6. Cryptogenic
  7. Infection via portal system (portal pyemia)
  8. No causes found in approximately one half of cases
  9. Incidence increased in patients with diabetes and metastatic cancer

- Amebic hepatic abscess is caused by the parasite *Entamoeba histolytica* (Fig. 183–1). Amebiasis is usually due to fecal-oral contamination and invades the intestinal mucosa gaining entry into the portal system to reach the liver (Fig. 183–2).
- Fungal (Fig. 183–3): usually seen in immunocompromised hosts

DIFFERENTIAL DIAGNOSIS
- Liver cyst (Fig. 183–4)
- Cholangitis, cholangiocarcinoma (see Fig. 187–2)
- Cholecystitis (see Fig. 186–1)
- Polycystic liver disease (Fig. 183–5)

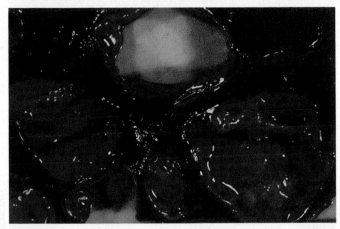

Fig 183–2
Human amebic liver abscess. Multiple abscesses, one cavitated, can be observed occupying virtually all lobes of the liver parenchyma, which is replaced by a semisolid material. (Courtesy of Dr. Jesús Aguirre García, Hospital General de México, Secretaría de Salud.)

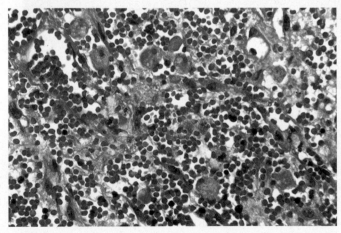

Fig 183–1
Entamoeba histolytica liver abscess. Multiple amebae with fine cytoplasm are present in a hemorrhagic, necrotic exudate. The nuclei are small with a small karyosome (nucleolus) and find nuclear chromatic (HANDE, ×1000).
(From Silverberg SG: Principles and Practice of Surgical Pathology and Cytopathology, 4th ed. Philadelphia, Churchill Livingstone, 2006.)

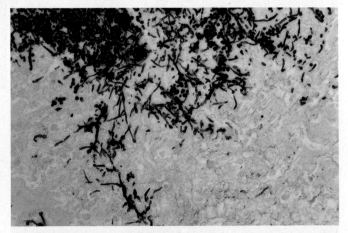

Fig 183–3
Candida liver abscess. A combination of budding yeast and pseudohyphae makes the most likely etiologic diagnosis candidiasis (GMS, ×45, *Candida albicans* isolated in culture).
(From Silverberg SG: Principles and Practice of Surgical Pathology and Cytopathology, 4th ed. Philadelphia, Churchill Livingstone, 2006.)

- Perforated viscus
- Mesentery ischemia (see Fig. 194–4)
- Pancreatitis (see Fig. 173–5)

WORKUP

- The workup of a liver abscess should focus on differentiating between amebic and pyogenic causes.

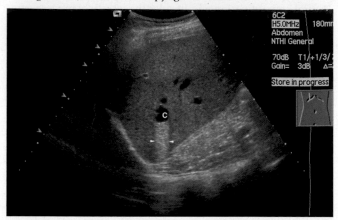

Fig 183–4

Increases sound transmission. The echoes (*arrowheads*) deep to this liver cyst appear brighter than those from the rest of the liver; this is because the cyst fluid attenuates less than the solid liver and so signals from beyond it are relatively overamplified. C = cyst. (From Grainger RG, Allison DJ, Adam A, Dixon AK [eds]: Grainger and Allison's Diagnostic Radiology, 4th ed. Philadelphia, Churchill Livingstone, 2001.)

- Features suggesting an amebic cause include travel to an endemic area, single abscess rather than multiple abscesses, subacute onset of symptoms, and absence of conditions predisposing to pyogenic liver abscess as highlighted under "Etiology."
- Laboratory studies (see below) are not specific but useful as adjunctive tests.
- CT is the preferred imaging modality but imaging studies cannot differentiate between the two.

LABORATORY TESTS

- CBC showing leukocytosis
- Liver function tests: alkaline phosphatase is most commonly elevated (95% to 100%); AST and ALT elevated in 50% of cases; elevated bilirubin (28% to 30%); decreased albumin
- PT (INR) prolonged (70%)
- Blood cultures positive in 50% of cases
- Aspiration (50% sterile)
- Stool samples for *E. histolytica* trophozoites (positive in 10% to 15% of amebic liver abscess cases)
- Serologic testing for *E. histolytica* does not differentiate acute from old infections

IMAGING STUDIES

- Chest x-ray is abnormal in 50% of the cases showing elevated right hemidiaphragm, subdiaphragmatic air fluid levels, pleural effusions, and consolidating infiltrates.
- Ultrasound (80% to 100% sensitivity in detecting abscesses) seen as round or oval hypoechogenic mass (Fig. 183–6).

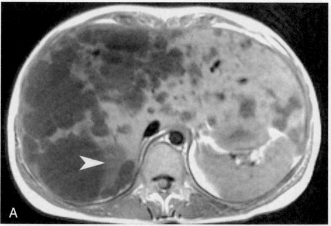

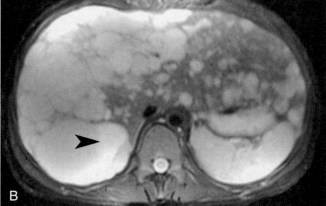

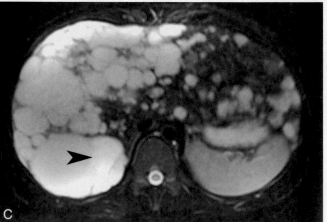

Fig 183–5

Polycystic liver disease. Multiple simple liver cysts are present and typically low signal on T1-weighted (**A**), and increased signal (greater than that of the spleen) on T2-weighted TE 60 milliseconds (**B**) and T2-weighted TE 120 milliseconds (**C**). Confusion may occur in the presence of hemorrhage, as this may increase the signal on T1-weighted images (*white arrowhead*). In these circumstances the lack of enhancement following IV Gd-DTPA may be diagnostic. (From Grainger RG, Allison DJ, Adam A, Dixon AK [eds]: Grainger and Allison's Diagnostic Radiology, 4th ed. Philadelphia, Churchill Livingstone, 2001.)

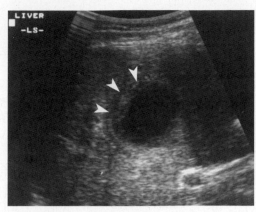

Fig 183–6
Liver abscess. An abscess, with typically reduced echoreflectivity and a thickened irregular wall (*arrowheads*).
(From Grainger RG, Allison DJ, Adam A, Dixon AK [eds]: Grainger and Allison's Diagnostic Radiology, 4th ed. Philadelphia, Churchill Livingstone, 2001.)

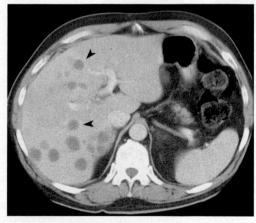

Fig 183–7
Liver abscess. Portal phase CT examination demonstrates multiple low attenuation lesions with ring enhancement (*arrowheads*). The appearances are often nonspecific on CT and often overlap with those of metastatic deposits.
(From Grainger RG, Allison DJ, Adam A, Dixon AK [eds]: Grainger and Allison's Diagnostic Radiology, 4th ed. Philadelphia, Churchill Livingstone, 2001.)

- CT scans are sensitive in detecting hepatic abscesses and contiguous organ extension (Fig. 183–7).
- Most liver abscesses are single; however, multiple liver abscesses are seen with systemic bacteremia.

TREATMENT
- The management of pyogenic liver abscess differs from that of amebic liver abscess.
- Medical management is the cornerstone of therapy in amebic liver abscess, whereas early intervention in the form of surgical therapy or catheter drainage and parenteral antibiotics is the rule in pyogenic liver abscess.
- Percutaneous drainage under CT or ultrasound guidance is essential in the treatment of pyogenic liver abscesses.
- Aspiration of hepatic amebic abscesses is not required unless there is no response to treatment or a pyogenic cause is being considered.

- Empirical broad-spectrum antibiotics are recommended initially until culture results are available.

B. ECHINOCOCCOSIS

DEFINITION
Echinococcosis is a chronic infection caused by the larval stage of several animal cestodes (flat worms) of the genus *Echinococcus*

PHYSICAL FINDINGS AND CLINICAL PRESENTATION
- Signs of an enlarging mass lesion in a visceral site such as the liver, lungs, kidneys, bone, or CNS
- Occasional cyst rupture causing allergic manifestations such as urticaria, angioedema, or anaphylaxis that bring the patient to medical attention
- Incidental discovery of cysts by abdominal or thoracic imaging studies performed for other reasons

CAUSE
- Four species of Echinococcus: *E. granulosus, E. multilocularis, E. oligarthrus,* and *E. vogeli.*
  1. *E. granulosus* is the cause of cystic hydatid disease.
  2. *E. multilocularis* and *E. vogeli* are the causes of alveolar and polycystic disease.
- The disease is transmitted to humans by infected canines (domestic or wild dogs, wolves, foxes) and seen most commonly in livestock-producing areas of the Middle East, Africa, Australia, New Zealand, Europe, and the Americas, including the southwestern United States. The life cycle of *Echinococcus granulosus* is shown in (Fig. 183–8)
- Eggs are present in the feces of infected canines; human infection occurs by ingestion of viable eggs in contaminated food. When humans ingest an egg of the dog tapeworm, *E. granulosus,* the larval form migrates to an organ, usually the liver or lung, where it develops into a hydatid cyst. A germinal layer of the hydatid cyst gives rise to brood capsules that eventually result in new cysts, called daughter cysts, producing an enlarging mass of increasingly complicated cysts. The final result resembles a giant balloon that is filled with myriads of tiny balloons (Fig. 183–9). Within each daughter cysts are numerous proctoscoleces, which have an invaginated head complete with hooklets (Fig. 183–10).
- It is common in many areas of the world, especially the Middle East.

DIFFERENTIAL DIAGNOSIS
- Liver neoplasms (see Fig. 182–2)
- Abscess (amebic or bacterial) (see Fig. 183–7)
- Congenital polycystic disease (see Fig. 183–5)

WORKUP
- Antibody assay
- Imaging study (CT scan, ultrasonography)
- Histologic examination of cyst or contents obtained by aspiration or resection (if possible) to confirm diagnosis

LABORATORY TESTS
Antibody assays (ELISA, latex agglutination, and Western blot): >90% sensitive and specific for liver cysts, but less accurate for cysts in other sites. A PCR assay is now available for problematic cases.

IMAGING STUDIES
Ultrasonography and/or CT scan
- Both are extremely sensitive for the detection of cysts, especially in the liver (Fig. 183–11).

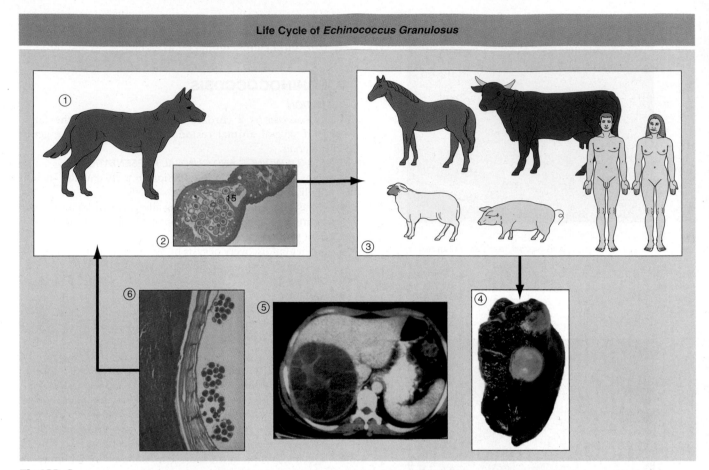

Life Cycle of *Echinococcus Granulosus*

Fig 183–8
Life cycle of *Echinococcus granulosus*. Adult tapeworms parasitize the small intestine of definitive hosts, mainly dogs (1). Parasite proglottids and eggs are shed with the feces (2), such eggs being infectious for intermediate hosts including humans (3). Hydatid cyst formation occurs predominantly in the liver (4), but also in lungs and other organs. Imaging techniques such as CT scanning (5) demonstrate well-delineated, fluid-filled, usually unilocular bladder-like lesions. Internal daughter cysts may be visible in larger cysts and are septated segments within the primary cyst. Histologically, the cyst by itself consists of a very thin inner germinal and nucleated layer with a predominantly syncytial structure (6). The germinal layer is externally protected by an acellular laminated layer of variable thickness. The endogenous formation of brood capsules and protoscolieces is a prerequisite for completion of the life cycle (6), which occurs when definitive hosts ingest protoscolex-containing hydatid cysts.
(From Cohen J, Powderly WG: Infectious Diseases, 2nd ed. St Louis, Mosby, 2004.)

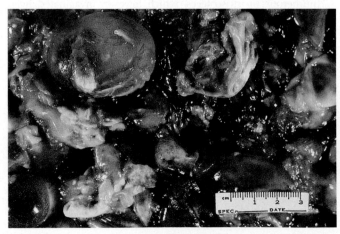

Fig 183–9
Echinococcal cyst of the liver. Eight liters of cysts and daughter cysts were present in a cyst that had slowly enlarged over a period of 10 to 20 years. Hydatid sand can be seen as granular material in the clear cyst fluid.
(From Silverberg SG: Principles and Practice of Surgical Pathology and Cytopathology, 4th ed. Philadelphia, Churchill Livingstone, 2006.)

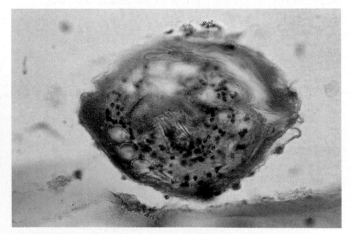

Fig 183–10
A protoscolex of *Echinococcus granulosus*, including the refractile hooklets, is demonstrated (HANDE, 2 ×50).
(From Silverberg SG: Principles and Practice of Surgical Pathology and Cytopathology, 4th ed. Philadelphia, Churchill Livingstone, 2006.)

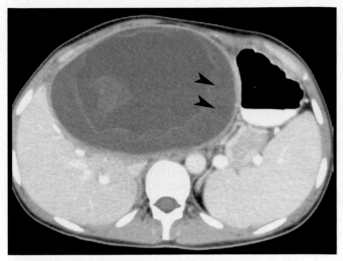

Fig 183–11
Hydatid disease. Portal phase CT demonstrates a large cystic structure with a discrete wall, separated internal membranes, and several "daughter cysts" (*arrowheads*).
(From Grainger RG, Allison DJ, Adam A, Dixon AK [eds]: Grainger and Allison's Diagnostic Radiology, 4th ed. Philadelphia, Churchill Livingstone, 2001.)

- Both lack specificity and are inadequate to establish the diagnosis of echinococcosis with certainty.

TREATMENT
- Treatment of choice for echinococcal cysts is surgical resection, when feasible.
- If resection is not feasible, perform percutaneous drainage with instillation of 95% ethanol to prevent dissemination of viable larve.
- Surgical therapy is followed by medical therapy with albendazole
- For echinococcosis confined to the liver: albendazole. Mebendazole if albendazole not available

C. VIRAL HEPATITIS

(1) Hepatitis A
DEFINITION
Hepatitis A is generally an acute self-limited infection of the liver by an enterically transmitted picorna virus (Fig. 183–12), hepatitis A virus (HAV). Infection may range from asymptomatic to fulminant hepatitis (Fig. 183–13).

PHYSICAL FINDINGS AND CLINICAL PRESENTATION
- Infection with HAV may have acute or subacute presentation, icteric or anicteric. Severity of illness seems to increase with age (90% of infection in children <5 years may be subclinical)
- There is a preicteric, prodromal phase of approximately 1-14 days; 15% no apparent prodrome. Symptoms are usually abrupt in onset and may include anorexia, malaise, nausea, vomiting, fever, headache, abdominal pain
- Less common symptoms are chills, myalgias, arthralgias, upper respiratory symptoms, constipation, diarrhea, pruritis, urticaria
- Jaundice occurs in >70% of patients
- The icteric phase is preceded by dark urine
- Bilirubinuria is typically followed a few days later by clay-colored stools and icterus

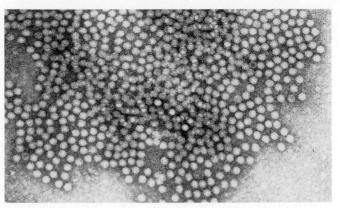

Fig 183–12
Hepatitis A virus. Note the vast number of virus particles present in a fecal extract.
(From Cohen J, Powderly WG: Infectious Diseases, 2nd ed. St Louis, Mosby, 2004.)

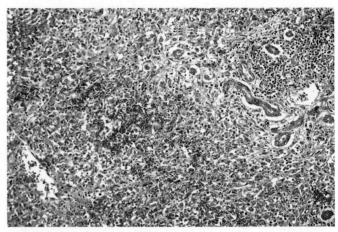

Fig 183–13
Acute viral hepatitis with massive necrosis. Note proliferated ductules and total dropping out of hepatocytes.
(From Silverberg SG: Principles and Practice of Surgical Pathology and Cytopathology, 4th ed. Philadelphia, Churchill Livingstone, 2006.)

PHYSICAL EXAMINATION
- Jaundice
- Hepatomegaly
- Splenomegaly
- Cervical lymphadenopathy
- Evanescent rash
- Petechie
- Cardiac arrhythmias

COMPLICATIONS
- Cholestasis
- Fulminant hepatitis
- Arthritis
- Myocarditis
- Optic neuritis
- Transverse myelitis
- Thrombocytopenic purpura
- Aplastic anemia
- Red cell aplasia
- Henoch-Schonlein purpura
- IgA dominant glomerulonephritis

CAUSE

- Caused by HAV, a 27-nm, nonenveloped, icosahedral, positive-stranded RNA virus
- Transmission is fecal-oral route, from person to person. Transmission requires close contact
- Parenteral transmission is considered rare
- Vertical transmission also reported

DIFFERENTIAL DIAGNOSIS

- Other hepatitis virus (B, C, D, E)
- Infectious mononucleosis
- Cytomegalovirus infection
- Herpes simplex virus infection
- Leptospirosis
- Brucellosis
- Drug-induced liver disease
- Ischemic hepatitis
- Autoimmune hepatitis

LABORATORY TESTS

- Diagnosis confirmed by IgM anti HAV; it is detectable in almost all infected patients at presentation and remains positive for 3 to 6 months. Figure 183-14 illustrates the course of acute hepatitis A
- A fourfold rise in titer of total antibody (IgM and IgG) to HAV confirms acute infection
- HAV detection in stool and body fluids by electron microscopy
- HAV RNA detection in stool, body fluids, serum, and liver tissue
- ALT and AST usually more than eight times normal in acute infection
- Bilirubin usually 5 to 15 times normal
- Alkaline phosphatase minimally elevated but higher level in cholestasis
- Albumin and prothrombin time are generally normal; if elevated may herald hepatic necrosis

TREATMENT

- Usually self-limited

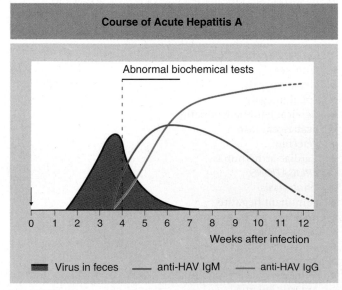

Course of Acute Hepatitis A

Abnormal biochemical tests

0 1 2 3 4 5 6 7 8 9 10 11 12
Weeks after infection

■ Virus in feces — anti-HAV IgM — anti-HAV IgG

Fig 183-14
Course of acute hepatitis A.
(From Cohen J, Powderly WG: Infectious Diseases, 2nd ed. St Louis, Mosby, 2004.)

- Supportive care
- Those with fulminant hepatitis may require hospitalization and treatment of associated complications
- Activity as tolerated
- Advise to avoid alcohol and hepatoxic drugs
- Patients with fulminant hepatitis should be assessed for liver transplantation

(2) Hepatitis B

DEFINITION

Hepatitis B is an acute infection of the liver parenchymal cells caused by the hepatitis B virus (HBV).

PHYSICAL FINDINGS AND CLINICAL PRESENTATION

- Often nonspecific symptoms
- Profound malaise
- Many asymptomatic cases
- Prodrome:
  1. 15% to 20% serum sickness (urticaria, rash, arthralgia) during early HBsAg
  2. HBsAg-Ab complex disease (arthritis, arteritis, glomerulonephritis)
- Hepatomegaly (87%) with RUQ tenderness
  1. Hepatic tenderness on palpation
  2. Splenomegaly: rare (10% to 15%)
- Jaundice, dark urine, with occasional pruritus
- Variable fever (when present, generally precedes jaundice and rapidly declines following onset of icteric phase)
- Spider angiomata: rare; resolves during recovery
- Rare polyarteritis nodosa, cryoglobulinemia

CAUSE

- Caused by hepatitis B virus (42-nm hepadnavirus with an outer surface coat [HBsAg], inner nucleocapsid core [HBcAg; HBeAg]; DNA polymerase; and partially double-stranded DNA genome)
- Transmission by parenteral route (needle use, tattooing, ear piercing, acupuncture, transfusion of blood and blood products, hemodialysis, sexual contact), perinatal transmission
- Infection may result from contact of infectious material with mucous membranes and open skin breaks (e.g., HBV is stable and can be transmitted from toothbrushes, utensils, razors, baby toys, various medical equipment [respirators, endoscopes])
- Oral intake of infectious material may result in infection through breaks in the oral mucosa
- Food or water virtually never found to be sources of HBV infection
- Infection occurring primarily in the liver, where necrosis probably results from cytotoxic T-cell response, direct cytopathic effect of HBcAg (core antigen), high-level HBsAg (surface antigen) expression, or co-infection with delta (D) hepatitis virus (RNA delta core within HBsAg envelope)
- Recovery (>90%):
  1. Fulminant hepatitis occurring in <1% (especially if coinfected with hepatitis D); 80% fatal
  2. Unusual (5%) prolonged acute disease for 4 to 12 months, with recovery
  3. Overall fatality increases with age and viral inoculation (e.g., transfusions)
- Chronic infection (1% to 2%):
  1. Persistent carrier state without hepatitis (HBsAg positive)

2. Chronic persistent hepatitis (CPH) (clinically well), or chronic active hepatitis (CAH) (HBsAg positive and HBeAg positive)

3. Cirrhosis

4. Hepatocellular carcinoma (especially after neonatal infection)

5. Chronic infection: more common following low-dose exposure and mild acute hepatitis, with earlier age of infection, in males, or if immunosuppressed

6. One third to one quarter of chronically infected will develop progressive liver disease (cirrhosis, hepatocellular carcinoma)

DIFFERENTIAL DIAGNOSIS

- Acute disease confused with other viral hepatitis infections (A, C, D, E)
- Any viral illness producing systemic disease and hepatitis (e.g., yellow fever, EBV, CMV, HIV, rubella, rubeola, coxsackie B, adenovirus, herpes simplex or zoster)
- Nonviral etiologies of hepatitis (e.g., leptospirosis, toxoplasmosis, alcoholic hepatitis, drug-induced [e.g., acetaminophen, INH], toxic hepatitis [carbon tetrachloride, benzene])

LABORATORY TESTS

- Diagnosis of acute HBV infection is best confirmed by IgM HBcAb in acute or early convalescent serum.
  1. Generally, IgM present during onset of jaundice
  2. Coexisting HBsAg
- HBsAg and IgG-HBcAb during acute jaundice are strongly suggestive of remote HBV infection and another etiology for current illness.
- HBsAb alone is suggestive of immunization response.
- With recovery, HBeAg is rapidly replaced by HBeAb in 2 to 3 months, and HBsAg is replaced by HBsAb in 5 to 6 months (Fig. 183–15).
- In chronic HBV hepatitis, HBsAg and HBeAg are persistent without corresponding Ab. Figure 183–16 illustrates the phases of chronic hepatitis B infection.

- In chronic carrier state, HBsAg is persistent, but HBeAg is replaced by HBe Ab.
- HBcAb develops in all outcomes.
- HBeAg correlation with highest infectivity; appearance of HBeAb heralds recovery.
- LFTs:
  1. ALT and AST: usually more than eight times normal (often 1000 U/L) at onset of jaundice (minimal acute ALT/AST rises often followed by chronic hepatitis or hepatocellular carcinoma)
  2. Bilirubin: variably elevated in icteric viral hepatitis
  3. Alkaline phosphatase: minimally elevated (one to three times normal) acutely
- Albumin and prothrombin time:
  1. Generally normal
  2. If abnormal, possible harbinger of impending hepatic necrosis (fulminant hepatitis)
- WBC and ESR: generally normal

IMAGING STUDIES

- Sonogram is useful to document rapid reduction in liver size during fulminant hepatitis or mass in hepatocellular carcinoma

TREATMENT

- Symptomatic is useful treatment as necessary
- Activity as tolerated
- High-calorie diet preferred; often best tolerated in morning
- In most cases of acute HBV infection no treatment necessary; >90% of adults will spontaneously clear infection
- Hospitalization advisable for any patient in danger from dehydration caused by poor oral intake, whose PT is prolonged, who has a rising bilirubin level >15 to 20 µg/dL, or who has any clinical evidence of hepatic failure
- IV therapy needed (rarely) for hydration during severe vomiting
- Treatment of chronic HBV infection consists of immune modulators (interferon alpha) and antiviral agents in the form of nucleoside analogues (e.g., lamivudine).

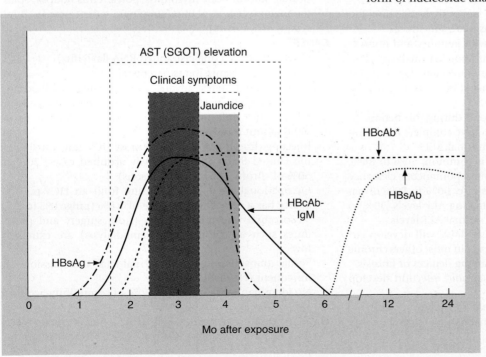

Fig 183–15
HBV surface antigen-antibody and core antibodies (note "core window").
$HB_CAb = HB_CAb$-IgM + HBCAb-IgG (combined).
(From Ravel R: Clinical laboratory medicine, 6th ed, St Louis, Mosby, 1995.)

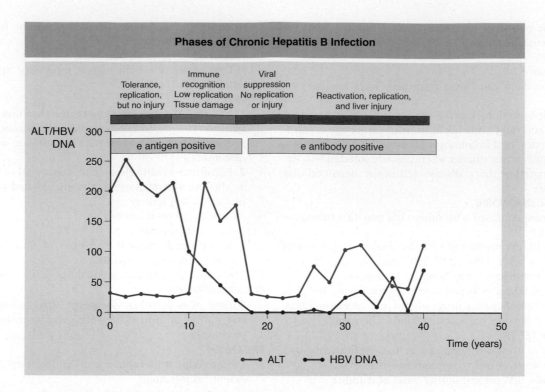

Fig 183–16
Phase of chronic hepatitis B infection. Initial infection is usually in childhood and has a long immune tolerant phase. Immune recognition then develops, which can allow inactivation of hepatitis B by either clearance of infected cells (with associated liver cell damage) or suppression of viral antigen expression on infected hepatocytes. This produces viral inactivation. In a significant proportion of patients in whom this has occurred, a third phase develops, where replication of HBV DNA again appearing in serum and increases the risk of chronic liver disease.
(From Cohen J, Powderly WG: Infectious Diseases, 2nd ed. St Louis, Mosby, 2004.)

(3) HEPATITIS C

DEFINITION
Hepatitis C is an acute liver parenchymal infection caused by hepatitis C virus (HCV).

PHYSICAL FINDINGS AND CLINICAL PRESENTATION
- Symptoms usually develop 7 to 8 weeks after infection (2 to 26 weeks), but 70% to 80% of cases are subclinical.
- 10% to 20% report acute illness with jaundice and nonspecific symptoms (abdominal pain, anorexia, malaise). Purpura (Fig. 183–17) and pulmonary infiltrates (Fig. 183–18) may be present in patients with hepatits C–associated cryoglobulinemia
- Fulminant hepatitis may rarely occur during this period.
- After acute infection, 15% to 25% have complete resolution (absence of HCV RNA in serum, normal ALT).
- Progression to chronic infection is common, 50% to 84%; 74% to 86% have persistent viremia; spontaneous clearance of viremia in chronic infection is rare. 60% to 70% of patients will have persistent or fluctuating ALT levels, 30% to 40% with chronic infection have normal ALT levels.
- 15% to 20% of those with chronic HCV will develop cirrhosis over a period of 20 to 30 years; in most others chronic infection leads to hepatitis and varying degrees of fibrosis.
- 0.4% to 2.5% of patients with chronic infection develop hepatocellular carcinoma.
- 25% of patients with chronic infection continue to have an asymptomatic course with normal LFTs and benign histology.
- In chronic HCV infection, extrahepatic sequela include a variety of immunologic and lymphoproliferative disorders (e.g., cryoglobulinemia [see Fig. 183–7], membranoproliferative glomerulonephritis, and possibly Sjögren's syndrome, autoimmune thyroiditis, polyarteritis nodosa, aplastic anemia, lichen planus, porphyria cutanea tarda, B-cell lymphoma, others).

CAUSE
- Caused by HCV (single-stranded RNA flavivirus)
- Most HCV transmission is parenteral
- In the United States, advances in screening of blood and blood products in 1990 and 1992 have made transfusion-related HCV infection rare (the risk is estimated to be 0.001%/unit transfused)
- Injecting-drug use accounts for most HCV transmission in the United States (60% of newly acquired cases, 20% to 50% of chronically infected persons)
- Occupational needlestick exposure from an HCV-positive source has a seroconversion rate of 1.8% (range 0% to 7%)
- Nosocomial transmission rates (from surgery and procedures such as colonoscopy, hemodialysis) are extremely low
- Sexual transmission and maternal-fetal transmission are infrequent (estimated at 5%)
- No identifiable risk in 40% to 50% of community-acquired HIV infection
- HCV infection may stimulate production of cytotoxic T lymphocytes and cytokines (inf-γ), which likely mediate hepatic necrosis

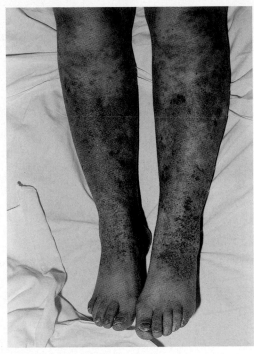

Fig 183–17
Purpura in a patient with hepatitis C–associated cryoglobulinemia. Raised purpuric lesions are present on the legs of this individual. The differential diagnosis of purpura and renal disease includes cryoglobuli- nemia, Henoch-Schönlein purpura, vasculitis, and endocarditis. (From Johnson RJ, Feehally J: Comprehensive Clinical Nephrology, 2nd ed. St Louis, Mosby, 2000.)

DIFFERENTIAL DIAGNOSIS
- Other hepatitis viruses (A, B, D, E)
- Other viral illnesses producing systemic disease (e.g., yellow fever, EBV, CMV, HIV, rubella, rubeola, coxsackie B, adeno- virus, HSV, HZV)
- Nonviral hepatitis (e.g., leptospirosis, toxoplasmosis, alco- holic hepatitis, drug-induced hepatitis [acetaminophen, INH], toxic hepatitis)

WORKUP
Laboratory tests
Diagnosis is often by exclusion, because it takes 6 weeks to 12 months to develop anti-HCV antibody (70% positive by 6 weeks, 90% positive by 6 months).

Diagnostic tests include serologic assays for antibodies and molecular tests for viral particles.

1. Enzyme immunoassay is the test for anti-HCV antibody (Fig. 183–19):
   - The current version can detect antibody within 4 to 10 weeks after infection
   - False-negative rate in low-risk populations is 0.5% to 1%
   - False-negatives also in immunocompromised persons, HIV-1, renal failure, HCV-associated essential mixed cryo- globulinemia
   - False-positives in autoimmune hepatitis, paraprotein- emia, and persons with no risk factors
2. Recombinant immunoblot is used to confirm positive en- zyme immunoassays:
   - Recommended only in low-risk settings

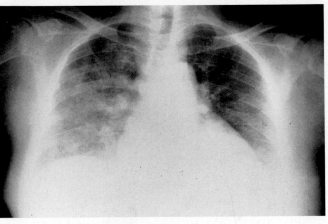

Fig 183–18
Chest radiograph showing nodular infiltrate in the lung secondary to cryoglobulinemic vasculitis in a patient with hepatitis C infection. (From Johnson RJ, Feehally J: Comprehensive Clinical Nephrology, 2nd ed. St Louis, Mosby, 2000.)

3. Qualitative and quantitative HCV RNA tests using PCR:
   - Lower limit of detection is <100 copies HCV RNA/mL
   - Used to confirm viremia and to assess response to treat- ment
   - Qualitative PCR useful in patients with negative enzyme immunoassay in whom infection is suspected
   - Quantitative tests use either branched-chain DNA or re- verse transcription PCR; the latter is more sensitive
4. Viral genotyping can distinguish among genotypes 1, 2, and 3, which is helpful in choosing therapy; most of these tests use PCR (NOTE: genotypes 1, 2, and 3 predominate in the United States and Europe [1 is especially common in North America])
5. LFTs:
   - ALT and AST may be elevated to more than eight times normal in acute infection; in chronic infection ALT may be normal or fluctuate
   - Bilirubin may be 5 to 10 times normal
   - Albumin and prothrombin time generally normal; if ab- normal, may be harbinger of impending hepatic necrosis
   - Liver biopsy with histologic staging is the gold standard for assessing the degree of disease activity and the likeli- hood of disease progression, and also help rule out other causes of liver disease.

IMAGING STUDIES
- Sonogram: useful in assessing rapid liver size reduction during fulminant hepatitis or mass in hepatocellular carcinoma

TREATMENT
- Supportive care
- Avoid hepatically metabolized drugs
- *Early* treatment with IFN-α-2b during acute HCV infection prevents chronic infection. The aim is to decrease viral load early in infection and allow the patient's immune system to control viral replication, thus preventing progression to chronic infection. The primary end point is sustained viro- logic response, with absence of HCV RNA in serum 24 weeks after completion of therapy.
- Mainstay for chronic hepatitis C therapy is interferon alpha and ribavarin.

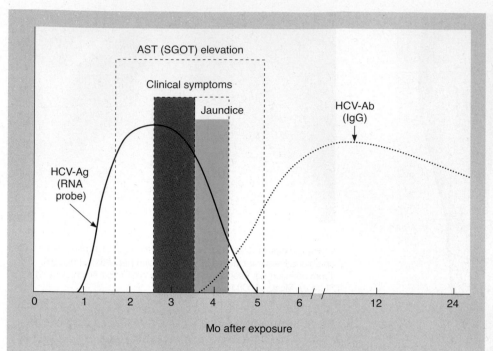

Fig 183–19
HCV antigen and antibody.
(From Ravel R: Clinical Laboratory Medicine, 6th ed. St Louis, Mosby, 1995.)

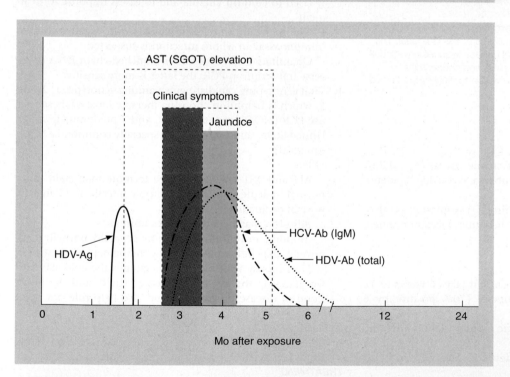

Fig 183–20
HDV antigen and antibodies.
(From Ravel R: Clinical Laboratory Medicine, 6th ed. St Louis, Mosby, 1995.)

(4) HEPATITIS D

- Hepatitis D is diagnosed by the presence of delta antigen or antibody to delta antigen (anti-HDV) in the patient's serum; it can cause either acute or chronic hepatitis.
- (Figure 183–20) describes serologic tests for hepatitis D infection.
- Acute hepatitis D can occur in two forms:
- Co-infection: simultaneous acute infection with hepatitis B and hepatitis D viruses; diagnosis is confirmed by the presence of anti-HDV and IgM anti-HBc (marker of acute hepatitis B).
- Superinfection: occurrence of acute delta infection in a chronic HBV carrier; diagnosis is made by presence of anti-HDV and HBsAg in the serum; IgM anti-HBc will be absent.
- Chronic hepatitis D is diagnosed by the presence in the serum of sustained high titers of anti-HDV and HBsAg; liver biopsy will confirm the diagnosis by demonstrating HDVAg in liver tissue.

Chapter 184 — Autoimmune hepatitis

DEFINITION
Autoimmune hepatitis is a chronic inflammatory condition of the liver, characterized by the presence of circulating autoantibodies. Three types have been described:

- Type 1 or "classic" autoimmune hepatitis is the most predominant form in the United States and worldwide (80%) and patients are positive for either antinuclear antibodies (ANA) or antismooth muscle antibodies (ASMA). Occurs across all age ranges and may be underdiagnosed in the elderly.
- Type 2 is rare in the United States and primarily affects young children. Type 2 is characterized by the presence of antibodies to liver/kidney microsomes (anti-LKM).
- Type 3 is characterized by antibodies to soluble liver antigen or liver-pancreas antigen (anti-SLA/LP). Occurs mostly in younger women (90%). Clinically indistinguishable from type 1. Designation of a type 3 autoimmune hepatitis has largely been abandoned.

CLINICAL PRESENTATION
- Varies from asymptomatic elevations of liver enzymes to advanced cirrhosis.
- Symptoms may include fatigue, anorexia, nausea, abdominal pain, pruritus, and arthralgia.
- Jaundice.
- Hepatomegaly/splenomegaly.
- Autoimmune findings may include arthritis, xerostomia, keratoconjunctivitis, cutaneous vasculitis, and erythema nodosum.
- For patients presenting with advanced disease: ascites, edema, abnormal bleeding, jaundice.

CAUSE
- Exact etiology unknown; liver histology demonstrates cell-mediated immune attack against hepatocytes.
- Presence of a variety of autoantibodies suggests an autoimmune mechanism.
- Strong genetic predisposition.

DIAGNOSIS
- Diagnosis is confirmed with liver biopsy (Fig. 184–1)

DIFFERENTIAL DIAGNOSIS
- Acute viral hepatitis (A, B, C, D, E, cytomegalovirus, Epstein-Barr, herpes) (see Fig. 183–13)
- Chronic viral hepatitis (B, C)
- Toxic hepatitis (alcohol, drugs)
- Primary biliary cirrhosis (see Fig. 179–3)
- Primary sclerosing cholangitis
- Hemochromatosis (see Fig. 180–4)
- Nonalcoholic steatohepatitis (see Fig. 181–1)
- SLE
- Wilson's disease (see Fig. 40–4)
- Alpha-$_1$ antitrypsin deficiency (see Fig. 131–2)

LABORATORY TESTS
- Aminotransferases generally elevated, may fluctuate.
- Bilirubin and alkaline phosphatase moderately elevated or normal.
- Hypergammaglobulinemia usually present.
- Circulating autoantibodies often present.
  1. Rheumatoid factor

2. Antinuclear antibodies (ANA)
   a. Present in two thirds of patients.
   b. Typical pattern is homogeneous or speckled.
   c. Titer does not correlate with the stage, activity, or prognosis.
3. Antismooth muscle antibodies (ASMA)
   a. Present in 87% of patients.
   b. Titer does not correlate with course or prognosis.
4. Antibodies to liver/kidney microsomes (anti-LKM)
   a. Typically found in patients who are ANA-negative and ASMA-negative.
   b. Found in <1/25 of patients in the United States
   c. Present in pediatric population and up to 20% of adults in Europe; also present in patients with drug-induced hepatitis.
5. Autoantibodies against soluble liver antigen and liver-pancreas antigen (anti-SLA/LP)
   a. Present in 10% to 30% of patients.
   b. Associated with higher rate of relapse after corticosteroid therapy.
   c. Several studies suggest that patients with anti-SLA/LP have a more severe course.

Hypoalbuminemia and prolonged prothrombin time with advanced disease.

There is a well-described overlap syndrome with primary biliary cirrhosis (7%), primary sclerosing cholangitis (6%), and autoimmune cholangitis (11%).

IMAGING STUDIES
- Ultrasound of liver and biliary tree to rule out obstruction or hepatic mass

TREATMENT
- Avoid alcohol and hepatotoxic medications.
- Liver transplantation is an option for end-stage disease.
- Supportive therapy for those in fulminant failure or end-stage cirrhosis at presentation and referral for transplantation evaluation
- Corticosteroids

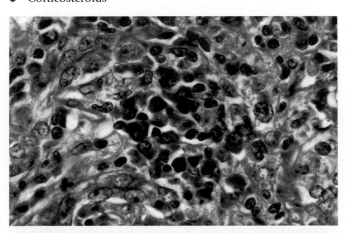

Fig 184–1
Autoimmune hepatitis with large numbers of plasma cells in the portal inflammatory infiltrate.
(From Silverberg SG: Principles and Practice of Surgical Pathology and Cytopathology, 4th ed. Philadelphia, Churchill Livingstone, 2006.))

GALLBLADDER AND BILE DUCTS

Chapter 185   Cholelithiasis

DEFINITION
Cholelithiasis is the presence of stones in the gallbladder (Fig. 185–1).

PHYSICAL FINDINGS AND CLINICAL PRESENTATION
- Physical examination is entirely normal unless patient is having a biliary colic; 80% of gallstones are asymptomatic.
- Typical symptoms of obstruction of the cystic duct include intermittent, severe, cramping pain affecting the RUQ.
- Pain occurs mostly after fatty meals or at night and may radiate to the back or right shoulder. It can last from a few minutes to several hours.

CAUSE
- 75% of gallstones contain cholesterol and are usually associated with obesity, female gender, diabetes mellitus; mixed stones are most common (80%), pure cholesterol stones account for only 10% of stones.
- 25% of gallstones are pigment stones (bilirubin, calcium, and variable organic material) associated with hemolysis and cirrhosis. These tend to be black pigment stones that are refractory to medical therapy.
- 50% of mixed-type stones are radiopaque.

DIFFERENTIAL DIAGNOSIS
- PUD (see Fig. 155–1)
- GERD (see Fig. 145–1)
- IBD (see Fig. 162–4)
- Pancreatitis (see Fig. 173–5)
- Neoplasms (see Fig. 187–1)
- Nonnuclear dyspepsia
- Inferior wall MI
- Hepatic abscess (see Fig. 183–7)

LABORATORY TESTS
Generally normal unless patient has biliary obstruction (elevated alkaline phosphatase, bilirubin).

IMAGING STUDIES
- Plain abdominal films may reveal opaque gallstones (Fig. 185–2).
- Ultrasound of the gallbladder (Fig. 185–3) will detect small stones and biliary sludge (sensitivity, 95%; specificity, 90%); the presence of a dilated gallbladder with thickened wall is suggestive of acute cholecystitis.
- Nuclear imaging (HIDA scan) (see Fig. 186–2) can be used when ultrasound is nondiagnostic to confirm suspected acute cholecystitis (>90% accuracy) if gallbladder does not visualize within 4 hours of injection and the radioisotope is excreted in the common bile duct.
- Common bile duct stones can be detected noninvasively by magnetic resonance cholangiopancreatography (MRCP) or invasively via endoscopic retrograde cholangiopancreatography (ERCP) and intraoperative cholangiography.

TREATMENT
- The management of gallstones is affected by the clinical presentation.
- Asymptomatic patients do not require therapeutic intervention.
- Surgical intervention is generally the ideal approach for symptomatic patients. Laparoscopic cholecystectomy is preferred over open cholecystectomy because of the shorter recovery period and lower mortality. Between 5% and 26% of patients undergoing elective laparoscopic cholecystectomy will require conversion to an open procedure. Most common reason is inability to clearly identify the biliary anatomy.

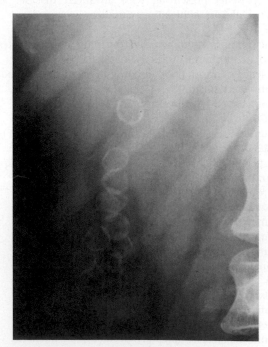

Fig 185–2
Cholelithiasis. Plain film showing faceted opaque gallstones.
(From Grainger RG, Allison DJ, Adam A, Dixon AK [eds]: Grainger and Allison's Diagnostic Radiology, 4th ed. Philadelphia, Churchill Livingstone, 2001.)

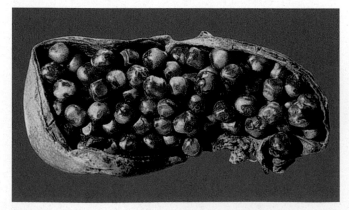

Fig 185–1
A gallbladder containing at least 50 mixed stones.
(From Forbes A, Misiewicz J, Compton C, et al: Atlas of Clinical Gastroenterology, 3rd ed. Edinburgh, Elsevier Mosby, 2005.)

- Laparoscopic cholecystectomy after endoscopic sphincterectomy is recommended for patients with common bile duct stones and residual gallbladder stones. Where possible, single-stage laparoscopic treatments with removal of duct stones and cholecystectomy during the same procedure are preferable.

- Patients who are not appropriate candidates for surgery because of coexisting illness or patients who refuse surgery can be treated with oral bile salts: ursodiol (Actigall), or chenodiol (Chenix) Candidates for oral bile salts are patients with cholesterol stones (radiolucent, noncalcified stones), with a diameter of ≤15 mm and having three or fewer stones. Candidates for medical therapy must have a functioning gallbladder and must have absence of calcifications on CT scans.

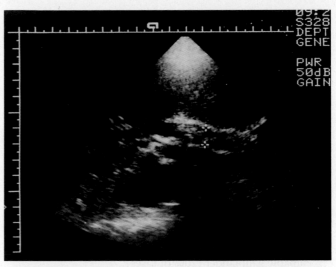

Fig 185–3
Calculi in the common bile duct, casting an acoustic shadow.
(From Grainger RG, Allison DJ, Adam A, Dixon AK [eds]: Grainger and Allison's Diagnostic Radiology, 4th ed. Philadelphia, Churchill Livingstone, 2001.)

Chapter 186   Cholecystitis

DEFINITION

Cholecystitis is an acute or chronic inflammation of the gall-bladder generally secondary to gallstones (>95% of cases).

PHYSICAL FINDINGS AND CLINICAL PRESENTATION

- Pain and tenderness in the right hypochondrium or epigastrium; pain possibly radiating to the infrascapular region
- Palpation of the RUQ eliciting marked tenderness and stoppage of inspired breath *(Murphy's sign)*
- Guarding
- Fever (33%)
- Jaundice (25% to 50% of patients): A cystic duct stone obstructing a common bile duct (see Fig. 186–3) can cause jaundice *(Mirizzi syndrome)*
- Palpable gallbladder (20% of cases)
- Nausea and vomiting (>70% of patients)
- Fever and chills (>25% of patients)
- Medical history often revealing ingestion of large, fatty meals before onset of pain in the epigastrium and RUQ

CAUSE

- Gallstones (>95% of cases)
- Ischemic damage to the gallbladder, critically ill patient (acalculous cholecystitis)
- Infectious agents, especially in patients with AIDS (CMV, *Cryptosporidium*)
- Strictures of the bile duct
- Neoplasms, primary or metastatic

DIFFERENTIAL DIAGNOSIS

- Hepatic: hepatitis, abscess (see Fig. 183–7), hepatic congestion, neoplasm (see Fig. 182–2), trauma
- Biliary: neoplasm (see Fig. 187–2), stricture
- Gastric: PUD, neoplasm, alcoholic gastritis, hiatal hernia (see Fig. 146–1)
- Pancreatic: pancreatitis (see Fig. 173–5), neoplasm (see Fig. 175–4), stone in the pancreatic duct or ampulla
- Renal: calculi (see Fig. 216–6), infection, inflammation, neoplasm (see Fig. 212–2), ruptured kidney
- Pulmonary: pneumonia, pulmonary infarction, right-sided pleurisy
- Intestinal: retrocecal appendicitis (see Fig. 161–1), intestinal obstruction (see Fig. 157–2), high fecal impaction
- Cardiac: myocardial ischemia (particularly involving the inferior wall), pericarditis
- Cutaneous: herpes zoster
- Trauma
- Fitz-Hugh-Curtis syndrome (perihepatitis) (see Fig. 250–2)
- Subphrenic abscess
- Dissecting aneurysm
- Nerve root irritation caused by osteoarthritis of the spine

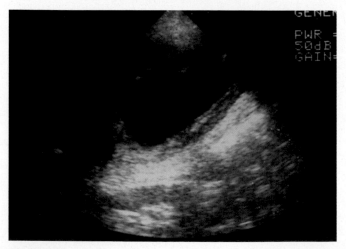

Fig 186–1
Thickened gallbladder wall in acute cholecystitis. The gallbladder contains echogenic calculi.
(From Grainger RG, Allison DJ, Adam A, Dixon AK [eds]: Grainger and Allison's Diagnostic Radiology, 4th ed. Philadelphia, Churchill Livingstone, 2001.)

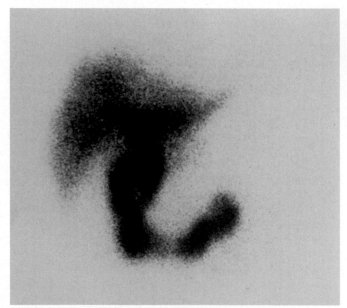

Fig 186–2
Acute cholecystitis. Following the intravenous administration of 200 MBq (5 mCi) of ^{99m}Tc-HIDA and a stimulus of CCK, the region of the liver and gallbladder is imaged. Intrahepatic bile ducts are visualized, as is excretion through the common duct into the small bowel. The gallbladder is not seen. This patient had gallstones demonstrated by ultrasound and confirmed at surgery. The pathologic diagnosis was acute cholecystitis.
(From Grainger RG, Allison DJ, Adam A, Dixon AK [eds]: Grainger and Allison's Diagnostic Radiology, 4th ed. Philadelphia, Churchill Livingstone, 2001.)

LABORATORY TESTS

- Leukocytosis (12,000 to 20,000) is present in >70% of patients.
- Elevated alkaline phosphatase, ALT, AST, bilirubin; bilirubin elevation >4 mg/dL is unusual and suggests presence of choledocholithiasis.
- Elevated amylase may be present (consider pancreatitis if serum amylase elevation exceeds 500 U).

IMAGING STUDIES

- Ultrasound of the gallbladder is the preferred initial test; it will demonstrate the presence of stones and also dilated gallbladder with thickened wall and surrounding edema in patients with acute cholecystitis (Fig. 186–1).
- Nuclear imaging (HIDA scan) is useful for diagnosis of cholecystitis when ultrasound is inconclusive: sensitivity and specificity exceed 90% for acute cholecystis. This test is only reliable when bilirubin is <5 mg/dL. A positive test will demonstrate obstruction of the cystic or common hepatic duct (Fig. 186–2); the test will not demonstrate the presence of stones.
- ERCP (Fig. 186–3) can be used in cases of suspected impacted hepatic or cystic duct stones.
- CT scan of the abdomen is useful in cases of suspected abscess, neoplasm, or pancreatitis.
- Plain film of the abdomen generally is not useful, because <25% of stones are radiopaque.

TREATMENT

- Cholecystectomy
- ERCP with sphincterectomy and stone extraction can be performed in conjunction with laparoscopic cholecystectomy for patients with choledochal lithiasis; approximately 7% to 15% of patients with cholelithiasis also have stones in the common bile duct.

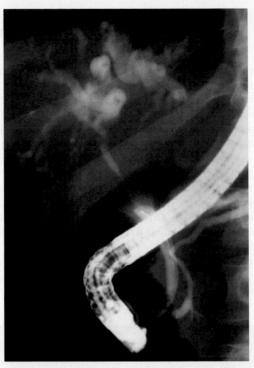

Fig 186–3
Mirizzi syndrome type I. ERCP shows compression of the common hepatic duct from a large stone impacted in the cystic duct.
(From Grainger RG, Allison DJ, Adam A, Dixon AK [eds]: Grainger and Allison's Diagnostic Radiology, 4th ed. Philadelphia, Churchill Livingstone, 2001.)

Chapter 187   Cholangiocarcinoma

- Rare tumor most often loced at the hepatic duct bifurcation (70% of cases).
- Clinical presentation: jaundice (90%), pruritus, abdominal pain, fever, weight loss
- Increased incidence in primary sclerosing cholangitis, prior biliary-enteric anastomosis, choledochal cysts, hepatolithiasis, exposure to nitosamines or dioxin, and infection with liver flukes.
- Labs: elevated bilirubin, elevated alkaline phospahtase
- Diagnosis: Diagnostic modalities include abdominal ultrasound (Fig. 187–1), CT scan (Fig. 187–2), PTC (Fig. 187–3), ERCP (Fig. 187–4), and fine needle aspiration biopsy (Fig. 187–5).
- Treatment: surgical resection, radiation therapy, chemotherapy. Survival is highly dependent on stage of disease at presentation.

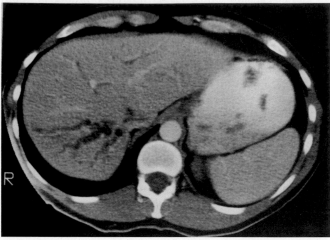

Fig 187–2
Contrast-enhanced CT demonstrating atrophy of the right lobe of the liver with hypertrophy of segments II, III, and IV. This patient has primary sclerosing cholangitis and has developed a cholangiocarcinoma of the right hepatic duct.
(From Grainger RG, Allison DJ, Adam A, Dixon AK [eds]: Grainger and Allison's Diagnostic Radiology, 4th ed. Philadelphia, Churchill Livingstone, 2001.)

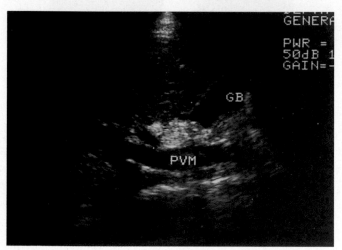

Fig 187–1
Cholangiocarcinoma. An echogenic mass is obstructing the common bile duct anterior to the main portal vein (PVM) and causing dilation of the intrahepatic ducts. GB = gallbladder. (Reproduced courtesy of Dr. P. Dawson.)

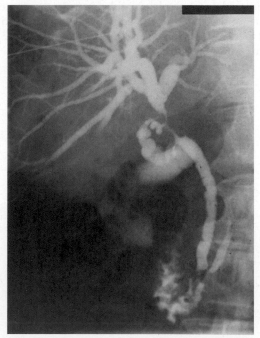

Fig 187–3
PTC in hilar tumor assessment. Relatively undistended ducts in a patient with a cholangiocarcinoma; a short stricture involves the junction of the common hepatic and common bile ducts.
(From Grainger RG, Allison DJ, Adam A, Dixon AK [eds]: Grainger and Allison's Diagnostic Radiology, 4th ed. Philadelphia, Churchill Livingstone, 2001.)

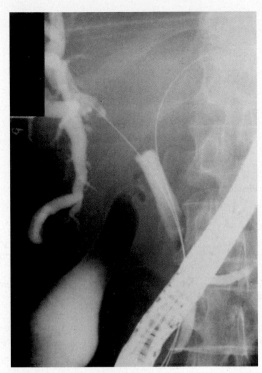

Fig 187–4

Klatskin tumor. Invasion of both lobes of the liver from a hilar cholangiocarcinoma. Wires have been placed endoscopically into both hepatic ducts in preparation of metal stenting.
(From Grainger RG, Allison DJ, Adam A, Dixon AK [eds]: Grainger and Allison's Diagnostic Radiology, 4th ed. Philadelphia, Churchill Livingstone, 2001.)

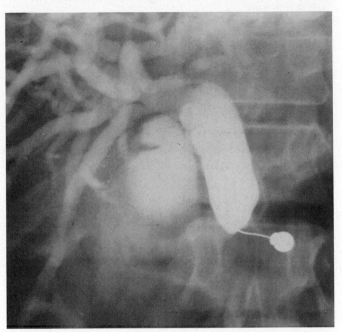

Fig 187–5

Fine-needle aspiration biopsy. An obstructing lesion is present in the lower common bile duct. A 22-guage needle has been inserted percutaneously. Cytology revealed a cholangiocarcinoma.
(From Grainger RG, Allison DJ, Adam A, Dixon AK [eds]: Grainger and Allison's Diagnostic Radiology, 4th ed. Philadelphia, Churchill Livingstone, 2001.)

GASTROINTESTINAL INFECTIONS

Chapter 188 | Viral gastroenteritis

- Epidemiologic and clinical characteristics of gastroenteritis viruses are described in (Table 188–1)
- Electron micrographs: enteric adenovirus (Fig. 188–1), rotavirus (Fig. 188–2), norovirus (Fig. 188–3)
- Treatment: supportive therapy, hydration (PO, IV), electrolyte replacement, antiperistaltic agents

TABLE 188–1 Epidemiologic and clinical characteristics of gastroenteritis viruses

Characteristic	Rotavirus	Enteric adenovirus	Astrovirus	Norovirus	Sapovirus
Age group	6-24 months	<2 years	<7 years	Adults and children	Children
Mode of transmission	Person-to-person, food, water	Person-to-person	Person-to-person, water, raw shellfish	Person-to-person, water, cold foods, raw shellfish	Person-to-person, water, cold foods, raw shellfish
Disease pattern	Endemic	Endemic	Endemic, outbreaks	Outbreaks, endemic	Endemic, outbreaks
Seasonality	Winter	No	Winter	No	No
Clinical characteristics	Dehydrating diarrhea; vomiting and fever very common	Prolonged diarrhea; vomiting and fever	Watery diarrhea, usually short	Acute vomiting, diarrhea, fever, myalgia, headache, usually short	Rotavirus-like illness in children
Prodrome (days)	2	3-10	1-2	1-2	1-3
Duration of illness (days)	3-8	>7	1-4	0.5-2.5	4
Outpatient prevalence (%)	5-10	4–8	7-8	10-25 endemic, 90 outbreaks	1-10
Inpatient prevalence (%)	35-40	5-20	3-5	Rare	3-5

From Cohen J, Powderly WG: Infectious Diseases, 2nd ed. St Louis, Mosby, 2004.

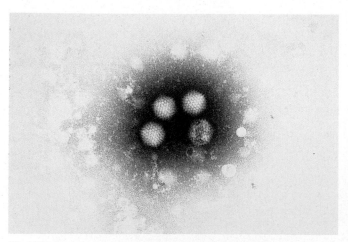

Fig 188–1
Epidemiologic and clinical characteristics of gastroenteritis viruses. (From Cohen J, Powderly WG: Infectious Diseases, 2nd ed. St Louis, Mosby, 2004.)

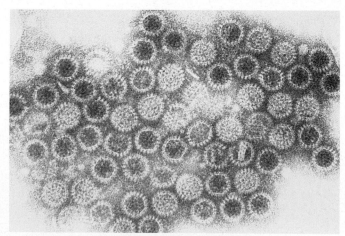

Fig 188–2
Rotavirus. Electron micrograph. (Courtesy of S. Spangenberger.)

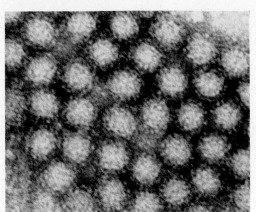

Fig 188 – 3
Norovirus. Electron micrograph.
(Courtesy of C. Humphrey [CDC].)

Chapter 189   Salmonellosis

DEFINITION
Salmonellosis is an infection caused by one of several serotypes of *Salmonella*.

PHYSICAL FINDINGS AND CLINICAL PRESENTATION
- Infections
  1. Localized to GI tract (gastroenteritis)
  2. Systemic (typhoid fever)
  3. Localized outside of GI tract
- Gastroenteritis
  1. Incubation period: 12 to 48 hours
  2. Nausea, vomiting
  3. Diarrhea, abdominal cramps
  4. Fever
  5. Bacteremia: Occurs mostly in the immunocompromised host or those with underlying conditions, including HIV infection
  6. Self-limited illness lasting 3 or 4 days
  7. Colonization of GI tract persistent for months, especially in those treated with antibiotics
- *Typhoid fever*
  1. Incubation period of few days to several weeks
  2. Prolonged fever, often with a stepwise-increasing temperature pattern
  3. Myalgias
  4. Headache, cough, sore throat
  5. Malaise, anorexia
  6. Abdominal pain
  7. Hepatosplenomegaly
  8. Diarrhea or constipation early in the course of illness
  9. *Rose spots* (faint, maculopapular, blanching lesions) sometimes seen on chest or abdomen (Fig. 189–1)
- Untreated disease
  1. Fever lasting 1 to 2 months
  2. Main complication: GI bleeding caused by perforation from ulceration of Peyer's patches in the ileum (Fig. 189–2), severe colitis, necrosis of lymphoid follicles (Fig. 189–3)
  3. Rare complications:
     a. Mental status changes
     b. Shock
  4. Relapse rate of approximately 10%
- Infections outside GI tract
  1. Can occur in virtually any location
  2. Usually occur in patients with underlying diseases
  3. Endocarditis, endovascular infections are caused by seeding of atherosclerotic plaques or aneurysms
  4. Hepatic (Fig. 189–4) or splenic abscesses in patients with underlying disease in these organs
  5. Urinary tract infections in patients with renal TB or schistosomiasis
  6. Salmonellae are a frequent cause of gram-negative meningitis in neonates
  7. Osteomyelitis in children with hemoglobinopathies (particularly sickle cell disease)

CAUSE
- More than 2000 serotypes of *Salmonella* exist, but only a few cause disease in humans.
- Some found only in humans are the cause of enteric fever.
  1. *S. typhi*
  2. *S. paratyphi*

Fig 189–1
Rose spots. In *Salmonella typhi* and *S. paratyphi* infections (enteric fever), classic rose spots of 1- to 3-mm in diameter can be found, especially on the abdominal wall, lower thorax, and back of the trunk. These are small erythematous macular lesions, which tend to come and go during infection.
(Courtesy of Anthony Bryceson.)

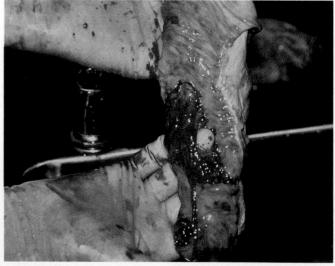

Fig 189–2
Perforating typhoid ulcer of the terminal ileum. This large, necrotic ulcer covered in dark brown slough is on the antimesentric side of the distal ileum. A gloved fingertip is seen within the large perforating ulcer that caused the patient's death.
(From Cohen J, Powderly WG: Infectious Diseases, 2nd ed. St Louis, Mosby, 2004.)

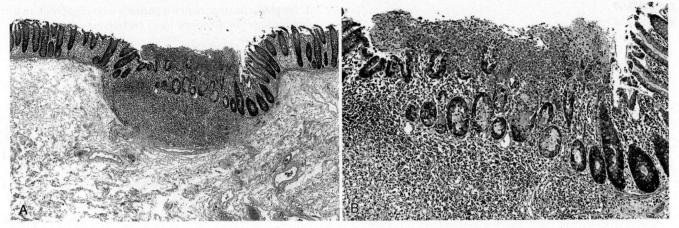

Fig 189–3
Salmonella colitis. (**A**) Severe colitis. (**B**) Necrosis involving a hyperplastic lymphoid follicle, a characteristic feature of Salmonella colitis.
(From Silverberg SG: Principles and Practice of Surgical Pathology and Cytopathology, 4th ed. Philadelphia, Churchill Livingstone, 2006.)

- Some responsible for gastroenteritis and frequently isolated from raw meat and poultry and uncooked or undercooked eggs.
  1. *S. typhimurium*
  2. *S. enteritidis*
- *S. cholerasuis* is a prototype organism that causes extraintestinal nontyphoidal disease.
- Transmission generally via ingestion of contaminated food or drink.
- Outbreaks of gastroenteritis related to contaminated poultry, meat, and dairy products.
- Typhoid fever is a systemic illness caused by serotypes exclusive to humans.
  1. Acquisition by ingestion of food or water contaminated by other humans
  2. Most cases in the United States are:
     a. Acquired during foreign travel
     b. Acquired by ingestion of food prepared by chronic carriers, many of whom have acquired the organism outside of the United States

DIFFERENTIAL DIAGNOSIS

- Other causes of prolonged fever:
  1. Malaria
  2. TB
  3. Brucellosis
  4. Amebic liver abscess
- Other causes of gastroenteritis:
  1. Bacterial: *Shigella, Yersinia, Campylobacter*
  2. Viral: Norwalk virus, rotavirus
  3. Parasitic: *Amoeba histolytica, Giardia lamblia*
  4. Toxic: enterotoxigenic *E. coli, Clostridium difficile*

WORKUP

- Typhoid fever
1. Cultures of blood, stool, urine; repeat if initially negative.
2. Blood cultures are more likely to be positive early in the course of illness.
3. Stool and urine cultures are more commonly positive in the second and third weeks of illness.

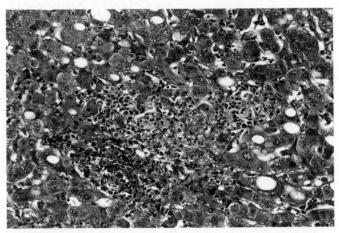

Fig 189–4
Typhoid fever. Numerous microabscesses are present in the liver due to hematogenous dissemination of the infection.
(From Silverberg SG: Principles and Practice of Surgical Pathology and Cytopathology, 4th ed. Philadelphia, Churchill Livingstone, 2006.)

4. Highest yield with bone marrow biopsy cultures:
   a. 90% positive
5. Serology using Widal's test is helpful in retrospect, showing a fourfold increase in convalescent titers.
- Gastroenteritis: stool cultures
- Extraintestinal localized infection:
  1. Blood cultures
  2. Cultures from the site of infection

LABORATORY TESTS

- Neutropenia is common
- Transaminitis is possible
- Culture to grow organism: blood, body fluids, biopsy specimens

IMAGING STUDIES

- Radiographs of bone may be suggestive of osteomyelitis.
- CT scan or sonogram of abdomen:
  1. May reveal hepatic or splenic abscesses
  2. May reveal aortic aneurysm

TREATMENT

- Typhoid fever:
  1. Ciprofloxacin 500 mg PO bid or 400 mg IV bid for 14 days
  2. Ceftriaxone 2 g IV qd for 14 days
  3. If sensitive, may switch therapy to TMP/SMX 1 to 2 DS tabs PO bid or amoxicillin 2 g PO q8h to complete 14 days
  4. Dexamethasone 3 mg IV initially, followed by 1 mg IV q6h for eight doses for patients with shock or mental status changes
- Gastroenteritis:
  1. Treatment generally not indicated for gastroenteritis alone because this illness is usually self-limited
  2. May prolong the carrier state

  3. Prophylactic treatment for patients who are at high risk of developing complications from bacteremia
     a. Neonates
     b. Patients with hemoglobinopathies
     c. Patients with atherosclerosis
     d. Patients with aneurysms
     e. Patients with prosthetic devices
     f. Immunocompromised patients
  4. Treatment can be oral or parenteral, with the same regimens used for typhoid, but only for 48 to 72 hours
- Intravascular infections require 6 weeks of parenteral therapy.
- Adequate hydration and electrolyte replacement in persons with diarrhea

Chapter 190 / Cholera

DEFINITION
Cholera is an acute diarrheal illness caused by *Vibrio cholere*.

PHYSICAL FINDINGS AND CLINICAL PRESENTATION
Infection may result in asymptomatic illness or a mild diarrhea. The classic illness is described as the abrupt onset of voluminous watery diarrhea, which may lead to severe dehydration (Fig. 190–1), acidosis, shock, and death. Vomiting may occur early in the illness, but fever and abdominal pain are usually absent. The typical "rice water" stools are pale with flecks of mucus and contain no blood. Muscle cramps may be prominent, and are the result of loss of fluid and electrolytes. Untreated illness results in hypovolemic shock, and death may occur in hours to days. With adequate fluid and electrolyte repletion, cholera is a self-limited illness that resolves in a few days. The use of antimicrobials can shorten the course of illness.

CAUSE
The organism responsible for this illness is one of several strains of *V. cholere*. Most infections result from the 01 serotype, the El Tor biotype. In the United States, one outbreak occurred from the ingestion of illegally imported crab, and sporadic infection has been associated with the consumption of contaminated shellfish in Gulf Coast states. Most cases are seen in returning travelers. Transmission during epidemics is the result of the ingestion of contaminated water and, in some instances, contaminated food.

DIFFERENTIAL DIAGNOSIS
- Mild illness may mimic gastroenteritis resulting from a variety of etiologies.
- Sudden, voluminous diarrhea causing marked dehydration is uncommon in other illnesses.

LABORATORY TESTS
- WBC may be elevated, and hemoglobin may be increased as a result of hemoconcentration.
- Elevated bun and creatinine suggests prerenal azotemia. Hypoglycemia may occur. Stool cultures on appropriate media may grow the organism. Wet mount of stool under dark field or phase contrast microscopy shows organisms with characteristic darting motility.

TREATMENT
The mainstay of therapy is adequate fluid and electrolyte replacement. This can usually be achieved using oral rehydration solutions containing salts and glucose (Fig. 190–2). Some patients may require intravenous fluid and electrolyte replacement.
- Antimicrobial therapy can decrease shedding of fluid and organisms and can shorten the course of illness: doxycycline, *or* SMX-TMP.

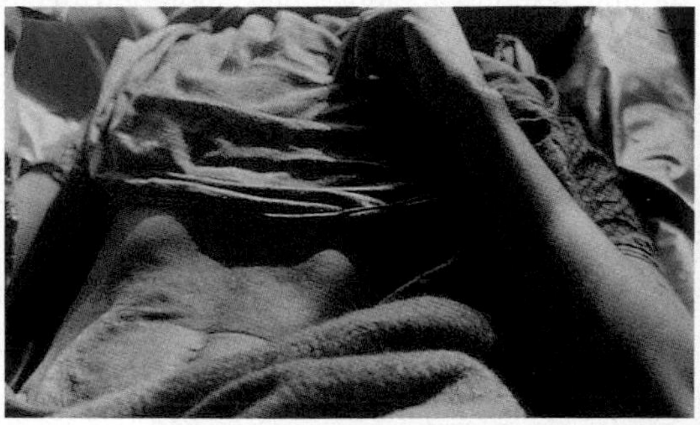

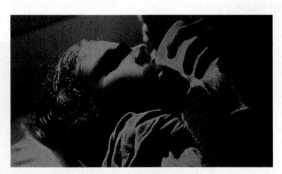

Fig 190–1
Severe dehydration from cholera. Decreased skin turgor in a severely dehydrated cholera patient.
(Courtesy of the International Centre for Diarrhoeal Disease Research, Bangladesh.)

Fig 190–2
Oral rehydration. The patient is immediately given ORS to correct her dehydration.
(Courtesy of the International Centre for Diarrhoeal Disease Research, Bangladesh.)

Chapter 191 Whipple's disease

DEFINITION

Whipple's disease is a multisystem illness characterized by malabsorption and its consequences, lymphadenopathy, arthritis, cardiac involvement, ocular symptoms and neurologic problems, caused by the gram-positive bacillus *Tropheryma whippelii*.

PHYSICAL FINDINGS AND CLINICAL PRESENTATION

Physical findings

- Abdominal distention, sometimes with tenderness and less commonly fullness or mass, which represents enlarged mesenteric lymph nodes
- Signs of weight loss, cachexia
- Clubbing
- Lymphadenopathy
- Inflamed joints
- Heart murmur or rub
- Sensory loss or motor weakness related to peripheral neuropathy
- Abnormal mental status examination
- Pallor

Clinical presentation

The disease may present with extraintestinal symptoms (e.g., arthralgia), but few clinicians will suspect the diagnosis unless or until GI symptoms are present. Weight loss, diarrhea, and arthropathies are found together in 75% of patients at time of presentation.

- The GI manifestations are those seen in malabsorption of any cause.

- Diarrhea: 5-10 semiformed, malodorous steatorrheic stools per day
- Abdominal bloating and cramps
- Anorexia
- Extraintestinal manifestations of malabsorption
  - Weight loss, fatigue
  - Anemia
  - Bleeding diathesis
  - Edema and ascites
  - Osteomalacia
- Extraintestinal involvement
  - Arthritis (intermittent, migratory, affecting small, large, and axial joints)
  - Pleuritic chest pain and cough
  - Pericarditis, endocarditis
  - Dementia, ophthalmoplegia, myoclonus, and many other neurologic symptoms, because any portion of the central nervous system may be a disease site
  - Fever

CAUSE AND PATHOGENESIS

- Infectious disease caused by *Tropheryma whippelii*, an actinobacter.
- The bacillus has never been cultured, nor has direct transmission from patient to patient ever been documented; however, the agent can be seen in tissue samples by electron microscopy and identified by polymerase chain reaction (PCR) (Fig. 191–1).
- Predictable response to appropriate antibiotic therapy confirms the pathogenic role of the infection.

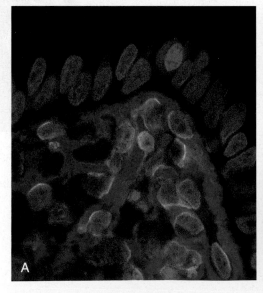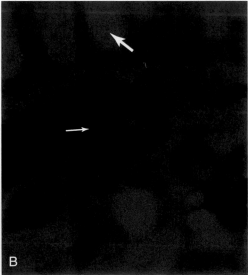

Fig 191–1
Fluorescence micrographs of a formalin fixed intestinal biopsy from a patient with Whipple's disease. (**A**) Confocal micrograph demonstrating hybridization of a fluorescent Tropheryma whippli rDNA probe (*blue*) to bacterial rRNA in a small intestine biopsy from a patient with Whipple's disease. Yo-pro dye (*green*) highlights cell nuclei and an anti-vimentin antibody (*red*) labels the cytoskeletal protein of human mesenchymal cells. Bacteria localize to the lamina propria and appear abundant in the extracellular spaces. Macrophages and polymorphonuclear leukocytes infiltrate the lamina propria of this enlarged villus. (**B**) Confocal micrograph of Whipple's disease intestine showing clumps of small bacillary bodies in the lamina propria stained with Yo-pro nucleic acid dye in green (*small arrow*), and a human epithelial cell nucleus (*large arrow*). The extremely small size of the Whipple bacillus makes detection difficult using standard methods.
(From Cohen J, Powderly WG: Infectious Diseases, 2nd ed. St Louis, Mosby, 2004.)

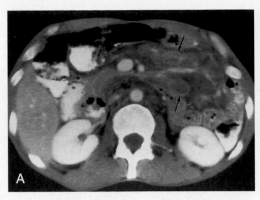
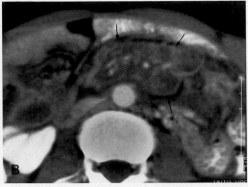

Fig 191–2
Whipple's disease. (**A**) Low-attenuation lymph nodes are seen within the small bowel mesentery (*arrows*). (**B**) In the mesenteric root the nodes become confluent (*arrows*) and are associated with increased attenuation of the mesenteric fat reflecting small bowel edema.
(From Grainger RG, Allison DJ, Adam A, Dixon AK [eds]: Grainger and Allison's Diagnostic Radiology, 4th ed. Philadelphia, Churchill Livingstone, 2001.)

- Tissue infiltration by macrophages is believed to be the mechanism of specific organ dysfunction and symptoms.
- Subtle defects of the cell-mediated immunity exist in active and inactive Whipple's disease that may predispose certain individuals to clinical manifestations. HLA-B27 positivity is found in 26% of patients (four times higher than expected).

DIFFERENTIAL DIAGNOSIS
Malabsorption/maldigestion
- Celiac disease
- *Mycobacterium avium-intracellulare* intestinal infection in patients with AIDS
- Intestinal lymphoma
- Abetalipoproteinemia
- Amyloidosis
- Systemic mastocytosis
- Radiation enteritis
- Crohn's disease
- Short bowel syndrome
- Pancreatic insufficiency
- Intestinal bacterial overgrowth
- Lactose deficiency
- Postgastrectomy syndrome
- Seronegative inflammatory arthritis
- Pericarditis and pleuritis
- Lymphadenitis
- Neurologic disorders

LABORATORY TESTS
- Anemia (iron, folate, or vitamin B_{12} deficiency)
- Hypokalemia
- Hypocalcemia
- Hypomagnesemia
- Hypoalbuminemia
- Prolonged prothrombin time
- Low serum carotene
- Low cholesterol
- Leukocytosis
- Steatorrhea demonstrated by a Sudan fecal fat stain
- 72-Hour stool collection demonstrating more than 7 g/24 hours of fat in the stool is impractical to perform, especially in ambulatory patients
- Defective d-xylose absorption

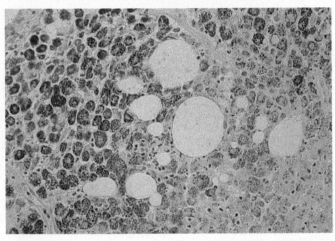

Fig 191–3
Section from a PAS-stained duodenal biopsy. There are numerous (pink-staining) PAS-positive macrophages in the lamina propria.
(From Cohen J, Powderly WG: Infectious Diseases, 2nd ed. St Louis, Mosby, 2004.)

IMAGING STUDIES
Small bowel x-rays after barium ingestion often show thickening of mucosal folds. CT scan may reveal low-attenuation lymph nodes and small bowel edema (Fig. 191–2)

BIOPSY
Infiltration of the intestinal lamina propria by PAS-positive macrophages (Fig. 191–3) containing gram-positive, acid-fast negative bacilli, associated with lymphatic dilation (diagnostic); PCR of the involved tissue in uncertain cases

TREATMENT
- Antibiotics: TMP/SMX DS bid for 6 to 12 months.
- Alternative antibiotics: penicillin alone, penicillin plus streptomycin, ampicillin, tetracycline, ceftriaxone.
- Treat specific vitamin, mineral, and nutrient deficiencies.
- In severely ill patients, oral therapy should be preceded by 2 weeks of parenteral therapy (e.g., ceftriaxone 2 g/day IV for 14 days).

Chapter 192   Mesenteric adenitis

DEFINITION

Acute mesenteric lymphadenitis is a syndrome of acute right lower quadrant abdominal pain associated with mesenteric lymph node enlargement and a normal appendix.

PHYSICAL FINDINGS AND CLINICAL PRESENTATION

- Abdominal pain of varying severity (mild ache to severe colic) beginning in upper abdomen or right lower quadrant, eventually localizes in right side but not in a precise location (unlike appendicitis)
- In *Yersinia* infection outbreaks, the symptoms include abdominal pain (84%), diarrhea (78%), fever (43%), anorexia (22%), nausea (13%), and vomiting (8%)

Physical Findings

- Other lymphadenopathy (20% of cases)
- Right lower quadrant tenderness (site of maximum tenderness may vary from one examination to the next)
- Guarding (rare)
- Mild fever

CAUSE AND PATHOGENESIS

- Reactive hyperplasia of lymph nodes that drain the ileocecal region, similar to that seen in inflammatory or allergic conditions. One study reported that approximately two thirds of cases are secondary (reactive) and one third are primary (no demonstrable associated inflammatory process).
- *Yersinia enterocolitica, Yersinia pseudotuberculosis* (Fig. 192–1), *Salmonella* species, *E. coli*, streptococci have been implicated with mesenteric adenitis.

DIFFERENTIAL DIAGNOSIS

- Acute appendicitis (see Fig. 161–1) (5% to 10% of patients admitted to hospitals with a diagnosis of appendicitis are discharged with a diagnosis of mesenteric adenitis)
- Crohn's disease

LABORATORY TESTS (see Fig. 162–5)

- CBC may show leukocytosis
- Abdominal sonography and helical appendiceal CT scan may be useful
- Laparotomy if appendicitis is suspected

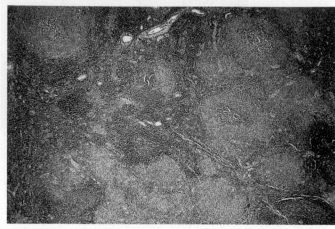

Fig 192–1

Yersinia mesenteric lymphadenitis. Multiple stellate granulomas with central necrosis replace a mesenteric lymph node. The inflammation extends into the surrounding perinodal fat. The preoperative diagnosis was acute suppurative appendicitis, but the appendix was macroscopically and microscopically normal (HANDE, ×5, *Yersinia pseudotuberculosis* isolated from cultures).
(From Silverberg SG: Principles and Practice of Surgical Pathology and Cytopathology, 4th ed. Philadelphia, Churchill Livingstone, 2006.)

| Chapter 193 | **Pseudomembranous colitis** |

DEFINITION

Pseudomembranous colitis is the occurrence of diarrhea and bowel inflammation (Fig. 193-1) associated with antibiotic use.

PHYSICAL FINDINGS AND CLINICAL PRESENTATION

- Abdominal tenderness (generalized or lower abdominal)
- Fever
- In patients with prolonged diarrhea, poor skin turgor, dry mucous membranes, and other signs of dehydration may be present

CAUSE

Risk factors for *C. difficile* (the major identifiable agent of antibiotic-induced diarrhea and colitis):

- Administration of antibiotics: can occur with any antibiotic, but occurs most frequently with clindamycin, ampicillin, and cephalosporins
- Prolonged hospitalization
- Advanced age
- Abdominal surgery
- Hospitalized, tube-fed patients are at risk for *C. difficile*–associated diarrhea. Clinicians should consider testing for *C. difficile* in tube-fed patients with diarrhea unrelated to the feeding solution

DIFFERENTIAL DIAGNOSIS

- GI bacterial infections (e.g., *Salmonella* [see Fig. 189-2], *Shigella*, *Campylobacter*, *Yersinia* [see Fig. 192-1])
- Enteric parasites (e.g., *Cryptosporidium*, *Entamoeba histolytica*)
- IBD (see Fig. 163-2)
- Celiac sprue (see Fig. 158-2)
- Irritable bowel syndrome
- Ischemic colitis
- Antibiotic intolerance (see Fig. 194-2)

LABORATORY TESTS

- *C. difficile* toxin can be detected by cytotoxin tissue-culture assay (gold standard for identifying *C. difficile* toxin in stool specimen). This test is difficult to perform and results are not available for 24 to 48 hours. A more useful test enzyme-linked immunoabsorbent assay (ELISA) for *C. difficile* toxins A and B. The latter is used most widely in the clinical setting. It has a sensitivity of 85% and a specificity of 100%.
- Fecal leukocytes (assessed by microscopy or lactoferrin assay) are generally present in stool samples.
- CBC usually reveals leukocytosis. A sudden increase in WBC to >30,000/mm³ may be indicative of fulminant colitis.
- Sigmoidoscopy (without cleansing enema) may be necessary when the clinical and laboratory diagnosis is inconclusive and the diarrhea persists. Biopsy (see Fig. 193-1) when diagnosis is unclear.
- In antibiotic-induced pseudomembranous colitis, the sigmoidoscopy often reveals raised white-yellow exudative plaques adherent to the colonic mucosa (Fig. 193-2)

IMAGING STUDIES

Abdominal film (flat plate and upright) is useful in patients presenting with abdominal pain or evidence of obstruction on physical examination. CT of abdomen may reveal edematous swollen haustra compressed together (accordion sign) (Fig. 193-3)

TREATMENT

- Discontinue offending antibiotic
- Fluid hydration and correct electrolyte abnormalities
- Metronidazole
- Vancomycin in cases resistant to metronidazole
- Cholestyramine in addition to metronidazole to control severe diarrhea (avoid use with vancomycin)

Fig 193-1
Biopsy appearance of *C. difficile*–associated pseudomembranous colitis.
(From Silverberg SG: Principles and Practice of Surgical Pathology and Cytopathology, 4th ed. Philadelphia, Churchill Livingstone, 2006.)

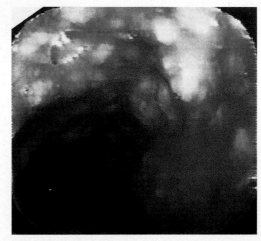

Fig 193-2
Endoscopic view of multiple pseudomembranes covering the colon in a patient with PMC.
(From Cohen J, Powderly WG: Infectious Diseases, 2nd ed. St Louis, Mosby, 2004.)

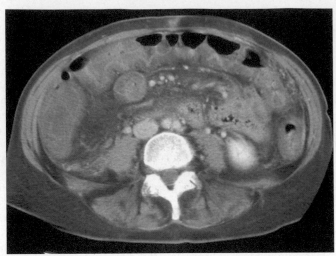

Fig 193–3
CT of pseudomembranous enterocolitis with the "accordion sign," where edematous swollen haustra are compressed together.
(Reproduced with the kind permission of Dr. A. McLean, St. Bartholomew's Hospital.)

VASCULAR

Chapter 194 · Mesenteric ischemia

DEFINITION
Acute mesenteric ischemia (AMI) is the sudden onset of intestinal hypoperfusion, caused by emboli, arterial or venous thrombosis, or by vasoconstriction due to low flow states.

PHYSICAL FINDINGS AND CLINICAL PRESENTATION
- The classic presentation is in the patient with risk factors, presenting with the rapid onset of severe periumbilical pain out of proportion to physical examination findings.
- Nausea and vomiting are commonly associated.
- Initial abdominal examination may be normal, with no rebound or guarding, or show minimal distention, or OB positive stool.
- Later in the course, the patient may present with gross distention, absence of bowel sounds, and peritoneal signs. In the elderly, mental status changes may be found.

CAUSE
The pathophysiologic mechanisms that cause AMI include:
- Mesenteric arterial embolism—typically from the left atrium, left ventricle or cardiac valves. The superior mesenteric artery is most commonly affected.
- Mesenteric arterial thrombosis—often in patients with prior progressive atherosclerotic stenoses, with superimposed abdominal trauma or infection.
- Mesenteric venous thrombosis (MVT) may occur in the setting of hypercoagulable states (acquired or inherited), blunt trauma, abdominal infection, portal hypertension, pancreatitis and portal malignancy.
- Non occlusive mesenteric ischemia (NOMI), usually occurs in the setting of atherosclerotic vascular disease, often in a patient with an acute cardiovascular disease process, who is being treated with drugs that reduce intestinal perfusion. This may include patients with recent cardiac surgery and dialysis patients. Cocaine use has also been a causative factor in a number of cases.

DIFFERENTIAL DIAGNOSIS
- Initially include other causes of abdominal pain of acute onset including perforated peptic ulcer, early appendicitis neoplasm (Fig. 194–1). Ultimately, the varied causes of peritonitis.

WORKUP
- Success of treatment is related to the duration of symptoms prior to diagnosis.
- Consider early laparotomy for diagnosis in cases with a high index of suspicion, where angiography is not available.

LABORATORY TEST(S)
- Laboratory test results are nonspecific, especially early in the course. Later they can include leukocytosis, acidosis, and elevated hematocrit due to hemoconcentration. Most abnormalities occur after progression to bowel necrosis.
- When a hypercoagulable state is suspected, work up may include proteins C and S, antithrombin III, and Factor V Leiden). This will likely not affect the diagnosis of AMI but may help guide long-term therapy.

IMAGING STUDIES
- The gold standard is mesenteric angiography (see Fig. 194–1).
- With strong clinical suspicion, workup should proceed directly to angiography, without delay for CT scan or other testing.
- Plain films are normal 25% of the time in the early stages. Suggestive findings may include ileus, thumbprinting (Fig. 194–2), bowel wall thickening, or intramural gas (Fig. 194–3). Intraluminal barium should not be used as it is rarely helpful in making a positive diagnosis, and will interfere with angiographic studies.
- Doppler ultrasound evaluation of intestinal blood flow is often limited by the presence of air filled loops of bowel.
- CT scan findings also are commonly nonspecific, and more often found late in the course. Portal venous gas or intramural

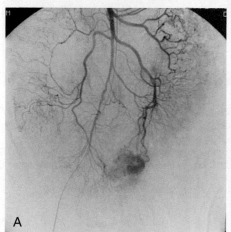 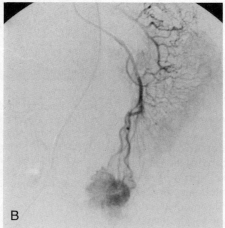 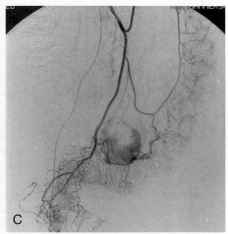

Fig 194–1
(**A**) A selective superior mesenteric artery angiogram demonstrates a vascular small bowel tumor in the left lower quadrant supplied by the last jejunal artery consistent with a leiomyoma. (**B**) A selective jejunal artery angiogram better demonstrates the vascular supply to this neoplasm. (**C**) A selective inferior mesenteric artery angiogram shows a significant supply to the same jejunal tumors from sigmoid artery branches, an important preoperative finding.
(From Grainger RG, Allison DJ, Adam A, Dixon AK [eds]: Grainger and Allison's Diagnostic Radiology, 4th ed. Philadelphia, Churchill Livingstone, 2001.)

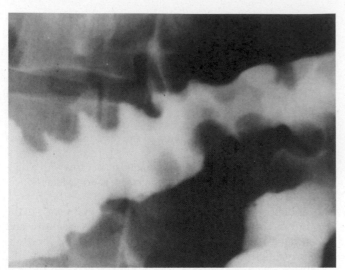

Fig 194–2
Thumbprinting in acute ischemic colitis at the splenic flexure.
(From Grainger RG, Allison DJ, Adam A, Dixon AK [eds]: Grainger and Allison's Diagnostic Radiology, 4th ed. Philadelphia, Churchill Livingstone, 2001.)

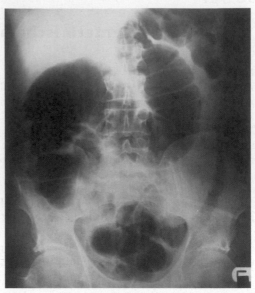

Fig 194–3
Ischemic colitis: supine. A thick-walled edematous descending colon outlined by gas. Slightly distended colon from cecum to splenic flexure, but with normal haustra and no evidence of abnormal mucosa.
(From Grainger RG, Allison DJ, Adam A, Dixon AK [eds]: Grainger and Allison's Diagnostic Radiology, 4th ed. Philadelphia, Churchill Livingstone, 2001.)

gas may be seen after the development of gangrene, but in many cases even at that advanced stage CT findings remain nonspecific.

- CT scanning has been found to be more useful in cases of mesenteric vein thrombosis causing AMI (Fig. 194–4), with sensitivity approaching 90%. It has also been found useful in monitoring the progress of patients with superior mesenteric venous thrombosis who are treated nonsurgically.
- MRA may prove to be useful, but significant data comparing this with angiography are needed.

TREATMENT
- The goal of treatment is to restore blood flow as rapidly as possible to ischemic bowel, before the occurrence of infarction.
- Initial management should include hemodynamic monitoring and support, correction of acidosis, administration of broad-spectrum antibiotics and gastric decompression via NG tube.
- Vasoconstricting agents should be avoided.
- Systemic anticoagulation may be started, although the timing of initiation is unclear.
- Signs of peritonitis mandate early laparotomy and resection of infarcted bowel.
- When work-up is positive for major superior mesenteric artery (SMA) embolus, embolectomy is considered standard treatment, in the absence of peritoneal signs. Depending on the location and degree of occlusion of the embolus, surgical revascularization, intra-arterial infusion of thrombolytics or vasodilators, or systemic anticoagulation may be considered.
- In cases of SMA thrombosis, emergency surgical revascularization is the treatment of choice.
- Angiography is needed to diagnose nonocclusive mesenteric ischemia before infarct, and should be followed by intra-arterial vasodilator infusion. This approach has been shown to significantly reduce mortality in this situation.

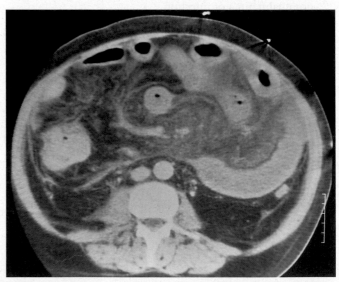

Fig 194–4
Mesenteric ischemia due to thrombosis of the superior mesenteric vein (not shown). Unenhanced CT shows diffuse haziness of the affected small bowel mesentery with effacement of the vascular markings, reflecting edema, hemorrhage, and venous congestion. Note also the thickened high-attenuation bowel wall due to intramural hemorrhage.
(From Grainger RG, Allison DJ, Adam A, Dixon AK [eds]: Grainger and Allison's Diagnostic Radiology, 4th ed. Philadelphia, Churchill Livingstone, 2001.)

- In patients with mesenteric vein thrombosis, treatment is dependent on the presence or absence of peritoneal signs. Laparotomy and resection of infarcted bowel in more advanced cases, or if there are no peritoneal signs anticoagulant therapy, immediately with heparin, and ultimately with warfarin, may be adequate.

Chapter 195 | **Portal vein thrombosis**

DEFINITION

Portal vein thrombosis is thrombotic occlusion of the portal vein.

PHYSICAL FINDINGS AND CLINICAL PRESENTATION

Upper GI hemorrhage (hematemesis and/or melena) caused by esophageal varices. If abdominal pain is present, mesenteric venous thrombosis should be suspected

CAUSE AND PATHOPHYSIOLOGY

Cause: In children: umbilical sepsis (pathophysiology unknown)

In adults:

1. Hypercoagulable states
   - Antiphospholipid syndrome
   - Neoplasm (common cause)
   - Paroxysmal nocturnal hemoglobinuria
   - Myeloproliferative diseases
   - Oral contraceptives
   - Polycythemia vera
   - Pregnancy
   - Protein S or C deficiency
   - Sickle cell disease
   - Thrombocytosis
2. Inflammatory diseases
   - Crohn's disease
   - Pancreatitis
   - Ulcerative colitis
3. Complications of medical intervention
   - Ambulatory dialysis
   - Chemoembolization
   - Liver transplantation
   - Partial hepatectomy
   - Sclerotherapy
   - Splenectomy
   - Transjugular intrahepatic portosystemic shunt
4. Infections
   - Appendicitis
   - Diverticulitis
   - Cholecystitis
5. Miscellaneous
   - Cirrhosis (common cause)
   - Bladder cancer

Pathophysiology: portal vein thrombosis results in portal hypertension leading to esophageal and gastrointestinal varices. The liver sustained by the hepatic artery maintains normal function.

WORKUP

- Esophagogastroscopy shows esophageal varices.
- Abdominal ultrasound (Fig. 195–1), CT (Fig. 195–2), or MRI (Fig. 195–3) may show the portal vein thrombosis.

TREATMENT

- Variceal sclerotherapy or banding
- Surgical mesocaval or splenorenal shunt

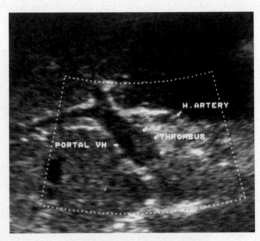

Fig 195–1

Portal venous thrombosis. Partial portal venous thrombosis is visible on B mode as echoreflective material on one side of the vein (*arrows*). Doppler examination is always required to assess patency as some thrombi are of reduced echoreflectivity and may not be visible on B mode.

(From Grainger RG, Allison DJ, Adam A, Dixon AK [eds]: Grainger and Allison's Diagnostic Radiology, 4th ed. Philadelphia, Churchill Livingstone, 2001.)

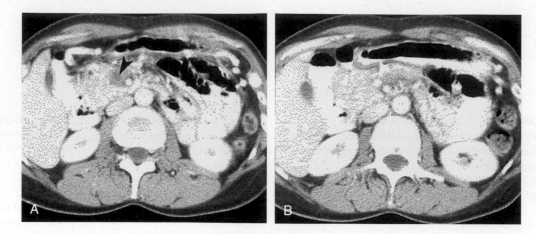

Fig 195–2
Portal vein thrombosis. Two adjacent CT (IV enhanced, portal phase) sections through the mesenteric root demonstrate a patent superior mesenteric vein (**B**, *white arrowhead*) which is occluded on the next section caranially (**A**, *black arrowhead*) just below the confluence with the splenic vein. Collateral veins are visible within and anterior to the pancreatic head.
(From Grainger RG, Allison DJ, Adam A, Dixon AK [eds]: Grainger and Allison's Diagnostic Radiology, 4th ed. Philadelphia, Churchill Livingstone, 2001.)

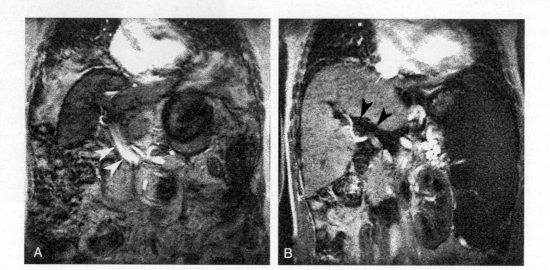

Fig 195–3
Portal vein thrombosis. (**A**) Flow-sensitive coronal magnetization prepared gradient-echo sections in two patients with cirrhosis and ascites demonstrate a patent portal vein (*white arrows*). (**B**) Completely occluded portal vein (*black arrows*). MRA using either time of flight or contrast-enhanced techniques can be diagnostic when Doppler US is equivocal or technically limited.
(From Grainger RG, Allison DJ, Adam A, Dixon AK [eds]: Grainger and Allison's Diagnostic Radiology, 4th ed. Philadelphia, Churchill Livingstone, 2001.)

Chapter 196 Budd-Chiari syndrome

DEFINITION

Budd-Chiari syndrome (BCS) is a rare disease defined by the obstruction of hepatic venous outflow anywhere from the small hepatic veins to the junction of the inferior vena cava and the right atrium. Primary BCS is defined by endoluminal obstruction as seen in thromboses or webs. Secondary BCS is when the obstruction is due to nonvascular invasion (malignancy or parasitic masses) or extrinsic compression (tumor, abscess, cysts).

CLINICAL PRESENTATION

Variable according to the degree, location, acuity of obstruction, and presence of collateral circulation

- Fulminant/acute: (uncommon) severe RUQ abdominal pain, fever, nausea, vomiting, jaundice, hepatomegaly, ascites, marked elevation in serum aminotransferases and drop in coagulation factors, and encephalopathy. Early recognition and treatment are essential to survival.
- Subacute/chronic: (more common) vague abdominal discomfort, gradual progression to hepatomegaly, portal hypertension with or without cirrhosis; late-onset ascites, lower extremity edema, esophageal varices, splenomegaly, coagulopathy, hepatorenal syndrome, and rarely, encephalopathy.
- Asymptomatic: usually discovered incidentally.

CAUSE

Myeloproliferative disease, often discovered in cases of initially idiopathic BCS, 20% to 53%

- Polycythemia vera, responsible for 10% to 40% of cases
- Essential thrombocytosis
- Myelofibrosis
  Hypercoagulable states, often coexist with other causes, up to 31%
- Protein C deficiency
- Protein S deficiency
- Antithrombin III deficiency
- Activated protein C resistance/factor V Leiden mutation
- Prothrombin gene mutation
- Methylene-tetrahydrofolate reductase mutation
- Antiphospholipid antibody syndrome
- Homocystinemia
- Pregnancy
- Oral contraceptive pills
- Sickle cell anemia
- Infection:
  - Liver abscess (amebic)
  - Filariasis
  - Schistosomiasis
  - Hydatid cyst (echinococcosis)
  - Syphilis
  - Tuberculosis
  - Aspergillosis
- Malignancy, <5%
  - Adrenal carcinoma
  - Ovarian
  - Bronchogenic
  - Renal-cell carcinoma
  - Hepatocellular carcinoma
  - Leiomyosarcoma
  - Metastatic cancer
- Other:
  - Sarcoid
  - Behçet's disease
  - Paroxysmal nocturnal hemoglobinuria
  - IVC membrane/congenital web
  - Abdominal trauma
  - Ulcerative colitis
  - Celiac disease
  - Dacarbazine therapy
  - Idiopathic

DIFFERENTIAL DIAGNOSIS

- Shock liver/ischemic hepatitis
- Viral hepatitis
- Toxic hepatitis
- Hepatic veno-occlusive disease (sinusoidal obstruction syndrome)
- Alcoholic hepatitis
- Cholecystitis
- Cardiac cirrhosis (i.e., chronic right-sided heart failure and anything causing it)
- Tricuspid regurgitation
- Right atrial myxoma
- Constrictive pericarditis
- Alcoholic cirrhosis
- Cirrhosis of other etiologies:
  - Wilson's disease
  - Hemochromatosis
  - Alpha-$_1$ antitrypsin deficiency
  - Autoimmune

LABORATORY TESTS

Assessment of liver injury and function:

- Serum aminotransferases, prothrombin time, albumin, bilirubin

Diagnostic tests (directed by history):

- CBC, bone marrow biopsy, viral hepatitis panel, alpha-$_1$ antitrypsin, serum iron, transferrin saturation, alkaline phosphatase, ceruloplasmin, toxicology screen, antismooth muscle antibody, antimitochondrial antibody, and double-stranded DNA antibody. Tests for hypercoagulable states (particularly protein C, protein S, and antithrombin deficiencies) may be difficult to interpret as many levels are abnormal because of liver dysfunction. Family studies may be the only way to identify a primary hypercoagulable disorder. Evaluation of ascitic fluid reveals a high serum-ascitic fluid albumin gradient (SAAG), mimicking the ascitic fluid in patients with cardiac disease.

IMAGING STUDIES

- Color and pulsed Doppler U/S (Fig. 196–1)—diagnostic sensitivity and specificity 85%-90%.
- MRI with gadolinium contrast—better than contrast-enhanced CT (Fig. 196–1), sensitivity/specificity of about 90%.

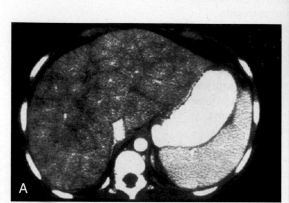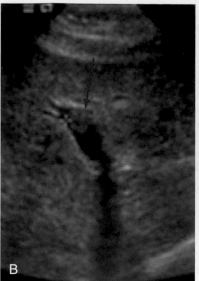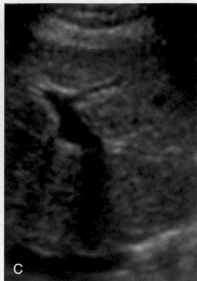

Fig 196–1

A, contrast computed tomography scan of the liver in a patient with Budd-Chiari syndrome. The hepatic veins are not visualized and there is centrilobular congestion (nutmeg liver). **B,** Thrombosis in the portal vein demonstrated by sonogram, which is no longer present after infusion of tissue plasminogen activator **(C).**

(From Young NS, Gerson SL, High KA [eds]: Clinical Hematology, St Louis, 2006, Mosby.)

- Venography is not essential for diagnosis, but when done with measurement of pressure gradients is mainly indicated to predict success of surgical shunt intervention. It confirms the classic spider web pattern caused by collateral venous flow, and look for BCS in cases of high clinical suspicion when initial studies are negative.
- Liver biopsy not necessary to diagnose BCS but may be helpful in patients with cirrhosis in whom the diagnosis remains uncertain and the differential still includes sinusoidal obstruction syndrome, cirrhosis of other origins, and malignancy. Of note, long-standing BCS is characterized by large, regenerative nodules in the liver that are indistinguishable from hepatocellular carcinoma on imaging.

TREATMENT

- Transjugular intrahepatic portosystemic shunt or stent placement in the hepatic vein have been shown in case studies to provide a "bridge" to orthotopic liver transplantation by correcting the hepatic outflow problem. These treatments are used sequentially.

- Orthotopic liver transplantation replaces the need for shunts or stents and in addition may correct the underlying coagulopathy causing thrombosis in the hepatic vein.
- Angioplasty and stenting, in situ thrombolysis, or removal of IVC webs to decompress the portal circulation, all combined with anticoagulation may be indicated for acute BCS in patients in stable condition.
- TIPSS (transjugular intrahepatic portosystemic stent shunt) may be a decompression option but can be especially hazardous in BCS patients because of the high prevalence of hepatic vein thromboses.
- Liver transplant may be indicated for fulminant BCS or patients that fail the previous therapies.

ENDOCRINE GASTROINTESTINAL DISORDERS

Chapter 197 **Carcinoid**

DEFINITION
Carcinoid syndrome is a symptom complex characterized by paroxysmal vasomotor disturbances, diarrhea, and broncho-spasm. It is caused by the action of amines and peptides (sero-tonin, bradykinin, histamine) produced by tumors arising from neuroendocrine cells. Sites of carcinoid tumors are described in (Table 197–1)

PHYSICAL FINDINGS AND CLINICAL PRESENTATION
- Cutaneous flushing (75% to 90%)
  1. The patient usually has red-purple flushes starting in the face (Fig. 197–1), then spreading to the neck and upper trunk.
  2. The flushing episodes last from a few minutes to hours (longer-lasting flushes may be associated with bronchial carcinoids).
  3. Flushing may be triggered by emotion, alcohol, or foods, or it may occur spontaneously.
  4. Dizziness, tachycardia, and hypotension may be associated with the cutaneous flushing.
- Diarrhea (>70%): often associated with abdominal bloat-ing and audible peristaltic rushes
- Intermittent bronchospasm (25%): characterized by severe dyspnea and wheezing
- Facial telangiectasia
- Tricuspid regurgitation from carcinoid heart lesions

CAUSE
- The carcinoid syndrome is caused by neoplasms originating from neuroendocrine cells (Fig. 197–2).
- Carcinoid tumors do not usually produce the syndrome un-less liver metastases are present or the primary tumor does not involve the GI tract.

DIFFERENTIAL DIAGNOSIS
The carcinoid syndrome must be distinguished from idiopathic flushing (IF); patients with IF more often are females, younger, and with a longer duration of symptoms; palpitations, syncope, and hypotension occur primarily in patients with IF.

TABLE 197–1 Sites of carcinoid tumors

Site	Incidence (%)
Appendix	40
Small bowel	25
Rectum	15
Bronchus	10
Colon	5
Stomach	<5
Duodenum	
Pancreas	<1
Ovary	
Testis	

From Besser CM, Thorner MO: Comprehensive Clinical Endocrinology, 3rd ed. St Louis, Mosby, 2002.

LABORATORY TESTS
- The biochemical marker for carcinoid syndrome is increased 24-hours urinary 5-hydroxyindoleacetic acid (5-HIAA), a metabolite of serotonin (5-hydroxytryptamine).
- False elevations can be seen with ingestion of certain foods (bananas, pineapples, eggplant, avocados, walnuts) and certain medications (acetaminophen, caffeine, guai-fenesin, reserpine); therefore, patients should be on a re-stricted diet and should avoid these medications when the test is ordered.
Liver function studies are an unreliable indicator of liver involvement.

IMAGING STUDIES
- Chest x-ray is useful to detect bronchial carcinoids (Fig. 197–3).
- CT scan of the abdomen (Fig. 197–4) or an octreotide scan (Fig. 197–5) are useful to detect metastases

TREATMENT
- Surgical resection of the tumor (Fig. 197–6) can be curative if the tumor is localized or palliative and results in pro-longed asymptomatic periods if metastases are present. Surgical manipulation of the tumor can, however, cause se-vere vasomotor abnormalities and bronchospasm (carci-noid crisis).
- Percutaneous embolization and ligation of the hepatic artery can decrease the bulk of the tumor in the liver and provide palliative treatment of tumors with hepatic metastases.
- Cytotoxic chemotherapy: combination chemotherapy with 5-fluorouracil and streptozotocin can be used in patients with unresectable or recurrent carcinoid tumors; however, it has only limited success.
- Control of clinical manifestations:
  1. Diarrhea usually responds to diphenoxylate with atropine
  2. Flushing can be controlled by the combination of H_1- and H_2-receptor antagonists
  3. Somatostatin analogue (SMS 201-995) is effective for both flushing and diarrhea in most patients.
  4. Severe bronchospasm can be treated with aminophylline and/or albuterol.
- Nutritional support: supplemental niacin therapy may be useful to prevent pellagra, because the tumor uses dietary tryptophan for serotonin synthesis, resulting in a nutritional deficiency in some patients.
- Subcutaneous somatostatin analogues (octreotide, lanreo-tide) have been used successfully for long-term control of symptoms in patients with unresectable neoplasms.
- Echocardiography and monitoring for right-sided CHF are recommended for patients with unresectable disease be-cause endocardial fibrosis, involving predominantly the endocardium, chordae, and valves of the right side of the heart, can occur.

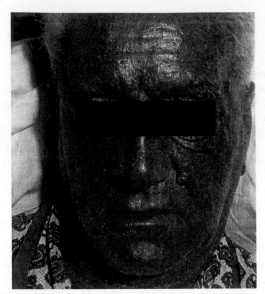

Fig 197–1
Carcinoid syndrome. Acute flushing can be seen.
(From Besser CM, Thorner MO: Comprehensive Clinical Endocrinology, 3rd ed. Mosby, 2002.)

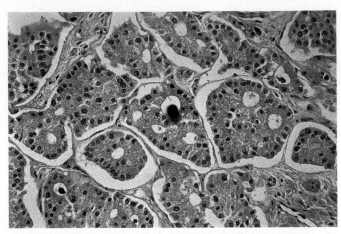

Fig 197–2
Carcinoid tumor. A high-power view shows both solid nests of cells and acinar structures with secretions. The secretions may stain positively with periodic acid-Schiff, mucicarmine, or Alcian blue. Note that the tumor cells have uniform round nuclei with a few coarse chromatin clumps. In typical carcinoid tumors, only minimal pleomorphism and hyperchromatism are found. Only a rare mitotic figure may be identified.
(From Silverberg SG: Principles and Practice of Surgical Pathology and Cytopathology, 4th ed. Philadelphia, Churchill Livingstone, 2006.)

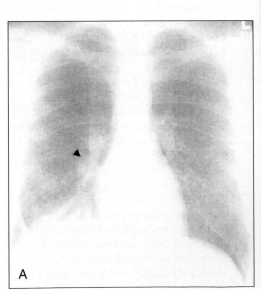
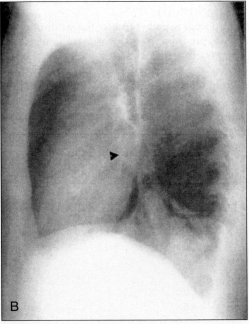

Fig 197–3
Carcinoid tumor. A 23-year-old man with history of recurring right lower-lobe "pneumonia." (**A, B**) Frontal and lateral chest radiographs show a right hilar mass (*arrowhead*). There is moderate right lower-lobe volume loss. Tubular opacities extending form the right inferior hilum represent dilated bronchi filled with impacted mucus. Biopsy showed a carcinoid tumor.
(From Grainger RG, Allison DJ, Adam A, Dixon AK [eds]: Grainger and Allison's Diagnostic Radiology, 4th ed. Philadelphia, Churchill Livingstone, 2001.)

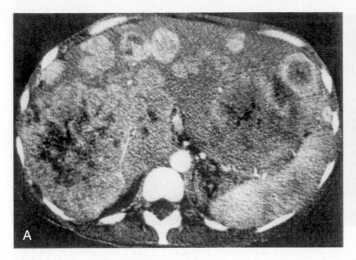
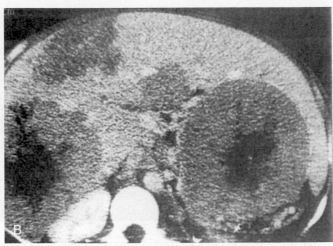

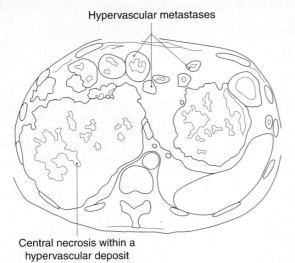
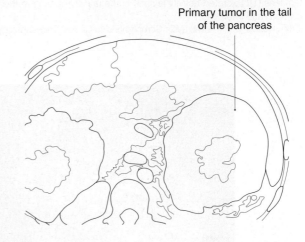

Hypervascular metastases

Primary tumor in the tail of the pancreas

Central necrosis within a hypervascular deposit

Fig 197–4

Liver metastases from a primary pancreatic carcinoid tumor: CT appearances. (**A**) The CT scan performed at 25 seconds following intravenous injection of contrast medium ("arterial" phase) shows typical hypervascular carcinoid liver metastases. The larger lesion in the right lobe shows central necrosis. (**B**) The CT scan performed at 75 seconds following intravenous injection of contrast medium ("portal venous" phase) shows that the vascular lesions have now become isodense with the normal liver parenchyma. The primary tumor in the tail of the pancreas in also clearly seen. As depicted here, carcinoid hepatic metastases are typically hypervascular and are optimally depicted during the arterial phase of a contrast-enhanced CT scan or MR image as they are isoattenuating when compared with adjacent hepatic parenchyma during the portal venous phase of enhancement.
(From Besser CM, Thorner MO: Comprehensive Clinical Endocrinology, 3rd ed. Mosby, 2002.)

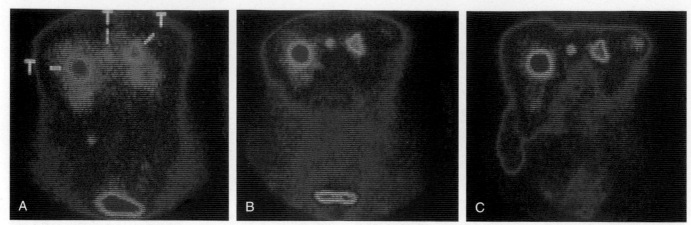

Fig 197–5

Metastatic carcinoid tumor. Indium (^{111}In)-labeled octreotide scans taken at (**A**) 10 minutes, (**B**) 4 hours, and (**C**) 21 hours show uptake in the metastases (T). Excreted activity is seen in the urinary bladder in the lower parts of (**A**) and (**B**). Note that on the delayed images the target-to-background ratio improves.

(From Besser CM, Thorner MO: Comprehensive Clinical Endocrinology, 3rd ed. Mosby, 2002.)

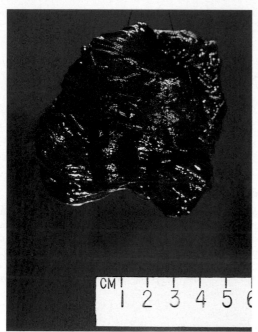

Fig 197–6

Carcinoid tumor of the distal duodenum. Two intramural masses bulge into the lumen, stretching the overlying mucosa. Pressure on the attenuated mucosa may result in ulceration and bleeding.

(From Silverberg SG: Principles and Practice of Surgical Pathology and Cytopathology, 4th ed. Philadelphia, Churchill Livingstone, 2006.)

Chapter 198 **Gastrinoma (Zollinger-Ellison syndrome)**

DEFINITION

Zollinger-Ellison (ZE) syndrome is a hypergastrinemic state caused by a pancreatic or extrapancreatic nonbeta islet cell tumor (gastrinoma) and resulting in peptic acid disease.

PHYSICAL FINDINGS AND CLINICAL PRESENTATION

- The vast majority of patients (95%) present with symptoms of peptic ulcer
- 60% of patients have symptoms related to gastroesophageal reflux disease
- One third of patients with ZE have diarrhea and, less commonly, steatorrhea.

The following circumstances warrant suspicion of ZE syndrome:

- Ulcers distal to the first portion of the duodenum
- Multiple peptic ulcers
- Ineffective treatment for peptic ulcer disease with the usual drug doses and schedules
- Peptic ulcer and diarrhea
- Familial history of peptic ulcer
- Patients with a personal or family history suggesting parathyroid or pituitary tumors of dysfunction
- Peptic ulcer and urinary tract calculi
- Patients with peptic ulcer who are negative for *H. pylori* and do not have a history of NSAID use

CAUSE

- The pathophysiologic manifestations of ZE syndrome are related to the effects of hypergastrinemia. Gastrin stimulates gastric acid secretion, which in turn is responsible for the development of duodenal ulcers and diarrhea. Gastrin also promotes gastric mucosal epithelial cell growth and resulting parietal cell hyperplasia.
- Gastrinomas are usually small (0.1-2 cm) but sometimes large (>20 cm) tumors.
- 60% of gastrinomas are malignant, with liver and regional lymph nodes the most common site of metastases. Histology is not a good predictor of the biology of gastrinomas.
- 60% of patients with multiple endocrine neoplasia-1 (MEN-1) have gastrinomas.
- 10% of patients with ZE syndrome have islet cell hyperplasia rather than gastrinomas; in 10% to 20% of patients with gastrinoma the tumors cannot be located because of small size.

DIFFERENTIAL DIAGNOSIS

- Peptic ulcer disease
- Gastroesophageal reflux disease

WORKUP

- Diagnosis of peptic ulcer
  - Endoscopy
  - UGI series (may also show prominent gastric rugal folds)
- Gastric acid secretion
  - Serum gastrin level (fasting) >150 pg/mL (causes of false-positive: pernicious anemia, renal failure, retained gastric antrum syndrome, diabetes mellitus, rheumatoid arthritis)
  - Provocative gastrin level tests
  - Secretin stimulation
  - Calcium stimulation
  - Standard test meal stimulation
- Gastrinoma localization
  - Arteriography (Fig. 198-1)
  - Abdominal sonography
  - Abdominal CT scan (see Fig. 198-1)
  - Abdominal MRI
  - Selective portal vein branch gastrin level
  - Octreotide scan (Fig. 198-2)

TREATMENT

- Surgical resection of the gastrinoma (NOTE: 90% of gastrinomas can be located, resulting in a 40% overall cure rate)
- Total gastrectomy or vagotomy (palliative in some patients)
- Medical treatment
  - Proton pump inhibitors (e.g., omeprazole or lansoprazole)
  - Somatostatin or octreotide
  - Chemotherapy for metastatic gastrinoma with streptozotocin, 5-FU, and doxorubicin

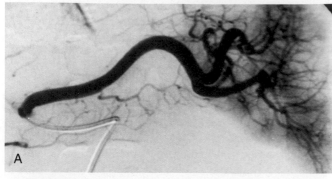

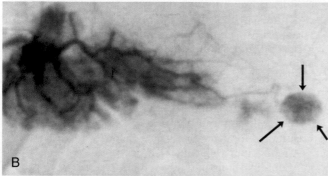

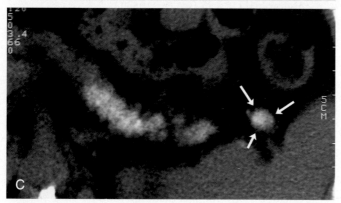

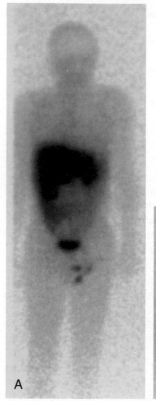

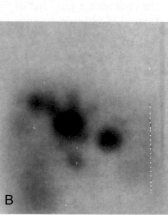

Fig 198–1

Selective pancreatic arteriography and arterially enhanced CT showing islet-cell tumor. (**A**) A celiac arteriogram shows no evidence of an islet-cell tumor—nor did the later films in this injection sequence. An oblique study (steep LAO) also failed to show a tumor. (**B**) A selective injection into the arteria pancreatica magna shows a small tumor at the tail of the pancreas (*arrows*). The fact that this is supplied by a pancreatic vessel suggest that it is a pancreatic tumor rather than a splenunculus. (**C**) Arterially enhanced CT shows the tumor to enhance (*arrows*). Note how the splenic parenchyma effectively surrounds this tumor, showing how it would be impossible to demonstrate it unobscured by the splenic blush on celiac or splenic arteriography, irrespective of the degree of obliquity of the patient or tube. This case emphasizes the vital importance of super-selective studies in the search for an islet-cell tumor.

(From Grainger RG, Allison DJ, Adam A, Dixon AK [eds]: *Grainger and Allison's Diagnostic Radiology*, 4th ed. Philadelphia, Churchill Livingstone, 2001.)

Fig 198–2

Somatostatin receptor scintigram of a patient with metastatic gastrinoma. **A**, whole-body scan at 24 hours after injection of ^{111}In octreotide shows metastatic tumor in the liver with primary tumor in the head of the pancreas. **B**, Detail of hepatic metastases with pancreatic primary.

(From Townsend CM, Beauchamp RD, Evers BM, Mattox KL (eds): *Sabiston Textbook of Surgery*, 17th ed. Philadelphia, WB Saunders, 2004.)

Chapter 199 **Glucagonoma**

In glucagonoma, the cardinal feature of the syndrome is necrotic migratory erythematous rash (Fig. 199–1). This usually starts in the groin with erythematous blotches that become eroded and then heal, leaving indurated pigmented areas. The rash migrates to the perineum, buttocks, and distal extremities. The underlying cause of the rash is unknown. This syndrome is very rare (1:20,000,000), and over 99% of cases result from pancreatic tumors that secrete glucagons. Over 75% of glucagonomas are malignant and over 50% of patients have metastases at the time of diagnosis. Figure 199–2 describes other gut hormone tumor syndromes.

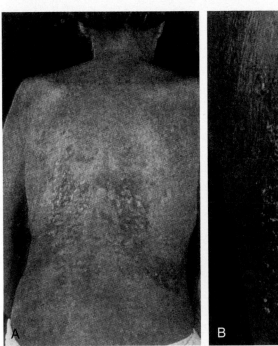 

Fig 199–1
Glucagonoma syndrome: necrolytic migratory erythema.
(From Besser CM, Thorner MO: Comprehensive Clinical Endocrinology, 3rd ed. Mosby, 2002.)

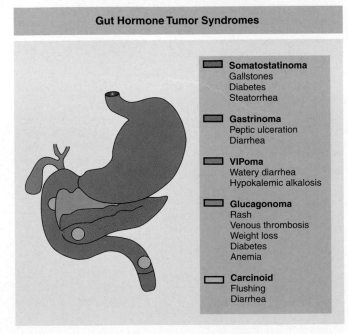

Gut Hormone Tumor Syndromes

Somatostatinoma
Gallstones
Diabetes
Steatorrhea

Gastrinoma
Peptic ulceration
Diarrhea

VIPoma
Watery diarrhea
Hypokalemic alkalosis

Glucagonoma
Rash
Venous thrombosis
Weight loss
Diabetes
Anemia

Carcinoid
Flushing
Diarrhea

Fig 199–2
Gut hormone tumor syndromes.
(From Besser CM, Thorner MO: Comprehensive Clinical Endocrinology, 3rd ed. Mosby, 2002.)

REFERENCES

Besser CM, Thorner MO: Comprehensive Clinical Endocrinology, 3rd ed. St Louis, Mosby, 2002.

Ferri F: Ferri's Clinical Advisor 2007. St Louis, Mosby, 2007.

Ferri F: Practical Guide to the Care of the Medical Patient, 7th ed. St Louis, Mosby, 2007.

Grainger RG, Allison DJ, Adam A, Dixon AK (eds): Grainger and Allison's Diagnostic Radiology, 4th ed. Philadelphia, Churchill Livingstone, 2001.

Townsend CM, Beauchamp RD, Evers BM, Mattox KL (eds): Sabiston Textbook of Surgery, 17th ed. Philadelphia, WB Saunders, 2004.

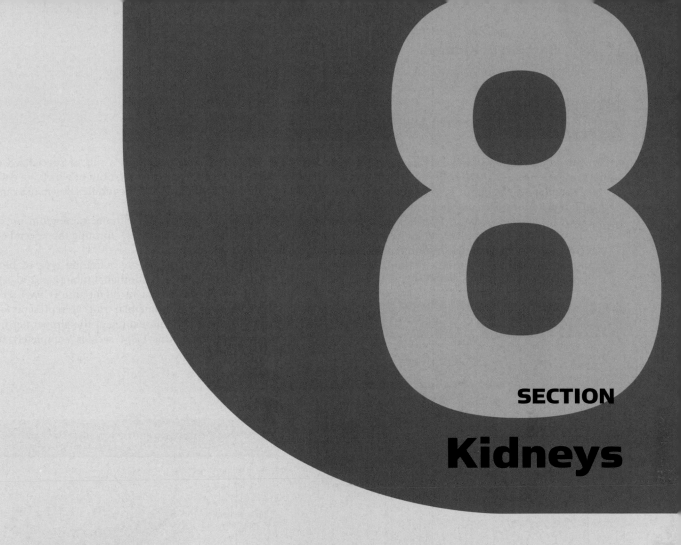

SECTION

Kidneys

Chapter 200: Normal anatomy
Chapter 201: Diagnostic tests and procedures
Chapter 202: Acute renal failure
Chapter 203: Chronic renal failure
Chapter 204: Glomerulonephritis
Chapter 205: Acute tubular necrosis
Chapter 206: IgA nephropathy
Chapter 207: Nephrotic syndrome

Chapter 208: Interstitial nephritis
Chapter 209: Amyloidosis
Chapter 210: Polycystic kidney disease
Chapter 211: Renal artery stenosis and thrombosis
Chapter 212: Neoplasms
Chapter 213: Pyelonephritis
Chapter 214: Hydronephrosis
Chapter 215: Rhabdomyolysis

Chapter 200 | Normal anatomy

- Structure of the kidney: the specific components of the kidneys are the nephrons, the collecting ducts, and a unique microvasculature. The kidneys of humans contain roughly 1 million nephrons. This number is already established during prenatal development; after birth, nephrons cannot be developed, and a lost nephron cannot be replaced. A nephron consists of a renal corpuscle (glomerulus) connected to a complicated and twisted tubule that finally drains into a collecting duct (Fig. 200–1).

- The glomerulus comprises a tuft of specialized capillaries attached to the mesangium, both of which are enclosed in a pouch-like extension of the tubule (Bowman's capsule; Figs. 200–2 and 200–3).

- The capillaries, together with the mesangium, are covered by epithelial cells (podocytes), forming the visceral epithelium of Bowman's capsule.

- Glomerular capillaries are a unique type of blood vessel made up of only an endothelial tube (Fig. 200–4).

- The glomerular basement membrane (GBM) serves as the skeleton of the glomerular tuft. It represents a complex folded sack with an opening at the glomerular hilum. The outer aspect of this GBM sack is completely filled with podocytes.

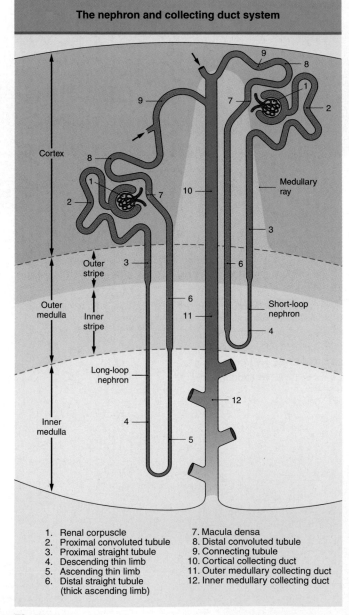

The nephron and collecting duct system

1. Renal corpuscle
2. Proximal convoluted tubule
3. Proximal straight tubule
4. Descending thin limb
5. Ascending thin limb
6. Distal straight tubule (thick ascending limb)
7. Macula densa
8. Distal convoluted tubule
9. Connecting tubule
10. Cortical collecting duct
11. Outer medullary collecting duct
12. Inner medullary collecting duct

Fig 200–1
Nephrons and the collecting duct system. Shown are a short-looped and long-looped nephron, together with a collecting duct (not drawn to scale). *Arrows* denote confluence of further nephrons.
(From Johnson RJ, Feehally J: Comprehensive Clinical Nephrology, 3rd ed. St. Louis, Mosby, 2007.)

Renal corpuscle and juxtaglomerular apparatus

AA	Afferent arteriole	PE	Parietal epithelium
MD	Macula densa	PO	Podocyte
EGM	Extraglomerular mesangium	M	Mesangium
EA	Efferent arteriole	E	Endothelium
N	Sympathetic nerve terminals	F	Foot process
GC	Granular cells	GBM	Glomerular basement membrane
SMC	Vascular smooth muscle cells	US	Urinary space

Fig 200–2
Renal corpuscle and juxtaglomerular apparatus.
(From Johnson RJ, Feehally J: Comprehensive Clinical Nephrology, 3rd ed. St. Louis, Mosby, 2007.)

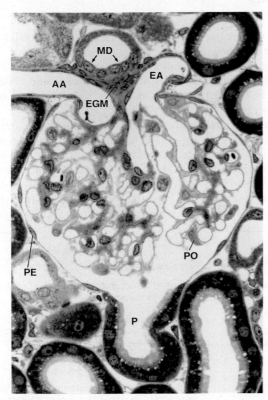

Fig 200–3

Longitudinal section through a glomerulus (rat). At the vascular pole, the afferent arteriole (AA), the efferent arteriole (EA), the extraglomerular mesangium (EGM), and the macula densa (MD) are seen. At the urinary pole, the parietal epithelium (PE) transforms into the proximal tubule (P) (light microscopy, ×390). PE, parietal epithelial cell; PO, podocyte.
(From Johnson RJ, Feehally J: Comprehensive Clinical Nephrology, 3rd ed. St. Louis, Mosby, 2007.)

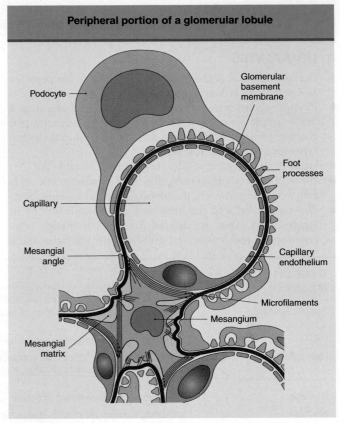

Peripheral portion of a glomerular lobule

Fig 200–4

Peripheral portion of a glomerular lobule. Shown are a capillary, the axial position of the mesangium, and the visceral epithelium (podocytes). At the capillary-mesangial interface, the capillary endothelium directly abuts the mesangium.
(From Johnson RJ, Feehally J: Comprehensive Clinical Nephrology, 3rd ed. St. Louis, Mosby, 2007.)

Chapter 201 — Diagnostic tests and procedures

A. URINALYSIS

- Urinalysis is one of the basic tests to evaluate the presence and severity of kidney and urinary tract disease.
- Physical parameters of importance in the evaluation of a urine sample are color, turbidity, odor, relative density, pH, glucose, protein, hemoglobin (dipstick for blood), leukocyte esterase, nitrites, and ketones.
- Urine dipstick testing results are described in Table 201–1.
- Urine microscopy is an integral part of urinalysis, and adds valuable information to the physicochemical investigation.
- The various cells of the urine sediment are illustrated in Figure 201–1. They are derived from the circulation (e.g., erythrocytes and leukocytes) and from the epithelia lining the urinary tract (e.g., renal tubular cells, uroepithelial cells, and squamous cells).
- Casts are elements with a cylindrical shape (Fig. 201–2) that form in the lumen of distal renal tubules and collecting ducts. Table 201–2 describes the clinical significance of urinary casts.
- Urine can also contain crystals; common types are illustrated in Figure 201–3. The finding in the urine of few uric acid, calcium oxalate, or calcium phosphate crystals is not uncommon. Usually, it is a finding without clinical importance because it reflects a transient supersaturation of the urine caused by the ingestion of some foods (e.g., meats [uric acid], spinach or chocolate [calcium oxalate], milk or

---

TABLE 201–1 Urine dipstick testing

Parameter	False-negative results	False-positive results
Specific gravity	Reduced values in the presence of glucose, urea, alkaline urine	Increased values in the presence of protein > 1 g/L, ketoacids
PH	Reduced values in the presence of formaldehyde	—
Hemoglobin	Ascorbic acid, high nitrite concentration, delayed examination, high density of urine, formaldehyde (0.5 g/L),	Myoglobin, microbial peroxidases, oxidizing detergents, hydrochloric acid
Glucose	Ascorbic acid, urinary tract infection	Oxidizing detergents, hydrochloric acid
Albumin	Immunoglobulin light chains, hydrochloric acid, tubular proteins, globulins, colored urine	Alkaline urine (pH 9), quaternary ammonium detergents, chlorhexidine, polyvinylpyrrolidone
Leukocyte esterase	isotonic urine, vitamin C (intake > 1 g/day), protein > 5 g/L, glucose > 20 g/L, mucous specimen, cephalosporins, nitrofurantoin; mercuric salts, trypsin inhibitor, oxalate, 1% boric acid	Oxidizing detergents, formaldehyde, sodium azidie, colored urine caused by beet ingestion, or bilirubin
Nitrites	No vegetables in diet, short bladder incubation time, vitamin C, gram-positive bacteria	Colored urine
Ketones	Improper storage	Free sulfhydryl groups (e.g., captopril) L-dopa, colored urine

From Johnson RJ, Feehally J: Comprehensive Clinical Nephrology, 3rd ed. St. Louis, Mosby, 2007.

TABLE 201–2 Clinical significance of urinary casts

Cast	Main clinical associations	Cast	Main clinical associations
Hyaline	Normal subject	Leukocyte	Acute pyelonephritis
	Renal disease		Acute interstitial nephritis
Granular	Renal disease		Proliferative glomerulonephritis
Waxy	Renal insufficiency	Epithelial	Acute tubular necrosis
	Rapidly progressive		Acute interstitial nephritis
	Glomerulonephritis		Glomerulonephritis
Fatty	Marked proteinuria	Myoglobin	Rhabdomyolysis
	Nephrotic syndrome		
Erythrocyte	Glomerular bleeding		
	Proliferative, necrotizing glomerulonephritis		
Hemoglobin	Glomerular bleeding		
	Proliferative, necrotizing glomerulonephritis		
	Hemoglobinuria		

From Johnson RJ, Feehally J: Comprehensive Clinical Nephrology, 3rd ed. St. Louis, Mosby, 2007.

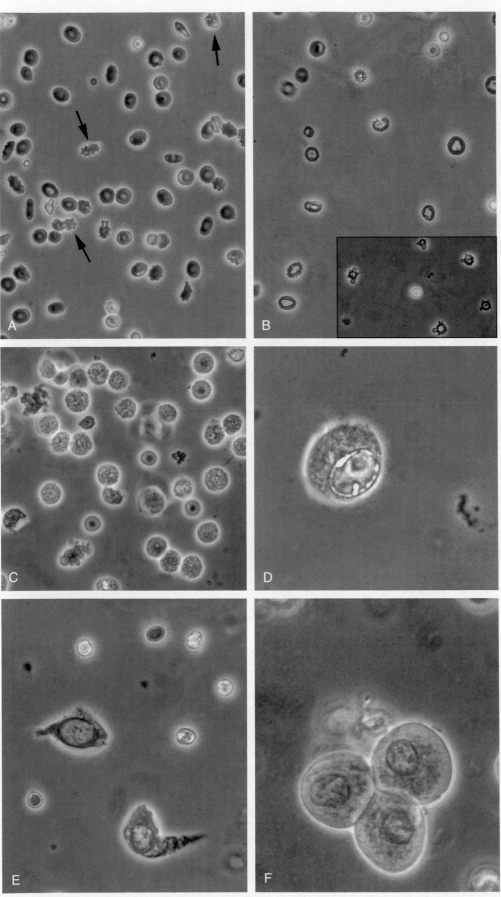

Fig 201–1
Urinary sediment cells. **A,** Isomorphic nonglomerular erythrocytes. The *arrows* indicate the so-called crenated erythrocytes, which are a frequent finding in nonglomerular hematuria. **B,** Dysmorphic glomerular erythrocytes. The dysmorphism is mainly caused by irregularities of the cell membrane. **Inset,** Acanthocytes, ring-formed cell bodies with one or more blebs of different sizes and shapes. These cells are the most reliable marker of glomerular bleeding. **C,** Neutrophils. Note their typical lobulated nucleus and granular cytoplasm. **D,** An ovoid renal tubular cell. The nucleus is large and the cytoplasm is granular. **E,** Two cells from the deep layers of the uroepithelium. **F,** Three cells from the superficial layers of the uroepithelium. Note the difference in shape and nucleus-to-cytoplasm ratio between the two types of uroepithelial cells (**A-E,** phase contrast microscopy, ×400). (From Johnson RJ, Feehally J: Comprehensive Clinical Nephrology, 3rd ed. St. Louis, Mosby, 2007.)

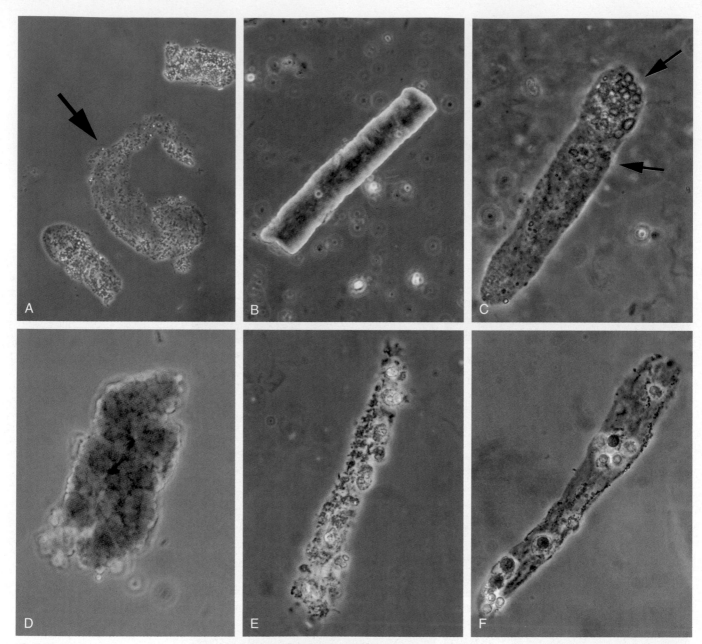

Fig 201-2

Casts. **A,** Finely granular cast *(arrow).* The two other elements shown are hyaline granular casts, which are also frequent in patients with a glomerular disease. **B,** Waxy cast. Note the typical appearance of melted wax and the hard edges. **C,** Erythrocyte cast. The *arrows* indicate the erythrocytes embedded in the matrix of the cast. **D,** Hemoglobin cast, identifiable by its typical brownish hue. **E,** Leukocyte cast. The polymorphonuclear leukocytes are easily identifiable because of their lobulated nucleus. **F,** Epithelial cast. It contains both large ovoid cells deriving from the proximal tubular segments (bottom) and smaller cells deriving from the distal tubular segments (top) (phase contrast microscopy; **A,** ×160; **B-F,** ×400). (From Johnson RJ, Feehally J: *Comprehensive Clinical Nephrology,* 3rd ed. St. Louis, Mosby, 2007.)

cheese [calcium phosphate]), or mild dehydration. However, such crystals may also be associated with pathologic conditions. For example, the presence of uric acid crystalluria in repeated samples may reflect hyperuricosuria, and large amounts of uric acid crystals may be associated with acute renal failure caused by uric acid nephropathy. Some crystals are always pathologic; this is the case with cholesterol, which is found in patients with marked proteinuria.

● Bacteria is a frequent finding, because urine is usually collected and handled under nonsterile conditions and examinations are often delayed. Urine infection can be suspected only if bacteria are found in noncontaminated freshly voided midstream urine, especially if numerous leukocytes are also present.

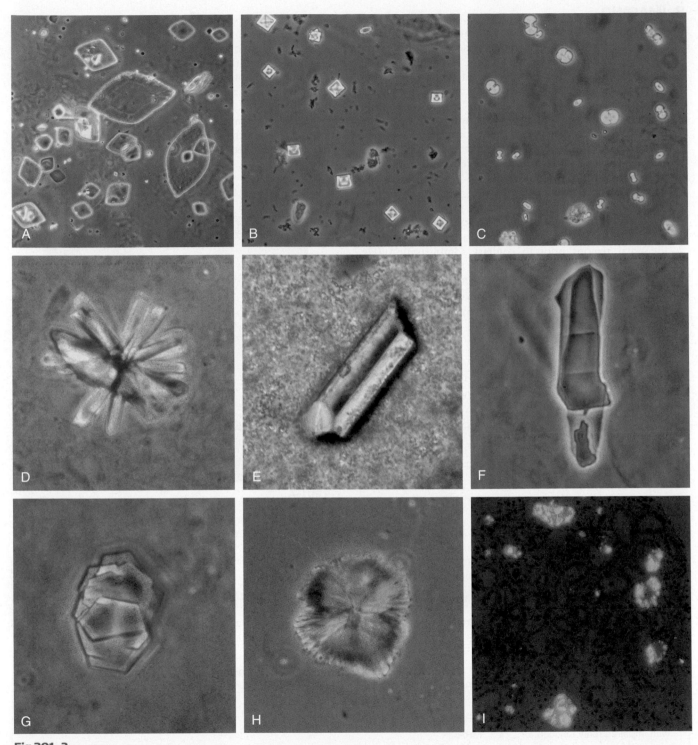

Fig 201–3
Crystals. **A,** Uric acid crystals. This rhomboid shape is the most frequent (phase contrast microscopy, ×400). **B,** Bihydrated calcium oxalate crystals. They have the typical appearance of a letter envelope. **C,** Different types of monohydrated types of monohydrated calcium oxalate crystals (phase contrast microscopy, ×400). **D,** A star-like calcium phosphate crystal. **E,** Triple phosphate crystal on the background of a massive amount of amorphous phosphate particles (phase contrast microscopy, ×400). **F,** Cholesterol crystal. **G,** Cystine crystals (phase contrast microscopy, ×400). **H,** Sulfadiazine crystal. This has a typical amber color and radial striations (phase contrast microscopy, ×400). **I,** Intratubular precipitation of monohydrated calcium crystals seen on renal histology. This phenomenon can be caused by drugs such as naftidrofuryl oxalate or vitamin C (polarized light, ×250)
(From Johnson RJ, Feehally J: Comprehensive Clinical Nephrology, 3rd ed. St. Louis, Mosby, 2007.)

B. IMAGING

- Renal failure associated with contrast administration has been reported as the third most common cause of in-hospital renal failure, after hypotension and surgery. In patients with serum creatinine >1.5 mg/dL, iodinated contrast should be used with caution because the risk of contrast-induced renal failure is increased.
- Box 201–1 describes risk factors for contrast nephrotoxicity. Proper hydration and the correct choice of imaging will minimize the time and cost of effective evaluation.
- The first-choice imaging techniques in common clinical situations are shown in Table 201–3.

Plain films and intravenous urography

- The typical urogram consists of a large plain film of the abdomen to include the region of the bladder (KUB—*k*idneys, *u*reter, *b*ladder) and one smaller film, a tomogram through the renal regions prior to contrast administration (Fig. 201–4).
- Plain films are used to assess for soft tissue masses, the bowel gas pattern, calcifications (Fig. 201–5), and renal location. IV urography (IVU; Fig. 201–6) is now only rarely used and has been replaced by computed tomography (CT) and ultrasound.
- Retrograde pyelography (Fig. 201–7) is performed when the ureters are poorly visualized on other imaging studies or when samples of urine need to be obtained from the kidney for cytology or culture.

Ultrasound

- Sonographic examination of the kidneys is relatively inexpensive and provides a rapid way to assess renal location, contour, and size (Fig. 201–8).

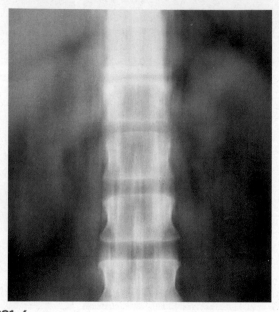

Fig 201–4
Scout tomogram of normal kidneys.
(From Johnson RJ, Feehally J: Comprehensive Clinical Nephrology, 3rd ed. St. Louis, Mosby, 2007.)

Box 201–1   Risk factors for contrast nephrotoxicity

Preexisting renal impairment (serum creatinine > 1.5 mg/dL)*
Diabetes*
Age > 75 yr
Fluid depletion
Myeloma
Concurrent nephrotoxic drugs
Uricosuria
Ionic contrast media

---

*The greatest risk is presented by the coincidence of diabetes and preexisting renal impairment.

TABLE 201–3   First-choice imaging techniques in renal disease

Renal failure, unknown cause	Ultrasound (US)
Hematuria	Intravenous urography (IVU) *or* US + plain radiograph of kidneys, ureter, and bladder (KUB)
Proteinuria, nephrotic syndrome	US
Hypertension	
with normal renal function	CT angiography including imaging of the adrenal glands
with impaired renal function	MRA
Renal artery stenosis	
with normal renal function	MRA
with impaired renal function	MRA
Renal infection	CT
Hydronephrosis detected by US	IVU (if renal function is preserved) or ^{99}Tc-DTPA renography
Retroperitoneal fibrosis	CT
Papillary necrosis	IVU
Cortical necrosis	Contrast-enhanced CT
Renal vein thrombosis	Contrast-enhanced CT
Renal infarction	Contrast-enhanced CT
Nephrocalcinosis	Noncontrast CT

CT, computed tomography; MRA, magnetic resonance angiography.
From Johnson RJ, Feehally J: Comprehensive Clinical Nephrology, 3rd ed. St. Louis, Mosby, 2007.

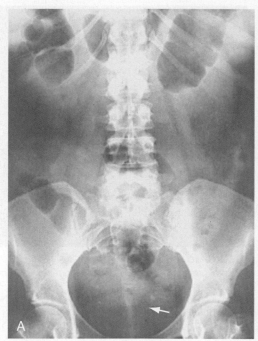
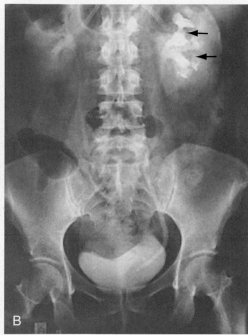

Fig 201–5

A, Plain radiograph (kidneys, ureter, and bladder) taken before contrast medium administration for an intravenous pyelogram shows a small radiopaque calculus shadow *(arrow)* at the left ureterovesical junction (UVJ). **B,** Subsequent delayed film at 40 minutes shows extravasation of the dye at the calyceal fornices *(arrows)* and columnization of the dye up to the left UVJ calculus.
(From Nseyo U, Weinman E, Lamm DL: Urology for Primary Care Physicians. Philadelphia, WB Saunders, 1999.)

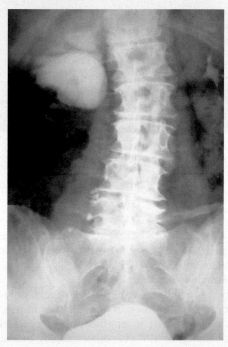

Fig 201–6

Intravenous urogram (IVU) demonstrating pelviureteric junction obstruction. The IVU was obtained in a previously asymptomatic adult to investigate nonspecific right-sided abdominal and back pain. There is unilateral (right-sided) dilation of the pelvicalyceal system, with abrupt tapering to a normal-sized ureter.
(From Johnson RJ, Feehally J: Comprehensive Clinical Nephrology, 3rd ed. St. Louis, Mosby, 2007.)

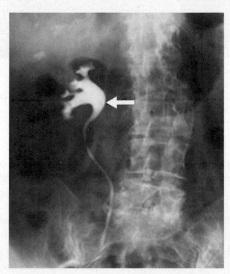

Fig 201–7

Retrograde pyelogram. The *arrow* indicates a small filling defect, which is a calculus in the renal pelvis. The remainder of the study is normal.
(From Johnson RJ, Feehally J: Comprehensive Clinical Nephrology, 3rd ed. St. Louis, Mosby, 2007.)

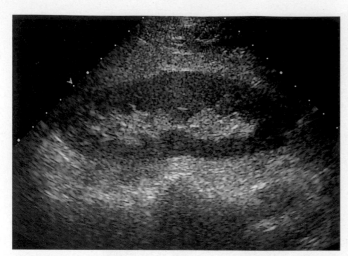

Fig 201–8
Normal sagittal renal ultrasound. The cortex is hypoechoic compared with the echogenic fat containing the renal sinus.
(From Johnson RJ, Feehally J: Comprehensive Clinical Nephrology, 3rd ed. St. Louis, Mosby, 2007.)

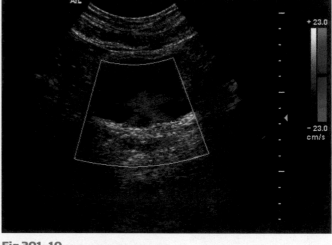

Fig 201–10
Bilateral ureteral jets detected with color Doppler ultrasound. This is a normal appearance.
(From Johnson RJ, Feehally J: Comprehensive Clinical Nephrology, 3rd ed. St. Louis, Mosby, 2007.)

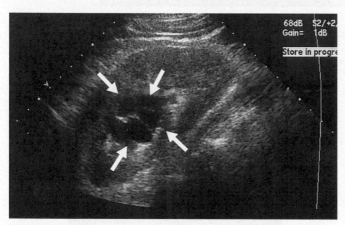

Fig 201–9
Sagittal renal ultrasound showing a complex cyst *(arrows)*.
(From Johnson RJ, Feehally J: Comprehensive Clinical Nephrology, 3rd ed. St. Louis, Mosby, 2007.)

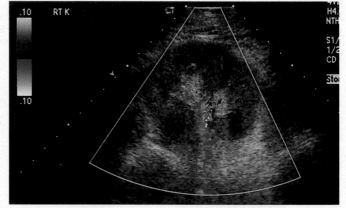

Fig 201–11
Transverse color Doppler ultrasound of the kidney. The artery is red and the vein is blue.
(From Johnson RJ, Feehally J: Comprehensive Clinical Nephrology, 3rd ed. St. Louis, Mosby, 2007.)

- Renal cysts can be identified as anechoic lesions and are a frequent coincidental finding during renal imaging.
- Differentiation into simple and complex cysts (Fig. 201–9) is required to plan intervention.
- Color flow Doppler evaluation in a well-hydrated patient can be used to identify a ureteral jet. The jet is produced when peristalsis propels urine into the bladder, with the incoming urine having a specific gravity higher relative to the urine already in the bladder (Fig. 201–10). Absence of the ureteral jet can indicate total ureteral obstruction. The color Doppler investigation of the kidneys provides a detailed evaluation of the renal vascular anatomy. The main renal arteries can be identified in most patients (Fig. 201–11).

Computed tomography
- CT examination of the kidneys is performed to evaluate suspect renal masses, locate ectopic kidneys to investigate

calculi (Fig. 201–12), assess retroperitoneal masses, and evaluate the extent of parenchymal involvement in patients with pyelonephritis (Fig. 201–13).

Magnetic resonance imaging
- Magnetic resonance imaging (MRI) should only rarely be the first examination used to evaluate the kidneys, but typically it is an adjunct to another imaging technique. The major advantage of MRI over other imaging modalities is its capability of direct multiplanar imaging (Fig. 201–14).
- MR angiography (MRA) can be performed with or without IV contrast administration, although contrast is preferred. The aorta and branch vessels are well demonstrated (Fig. 201–15). MRA is performed to evaluate the renal arteries for stenosis (Fig. 201–16) and is less invasive than angiography.

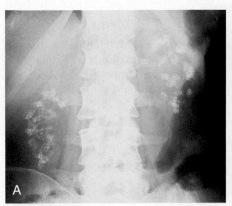
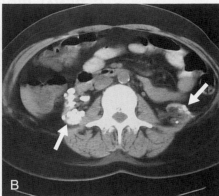
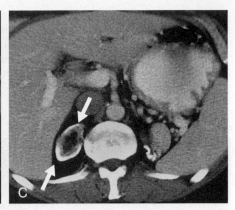

Fig 201–12

Nephrocalcinosis. **A,** Plain film showing bilateral medullary nephrocalcinosis in a patient with distal renal tubular acidosis. **B,** Noncontrast CT scan in a patient with hereditary oxalosis and dense bilateral renal calcification. The left kidney is atrophic. **C,** CT scan showing cortical nephrocalcinosis in the right kidney following cortical necrosis.

(From Johnson RJ, Feehally J: Comprehensive Clinical Nephrology, 3rd ed. St. Louis, Mosby, 2007.)

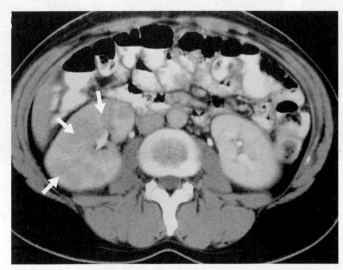

Fig 201–13

Acute pyelonephritis. Contrast CT scan shows areas of lower density caused by infection and edema *(arrows).*

(Courtesy of W. Bush)

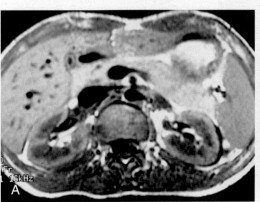
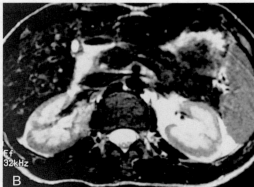
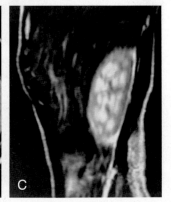

Fig 201–14

Normal MR images through the kidneys. **A,** T1-weighted image. Note the distinct corticomedullary differentiation. **B,** Fast spin-echo (FSE) image. The urine in the collecting tubules causes the high signal within the renal pelvis on this sequence. **C,** FSE for normal sagittal image of the right kidney.

(From Johnson RJ, Feehally J: Comprehensive Clinical Nephrology, 3rd ed. St. Louis, Mosby, 2007.)

Angiography

- Angiography is now most often performed for therapeutic intervention such as embolotherapy or angioplasty. Diagnostic angiography is now used most often for evaluation of the renal arteries to assess possible stenosis and, in many situations, correct it with angioplasty (Fig. 201–17).

C. RENAL BIOPSY

- The introduction of renal biopsy in the 1950s transformed the study of renal disease, particularly glomerular disease, by providing the pathologic information that formed the basis for classification of disease that is still in current use and offers many insights into pathogenesis.

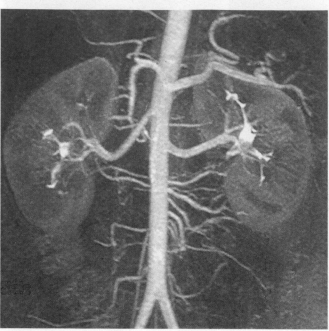

Fig 201–15
MR angiography. This coronal three-dimensional image following contrast administration shows normal renal arteries.
(From Johnson RJ, Feehally J: Comprehensive Clinical Nephrology, 3rd ed. St. Louis, Mosby, 2007.)

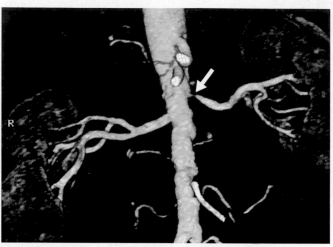

Fig 201–16
MR angiography. This coronal three-dimensional image shows left renal artery stenosis (arrow).
(From Johnson RJ, Feehally J: Comprehensive Clinical Nephrology, 3rd ed. St. Louis, Mosby, 2007.)

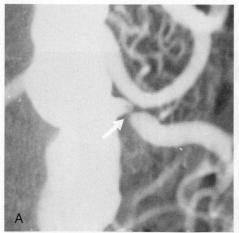
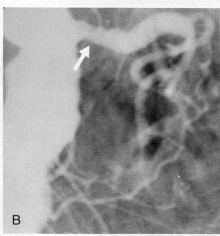

Fig 201–17
Left renal artery stenosis and angioplasty.
A, Aortogram demonstrating a tight left renal artery stenosis (arrow). **B,** Postangioplasty image with marked improvement of the stenosis (arrow).
(Courtesy of Dr. Harold Mitty.)

- Four groups of patients benefit most from the findings of renal biopsy: those with nephritic syndrome, those with renal disease in the setting of a systemic disorder, those with acute renal failure, and those with a renal transplant.
- Workup for renal biopsy (Fig. 201–18) is required to exclude problems that may jeopardize the safety of the procedure and to identify contraindications to biopsy (Table 201–4).
- The biopsy should be performed under ultrasound control using a needle biopsy gun (Fig. 201–19). Local anesthetic is infiltrated down to the capsule of the kidney, but not into the kidney itself (Fig. 201–20). The needle is advanced under ultrasound control (the ultrasound probe should be

placed in a sterile sleeve; Fig. 201–21) to just short of the renal capsule. The movement of the kidney relative to the probe should be watched during some deep respiratory cycles and the patient told to hold his or her breath so that the kidney is in the correct position to biopsy the lower pole (Fig. 201–22). The biopsy gun is then fired and the needle withdrawn. The specimen of renal tissue is recovered (Fig. 201–23) and handed to the attending pathologist or technician.

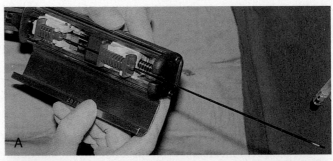
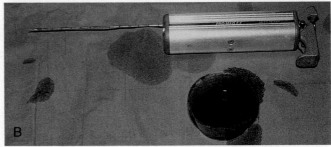

Fig 201–19
Renal biopsy gun. **A,** A 16-gauge needle is loaded in the gun. **B,** The loaded gun is cocked. The trigger mechanism is on the right. (From Johnson RJ, Feehally J: Comprehensive Clinical Nephrology, 3rd ed. St. Louis, Mosby, 2007.)

TABLE 201–4 Contraindications to renal biopsy*

Kidney status	Patient status
Multiple cysts	Uncontrolled blood pressure
Solitary kidney	Uncontrolled bleeding diathesis
Acute pyelonephritis, perinephric abscess	Uremia
Renal neoplasm	Obesity
	Uncooperative patient

Most contraindications to renal biopsy are relative rather than absolute; when clinical circumstances necessitate urgent biopsy they may be overridden, apart from uncontrolled bleeding diathesis.
From Johnson RJ, Feehally J: Comprehensive Clinical Nephrology, 3rd ed. St. Louis, Mosby, 2007.

Workup for renal biopsy

Assessments

Renal imaging: two normal size, unscarred, unobstructed kidneys

Blood pressure: diastolic BP < 95 mm Hg

Urine culture: sterile

Coagulation status
Drug therapy: stop aspirin/NSAID 5 days before biopsy
Platelet count: > 100 × 10⁹/L
Prothrombin time: < 1.2 times control
Activated partial thromboplastin time (APTT): < 1.2 times control (if prolonged exclude lupus anticoagulant)
Bleeding time (measure if BUN > 60 mg/dL (urea > 20 mmol/L) and high risk): < 10 min (if prolonged give DDAVP 0.4 µg/kg 2–3 h before biopsy)

Renal biopsy

Fig 201–18
Workup for renal biopsy. BP, blood pressure; BUN, blood urea nitrogen; DDAVP, desmopressin; NSAID, nonsteroidal anti-inflammatory drug. (From Johnson RJ, Feehally J: Comprehensive Clinical Nephrology, 3rd ed. St. Louis, Mosby, 2007.)

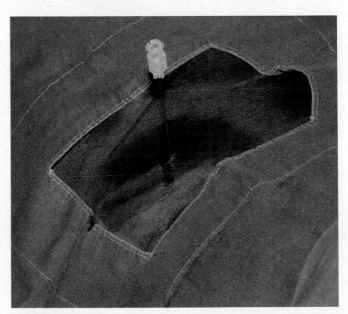

Fig 201–20
Renal biopsy. The skin has been cleaned with Betadine, the lower pole of the left kidney identified, and the skin marked appropriately. A fine needle has been inserted for local anesthetic infiltration. (From Johnson RJ, Feehally J: Comprehensive Clinical Nephrology, 3rd ed. St. Louis, Mosby, 2007.)

- In glomerulonephritis (GN), the pathologist will classify the different patterns of histologic injury seen on renal biopsy by examining the specimen with light microscopy, immunofluorescence, and electron microscopy. This classification is not ideal because it cannot always be assumed that one histologic pattern has a single cause or a single clinical presentation. Furthermore, one cause may produce a variety of histologic patterns (e.g., the varied glomerular disease seen in association with hepatitis B infection or lupus).

- When evaluating renal biopsy specimens, it is more helpful to regard the renal biopsy appearance as a pattern rather than a disease. In GN, the dominant histologic lesions are in the glomeruli (Fig. 201–24). GN is described as focal (only some glomeruli are involved) or diffuse. In any individual glomerulus, injury may be segmental (affecting only part of any glomerulus) or global. Indirect immunofluorescence and immunoperoxidase staining are both used to identify immune reactants (Fig. 201–25).

- Electron microscopy is valuable for defining the anatomy of the basement membranes and for localizing the site of immune deposits, which are usually homogeneous and electron-dense (Fig. 201–26).

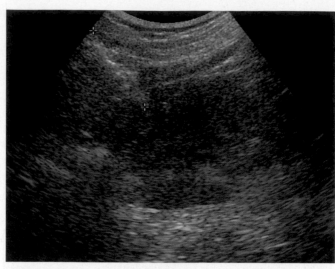

Fig 201–22
Renal biopsy—ultrasound appearance of the lower pole of the left kidney with biopsy entering.
(From Johnson RJ, Feehally J: Comprehensive Clinical Nephrology, 3rd ed. St. Louis, Mosby, 2007.)

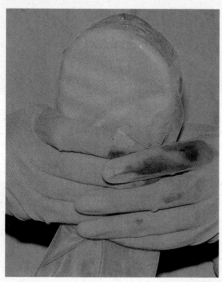

Fig 201–21
The ultrasound probe for renal biopsy. The probe is mounted in a sterile stocking for use during the biopsy.
(From Johnson RJ, Feehally J: Comprehensive Clinical Nephrology, 3rd ed. St. Louis, Mosby, 2007.)

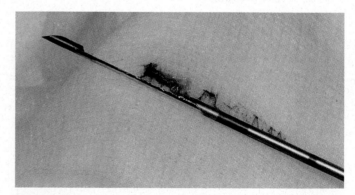

Fig 201–23
Renal biopsy specimen. Shown are the tip of biopsy the needle and the core of tissue obtained at biopsy. This core is only one half the length of the needle.
(From Johnson RJ, Feehally J: Comprehensive Clinical Nephrology, 3rd ed. St. Louis, Mosby, 2007.)

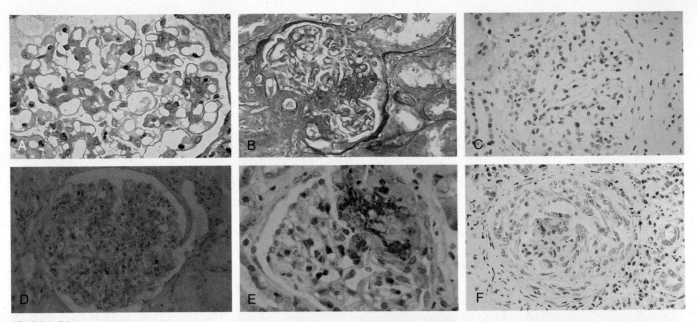

Fig 201–24
Pathology of glomerular disease shown by light microscopy. These characteristic patterns of glomerular disease illustrate the range of histologic appearances and the descriptive terms used. **A,** Normal glomerulus, minimal change disease. **B,** Segmental sclerosis, focal segmental glomerulo-sclerosis. **C,** Diffuse mesangial hypercellularity. **D,** Diffuse endocapillary hypercellularity, poststreptococcal glomerulonephritis. **E,** Segmental necrosis, renal vasculitis. **F,** Crescent formation, antiglomerular basement membrane disease.
(From Johnson RJ, Feehally J: Comprehensive Clinical Nephrology, 3rd ed. St. Louis, Mosby, 2007.)

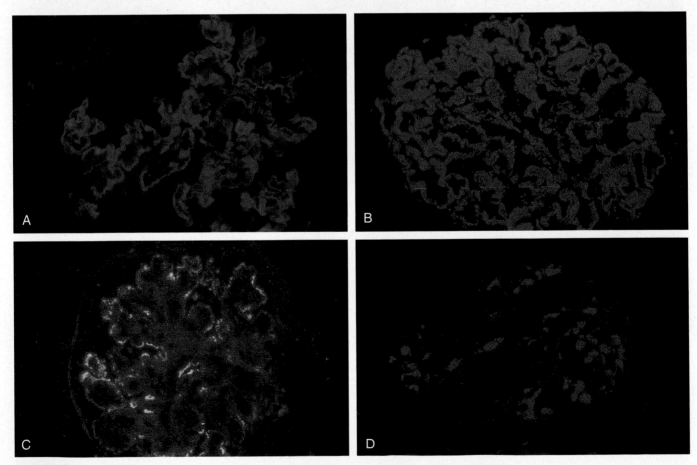

Fig 201–25
Pathology of glomerular disease showing common patterns of glomerular staining found by immunofluorescence microscopy. **A,** Linear capillary wall IgG, antiglomerular basement membrane disease. **B,** Fine granular capillary wall IgG, membranous nephropathy. **C,** Coarse granular capillary wall IgG, membranoproliferative GN type I. **D,** Granular mesangial IgA, IgA nephropathy.
(From Johnson RJ, Feehally J: Comprehensive Clinical Nephrology, 3rd ed. St. Louis, Mosby, 2007.)

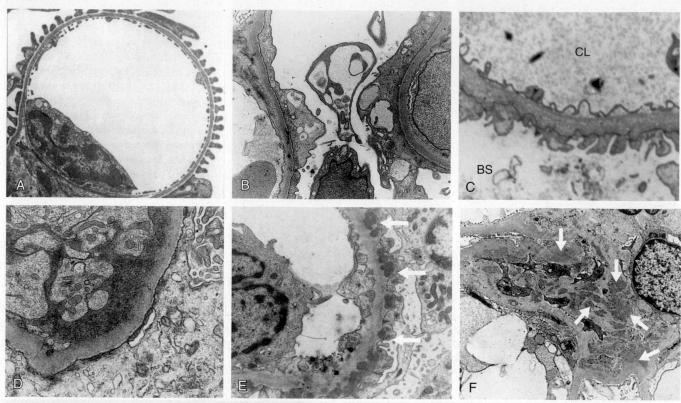

Fig 201–26
Ultrastructural pathology of glomerular disease. Some characteristic patterns of electron-dense deposits (EDD) and glomerular basement membrane (GBM) abnormalities seen in glomerular disease are shown. **A,** Normal. **B,** Foot process effacement, minimal change disease. **C,** GBM thickening and splitting, Alport's syndrome. **D,** Subendothelial EDD, membranoproliferative glomerulonephritis (MPGN) type I. **E,** Subepithelial EDD *(arrows),* membranous nephropathy. **F,** Mesangial EDD *(arrows),* IgA nephropathy.
(From Johnson RJ, Feehally J: Comprehensive Clinical Nephrology, 3rd ed. St. Louis, Mosby, 2007.)

Chapter 202 / Acute renal failure

DEFINITION

Acute renal failure (ARF) is the rapid impairment of renal function, resulting in retention of products in the blood that are normally excreted by the kidneys.

PHYSICAL FINDINGS AND CLINICAL PRESENTATION

The physical examination should focus on volume status. The physical findings noted here vary with the duration and rapidity of onset of renal failure.

- Peripheral edema (Fig. 202–1)
- Skin pallor, ecchymoses
- Oliguria (however, patients can have nonoliguric renal failure), anuria
- Delirium, lethargy, myoclonus, seizures
- Back pain, fasciculations, muscle cramps
- Tachypnea, tachycardia
- Weakness, anorexia, generalized malaise, nausea

CAUSE

- Prerenal: inadequate perfusion caused by hypovolemia, congestive heart failure (CHF), cirrhosis, sepsis. Of community-acquired cases of ARF, 60% are caused by prerenal conditions.
- Postrenal: outlet obstruction from prostatic enlargement, ureteral obstruction (stones), bilateral renal vein occlusion. Postrenal causes account for 5% to 15% of community-acquired ARF.
- Intrinsic renal: glomerulonephritis, acute tubular necrosis, drug toxicity (Fig. 202–2), contrast nephropathy
- Causes of acute renal failure and evaluation are described in Table 202–1.

LABORATORY TESTS

- Elevated serum creatinine: the rate of rise of creatinine is approximately 1 mg/dL/day in complete renal failure.
- Elevated blood urea nitrogen (BUN): BUN/creatinine ratio is >20:1 in prerenal azotemia, postrenal azotemia, and acute glomerulonephritis; it is <20:1 in acute interstitial nephritis and acute tubular necrosis

- Electrolytes (potassium, phosphate) are elevated; bicarbonate level and calcium are decreased.
- Complete blood count (CBC) may reveal anemia because of decreased erythropoietin production, hemoconcentration, or hemolysis.
- Urinalysis may reveal the presence of hematuria (GN), proteinuria (nephrotic syndrome), casts (see Fig. 201–1) (e.g., granular casts in acute tubular necrosis (ATN), red blood cell (RBC) casts in acute GN, white blood cell (WBC) casts in acute interstitial nephritis), eosinophiluria (acute interstitial nephritis). Urine chemistry in the differential diagnosis of ARF is described in Table 202–2.
- Urinary sodium and urinary creatinine should also be obtained to calculate the fractional excretion of sodium (FE_{Na}):

$$\frac{\text{urine sodium/plasma sodium}}{\text{urine creatinine/plasma creatinine}} \times 100$$

The fractional excretion of sodium is <1 in prerenal failure and >1 in intrinsic renal failure in patients with a urine output of less than 400 mL/day.

- Urinary osmolarity is 250 to 300 mOsm/kg in ATN, <400 mOsm/kg in postrenal azotemia, and >500 mOsm/kg in prerenal azotemia and acute glomerulonephritis.
- Additional useful studies are blood cultures for patients suspected of sepsis, liver function tests (LFTs), immunoglobulins, and protein immunoelectrophoresis in patients suspected of myeloma, and creatinine kinase in patients with suspected rhabdomyolysis.

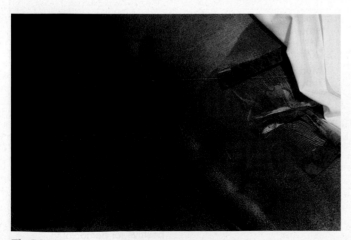

Fig 202–1
Fluid overload in acute renal failure (ARF). Gross pitting flank edema in a patient with ARF in whom femoral venous access has just been established to initiate hemodialysis.
(From Johnson RJ, Feehally J: Comprehensive Clinical Nephrology, 3rd ed. St. Louis, Mosby, 2007.)

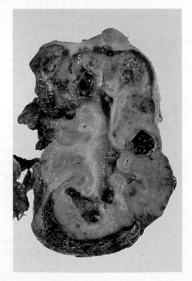

Fig 202–2
Papillary necrosis—autopsy macroscopic appearance of papillary necrosis in a patient with long-standing analgesic nephropathy.
(From Johnson RJ, Feehally J: Comprehensive Clinical Nephrology, 3rd ed. St. Louis, Mosby, 2007.)

TABLE 202–1 Evaluation for the cause of acute renal failure (ARF)

Cause of acute renal failure	Suggestive clinical features	Typical urinalysis*	Confirmatory tests
Prerenal ARF	Evidence of true volume depletion (thirst, postural or absolute hypotension and tachycardia, low jugular vein pressure, dry mucous membranes and axillae, weight loss, fluid output > input) or decreased effective circulatory volume (e.g., heart failure, liver failure), treatment with NSAIDs or ACE inhibitor	Hyaline casts; $FE_{Na} < 10$ mmol/L; SG > 1.018	Occasionally requires invasive hemodynamic monitoring; rapid resolution of ARF on restoration of renal perfusion
Intrinsic renal ARF			
Diseases involving large renal vessels			
Renal artery thrombosis	History of atrial fibrillation or recent myocardial infarct, nausea, vomiting, flank or abdominal pain	Mild proteinuria; occasionally, red blood cells	Elevated lactate dehydrogenase with normal transaminases, renal arteriogram
Atheroembolism	Age usually >50 yr, recent manipulation of aorta, retinal plaques, subcutaneous nodules, palpable purpura, livedo reticularis, vasculopathy, hypertension	Often normal; eosinophiluria; rarely, casts	Eosinophilia, hypocomplementemia, skin biopsy, renal biopsy
Renal vein thrombosis	Evidence of nephrotic syndrome or pulmonary embolism, flank pain	Proteinuria, hematuria	Inferior venacavogram and selective renal venogram; Doppler flow studies; MRI
Diseases of small vessels and glomeruli			
Glomerulonephritis or vasculitis	Compatible clinical history (e.g., recent infection) sinusitis, lung hemorrhage, rash or skin ulcers, arthralgias, hypertension, edema	Red blood cell or granular casts, red blood cells, white blood cells, mild proteinuria	Low C3, antineutrophil cytoplasmic antibodies, antiglomerular basement membrane antibodies, antinuclear antibodies, antistreptolysin 0, anti-DNase, cryoglobulins, renal biopsy
HUS or TTP	Compatible clinical history (e.g., recent gastrointestinal infection, cyclosporine, fever, pallor, ecchymoses, neurologic abnormalities	May be normal, red blood cells, mild proteinuria; rarely, red blood cell or granular casts	Anemia, thrombocytopenia, schistocytes on blood smear, increased lactate dehydrogenase, renal biopsy
Malignant hypertension	Severe hypertension with headaches, cardiac failure, retinopathy, neurologic dysfunction, papilledema	Red blood cells, red blood cell casts, proteinuria	LVH by echocardiography or electrocardiography, resolution of ARF with control of blood pressure
ARF mediated by ischemia or toxin (ATN)			
Ischemia	Recent hemorrhage, hypotension (e.g., cardiac arrest), surgery	Muddy brown granular or tubule epithelial cell casts, $FE_{Na} > 1\%$, $U_{Na} > 20$ mmol/L, SG = 1.010	Clinical assessment and urinalysis usually sufficient for diagnosis
Exogenous toxins	Recent radiocontrast study, nephrotoxic antibiotics or anticancer agents often coexistent with volume depletion, sepsis, or chronic renal insufficiency	Muddy brown granular or tubular epithelial cell casts, $FE_{Na} > 1\%$, $U_{Na} > 20$ mmol/L, SG = 1.010	Clinical assessment and urinalysis usually sufficient for diagnosis
Endogenous toxins	History suggestive of rhabdomyolysis (seizures, coma, ethanol abuse, trauma)	Urine supernatant tests positive for heme	Hyperkalemia, hyperphosphatemia, hypocalcemia, increased circulating myoglobin, creatine kinase MM, uric acid
	History suggestive of hemolysis (blood transfusion)	Urine supernatant pink and positive for heme	Hyperkalemia, hyperphosphatemia, hypocalcemia, hyperuricemia, pink plasma positive for hemoglobin

Clinical features, typical urinalysis and confirmatory tests for diagnosis of common causes of ARF.

ACE, angiotensin-converting enzyme; ATN, acute tubular necrosis; FE_{Na}, fractional excretion of sodium; HUS, hemolytic-uremic syndrome; LVH, left ventricular hypertrophy; NSAIDs, nonsteroidal anti-inflammatory drugs; TTP, thrombotic thrombocytopenic purpura; U_{NA}, urine Na^+ concentration; SG, specific gravity.

TABLE 202–1 Evaluation for the cause of acute renal failure (ARF)—cont'd

Cause of acute renal failure	Suggestive clinical features	Typical urinalysis*	Confirmatory tests
Endogenous toxins (cont'd)	History suggestive of tumor lysis (recent chemotherapy), myeloma (bone pain), or ethylene glycol ingestion	Uric acid crystals, dipstick-negative proteinuria, oxalate crystals, respectively	Hyperuricemia, hyperkalemia, hyperphosphatemia (for tumor lysis); circulating or urinary monoclonal band (for myeloma); toxicology screen, acidosis. osmolal gap (for ethylene glycol)
Acute diseases of the tubulointerstitium			
Allergic interstitial nephritis	Recent ingestion of drug and fever, rash, or arthralgias	White blood cell casts, white blood cells (frequently eosinophiluria), red blood cells, rarely red blood cell casts, proteinuria (occasionally nephrotic)	Systemic eosinophilia, skin biopsy of rash area (leukocytoclastic vasculitis), renal biopsy
Acute bilateral pyelonephritis	Flank pain and tenderness, toxic state, febrile	Leukocytes, proteinuria, red blood cells, bacteria	Urine and blood cultures
Postrenal ARF	Abdominal or flank pain, palpable bladder	Frequently normal; hematuria if stones, hemorrhage, malignancy, or prostatic hypertrophy	Plain film, renal ultrasonography, retrograde or anterograde pyelography, CT

TABLE 202–2 Urine chemistry in the differential diagnosis of acute renal failure

Urine chemistry	Prerenal acute renal failure*	Ischemic intrinsic acute renal failure[†]
Urine osmolality, U_{osm} (mOsm/kg H_2O)	>500	<250
Urine to plasma osmolality	>1.5	<1.1
Urine specific gravity	>1.018	<1.012
Plasma blood urea nitrogen-to-creatinine ratio	>20	<10-15
Urinary urea nitrogen-to-plasma urea nitrogen ratio	>8	<3
Urinary creatinine-to-plasma creatinine ratio	>40	<20
Urinary Na^+ concentration (mmol/L)	<10	>20
Fractional excretion of Na^+ (%)[‡]	<1	>2
Renal failure index[§] $U_{Na}/U_{cr}/P_{cr}$	<1	>1
Urine sediment	Hyaline casts	Muddy brown granular casts

*Parameters suggesting prerenal failure are sometimes seen with nonoliguric acute tubular necrosis (ATN), acute glomerulonephritis, and early obstruction.
[†]Parameters suggesting ATN may be misleading in prerenal failure in older patients, in those with preexisting renal impairment, and following diuretic administration.
[‡](Urine Na^+/plasma Na^+)/(urine creatinine/plasma creatinine) × 100.
[§]Urine Na^+/(urine creatinine/plasma creatinine) × 100.
From Johnson RJ, Feehally J: Comprehensive Clinical Nephrology, 3rd ed. St. Louis, Mosby, 2007.

- Renal biopsy may be indicated in patients with intrinsic renal failure when considering specific therapy; major uses of renal biopsy are differential diagnosis of nephrotic syndrome, differentiation of lupus vasculitis from other vasculitides and of lupus membranous glomerulopathy, from idiopathic membranous glomerulopathy, confirmation of hereditary nephropathies on the basis of the ultrastructure, diagnosis of rapidly progressing glomerulonephritis, differentiation of allergic interstitial nephritis from ATN, and differentiation of primary glomerulonephritis syndromes. The biopsy may be performed percutaneously or by an open method. The percutaneous approach is favored and generally yields adequate tissue in more than 90% of cases. Open biopsy is generally reserved for uncooperative patients, those with a solitary kidney, and patients at risk for uncontrolled bleeding.

IMAGING STUDIES

- Chest x-ray is useful to evaluate for fluid overload (Fig. 202–3) and for pulmonary renal syndromes (Goodpasture's syndrome, Wegener's granulomatosis).
- Ultrasound of kidneys (see Fig. 201–8) is used to evaluate for kidney size (useful to distinguish ARF from chronic renal failure [CRF]), presence of obstruction, and renal vascular status (with Doppler evaluation).
- Anterograde and/or retrograde pyelography (see Fig. 201–7) can be used for ruling out obstruction; useful in patients at high risk of obstruction
- ECG : hypocalcemia (Fig. 202–4), hyperkalemia (Fig. 202–5)

TREATMENT

- Stop all nephrotoxic medications.
- Modify diet to supply adequate calories while minimizing accumulation of toxins; control fluid balance appropriately.
- Daily weight
- Monitoring of renal function and electrolytes.
- Modification of dosages of renally excreted drugs
- Treatment is variable with cause of ARF:

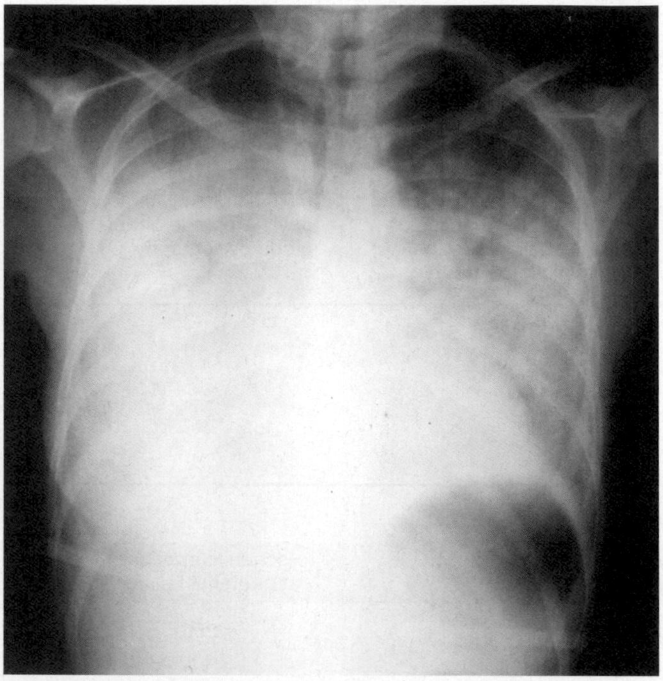

Fig 202–3
Fluid overload in acute renal failure—severe pulmonary edema.
(From Johnson RJ, Feehally J: Comprehensive Clinical Nephrology, 3rd ed. St. Louis, Mosby, 2007.)

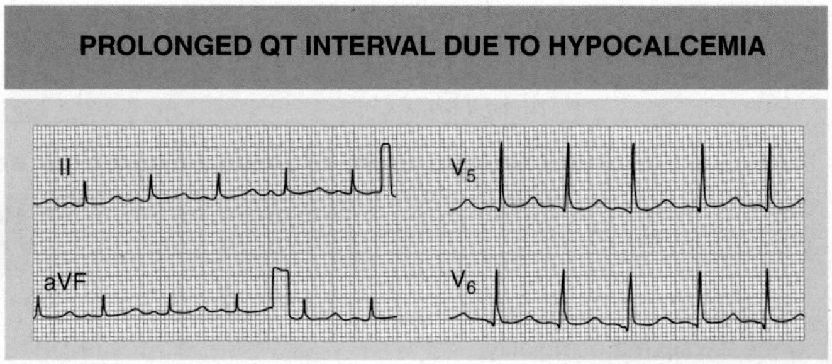

PROLONGED QT INTERVAL DUE TO HYPOCALCEMIA

II V_5

aVF V_6

Fig 202–4
Four ECG leads showing a prolonged QT interval caused by hypocalcemia.
(From Crawford MH, DiMarco JP, Paulus WJ [eds]: Cardiology, 2nd ed. St. Louis, 2004, Mosby.)

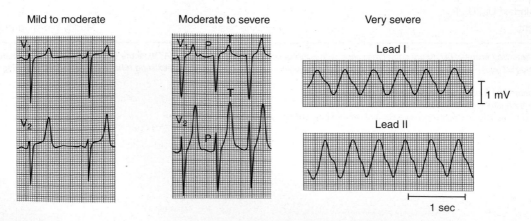

Mild to moderate   Moderate to severe   Very severe

Lead I   1 mV

Lead II

1 sec

Fig 202–5
The earliest change with hyperkalemia is peaking ("tenting") of the T waves. With progressive increases in serum potassium, the QRS complexes widen, the P waves decrease in kmplitude and may disappear, and finally, a sine wave pattern leads to asystole.
(From Goldberger AL [ed]: Clinical Electrocardiography, 6th ed. St. Louis, Mosby, 1999.)

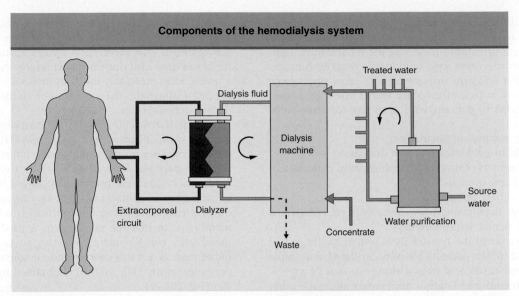

Components of the hemodialysis system

Fig 202–6
Components of the hemodialysis system.
(From Johnson RJ, Feehally J: Comprehensive Clinical Nephrology, 3rd ed. St. Louis, Mosby, 2007.)

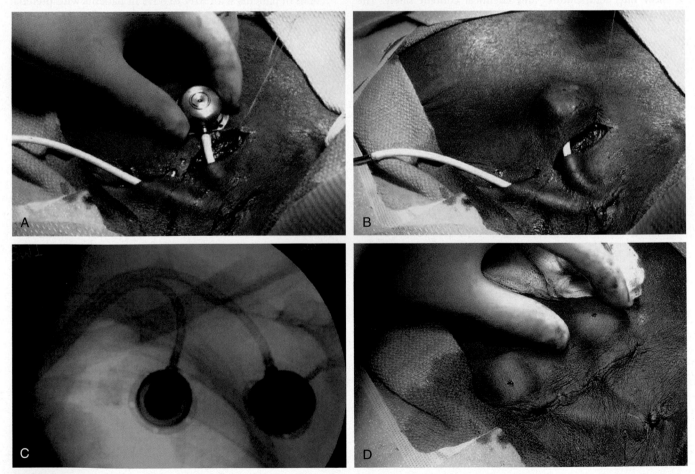

Fig 202–7
Implantation of the LifeSite hemodialysis access system (Vasca, Tewksbury, Mass). Cannulae are inserted over guidewires advanced into the inferior vena cava under fluoroscopic control. **A,** After cutting cannula to appropriate length, the cannula is connected to the LifeSite valve. **B,** Valve is placed in tissue pocket; the flat base is secured to the underlying fascia to reduce risk of valve rotation or migration. **C,** Fluoroscopy of LifeSite valves confirms proper placement. **D,** Subcutaneous tissue and skin are closed. The LifeSite system is immediately ready for access by simple cannulation with a 14-gauge needle.
(From Johnson RJ, Feehally J: Comprehensive Clinical Nephrology, 3rd ed. St. Louis, Mosby, 2007.)

1. Prerenal: IV volume expansion in hypovolemic patients
2. Intrinsic renal: discontinuation of any potential toxins and treatment of condition causing the renal failure. Low-dose dopamine is often used to influence renal dysfunction and may offer transient improvement in renal physiology; however, there is lack of evidence that it offers significant clinical benefits to patients with or at risk for acute renal failure.
3. Postrenal: removal of obstruction
- General indications for initiation of dialysis:
1. Florid symptoms of uremia (encephalopathy, pericarditis)
2. Severe volume overload
3. Severe acid-base imbalance
4. Significant derangement in electrolyte concentrations (e.g., hyperkalemia, hyponatremia)
- The components of the hemodialysis system are illustrated in Figure 202–6. The patient's blood is circulated in a simple extracorporeal circuit and passed along one side of a semipermeable membrane. Dialysis fluid passes along the other side of the membrane in the opposite direction (countercurrent) to optimize diffusion gradients. The main role of the dialysis machine is to supply dialysis fluid with the intended flow rate, temperature, and chemical content safely. The machine mixes a preprepared concentrate of electrolytes with treated water to produce dialysis fluid. It also removes a prescribed volume of ultrafiltrate during the dialysis session. The development of fully implantable, subcutaneous, vascular access devices is a relatively recent innovation in vascular access. The LifeSite hemodialysis access system (Vasca, Tewksbury, Mass) consists of two titanium alloy subcutaneous valves with connecting silicone cannulae, one for blood draw and one for blood return, that are placed in a central vein, preferably the right internal jugular vein. Figure 202–7 illustrates the implantation of the LifeSite hemodialysis access system.
- Peritoneal dialysis (PD) should not be thought of as a technique in competition with hemodialysis (HD) but rather as a complementary modality that can be offered to the patient with end-stage renal disease (ESRD) with some residual renal function. The basic principle of dialysis is the separation of substances in solution by their varying rates of diffusion down a concentration gradient through a semipermeable membrane. In PD, the peritoneum is used as the porous membrane. Fluid removal is along an osmotic gradient rather than as a result of a pressure gradient. Access to the peritoneal cavity (Fig. 202–8) is obtained by use of a catheter (Fig. 202–9).
- Renal function recovery (ability to discontinue dialysis) varies from 50% to 75% in survivors of ARF.
- Overall mortality rate in ARF is almost 50%, varying from 60% in patients with ATN to 35% in patients with prerenal or postrenal ARF.
- The combination of acute renal failure and sepsis is associated with a 70% mortality rate.

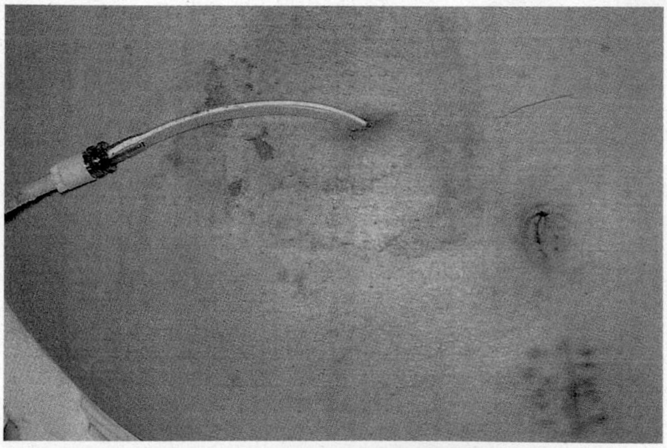

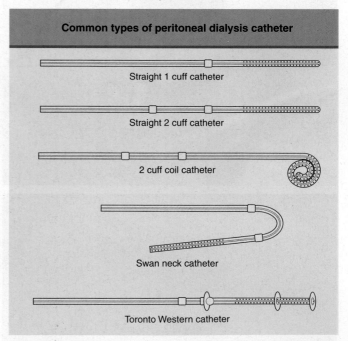

Common types of peritoneal dialysis catheter

Straight 1 cuff catheter

Straight 2 cuff catheter

2 cuff coil catheter

Swan neck catheter

Toronto Western catheter

Fig 202–8
A recently implanted peritoneal dialysis catheter in situ.
(From Johnson RJ, Feehally J: Comprehensive Clinical Nephrology, 3rd ed. St. Louis, Mosby, 2007.)

Fig 202–9
Common types of peritoneal catheters.
(From Johnson RJ, Feehally J: Comprehensive Clinical Nephrology, 3rd ed. St. Louis, Mosby, 2007.)

Chapter 203 | Chronic renal failure

DEFINITION

CRF is a progressive decrease in renal function (CFR < 60 mL/min for 3 months or longer) with subsequent accumulation of waste products in the blood, electrolyte abnormalities, and anemia.

PHYSICAL FINDINGS AND CLINICAL PRESENTATION

- Skin pallor, nodular prurigo (Fig. 203–1), ecchymoses, diffuse brown pigmentation (Fig. 203–2), pseudoporphyria (Fig. 203–3)
- Edema
- Hypertension
- Emotional lability and depression
- Malnutrition (Fig. 203–4), muscle wasting (Fig. 203–5)
- The clinical presentation varies with the degree of renal failure and its underlying cause. Common symptoms are generalized fatigue, nausea, anorexia, pruritus, insomnia, taste disturbances, and muscle weakness.
- Extraskeletal calcifications are frequently encountered in patients with advanced renal insufficiency (Fig. 203–6) and are aggravated by persistent elevation of the calcium phosphate product. Calciphylaxis, calcific uremic arteriolopathy, is a severe form of vascular calcification and is found far less

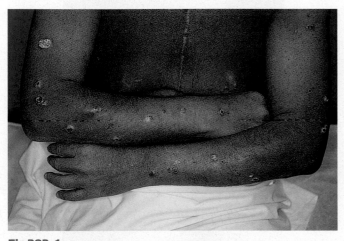

Fig 203–1
Prurigo nodularis developed in this patient with chronic renal failure on hemodialysis.
(From Callen JP, Greer KE, Paller AS, Swinyer LJ: Color Atlas of Dermatology, 2nd ed. Philadelphia, WB Saunders, 2000.)

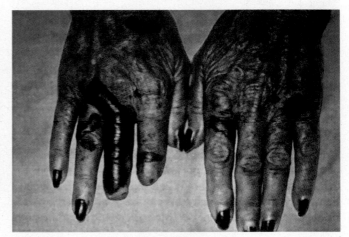

Fig 203–3
Pseudoporphyria in a patient with chronic renal failure. This condition is also known as bullous dermatosis of renal failure.
(From Callen JP, Greer KE, Paller AS, Swinyer LJ: Color Atlas of Dermatology, 2nd ed. Philadelphia, WB Saunders, 2000.)

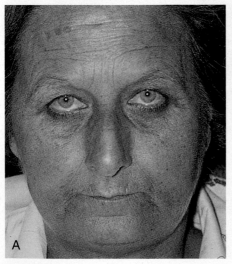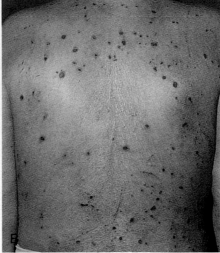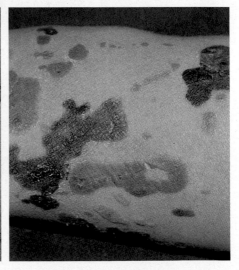

Fig 203–2
Dermatologic manifestations in chronic renal failure. **A,** Pigmentation. A diffuse brown pigmentation is typical of long-standing renal failure; it may be caused by retention of β-melanocyte-stimulating hormone. **B,** Nodular prurigo. Extensive nodular prurigo is associated with severe pruritus (note the scratch marks) in a man with advanced renal failure shortly before the initiation of renal replacement therapy. **C,** Pseudoporphyria; bullous eruption in a patient on regular dialysis. The bullae are hemorrhagic in this individual because of a coincidental thrombocytopenia.
(From Johnson RJ, Feehally J: Comprehensive Clinical Nephrology, 3rd ed. St. Louis, Mosby, 2007.)

commonly in patients with chronic kidney disease than arterial or cardiac valvular calcification. The syndrome is characterized by the development of painful nodules in the lower extremities, trunk, buttocks, or other areas that then become mottled or violaceous, indurated, and ultimately ulcerated (Fig. 203–7).

CAUSE
- Diabetes (37%), hypertension (30%), chronic glomerulonephritis (12%)
- Polycystic kidney disease

- Tubular interstitial nephritis (e.g., drug hypersensitivity, analgesic nephropathy), obstructive nephropathies (e.g., nephrolithiasis, prostatic disease)
- Vascular diseases (e.g., renal artery stenosis, hypertensive nephrosclerosis)

LABORATORY TESTS
- Elevated BUN, creatinine, creatinine clearance
- Urinalysis: may reveal proteinuria, RBC casts
- Serum chemistry: elevated BUN and creatinine, hyperkalemia, hyperuricemia, hypocalcemia, hyperphosphatemia, hyperglycemia, decreased bicarbonate

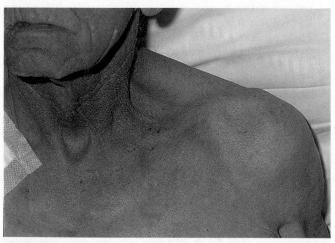

Fig 203–4
A severely malnourished hemodialysis patient. Shown is muscle wasting around the clavicle and shoulder.
(From Johnson RJ, Feehally J: Comprehensive Clinical Nephrology, 3rd ed. St. Louis, Mosby, 2007.)

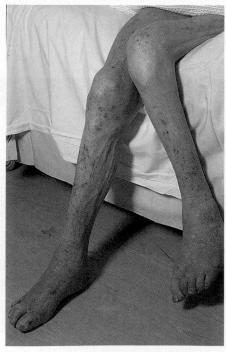

Fig 203–5
A severely malnourished hemodialysis patient. There is marked wasting of the quadriceps and calf muscles.
(From Johnson RJ, Feehally J: Comprehensive Clinical Nephrology, 3rd ed. St. Louis, Mosby, 2007.)

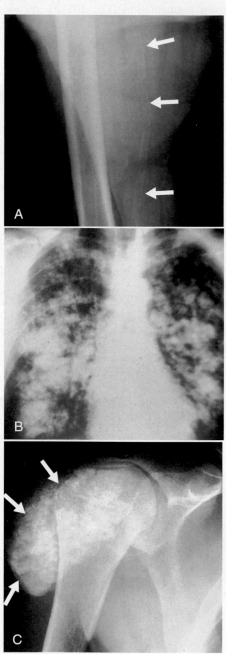

Fig 203–6
Extraskeletal calcification in chronic renal failure. **A,** Arterial calcification *(arrows)*. **B,** Pulmonary calcification. **C,** Periarticular calcification *(arrows)*.
(From Johnson RJ, Feehally J: Comprehensive Clinical Nephrology, 3rd ed. St. Louis, Mosby, 2007.)

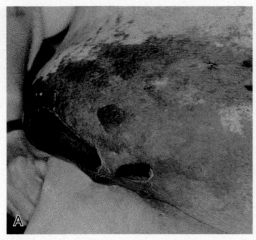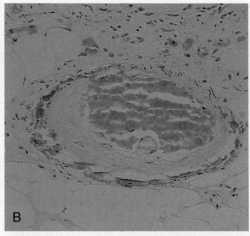

Fig 203-7
Calciphylaxis. **A,** Calciphylaxis may involve the trunk or extremities as violaceous skin lesions that progress to ulceration. **B,** Skin biopsy showing thrombosis of calcified blood vessel.
(From Johnson RJ, Feehally J: Comprehensive Clinical Nephrology, 3rd ed. St. Louis, Mosby, 2007.)

- Measure urinary protein excretion. The finding of a ratio of protein to creatinine of more than 1000 mg/g suggests the presence of glomerular disease
- Special studies: serum and urine immunoelectrophoresis (in suspected multiple myeloma), antinuclear antibody (ANA; in suspected systemic lupus erythematosus [SLE])
- Cystatin C is a cysteine proteinase inhibitor produced by all nucleated cells that is freely filtered at the glomerulus but not secreted by tubular cells. Given these characteristics, it may be superior to creatinine concentration in kidney disease and as a marker of acute kidney injury.

IMAGING STUDIES
- Ultrasound of kidneys to measure kidney size and to rule out obstruction (Fig. 203-8)
- Chest x-ray: to rule out CHF, pericardial effusion (Fig. 203-9)

TREATMENT
- Restrict sodium (approximately 100 mmol/day), potassium (≤60 mmol/day), and phosphate (<800 mg/day).
- Adjust drug doses to correct for prolonged half-lives.
- Restrict fluid if significant edema is present.
- Provide adequate nutrition and calories (147 to 168 kJ/kg/day in energy intake, chiefly from carbohydrates and polyunsaturated fats). Protein restriction (≤0.8 g/kg/day) may slow deterioration of renal function; however, recent studies have not confirmed this benefit.
- Avoid radiocontrast agents. Hydration with sodium bicarbonate before contrast exposure is more effective than hydration with sodium chloride for prophylaxis of contrast-induced renal failure.
- Angiotensin-converting enzyme (ACE) inhibitors and angiotensin receptor blockers (ARBs) are useful in reducing proteinuria and slowing the progression of chronic renal disease, especially in hypertensive diabetic patients. A systolic blood pressure between 110 and 129 mm Hg may be beneficial in patients with urine protein excretion >1.0 g/day. Systolic blood pressure (BP) <110 mm Hg may be associated with a higher risk for kidney disease progression.
- Initiation of dialysis
  1. Urgent indications: uremic pericarditis, neuropathy, neuromuscular abnormalities, CHF, hyperkalemia, seizures.
  2. Judgmental indications: creatinine clearance 10 to 15 mL/min; progressive anorexia, weight loss, reversal of sleep pattern, pruritus, uncontrolled fluid gain with hypertension, signs of CHF
- Erythropoietin for anemia: 2000 to 3000 U three times weekly, IV or SC, to maintain hematocrit (Hct) at approximately 30%.
- Diuretics for significant fluid overload (loop diuretics are preferred).
- Correction of hypertension to at least 130/85 mm Hg with ACE inhibitors (avoid in patients with significant hyperkalemia). ARBs, and/or nondihydropyridine calcium channel blockers (verapamil, diltiazem) can be used in patients intolerant to ACE inhibitors or when other agents are needed to control blood pressure
- Correction of electrolyte abnormalities (e.g., calcium chloride, glucose, sodium polystyrene sulfonate for hyperkalemia), sodium bicarbonate in patients with severe metabolic acidosis
- Lipid-lowering agents in patients with dyslipidemia; target low-density lipoprotein (LDL) cholesterol is <100 mg/dL.
- Control of renal osteodystrophy with calcium supplementation and vitamin D
- Sevelamer is a useful phosphate binder to reduce serum phosphate levels.
- Kidney transplantation in select patients improves survival. The 2-year kidney graft survival rate for living related donor transplantations is more than 80%, whereas the 2-year graft survival rate for cadaveric donor transplantation is approximately 70%.

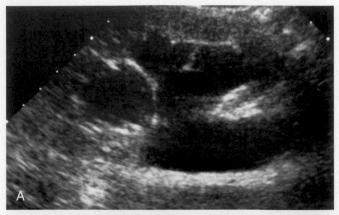

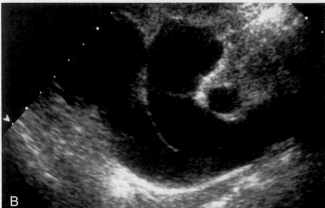

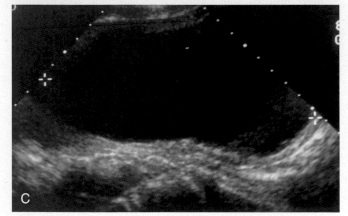

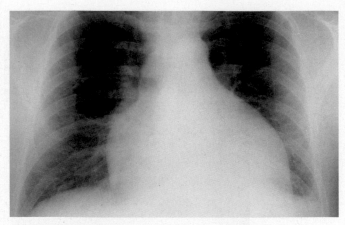

Fig 203–9
Pericardial effusion. Chest radiograph shows a large pericardial effusion.
(From Johnson RJ, Feehally J: Comprehensive Clinical Nephrology, 3rd ed. St. Louis, Mosby, 2007.)

Fig 203–8
Obstructive renal failure in a man with benign prostatic hypertrophy.
A, B, Longitudinal ultrasound images show marked pelvicalyceal dilation in both kidneys and a large postvoid bladder residue **(C)**.
(From Grainger RG, Allison DJ, Adam A, Dixon AK [eds]: Grainger & Allison's Diagnostic Radiology, 4th ed. London, Harcourt, 2001.)

Chapter 204 / Glomerulonephritis

DEFINITION
Acute glomerulonephritis is an immunologically mediated inflammation primarily involving the glomerulus that can result in damage to the basement membrane, mesangium, or capillary endothelium.

PHYSICAL FINDINGS AND CLINICAL PRESENTATION
- Edema (peripheral, periorbital, or pulmonary)
- Joint pains, oral ulcers, malar rash (frequently seen with lupus nephritis)
- Dark urine
- Hypertension
- Findings of palpable purpura in patients with Henoch-Schönlein purpura
- Heart murmurs may indicate endocarditis.
- Impetigo, skin pallor, tenderness in the abdomen and/or back; pharyngeal erythema may be present.

CAUSE
Acute glomerulonephritis may be caused by primary renal disease or a systemic disease. A number of pathogenic processes (e.g., antibody deposition, cell-mediated immune mechanisms, complement activation, hemodynamic alterations) have been implicated in the pathogenesis of glomerular inflammation. Medical disorders generally associated with glomerulonephritis include the following:
- Post–group A β-hemolytic *Streptococcus* infection (other infectious causes, including endocarditis and visceral abscess)
- Collagen-vascular diseases (SLE; Fig. 204–1)
- Vasculitis (Wegener's granulomatosis, polyarteritis nodosa)
- Idiopathic glomerulonephritis (membranoproliferative (Fig. 204–2), idiopathic, crescentic, IgA nephropathy)
- Goodpasture's syndrome
- Other cryoglobulinemia (Henoch-Schönlein purpura)
- Drug-induced (gold, penicillamine)

DIFFERENTIAL DIAGNOSIS
- Cirrhosis with edema and ascites
- CHF
- Acute interstitial nephritis
- Severe hypertension
- Hemolytic-uremic syndrome
- SLE, diabetes mellitus, amyloidosis, preeclampsia, scleroderma renal crisis

LABORATORY TESTS
- Urinalysis (hematuria [dysmorphic erythrocytes and red cell casts], proteinuria)
- Serum creatinine (to estimate glomerular filtration rate [GFR]), BUN
- 24-hour urine for protein excretion and creatinine clearance (to document degree of renal dysfunction and amount of proteinuria). Proteinuria in acute glomerulonephritis typically ranges from 500 mg/day to 3 g/day but nephrotic-range proteinuria (>3.5 g/day) may be present.
- Streptococcal tests (Streptozyme), antistreptolysin O (ASO) quantitative titer (highest in 3 to 5 weeks); ASO titer, however, is not related to the severity of renal disease, duration, or prognosis.
- Additional useful tests depending on the history: anti-DNA antibodies (rule out SLE), CH_{50} level (if elevated, obtain C3, C4 levels), triglycerides, cryoglobulins, hepatitis B and C serologies, ANCA (antineutrophil cytoplasmic antibody), c-ANCA (in suspected cases of Wegener's granulomatosis), p-ANCA found in pauci-immune (lack of immune deposits) idiopathic rapidly progressive glomerulonephritis, with or without systemic vasculitis, anti-GBM antibodies
- Hct (decrease in glomerulonephritis), platelet count (thrombocytopenia in cases of lupus nephritis)
- Anti-GBM antibody (in Goodpasture's syndrome)
- Blood cultures are indicated in all febrile patients.

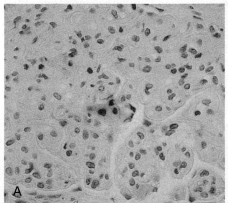
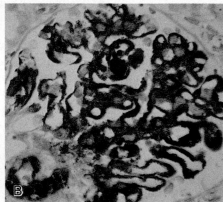
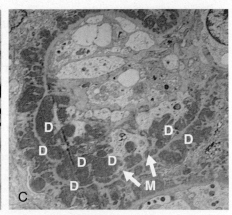

Fig 204–1
WHO class IV lupus nephritis (diffuse proliferative), present in 35% to 60% of biopsies. **A,** The tuft is increased in size by a diffuse increase in matrix and an excess of cells; capillary walls are irregularly thickened (H&E). **B,** Dense irregular aggregates of IgG along the peripheral capillary walls are shown by immunoperoxidase stain. **C,** Electron microscopy shows the immune aggregates as electron-dense masses (D) at subendothelial and subepithelial sites, with the lighter capillary basement membrane (M) *(arrows)* between them.
(From Johnson RJ, Feehally J: Comprehensive Clinical Nephrology, 3rd ed. St. Louis, Mosby, 2007.)

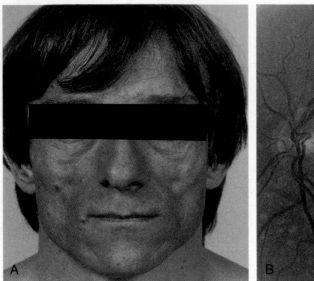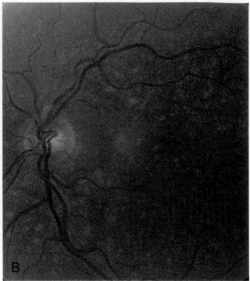

Fig 204-2
Membranoproliferative glomerulonephritis type II. **A,** Partial lipodystrophy; note the absence of subcutaneous fat from the face.
B, Drusen bodies in the retina.
(Courtesy of Dr. C. D. Short.)

IMAGING STUDIES
- Chest x-ray: pulmonary congestion, Wegener's granulomatosis, Goodpasture's syndrome
- Renal ultrasound if GFR is depressed to evaluate renal size and determine extent of fibrosis. A kidney size smaller than 9 cm is suggestive of extensive scarring and low likelihood of reversibility.
- Echocardiography in patients with new cardiac murmurs or positive blood cultures to rule out endocarditis and pericardial effusion
- Renal biopsy and light, electron, and immunofluorescent microscopy to confirm diagnosis (Fig. 204–3)
- Kidney biopsy: generally reveals a granular pattern in poststreptococcal glomerulonephritis (Fig. 204–4), linear pattern in Goodpasture's syndrome; absence of immune deposits suggests vasculitis.
- Renal biopsy: although helpful to define the cause of glomerulonephritis, not usually essential. It is useful to determine the degrees of inflammation and fibrosis. It is also especially important for patients with rapidly progressive GN (RPGN) for whom prompt diagnosis and treatment are essential.
- Immunofluorescence: generally reveals C3; negative immunofluorescence suggests Wegener's granulomatosis, idiopathic crescentic glomerulonephritis, polyarteritis nodosa
- Angiography or biopsy of other affected organs if systemic vasculitis is suspected

TREATMENT
- Correction of electrolyte abnormalities (hypocalcemia, hyperkalemia) and acidosis (if present)
- Treatment of streptococcal infection with penicillin (or erythromycin for penicillin-allergic patients)
- Furosemide in patients with significant hypertension and/or edema
- Immunosuppressive treatment in patients with heavy proteinuria or rapidly decreasing glomerular filtration rate (high-dose corticosteroids, cyclosporine, cyclophosphamide); corticosteroids, however, are generally not useful in poststreptococcal glomerulonephritis
- Fish oil (omega-3 fatty acids), 12 g/day: may prevent or slow down loss of renal function in patients with IgA nephropathy
- Plasma exchange therapy and immunosuppressive drugs (prednisone and cyclophosphamide): effective in Goodpasture's syndrome
- Short-term therapy with IV cyclophosphamide followed by maintenance therapy with mycophenolate mofetil or azathioprine is more efficacious and safer than long-term therapy with IV cyclophosphamide in patients with proliferative lupus nephritis.

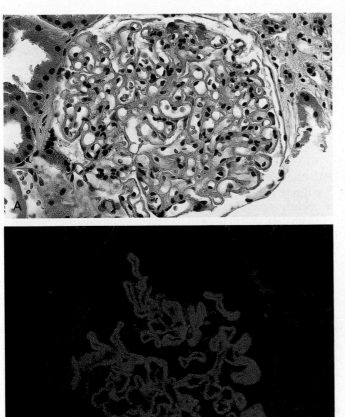

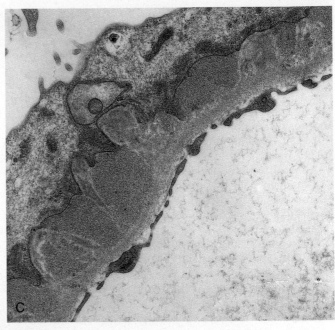

Fig 204-3

A, Membranous glomerulopathy with diffusely thickened peripheral walls. **B,** Immunofluorescence for IgG-granular peripheral capillary wall staining typical of membranous glomerulonephritis. **C,** Regularly disposed epimembranous immune complexes surrounded by protrusions of basement membrane material (spikes) (**A, B,** ×500; **C,** transmission electron microscopy, uranyl acetate and lead citrate, ×15,500).
(**A** from Silverberg SG, Frable WJ, Wick MR, et al [eds]: Principles and Practice of Surgical Pathology and Cytopathology, 4th ed. Philadelphia, Elsevier, 2006.)

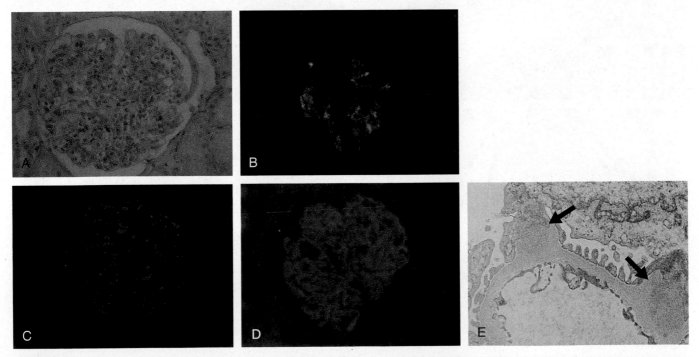

Fig 204-4

Poststreptococcal glomerulonephritis. **A,** A diffuse proliferative and exudative glomerulonephritis can be seen by light microscopy. Immunofluorescence shows the mesangial **(B)**, starry sky **(C)**, and garland **(D)** patterns. **E,** Electron microscopy demonstrates large subepithelial "humps" *(arrows)* beneath effaced foot processes.
(**E** courtesy of L. de Moura.)

Chapter 205 Acute tubular necrosis

DEFINITION

Acute tubular necrosis refers to intrinsic tubular damage induced by hypoperfusion to renal parenchymal cells, particularly tubular epithelium, that results in sodium loss and $FE_{Na} > 1\%$ (fractional excretion of sodium).

PHYSICAL FINDINGS AND CLINICAL PRESENTATION

- No apparent physical findings
- Clinical features include recent hemorrhage, hypotension, or surgery, thereby suggesting ischemic ARF. Recent radiocontrast study, nephrotoxic drugs, history suggestive of rhabdomyolysis, hemolysis, or myeloma may suggest toxin-mediated ARF.
- Three phases of ischemic ARF:
  1. Initiation phase (hours to days): renal hypoperfusion, evolving ischemia.
  2. Maintenance phase (1-2 weeks): renal cell injury established, GFR stabilizes at its nadir (5 to 10 mL/min), urine output at its lowest, uremic complications arise

3. Recovery phase (after 2 weeks): renal parenchymal cell repair and regeneration, gradual return of GFR to premorbid levels; may be complicated by a marked diuretic phase caused by excretion of retained salt and water and other solutes, continued use of diuretics, or delayed recovery of epithelial cell function (solute and water reabsorption) relative to glomerular filtration

PATHOLOGIC FINDINGS

See Figure 205-1.

- Ischemic ARF: patchy and focal necrosis of tubule epithelium with detachment from its basement membrane and occlusion of tubule lumens with casts composed of epithelial cells, cellular debris, Tamm-Horsfall mucoprotein (represents the matrix of all urinary casts), and pigments. Also present is leukocyte accumulation in the vasa recta (capillaries that return the NaCl and water reabsorbed in the loop of Henle and medullary collecting tubule to the systemic circulation). Morphology of glomeruli and renal vasculature remain normal. Necrosis is

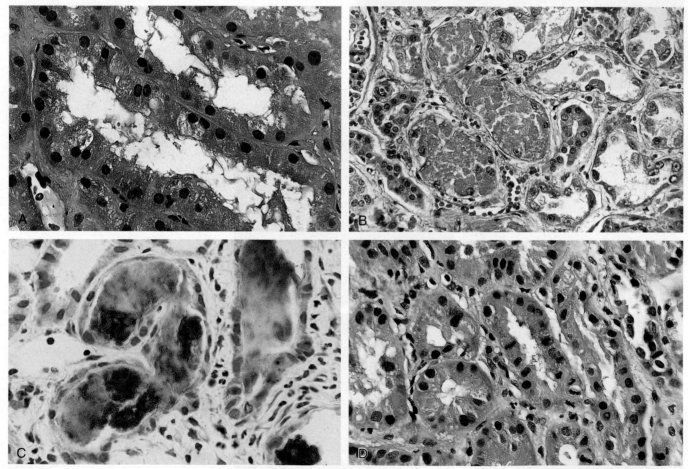

Fig 205-1

Acute tubular necrosis. **A,** Subtle early changes of acute tubular necrosis. **B,** Overt selective proximal tubular necrosis in nephrotoxic type of acute tubular necrosis. **C,** Myoglobulin casts and tubular simplification. **D,** Evidence of tubular regeneration with several mitotic figures in tubular cells (**A-C,** ×500; **D,** ×350).

(From Silverberg SG, Frable WJ, Wick MR, et al [eds]: Principles and Practice of Surgical Pathology and Cytopathology, 4th ed. Philadelphia, Elsevier, 2006.)

most severe in the pars recta (straight portion of proximal tubule and thick ascending limb of loop of Henle).
- Nephrotoxic ARF: morphologic changes in convoluted and straight portion of proximal tubule. Tubule cell necrosis is less pronounced than in ischemic ARF.

CAUSE
- Hypotension or shock
- Prolonged prerenal azotemia
- Postoperative sepsis syndrome
- Rhabdomyolysis
- Hemolysis (hypercalcemia, hemoglobin, urate, oxalate, myeloma light chains),
- Antimicrobial drugs (acyclovir, foscarnet, aminoglycosides, amphotericin B, pentamidine)
- Radiocontrast (contrast nephropathy)
- Chemotherapy (cisplatin, ifosfamide)

DIFFERENTIAL DIAGNOSIS
- Allergic interstitial nephritis
- Acute bilateral pyelonephritis

LABORATORY TESTS
- Urinalysis: urine microscopy reveals muddy brown casts (Fig. 205–2).
- Urinalysis for specific gravity (SG), U_{Na}, P_{Cr}, P_{Na}, U_{Cr}
- Calculate fractional excretion of sodium;

$$(FE_{Na}) = [(U_{Na} \times P_{Cr})/(P_{Na} \times U_{Cr})] \times 100$$

LABORATORY FINDINGS
- $FE_{Na} > 1\%$
- $U_{Na} > 20$ mmol/L
- SG < 1.015

IMAGING STUDIES
- Generally not necessary

TREATMENT
- Should focus on providing cause-specific supportive care or correction of primary hemodynamic abnormality
- No specific therapies for established ATN
- Peritoneal or hemodialysis for replacement of renal function until regeneration and repair restore renal function

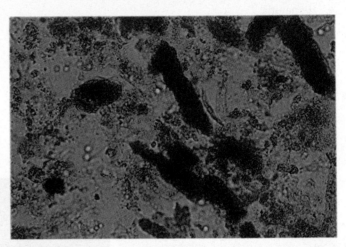

Fig 205–2
Muddy brown casts in acute tubular necrosis (ATN). Urine microscopy shows the typical muddy brown casts of ATN.
(Courtesy of Dr. Michael Ryan.)

Chapter 206 / IgA nephropathy

DEFINITION

IgA nephropathy (Buerger's disease) is a mesangial proliferative glomerulonephritis characterized by diffuse mesangial deposition of IgA. It is the most frequent form of idiopathic glomerulonephritis worldwide.

PHYSICAL FINDINGS AND CLINICAL PRESENTATION

- Hematuria
- Proteinuria
- Hypertension

CAUSE

- Abnormal; antigenic stimulation of mucosal IgA production and subsequent immune complex deposition in the glomeruli

DIFFERENTIAL DIAGNOSIS

- Henoch-Schönlein purpura glomerulonephritis
- Poststreptococcal glomerulonephritis

LABORATORY TESTS

- Kidney biopsy: presence of glomerular IgA deposits either as the dominant or co-dominant immunoglobulin on immunofluorescence microscopy establishes the diagnosis (Fig. 206-1)
- Elevated serum creatinine
- Urinalysis: hematuria, proteinuria

TREATMENT

- Aggressive lowering of blood pressure
- Tonsillectomy reduces the frequency of episodic hematuria when recurrent tonsillitis is the provoking infection.
- Corticosteroids, omega-3 fish oil, cytotoxic agents (in crescenteric IgA nephropathy)

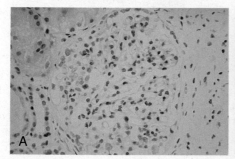  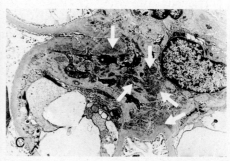

Fig 206-1

Renal pathology in IgA nephropathy. **A,** Light microscopy, diffuse mesangial hypercellularity (H&E, ×300). **B,** Immunofluorescence microscopy, diffuse mesangial IgA (indirect immunofluorescence with FITC-anti IgA, ×300). **C,** Electron microscopy, mesangial electron-dense deposits. The deposits are shown by *arrows* (electron micrograph, ×16,000).
(From Johnson RJ, Feehally J: Comprehensive Clinical Nephrology, 3rd ed, St. Louis, Mosby, 2007.)
(**A, C,** Micrographs courtesy of Prof. P. Furness; **B,** Courtesy of Chapman & Hall.)

Chapter 207 | Nephrotic syndrome

DEFINITION

Nephrotic syndrome is a renal disorder characterized by high urine protein excretion ($>3.5g/1.73$ $m^3/24$ hr), peripheral edema, and metabolic abnormalities (hypoalbuminemia, hypercholesterolemia).

PHYSICAL FINDINGS AND CLINICAL PRESENTATION

- Periorbital edema (Fig. 207–1)
- Peripheral edema (Fig. 207–2)

- Ascites, anasarca
- Hypertension
- Pleural effusion
- Xanthelasma (Fig. 207–3)
- Nails with Muehrcke's lines (Fig. 207–4)
- Typically, patients present with severe peripheral edema, exertional dyspnea, and abdominal fullness secondary to ascites. There is a significant amount of weight gain in most patients.

CAUSE

- Membranous glomerulonephritis is the most common cause of nephrotic syndrome.

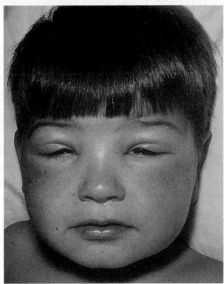

Fig 207–1
Periorbital edema in the early morning in a nephrotic child. The edema resolves during the day under the influence of gravity.
(From Johnson RJ, Feehally J: Comprehensive Clinical Nephrology, 3rd ed. St. Louis, Mosby, 2007.)

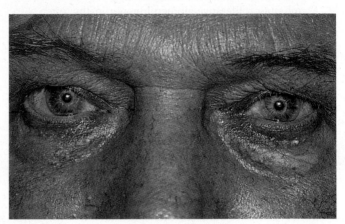

Fig 207–3
Xanthelasma in nephrotic syndrome. These prominent xanthelasma developed within a period of two months in a patient with recent onset of severe nephrotic syndrome and serum cholesterol 550 mg/dL (14.2 mmol/L).
(From Johnson RJ, Feehally J: Comprehensive Clinical Nephrology, 3rd ed. St. Louis, Mosby, 2007.)

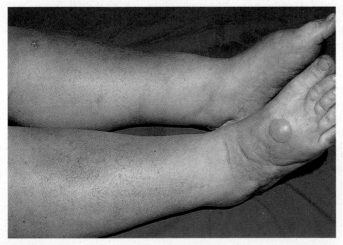

Fig 207–2
Nephrotic edema. Severe peripheral edema in nephrotic syndrome; note the blisters caused by intradermal fluid.
(From Johnson RJ, Feehally J: Comprehensive Clinical Nephrology, 3rd ed. St. Louis, Mosby, 2007.)

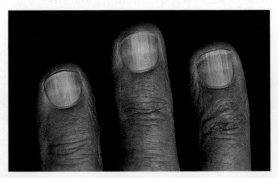

Fig 207–4
Muehrcke's bands in nephrotic syndrome. The white band grew during a transient period of hypoalbuminemia caused by the nephrotic syndrome.
(From Johnson RJ, Feehally J: Comprehensive Clinical Nephrology, 3rd ed. St. Louis, Mosby, 2007.)

- Idiopathic (may be secondary to the following glomerular diseases: minimal change disease [nail disease, lipoid nephrosis], focal segmental glomerular sclerosis, membranous nephropathy, membranoproliferative glomerular nephropathy)
- Associated with systemic diseases (diabetes mellitus, SLE, amyloidosis). Amyloidosis and dysproteinemias should be considered in patients older than 40 years.
- Majority of children with nephrotic syndrome have minimal change disease (this form also associated with allergy, nonsteroidals, and Hodgkin's disease)
- Focal glomerular disease: can be associated with HIV infection, heroin abuse. A more severe form of nephrotic syndrome associated with rapid progression to end-stage renal failure within months can also occur in HIV seropositive patients and is known as collapsing glomerulopathy.
- Membranous nephropathy: can occur with Hodgkin's lymphoma, carcinomas, SLE, gold therapy
- Membranoproliferative glomerulonephropathy: often associated with upper respiratory infections

DIFFERENTIAL DIAGNOSIS
- Other edema states (CHF, cirrhosis)
- Primary renal disease (e.g., focal glomerulonephritis, membranoproliferative glomerulonephritis)
- Carcinoma, infections
- Malignant hypertension
- Polyarteritis nodosa
- Serum sickness
- Toxemia of pregnancy

LABORATORY TESTS
- Urinalysis reveals proteinuria. The presence of hematuria, cellular casts, and pyuria is suggestive of nephritic syndrome. Oval fat bodies (tubular epithelial cells with cholesterol esters) (Fig. 207–5) are also found in the urine in patients with nephrotic syndrome.
- 24-hour urine protein excretion is >3.5 g/1.73 m^3/24 hr.
- Abnormalities of blood chemistries include serum albumin <3 g/dL, decreased total protein, elevated serum cholesterol, glucose, and azotemia.
- Additional tests in patients with nephrotic syndromes depending on the history and physical examination are ANA, serum and urine immunoelectrophoresis, C3, C4, CH_{50}, lactate dehydrogenase (LDH), liver enzymes, alkaline phosphatase, hepatitis B and C screening, and HIV.

IMAGING STUDIES
- Ultrasound of kidneys
- Chest x-ray

TREATMENT
- Bed rest as tolerated, avoidance of nephrotoxic drugs, low-fat diet, fluid restriction in hyponatremic patients; normal protein intake unless urinary protein loss exceeds 10 g/24 hr (some patients may require additional dietary protein to prevent negative nitrogen balance and significant protein malnutrition).
- Improved urinary protein excretion and serum lipid changes have been observed with a low-fat soy protein diet providing 0.7 g of protein/kg/day. However, because of increased risk of malnutrition, many nephrologists recommend normal protein intake.
- Strict sodium restriction to help manage peripheral edema
- Close monitoring of patients for development of peripheral venous thrombosis and renal vein thrombosis because of hypercoagulable state secondary to loss of antithrombin III and other proteins involved in the clotting mechanism
- Furosemide is useful for severe edema.
- Use of ACE inhibitors to reduce proteinuria is generally indicated, even in normotensive patients.
- Anticoagulant therapy should be administered as long as patients have nephrotic proteinuria, an albumin level <20 g/L, or both.

The mainstay of therapy is treatment of the underlying disorder:
- Minimal change disease generally responds to prednisone. Relapses can occur when corticosteroids are discontinued. In these individuals, cyclophosphamide and chlorambucil may be useful.
- Focal and segmental glomerulosclerosis: corticosteroid therapy is also recommended. However, response rate is approximately 35% to 40%, and most patients progress to end-stage renal disease within 3 years.
- Membranous glomerulonephritis: prednisone, may be useful in inducing remission. Cytotoxic agents can be added if there is poor response to prednisone.
- Membranoproliferative glomerulonephritis: most patients are treated with steroid therapy and antiplatelet drugs. Despite treatment, the majority of patients will progress to end-stage renal disease within 5 years.

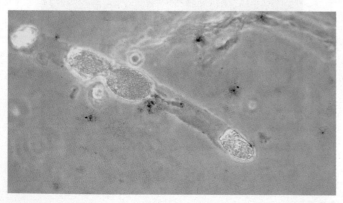

Fig 207–5
Fat in the urine. A hyaline cast containing oval fat bodies, which are tubular epithelial cells full of fat. Oval fat bodies often appear brown in color.
(From Johnson RJ, Feehally J: Comprehensive Clinical Nephrology, 3rd ed. St. Louis, Mosby, 2007.)

Chapter 208 / Interstitial nephritis

DEFINITION

Interstitial nephritis refers to a group of disorders primarily affecting the interstitium and renal tubules. Interstitial nephritis may be acute or chronic.

PHYSICAL FINDINGS AND CLINICAL PRESENTATION

Acute interstitial nephritis (AIN)

- Patients usually asymptomatic and found to have a sudden decrease in renal function
- Characteristically occurs over several days to weeks after an infection or initiation of a new medication
- Classic triad—fever, rash (Fig. 208–1), and arthralgias
- Lumbar flank pain
- Gross hematuria
- Usually oliguric

Chronic interstitial nephritis (CIN)

- Usually present with symptoms related to the underlying cause (e.g., sarcoidosis, multiple myeloma, urate nephropathy)
- Symptoms of renal failure (e.g., weakness, nausea, pruritus)
- Hypertension

CAUSE

- AIN is usually caused by drugs or infection, or is associated with immune or neoplastic disorders.
- Common drugs include penicillin, methicillin, rifampin, cephalosporins, trimethoprim-sulfamethoxazole, ciprofloxacin, nonsteroidal anti-inflammatory drugs (NSAIDs), thiazides, furosemide, triamterene, allopurinol, phenytoin, captopril, and cimetidine.
- Infection (e.g., *Streptococcus*, *Legionella*, *Corynebacterium diphtheriae*, *Yersinia*, *Salmonella*, HIV, Epstein-Barr virus [EBV], cytomegalovirus [CMV], *Mycoplasma*, *Rickettsia*, and *Mycobacterium tuberculosis*)
- Autoimmune causes of AIN include Sjögren's syndrome, SLE, and Wegener's granulomatosis.
- Common causes of CIN include polycystic kidney disease, urate nephropathy, analgesic nephropathy, sarcoidosis, multiple myeloma, lead nephropathy, hypercalcemia, and Balkan nephropathy.

DIAGNOSIS

Renal biopsy (Fig. 208–2) is the only definitive method of establishing the diagnosis of interstitial nephritis. All other laboratory tests provide supportive evidence of interstitial nephritis.

DIFFERENTIAL DIAGNOSIS

The differential diagnosis includes the diseases listed under "Cause."

LABORATORY TESTS

- CBC showing anemia and eosinophilia
- BUN and creatinine are elevated and typically represent the first clue of interstitial nephritis.
- Electrolytes, calcium, and phosphorus
- Uric acid
- Elevated IgE level
- Urinalysis reveals hematuria and pyuria.
- Eosinophiluria by Hansen stain is suggestive of allergic interstitial nephritis.
- Proteinuria, <3 g/24 hr

IMAGING STUDIES

- Ultrasound of the kidneys shows normal-size kidneys in AIN and small contracted kidneys in CIN.

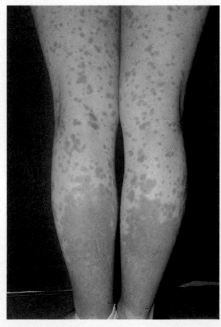

Fig 208–1
Maculopapular rash in a patient with drug-induced acute interstitial nephritis (AIN). Such cutaneous lesions occur in about 40% of patients with drug-induced AIN, but they can also be seen in patients with drug-induced acute tubular necrosis.
(From Johnson RJ, Feehally J: Comprehensive Clinical Nephrology, 3rd ed. St. Louis, Mosby, 2007.)

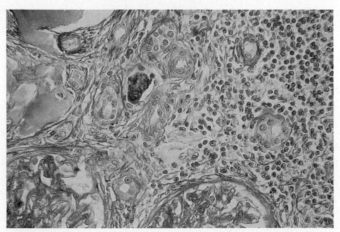

Fig 208–2
Drug-induced acute interstitial nephritis. On light microscopy, the characteristic feature is of an interstitial infiltration with mononuclear cells, with normal glomeruli. It is usually associated with interstitial edema and with tubular lesions.
(Courtesy of Dr. B. Mougenot.)

- Intravenous pyelography (IVP) findings are similar to ultrasound findings.
- Renal biopsy in AIN reveals infiltration of inflammatory cells into the interstitium with interstitial edema and sparing of the glomeruli. In CIN, fibrotic scar tissue replaces the cellular infiltrate.

TREATMENT

- Low-protein, low-potassium, low-sodium diet
- Correction of underlying electrolyte abnormalities
- IV hydration for hypercalcemia

- Corticosteroids are used in patients with drug-induced AIN not responding to withdrawal of the offending medication within 3 to 4 days.
- Cyclophosphamide may be added as a second agent for patients not responding to corticosteroids.
- Combined therapy is generally continued for 6 weeks.
- Treatment of chronic interstitial nephritis is directed at the underlying cause (e.g., corticosteroids for sarcoidosis, EDTA in lead nephropathy).

Chapter 209 Amyloidosis

DEFINITION

Amyloidosis is a generic term describing the deposition of amyloid fibrils in body tissues. Amyloid is an amorphous, eosinophilic material; it is birefringent and usually extracellular. Electron microscopy reveals nonbranching fibrils that are soluble and relatively resistant to proteolytic digestion. Table 209–1 describes the characteristics of systemic amyloidoses.

PHYSICAL FINDINGS AND CLINICAL PRESENTATION

- Findings are variable with organ system involvement. Shrunken flexor tendons in the hands (Fig. 209–1), symmetrical polyarthritis, peripheral neuropathy, and carpal tunnel syndrome may be present with joint involvement.
- Signs and symptoms of nephrotic syndrome may be present with renal involvement.
- Fatigue and dyspnea may occur with pulmonary involvement.
- Diarrhea, macroglossia (20% of patients; Fig. 209–2), malabsorption, hepatomegaly, and weight loss may occur with GI involvement.
- Cardiac involvement is common and can lead to predominantly right-sided CHF, jugular venous distention (JVD), peripheral edema, and hepatomegaly.
- Vascular involvement can result in easy bleeding and periorbital purpura (raccoon eyes) or purpuric macules (Fig. 209–3).

CAUSE

In patients with amyloidosis, a soluble circulating protein (serum amyloid P [SAP]) is deposited in tissues as insoluble beta-pleated sheets. The source of amyloid protein is a population of monoclonal plasma cells in the bone marrow. There are several chemically documented amyloidoses that can be principally subdivided into the following:

1. Acquired systemic amyloidosis (immunoglobulin light chain, multiple myeloma, hemodialysis amyloidosis)

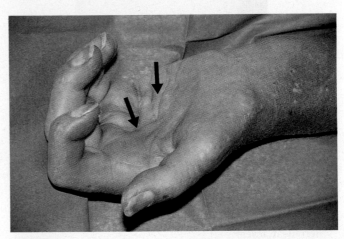

Fig 209–1

Hand involvement in Aβ_2M-amyloidosis. The hand of this long-term hemodialysis patient shows maximal extension. Note the prominence of shrunken flexor tendons (arrows). This is also known as the guitar string sign.
(From Johnson RJ, Feehally J: Comprehensive Clinical Nephrology, 3rd ed. St. Louis, Mosby, 2007.)

TABLE 209–1 Characteristics of systemic amyloidosis (AL)

Feature	Light-chain related AL	Secondary-reactive AA	Dialysis-associated Aβ2-M	Familial
Underlying disease	Almost always associated with monoclonal protein	Usually associated with chronic infection or inflammatory disease	Usually occurs after long-term dialysis	Usually related to altered protein, most frequently transthyretin
Major clinical presentation	Cardiac, renal, gastrointestinal, carpal tunnel	Renal	Chronic arthralgias, destructive arthropathy, carpal tunnel syndrome	Dependent on family, but commonly neuropathic
Renal	Expected	Expected	Already on dialysis	
Hepatic	Usually	Usually	Uncommon	
Spleen	Often	Often	Uncommon	
Cardiac	Frequently impaired	Deposits common, but impairment very rare	Uncommon	
Periarticular	Occurs; carpal tunnel common	Rare	Expected, carpal tunnel common	
Neurologic	Common, often autonomic	Rare		
Macroglossia	12%-15%	No	One case reported	
Cutaneous findings	Clinical lesions 10%-40%, subclinical deposits frequent	Clinical lesions rare, subclinical deposits frequent	Clinical skin lesions rare, subclinical deposits occasionally	Syndrome dependent; clinical lesions occur in several, subclinical deposits expected in some syndromes

From Callen JP, Jorizzo JL, Bolognia JL, et al: Dermatological Signs of Internal Disease, 3rd ed. Philadelphia, WB Saunders, 2003.

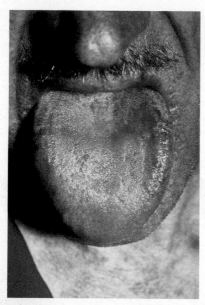

Fig 209-2
Primary systemic amyloidosis.
(Courtesy of Dr. R. A. Marsden, St. George's Hospital, London.)

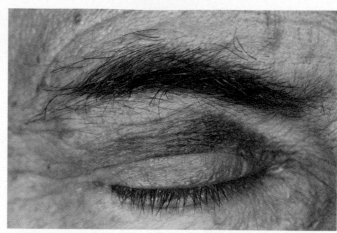

Fig 209-3
Skin involvement in AL-amyloidosis. Noninfiltrated purpuric macule of the superior eyebrow is very typical of AL-amyloidosis.
(From Johnson RJ, Feehally J: Comprehensive Clinical Nephrology, 3rd ed, Mosby, St. Louis, 2007.)

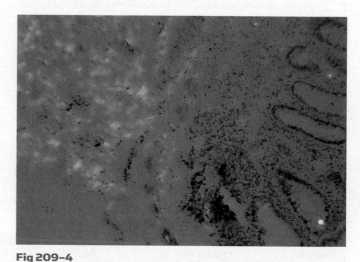

Fig 209-4
Rectal biopsy positive for amyloidosis. The tissue has been stained with Congo red and examined by polarized light. Note the apple-green birefringence.
(From Hochberg MC, Silman AJ, Smolen JS, et al (eds): Rheumatology, 3rd ed. St. Louis, Mosby, 2003.)

2. Heredofamilial systemic (polyneuropathy, familial Mediterranean fever)
3. Organ limited (Alzheimer's disease)
4. Localized endocrine (pancreatic islet, medullary thyroid carcinoma)

DIFFERENTIAL DIAGNOSIS

This is variable, depending on the organ involvement:

- Renal involvement (toxin- or drug-induced necrosis, glomerulonephritis, renal vein thrombosis)
- Interstitial lung disease (sarcoidosis, connective tissue disease, infectious causes)
- Restrictive cardiac (endomyocardial fibrosis, viral myocarditis)
- Carpal tunnel (rheumatoid arthritis, hypothyroidism, overuse)
- Mental status changes (multi-infarct dementia)
- Peripheral neuropathy (alcohol abuse, vitamin deficiencies, diabetes mellitus)

LABORATORY TESTS

- Initial laboratory evaluation should include CBC, thyroid-stimulating hormone (TSH), renal function studies, alanine aminotransferase (ALT), aspartate transaminase (AST), alkaline phosphatase, bilirubin, urinalysis, and serum and urine protein immunoelectrophoresis.
- Various laboratory abnormalities include proteinuria (found in more than 70% of cases), anemia, renal insufficiency, liver function abnormalities, hypothyroidism (10% to 20% of patients), and elevated monoclonal proteins. The finding of a monoclonal light chain in the serum or urine is useful for diagnosis.
- Diagnostic approach is aimed at demonstration of amyloid deposits in tissues. This may be accomplished with rectal biopsy (positive in more than 60% of cases; Fig. 209-4). Renal, myocardial, and bone marrow biopsies are

other options. Abdominal fat pad biopsy can also be diagnostic (Fig. 209-5); however, its yield is low and it should generally be reserved for evaluation of patients with peripheral neuropathy who also have findings associated with systemic amyloidosis.

- DNA analysis is necessary for the diagnosis of hereditary amyloidosis.

IMAGING STUDIES

- Chest x-ray may reveal hilar adenopathy and mediastinal adenopathy.
- Two-dimensional Doppler echocardiography to study diagnostic filling is useful to evaluate for cardiac involvement.
- Nuclear imaging with technetium-labeled aprotinin may detect cardiac amyloidosis. SAP scintigraphy has high sensitivity for the detection of amyloid deposits in the liver, spleen, kidneys, adrenal glands, and bones.

TREATMENT

- Therapy is variable, depending on the type of amyloidosis. Amyloidosis associated with plasma cell disorders may be treated with melphalan and prednisone, along with colchicine. Colchicine may also be effective in renal amyloidosis.
- Treatment of amyloid light-chain amyloidosis with high-dose melphalan and stem cell transplantation may result in hematologic remission and improved 5-year survival.
- Promising results have been found with the use of a molecule known as CPHPC given IV or SC in amyloidosis. This molecule has been shown to be effective in reducing circulating levels of SAP.
- Renal transplantation is generally needed in patients with renal amyloidosis. Peritoneal dialysis in place of hemodialysis in patients with renal failure may improve hemodialysis amyloidosis by clearing beta$_2$-microglobulin.
- In reactive amyloidosis, eradication of the predisposing disease slows and can occasionally reverse the progression of amyloid disease. Survival of 5 to 10 years after diagnosis is not uncommon.
- Patients with familial amyloidotic polyneuropathy generally have a prolonged course lasting 10 to 15 years.
- Amyloidosis associated with immunocytic processes carries the worst prognosis (life expectancy, less than 1 year).
- The progression of amyloidosis associated with renal hemodialysis can be improved with newer dialysis membranes that can pass beta$_2$-microglobulin.
- Median survival in patients with overt CHF is approximately 6 months, 30 months without CHF.

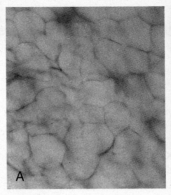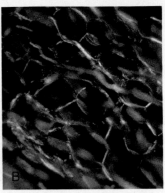

Fig 209–5

Amyloidosis in subcutaneous fat. Subcutaneous abdominal fat is obtained by needle aspiration. Regular light microscopy **(A)** is compared with polarized microscopy **(B)** after staining with Congo red. (Courtesy of the American College of Rheumatology, Atlanta, teaching slide collection.)

Chapter 210   Polycystic kidney disease

DEFINITION

Polycystic kidney disease refers to a systemic hereditary disorder characterized by the formation of cysts (Fig. 210–1) in the cortex and medulla of both kidneys (Fig. 210–2). Extrarenal manifestations include aneurysms (Fig. 210–3), and arachnoid cysts (Fig. 210–4).

PHYSICAL FINDINGS AND CLINICAL PRESENTATION

- Usually presents in the third to fourth decade of life
- Pain (abdominal, flank, or back)
- Palpable flank mass
- Hypertension
- Headache
- Nocturia
- Hematuria
- Nephrolithiasis (20%)
- Urinary tract infection

CAUSE

- Approximately 90% of cases are inherited as an autosomal dominant trait.
- Spontaneous mutations occur in 10% of cases.
- The abnormal gene in the majority of cases has been located to the short arm of chromosome 16. In the minority of cases the defect is located on chromosome 4.
- All cysts develop from preexisting renal tubules segments and only a small portion of the nephrons (1%) undergo cystic formation (see Fig. 210–1).

DIAGNOSIS

A person is considered to have polycystic kidney disease if three or more cysts are noted in both kidneys and there is a positive family member with autosomal dominant polycystic kidney disease (ADPKD).

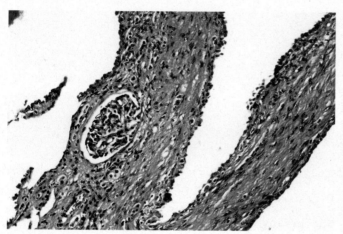

Fig 210–1
Adult polycystic kidney disease. These are photomicrographs of cysts with septa containing normal renal elements.
(From Silverberg SG, Frable WJ, Wick MR, et al [eds]: Principles and Practice of Surgical Pathology and Cytopathology, 4th ed. Philadelphia, Elsevier, 2006.)

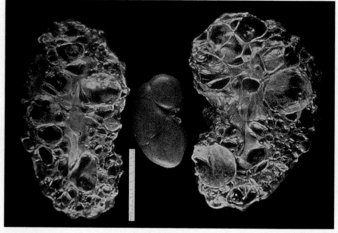

Fig 210–2
Markedly enlarged polycystic kidneys from a patient with autosomal dominant polycystic kidney disease (ADPKD) in comparison with a normal kidney in the middle.
(From Johnson RJ, Feehally J: Comprehensive Clinical Nephrology, 3rd ed. St. Louis, Mosby, 2007.)

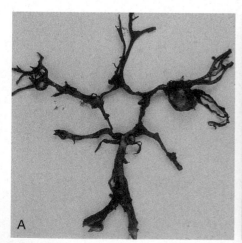

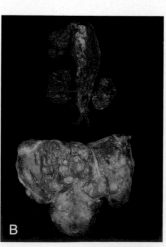

Fig 210–3
Vascular manifestations of autosomal dominant polycystic kidney disease. **A,** Gross specimen demonstrating bilateral aneurysms of the middle cerebral arteries. **B,** Gross specimen demonstrating a thoracic aortic dissection extending into the abdominal aorta in a patient with autosomal dominant polycystic kidney and liver disease.
(From Johnson RJ, Feehally J: Comprehensive Clinical Nephrology, 3rd ed. St. Louis, Mosby, 2007.)

A

B

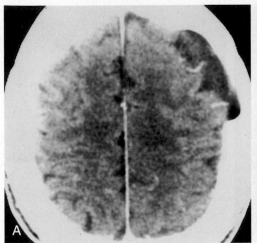
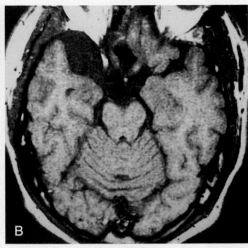

Fig 210–4
Extrarenal manifestations of autosomal dominant polycystic kidney
disease. Arachnoid cysts are demonstrated by CT **(A)** and MRI **(B)**.
(From Johnson RJ, Feehally J: Comprehensive Clinical Nephrology, 3rd
ed. St. Louis, Mosby, 2007.)

DIFFERENTIAL DIAGNOSIS
- Simple cysts (Fig. 210–5)
- Medullary sponge kidney (Fig. 210–6)
- Tuberous sclerosis (Fig. 210–7)
- von Hippel-Lindau disease
- Hydatid disease of kidneys (Fig. 210–8)
- Renal abscess (Fig. 210–9)
- Table 210–1 describes the differential features of adult renal cystic disease.

LABORATORY TESTS
- Hemoglobin and hematocrit are elevated because of in-creased secretion of erythropoietin from functioning renal cysts. This also explains the relatively mild anemia found in patients with ADPKD and renal insufficiency.
- Electrolyte abnormalities commonly seen in any patient with renal insufficiency may be present.
- BUN and creatinine may be elevated.
- Urinalysis can show microscopic hematuria, WBC casts in pyelonephritis, or proteinuria (seldom >1 g/24 hr).
- Increased erythropoietin level
- Patients with a strong positive family history of ADPKD and no cysts detected by imaging studies can undergo genetic linkage analysis for additional evaluation.

IMAGING STUDIES
- Abdominal renal ultrasound (Fig. 210–10) is the easiest and more cost-efficient test for renal cysts. Renal ultrasound can detect cysts from 1 to 1.5 cm.
- Abdominal CT scanning (Fig. 210–11) is more sensitive than ultrasound and can detect cysts as small as 0.5 cm.
- Both studies can detect associated hepatic, splenic, and pan-creatic cysts.
- MRI is more sensitive than ultrasound and may help in dis-tinguishing renal cell carcinomas from simple cysts.

TREATMENT
- Nephrolithiasis is treated in a similar manner, with IV or PO hydration. If stones remain lodged, lithotripsy or percutane-ous nephrostolithotomy can be done.
- Hypertension treatment is initiated with salt restriction, weight loss, and daily walking exercise.
- Avoidance of physical contact sports is advised.

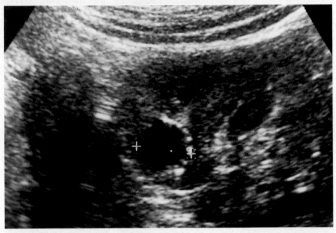

Fig 210–5
Ultrasound of a renal cyst. Ultrasound demonstrates a well-defined le-
sion with no internal echoes and enhanced through transmission.
There are fine foci of linear calcification in the wall, making the lesion
Bosniak class II.
(From Grainger RG, Allison DJ, Adam A, Dixon AK [eds]: Grainger &
Allison's Diagnostic Radiology, 4th ed. London, Harcourt, 2001.)

- Kidney infections should be treated with antibiotics known to penetrate the cyst (e.g., trimethoprim-sulfamethoxazole or ciprofloxacin).
- Angiotensin-converting enzyme inhibitors are effective in the treatment of hypertension associated with ADPKD.
- Calcium channel blockers can be used with or without ACE inhibitors in the treatment of hypertension.
- Alpha blockers and diuretics can be added as adjunctive therapy for hypertension.
- Blood pressure lower than 130/85 mm Hg is the goal for patients with renal disease. If there is more than 1 g of uri-nary protein/24 hr, the target blood pressure is lower than 125/75 mm Hg.
- Dialysis for end-stage renal failure
- Renal transplantation
- Cystic decompression in patients with intractable pain caused by enlarging cysts

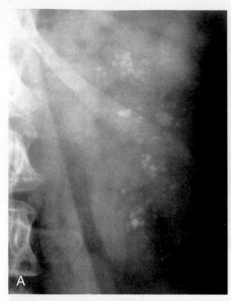
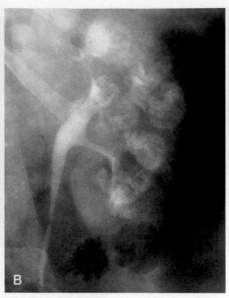
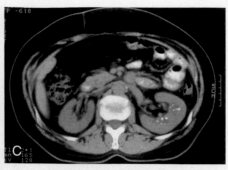

Fig 210–6
Radiologic findings in medullary sponge kidney in a 52-year-old symptomatic woman. **A,** Preliminary film shows medullary nephrolithiases.
B, Ten-minute film from an excretory urograph shows clusters of rounded densities in the papillae amidst discrete linear opacities (paintbrush appearance). **C,** Nonenhanced CT reveals densely echogenic foci in the medulla.
(From Johnson RJ, Feehally J: Comprehensive Clinical Nephrology, 3rd ed. St. Louis, Mosby, 2007.)

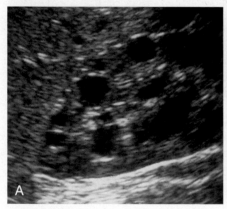
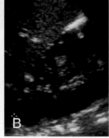

Fig 210–7
Tuberous sclerosis. **A,** Longitudinal ultrasound scan of the right kidney. The left kidney had a similar appearance. Both kidneys contain multiple cysts of varying sizes. The appearances on ultrasound are indistinguishable from autosomal dominant polycystic kidney disease. This child also had the skin stigmata of tuberose sclerosis. **B,** Longitudinal ultrasound scan of the right kidney in another patient. The left kidney had a similar appearance. This shows the more usual appearances of tuberose sclerosis in the kidney, with the small echogenic foci of the angiomyolipomas.
(From Grainger RG, Allison DJ, Adam A, Dixon AK [eds]: Grainger & Allison's Diagnostic Radiology, 4th ed. London, Harcourt, 2001.)

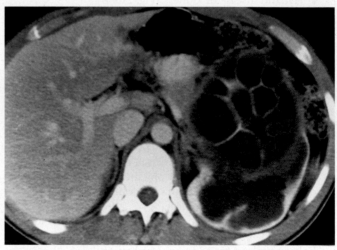

Fig 210–8
Hydatid disease of the kidney. There is a cystic mass in the left kidney with a multiloculated internal appearance from the presence of many daughter cysts. The mass is causing marked pelvicaliceal dilation.
(From Grainger RG, Allison DJ, Adam A, Dixon AK [eds]: Grainger & Allison's Diagnostic Radiology, 4th ed. London, Harcourt, 2001.)

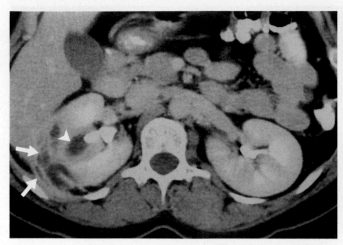

Fig 210–9
Renal abscess. Contrast CT scan shows an abscess in the medulla of the kidney *(arrowhead),* with penetration and extension into the perinephric space *(arrows).* (Courtesy of L. Towner.)

TABLE 210–1 Differential features of adult renal cystic disease

Feature	Simple cysts	ADPKD	MSK	VHL	TSC	Acquired cystic disease
Age at clinical onset (yr)	>40	30-40	20-40	30-40	10-30	Chronic renal failure
Cysts	Single, multiple	Multiple	Multiple	Few, bilateral	Multiple	Multiple
Cyst infection	Uncommon	Common	Common	Uncommon	Uncommon	Uncommon
Tumors	No	Rare	No	RCC, often bilateral	Astrocytoma, renal angiomyolipoma	Common
BP	Normal, increased	Increased	Normal	Normal, increased	Normal, increased	Normal, increased
Renal function	Normal	Normal, impaired	Normal	Normal	Normal, impaired	Impaired, ESRD
Nephrolithiasis	No	Common	Common	No	No	No
Liver cysts	No	Common	No	Rare	No	No
Pancreas cysts	No	Few	No	Multiple	No	No
CNS involvement	No	Aneurysms	No	Hemangio-blastomas	Seizures, mental retardation	No
Skin lesions	No	No	No	No		No

ADPKD, autosomal dominant polycystic kidney disease; BP, blood pressure; ESRD, end-stage renal disease; MSK, medullary sponge kidney; RCC, renal cell carcinoma; VHL, von Hippel-Lindau; TSC, tuberous sclerosis complex.
From Johnson RJ, Feehally J: Comprehensive Clinical Nephrology, 3rd ed. St. Louis, Mosby, 2007.

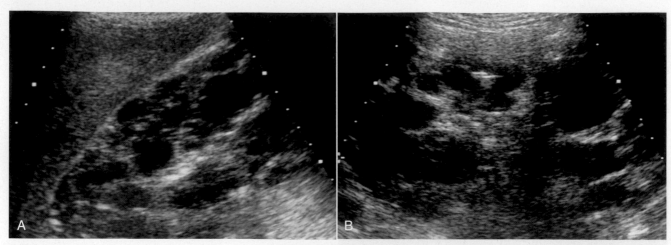

Fig 210–10

Ultrasound images of autosomal dominant polycystic kidney disease. Longitudinal images of the upper right **(A)** and left **(B)** kidneys show that the kidneys are enlarged, with normal architecture replaced by multiple cysts at varying sites.
(From Grainger RG, Allison DJ, Adam A, Dixon AK [eds]: Grainger & Allison's Diagnostic Radiology, 4th ed. London, Harcourt, 2001.)

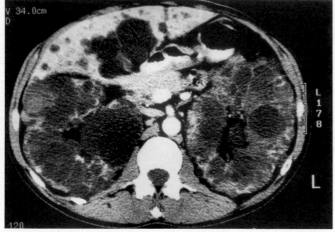

Fig 210–11

CT scans of autosomal dominant polycystic kidney disease. Enhanced CT scan shows markedly enlarged kidneys containing multiple cysts and cysts in the liver.
(From Grainger RG, Allison DJ, Adam A, Dixon AK [eds]: Grainger & Allison's Diagnostic Radiology, 4th ed. London, Harcourt, 2001.)

Chapter 211 | Renal artery stenosis and thrombosis

DEFINITION

Renal artery stenosis is the narrowing or occlusion of a renal artery, which can occur acutely (thrombosis or embolism) and cause renal infarction, or progressively (e.g., atheroma or fibromuscular dysphasia) and cause renovascular hypertension and/or lead to ischemic nephropathy. In addition, renal athero-embolism caused by showers of cholesterol microemboli can lead to progressive renal failure if sustained or recurrent.

PHYSICAL FINDINGS AND CLINICAL PRESENTATION

Acute renal artery occlusion

- Flank or abdominal pain
- Fever
- Nausea or vomiting
- Leukocytosis
- Hematuria (microscopic or gross)
- Elevated AST, LDH, alkaline phosphatase
- Oliguric renal failure if occlusion is bilateral; normal or near-normal renal function in unilateral occlusion

Cholesterol emboli

- Multisystem manifestations resembling vasculitis (visual disturbance, painful distal extremities, abdominal pain, signs of organ or limb ischemia). Laboratory findings include eosinophiluria, proteinuria, renal failure, elevated erythrocyte sedimentation rate (ESR).

Progressive renal artery stenosis

- Hypertension in a young person without a family history (fibromuscular dysplasia; Fig. 211–1)
- Hypertension in a middle-aged person with other evidence of atheromatous disease
- Abdominal bruit (40% of cases)
- Renal failure
- Hypertensive retinopathy

- Pulmonary edema in a hypertensive patient
- Hypokalemia
- Renal failure following the administration of an ACE inhibitor (if bilateral renal artery stenosis present)

CAUSE AND PATHOGENESIS

Cause of renal artery thrombosis

- Atherosclerosis
- Fibromuscular dysphasia
- Arteritis
- Aneurysm
- Arteriography
- Syphilis
- Hypercoagulable state (Fig. 211–2)
- Complication of renal transplantation (role of cyclosporine)
- Trauma (Fig. 211–3)

Cause of renal artery embolism

- Cardiac conditions (90%)
- Myocardial infarction
- Atrial fibrillation
- Cardiomyopathy
- Endocarditis
- Paradoxical emboli from deep venous thrombosis (DVT) in patient with cardiac septal defect
- Atheromatous plaques (cholesterol emboli)

Pathogenesis Renal hypoperfusion or ischemia produces an increase in plasma renin that stimulates the conversion of angiotensin I to angiotensin II, causing vasoconstriction and aldosterone secretion, sodium retention, and potassium wasting. Hypertension develops and can be self-sustaining after some time, even in the case of unilateral renal artery stenosis because of hypertensive damage to the other kidney.

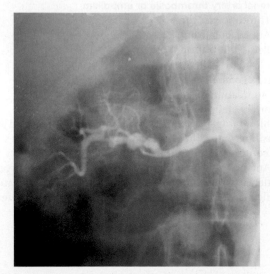

Fig 211–1
Fibromuscular dysplasia. This selective right renal arteriogram demonstrates typical beaded appearance.
(Courtesy of Dr. Harold Mitty.)

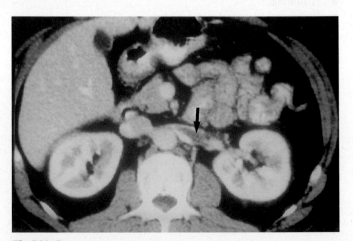

Fig 211–2
Renal vein thrombus in a patient with nephrotic syndrome. Contrast-enhanced CT scan at the level of the renal veins shows thrombus in the left renal vein (arrow).
(From Grainger RG, Allison DJ, Adam A, Dixon AK [eds]: Grainger & Allison's Diagnostic Radiology, 4th ed. London, Harcourt, 2001.)

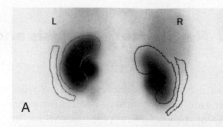

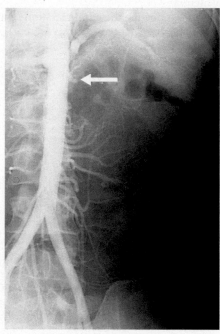

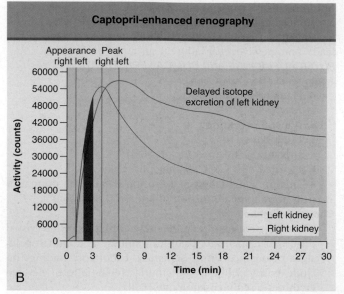

Fig 211–3
Acute renal artery occlusion caused by trauma. An aortogram shows the stump of the left renal artery *(arrow)* after the patient fell off his motorcycle.
(Courtesy of Dr. J. Reidy.)

Fig 211–4
Captopril-enhanced renography. **A,** Scan in a patient with newly developing hypertension. **B,** Renogram demonstrates delayed arrival and excretion of isotope (MAG3) in the affected left kidney.
(From Johnson RJ, Feehally J: Comprehensive Clinical Nephrology, 3rd ed. St. Louis, Mosby, 2007.)

LABORATORY TESTS
● Creatinine
● Potassium level
● Urinalysis
● Peripheral plasma renin activity
● Captopril test (stimulation of excessive renin secretion)
IMAGING STUDIES
● Renal scan (70% sensitivity, 79% specificity)
● Captopril renal scan (85% sensitivity, 90% specificity; Fig. 211–4)
● Intravenous digital subtraction angiography (88% sensitivity, 90% specificity) is the reference standard for anatomic diagnosis of renal artery stenosis (Fig. 211–5).
● Magnetic resonance angiography (Fig. 211–6)
● CT (see Fig. 211–2)

TREATMENT
Acute renal artery thrombosis or embolism
● Thrombolytic therapy
● Anticoagulation
● Revascularization (surgery)
● Blood pressure control
Cholesterol emboli
● No treatment, statins
Renal artery stenosis
● Blood pressure control: role of ACE inhibitors and angiotensin receptor blockers is controversial, but neither should be continued if renal function worsens.
● Angioplasty or revascularization should be reserved for patients whose blood pressure control with medication is difficult and for patients with progressive renal failure.

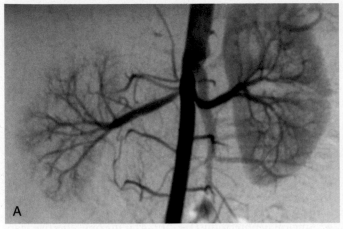

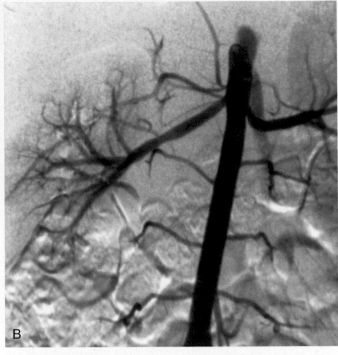

Fig 211–5
A, Angiogram demonstrating right renal artery stenosis as the cause of the functional abnormality. **B,** Postdilation angiogram.
(From Grainger RG, Allison DJ, Adam A, Dixon AK [eds]: Grainger & Allison's Diagnostic Radiology, 4th ed. London, Harcourt, 2001.)

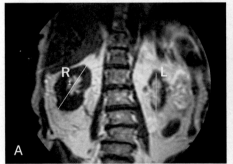

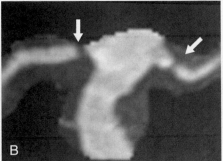

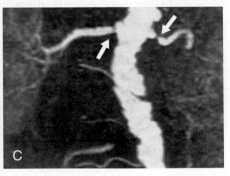

Fig 211–6
Magnetic resonance angiogram in renal failure in an older woman with renal failure (serum creatinine, 2.5 mg/dL) and severe hypertension. **A,** Severe discrepancy in kidney size with a small left kidney. **B,** Gadolinium-enhanced aortography illustrating high-grade, bilateral, renal artery stenotic lesions *(arrows)*. **C,** Extensive aortic and iliac disease, bilateral renal artery stenoses *(arrows),* and markedly diminished filtration on the left side.
(From Johnson RJ, Feehally J: Comprehensive Clinical Nephrology, 3rd ed. St. Louis, Mosby, 2007.)

Chapter 212 / Neoplasms

A. RENAL CELL ADENOCARCINOMA

DEFINITION

Renal cell adenocarcinoma (RCA) is a primary adenocarcinoma originating in the renal parenchyma from the malignant transformation of proximal renal tubular epithelial cells.

PHYSICAL FINDINGS AND CLINICAL PRESENTATION

Presenting findings in RCA patients:

- Hematuria: 50% to 60%
- Elevated ESR: 50% to 60%
- Abdominal mass: 25% to 45%
- Anemia: 20% to 40%
- Flank pain: 35% to 40%
- Hypertension: 20% to 40%
- Weight loss: 30% to 35%
- Fever: 5% to 15%
- Hepatic dysfunction: 10% to 15%
- Classic triad (hematuria, abdominal mass, flank pain): 5% to 10%
- Hypercalcemia: 3% to 6%
- Erythrocytosis: 3% to 4%
- Varicocele: 2% to 3%

CAUSE

Hereditary forms

- Familial renal carcinoma
- Renal carcinoma associated with von Hippel-Lindau disease
- Hereditary papillary renal cell carcinoma

Risk factors

- Cigarette smoking
- Obesity
- Use of diuretics
- Phenacetin-containing analgesics
- Asbestos exposure
- Gasoline and other petroleum products
- Lead
- Cadmium
- Thorotrast
- Role of the *VHL* gene located on chromosome 3

DIFFERENTIAL DIAGNOSIS

- Transitional cell carcinomas of the renal pelvis (8% of all renal cancers)
- Wilms' tumor (Fig. 212–1)
- Renal cysts (see Figs. 210–5, 210–6, 210–11)
- Retroperitoneal tumors
- Renal abscess (see Fig. 210–9)

LABORATORY TESTS

- CBC: anemia or erythrocytosis
- Elevated ESR
- Nonmetastatic hepatic dysfunction with elevated alkaline phosphatase, prolonged prothrombin time, hypoalbuminemia
- Hypercalcemia (secondary to parathyroid related protein)
- Other: elevated ferritin, elevated insulin and glucagon levels, elevated alpha-fetoprotein, elevated beta–human chorionic gonadotropin

IMAGING STUDIES

- Renal ultrasound (Fig. 212–2)
- Abdominal CT scan with contrast (Fig. 212–3)
- MRI
- Renal arteriogram

COMMON SITES OF METASTASES

- Lung: 50% to 60%
- Bone: 30% to 40%
- Regional nodes: 15% to 30%

TREATMENT

Surgery

- Surgical nephrectomy (Fig. 212–4) is the only effective management for stages I, II, and some stage III tumors.
- Various forms of partial nephrectomy may be available for patients with bilateral cancers or with a solitary kidney.

The role of nephrectomy in patients with metastatic renal cell carcinoma is controversial and should probably be reserved for patients who have a solitary metastasis amenable to surgical resection.

Other treatment

- Angioinfarction (for palliation)
- Radiotherapy (for palliation)

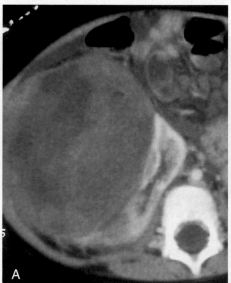
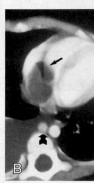

Fig 212–1

Wilms' tumor. **A,** Axial CT scan of the abdomen after IV contrast enhancement in a 2½-year-old boy showing a large mass arising from the right kidney that is of heterogenous attenuation. The mass is seen to displace the normal enhancing renal parenchyma to the left. **B,** Thoracic CT tumor thrombus was seen to extend from the inferior vena cava into the right atrium, causing a filling defect within the heart (long thin arrow). Note an enlarged azygos vein (short arrow) adjacent to the aorta and a large right pleural effusion.
(From Grainger RG, Allison DJ, Adam A, Dixon AK [eds]: Grainger & Allison's Diagnostic Radiology, 4th ed. London, Harcourt, 2001.)

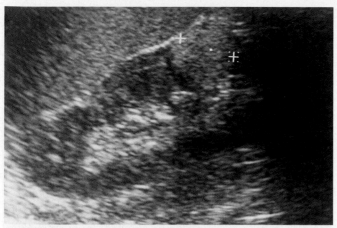

Fig 212–2
Renal cell carcinoma. Ultrasound demonstrates a 17-mm hyperreflective mass in the left kidney with posterior shadowing.
(From Grainger RG, Allison DJ, Adam A, Dixon AK [eds]: Grainger & Allison's Diagnostic Radiology, 4th ed. London, Harcourt, 2001.)

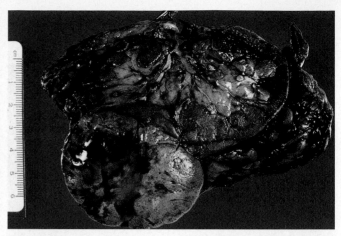

Fig 212–4
Clear renal cell carcinoma, characteristic gross appearance with variegated color that includes bright yellow areas, hemorrhage, and necrosis. In this example, the tumor bulges into the perinephric fat; despite this appearance, the tumor is categorized as T2 (confined to the kidney) unless invasion of the fat is demonstrated histologically.
(From Silverberg SG, Frable WJ, Wick MR, et al [eds]: Principles and Practice of Surgical Pathology and Cytopathology, 4th ed. Philadelphia, Elsevier, 2006.)

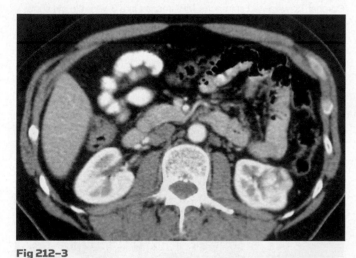

Fig 212–3
Renal cell carcinoma. CT scan demonstrates a peripherally enhancing tumor in the lower pole of the left kidney with loss of the normal smooth renal contour. The tumor was stage T1 N0 M0 and was removed following a partial nephrectomy.
(From Grainger RG, Allison DJ, Adam A, Dixon AK [eds]: Grainger & Allison's Diagnostic Radiology, 4th ed. London, Harcourt, 2001.)

- Chemotherapy (only 5% response rate)
- Hormonal therapy (high-dose progesterone may achieve a 15% to 20% response rate)
- Immunotherapy: interleukin-2 may achieve a 15% to 30% response rate; alpha, beta, and gamma interferons are somewhat less effective.
- Antivascular endothelial growth factor antibody bevacizumab slows disease progression in metastatic renal cancer.

B. NEPHROBLASTOMA (WILMS' TUMOR)

DEFINITION
This is a malignant renal tumor derived from a primitive metanephric blastoma. Most tumors are unicentric, but some are multifocal in one or both kidneys. Associated anomalies may be present.

PHYSICAL FINDINGS AND CLINICAL PRESENTATION
- Wilms' tumor often is discovered when a parent notices a mass while bathing or dressing a child, most commonly a child who is about 3 years old, or during a routine physical examination. The mass is unilateral, firm, and nontender, below the costal margin.
- Abdominal swelling and/or pain
- Nausea
- Vomiting
- Constipation
- Loss of appetite
- Fever of unknown origin
- Night sweats
- Hematuria (less common than in adult renal malignancies)
- Malaise
- High blood pressure triggered when the tumor obstructs the renal artery
- Varicocele
- Signs of associated syndromes

CAUSE AND PATHOGENESIS
- Three cell types (Fig. 212–5)—blastomal, stromal, and epithelial—may be present. Structural diversity is characteristic.

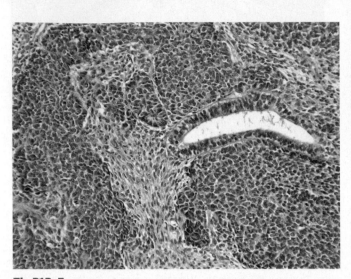

Fig 212–5
Nephroblastoma. Characteristic triphasic histology includes epithelial, blasternal, and mesenchymal components.
(From Silverberg SG, Frable WJ, Wick MR, et al [eds]: Principles and Practice of Surgical Pathology and Cytopathology, 4th ed. Philadelphia, Elsevier, 2006.)

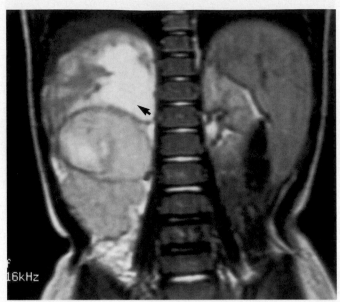

Fig 212–6
Coronal T2-weighted spin-echo MRI images in a 3-year-old girl showing a large right-sided Wilms' tumor affecting the lower pole of the right kidney, with obstruction to drainage and hydronephrosis evident superiorly (arrow). The left kidney was normal.
(From Grainger RG, Allison DJ, Adam A, Dixon AK [eds]: Grainger & Allison's Diagnostic Radiology, 4th ed. London, Harcourt, 2001.)

DIFFERENTIAL DIAGNOSIS
- Other renal malignancies:
  1. Renal cell carcinoma (see Fig. 212–3)
  2. Transitional cell carcinoma
  3. Lymphoma
  4. Clear cell sarcoma
  5. Rhabdoid tumor of the kidney
- Renal cyst (see Fig. 210–5)
- Renal abscess (see Fig. 210–9)
- Other intra-abdominal or retroperitoneal tumors

LABORATORY TESTS
- CBC
- Transaminases (ALT, AST)
- Alkaline phosphatase
- BUN and creatinine
- Serum calcium
- Urinalysis

IMAGING STUDIES
- Renal ultrasound to confirm existence of a solid mass in a kidney
- Abdominal CT scan with contrast (see Fig. 212–1)
- MRI of the kidneys (Fig. 212–6)

TREATMENT
- Surgical resection (Fig. 212–7) and surgical staging
- Radiation therapy and chemotherapy

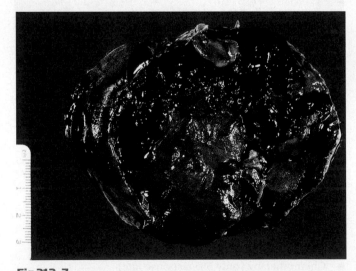

Fig 212–7
Nephroblastoma; typical gross appearance of a bulging red-tan tumor with areas of hemorrhage and necrosis.
(From Silverberg SG, Frable WJ, Wick MR, et al [eds]: Principles and Practice of Surgical Pathology and Cytopathology, 4th ed. Philadelphia, Elsevier, 2006.)

Chapter 213 Pyelonephritis

DEFINITION
Pyelonephritis is an infection, usually bacterial in origin, of the upper urinary tract (Fig. 213–1).

PHYSICAL FINDINGS AND CLINICAL PRESENTATION
- Fever
- Rigors
- Chills
- Flank pain
- Dysuria
- Polyuria
- Hematuria
- Toxic feeling and appearance
- Nausea and vomiting
- Headache
- Diarrhea
- Physical examination notable:
  1. Costovertebral angle tenderness
  2. Exquisite flank pain

CAUSE
- Gram-negative bacilli such as *Escherichia coli* and *Klebsiella* spp. in more than 95% of cases
- Other, more unusual gram-negative organisms, especially with instrumentation of the urinary system
- Resistant gram-negative organisms or even fungi in hospitalized patients with indwelling catheters
- Gram-positive organisms such as enterococci
- *Staphylococcus aureus:* presence in urine indicates hematogenous origin
- Viruses: rare, but usually limited to the lower tract
- *Candida albicans* (Emphysematous pyelonephritis, see Fig. 213–4)

DIFFERENTIAL DIAGNOSIS
- Nephrolithiasis (see Fig. 216–3)
- Appendicitis
- Ovarian cyst torsion or rupture
- Acute glomerulonephritis
- Pelvic inflammatory disease (PID)
- Endometritis
- Other causes of acute abdomen
- Perinephric abscess
- Hydronephrosis (see Fig. 214–3)

LABORATORY TESTS
- CBC with differential
- Renal panel
- Blood cultures
- Urine cultures
- Urinalysis
- Gram stain of urine

DIAGNOSTIC IMAGING
- Urgent renal sonography (Fig. 213–2) if obstruction or closed space infection suspected
- CT scanning (Fig. 213–3) may better define the extent of collections of pus.

TREATMENT
- Antibiotic therapy should be initiated after cultures are obtained and guided by the results of culture and sensitivity testing.
- Prompt drainage with nephrostomy tube placement for obstruction
- Surgical drainage of large collections of pus to control infection
- Diabetic patients, as well as those with indwelling catheters, are especially prone to complicated infections and abscess formation (Fig. 213–4).

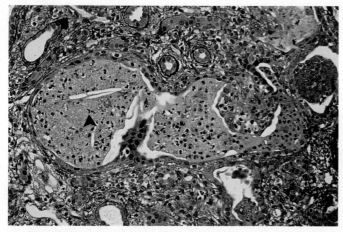

Fig 213–1
Acute pyelonephritis. Renal tissue shows a dilated tubule with neutrophils enmeshed in proteinaceous debris (pus casts; *arrowhead*) with adjacent interstitial inflammation.
(Courtesy of C. Alpers.)

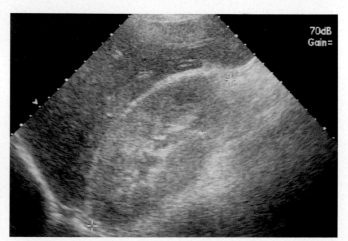

Fig 213–2
Acute pyelonephritis. Ultrasound demonstrates an enlarged echogenic kidney; bipolar length of kidney = 12.9 cm.
(From Johnson RJ, Feehally J: Comprehensive Clinical Nephrology, 3rd ed. St. Louis, Mosby, 2007.)

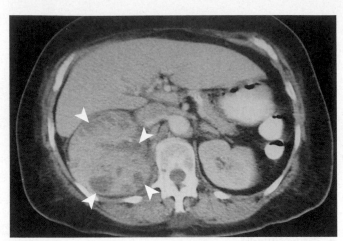

Fig 213–3

Acute pyelonephritis. CT scan obtained 24 hours after image shown in Figure 213-2 demonstrates multiple nonenhancing abscesses *(arrowheads)*.

(From Johnson RJ, Feehally J: Comprehensive Clinical Nephrology, 3rd ed. St. Louis, Mosby, 2007.)

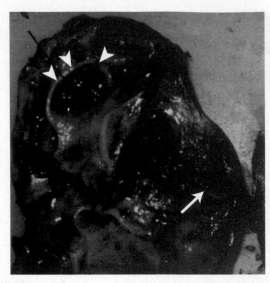

Fig 213–4

Emphysematous pyelonephritis. Shown are cortical necrosis *(solid arrow),* diffuse cortical hemorrhage *(open arrow),* and dilation of the collecting system *(arrowheads)* in a nephrectomy specimen from a diabetic patient who received combined medical-surgical therapy and survived emphysematous pyelonephritis caused by an unusual pathogen, *Candida albicans*

(From Cohen J, Powderly WG: Infectious Diseases, 2nd ed. St. Louis, Mosby, 2004.)

Chapter 214 Hydronephrosis

DEFINITION
Hydronephrosis is dilation of the renal pyelocalyceal system, most often as a result of impairment of urinary flow.

CLINICAL PRESENTATION

History
- Pain is caused by distention of the collecting system or renal capsule and is more related to the rate of onset than the degree of obstruction. It can vary in location from flank to lower abdomen to testes/labia. Pain in the flank occurring only on micturition is highly suggestive of vesicoureteral reflux.
- Anuria can occur with total obstruction of urinary flow (bilateral hydronephrosis or unilateral if only one kidney is present).
- Polyuria or nocturia can occur with chronic (incomplete) obstruction because of deleterious effects on renal concentrating ability (nephrogenic diabetes insipidus).
- Urinary frequency, hesitancy, postvoid dribbling, and difficulty initiating stream are all symptoms that can occur with obstruction at or below the bladder (e.g., prostatic hyperplasia).
- Chronic urinary infections can either result from chronic urinary obstruction (organisms favoring growth with stasis of urine) or lead to conditions (e.g., urine pH changes) that favor stone formation and subsequent obstruction.

Physical examination
- Hypertension can be caused by increased renin release in acute or subacute obstruction.
- Fever or CVA tenderness can suggest urinary tract infection.
- Palpate bladder and kidneys to detect if distention present.
- Rectal examination to evaluate prostate for size and nodularity and also to check rectal sphincter tone.
- Pelvic examination to assess for vaginal anatomy, pelvic mass, or pelvic inflammatory disease (PID).
- Penile examination to rule out meatal stenosis or phimosis.
- Bladder catheterization to assess postvoid residual volume if urinary tract obstruction is considered. Should rule out postrenal obstruction in unexplained acute renal failure.

CAUSE

Mechanical impairments
Congenital:
- Ureteropelvic junction narrowing
- Ureterovesical junction narrowing
- Ureterocele
- Retrocaval ureter
- Bladder neck obstruction
- Urethral valve
- Urethral stricture
- Meatal stenosis

Acquired:
- Intrinsic to urinary tract
- Calculi (see Fig. 216–6)
- Inflammation
- Trauma
- Sloughed papillae
- Ureteral tumor
- Blood clots
- Prostatic hypertrophy (see Fig. 218–1) or cancer (see Fig. 220–4)

- Bladder cancer
- Urethral stricture
- Phimosis
- Extrinsic to urinary tract
- Gravid uterus
- Retroperitoneal fibrosis (Fig. 214–1) or tumor (e.g., lymphoma)
- Aortic aneurysm
- Uterine fibroids
- Trauma (surgical or nonsurgical)
- Pelvic inflammatory disease
- Pelvic malignancies (e.g., prostate, colorectal, cervical, uterine)

Functional impairments
- Neurogenic bladder (often with adynamic ureter) can occur with spinal cord disease or diabetic neuropathy.
- Pharmacologic agents such as alpha-adrenergic antagonists and anticholinergic drugs can inhibit bladder emptying.
- Vesicoureteral reflux may occur.
- Pregnancy can cause hydroureter and hydronephrosis (right more often than left) as early as the second month. Hormonal effects on ureteral tone combine with mechanical factors.

DIFFERENTIAL DIAGNOSIS
- Urinary stones (see Fig. 216–9)
- Neoplastic disease (see Fig. 212–3)
- Prostatic hypertrophy (see Fig. 218–2)
- Neurologic disease
- Urinary reflux
- Urinary tract infection
- Medication effects
- Trauma
- Congenital abnormality of urinary tract

LABORATORY TESTS
- Serum BUN and creatinine to assess for renal insufficiency (usually implies bilateral obstruction or unilateral obstruction of a solitary kidney)

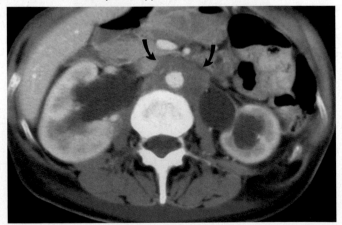

Fig 214–1
Retroperitoneal fibrosis causing renal failure. This enhanced CT scan shows the periaortic soft tissue mass *(arrows)* and marked bilateral pelvicaliceal dilation.
(From Grainger RG, Allison DJ, Adam A, Dixon AK [eds]: Grainger & Allison's Diagnostic Radiology, 4th ed. London, Harcourt, 2001.)

- Electrolytes may reveal hypernatremia (if nephrogenic diabetes insipidus), hyperkalemia (from renal failure and effects on tubular function), or distal renal tubular acidosis.
- Urinalysis and examination of sediment may reveal WBCs, RBCs, or bacteria in the appropriate setting (e.g., infection, stones), but often the sediment is normal in obstructive renal disease.

IMAGING STUDIES

- Abdominal plain film of kidneys, ureters, and bladder (see Fig. 201–5) are used to look for nephrocalcinosis or a radiopaque stone.
- Assess kidney and bladder size with ultrasound (Fig. 214–2), contour of pyelocalyces and ureters. Ultrasound is about 90% sensitive and specific for hydronephrosis and is noninvasive, so it will not worsen preexisting renal insufficiency.
- Intravenous pyelography (IVP) (see Fig. 201–6) helps localize the site of obstruction when hydronephrosis is seen on ultrasound, but the contrast may have deleterious effects on the kidneys if there is renal insufficiency.
- Antegrade or retrograde urograms can be performed if renal failure is a concern with IVP, and either of these two procedures could be extended to provide relief of the obstruction.
- Abdominal CT scanning (Fig. 214–3) provides excellent localization of the site of obstruction.
- Voiding cystourethrogram is helpful in diagnosing vesicoureteral reflux and obstructions of the bladder neck or urethra.
- Magnetic resonance urography may be useful if contrast studies are not feasible or other studies are nondiagnostic.

TREATMENT

- Urgent treatment is required if urinary tract obstruction is associated with urinary tract infection, acute renal failure, or uncontrollable pain.

- Conservative management of calculi with IV fluid, IV antibiotics (if evidence of infection), and aggressive analgesia may be enough to treat acute unilateral urinary tract obstruction, depending on the size (90% of stones smaller than 5 mm will pass spontaneously).
- Urethral catheterization is adequate to relieve most obstructions at or distal to the bladder, but occasionally a suprapubic catheter will be required (e.g., impassable urethral stricture or urethral injury). Neurogenic bladder may require intermittent clean catheterization if frequent voiding and pharmacologic treatments are ineffective.
- Nephrostomy tube can be placed percutaneously to facilitate urinary drainage.
- Extracorporeal shock wave lithotripsy (ESWL) is used to fragment large stones to facilitate spontaneous passage or subsequent extraction (*note*: ESWL is contraindicated in pregnancy).
- Nephroscopy is performed for extraction of proximal stones under direct vision.
- Cystoscopy with ureteroscopy is used for removal of distal ureteral stones using a loop or basket, with or without fragmentation by ultrasonic or laser lithotripsy.
- Ureteral stents can be used for extrinsic and some intrinsic ureteral obstructions.
- Urethral dilation or internal urethrotomy can be used for urethral strictures.
- Nephrectomy or ureteral diversion may be required in severe cases (e.g., malignancy).
- Ureterovesical reimplantation can be used for reflux disease.
- Transurethral retrograde prostatectomy (TURP) is used for severe obstruction from benign prostatic hypertrophy (BPH).
- IV fluid and electrolyte replacement is needed; the patient must be monitored closely during the postobstructive diuresis (usually lasting several days to a week).
- Antibiotics in suspected infection

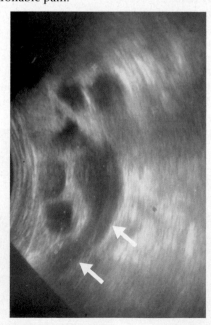

Fig 214–2
Renal ultrasound scan of a patient with obstruction of the urinary tract causing hydronephrosis. The kidney is hydronephrotic, with dilation of the pelvicaliceal system; dilation of the upper ureter is also clearly seen (*arrows*)
(From Johnson RJ, Feehally J: Comprehensive Clinical Nephrology, 3rd ed. St. Louis, Mosby, 2007.)

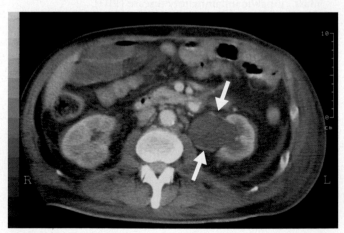

Fig 214–3
CT scan of the abdomen showing a grossly hydronephrotic kidney on the left (*arrows* mark dilated renal pelvis). Dilated loops of small bowel are seen in the right hypochondrium. Sequential sections demonstrated that the ureter was dilated along its length and that there was a pelvic mass, which was responsible for both bowel and left ureteric construction. The mass was subsequently shown to originate from a carcinoma of the colon.
(From Johnson RJ, Feehally J: Comprehensive Clinical Nephrology, 3rd ed. St. Louis, Mosby, 2007.)

Chapter 215 | Rhabdomyolysis

DEFINITION
Rhabdomyolysis is the dissolution or disintegration of muscle (Fig. 215–1) that causes membrane lysis and leakage of muscle constituents, resulting in the excretion of myoglobin in the urine. Renal damage can occur as a result of tubular obstruction by myoglobin, as well as hypovolemia.

PHYSICAL FINDINGS AND CLINICAL PRESENTATION
- Variable muscle tenderness
- Weakness
- Muscular rigidity
- Fever
- Altered consciousness
- Muscle swelling
- Malaise
- Dark urine

CAUSE
- Exertion (exercise-induced)
- Electrical injury
- Drug-induced (statins, combination of statins with fibrates, amphetamines, haloperidol)
- Compartment syndrome
- Multiple trauma
- Malignant hyperthermia
- Limb ischemia
- Reperfusion after revascularization procedures for ischemia (Fig. 215–2)

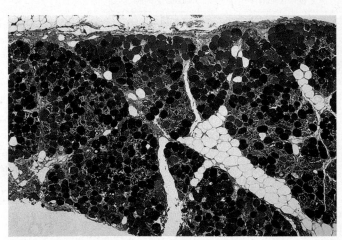

Fig 215–1
Alcohol-related rhabdomyolysis with widespread muscle fiber necrosis. (From Silverberg SG, Frable WJ, Wick MR, et al [eds]: Principles and Practice of Surgical Pathology and Cytopathology, 4th ed. Philadelphia, Elsevier, 2006.)

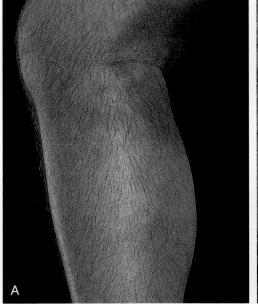 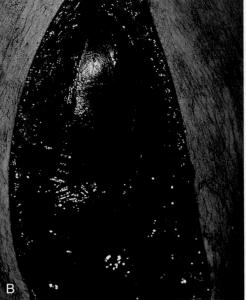

Fig 215–2
Compartment syndrome. **A,** Severe calf swelling caused by anterior and posterior compartment syndromes following ischemia-reperfusion.
B, Appearance following emergency fasciotomy; note edematous muscle and hematoma.
(Courtesy of M. J. Allen.)

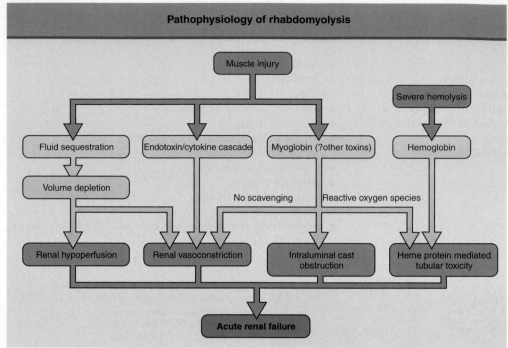

Fig 215-3
Pathophysiology of rhabdomyolysis. Renal impairment is caused by multiple factors, including volume depletion, renal vasoconstriction, direct tubular cell toxicity, and intraluminal obstructing casts.
(From Johnson RJ, Feehally J: Comprehensive Clinical Nephrology, 3rd ed. St. Louis, Mosby, 2007.)

- Extensive surgical (spinal) dissection
- Tourniquet ischemia
- Prolonged static positioning during surgery
- Infectious and inflammatory myositis
- Metabolic myopathies
- Hypovolemia and urinary acidification are important precipitating causes in the development of acute renal failure.
- Sickle cell trait is a predisposing condition.
- Figure 215–3 illustrates the pathophysiology of rhabdomyolysis.

LABORATORY TESTS
- Screening for myoglobinuria with a simple urine dipstick test using orthotoluidine or benzidine
- BUN, creatinine
- Increased creatine phosphokinase (CPK)
- Hyperkalemia
- Hypocalcemia
- Hyperphosphatemia
- Increased urinary myoglobin
- Pigmented granular casts
- Hyperuricemia

TREATMENT
- Early, aggressive high-volume IV fluid replacement with mannitol, to induce diuresis to prevent acute renal failure
- Treatment of electrolyte imbalances
- Alkalinization of urine is controversial but appears helpful in research models.

REFERENCES

Ferri F: Ferri's Clinical Advisor 2007. St. Louis, Mosby, 2007.

Ferri F: Practical Guide to the Care of the Medical Patient, 7th ed. St. Louis, Mosby, 2007.

Grainger RG, Allison DJ, Adam A, Dixon AK (eds): Grainger & Allison's Diagnostic Radiology, 4th ed. London, Harcourt, 2001.

Johnson RJ, Feehally J: Comprehensive Clinical Nephrology, 3rd ed. St. Louis, Mosby, 2007.

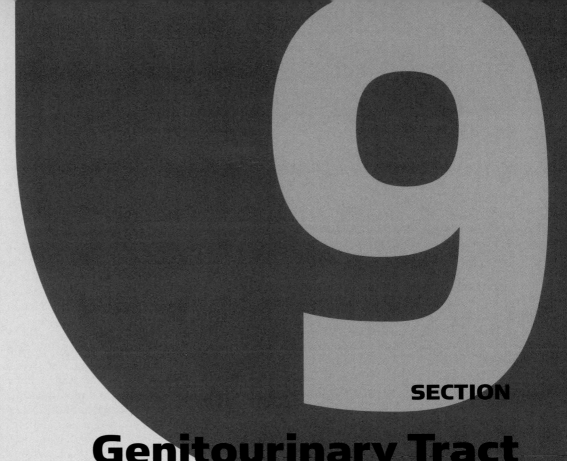

SECTION

Genitourinary Tract

Ureters
Chapter 216: Urolithiasis

Bladder
Chapter 217: Bladder carcinoma

Prostate
Chapter 218: Benign prostatic hyperplasia
Chapter 219: Prostatitis
Chapter 220: Prostate cancer

Testicles
Chapter 221: Hydrocele
Chapter 222: Varicocele
Chapter 223: Epididymitis
Chapter 224: Testicular neoplasms
Chapter 225: Testicular torsion

Vulva, urethra, penis
Chapter 226: Diseases of the genital skin
Chapter 227: Urethritis, gonococcal
Chapter 228: Urethritis, nongonococcal
Chapter 229: Hypospadias
Chapter 230: Peyronie's disease

URETERS

Chapter 216 **Urolithiasis**

DEFINITION
Urolithiasis is the presence of calculi within the urinary tract. The five major types of urinary stones are calcium oxalate (>50%) (Fig. 216–1), calcium phosphate (10% to 20%), uric acid (8%), struvite (15%), and cystine (3%)(Fig. 216–2).

PHYSICAL FINDINGS AND CLINICAL PRESENTATION
Stones may be asymptomatic or may cause the following signs and symptoms from obstruction:
- Sudden onset of flank tenderness
- Nausea and vomiting
- Patient in constant movement, attempting to lessen the pain (patients with an acute abdomen are usually still because movement exacerbates the pain)
- Pain may be referred to the testes or labium (progression of stone down the urinary ureter).

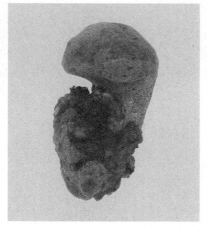

Fig 216–1
Ureteral calculus. A 1-cm wide calcium oxalate stone provoked ureteral colic and required surgical removal.
(From Johnson RJ, Feehally J: Comprehensive Clinical Nephrology, 3rd ed. St. Louis, Mosby, 2007.)

- Fever and chills accompanying the acute colic if there is superimposed infection
- Pain may radiate anteriorly over to the abdomen and result in intestinal ileus.
- Untreated chronic obstruction from stones can result in severe damage to the involved kidney (Fig. 216–3).

CAUSE
- Increased absorption of calcium in the small bowel: type I absorptive hypercalciuria (independent of calcium intake)
- Idiopathic hypercalciuria nephrolithiasis is the most common diagnosis for patients with calcium stones; the diagnosis is made only if there is no hypercalcemia and no known cause for hypercalciuria
- Increased vitamin D synthesis (e.g., secondary to renal phosphate loss: type III absorptive hypercalciuria)
- Renal tubular malfunction with inadequate reabsorption of calcium and resulting hypercalciuria
- Heterozygous mutations in the *NPT2a* gene result in hypophosphatemia and urinary phosphate loss
- Hyperparathyroidism with resulting hypercalcemia
- Elevated uric acid level (metabolic defects, dietary excess)
- Chronic diarrhea (e.g., inflammatory bowel disease) with increased oxalate absorption
- Type I (distal tubule) renal tubular acidosis (<1% of calcium stones)
- Chronic hydrochlorothiazide treatment
- Chronic infections with urease-producing organisms (e.g., *Proteus, Providencia, Pseudomonas, Klebsiella*). Struvite, or magnesium ammonium phosphate crystals, is produced when the urinary tract is colonized by bacteria, producing elevated concentrations of ammonia.
- Abnormal excretion of cystine
- Chemotherapy for malignancies

DIFFERENTIAL DIAGNOSIS
- Urinary tract infection
- Pyelonephritis
- Diverticulitis

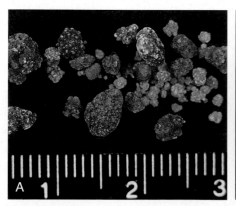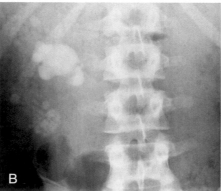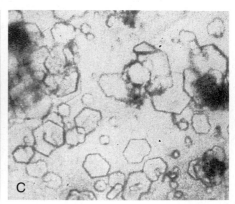

Fig 216–2
Cystinuria. **A,** Both rough and smooth cystine calculi. **B,** Plain radiograph of a cystine calculus in the right renal pelvis and further multiple parenchymal calculi. **C,** Urine microscopy showing characteristic flat hexagonal crystals.
(From Johnson RJ, Feehally J: Comprehensive Clinical Nephrology, 3rd ed. St. Louis, Mosby, 2007.)

- Pelvic inflammatory disease (PID)
- Ovarian pathology
- Factitious (drug addicts)
- Appendicitis
- Small bowel obstruction
- Ectopic pregnancy

LABORATORY TESTS

- Urinalysis: note presence of urine crystals (Fig. 216–4). Hematuria may be present; however, its absence does not exclude urinary stones. Evaluation of urinary pH is of value in identification of type of stone (pH >7.5 is associated with struvite stones, whereas pH <5 generally is seen with uric acid or with cystine stones).
- Stone analysis should be performed on recovered stones.
- Urine culture and senstivity (C&S) should be performed for all patients.
- Serum chemistries should include calcium, electrolytes, phosphate, and uric acid.
- Additional tests: 24-hour urine collection for calcium, uric acid, phosphate, oxalate, and citrate excretion is generally reserved for patients with recurrent stones.
- Table 216–1 describes key laboratory tests for renal stones.

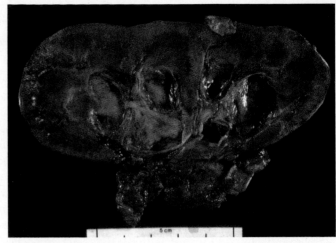

Fig 216-3

Autopsy specimen of a kidney showing the early effects of ureteral obstruction. The kidney is enlarged and edematous, with pelvicaliceal dilation. There is good preservation of the renal parenchyma.
(From Johnson RJ, Feehally J: Comprehensive Clinical Nephrology, 3rd ed. St. Louis, Mosby, 2007.)

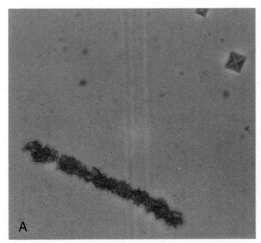

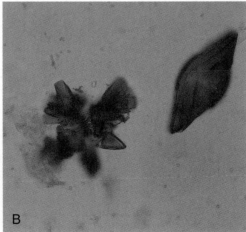

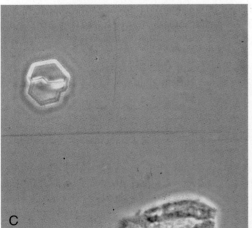

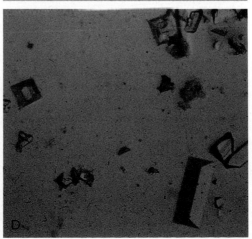

Fig 216-4

Urine crystals. **A,** Oxalate crystals—a pseudocast of calcium oxalate crystals accompanied by crystals of calcium oxalate dihydrate. **B,** Uric acid crystals—complex crystals suggestive of acute uric acid nephropathy or uric acid nephrolithiasis. **C,** A typical hexagonal cystine crystal. A single crystal provides a definitive diagnosis of cystinuria. **D,** Coffin lid crystals of magnesium ammonium phosphate (struvite).
(Courtesy of Dr. Patrick Fleet.)

TABLE 216–1 Key laboratory tests for renal stones

Finding	Clinical implication or type
Dipstick	
pH	Provides clue as to type of stone present:
	Acidic—uric acid or cystine crystals
	Alkaline—phosphates, struvite
Blood	Must confirm by microscopy
Leukocytes	Signifies infection or inflammation
Nitrites	Infection with urease-producing organisms
Microscopy	
RBCs	May not have hematuria with complete obstruction
WBCs	Signifies infection or inflammation
Crystals	Oxalate—bipyramids or dumbbells
	Phosphate—splinter-like
	Struvite—"coffin lids"
	Uric acid—amorphous powder
	Cystine—hexagonal
Culture	Definitive diagnosis of associated infection
24-hour urine—calcium, magnesium, oxalate, phosphate, creatinine	Determine cause in recurrent stone formers
Blood	
CBC	Leukocytosis—infection
Serum creatinine	Marker of renal function; required for IVP
Other (order selectively)	Calcium
	Uric acid
	PTH
	Magnesium

CBC, complete blood count; IVP, intravenous pyelography; PTH, parathyroid hormone; RBC, red blood cell; WBC, white blood cell.
From Nseyo U, Weinman E, Lamm DL: Urology for Primary Care Physicians. Philadelphia, WB Saunders, 1999.

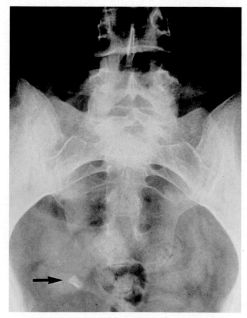

Fig 216–5
Kidney, ureter, and bladder (KUB) radiograph in a patient presenting with hematuria shows a radiopaque shadow *(arrow)* along the course of the distal right ureter that proved to be a calculus.
(From Nseyo U, Weinman E, Lamm DL: Urology for Primary Care Physicians. Philadelphia, WB Saunders, 1999.)

IMAGING STUDIES
- Plain films of the abdomen can identify radiopaque stones (calcium, uric acid stones) (Fig. 216–5).
- Renal sonogram (Fig. 216–6) may be helpful.
- Intravenous urography (IVU) (Fig. 216–7) or retrograde pyelography (Fig. 216–8) can demonstrate the size and location of the stone, as well as degree of obstruction.
- CT (Fig. 216–9). Unenhanced (noncontrast) helical CT scan does not require contrast medium and can visualize the calculus (identified by the rim sign or halo representing the edematous ureteral wall around the stone). It is fast, accurate (sensitivity 15% to 100%, specificity 94% to 96%), and readily identifies all stone types in all locations. This modality is being used increasingly in the initial assessment of renal colic.

TREATMENT
- Increase in water or other fluid intake (doubling of previous fluid intake unless patient has a history of congestive heart failure [CHF] or fluid overload)
- Normal dietary calcium intake is recommended. If one does not consume enough calcium, less is available to bind to dietary oxalate; as a result, more oxalate reaches the colon, is absorbed into the bloodstream, and is excreted as calcium oxalate, setting the stage for calcium urolithiasis.

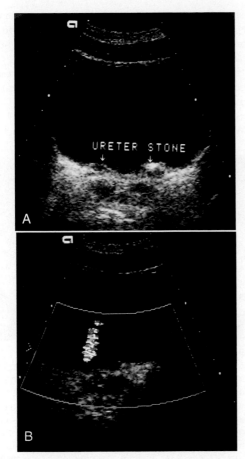

Fig 216–6
Left ureterovesical (UV) stone causing total obstruction of urine flow.
A, Transverse ultrasound of urine-filled bladder indicates calculus
(stone) in left UV junction (UVJ). Note normal right UVJ. **B,** Color Doppler of bladder demonstrates a patent right ureter as indicated by 'jet'
and absence of patent ureter on left.
(From Nseyo U, Weinman E, Lamm DL: Urology for Primary Care Physicians. Philadelphia, WB Saunders, 1999.)

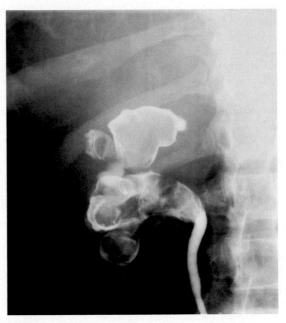

Fig 216–8
Retrograde pyelogram at time of percutaneous nephrolithotomy show-
ing lucent matrix filling the pelvicaliceal system.
(From Grainger RG, Allison DJ, Adam A, Dixon AK [eds]: Grainger &
Allison's Diagnostic Radiology, 4th ed. London, Harcourt, 2001.)

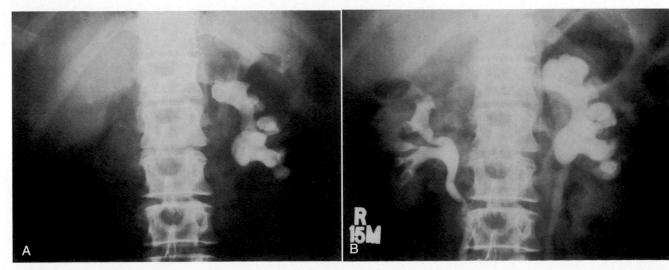

Fig 216–7
Plain film **(A)** and 15-minute intravenous urography (IVU) film **(B)** of a left staghorn calculus. Contrast medium in **B** completely hides the stone.
There is loss of parenchyma on the left, and the right kidney shows compensatory hypertrophy.
(From Grainger RG, Allison DJ, Adam A, Dixon AK [eds]: Grainger & Allison's Diagnostic Radiology, 4th ed. London, Harcourt, 2001.)

- Sodium restriction (to decrease calcium excretion), decreased protein intake to 1 g/kg/day (to decrease uric acid, calcium, and oxalate excretion)
- Increase in bran consumption (may decrease bowel transit time with increased binding of calcium and subsequent decrease in urinary calcium)
- Pain control (use of narcotics is often necessary because of the severity of pain)
- Specific therapy tailored to the stone type:

  1. Uric acid calculi: control of hyperuricosuria with allopurinol, 100 to 300 mg/day; increase urinary pH with potassium citrate, 10-mEq tablets three times daily.

  2. Calcium stones

     a. Hydrochlorothiazide (HCTZ), 25 to 50 mg daily, in patients with type I absorptive hypercalciuria

     b. Decrease bowel absorption of calcium with cellulose phosphate, 10 g/day, in patients with type I absorptive hypercalciuria

     c. Orthophosphates to inhibit vitamin B synthesis in patients with type III absorptive hypercalciuria

     d. Potassium citrate supplementation in patients with hypocitraturic calcium nephrolithiasis

     e. Purine dietary restrictions or allopurinol in patients with hyperuricosuric calcium nephrolithiasis

  3. Struvite stones

     a. Most of the stones are large and cause obstruction and bleeding.

     b. Extracorporeal shock wave lithotripsy (ESWL) and percutaneous nephrolithotomy are generally necessary.

     c. Prolonged use of antibiotics directed against the predominant urinary tract organism may be beneficial to prevent recurrence.

  4. Cystine stones: hydration and alkalization of the urine to pH >6.5, penicillamine, and tiopronin can also be used to reduce the formation of cystine; captopril is also beneficial and causes fewer side effects.

- Surgical treatment in patients with severe pain unresponsive to medication and patients with persistent fever or nausea or significant impediment of urine flow:

  1. Ureteroscopic stone extraction

  2. ESWL for most renal stones

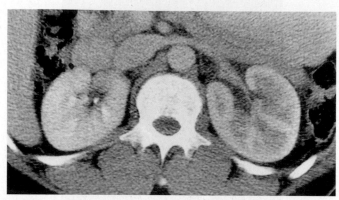

Fig 216–9
CT scan of obstructive nephrogram in patient with obstructing left ureteric stone 90 seconds after injection of contrast material. There is a normal equilibrium phase nephrogram in the right kidney, with a small amount of excreted contrast material in central collecting system. The obstructed left kidney shows persistence of the cortical-medullary nephrogram phase, reflecting delayed nephron transit of contrast material.
(From Grainger RG, Allison DJ, Adam A, Dixon AK [eds]: Grainger & Allison's Diagnostic Radiology, 4th ed. London, Harcourt, 2001.)

BLADDER

Chapter 217 — Bladder carcinoma

DEFINITION

Bladder cancer is a heterogeneous spectrum of neoplasms ranging from non–life-threatening, low-grade, superficial papillary lesions to high-grade invasive tumors, which often have metastasized at the time of presentation. It is a field change disease in which the entire urothelium from the renal pelvis to the urethra may be susceptible to malignant transformation.

- Types: transitional cell carcinoma (TCCa), squamous cell carcinoma, adenocarcinoma

PHYSICAL FINDINGS AND CLINICAL PRESENTATION

- Gross painless hematuria
- Microhematuria
- Frequency, urgency, occasional dysuria
- With locally invasive to distant metastatic disease, the presentation can include:
  - Abdominal pain
  - Flank pain
  - Lymphedema
  - Renal failure
  - Anorexia
  - Bone pain

CAUSE

Bladder cancer is a potentially preventable disease associated with specific causative factors:

- Cigarette smoking is associated with 25% to 65% of cases. The risk of developing a TCCa is two to four times higher in smokers than in nonsmokers, and that risk persists for many years, being equal to nonsmokers only after 12 to 15 years of smoking abstinence. Smoking tobacco is associated with tumors characterized by higher histologic grade, increased tumor stage, increase in the numbers of tumor present, and increased tumor size.
- Occupational exposures: dye workers, textile workers, tire and rubber workers, petroleum workers
- Chemical exposure: *o*-toluidine, 2-naphthylamine, benzidine, 4-aminobiphenyl, and nitrosamines
- Exposure to human papilloma virus (HPV) type 16
- Squamous carcinomas are associated with:
  - Schistosomiasis
  - Urinary calculi
  - Indwelling catheters
  - Bladder diverticula
  - Miscellaneous causes:
  - Phenacetin abuse
  - Cyclophosphamide
  - Pelvic irradiation
  - Tuberculosis
- Adenocarcinomas are associated with:
  - Exstrophy
  - Endometriosis
  - Neurogenic bladder
  - Urachal abnormalities
  - As a secondary site for distant metastases from other organs (i.e., colon cancer)

DIAGNOSIS

- History and physical examination
- Urinalysis
- Cystoscopy (Fig. 217–1) with bladder barbotage and biopsy
- Transurethral resection of bladder tumor(s)

DIFFERENTIAL DIAGNOSIS

- Urinary tract infection
- Frequency-urgency syndrome
- Interstitial cystitis
- Stone disease
- Endometriosis
- Neurogenic bladder

LABORATORY TESTS

- Urine cytology.
- Urine telomerase: telomerase activity in voided urine or bladder washings determined by the telomeric repeat amplification protocol (TRAP) assay. This test has been reported to detect the presence of bladder tumors in men accurately. It represents a potentially useful noninvasive diagnostic innovation for bladder cancer detection in high-risk groups such as habitual smokers or symptomatic patients.

IMAGING STUDIES

- CT and cystography (Fig. 217–2), MRI (Fig. 217–3)
- One or a combination of studies can be used..

TREATMENT

- Initially, transurethral resection of bladder tumor (TURBT)
- Loop biopsy of the prostatic urethra if high-grade TCCa is suspected
- If superficial disease, follow-up protocol with repeat TURBT and/or the use of intravesical agents is recommended.
- For advanced bladder cancer, radical cystectomy with urethrectomy (unless orthotopic diversion is planned) and ileal loop conduit or orthotopic diversion

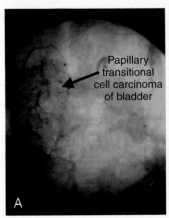
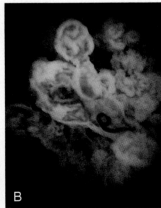

Papillary transitional cell carcinoma of bladder

Fig 217–1
Cystoscopic views of papillary transitional cell carcinoma of the bladder. **A,** Low magnification. **B,** High magnification.
(From Townsend CM, Beauchamp RD, Evers BM, Mattox KL [eds]: Sabiston Textbook of Surgery, 17th ed. Philadelphia, WB Saunders, 2004.)

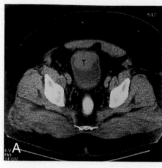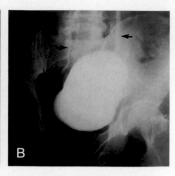

Fig 217–2

Transitional cell carcinoma of the bladder. **A,** CT scan. **B,** Cystogram study. A large polypoid tumor (T) is seen on the CT scan but because of the dense concentration of contrast medium, the tumor is not detected on cystogram study. A cystogram, however, does demonstrate bilateral ureteric reflux *(arrows)*.

(From Grainger RG, Allison DJ, Adam A, Dixon AK [eds]: Grainger & Allison's Diagnostic Radiology, 4th ed. London, Harcourt, 2001.)

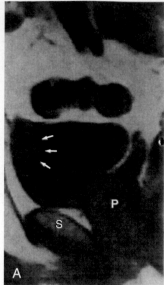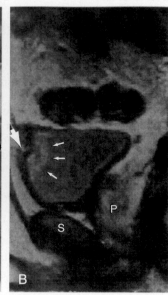

Fig 217–3

Transitional cell carcinoma of the urinary bladder, MRI study: **A,** T1-weighted image. **B,** T2-weighted image. On the T1-weighted image, the papillary component of the tumor *(small white arrows)* is well contrasted against the lower-signal-intensity urine within the urinary bladder. The tumor volume is less clearly seen on the T2-weighted image, but the interruption of the muscular wall anteriorly *(large white arrow)* indicates deep bladder-wall invasion. P, prostate gland; S, symphysis pubis.

(From Grainger RG, Allison DJ, Adam A, Dixon AK [eds]: Grainger & Allison's Diagnostic Radiology, 4th ed. London, Harcourt, 2001.)

PROSTATE

Chapter 218 **Benign prostatic hyperplasia**

DEFINITION

Benign prostatic hyperplasia (BPH) is the benign growth of the prostate, generally originating in the periureteral and transition zones, with subsequent obstructive and irritative voiding symptoms.

PHYSICAL FINDINGS AND CLINICAL PRESENTATION

- Digital rectal examination (DRE) reveals enlargement of the prostate.
- Focal enlargement may be indicative of malignancy.
- There is poor correlation between the size of the prostate and symptoms (BPH may be asymptomatic if it does not encroach on the urethral lumen).
- Most patients with BPH complain of difficulty in initiating urination (hesitancy), decrease in caliber and force of stream, incomplete emptying of bladder, often resulting in double voiding (need to urinate again a few minutes after voiding), postvoid "dribbling," and nocturia.

CAUSE

- Multifactorial; a functioning testicle is necessary for development of BPH (as evidenced by the absence in males who were castrated before puberty).

DIFFERENTIAL DIAGNOSIS

- Prostatitis
- Prostate cancer
- Strictures (urethral)
- Medication interfering with the muscle fibers in the prostate and also with bladder function

LABORATORY TESTS

- Prostate-specific antigen (PSA)
- Urinalysis, urine C&S to rule out infection (if suspected)
- Blood urea nitrogen (BUN) and creatinine to rule out postrenal insufficiency

IMAGING STUDIES

- Transrectal ultrasound may be indicated in patients with palpable nodules or significant elevation of PSA. It is also useful to estimate prostate size. Prostatic hyperplasia may be noted on intravenous urography (IVU; Fig. 218–1), ultrasound (Fig. 218–2), or MRI (Fig. 218–3).

TREATMENT

- Avoidance of caffeine or any other foods that may exacerbate symptoms
- Avoidance of medications that may exacerbate symptoms (e.g., most cold and allergy remedies)
- Asymptomatic patients with prostate enlargement caused by BPH generally do not require treatment. Patients with mild to moderate symptoms are candidates for pharmacologic

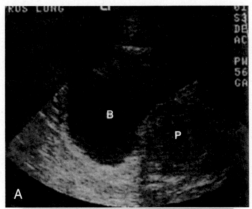

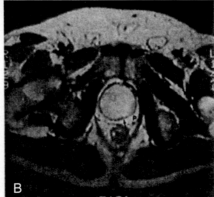

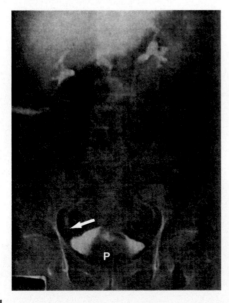

Fig 218–1

Patient with an enlarged prostate gland, intravenous urography (IVU) and coronal plane T2-weighted MRI. On the IVU study, the enlarged prostate gland (P) elevates the bladder floor and causes a J-hooking (fish-hooking) deformity of the distal ureters *(arrow)*. No obstruction is seen.

(From Grainger RG, Allison DJ, Adam A, Dixon AK [eds]: Grainger & Allison's Diagnostic Radiology, 4th ed. London, Harcourt, 2001.)

Fig 218–2

Benign prostatic nodular hyperplasia. **A,** Ultrasound (US; suprapubic abdominal approach). **B,** T2-weighted MRI. On US, the prostate demonstrates uniform low-level acoustic reflectivity, whereas on the MRI scan the adenomatous enlargement of the prostate and the peripheral zone can be distinguished. The two are separated by a low-intensity surgical pseudocapsule *(arrow)*. P, prostate, B, bladder.

(From Grainger RG, Allison DJ, Adam A, Dixon AK [eds]: Grainger & Allison's Diagnostic Radiology, 4th ed. London, Harcourt, 2001.)

treatment (see below). For those patients who have specific complications from BPH, prostate surgery is usually the most appropriate form of treatment. However, surgery may result in significant complications (e.g., incontinence, infection).

- Transurethral resection of the prostate (TURP) is the most commonly used surgical procedure for BPH. Other invasive treatment modalities include transurethral incision of the prostate (TUIP), laser therapy, and balloon dilation.

- The dietary supplement saw palmetto is available without a prescription to relieve BPH symptoms in patients with mild obstruction, however, clinical trials have failed to show significant efficacy.

- Alpha blockers (tamsulosin, alfuzosin, doxazosin, terazosin) relax smooth muscle of the bladder neck and prostate and can increase peak urinary flow rate. They have no effect on the size of the prostate. Alpha$_1$ blockers are useful in symptomatic patients to relieve symptoms of obstruction by causing relaxation of smooth muscle tone in the prostatic capsule and urethra and bladder neck.

- Hormonal manipulation with 5-alpha-reductase inhibitors that blocks conversion of testosterone to dihydrotestosterone (finasteride, dutasteride) can reduce the size of the prostate.

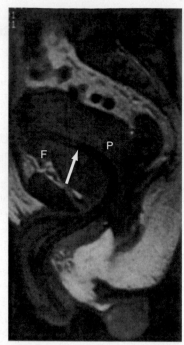

Fig 218–3
Benign nodular hyperplasia, proton density T1-weighted image. The prostate gland (P) is markedly enlarged. A Foley catheter (*arrow*) seen in place. The inflated Foley balloon (F) demarcates the level of the bladder neck.
(From Grainger RG, Allison DJ, Adam A, Dixon AK [eds]: Grainger & Allison's Diagnostic Radiology, 4th ed. London, Harcourt, 2001.)

Chapter 219 Prostatitis

DEFINITION

Prostatitis refers to inflammation of the prostate gland. There are four major categories (Table 219–1):

- Acute bacterial prostatitis (type I)
- Chronic bacterial prostatitis (type II)
- Chronic prostatitis/chronic pelvic pain syndrome (CP/CPPS) (type III): subdivided into type IIIA (inflammatory) and IIIB (noninflammatory)
- Asymptomatic inflammatory prostatitis (type IV)

PHYSICAL FINDINGS AND CLINICAL PRESENTATION

Acute bacterial prostatitis

- Sudden or rapidly progressive onset of:
  1. Dysuria
  2. Frequency
  3. Urgency
  4. Nocturia
  5. Perineal pain that may radiate to the back, rectum, or penis
- Hematuria or a purulent urethral discharge may occur.
- Occasionally, urinary retention complicates the course.
- Fever, chills, and signs of sepsis can also be parts of the clinical picture.
- On rectal examination the prostate is typically tender.

Chronic bacterial prostatitis

- Characterized by positive culture of expressed prostatic secretions; may cause symptoms such as suprapubic, low back, or perineal pain, mild urgency, frequency, and dysuria with urination, and may be associated with recurrent urinary tract infections
- May be asymptomatic when the infection is confined to the prostate.
- May present as an increase in severity of baseline symptoms of benign prostatic hypertrophy.
- When cystitis is also present, urinary frequency, urgency, and burning may be reported.
- Hematuria may be a presenting complaint.
- In older men, new onset of urinary incontinence may be noted.

Chronic prostatitis–chronic pelvic pain syndrome

- Presents similarly with pain in the pelvic region lasting more than 3 months. Symptoms also can include pain in the suprapubic region, low back, penis, testes, or scrotum.
- The symptoms can be of variable severity and may include lower urinary tract symptoms, sexual dysfunction, and reduced quality of life.

CAUSE

Acute bacterial prostatitis

- Acute usually gram-negative infection of the prostate gland
  1. Generally associated with cystitis
  2. Resulting from the ascent of bacteria in the urethra
- Occasionally, the route of infection is hematogenous or lymphatogenous spread of rectal bacteria.
- The condition is seen in young or middle-aged men.

Chronic bacterial prostatitis

- Often asymptomatic
- Exacerbation of symptoms of benign prostatic hypertrophy caused by the same mechanism as acute bacterial prostatitis

Chronic prostatitis–chronic pelvic pain syndrome

- Type IIIA: refers to symptoms of prostatic inflammation associated with the presence of white blood cells (WBCs) in prostatic secretions with no identifiable bacterial organism. *Chlamydia* infection may be causative factor in some cases.
- Type IIIB: refers to symptoms of prostatic inflammation with no or few WBCs in the prostatic secretion. Its cause is unknown. Spasm in the bladder neck or urethra may be responsible for the symptoms.

DIFFERENTIAL DIAGNOSIS

- Benign prostatic hypertrophy with lower urinary tract symptoms
- Prostate cancer
- Also see differential diagnosis of hematuria.

TABLE 219–1 National Institutes of Health consensus classification of prostatitis syndromes

Category	Characteristic clinical features	Bacteriuria	Inflammation*
I. Acute bacterial	Acute urinary tract infection (UTI)		+
II. Chronic bacterial	Recurrent UTI caused by same organism	+	+
III. Chronic prostatitis–chronic pelvic pain syndrome	Primarily pain complaints, but also voiding complaints and sexual dysfunction		
A. Inflammatory subtype†		−	+
B. Noninflammatory subtype‡		−	−
IV. Asymptomatic	Diagnosed during evaluation of other genitourinary complaints	−	+

*Objective evidence of an inflammatory response in expressed prostatic secretion, postprostate massage, urine, or semen or by histology.
†Formerly termed nonbacterial prostatitis.
‡Formerly termed prostatodynia.
From Cohen J, Powderly WG: Infectious Diseases, 2nd ed. St. Louis, Mosby, 2004.

LABORATORY TESTS
- Urinalysis
- Urine culture and sensitivity
- Cell count and culture of expressed prostatic secretions (Fig. 219–1)
- PSA is not used to diagnose prostatitis; however, a rapid rise over baseline should raise the possibility of prostatitis even in the absence of symptoms. In such cases, a follow-up PSA after treatment of prostatitis is appropriate.
- Complete blood count (CBC) and blood cultures if fever, chills, or signs of sepsis exist.
- If hematuria is present, a workup to rule out a urologic malignancy should be considered if the hematuria does not clear after treatment of prostatitis.

TREATMENT

Acute bacterial prostatitis
- Culture-guided antibiotic therapy for 4 weeks (beginning with a few days of intravenous antibiotics if the infection is serious or if the patient is bacteremic)

Chronic bacterial prostatitis
- Trimethoprim-sulfamethoxazole (TMP-SMX) is first-line choice for 4 weeks if the organism is sensitive.
- Second-line choice for treatment failure or organisms resistant to TMP-SMX is a fluoroquinolone (Ciprofloxacin).
- Patient with refractory infection or with multiple relapses may be offered long-term suppressive therapy.

Chronic prostatitis–chronic pelvic pain syndrome
- No specific treatment
- Antibiotics are not effective
- A trial of treatment with an alpha-adrenergic blocker (terazosin, doxazosin, or tamsulosin) may be considered, but recent trials have failed to show a significant reduction in symptoms.
- Any underlying bladder pathology should be ruled out by cystoscopy and treated if identified.

MEARES AND STAMEY LOCALIZATION TECHNIQUE

1. Approximately 30 minutes before taking the specimen, the patient should drink 400 mL of liquid (two glasses). The test starts when the patient wants to void.
2. The lids of four sterile specimen containers, which are marked VB_1, VB_2, EPS, and VB_3, should be removed. Place the uncovered specimen containers on a flat surface and maintain sterility.
3. Hands are washed.
4. Expose the penis and retract the foreskin so that the glans is exposed. The foreskin should be retracted throughout.
5. Cleanse the glans with a soap solution, remove the soap with sterile gauze or cotton and dry the glans.
6. Urinate 10–15 mL into the first container marked VB_1.
7. Urinate 100–200 mL into the toilet bowl or vessel and without interrupting the urine stream, urinate 10–15 mL into the second container marked VB_2.
8. The patient bends forward and holds the sterile specimen container (EPS) to catch the prostate secretion.
9. The physician massages the prostate until several drops of prostate secretion (EPS) are obtained.
10. If no EPS can be collected during massage, a drop may be present at the orifice of the urethra and this drop should be taken with a 10 µL calibrated loop and cultured.
11. Immediately after prostatic massage, the patient urinates 10–15 mL of urine into the container marked VB_3.

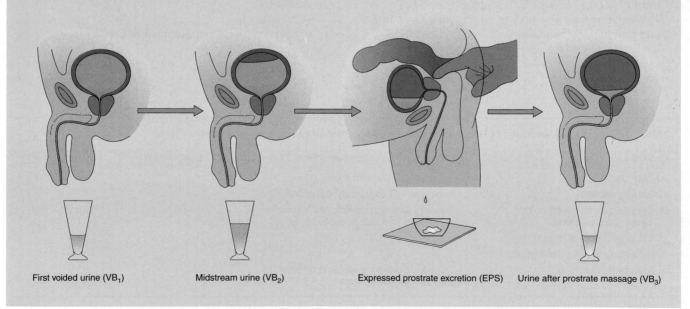

First voided urine (VB_1)   Midstream urine (VB_2)   Expressed prostrate excretion (EPS)   Urine after prostrate massage (VB_3)

Fig 219–1
Meares and Stamey localization technique to diagnose chronic bacterial prostatitis. Prostate secretion can be more readily obtained if the patient has not ejaculated for approximately 3 to 5 days before the examination.
(From Cohen J, Powderly WG: Infectious Diseases, 2nd ed. St. Louis, Mosby, 2004.

DEFINITION AND CLASSIFICATION

Prostate cancer is a neoplasm involving the prostate; various classifications have been developed to evaluate malignancy potential and prognosis:

- The degree of malignancy varies with the stage.
  Stage A: Confined to the prostate, no nodule palpable
  Stage B: Palpable nodule confined to the gland
  Stage C: Local extension
  Stage D: Regional lymph nodes or distant metastases
- In the Gleason classification, two histologic patterns are independently assigned numbers 1 to 5 (best to least differentiated). These numbers are added to give a total tumor score between 2 and 10. Prognosis is best for highly differentiated tumors (e.g., Gleason score 2 to 4) as compared with most poorly differentiated tumors (Gleason score 7 to 10).
- Another commonly used classification is the tumor-node-metastasis (TNM) classification of prostate cancer.

PHYSICAL FINDINGS AND CLINICAL PRESENTATION

- Generally silent disease until it reaches advanced stages
- Bone pain and pathologic fractures may be initial symptoms of prostate cancer.
- Local growth can cause symptoms of outflow obstruction.
- DRE may reveal an area of increased firmness; 10% of patients will have a negative DRE.
- Prostate may be hard, fixed, with extension of tumor to the seminal vesicles in advanced stages.

DIFFERENTIAL DIAGNOSIS

- Benign prostatic hyperplasia
- Prostatitis
- Prostate stones

LABORATORY TESTS

- Measurement of PSA
- Prostatic acid phosphatase (PAP) can be used for evaluation of nonlocalized disease.

- Transrectal biopsy and fine-needle aspiration of prostate can confirm the diagnosis (Fig. 220–1).

IMAGING STUDIES

- Bone scan is useful to evaluate bone metastasis (Fig. 220–2). Osteoblastic lesions may be present on plain films (Fig. 220–3).
- CT scan, MRI, and transrectal ultrasonography (Fig. 220–4) may be useful in select patients to assess extent of prostate cancer.

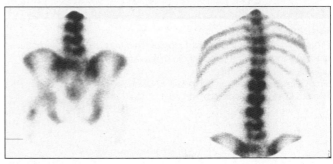

Fig 220–2
Technetium bone scan. Increased tracer activity throughout the axial skeleton is secondary to metastatic prostate cancer.
(From Hochberg MC, Silman AJ, Smolen JS, et al [eds]: Rheumatology, 3rd ed. St. Louis, Mosby, 2003.)

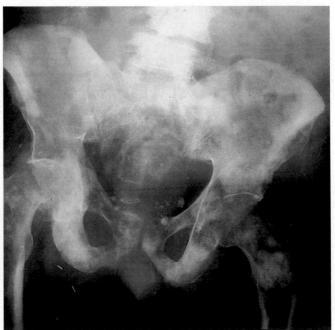

Fig 220–3
Metastatic prostate cancer—plain radiograph demonstrating osteoblastic lesions replacing lower lumbar vertebral bodies and most of the bony pelvis.
(From Hochberg MC, Silman AJ, Smolen JS, et al [eds]: Rheumatology, 3rd ed. St. Louis, Mosby, 2003.)

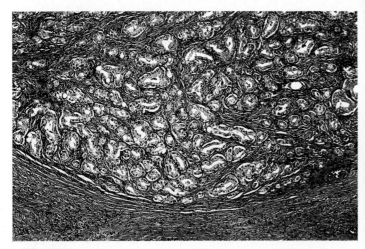

Fig 220–1
Well-differentiated Gleason grade 2 + 2 = score of 4 adenocarcinoma.
(From Silverberg SG, Frable WJ, Wick MR, et al [eds]: Principles and Practice of Surgical Pathology and Cytopathology, 4th ed. Philadelphia, Elsevier, 2006.)

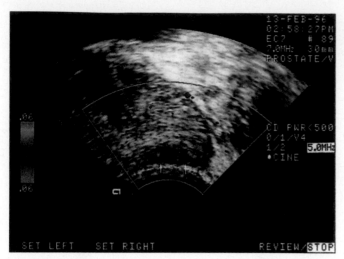

Fig 220-4
Prostatic carcinoma with color Doppler. This transverse image of the left midgland shows a hypoechoic mass *(arrows)* with increased color flow.
(From Grainger RG, Allison DJ, Adam A, Dixon AK [eds]: Grainger & Allison's Diagnostic Radiology, 4th ed. London, Harcourt, 2001.)

TREATMENT

- Therapeutic approach varies with the following:
  1. Stage of the tumor
  2. Patient's life expectancy
  3. General medical condition
  4. Patient's treatment preference (e.g., patient may be opposed to orchiectomy)
- The optimal treatment of clinically localized prostate cancer is unclear.
  1. Radical prostatectomy is generally performed in patients with localized prostate cancer and a life expectancy of more than 10 years.
  2. Radiation therapy (external beam irradiation or brachytherapy with implantation of radioactive pellets [iodine-125 or palladium-103 seeds] into the prostate gland) represents an alternative in patients with localized prostate cancer, especially poor surgical candidates or patients with a high-grade malignancy.
  3. Watchful waiting is reasonable in patients who are too old or too ill to survive longer than 10 years. If the cancer progresses to the point where it becomes symptomatic, palliation can be attempted with several methods.
- Patients with advanced disease and a projected life expectancy of less than 10 years are candidates for radiation therapy and hormonal therapy (diethylstibestrol [DES], luteinizing hormone–releasing hormone [LHRH] analogues, antiandrogens, bilateral orchiectomy).
- Recommended treatment of patients with regional metastatic prostate cancer with projected life expectancy of 10 years or more includes radiation and hormone therapy.
- Androgen-deprivation therapy (ADT) with a gonadotropin-releasing hormone agonist is the mainstay of treatment for metastatic prostate cancer.
- Docetaxel plus prednisone or docetaxel plus estramustine can be used in metastatic hormone-refractory prostate cancer.

TESTICLES

Chapter 221   Hydrocele

DEFINITION

A hydrocele is a fluid collection in a serous scrotal space, usually between the layers of the tunica vaginalis. Figure 221–1 illustrates the gross anatomy of a normal scrotum. A hydrocele that fills with fluid from the peritoneum is termed *communicating*.

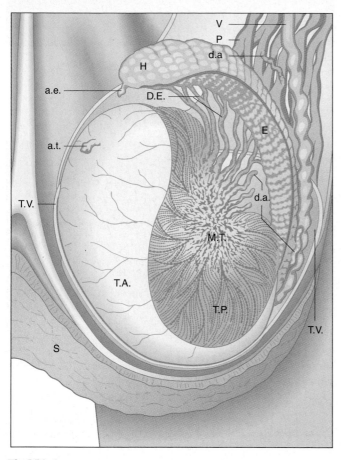

Fig 221–1

Gross anatomy of the scrotal contents. The anterolateral aspect of the scrotal sac (S), tunica vaginalis (T.V.), testis, and epididymis have been cut away. The epididymis has been lifted away from the testis to demonstrate the intervening structures better. Although the spermatic artery is not shown, other structures of the spermatic cord, vas deferens (V), and pampiniform venous plexus (P) are seen at the top. The firm white tunica albuginea (T.A.) has been cut away to demonstrate testicular parenchyma (T.P.), which is composed of tiny coiled seminiferous tubules separated by thin fibrous septa. The tubules drain into the fibrous mediastinum testis (M.T.) and pass to the head of the epididymis (H) via several ductuli efferentes (D.E.). The duct of the epididymis is tightly coiled in the body of the epididymis (E). The tail of the epididymis lies behind the testis, where it joins the vas deferens (V). Embryologic remnants shown are the appendix epididymis (a.e.), appendix testis (a.t.), and the rarely noted remnants of mesonephric ductules, the ductuli aberrantes (d.a.), which may be found in a variety of locations.
(From Wheeler JE, Rudy FR. The testis, paratesticular structures, and male external genitalia. In Silverberg SG, Frable WJ, Wick MR, et al [eds]: Principles and Practice of Surgical Pathology and Cytopathology, 4th ed. Philadelphia, Elsevier, 2006.)

This is distinguished from a *noncommunicating* hydrocele by history of variation in size throughout the day and palpation of a thickened cord above the testicle on the affected side. A communicating hydrocele is basically a small inguinal hernia in which fluid, but not peritoneal structures, traverses the processus vaginalis.

PHYSICAL FINDINGS AND CLINICAL PRESENTATION

Symptoms
- Scrotal enlargement (Fig. 221–2)
- Scrotal heaviness or discomfort radiating to the inguinal area
- Back pain

Physical findings
- Scrotal distention (testicle may be difficult to palpate)
- Transillumination (Fig. 221–3)

CAUSE

- Hydroceles may occur as a congenital abnormality in which the processus vaginalis fails to close. In this case, an inguinal hernia is almost always associated with the malformation.
- Congenital hydroceles are usually diagnosed in infants and children. In adults, hydroceles are more frequently caused by infection, tumor, or trauma.
- Infection of the epididymis often results in the development of a secondary hydrocele in adults.
- Tropical infections such as filariasis may also produce hydroceles.

DIFFERENTIAL DIAGNOSIS

- Spermatocele
- Inguinoscrotal hernia
- Testicular tumor (see Fig. 223–2)
- Varicocele (see Fig. 222–1)
- Epididymitis (see Fig. 223–3)
- Epididymal cyst (see Fig. 223–1)

IMAGING STUDIES

- Scrotal ultrasound (useful to rule out a testicular tumor as the cause of the hydrocele)

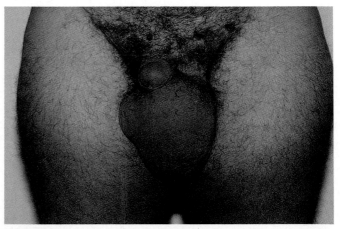

Fig 221–2

Hydrocele.
(From Swartz MH: Textbook of Physical Diagnosis, 5th ed. Philadelphia, 2006, WB Saunders, 2006.)

- (Figure 221–4 shows a sonogram of a normal testis. A sonogram of a hydrocele is shown in Figure 221–5.
- The acute development of a hydrocele might be associated with the onset of epididymitis, testicular tumor, trauma, and torsion of a testicular appendage (see Fig. 225–1). An ultrasound of the scrotum may provide important diagnostic information.

TREATMENT

- No treatment if asymptomatic and testicle is thought to be normal
- Surgical repair. Communicating hydroceles should be repaired in the same manner as an indirect hernia. The indications for repair of a noncommunicating hydrocele include failure to resolve and increase in size to one that is large and tense.

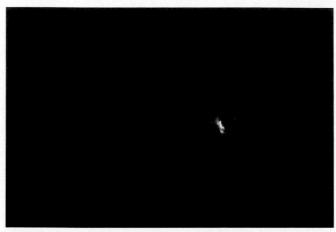

Fig 221–3
Transilluminated hydrocele.
(From Swartz MH: Textbook of Physical Diagnosis, 5th ed. Philadelphia, 2006, WB Saunders, 2006.)

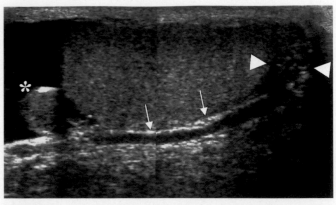

Fig 221–4
Normal testis—montage longitudinal ultrasound view showing tail *(arrowheads),* body *(arrows),* and appendix *(asterisk)* of the epididymis. (From Grainger RG, Allison DJ, Adam A, Dixon AK [eds]: Grainger & Allison's Diagnostic Radiology, 4th ed. London, Harcourt, 2001.)

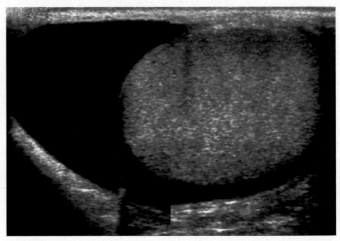

Fig 221–5
Longitudinal ultrasound view of normal testis and moderate sized hydrocele.
(From Grainger RG, Allison DJ, Adam A, Dixon AK [eds]: Grainger & Allison's Diagnostic Radiology, 4th ed. London, Harcourt, 2001.)

Chapter 222 | Varicocele

- A varicocele is caused by dilation of veins that drain into the internal spermatic veins, usually secondary to incompetent internal spermatic vein valves.
- Physical examination reveals dilated tortuous veins lying posterior to and above the testis (Fig. 222–1)
- Differential diagnosis
  - Hydrocele (see Fig. 221–2)
  - Testicular tumor (see Fig. 223–2)
  - Inguinoscrotal hernia
  - Epididymitis (see Fig. 223–3)

- Imaging: ultrasound (Fig. 222–2) can be performed when diagnosis is uncertain or there is suspicion of a mass.
- Treatment: surgical ligation for the dilated internal spermatic veins in symptomatic patients or when infertility is present

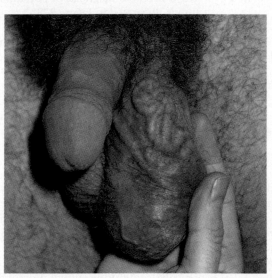

Fig 222–1
Varicocele.
(From Swartz MH: Textbook of Physical Diagnosis, 5th ed. Philadelphia, 2006, WB Saunders, 2006.)

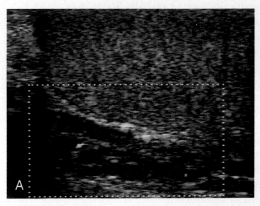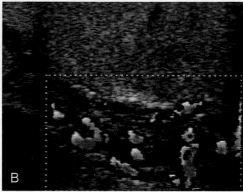

Fig 222–2
Ultrasound of an asymptomatic left varicocele. At rest **(A)**, there is little detectable flow on color Doppler. During Valsalva maneuver, the flow is enhanced **(B)**.
(From Grainger RG, Allison DJ, Adam A, Dixon AK [eds]: Grainger & Allison's Diagnostic Radiology, 4th ed. London, Harcourt, 2001.)

Chapter 223 Epididymitis

DEFINITION
Epididymitis is an inflammatory reaction of the epididymis caused by an infectious agent or local trauma.

PHYSICAL FINDINGS AND CLINICAL PRESENTATION
- Tender swelling of the scrotum with erythema, usually unilateral testicular pain and tenderness
- Dysuria and/or urethral discharge
- Fever and signs of systemic illness (less common)
- Pain and redness on scrotal examination
- Hydrocele or even epididymo-orchitis, especially late
- Chronic draining scrotal sinuses, with a beadlike enlargement of the vas deferens in tuberculous disease

CAUSE
- In young sexually active men, the most common infectious agents isolated are *Neisseria gonorrhoeae* and *Chlamydia trachomatis*.
- In men older than 35 years or with underlying urologic disease:
  1. Gram-negative aerobic rods are predominant.
  2. Similar organisms are found in men following invasive urologic procedures.
  3. Gram-positive cocci are rarely seen in these groups.
  4. Mycobacteria are also a cause of epididymitis.
- Young prepubertal boys may present with epididymitis caused by coliform bacteria, almost always a complication of underlying urologic disease such as reflux.
- In AIDS patients, cytomegalovirus (CMV) and *Salmonella* epididymitis have been described. CMV may have a negative urine culture. Toxoplasmosis should also be considered as a cause of epididymitis in AIDS patients.

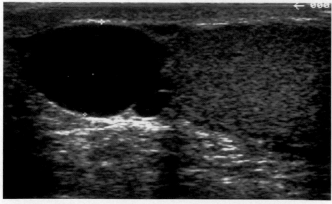

Fig 223–1
Ultrasound of epididymal cyst in head of epididymis.
(From Grainger RG, Allison DJ, Adam A, Dixon AK [eds]: Grainger & Allison's Diagnostic Radiology, 4th ed. London, Harcourt, 2001.)

DIFFERENTIAL DIAGNOSIS
- Orchitis
- Testicular torsion (see Fig. 225–1), trauma, or tumor (see Fig. 224–4),
- Epididymal cyst (Fig. 223–1)
- Hydrocele (see Fig. 221–5)
- Varicocele (see Fig. 222–2)
- Spermatocele
- Testicular torsion should be considered in all cases.
- Table 223–1 describes common intrascrotal conditions. The differential diagnosis of physical findings in acute scrotum is illustrated in Figure 223–2.

WORKUP
- Consideration of a full assessment of the urologic tract in patients with bacterial infection, especially if recurrent
- Imaging with sonography (Fig. 223–3)
- If discharge is present: cultures and Gram stain smear of urethral exudate
- In homosexual men: gonococcal cultures of the throat and rectum possibly of value
- If testicular torsion a consideration: radionuclear imaging (see Fig. 225–3)
- Examination of first-void uncentrifuged urine for leukocytes if the urethral Gram stain is negative. A culture and Gram-stained smear of this urine specimen should be performed along with nucleic acid amplification studies (ligase chain reaction [LCR]) from urine samples for gonorrhea and *Chlamydia* spp.

LABORATORY TESTS
- Urinalysis and urine culture if dysuria is present or urinary tract infection is suspected
- VDRL chlamydia serology in sexually active men
- Purified protein derivative (PPD) placed and chest x-ray if TB suspected
- Rarely, biopsy to ensure the diagnosis of tuberculous epididymitis
- HIV testing and counseling

TREATMENT
- Ice packs and scrotal elevation for relief of pain
- Analgesia with acetaminophen with or without codeine or nonsteroidal anti-inflammatory drugs (NSAIDs).
- Antibiotics to cover suspected pathogens
  - In sexually active men, doxycycline
  - Best treatment for older men with gram-negative bacteriuria: ofloxacin or levofloxacin
  - *Pseudomonas* covered by ciprofloxacin
- Surgical aspiration of local abscesses or even open surgical drainage
- Repair of underlying structural defects is considered, especially if infections are severe or recur.
- Surgical repair of reflux in young boys should be undertaken promptly and at a young age when possible.
- Sex partners of patient should be referred for evaluation and treatment.

TABLE 223-1 Common intrascrotal conditions

	Testicular torsion	Epididymitis	Testis tumor
Symptoms			
Age	Neonate-early 20s	Childhood-old age	15-35 yr
Pain			
Nature	Sudden	Progressive	Absent or gradual
Degree	Severe	Variable	Absent or mild
Nausea, vomiting	Yes	No	No
Physical Examination			
Testes	Swollen, tender	May be swollen	Hard mass
Epididymides	Swollen, tender	Swollen, tender	Normal
Spermatic cord	Shortened	Thickened, may be tender	
Urinalysis	Normal	Pyuria, bacteriuria	Normal

From Nseyo U, Weinman E, Lamm DL: Urology for Primary Care Physicians. Philadelphia, WB Saunders, 1999.

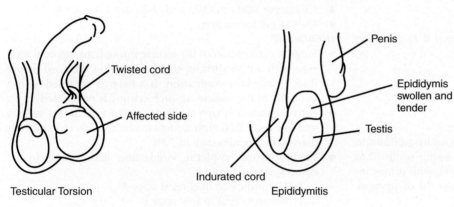

Testicular Torsion

Epididymitis

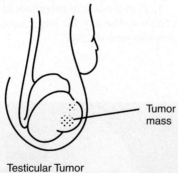

Testicular Tumor

Fig 223–2
Physical findings in acute scrotum. **Upper left,** Testicular torsion. **Upper right,** Epididymitis. **Lower,** Testicular tumor. Scrotal examination, which begins with palpation of the scrotal contents, should be performed in the following order: (1) testes, (2) epididymides, (3) spermatic cord structures, and (4) inguinal ring.
(From Nseyo U, Weinman E, Lamm DL: Urology for Primary Care Physicians. Philadelphia, WB Saunders, 1999.)

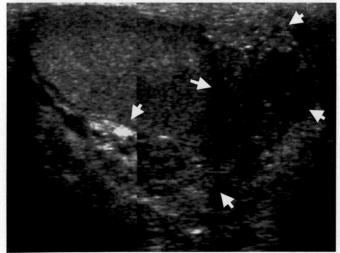

Fig 223–3
Ultrasound of acute bacterial epididymitis. The body and tail of the epididymis *(arrows)* are heterogeneous and enlarged. The testis is normal. (From Grainger RG, Allison DJ, Adam A, Dixon AK [eds]: Grainger & Allison's Diagnostic Radiology, 4th ed. London, Harcourt, 2001.)

Chapter 224 **Testicular neoplasms**

DEFINITION

Testicular neoplasms are primary cancers originating in a testis.

PHYSICAL FINDINGS AND CLINICAL PRESENTATION

- Any mass within the testicle should be considered cancer until proved otherwise. It may be found by the patient who brings it to the attention of a physician or by a physician on a routine examination.
- Symptoms other than scrotal or testicular swelling are typically absent unless the cancer has metastasized. Occasionally, a patient may complain of scrotal fullness or heaviness.
- Testicular palpation should be performed with two hands. Transillumination (see Fig. 221–3) may distinguish a solid mass (e.g., cancer) and a fluid-filled lesion (e.g., hydrocele or spermatocele). The mass is nontender, indeed less sensitive than a normal testicle.

CAUSE AND PATHOLOGY

- Cryptorchidism (undescended testes), even if corrected by orchiopexy
- Pathology: Cell type—frequency, %
  - Seminoma (Fig. 224–1)—42
  - Embryonal cell carcinoma—26
  - Teratocarcinoma—26
  - Teratoma (Fig. 224–2)—5

The clinical stages consist of stage A, with tumor confined to the testis and cord structures; stage B, with tumor confined to the retroperitoneal lymph nodes; and stage C, with tumor involving the abdominal viscera or disease above the diaphragm.

DIFFERENTIAL DIAGNOSIS

- Spermatocele
- Varicocele (see Fig. 222–1)
- Hydrocele (see Fig. 221–3)
- Epididymitis (see Fig. 223–2)
- Epidermoid cyst of the testicle (see Fig. 223–1)
- Epididymis tumors

LABORATORY TESTS

- Serum human chorionic gonadotropin (hCG)
- Serum alpha-fetoprotein (AFP)

One or both of these tumor markers will be elevated in 70% of cases of testicular cancer.

IMAGING STUDIES

- Ultrasound (Figs. 224–3 and 224–4)
- CT scan or MRI of pelvis and abdomen for staging
- Chest x-ray for staging

TREATMENT

- Surgical exploration of the testicle through an inguinal incision with a noncrushing clamp placed on the cord before direct testicular examination. If a mass is confined within the body of the testicle, an orchiectomy is performed.
- Retroperitoneal lymph node dissection for clinical stage A and low stage B (lymph nodes smaller than 6 cm in greatest diameter) provides cure in 70%
- Chemotherapy: cisplatin, vinblastine, and bleomycin are commonly used agents
  1. Not indicated in clinical stage A
  2. Controversial in low stage B
  3. Cornerstone of treatment in high stage B or stage C
- Radiation therapy for stage A and low stage B seminoma provides cure in 85%

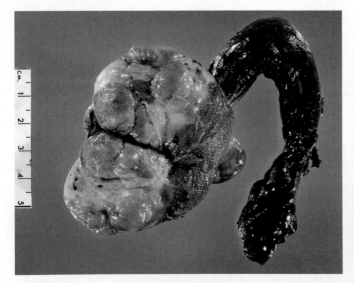

Fig 224–1
Classic seminoma—grossly, a homogeneous fleshy mass, with bulging cut surface, replacing the testicular parenchyma.
(From Silverberg SG, Frable WJ, Wick MR, et al [eds]: Principles and Practice of Surgical Pathology and Cytopathology, 4th ed. Philadelphia, Elsevier, 2006.)

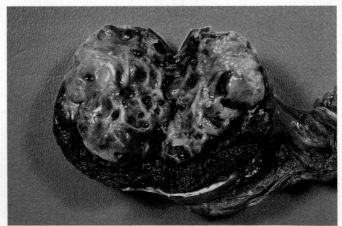

Fig 224–2
Teratoma occurring in an adult. The tumor shows multiple cystic and solid areas. (From Wheeler JE, Rudy FR. The testis, paratesticular structures, and male external genitalia. In Silverberg SG [ed]: Principles and Practice of Surgical Pathology and Cytopathology, 4th ed. Elsevier, 2006.

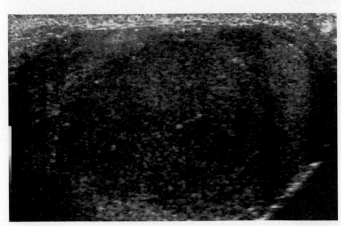

Fig 224–3
Seminoma, longitudinal ultrasound view. The slightly hyporeflective lesion is almost replacing the entire testis. Microcalcifications are seen in the normal and abnormal parenchyma.
(From Grainger RG, Allison DJ, Adam A, Dixon AK [eds]: Grainger & Allison's Diagnostic Radiology, 4th ed. London, Harcourt, 2001.)

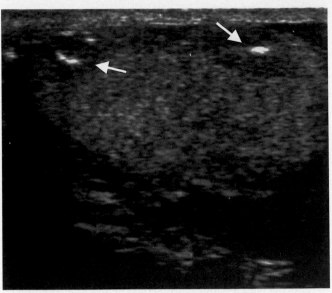

Fig 224–4
Ultrasound of teratoma. The malignancy is multifocal with macrocalcifications (arrows).
(From Grainger RG, Allison DJ, Adam A, Dixon AK [eds]: Grainger & Allison's Diagnostic Radiology, 4th ed. London, Harcourt, 2001.)

Chapter 225   Testicular torsion

DEFINITION

Testicular torsion is a twisting of the spermatic cord (Fig. 225–1) leading to cessation of testicular blood flow, ischemia, and infarction (Fig. 225–2) if left untreated.

PHYSICAL FINDINGS AND CLINICAL PRESENTATION

- Typical sequence is sudden onset of hemiscrotal pain, then swelling, nausea, and vomiting without fever or urinary symptoms.
- Physical examination may reveal a tender firm testis, high-riding testis, horizontal lie of testis, absent cremasteric reflex, and no pain with elevation of testis.
- Painless testicular swelling occurs in 10% of patients.
- One out of three patients reports previous episodes of spontaneously remitting scrotal pain.
- In the neonate, testicular torsion should be presumed in patients with a painless, discolored hemiscrotal swelling.
- In rare cases, torsion may involve an undescended testicle. In such cases, an empty hemiscrotum is palpated together with a tender lump in the inguinal area.

CAUSE

There are two types of testicular torsion:
- Extravaginal, caused by nonadherence of the tunica vaginalis to the dartos layer
- Intravaginal, caused by malrotation of the spermatic cord with the tunica vaginalis

DIAGNOSIS

Diagnosis is made mainly by clinical suspicion. Color Doppler ultrasound evaluation or a nuclear testicular scan may help with the diagnosis.

DIFFERENTIAL DIAGNOSIS

- Torsion of the testicular appendages
- Testicular tumor (see Figs. 224–1, 224–4)
- Epididymitis (Fig. 225–3)
- Incarcerated inguinoscrotal hernia
- Orchitis
- Spermatocele
- Hydrocele (see Fig. 221–3)
- Varicocele (see Fig. 222–1)
- Table 225–1 describes the differential diagnosis of acute scrotum.

IMAGING STUDIES

- Radionuclide scrotal scanning (technetium-99m): cold testicle (Fig. 225–4)
- Doppler ultrasonic stethoscope (Doppler flowmetry)

TREATMENT

- Surgical derotation of the spermatic cord followed by bilateral testicular fixation with nonabsorbable sutures
- If the affected testis is nonviable, orchiectomy of the affected testis and orchiopexy of the contralateral side are performed.

PROGNOSIS

- There is an 80% testicular salvage rate if detorsion occurs within 12 hours of onset.
- After 24 hours, irreversible testicular infarction is expected.
- Because the contralateral testes can be affected (immunologic process), when treatment is delayed and return of blood flow does not occur after detorsion, some recommend orchiectomy of the infarcted testicle.

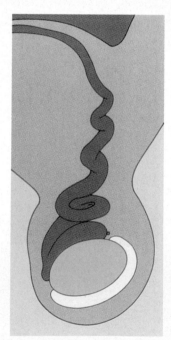

Fig 225–1
Torsion of the spermatic cord.
(From Zitelli BJ, Davis HW: Atlas of Pediatric Physical Diagnosis, 4th ed. St. Louis, Mosby, 2002.)

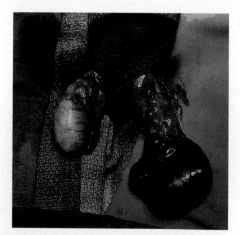

Fig 225–2
Surgical exploration and detorsion of left spermatic cord. Right testis also shows bell and clapper deformity.
(From Zitelli BJ, Davis HW: Atlas of Pediatric Physical Diagnosis, 4th ed. St. Louis, Mosby, 2002.)

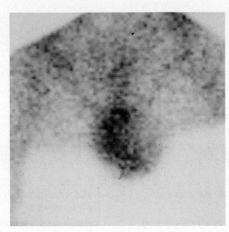

Fig 225-3
Nuclear blood flow scan showing increased flow to the right testis resulting from epididymitis.
(From Zitelli BJ, Davis HW: Atlas of Pediatric Physical Diagnosis, 4th ed. St. Louis, Mosby, 2002.)

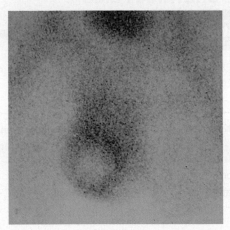

Fig 225-4
Nuclear blood flow scan showing the classic bull's eye configuration of a missed torsion of the right testis.
(From Zitelli BJ, Davis HW: Atlas of Pediatric Physical Diagnosis, 4th ed. St. Louis, Mosby, 2002.)

TABLE 225-1 Acute scrotum: differential diagnosis

	Torsion*	Epididymitis	Tumor
Age	Birth to 20 yr	Puberty to old age	15-35 yr
Pain			
Onset	Sudden	Rapid	Gradual
Degree	Severe	Increasing severity	Mild or absent†
Nausea, vomiting	Yes	No	No
Examination			
Testes	Swollen together and both tender	Normal early	Mass
Epididymis		Swollen, tender	Normal
Spermatic cord	Shortened	Thickened, often tender, as high as inguinal canal	Normal
Urinalysis	Normal	Often infection	Normal

*Testes and appendices of testes and epididymis.
†Present in 30% of patients with testis tumor.
From Nseyo U, Weinman E, Lamm DL: Urology for Primary Care Physicians. Philadelphia, WB Saunders, 1999.

VULVA, URETHRA, PENIS

Chapter 226 — Diseases of the genital skin

- Table 226–1 describes the differential diagnosis of cutaneous genital lesions.
- An algorithm for the evaluation of patients with genital lesions or ulcers is shown in Figure 226–1.

TABLE 226-1 Differential diagnosis of cutaneous genital lesions.

Category	Lesion	Usual morphology	Comments
Flat lesions			
Erythematous	Contact dermatitis	Red edematous patch, may be vesicular	Recent contact with an irritant or allergen
	Seborrheic dermatitis	Ill-defined, erythematous, scaly patches or plaques with crusting	Idiopathic inflammation of the sebaceous glands
	Tinea cruris (dermatophytosis)	Well-demarcated scaling plaques, with an erythematous border, over inner thighs	See Section 1, Chapter 26
	Psoriasis	Well-demarcated erythematous plaques with scales on keratinized skin, and without scales on nonkeratinized skin	Typically involves the scalp, elbows, knees, back and buttocks
	Candidal balanitis	Red papules or plaques on penile shaft	See Section 1, Chapter 26
	Plasma cell (Zoon's) balanitis	Glistening, moist, erythematous patch over glans penis or coronal sulcus	Benign chronic balanitis
Hyperpigmented	Pigmented nevi	Well-demarcated lesions with regular borders and homogeneous pigmentation	Biopsy to rule out malignant melanoma
Hypopigmented	Lichen sclerosis	Hypopigmented plaques of atrophic skin with progressive scarring over vulva or penis (balanitis xerotica obliterans)	Benign chronic dystrophic disease, more common in postmenopausal women
	Lichen planus	Reticulated, white branching striae on nonkeratinized skin	Presents as inflammatory papules on keratinized skin
	Vitiligo	Depigmented well-demarcated patches with no skin surface changes	Absence of melanocytes, possibly autoimmune
	Postinflammatory hypopigmentation	Flat ill-defined demarcated patches with partial or total loss of pigment	Follows healing of some inflammatory lesions
Raised lesions			
Normal pigmentation	Genital warts	Cauliflower-like (condylomata acuminate), flat-topped, or rounded papules	See Figs. 226–9, 226–10
	Secondary syphilis	Moist, hypertrophic, flat-topped papules (condylomata lata)	May also be ulcerative; see Figs. 226–13, 226–14
	Molluscum contagiosum	Smooth, firm, shiny umbilicated nodules	See Section 1, Chapter 27
	Pearly penile papules	Crownlike arrangement of dome-shaped papules around corona of the penis	Benign angiofibromas usually appearing in adolescence
	Prominent sebaceous (Tyson's) glands	Clustered pale papules on corona and inner surface of prepuce	Aberrant sebaceous glands, normal anatomic variant
	Cysts	Dome-shaped nodules or papules	Common benign growths
	Fordyce spots	Purplish or reddish telangiectatic papules on scrotum, penis, or vulva	Occurs in late puberty, normal anatomic variant
	Sclerosing lymphangitis	Firm translucent cord encircling penis proximal to the corona	Result of trauma or friction
Erythematous	Scabies	Elongated papules (female's burrow) with surrounding excoriation	Look for corresponding lesions on wrists or in finger webs; see Section 1, Chapter 29
	Hidradenitis suppurativa	Tender inflamed nodules at base of hair follicles	Recurrent abscesses of apocrine gland
	Pyogenic granulomas	Pedunculated vascular masses usually on scrotum	Benign tumors

From Cohen J, Powderly WG: Infectious Diseases, 2nd ed. St. Louis, Mosby, 2004.

TABLE 226-1 Differential diagnosis of cutaneous genital lesions—cont'd

Category	Lesion	Usual morphology	Comments
Hyperpigmented	Seborrheic keratosis	Brown, keratotic, verrucous lesions	Benign lesions usually occurring after age 40 yr
	Lichen planus	Pruritic, flat-topped violaceous papules on keratinized skin	Idiopathic, inflammatory eruption, often associated with oral lesions
	Squamous cell carcinoma in situ (three forms)	Large, red-brown scaly or crusted verrucous lesion, usually solitary	Bowen's disease
		Smaller, flat verrucous lesions, usually multifocal	Bowenoid papulosis
		Erythematous, raised, irregular plaques	Erythroplasia of Queyrat
	Kaposi's sarcoma	Violaceous indurated plaques or nodules	
Ulcerative lesions			
Nonvenereal diseases	Aphthous ulcers	Painful irregular ulcers with erythematous borders and white fibrin base	Commonly associated with oral ulcer
	Behçet's syndrome	Painful, shallow, irregular ulcers with erythematous borders and white fibrin base on glans penis or labia minora	Associated with oral ulcers, uveitis, arthritis, vasculitis, or chronic meningoencephalitis

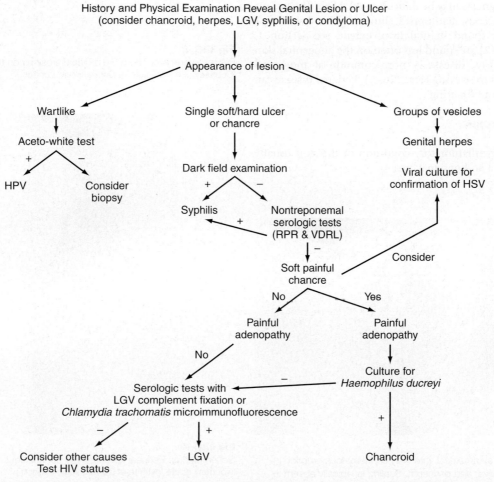

Fig 226–1

Algorithm for evaluation of patients with genital lesions or ulcers. HIV, human immunodeficiency virus; HSV, herpes simplex virus; HPV, human papillomavirus; LGV, lymphogranuloma venereum; RPR, rapid plasma reagin; VDRL, Venereal Disease Research Laboratory. (From Nseyo U, Weinman E, Lamm DL: Urology for Primary Care Physicians. Philadelphia, WB Saunders, 1999.)

A. INFLAMMATORY DERMATOSES

(1) Psoriasis

Flexural psoriasis is the most common pattern seen in the ano-genital region, with extension into the genitocrural folds (Fig. 226–2). There are often clinical difficulties in distinguishing between psoriasis and seborrheic eczema. Histology is often unhelpful, because the changes can be nonspecific. The typical features of psoriasis are rarely evident and the presence of secondary spongiosis may be misleading. For additional information on psoriasis, see Section 1, Chapter 7.

(2) Reiter's syndrome

Reiter's syndrome represents a triad of polyarthritis associated with urethritis and nongonococcal conjunctivitis. Additional information on Reiter's syndrome can be found in Section 12, Chapter •••. In the genitalia, circinate balanitis, presenting as a moist superficial erosion, 2 to 4 mm across, may affect the glans penis and meatus (Fig. 226–3). Superficial ulceration of the oral mucosa may also occur, together with reddening and a granular appearance of the surrounding mucous membrane.

(3) Lichen planus

Anogenital lesions may be found in up to 40% of patients with generalized disease. In some patients, however, the disease is restricted to the genitalia and/or the perineal region and these instances, the diagnosis may be difficult to establish. The lesions are typical, violaceous, flat-topped shiny papules. Wickham's striae (frequently found in oral involvement; see Section 1, Chapter 8, Fig. 8–2) are found less often on the anogenital skin (Fig. 226–4). Erosive disease is more common at anogenital sites and can lead to scarring (Fig. 226–5). Perianal disease can lead to deep painful fissuring.

(4) Lichen sclerosus

DEFINITION

Thus is a chronic inflammatory condition of the skin usually affecting the vulva and perianal area.

PHYSICAL FINDINGS AND CLINICAL PRESENTATION

- Erythema may be the only initial sign. A characteristic finding is the presence of ivory white atrophic lesions on the involved area.

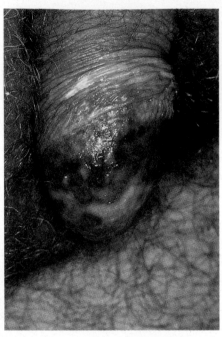

Fig 226–3
Reiter's syndrome. There are multiple erosions on the glans penis. (Courtesy of the Institute of Dermatology, London.)

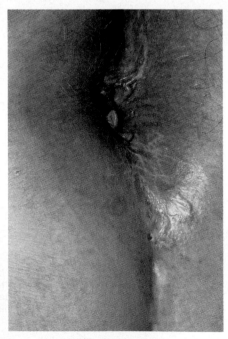

Fig 226–4
Lichen planus. Perineal lesions show conspicuous striae. (Courtesy of the Institute of Dermatology, London.)

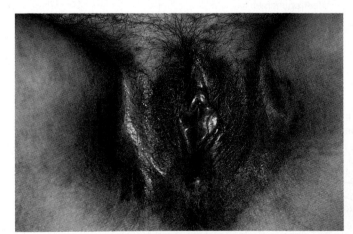

Fig 226–2
Psoriasis. Note the symmetrical, intensely erythematous eruption involving the groin, vulva, and perineum. Scaling is typically absent in flexural disease. The sharply demarcated border is characteristic. (Courtesy of the Institute of Dermatology, London.)

- Close inspection of the affected area will reveal the presence of white to brown follicular plugs on the surface (dells).
- When the genitals are involved, the white, parchment-like skin assumes an hourglass configuration around the introital and perianal areas (keyhole distribution; Fig. 226–6).

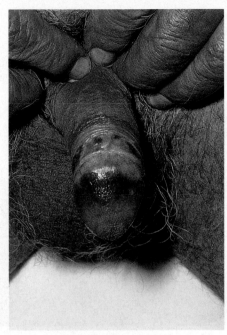

Fig 226–5
Erosive lichen planus. There is extensive erosion of the glans penis. (Courtesy of the Institute of Dermatology, London.)

Inflammation, urethral stricture (Fig. 226–7), subepithelial hemorrhages, and chronic ulceration may develop.

- Dyspareunia, genital bleeding, and anal bleeding are common.

CAUSE

- Unknown. There may be an autoimmune association and a genetic familial component.

DIFFERENTIAL DIAGNOSIS

- Localized scleroderma (morphea)
- Cutaneous discoid lupus erythematosus
- Atrophic lichen planus
- Psoriasis

WORKUP

- Diagnosis is based on close examination of the lesions for the presence of ivory white atrophic lesions and typical location.

LABORATORY TESTS

- Punch or deep shave biopsy can be used to confirm the diagnosis when in doubt.

TREATMENT

- Application of clobetasol propionate, 0.05% topically, twice daily for up to 4 weeks is usually effective.
- Lubricants (e.g., urea [Nutraplus] cream) are useful to soothe dry tissues.
- Hydroxyzine, 25 mg, at bedtime is effective in decreasing nocturnal itching.
- Intralesional steroids, etretinate, and surgical management are usually reserved for refractory cases.

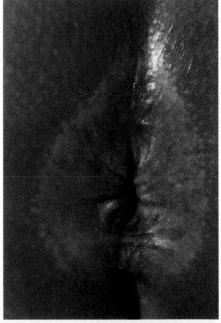

Fig 226–6
Lichen sclerosus. Perianal disease is often present in addition to vulval involvement, giving rise to the so-called hourglass distribution. (Courtesy of the Institute of Dermatology, London.)

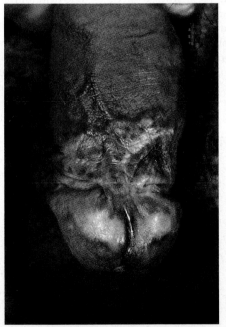

Fig 226–7
Lichen sclerosus. In males, lesions of the foreskin and glans may be complicated by urethral stricture (so-called balanitis xerotica obliterans). (Courtesy of the Institute of Dermatology, London.)

B. INFECTIOUS DISEASES

(1) ERYTHRASMA

This is a superficial infection of the skin at the flexural sites and is common in the inguinal and genitocrural folds (Fig. 226–8). The organism involved is an aerobic, Gram-positive organism, *Corynebacterium minutissimum*. The organism normally lives in the skin but causes disease as a result of a warm and humid environment. Obesity, heat, friction, diabetes mellitus, and immunosuppression are all contributory factors. The affected areas are covered with red-brown scaly plaques with well-demarcated edges. The rash is usually asymptomatic or mildly itchy.

DIAGNOSIS

The affected areas fluoresce coral pink under Wood's light.

(2) CONDYLOMA ACUMINATUM

Anogenital warts are most common in young, sexually active patients. Genital warts are the most common viral sexually transmitted disease (STD) in the United States, with up to 24 million Americans carrying the viruses that cause them.

- Genital warts
  - Generally pale pink with several projections and a broad base. They may coalesce in the perineal area to form masses with a cauliflower-like appearance (Fig. 226–9).
  - On cervical epithelium can produce subclinical changes that may be noted on PAP smear or colposcopy (Fig. 226–10).
  - Usually caused by HPV type 6 or 11

TREATMENT

- Can be effectively treated with 20% podophyllin resin in compound tincture of benzoin applied with a cotton tip applicator by the treating physician and allowed to air-dry. The treatment can be repeated weekly if necessary.
- Podofilox (0.5% gel) is now available for application by the patient. Local adverse effects include pain, burning, and inflammation at the site.
- Cryosurgery with liquid nitrogen delivered with a probe or as a spray is effective for treating smaller genital warts.
- Carbon dioxide laser can also be used for treating primary or recurrent genital warts (cure rate more than 90%).
- Imiquimod cream 5% is a patient-applied immune response modifier effective in the treatment of external genital and perianal warts (complete clearing of genital warts in more than 70% of women and more than 30% of men in 4 to 16 weeks). Sexual contact should be avoided while the cream is on the skin. It is applied three times/wk before normal sleeping hours and is left on the skin for 6 to 10 hours.

(3) SYPHILIS

DEFINITION

Syphilis is a sexually transmitted treponemal disease, acute and chronic, characterized by primary skin lesions, secondary eruption involving skin and mucous membranes, long periods of

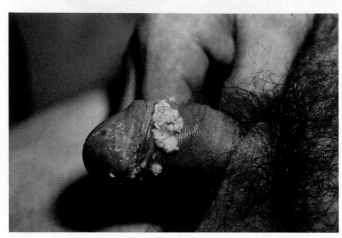

Fig 226–9
Condyloma acuminatum. In this patient, the lesions have a typical filiform appearance.
(Courtesy of the Department of Genitourinary Medicine, St. Thomas Hospital, London.)

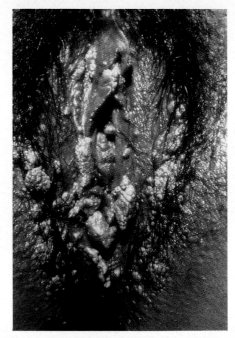

Fig 226–10
Condyloma acuminatum. There is very extensive disease. The patient is at considerable risk of developing cervical disease.
(Courtesy of Dr. R. A. Marsden, St George's Hospital, London.)

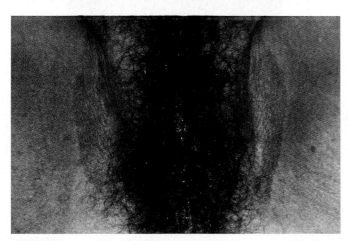

Fig 226–8
Erythrasma. The flexural distribution and sharply demarcated border are characteristic features.
(Courtesy of the Institute of Dermatology, London.)

latency, and late lesions of skin, bone, viscera, central nervous system (CNS), and cardiovascular system.

PHYSICAL FINDINGS AND CLINICAL PRESENTATION

Primary syphilis

- Characteristic lesion is a painless chancre on the genitalia, mouth, or anus; atypical primary lesions may occur. It usually appears 3 weeks after exposure and may spontaneously involute.
- The typical initial lesion (or chancre) is seen more often on the glans penis (especially the coronal sulcus), the shaft or prepuce, or on the labia, and usually develops 20 to 30 days after exposure to an infectious lesion (Fig. 226–11).
- The chancre appears as an indurated, punched-out, painless ulcer (Fig. 226–12). It is usually accompanied by painless lymphadenopathy. This resolves without scarring after 1 to 5 weeks.

Secondary syphilis

- The secondary cutaneous lesions (syphilids), which are highly infectious, may mimic almost any skin disorder and present 6 to 8 weeks after the appearance of the chancre. They develop insidiously (in up to 80% of patients) with a papular (Fig. 226–13), roseolar, or macular erythematous rash on the head, face, and neck followed by a polymorphic papular eruption (Fig. 226–14). The macules measure 5 to 10 mm in diameter, are not pruritic and occur especially on the trunk, abdomen, and limbs, especially the palms and soles. 60% to 80% of patients have maculopapular lesions on their palms and soles. It is common to

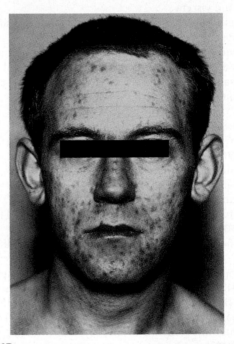

Fig 226–13
Secondary syphilis. The face is commonly affected. Note the numerous papules.
(Courtesy of Dr. R. N. Thin, St. Thomas Hospital, London.)

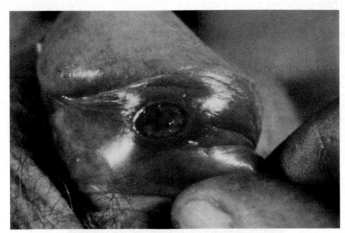

Fig 226–11
Primary chancre. The chancre is a painless ulcer with an indurated edge. The base is yellow and harbors large numbers of spirochetes.
(Courtesy of Dr. F. Lim, MD, King's College Hospital, London.)

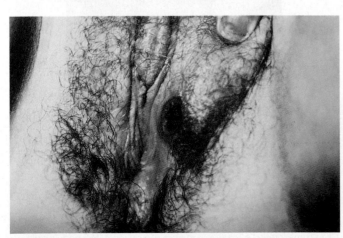

Fig 226–12
Primary syphilis. A typical chancre is present on the left labium majus.
(Courtesy of Dr. R. N. Thin, St. Thomas Hospital, London.)

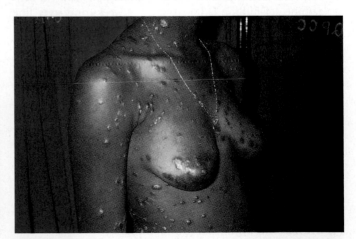

Fig 226–14
Secondary syphilis. Note the widespread papules and nodules, many of which have a hypertrophic appearance.
(Courtesy of Dr. C. Furlonge, Port of Spain, Trinidad.)

have constitutional symptoms, flulike symptoms; may begin about 4 to 6 weeks after appearance of primary lesion. Manifestations may resolve in 1 week to 12 months.
- Condylomata lata intertriginous papules form at areas of friction and moisture, such as the vulva.
- 21% to 58% have mucocutaneous or mucosal lesions (pharyngitis, tonsillitis, mucous patch lesion on oral and genital mucosa).

Early latent (less than 1 year)
- Generally asymptomatic

Late latent (more than 1 year)
- Characterized by gummas (nodular, ulcerative lesions) that can involve the skin, mucous membranes, skeletal system, and viscera
- Manifestations of cardiovascular syphilis include aortitis, aneurysm, or aortic regurgitation.
- Neurosyphilis may be asymptomatic or symptomatic. Tabes dorsalis, meningovascular syphilis, general paralysis, or insanity may occur. Iritis, choroidoretinitis, and leukoplakia may also occur.

CAUSE
- *Treponema pallidum*, a spirochete
- Spread by sexual intercourse or intrauterine transfer

DIFFERENTIAL DIAGNOSIS
- Genital herpes (see Fig. 226–27)
- Chancroid (see Fig. 226–18)
- Granuloma inguinale (see Fig. 226–15)
- Lymphogranuloma venereum (see Fig. 226–21)

LABORATORY TESTS
- Dark-field microscopy of fluid from lesion to look for treponema
- Serologic testing, nontreponemal (VDRL, rapid plasma reagin [RPR]) and treponemal (fluorescent treponemal antibody [FTA], major histocompatibility antigen [MHA])
- Lumbar puncture for cerebrospinal fluid (CSF) VDRL in patients with evidence of latent syphilis

TREATMENT
- Early (primary, secondary, early latent): penicillin G benzathine 2.4 million U IM × 1 or doxycycline 100 mg PO twice daily × 14 days
- Late (late latent, cardiovascular, gumma): penicillin G benzathine 2.4 million U IM weekly × 3 weeks or doxycycline 100 mg PO twice daily × 4 weeks
- Neurosyphilis: aqueous crystalline penicillin G 18 to 24 million U/day, administered as 3 to 4 million U IV every 4 hours × 10 to 14 days or procaine penicillin 2.4 million U IM/day plus probenecid 500 mg PO four times daily, both for 10 to 14 days
- Congenital syphilis: aqueous crystalline penicillin G 50,000 U/kg/dose IV every 12 hours × first 7 days of life and every 8 hours after that for total of 10 days, or procaine penicillin G 50,000 U/kg/dose IM/day × 10 days
- Latent syphilis in penicillin-allergic patient: doxycycline 100 mg PO twice daily or tetracycline 500 mg four times daily for 28 days

(4) Granuloma inguinale (donovanosis)

DEFINITION

Granuloma inguinale is caused by a gram-negative bacterium, *Calymmatobacterium granulomatis*, that may be sexually transmit-

ted, possibly by anal intercourse. It can also be spread through close, chronic nonsexual contact.

PHYSICAL FINDINGS AND CLINICAL PRESENTATION
- The initial presentation in females is usually of one or more indurated papules or nodules on the inner aspect of the labia, the fourchette, or around the clitoris (Fig. 226–15). The indurated nodule is usually painless. In males, the glans, prepuce, coronal sulcus, or shaft is affected. The papules ulcerate irregularly and extend widely if untreated. The base of the ulcer is beefy and the margins are undermined and indurated (Fig. 226–16). Spread by contiguous kissing areas may sometimes occur.
- Pathogenic features are as follows:
  1. Large infected mononuclear cell containing many Donovan bodies (Fig. 226–17)
  2. Intracytoplasmic location

CAUSE
- *C. granulomatis* is a gram-negative bacillus that reproduces in polymorphonuclear neutrophils (PMNs), plasma cells, and histiocytes, causing the infected cells to rupture.

DIFFERENTIAL DIAGNOSIS
- Carcinoma (see Fig. 226–30)
- Syphilis (see Fig. 226–11)
- Condylomata lata (see Fig. 226–9)
- Amebiasis: necrotic ulceration
- Lymphogranuloma venereum (see Fig. 226–21)
- Chancroid (see Fig. 226–18)
- Genital herpes (see Fig. 226–27)

WORKUP
- Check for clinical manifestations.
  1. Lesions bleed easily.

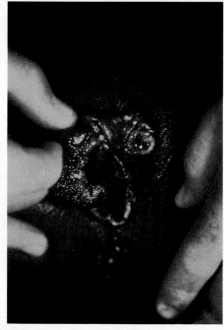

Fig 226–15
Granuloma inguinale, early lesion showing an ulcerated papule adjacent to the clitoris.
(Courtesy of Dr. J. Lawson, University of Newcastle-upon-Tyne, Newcastle-upon-Tyne, England.)

2. Lesions are sharply defined and painless.

3. Secondary infection may ensue.

4. Inguinal involvement may cause pseudobuboes.

5. Elephantiasis can result from obstruction of lymphatics.

6. Suppuration and sinus formation are rare in female patients.

- Screen for other sexually transmitted diseases.
- Exclude other causes of lesions.
- Obtain stained preparation from lesion.

LABORATORY TESTS

- Wright stain: observation of Donovan bodies (intracellular bacteria); organisms in vacuoles within macrophages

TREATMENT

- Recommended regimens
  - Doxycycline
  - Trimethoprim-sulfamethoxazole

- Alternative regimens
  - Ciprofloxacin
  - Erythromycin base
  - Azithromycin

(5) Chancroid

DEFINITION

Chancroid is a sexually transmitted disease characterized by painful genital ulcerations and inflammatory inguinal adenopathy.

PHYSICAL FINDINGS AND CLINICAL PRESENTATION

- The initial lesion is usually a transient vesicular tender papule, which rapidly ulcerates with copious suppuration. The ulcer is sharply circumscribed, with an undetermined edge, and is typically not indurated. These lesions appear much more commonly in the male, usually on the penis (Fig. 226–18). The prepuce, coronal sulcus, frenulum, and glans are the most favored sites. Lesions in the female are seen on the fourchette, labia, or around the clitoris. The ulcers are tender and especially painful when in contact with urine.
- Lymphadenitis occurs in about 50% of cases approximately 1 week after the genital lesion and usually, in 50% of these, suppuration (bubo formation) follows.
- Unilateral lymphadenopathy develops 1 week later in 50% of patients.

CAUSE

- *Haemophilus ducreyi,* a bacillus (Fig. 226–19)

DIFFERENTIAL DIAGNOSIS

- Genital herpes (see Fig. 226–27)
- Granuloma inguinale (see Fig. 226–15)
- Lymphogranuloma venereum (see Fig. 226–21)
- Syphilis (see Fig. 226–11)

WORKUP

- Diagnosis based on history and physical examination is often inadequate. Syphilis must be ruled out in women because of the consequences of inappropriate therapy in pregnant women. Base initial diagnosis and treatment recommendations on clinical impression of appearance of ulcer and most likely diagnosis for population. Definitive

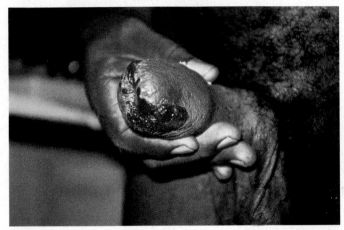

Fig 226–16
Granuloma inguinale. In this patient, there is extensive ulceration of the glans penis. Note the typical beefy appearance.
(Courtesy of Dr. C. Furlonge, Port of Spain, Trinidad.)

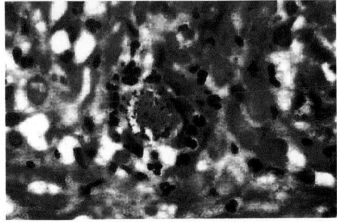

Fig 226–17
Granuloma inguinale. The histiocytes contain characteristic Donovan bodies (Warthin-Starry stain).
(Courtesy of Dr. W. Grayson, University of Witwatersrand, Johannesburg, South Africa.)

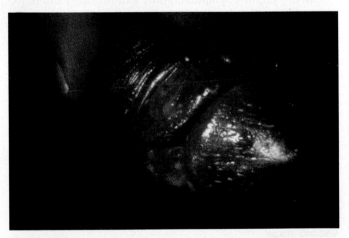

Fig 226–18
Chancroid, irregular ulcer extending along the coronal sulcus of the penis.
(Courtesy of Dr. R. A. Marsden, St. George's Hospital, London.)

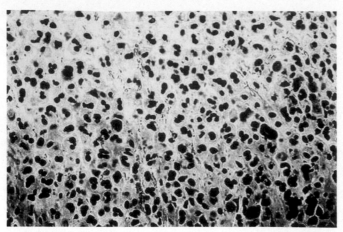

Fig 226–19
Chancroid. Note the coccobacilli growing in chains.
(From McKee PH, Calonje E, Granter SR [eds]: Pathology of the Skin With Clinical Correlations, 3rd ed. St. Louis, Mosby, 2005.)

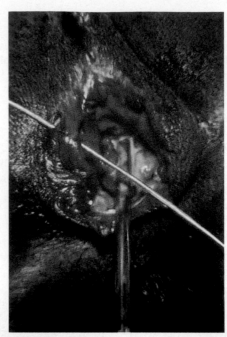

Fig 226–20
Lymphogranuloma venereum. Note the ulcer on the right labium majus.
(Courtesy of Dr. S. Lucas, St. Thomas Hospital, London.)

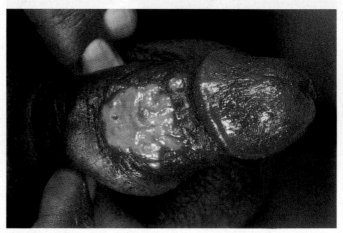

Fig 226–21
Lymphogranuloma venereum. There is an ulcer on the penile shaft covered with necrotic debris.
(Courtesy of the Institute of Dermatology, London.)

diagnosis is made by isolation of organism from ulcers by culture or Gram stain.

LABORATORY TESTS
- Dark-field microscopy, RPR, herpes simplex virus (HSV) serology or cultures, *H. ducreyi* culture, HIV testing recommended

TREATMENT

Acute general treatment
- Azithromycin , ceftriaxone , ciprofloxacin, or erythromycin
- Fluctuant nodes should be aspirated through healthy adjacent skin to prevent formation of draining sinus. Incision and drainage (I&D) not recommended, delays healing; use warm compresses to remove necrotic material.
- All sexual partners should be treated with a 10-day course of one of the previous regimens. Patients should be re-examined 3 to 7 days after initiation of therapy. Ulcers should improve symptomatically within 3 days and objectively within 7 days after initiation of successful therapy.

(6) Lymphogranuloma venereum

DEFINITION
Lymphogranuloma venereum (LGV) is a sexually transmitted, systemic disease caused by *Chlamydia trachomatis*.

PHYSICAL FINDINGS AND CLINICAL PRESENTATION

Primary stage
- Primary lesion caused by multiplication of organism at site of infection
- The initial lesion develops 3 to 30 days after contact as a small, transient, frequently asymptomatic papulovesicle or shallow ulcer on the penis, scrotum, rectum, vulva, vagina, and/or cervix (Figs. 226–20 and 226–21). The most commonly affected site on the vulva is the fourchette.

Second stage
- Inguinal syndrome: characteristic inguinal adenopathy
- Begins 1 to 4 weeks after primary lesion
- Syndrome is the most frequent clinical sign of the disease

- Unilateral inguinal adenopathy in 70% of cases
- Symptoms: painful, extensive adenitis (bubo) (Fig. 226–22) and suppuration may occur, with numerous sinus tracts.
- Groove sign signaling femoral and inguinal node involvement (20%); most often seen in men
- Involvement of deep iliac and retroperitoneal lymph nodes in women may present as a pelvic mass.

Third stage (anogenital syndrome)
- Subacute: proctocolitis
- Late: tissue destruction or scarring, sinuses, abscesses, fistulas, strictures of perineum, elephantiasis

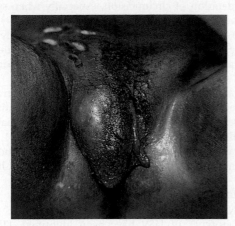

Fig 226–22
Lymphogranuloma venereum causing unilateral vulvar lymphedema and inguinal buboes.
(From Cohen J, Powderly WG: Infectious Diseases, 2nd ed. St. Louis, Mosby, 2004.)

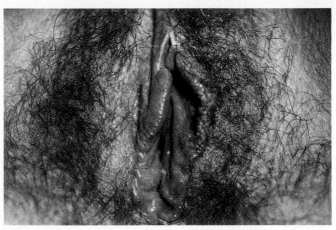

Fig 226–23
Typical *Candida* vulvovaginitis with bilateral symmetrical erythema and edema of vestibule and labia.
(From Cohen J, Powderly WG: Infectious Diseases, 2nd ed. St. Louis, Mosby, 2004.)

CAUSE
- *Chlamydia trachomatis* is the causative agent. There are three serotypes—L1, L2, and L3.

DIFFERENTIAL DIAGNOSIS
  - Inguinal adenitis, suppurative adenitis, retroperitoneal adenitis, proctitis, schistosomiasis
    - Granuloma inguinale(see Fig. 226–15)
    - Syphilis (see Fig. 226–11).

LABORATORY TESTS
- Positive Frei test
  1. Intradermal chlamydial antigen
  2. Nonspecific for all *Chlamydia*
  3. No longer available (historical significance only)
- Complement fixation test:
  1. Titer >1:64 in active infection
  2. Convalescent titers no difference
- Cell culture of *Chlamydia*: aspiration of fluctuant node yields highest rates of recovery
- CBC: mild leukocytosis with lymphocytosis or monocytosis
- Elevated sedimentation rate
- VDRL and HIV screening to rule out other STDs

IMAGING STUDIES
- CT scan for retroperitoneal adenitis

TREATMENT
- Doxycycline
- Erythromycin
- Sulfisoxazole
- Surgical: aspirate fluctuant nodes, incise and drain abscesses

(7) Candidal infections
VULVOVAGINAL CANDIDIASIS (MONILIASIS)
DEFINITION
Vulvovaginal candidiasis is an inflammatory process involving the vulva or the vagina and is caused by superficial invasion of epithelial cells by *Candida* species.

PHYSICAL FINDINGS AND CLINICAL PRESENTATION
- Vulvar pruritus with vaginal discharge that typically resembles cottage cheese.

- Erythema and edema of labia and vulvar skin (Fig 226–23); possible discrete pustulopapular peripheral lesions (satellite lesions).
- Vagina may be erythematous with an adherent, whitish discharge.
- Cervix may appear normal.
- Symptoms characteristically exacerbated in the week preceding menses with some relief after onset of menstrual flow.

CAUSE
- *Candida* are dimorphic fungi (spores and mycelial forms).
- *C. albicans* is responsible for 85% to 90% of vaginal yeast infections.
- *C. glabrata* and *C. tropicalis* (non-*albicans* species) also cause vaginitis and may be more resistant to conventional therapy.

DIFFERENTIAL DIAGNOSIS
- Bacterial vaginosis
- Trichomoniasis

WORKUP
- Usually normal vaginal pH (<4.5).
- Budding yeast forms or mycelia will appear in as many as 80% of cases. Saline wet preparation of vaginal secretions usually is normal; may be increased in inflammatory cells in severe cases.
- Whiff test negative (KOH).
- 10% KCl useful and more sensitive than wet mount for microscopic identification
- Can make a presumptive diagnosis based on symptomatology in the absence of microscopy-proven fungal elements if the pH and wet preparation are normal. Fungal culture is recommended to confirm diagnosis.
- In chronic or recurrent cases, burning replaces itching as prominent symptom. Confirm diagnosis with direct microscopy and culture. Many may actually have chronic or atrophic dermatitis. Test for HIV.

LABORATORY TESTS
- If sending cultures, send on Nickerson's media or semi-quantitative slide-stix cultures. There is no reliable serologic technique for diagnosis.

TREATMENT
- Topical buconazole, miconazole, tioconazole, terconazole, or clotrimazole vaginal cream
- Oral fluconazole, 150 mg PO, single dose

BALANITIS

DEFINITION
- Balanitis is an inflammation of the superficial tissues of the penile head (Fig. 226–24).

PHYSICAL FINDINGS AND CLINICAL PRESENTATION
- Itching and tenderness
- Pain, dysuria, and local edema
- Rarely, ulceration and lymph node enlargement
- Severe ulcerations leading to superimposed bacterial infections
- Inability to void: unusual, but a more distressing and serious complication

CAUSE
- Poor hygiene, causing erosion of tissue with erythema and promoting growth of *C. albicans*
- Sexual contact, urinary catheters, and trauma
- Allergic reactions to condoms or medications

DIFFERENTIAL DIAGNOSIS
- Leukoplakia
- Reiter's syndrome (see Fig. 226–3)
- Lichen planus (see Fig. 226–5)
- Psoriasis
- Carcinoma of the penis (see Fig. 226–28)
- Nodular scabies

LABORATORY TESTS
- VDRL
- Serum glucose
- Wet mount
- KOH prepration
- Microbial culture

TREATMENT
- Maintenance of meticulous hygiene
- Retraction and bathing of prepuce several times a day
- Warm sitz baths to ease edema and erythema

- Consideration of circumcision, especially when symptoms are severe or recurrent
- With Foley catheters, strict catheter care is strongly advised.
- Analgesics, such as acetaminophen and/or codeine
- Clotrimazole, 1% cream, applied topically twice daily to affected areas
- Referral for surgical evaluation for circumcision if symptoms are recurrent, especially if phimosis or meatitis occurs

Note: Severe phimosis with an inability to void may require prompt slit drainage.
- Referral for biopsy to rule out other diagnosis such as premalignant or malignant lesions if lesions are not healing

(8) Genital herpes

CAUSE AND CLINICAL PRESENTATION
- Two serotypes of HSV have been identified, HSV-1 and HSV-2; most cases of genital herpes are caused by HSV-2 (Fig. 226–25).
- Approximately 30 million people in the United States may have genital HSV infection. Most infected people never recognize signs suggestive of genital herpes; some have symptoms shortly after infection and never again.
- The first episode may result in severe local symptoms such as painful bilateral genital ulcers (Fig. 226–26) or vesicles (Fig. 226–27), inguinal adenopathy, along with fever, malaise, and myalgia.
- The classic appearance is that of vesicles or ulcers in various stages of development.
- A prodrome of itching or burning is common for recurrent herpes.

TREATMENT
- First clinical episode of genital herpes:
  - Acyclovir 400 mg PO three times daily for 7 to 10 days, *or*
  - Famciclovir 250 mg PO three times daily for 7 to 10 days, *or*
  - Valacyclovir 1 g PO twice daily for 7 to 10 days

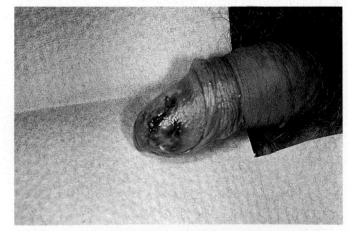

Fig 226–24
Candidal balanitis. Note the erythema with erosion and the small white pustule at the margin of the lesion.
(Courtesy of Dr. C. Furlonge, Port of Spain, Trinidad.)

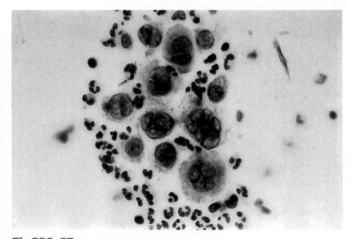

Fig 226–25
Herpes virus in cervical vaginal smear. Multinucleated giant cells with ground glass nuclear inclusions (Papanicolaou, ×600).
(From Silverberg SG, Frable WJ, Wick MR, et al [eds]: Principles and Practice of Surgical Pathology and Cytopathology, 4th ed. Philadelphia, Elsevier, 2006.)

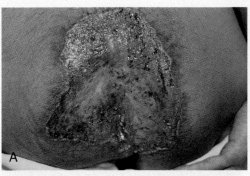
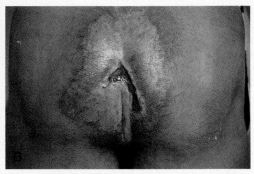

Fig 226–26
Severe perianal acyclovir-resistant herpes simplex virus 2 infection. **A,** Untreated appearance. **B,** Healing and re-epithelialization after treatment with foscarnet and institution of highly active antiretroviral therapy (HAART).
(From Cohen J, Powderly WG: Infectious Diseases, 2nd ed. St. Louis, Mosby, 2004.)

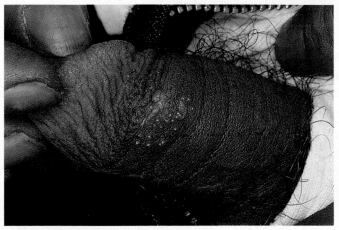

Fig 226–27
Herpes simplex virus type 2 infection.
(From Swartz MH: Textbook of Physical Diagnosis, 5th ed. Philadelphia, 2006, WB Saunders, 2006.)

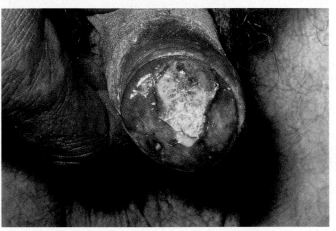

Fig 226–28
Intraepithelial neoplasia. This patient presented with multiple ulcerated lesions and a thick scaly plaque.
(Courtesy of the Institute of Dermatology, London.)

C. EPITHELIAL LESIONS

(1) Intraepithelial neoplasia

In this text, the term *intraepithelial neoplasia* is restricted to squamous intraepithelial neoplasia and does not exclude extramammary Paget's disease or melanoma in situ. Older terms such as Bowen's disease, erythroplasia of Queyrat, bowenoid papulosis, and severe dysplasia were replaced with newer terminology in 1986. Vulvar intraepithelial neoplasia (VIN) can be classified as VIN-1, mild dysplasia, VIN-2, moderate dysplasia, and VIN-3, severe dysplasia or carcinoma in situ. The morphology of the lesions ranges from papules to plaques, which may be skin-colored, white, erythematous, or pigmented (Figs. 226–28 and 226–29). The main presenting symptom is pruritus. In male patients, lesions often mimic the appearance of lichen planus, appearing as violaceous papules or as erythematous velvety plaques. Multifocal disease is strongly associated with the oncogenic papilloma viruses, particularly HPV-16 and HPV-18, and almost exclusively occurs in smokers.

(2) Vulva squamous cell carcinoma

The great majority of vulval squamous cell carcinomas (SCCs) develop on the labia, with a particular predilection for the labia majora. The second most common site is the clitoris. Patients

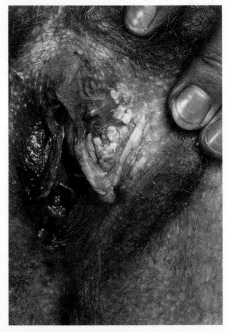

Fig 226–29
Intraepithelial neoplasia. There is an erythematous plaque with focal scaling.
(Courtesy of the Institute of Dermatology, London.)

present with a mass that is sometimes associated with pruritus, ulceration, bleeding, discharge. or pain (Fig. 226–30). Vulvar SCC usually spreads via lymphatics to inguinal, femoral and pelvic lymph nodes. Up to 30% of patients have inguinal node spread at the time of presentation. For additional information on squamous cell carcinoma, see Section 1, Chapter 22.

(3) Verrucous carcinoma

This is a low-grade, slow growing SCC. The tumor presents as a warty exophytic plaque (Fig. 226–31). Verrucous carcinoma of the penis and vulva may arise on the background of lichen sclerosus or lichen planus.

DIAGNOSIS

● Biopsy

TREATMENT

● Surgical excision

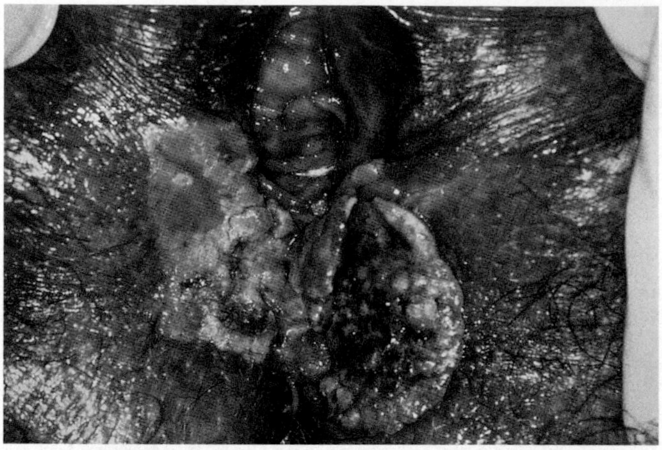

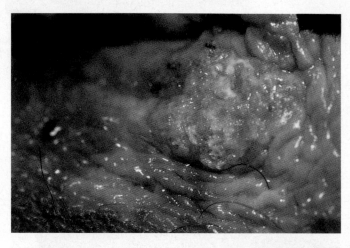

Fig 226–30
Vulval squamous cell carcinoma. This tumor arose against a background of long-standing carcinoma in situ (Bowen's disease). (Courtesy of the Institute of Dermatology, London.)

Fig 226–31
Verrucous carcinoma. Note the keratotic warty tumor mass. (Courtesy of the Institute of Dermatology, London.)

Chapter 227 **Urethritis, gonococcal**

DEFINITION

Gonococcal urethritis (GCU) is a well-defined clinical syndrome manifested by dysuria, a urethral discharge, or both.

PHYSICAL FINDINGS AND CLINICAL PRESENTATION

Symptoms

- Urethral discharge and dysuria are the most common symptoms.
- There is complaint of urethral itching.
- Prostatic involvement can cause frequency, urgency, and nocturia. It can involve the epididymis through spreading down the vas deferens, causing acute epididymitis.

Incubation period and duration

- 3 to 10 days
- Without treatment, urethritis persists for 3 to 7 weeks, with 95% of men becoming asymptomatic after 3 months. GCU is asymptomatic in up to 60% of contacts.

Signs

- Yellow-brown discharge (Fig. 227–1)
- Meatal edema
- Urethral tenderness to palpation
- Rectal bleeding with pus seen with gonococcal proctitis
- Periurethritis leading to urethral stenosis can occur.
- Disseminated infection can occur. Pustules may be noted on feet and hands (Fig. 227–2).
- Tenosynovitis and arthritis can occur.
- Rarely, hepatitis, myocarditis, endocarditis, and meningitis can occur.

DIFFERENTIAL DIAGNOSIS

- Nongonococcal urethritis (NGU)
- Herpes simplex virus (see Fig. 226–27)

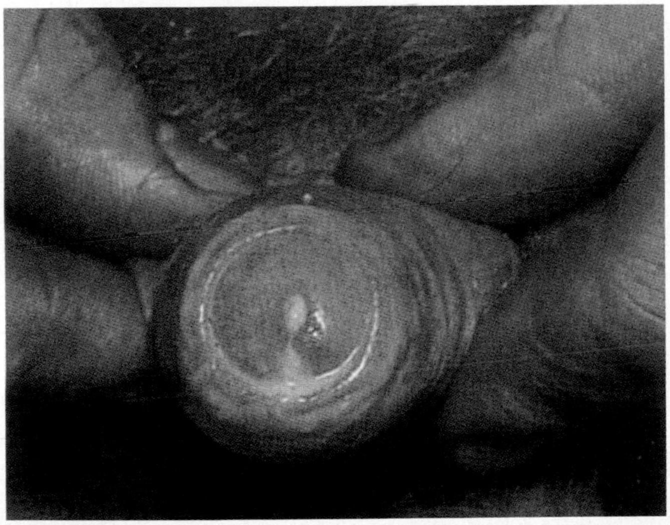

LABORATORY TESTS

- Calcium alginate or rayon swab on a metal shaft (*not* cotton-tipped swabs, which are bactericidal) of the urethra should be done from 2 to 4 hours after voiding to prevent bacterial washout with voiding.
- Cultures of the pharynx and rectum when indicated
- Gram staining should be done (Fig. 227–3) using modified Thayer-Martin medium.
- On examination of the urethral smear, the presence of small numbers of PMNs provides objective evidence of urethritis. The complete absence of PMNs on a urethral smear argues

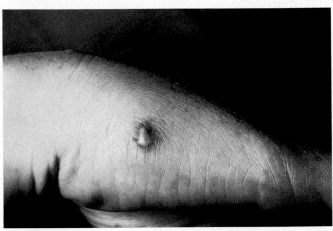

Fig 227–2
Gonococcemia. Pustules are commonly found on the hands and feet. (Courtesy of Dr. R. N. Thin, St. Thomas Hospital, London.)

Fig 227–1
Purulent penile discharge of gonorrhea.
(From Swartz MH: Textbook of Physical Diagnosis, 5th ed. Philadelphia, 2006, WB Saunders, 2006.)

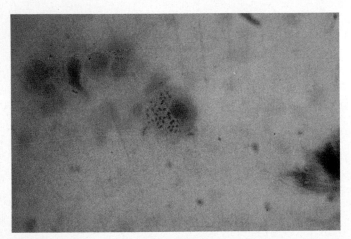

Fig 227–3
Gram stain of urethral discharge from a male who has gonorrhea. Note the intracellular gram-negative diplococci with neutrophils.
(From Cohen J, Powderly WG: Infectious Diseases, 2nd ed. St. Louis, Mosby, 2004.)

against urethritis. If in addition to the PMNs there are gram-negative intracellular diplococci, the diagnosis of gonorrhea is established.

- Table 227–1 compares various diagnostic tests for gonococcal urethritis.

TREATMENT

- Ceftriaxone IM plus doxycycline
- Alternative therapy: ciprofloxacin or ofloxacin followed by doxycycline

TABLE 227–1 Diagnostic tests for *Neisseria gonorrhoeae*

Test	Sensitivity (%)	Specificity (%)	Comment
Gram stain*	95 (symptomatic) 60 (asymptomatic)	98	Results available immediately
Culture†	90-97	98-99	Requires careful handling and proper j Facilities
DNA probe†	85	98-99	Can test for *Chlamydia trachomatis* with same swab
DNA amplification†	95	98-99	Can use first-voided portion of urine or urethral swab with equal performance, and test for *C. trachomatis* with same specimen

Sensitivity and specificity are given for the diagnosis of urethritis in men, using urethral specimens unless otherwise stated.
*Compared with culture.
†Compared with enhanced reference standard comprising culture and DNA amplification or probe competition assay.
From Cohen J, Powderly WG: Infectious Diseases, 2nd ed. St. Louis, Mosby, 2004.

Chapter 228 Urethritis, nongonococcal

DEFINITION

Nongonococcal urethritis is urethral inflammation caused by several organisms.

PHYSICAL FINDINGS AND CLINICAL PRESENTATION

Incubation period
- 2 to 35 days

Symptoms
- Dysuria, whitish to clear urethral discharge, and urethral itching
- The onset of symptoms in NGU is less acute than GCU.

Signs
- Whitish to clear urethral discharge, meatal edema, and erythema
- Infected women manifest pyuria, and the disease can present as acute urethral syndrome.

COMPLICATIONS

- Epididymitis in heterosexual men may be linked to nonbacterial prostatitis, proctitis in homosexual men, and Reiter's syndrome.

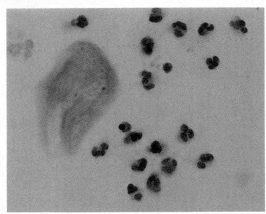

Fig 228–1
Nongonococcal urethritis—Gram-stained smear of urethral discharge containing many polymorphonuclear neutrophils but no visible bacteria. (From Cohen J, Powderly WG: Infectious Diseases, 2nd ed. St. Louis, Mosby, 2004.)

CAUSE

- Most common agent is *Chlamydia* spp., an obligate intracellular parasite possessing both DNA and RNA, replicating by binary fission. It causes 20% to 50% of NGU cases. Two species exist:
  1. *Chlamydia psittaci*
  2. *Chlamydia trachomatis* with its 15 serotypes
     a. Serotypes A to C cause hyperendemic blinding trachoma.
     b. Serotypes D to K cause genital tract infection.
     c. Serotypes L1 to L3 cause lymphogranuloma venereum.
- Other causes of NGU: *Ureaplasma urealyticum* (causes 15% to 30% of NGU cases), *Trichomonas vaginalis*, and herpes simplex virus. The cause of 20% of NGU cases has not been identified.
- Asymptomatic infection occurs in 28% of the contacts of women with chlamydial cervical infection.

DIFFERENTIAL DIAGNOSIS

- GCU (see Fig. 227–1)
- Herpes simplex virus (see Fig. 226–27)
- Trichomoniasis

LABORATORY TESTS

- Requires demonstration of urethritis and exclusion of infection with *N. gonorrhoeae*.
- The appearance of PMNs on urethral smear confirms the diagnosis of urethritis (Fig. 228–1). Because *Chlamydia* is an intracellular parasite of the columnar epithelium, the best specimen for culture is an endourethral swab taken from an area 2 to 4 cm inside the urethra. The organism can only be grown in tissue culture, which is expensive.
- New techniques have been developed and are useful in making the diagnosis: nucleic acid hybridization, enzyme-linked immunosorbent assay (ELISA), and direct immunofluorescence.
- For culture, a Dacron-tipped swab is used; avoid calcium alginate or cotton swabs.
- Table 228–1 compares diagnostic tests for *Chlamydia trachomatis*

TABLE 228–1 Diagnostic tests for *Chlamydia trachomatis*

Test	Sensitivity (%)	Specificity (%)	Comment
EIA*	70-90	95-99	Readily done in high volume
DFA*	70-95	95-99	Depends on skill of microscopist; not amenable to high volume
Culture†	65-80	>99	Requires expert laboratory
DNA probe†	85-93	98-99	Can test for Neisseria *gonorrhoeae* with same swab
DNA amplification (PCR, others)†	94-99	98-99	Can use first-voided portion of urine or urethral swab with equal effectiveness, and test for *N. gonorrhoeae* with same specimen

Sensitivity and specificity are given for the diagnosis of urethritis in men, using urethral specimens unless otherwise stated.
*Compared with culture.
†Compared with enhanced reference standard comprising DNA amplification plus culture or DFA test.
DFA, direct fluorescent antibody; EIA, enzyme immunoassay; PCR, polymerase chain reaction.
From Cohen J, Powderly WG: Infectious Diseases, 2nd ed. St. Louis, Mosby, 2004.

TREATMENT

Because it is impossible to differentiate among the common causes of NGU, the condition is treated syndromically, including in the initial treatment regimen those drugs effective against the common causative agents.

- Recommended: doxycycline
- Alternative regimens: azithromycin, erythromycin, or ofloxacin

Chapter 229 | Hypospadias

DEFINITION

Hypospadias is a developmental abnormality of the penis characterized by the following:

- Abnormal ventral opening of the urethral meatus anywhere from the ventral aspect of the glans penis to the perineum
- Ventral curvature of the penis (chordee)
- Dorsal foreskin hood

PHYSICAL FINDINGS AND CLINICAL PRESENTATION

See Figure 229–1.

- Genetics: normal karyotypes are seen with glandular hypospadias; abnormal karyotypes are noted in more severe forms of hypospadias.
- Cryptorchidism: 8% to 9% occurrence
- Inguinal hernia: 9% to 10% occurrence
- Hydrocele: 9% to 16% occurrence

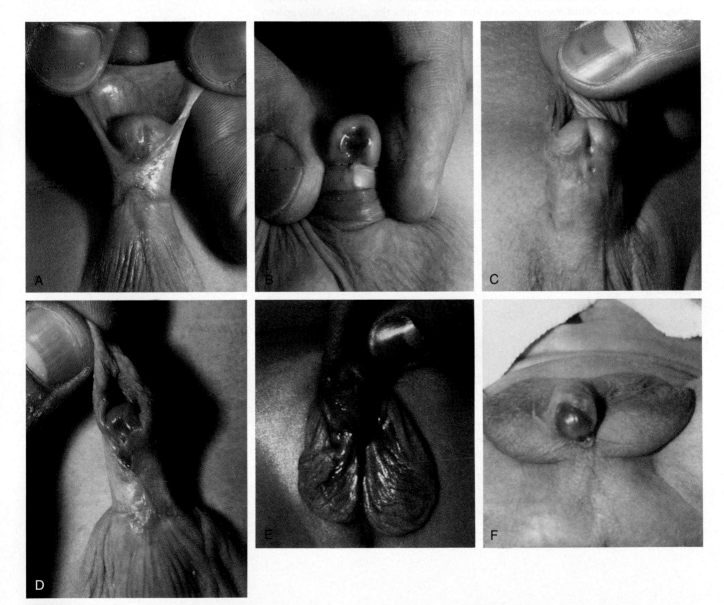

Fig 229–1

The various forms of hypospadias, revealing location of the meatus. **A,** The typical appearance of the dorsal hood prepuce seen in association with hypospadias. **B,** Glandular hypospadias. **C,** Subcoronal hypospadias. **D,** Midshaft hypospadias. **E,** Scrotal hypospadias with bifid scrotum but without chordee. **F,** Perineal hypospadias with chordee.

(From Zitelli BJ, Davis HW: Atlas of Pediatric Physical Diagnosis, 4th ed. St. Louis, Mosby, 2002.)

Penile curvature (chordee)

Three theories:

- Abnormal development of the urethral plate
- Abnormal fibrotic mesenchymal tissue at the urethral meatus
- Corporal disproportion

CAUSE

- Multifactorial
- Endocrine factors
  1. Abnormal androgen production
  2. Limited androgen sensitivity in the target tissues
  3. Premature cessation of androgenic stimulation secondary to Leydig cell dysfunction
  4. 5-Alpha-reductase deficiency: autosomal recessive disorder in 46,XY males characterized by severe perineoscrotal hypospadias, a blind vaginal pouch that opens into the urogenital sinus or the urethra, testes, epididymides, vas deferens, seminal vesicles, and ejaculatory ducts that terminate in a blind-ended vagina, a female habitus with normal axillary and pubic hair but absence of female urogenital structures, failure of female breast development at adolescence, normal male plasma testosterone, and variable masculinization during adolescence. A failure of dihydrotestosterone formation in the male embryo is responsible for the phenotype (Fig. 229–2)
- Arrested development

DIAGNOSIS

- Made by observation and examination

LABORATORY TESTS

- Intersex evaluation should be undertaken if there is associated cryptorchidism.
- The evaluation should include ultrasound, genitographic studies, chromosomal, gonadal, biochemical, and molecular studies.

TREATMENT

Designation and classification

- Anterior: 33%
- Middle: 25%
- Posterior: 41%

Special considerations

- The major reason for operating on any hypospadias patient is to correct deformities that interfere with the function of urination and procreation
- Other reasons for interventions: cosmetic concerns
- The American Academy of Pediatrics recommends that the best time for surgical intervention is at 6 to 12 months of age.

Hormonal manipulation

- Controversial
- hCG is given before the repair of proximal hypospadias.
- The effect of hCG administration is decreased hypospadias and chordee severity in all patients, and increased vascularity and thickness of the proximal corpus spongiosum.
- Application of topical testosterone increases mean penile circumference and length without any lasting side effects.
- Prepubertal exogenous testosterone does not adversely effect ultimate penile growth.

Surgical procedures

There is no single universally acceptable applicable technique for hypospadias repair.

- Orthoplasty (correcting penile curvature)
- Urethroplasty
- Meatoplasty
- Glanuloplasty
- Skin coverage

Types of repair

- Anterior hypospadias: meatal advancement and glanduloplasty (MAGPI), Thiersch-Duplay urethroplasty, glans approximation procedure (GAP), tubularized incised plate (TIP) urethroplasty, Mathieu perimeatal flap, Mustarde technique, megameatus intact prepuce (MIP), pyramid procedure
- Midlevel hypospadias: TIP, Mathieu flap, onlay island flap (OIF), King procedure
- Posterior hypospadias:
1. One-stage repair: OIF, double-onlay preputial flap, pedicled preputial flap, transverse preputial island flap (TPIF)
2. Two-stage repair: orthoplasty to correct chordee followed 6 months or more later by Thiersch-Duplay urethroplasty, bladder and/or buccal mucosal hypospadias repair

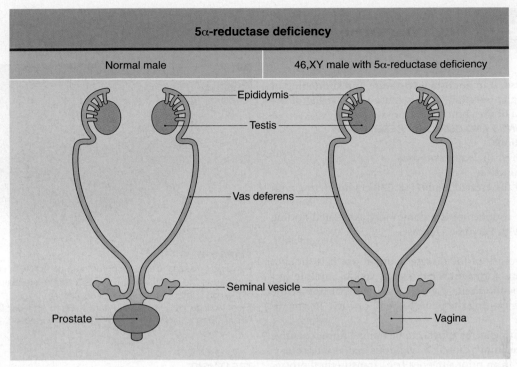

5α-reductase deficiency

Normal male	46,XY male with 5α-reductase deficiency

Epididymis

Testis

Vas deferens

Seminal vesicle

Prostate

Vagina

Fig 229–2
The urogenital tract in a normal man is compared with that in a 46,XY male with 5-alpha-reductase deficiency.
(From Besser CM, Thorner MO: Comprehensive Clinical Endocrinology, 3rd ed. St. Louis, Mosby, 2002)

Chapter 230   Peyronie's disease

DEFINITION

Peyronie's disease is an abnormal curvature and shortening of the penis during an erection. This is caused by scarring of the tunica albuginea of the corpora cavernosa.

PHYSICAL FINDINGS AND CLINICAL PRESENTATION

- Painful erections
- Tenderness over the scar tissue area
- Erectile dysfunction
- Curvature of the erected penis (Fig. 230–1) interfering with penetration
- Dupuytren's contracture is a commonly associated finding in patients with Peyronie's disease.

CAUSE

- The specific cause of the disease is unknown. It is thought that scar tissue forms on the dorsal or ventral midline surface of the penile shaft. The scar restricts expansion at the involved site, causing the penis to bend or curve in one direction.
- The precipitating factor appears to be trauma from repetitive microvascular injury caused by vigorous sexual intercourse, accidents, or from prior surgeries (e.g., transurethral prostatectomy or radical prostatectomy, cystoscopy).

DIFFERENTIAL DIAGNOSIS

- The history differentiates congenital from acquired curvature of the penis. A cavernogram (Fig. 230–2) will reveal stricture of the corpora cavernosa.
- Other causes of erectile dysfunction must be excluded, including metabolic, diabetes, thyroid, renal, hypogonadism, and hyperprolactinemia.

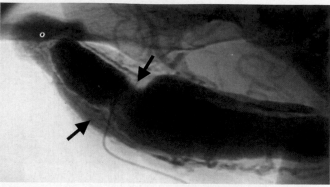

Fig 230–2

Peyronie's disease. Cavernosogram in a patient with erectile failure confined to the distal penis. There is a circumferential stricture *(arrows)* of the mid shafts of both corpora cavernosa.
(From Grainger RG, Allison DJ, Adam A, Dixon AK [eds]: Grainger & Allison's Diagnostic Radiology, 4th ed. London, Harcourt, 2001.)

TREATMENT

Nonpharmacologic therapy: A conservative approach of reassurance and observation is taken at first because the disease process may be self-limited.

Other: Although not substantiated by direct randomized, controlled clinical trials, the following treatment modalities are commonly used:

- Vitamin E, 400 mg twice daily
- Para-aminobenzoic acid, 12 g/day
- Colchicine, 0.6 mg twice daily, for 2 to 3 weeks
- Fexofenadine, 60 mg twice daily, for 3 months
- Steroid injection into the scar tissue
- Collagenase injection into the scar tissue
- Radiation to the scar tissue area

In patients who have progressed to intractable pain with erection or erectile dysfunction, surgical treatment with excision of the plaque and skin grafting may be indicated.

REFERENCES

Ferri F: Ferri's Clinical Advisor 2007. St. Louis, Mosby, 2007.

Ferri F: Practical Guide to the Care of the Medical Patient, 7th ed. St. Louis, Mosby, 2007.

Grainger RG, Allison DJ, Adam A, Dixon AK (eds): Grainger & Allison's Diagnostic Radiology, 4th ed. London, Harcourt, 2001.

Nseyo U, Weinman E, Lamm DL: Urology for Primary Care Physicians. Philadelphia, WB Saunders, 1999.

Townsend CM, Beauchamp RD, Evers BM, Mattox KL (eds): Sabiston Textbook of Surgery, 17th ed. Philadelphia, WB Saunders, 2004.

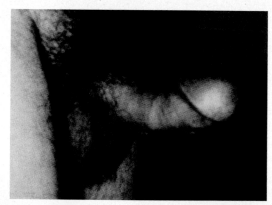

Fig 230–1

Peyronie's disease.
(From Swartz MH: Textbook of Physical Diagnosis, 5th ed. Philadelphia, 2006, WB Saunders, 2006.)

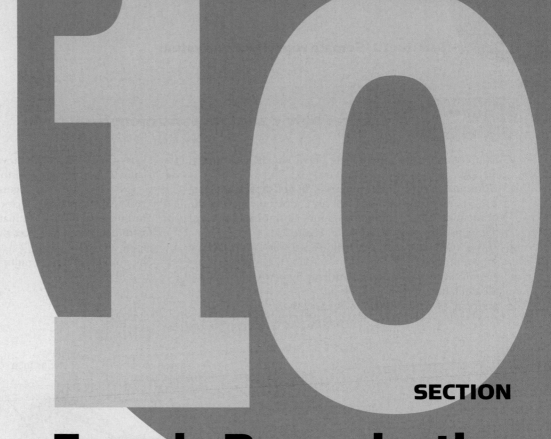

SECTION

Female Reproductive System

Chapter 231: Clinical pelvic anatomy and menstrual cycle
Chapter 232: Diagnostic tests and procedures
Chapter 233: Endometriosis
Chapter 234: Contraception

Vulva, Vagina
Chapter 235: Vaginosis, bacterial
Chapter 236: Vulvovaginitis, fungal
Chapter 237: Vulvovaginitis, trichomonas
Chapter 238: Vulvovaginitis, estrogen deficient (atrophic vaginitis)
Chapter 239: Vulvar cancer

Cervix
Chapter 240: Cervicitis
Chapter 241: Cervical dysplasia
Chapter 242: Cervical cancer

Uterus
Chapter 243: Uterine prolapse
Chapter 244: Uterine myomas
Chapter 245: Uterine polyps
Chapter 246: Endometrial cancer

Ovaries
Chapter 247: Benign ovarian lesions
Chapter 248: Polycystic ovary syndrome
Chapter 249: Ovarian cancer

Infections
Chapter 250: Pelvic inflammatory disease

Breasts
Chapter 251: Fibrocystic breast disease
Chapter 252: Breast abscess
Chapter 253: Breast cancer
Chapter 254: Paget's disease of the breast

Pregnancy
Chapter 255: Physiologic changes and prenatal monitoring
Chapter 256: Normal labor and delivery
Chapter 257: Abnormal labor
Chapter 258: Ectopic pregnancy
Chapter 259: Preeclampsia
Chapter 260: Abruptio placentae
Chapter 261: Placenta previa
Chapter 262: Hydatidiform mole

Chapter 231 Clinical pelvic anatomy and menstrual cycle

- Figure 231–1 shows the female pelvic organs in a frontal section
- Hormonal events in the ovarian cycle are shown in Figure 231–2, and Figure 231–3 shows an endoscopic view of the ovary immediately prior to ovulation. Hormonal changes of the menstrual cycle are shown in Figure 231–4.
- The normal vulva and the major anatomic landmarks are shown in Figure 231–5.
- Figure 231–6 shows an imperforate hymen with resulting accumulation of menstrual blood
- A septate hymen is shown in Figure 231–7.

- Signs of sexual abuse are shown in Figures 231–8 and 231–9.
- Figure 231–10 reveals a Bartholin's gland abscess.
- A cystocele is shown in Figure 231–11.
- Figure 231–12 shows a rectocele.
- The bimanual pelvic examination is shown in Figure 231–13. Instruments used for gynecologic examination are shown in Figure 231–14.
- The normal cervix of a nulliparous woman is shown in Figure 231–15.

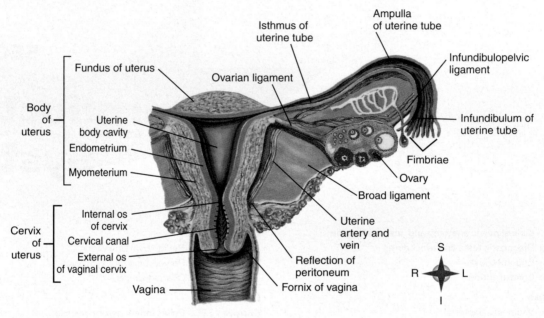

Fig 231–1
Female pelvic organs in a frontal section. The entire uterus is shown, with the upper portion of the vagina and the left uterine tube and ovary. (From Thibodeau GA, Patton KP: Anatomy and Physiology, 4th ed. St Louis, Mosby, 1999.)

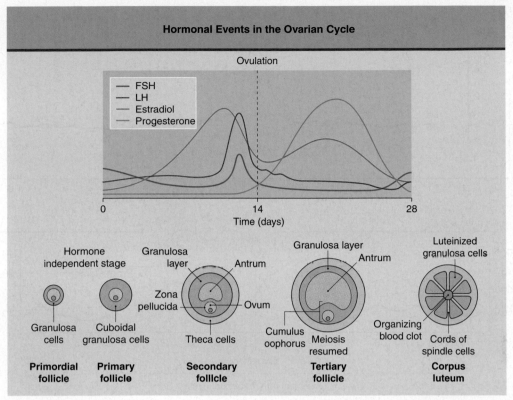

Hormonal Events in the Ovarian Cycle

Ovulation

— FSH
— LH
— Estradiol
— Progesterone

Time (days)

0   14   28

Hormone
independent stage

Granulosa
layer

Antrum

Granulosa layer

Antrum

Luteinized
granulosa cells

Zona
pellucida

Ovum

Granulosa
cells

Cuboidal
granulosa cells

Theca cells

Cumulus
oophorus

Meiosis
resumed

Organizing
blood clot

Cords of
spindle cells

**Primordial
follicle**

**Primary
follicle**

**Secondary
follicle**

**Tertiary
follicle**

**Corpus
luteum**

Fig 231-2
Hormonal events in the ovarian cycle. FSH, follicle-stimulating hormone; LH, luteinizing hormone.
(From Besser CM, Thorner MO: Comprehensive Clinical Endocrinology, 3rd ed. St Louis, Mosby, 2002.)

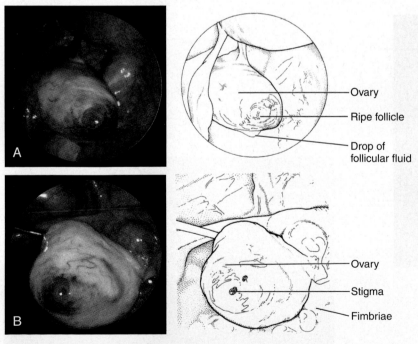

A

B

Fig 231-3
Ovulation of the cumulus–oocyte complex. Endoscopic
view of the ovary immediately prior to ovulation (**A**) and
following ovulation (**B**).
(Courtesy of Prof. H. Frangenheim and Dr. M. R. Darling.)

Ovary

Ripe follicle

Drop of
follicular fluid

Ovary

Stigma

Fimbriae

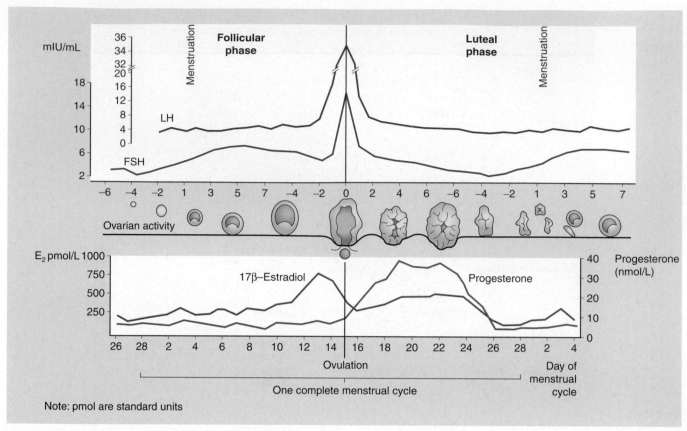

Fig 231–4
Hormonal changes of the menstrual cycle.
(From Black M, McKay M: Obstetrics and Gynaecological Dermatology, 2nd ed. St Louis, Mosby, 2002.)

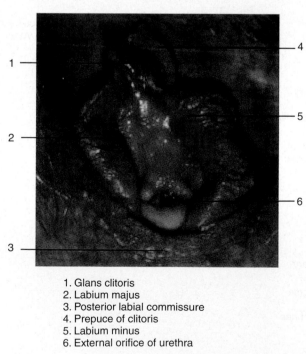

1. Glans clitoris
2. Labium majus
3. Posterior labial commissure
4. Prepuce of clitoris
5. Labium minus
6. External orifice of urethra

Fig 231–5
Normal vulva showing the major anatomic landmarks.
(From McKee PH, Calonje E, Granter SR [eds]: Pathology of the Skin With Clinical Correlations, 3rd ed. St Louis, 2005, Mosby.)

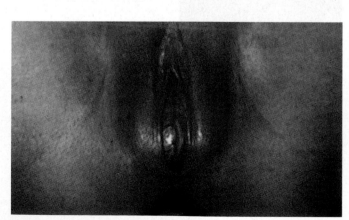

Fig 231–6
Imperforate hymen resulting in the accumulation of menstrual blood.
(From Black M, McKay M: Obstetrics and Gynaecological Dermatology, 2nd ed. St Louis, Mosby, 2002.)

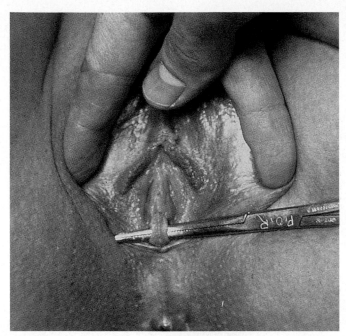

Fig 231–7
Septate hymen.
(From Black M, McKay M: Obstetrics and Gynaecological Dermatology, 2nd ed. St Louis, Mosby, 2002.)

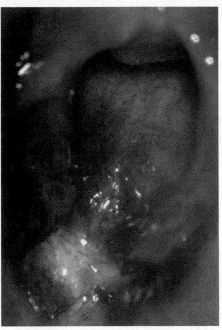

Fig 231–9
Sexual abuse. Same child as in Figure 231-8 (supine position) 2 years later with a healed scar at the 6-o'clock position.
(From Black M, McKay M: Obstetrics and Gynecological Dermatology, 2nd ed. St Louis, Mosby, 2002.)

Fig 231–8
Sexual abuse. A 5-year-old girl with a typical keyhole deformity of the hymenal ring at the 6-o'clock position resulting from penetration, laceration, and scarring.
(From Black M, McKay M: Obstetrics and Gynaecological Dermatology, 2nd ed. St Louis, Mosby, 2002.)

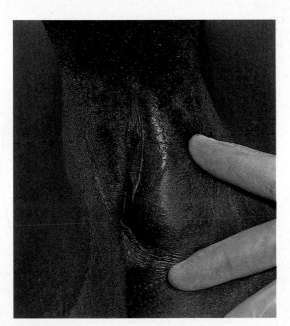

Fig 231–10
Bartholin's gland abscess.
(From Swartz MH: Textbook of Physical Diagnosis, 5th ed. Philadelphia, 2006, WB Saunders.)

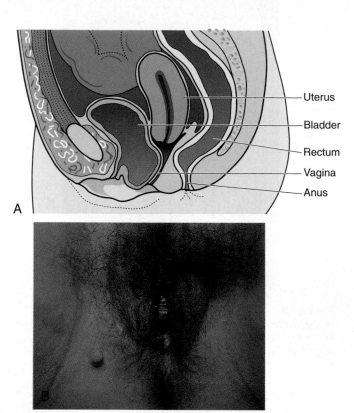

Fig 231–11
Cystocele.
(From Drife J, Magowan B: Clinical Obstetrics and Gynaecology. Edinburgh, WB Saunders, 2004.)

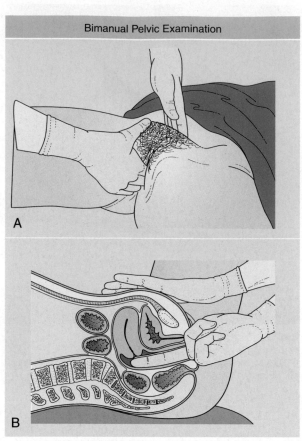

Fig 231–13
Bimanual examination in the dorsal position. The fingers in the vagina steady the pelvic organs, and the structures palpable in the midline are felt between the abdominal hand and the vaginal fingers.
(From Greer IA, Cameron IT, Kitchener HC, Prentice A: Mosby's Color Atlas and Text of Obstetrics and Gynaecology. London, Harcourt, 2001.)

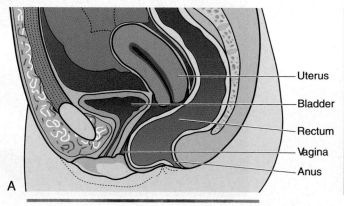
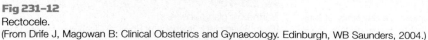

Fig 231–12
Rectocele.
(From Drife J, Magowan B: Clinical Obstetrics and Gynaecology. Edinburgh, WB Saunders, 2004.)

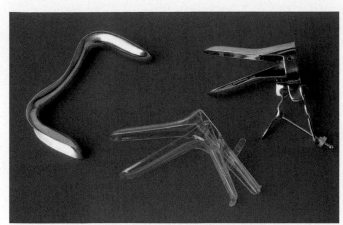

Fig 231–14
Speculae used for gynecologic examination. *Top:* Sim's speculum; *middle* and *bottom:* plastic and metal bivalve speculae.
(From Greer IA, Cameron IT, Kitchener HO, Prentice A: Mosby's Color Atlas and Text of Obstetrics and Gynaecology. London, Harcourt, 2001.)

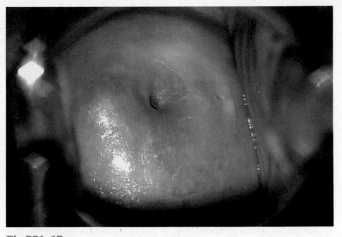

Fig 231–15
A normal cervix. Note the round external cervical os in a nulliparous woman.
(From Swartz MH: Textbook of Physical Diagnosis, 5th ed. Philadelphia, 2006, WB Saunders.)

Chapter 232 | Diagnostic tests and procedures

A. PAP SMEAR

- After the patient is positioned in the dorsal lithotomy position, choose a speculum that allows visualization of the entire cervix. Note any abnormalities of the cervix at this time.
- The choice of sampling devices depends on personal preference as well as on the ectocervix. Some physicians advocate sampling the posterior fornix to obtain desquamated cells from the cervix and endometrial cavity; however, a well-sampled endocervix and ectocervix generally provide an adequate smear.
- With an Ayres spatula (Fig. 232–1) or a similar device, the entire transition zone is sampled by rotating the spatula 360° around the cervix. The specimen can be left on the spatula until all sampling is completed or it can be smeared onto a slide that is then immediately fixed.

- The endocervix is sampled with a cotton-tipped applicator or cervical brush. The latter should generally be avoided in pregnancy. Insert the cotton-tipped applicator or cervical brush into the os and gently rotate. One half-turn is usually sufficient to sample the endocervix (Fig. 232–2).
- The samples should be spread thinly and evenly onto the glass slide. One or two slides may be used. The ectocervical spatula should be smeared across the slide, and both sides of the spatula should be sampled.
- The endocervical sample is placed by rolling the applicator across the slide using gentle pressure; rubbing the applicator back and forth results in a less desirable specimen. Figure 232–3 shows normal squamous cells. Figure 232–4 shows a low-grade squamous intraepithelial lesion, and Figure 232–5 shows a high-grade squamous intraepithelial lesion.

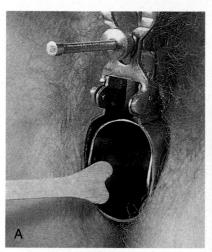
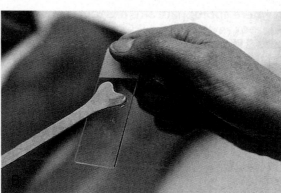

Fig 232–1
(**A**) A cervical smear is taken using an Ayres spatula. (**B**) The material obtained is plated on to a glass slide and fixed.
(From Symonds EM, Symonds IM: Essential Obstetrics and Gynaecology, 4th ed. Edinburgh, Churchill Livingstone, 2004.)

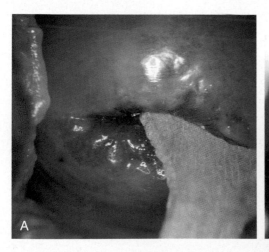
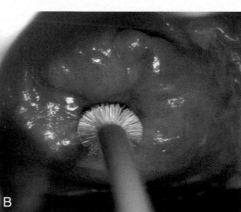

Fig 232–2
Cervical sampling with spatula and brush.
(From Apgar BS, Brotzman GL, Spitzer M: Colposcopy, Principles and Practice, An Integrated Textbook and Atlas. Philadelphia, WB Saunders, 2002.)

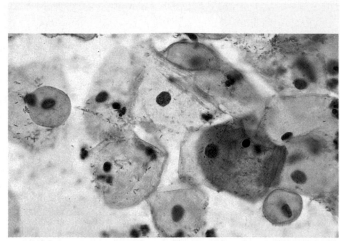

Fig 232-3
Normal squamous cells and inflammatory cells (Pap stain). (Courtesy of Dr. William H. Rogers.)

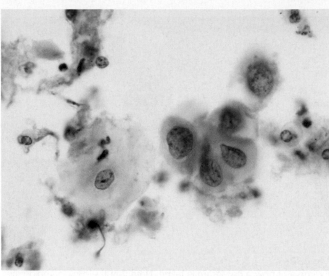

Fig 232-5
A ThinPrep Papanicolaou test showing a high-grade squamous intraepithelial lesion. Note that although hyperchromasia is slight to absent, the chromatin is irregularly distributed and the nuclear outlines are markedly irregular, ensuring the abnormal diagnosis (magnification, ×600).
(From Apgar BS, Brotzman GL, Spitzer M: Colposcopy, Principles and Practice, An Integrated Textbook and Atlas. Philadelphia, WB Saunders, 2002.)

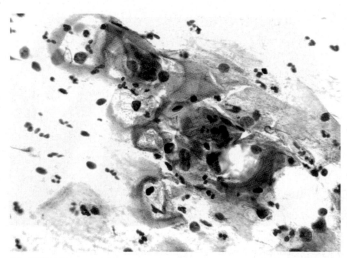

Fig 232-4
Papanicolaou smear classified as an epithelial cell abnormality, low-grade squamous intraepithelial lesion. Some koilocytes are evident in this smear, characterized by slightly enlarged nuclei with somewhat irregular nuclear outlines and distinctive perinuclear haloes. Two binucleated squamous cells are also present.
(From Apgar BS, Brotzman GL, Spitzer M: Colposcopy, Principles and Practice, An Integrated Textbook and Atlas. Philadelphia, WB Saunders, 2002.)

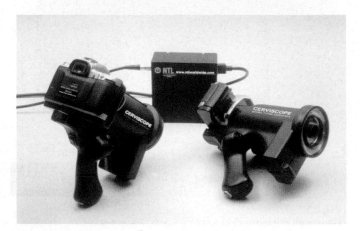

Fig 232-6
Example of a cerviscope, power supply, and power cable.
(From Apgar BS, Brotzman GL, Spitzer M: Colposcopy, Principles and Practice, An Integrated Textbook and Atlas. Philadelphia, WB Saunders, 2002.)

B. CERVICOGRAPHY

Adjunctive test to increase the sensitivity and specificity of the Pap smear for detection of precancerous and invasive cervical lesions. It uses an optical instrument known as a cerviscope (Fig. 232-6) to take a picture of the cervix for permanent documentation of the cervical findings (Figs. 232-7 and 232-8). Cervigrams are cervicograph slides projected on a screen and observed by the evaluator from a distance of 3 feet (Fig. 232-9). A lesion detected on a cervigram is shown in Figure 232-10.

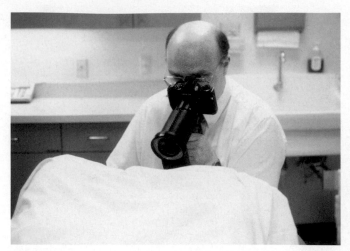

Fig 232–7

Example of how a cervigram is taken. Note that the clinician holds the cerviscope in the left hand. The trigger release is located on the handle so the right hand does not need to be used to snap the picture.
(From Apgar BS, Brotzman GL, Spitzer M: Colposcopy, Principles and Practice, An Integrated Textbook and Atlas. Philadelphia, WB Saunders, 2002.)

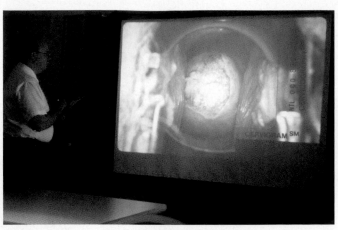

Fig 232–9

The evaluation process. The evaluator stands 3 feet from the screen, giving a magnified, panoramic view of the cervix.
(From Apgar BS, Brotzman GL, Spitzer M: Colposcopy, Principles and Practice, An Integrated Textbook and Atlas. Philadelphia, WB Saunders, 2002.)

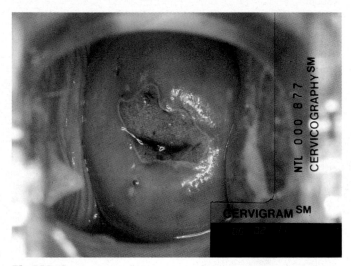

Fig 232–8

Cervigram demonstrating a normal cervix. Patient and clinic identifier information is located on the right side of the slide, resulting from camera databack impression on the film when the image is obtained.
(From Apgar BS, Brotzman GL, Spitzer M: Colposcopy, Principles and Practice, An Integrated Textbook and Atlas. Philadelphia, WB Saunders, 2002.)

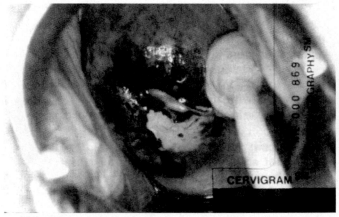

Fig 232–10

P2 cervigram. Lesion noted at 6 o'clock with sharp margins and dense, acetowhite epithelium.
(From Apgar BS, Brotzman GL, Spitzer M: Colposcopy, Principles and Practice, An Integrated Textbook and Atlas. Philadelphia, WB Saunders, 2002.)

C. COLPOSCOPY

- A colposcope is a binocular microscope (Fig. 232–11) with magnification from ×6 to ×40 and a variable-intensity light source to allow visualization of the lower genital tract.
- The patient is placed in the lithotomy position, and the largest speculum that can comfortably be inserted is used to visualize the cervix and upper vagina.
- The entire cervix and transition zone must be clearly visualized. Inability to visualize the entire squamocolumnar junction results in an unsatisfactory colposcopy.

- Once abnormal tissue has been identified, colposcopic biopsy can be performed using a cervical biopsy punch. If needed, multiple biopsies can be obtained. Figure 232–12 shows condyloma acuminate. Cervical intraepithelial neoplasia is shown in Figure 232–13.

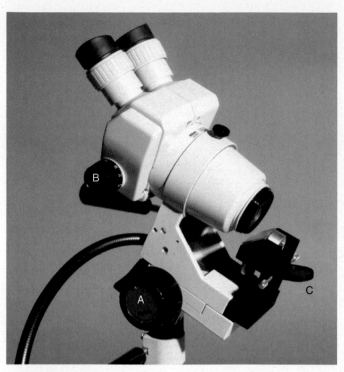

Fig 232-11
Close-up of colposcope head with the fine focus knob noted at the base of the head (**A**) and the zoom focus noted near the oculars (**B**). The green filter (**C**) flips up to provide green-light examination of the genital skin.
(From Apgar BS, Brotzman GL, Spitzer M: Colposcopy, Principles and Practice, An Integrated Textbook and Atlas. Philadelphia, WB Saunders, 2002.)

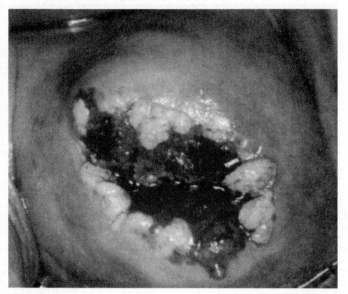

Fig 232 -12
Condyloma acuminata: Exophytic, warty lesions caused by human papillomavirus infection; they may display exaggerated vessel patterns; lesions are often multifocal and can be located both within and outside the transformation zone; some are subclinical and are manifested by subtle, minimally raised areas of acetowhite epithelium.
(From Apgar BS, Brotzman GL, Spitzer M: Colposcopy, Principles and Practice, An Integrated Textbook and Atlas. Philadelphia, WB Saunders, 2002.)

D. HYSTEROSCOPY

- Indications
  - Abnormal uterine bleeding, whether premenopausal or postmenopausal
  - Infertility
  - Retained or lost intrauterine device (IUD)
  - Abnormal radiologic studies, i.e., hysterosalpingogram or sonogram
- Benefits
  - Diagnosis and treatment of polyps, myomas, septa, adhesions, adenomyosis, polypoid endometrial hyperplasia, carcinoma, and IUDs
  - Directed tissue sampling

E. ABDOMINAL-PELVIC LAPAROSCOPY

- Indication:
  - Female sterilization
  - Evaluation of infertility
  - Tubal ligation
  - Treatment and evaluation of pelvic pain, ectopic pregnancy, endometriosis, adhesions, chronic pulmonary inflammatory disease (PID)
  - Ovarian biopsy, lymph node biopsy, retropubic bladder suspension

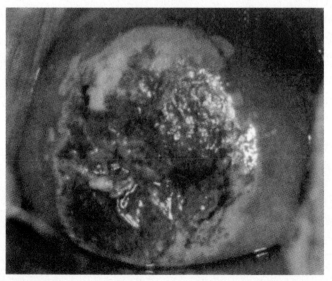

Fig 232-13
Cervical intraepithelial neoplasia (CIN): The histologic description of the three grades of precancerous lesions of the cervix—CIN 1, CIN 2, and CIN 3; the degree of CIN represents the amount of abnormal cellular change in the epithelial layers.
(From Apgar BS, Brotzman GL, Spitzer M: Colposcopy, Principles and Practice, An Integrated Textbook and Atlas. Philadelphia, WB Saunders, 2002.)

F. FISH

Fluorescence in situ hybridization (FISH) technique used to rapidly analyze amniocentesis fluid to exclude chromosomal abnormalities such as trisomy 21 (Fig. 232–14).

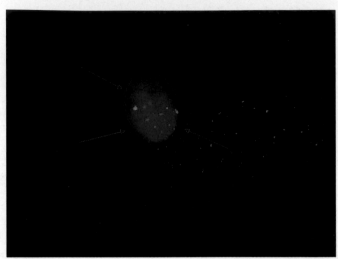

Fig 232–14
FISH. Probes to chromosome 21 appear red in this cell, demonstrating trisomy 21.
(From Drife J, Magowan B: Clinical Obstetrics and Gynaecology. Edinburgh, WB Saunders, 2004.)

Chapter 233 **Endometriosis**

DEFINITION

Endometriosis is defined as the presence of functioning endometrial glands and stroma outside the uterine cavity (Fig. 233–1).

PHYSICAL FINDINGS AND CLINICAL PRESENTATION

- Classic triad is dysmenorrhea, dyspareunia, and infertility.
- Presence of pelvic pain *not correlated* with the total area of endometriosis, type of lesion, or volume of disease, but it *is correlated* with the depth of infiltration.
- Other symptoms include: abnormal bleeding (premenstrual spotting, menorrhagia), cyclic abdominal pain, intermittent constipation/diarrhea, dyschezia, dysuria, hematuria, urinary frequency
- Rare manifestations: catamenial hemothorax, bloody pleural effusion, massive ascites occurring during menses
- Most severe discomfort is associated with lesions >1 cm in depth
- Bimanual examination may reveal tender uterosacral ligaments, cul-de-sac nodularity, induration of the rectovaginal septum, fixed retroversion of the uterus, adnexal mass, and generalized or localized tenderness.

CAUSE

- Reflux and direct implantation theory: retrograde menstruation with implantation of viable endometrial cells to surrounding pelvic structures
- Celomic metaplasia theory: transformation of multipotential cells of the coelomic epithelium into endometrium-like cells
- Vascular dissemination theory: transport of endometrial cells to distant sites via the uterine vascular and lymphatic systems
- Autoimmune disease theory: disorder of immune surveillance allows growth of endometrial implants

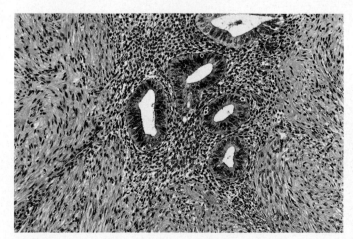

Fig 233–1

Endometriosis. Endometrial-type glands and stroma are present in the muscularis of the fallopian tube.
(From Silverberg SG: Principles and Practice of Surgical Pathology and Cytopathology, 4th ed. Edinburgh, Churchill Livingstone, 2006.)

DIFFERENTIAL DIAGNOSIS

- Ectopic pregnancy
- Acute appendicitis
- Chronic appendicitis
- PID
- Pelvic adhesions
- Hemorrhagic cyst
- Hernia
- Psychological disorder
- Irritable bowel syndrome
- Uterine leiomyomata
- Adenomyosis
- Nerve entrapment syndrome
- Scoliosis
- Muscular/skeletal strain
- Interstitial cystitis

LABORATORY TESTS

- Cancer antigen 125 (CA125)
  - CA 125 value >35 U/ml: positive predictive value of 0.58 and a negative predictive value of 0.96 for the presence of endometriosis
  - Also elevated in ovarian epithelial neoplasm, myomas, adenomyosis, acute PID, ovarian cysts, pancreatitis, chronic liver disease, menstruation, and pregnancy

IMAGING STUDIES

- Ultrasound: for evaluating adnexal mass; cannot reliably distinguish endometriomas from other benign or malignant ovarian conditions
- MRI: highly accurate in detecting endometriomas; limited sensitivity in detecting diffuse pelvic endometriosis
- Laparoscopy (Fig. 233–2) will confirm diagnosis

TREATMENT

- Expectant management (observation for 5 to 12 months) for early-stage endometriosis-associated infertility
- Nonsteroidal anti-inflammatory drugs (NSAIDs) for symptomatic relief of dysmenorrhea
- Pharmacologic management: estrogen-progesterone, progestins, gonadotropin-releasing hormone (GnRH) agonists
- Alternative therapy for inhibition of estrogen action currently under investigation are aromatase inhibitors, raloxifene, anastrozole, letrozole

SURGICAL MANAGEMENT

Conservative

- Directed at enhancing fertility or treating pain unresponsive to first-line medical treatment
- Usually accomplished through laparoscopy
- Removal or destruction of endometriotic implants by excision, electrocautery, or laser
- Cystectomy for endometrioma
- Laparoscopic uterosacral nerve ablation (LUNA) for midline pain such as dysmenorrhea or dyspareunia
- Unless pregnancy is desired, patient is usually started on GnRH agonist therapy immediately after surgery
- For those desiring pregnancy, surgery alone results in significant increase in fertility

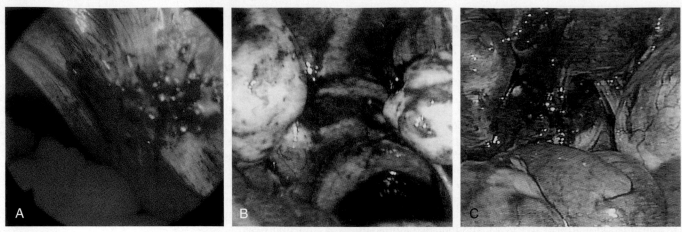

Fig 233–2
Peritoneal appearances of endometriosis. Laparoscopic views show (**A**) clear blisters ("sago" granules), "blood blisters," yellow brown patches, "powder burns," atypical vascularity and telangiectasia; (**B**) bilateral endometriomas; (**C**) severe endometriosis with adhesions.
Parts (**B**) and (**C**) courtesy of Karl Storz Endoscopy (UK) Ltd.

Definitive

- Directed at relieving endometriosis-associated pain
- Total abdominal hysterectomy with bilateral salpingo-oophorectomy and complete excision or ablation of endometriosis
- Thorough abdominal exploration to ensure removal of all disease
- Must be prepared to manage possible gastrointestinal (GI) and urinary tract endometriosis
- 90% effective in pain relief
- Estrogen replacement therapy (ERT) to be considered in all women undergoing definitive surgical management; after ERT, recurrence rate of 0% to 5% in women with endometriosis confined to the pelvis but 18% in women with bowel involvement

MANAGEMENT OF ENDOMETRIOSIS-ASSOCIATED INFERTILITY
Conservative Surgery

- Yields significantly increased pregnancy rate than does expectant management, in part because of correction of mechanical factors such as adhesions
- Assisted reproductive technologies
  - Can be used to circumvent unknown mechanism of endometriosis-associated infertility
  - Superovulation with clomiphene citrate or human menopausal gonadotropins; clomiphene citrate results in threefold pregnancy rate over either danazol or expectant management
  - Further improvement with intrauterine insemination combined with superovulation
  - In vitro fertilization if above mentioned unsuccessful

Chapter 234 Contraception

DEFINITION

Contraception refers to the various options that a sexually active couple has to prevent pregnancy. These options can be either medical or nonmedical and used by men or women or both. The options are as follows:

- No contraception: failure rate 85% both typical and perfect use
- Abstinence
  1. 12.4% of unmarried men
  2. 13.2% of unmarried women
  3. More frequently practiced before age 17 years
  4. No intercourse experienced by 13% of women ages 30 to 34 years
  5. Failure rate 0%
- Withdrawal
  1. Used in only 2% of sexually active women
  2. Failure rate with perfect use, 4%; with typical use, 19%
- Rhythm method (natural family planning)
  1. Failure rate with perfect use, 1% to 9%; with typical use, 20%
  2. Symptothermal type: mucus method and ovulation pain combined with basal body temperature
  3. Ovulation (Billings' method): takes into account mucus quality
  4. Basal body temperature method: uses biphasic temperature chart
  5. Lactation amenorrhea method: effective in fully breastfeeding women, especially 70 to 100 days after delivery; depends on number of feedings per day
- Barriers
  1. Diaphragm and cervical cap (Figs. 234–1 and 234–2): failure rate 5% to 9% in nulliparous women, 20% in multiparous women
  2. Female condom (Fig. 234–3): failure rate with perfect use, 5.1%; with typical use, 12.4%; U.S. Food and Drug Administration (FDA) labeling states 25% failure rate
  3. Male condom: failure rate with perfect use, 3%, with typical use, 12%
  4. Spermicides (aerosols, foam, jellies, creams, tabs): failure rate with perfect use, 3%; with typical use, 21%
- Oral contraceptives
  1. Failure rate with perfect use, <1%; with typical use, 3%
  2. Come in combinations of estrogen/progestin or as progestin only
- Hormonal implants and injectables
  1. Norplant
     a. Most typically used in the United States
     b. Failure rate in first 5 years: 1%
     c. Failure rate after 6 years: 2%
     d. May be extended to 7 years use
  2. Depo-Provera: failure rate 0.3% in first year of use
  3. Lunelle: failure rate 0.2% in first year
  4. Etonogestrel implant: 2-year cumulative pregnancy rate 0%
  5. Jadelle implant

- Mini pill (progesterone only pill)
  1. Failure rate with typical use, 1.1% to 13.2%
  2. With perfect use, 5 pregnancies/1000 women
- Emergency postcoital contraception
  1. Decreases pregnancy rate by 75% with women treated immediately postcoitally
  2. Involves hormonal use or IUD insertion
- IUD (available over the counter [OTC] in some states) (Fig. 234–4)
  1. Progestasert: failure rate with perfect use, 2%; with typical use, 3%
  2. Copper T (380-A): failure rate with perfect use, 0.8%; with typical use, 3%
  3. Levonorgestrel Intrauterine System (Mirena)
     a. 1-year failure rate, 1%
     b. 5-year cumulative failure rate, 0.71/100 women
- Female sterilization (tubal ligation) (Fig. 234–5): failure rate with perfect use, 0.2%; with typical use, 3%
- Male sterilization (vasectomy) (Fig. 234–6): failure rate of 0.1% in first year
- Vaginal ring (Nuva ring): failure rate pearl index 0.77
- Contraceptive patch (Orthoevra): failure rate 0.4% to 0.7%

WORKUP

- Thorough medical history
- Thorough surgical history
- Obstetric history (fertility desired?)

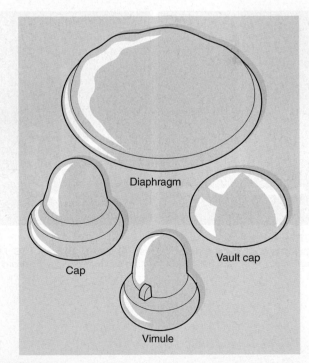

Fig 234–1
Female barrier methods of contraception. D, diaphragm; Va, vault cap; Vi, vimule; C, cervical cap.
(From Drife J, Magowan B: Clinical Obstetrics and Gynaecology. Edinburgh, WB Saunders, 2004.)

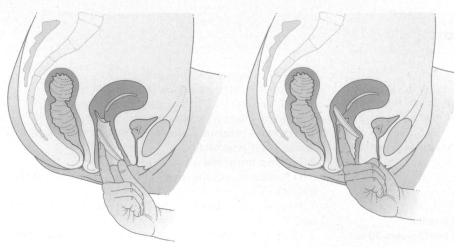

Fig 234–2
Insertion of a vaginal diaphragm to cover the cervix and anterior vaginal wall.
(From Symonds EM, Symonds IM: Essential Obstetrics and Gynecology, 4th ed. Edinburgh, Churchill Livingstone, 2004.)

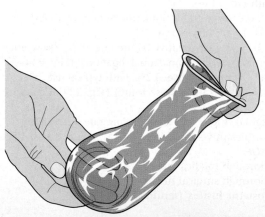

Fig 234–3
Female condom.
(From Drife J, Magowan B: Clinical Obstetrics and Gynaecology. Edinburgh, WB Saunders, 2004.)

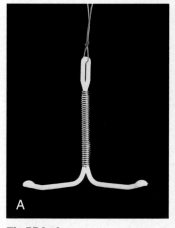 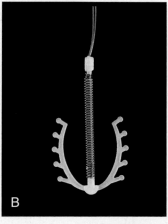 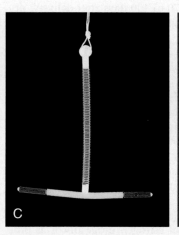 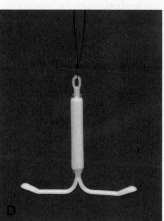

Fig 234–4
Intrauterine contraceptive devices (IUDs). (**A**) Mirena; (**B**) Nova T; (**C**) Multiload; (**D**) Orythogynae T.
(From Drife J, Magowan B: Clinical Obstetrics and Gynaecology. Edinburgh, WB Saunders, 2004.)

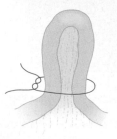 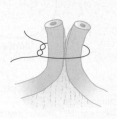 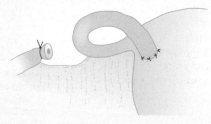

Madlener   Pomeroy   Burial of tubal stumps

Fig 234–5
Sterilization by tubal ligation.
(From Symonds EM, Symonds IM: Essential Obstetrics and Gynaecology, 4th ed. Edinburgh, Churchill Livingstone, 2004.)

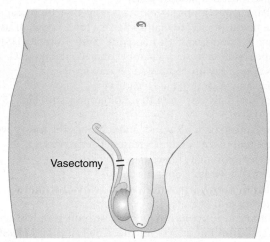

Fig 234-6
Vasectomy involves excision of a segment of the vas deferens.
(From Symonds EM, Symonds IM: Essential Obstetrics and Gynaecology,
4th ed. Edinburgh, Churchill Livingstone, 2004.)

- Gynecologic history, including:
  1. History of previous sexually transmitted diseases
  2. Number of partners
  3. Previous difficulties with contraception
  4. Frequency of intercourse
- Family history

LABORATORY TESTS
- Pap smear
- Cultures, aerobic and *Chlamydia*
- Pregnancy test if suspected pregnancy
- Lipid profile if family history of premature vascular event

TREATMENT
- Male condoms
  1. 95% latex (rubber), 5% skin or natural membrane
  2. Proper use: place on an erect penis and leave ½-inch empty space at the tip of the condom; use with non–oil-based lubricants
  3. Effectiveness increased when used with spermicides
- Female condoms
  1. Composed of polyurethane, with one end open and one end closed
  2. Proper use: place closed end over cervix, open end hanging out of vagina to cover penis and scrotum
  3. Highly effective against human immunodeficiency virus (HIV)
- Spermicides
  1. Types: nonoxynol, octoxynol
  2. Forms: jellies, creams, foams, suppositories, tablets, soluble films
  3. Proper use: put in immediately before intercourse; may be used with other barrier methods
- Diaphragm and cervical cap
  1. Must be fitted by practitioner, used with contraceptive gels, and refitted with weight gain or loss
  2. Diaphragm sizes: 50 to 95 mm; cervical cap sizes: 22, 25, 28, and 31 mm
  3. Proper use of diaphragm: put in immediately before intercourse and keep in for 6 hours after intercourse; must not remain in the vagina for longer than 24 hours
  4. Proper use of cervical cap: fit over the cervix exactly; must not remain in place for longer than 48 hours
- Lactation amenorrhea method
  1. Depends on number of breast-feedings per day; effective as birth control for 6 months if 15 or more feedings, lasting 10 minutes each, are accomplished daily
  2. Not a common practice in the United States
- Withdrawal
  1. Withdrawal of the penis from the vagina before ejaculation
  2. Dependent on self-control
- Rhythm method
  1. Dependent on awareness of physiology of male and female reproductive tracts
  2. Sperm viable in vagina for 2 to 7 days
  3. Ovum life span 24 hours
- Sterilization
  1. Male
     a. Vasectomy (see Fig. 234–6) to interrupt vas deferens and block passage of sperm to seminal ejaculate
     b. Scalpel and nonscalpel techniques available
     c. More easily performed procedure than female sterilization and does not require general anesthesia
  2. Female
     a. Leading method of birth control in the United States in women older than 30 years
     b. Interrupts fallopian tubes, blocking passage of ovum proximally and sperm distally through tube
     c. Several types; modified Pomeroy done during cesarean section or laparoscopic done in nonpregnant females most common
     d. Essure-tubal occlusion through hysteroscopic placement of micro-inserts into the fallopian tubes.
- Combination oral contraceptives
  1. Taken daily for 21 days, pill-free interval of 7 days
  2. Less than 50 μg ethynyl estradiol in most common combination oral contraceptives; progestins most commonly used in combination pills are norethindrone, levonorgestrel, norgestrel, norethindrone acetate, ethynodiol diacetate, norgestimate, or desogestrel; triphasic combination oral contraceptives (give varying doses of progestin and estrogens throughout cycle); monophasic oral contraceptives: offer same dose of progestin and estrogen throughout cycle, taken daily at same time; estrophasic pill (constant progesterone with variation of estrogen throughout the cycle)
  3. If pill taken with antibiotics, efficacy affected by inadequate gastrointestinal absorption in most cases; only rifampin truly reduces pill's effectiveness
  4. Increased body weight decreases effectiveness
- Mini pill
  1. Progestin only; taken without a break
  2. Causes much irregular bleeding because of the lack of estrogen effect on the lining of the uterus
- Hormonal implants and injectables

1. Norplant
   a. Progestin only; inserted under the skin
   b. Six levonorgestrel implants placed subcutaneously in upper inner arm effective for 5 years
2. Depo-Provera
   a. Medroxyprogesterone acetate given every 3 months in intramuscular injection form
   b. Major side effect: irregular bleeding
   c. Fertility return possibly delayed up to 18 months after discontinuation
3. Lunelle: monthly injectable administered intramuscularly. Contains 0.5 mL aqueous, 5 mg estradiol cypionate, and 25 mg medroxyprogesterone acetate
4. Etonogestrel implant: single-rod release etonogestrel for 3 years placed subdermally

● Postcoital contraception
   1. Done on emergency basis, usually secondary to noncompliance with birth control or failure of birth control (e.g., condom breakage) at the time of ovulation
   2. Methods:
      a. IUD insertion within 7 days of coitus
      b. Hormonal methods (combination pills and danazol) given within 48 hours of coitus

● IUD
   1. Device inserted into uterus to prevent sperm and ovum from uniting in fallopian tube

2. Types available in the United States:
   a. Progestasert: a T-shaped device that is an ethylene vinyl acetate copolymer T; vertical stem contains 38 mg progesterone and must be changed yearly
   b. ParaGard (Copper T/380-A): a polyethylene T wrapped with a fine copper wire that is effective for 10 years of use

● Mirena Levonorgestrel Intrauterine System (LNGIUS): a T-shaped system with a chamber that contains LNG. Releases 20 μg/day; is effective for 5 years

● Vaginal ring (brand name Nuvaring)
   1. Provides daily dose of 120 μg of etonogestrel and 15 μg ethinyl estradiol
   2. Stays in vagina for 3 weeks and removed the fourth week
   3. Increased body weight decreases effectiveness

● Contraceptive patch (brand name Evra)
   1. Provides low daily dose of steroids
   2. Releases a progestin and estrogen (ethinyl estradiol)
   3. Patch size 20 cm^2
   4. Each patch contains 6 mg norelgestronin and delivers an estimated continuous systemic dose of 150 μg norelgestronin and 20 μg of ethinyl estradiol; common dose 250 μg/day progestin and 25 μg/day estrogen
   5. Worn 3 of 4 weeks
   6. Increased body weight decreases effectiveness

VULVA/VAGINA

Chapter 235 **Vaginosis, bacterial**

DEFINITION

Bacterial vaginosis (BV) is a thin, gray, homogeneous, malodorous vaginal discharge (Fig. 235–1) that results from a shift in the vaginal flora from a predominance of lactobacilli to high concentrations of anaerobic bacteria.

PHYSICAL FINDINGS AND CLINICAL PRESENTATION

- 50% of patients are asymptomatic.
- A thin, dark, or dull gray homogeneous discharge that adheres to the vaginal walls
- An offensive, "fishy" odor that is accentuated after intercourse or menses
- Pruritus (only in 13%)

CAUSE

- *Gardnerella vaginalis* is detected in 40% to 50% of vaginal secretions.
  1. Increase in vaginal pH caused by decrease in hydrogen peroxide lactobacilli
  2. Anaerobes predominate and produce amines
- Amines, when alkalinized by semen, menstrual blood, the use of alkaline douches, or the addition of 10% KOH, volatilize and cause the unpleasant "fishy" odor.
- In BV:
  1. *Bacteroides* (anaerobes) species are increased 1000× the usual concentration.
  2. *G. vaginalis* are 100× normal.
  3. *Peptostreptococcus* are 10× normal.
  4. *Mycoplasma hominis* and Enterobacteriacea members are present in increased concentrations.

DIFFERENTIAL DIAGNOSIS

- Trichomonas vaginalis (see Fig. 237–1)
- Fungal vulvovaginitis (see Fig. 236–1)
- Atrophic vaginitis (see Fig. 238–1)

WORKUP

Seattle Group Criteria

- Detecting three of the four following signs will diagnose 90% correctly, with <10% false positives:
  1. Thin, gray, homogeneous, malodorous discharge that adheres to the vaginal walls
  2. Elevated pH >4.5
  3. Positive KOH whiff test
  4. Clue cells present on wet mount (Fig. 235–2)
- Cultures are unnecessary.
- Pap smear will not identify *G. vaginalis*.
- Gram stain of vaginal secretions will reveal clue cells and abnormal mixed bacteria
- Figure 235–3 shows a diagnostic algorithm in patients with dysuria and/or urethral and/or vaginal discharge.
- Table 235–1 shows characteristics of common vaginal discharges

TREATMENT

1. Metronidazole 500 mg PO bid for 7 days
2. 0.75% metronidazole gel in vagina bid for 5 days
3. 2% clindamycin cream qd for 7 days

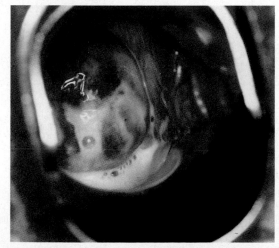

Fig 235–1
Bacterial vaginosis. BV is due to an overgrowth of anaerobic bacteria, genital mycoplasmas, and *Gardnerella vaginalis*. The discharge is milky white and adherent to the vaginal walls, and may be frothy.
(From Drife J, Magowan B: Clinical Obstetrics and Gynaecology. Edinburgh, WB Saunders, 2004.)

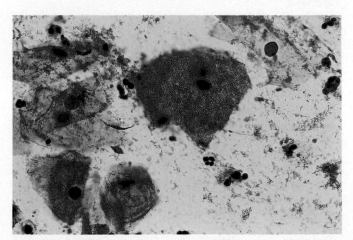

Fig 235–2
Bacterial vaginitis, cervical vaginal smear. Squamous cell covered with small coccobacillary organisms with many additional organisms in the background. These cells are referred to as "clue" cells, indicating a bacterial overgrowth of mixed-type vaginal flora (Papanicolaou, ×600).
(From Silverberg SG: Principles and Practice of Surgical Pathology and Cytopathology, 4th ed. Edinburgh, Churchill Livingstone, 2006.)

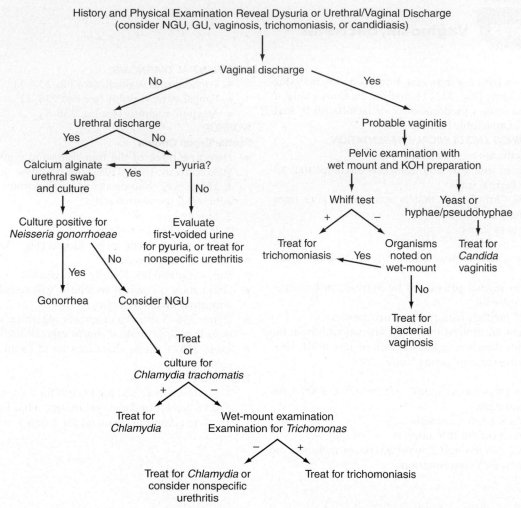

History and Physical Examination Reveal Dysuria or Urethral/Vaginal Discharge
(consider NGU, GU, vaginosis, trichomoniasis, or candidiasis)

Fig 235-3
Evaluation of patients with dysuria and/or urethral/vaginal discharge. NGU, nongonococcal urethritis; GU, gonococcal urethritis; KOH, potassium hydroxide.
(From Nseyo U, Weinman E, Lamm DL: Urology for Primary Care Physicians. Philadelphia, WB Saunders, 1999.)

TABLE 235–1 Characteristics of common vaginal discharges

Feature	Physiologic Discharge	Nonspecific Vaginitis	*Trichomonas*	*Candida*	Gonococcal
Color	White	Gray	Grayish-yellow	White	Greenish-yellow
Fishy odor	Absent	Present	Present	Absent	Absent
Consistency	Nonhomogeneous	Homogeneous	Purulent, often with bubbles	Cottage cheese-like	Mucopurulent
Location	Dependent	Adherent to walls	Often pooled in fornix	Adherent to walls	Adherent to walls
Discharge at introitus	Rare	Common	Common	Common	Common
Vulva	Normal	Normal	Edematous	Erythematous	Erythematous
Vaginal mucosa	Normal	Normal	Usually normal	Erythematous	Normal
Cervix	Normal	Normal	May show red spots	Patches of discharge	Pus in os

Swartz MH: Textbook of Physical Diagnosis, ed 5, Philadelphia, 2006, Saunders

Chapter 236 | Vulvovaginitis, fungal

DEFINITION

Fungal vulvovaginitis is the inflammation of vulva and vagina caused by *Candida* spp.

PHYSICAL FINDINGS AND CLINICAL PRESENTATION

- Intense vulvar and vaginal pruritus
- Edema and erythema of vulva
- Thick, curdlike vaginal discharge (Fig. 236–1)
- Adherent, dry, white, curdy patches attached to vaginal mucosa

CAUSE

- *Candida albicans* is responsible for 80% to 95% of vaginal fungal infections.
- *Candida tropicalis* and *Torulopsis glabrata (Candida glabrata)* are the most common non-*albicans Candida* species that can induce vaginitis.

PREDISPOSING HOST FACTORS

- Pregnancy
- Oral contraceptives (high estrogen)
- Diabetes mellitus
- Antibiotics
- Immunosuppression
- Tight, poorly ventilated, nylon underclothing, with increased local perineal moisture and temperature

DIFFERENTIAL DIAGNOSIS

- Bacterial vaginosis (see Fig. 235–1)
- *Trichomonas vaginitis* (see Fig. 237–2)
- Atrophic vaginitis (see Fig. 238–1)

LABORATORY TESTS

- Speculum examination (see Fig. 236–1)
- Hyphae or budding spores on 10% KOH preparation (positive in 50% to 70% of individuals with yeast infection)
- Culture, especially recurrence for identification

TREATMENT

- Cure rate of the various azole derivatives 85% to 90%; little evidence of superiority of one azole agent over another

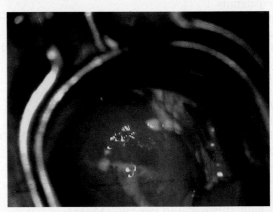

Fig 236–1
Candida Infection. Although candida may present with these "typical" white plaques, the discharge is sometimes minimal.
(From Drife J, Magowan B: Clinical Obstetrics and Gynaecology. Edinburgh, WB Saunders, 2004.)

Chapter 237 Vulvovaginitis, trichomonas

DEFINITION

Trichomonas vulvovaginitis is the inflammation of vulva and vagina caused by *Trichomonas* spp.

PHYSICAL FINDINGS AND CLINICAL PRESENTATION

- Profuse, yellow, malodorous vaginal discharge and severe vaginal itching
- Vulvar itching
- Dysuria
- Dyspareunia
- Intense erythema of the vaginal mucosa
- Cervical petechiae ("strawberry cervix")
- Asymptomatic in approximately 50% of women and 90% of men

CAUSE

Single-cell parasite known as *trichomonad*

RISK FACTORS

- Multiple sexual partners
- History of previous sexually transmitted diseases (STDs)

DIFFERENTIAL DIAGNOSIS

- Bacterial vaginosis (see Fig. 235–1)
- Fungal vulvovaginitis (see Fig. 236–1)
- Cervicitis (see Fig. 240–1)
- Atrophic vulvovaginitis (see Fig. 238–1)

WORKUP

- Pelvic examination
- Speculum examination
- Mobile trichomonads (Fig. 237–1) seen on normal saline preparation (Fig. 237–2): 70% sensitivity
- Elevated pH (>5) of vaginal discharge
- Culture is most sensitive commercially available method
- A large number of inflammatory cells on normal saline preparation

LABORATORY TESTS

- Culture (modified Diamond media): 90% sensitivity
- Direct enzyme immunoassay
- Fluorescein-conjugated monoclonal antibody test
- Pap test 40% detected

TREATMENT

- Tinidazole single 2 g oral dose in both sexes
- Metronidazole 2 g PO × 1 or 500 mg PO bid × 7 days

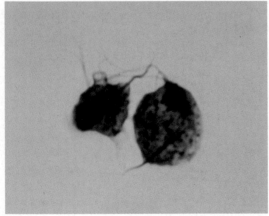

Fig 237–1
Trichomonas vaginalis. Trophozoites showing axostyle, flagella and part of the undulating membrane (smaller organism) (Giemsa stain). There is no known cyst form for this organism. From Cohen J, Powderly WG: Infectious Diseases, 2nd ed. St Louis, Mosby, 2004.)

Fig 237–2
Trichomonal infection. Saline mount of *Trichomonas vaginalis (arrow);* characteristic ovoid shape and flagella can be seen.
(From Cohen J, Powderly WG: Infectious Diseases, 2nd ed. St Louis, Mosby, 2004.)

Chapter 238	Vulvovaginitis, estrogen deficient (atrophic vaginitis)

DEFINITION
Estrogen-deficient vulvovaginitis is the irritation and/or inflammation of the vulva and vagina because of progressive thinning and atrophic changes secondary to estrogen deficiency.

PHYSICAL FINDINGS AND CLINICAL PRESENTATION
- Thinning of pubic hair, labia minora and majora
- Decreased secretions from the vestibular glands, with vaginal dryness (Fig. 238–1)
- Regression of subcutaneous fat
- Vulvar and vaginal itching
- Dyspareunia
- Dysuria and urinary frequency
- Vaginal spotting

CAUSE
  Estrogen deficiency

DIFFERENTIAL DIAGNOSIS
- Infectious vulvovaginitis (see Fig. 236–1)
- Squamous cell hyperplasia
- Lichen sclerosus
- Vulva malignancy (see Fig. 239–2)
- Vaginal malignancy
- Cervical and endometrial malignancy

WORKUP
- Pelvic examination
- Speculum examination
- Pap smear
- Possible endometrial biopsy if bleeding

LABORATORY TESTS
Follicle-stimulating hormone (FSH) and estradiol: generally after menopause, estradiol <15 pg and FSH >40 mIU/mL

TREATMENT
- Estrogen replacement

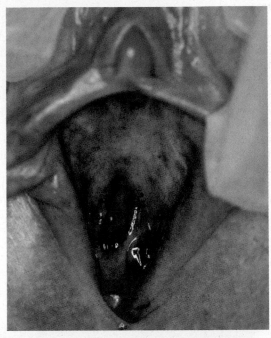

Fig 238–1
Atrophic vulva. Slightly enlarged clitoris owing to loss of estrogen, with a pale, thin vulvar vestibule.
(From Apgar BS, Brotzman GL, Spitzer M: Colposcopy, Principles and Practice, An Integrated Textbook and Atlas. Philadelphia, WB Saunders, 2002.)

Chapter 239 Vulvar cancer

DEFINITION

Vulvar cancer is an abnormal cell proliferation arising on the vulva and exhibiting malignant potential. The majority are of squamous cell origin; however, other types include adenocarcinoma, basal cell carcinoma, sarcoma, and melanoma.

PHYSICAL FINDINGS AND CLINICAL PRESENTATION

- Vulvar pruritus or pain may be present.
- May produce a malodor or discharge or present as bleeding
- Raised lesion, may have fleshy, ulcerated, leukoplakic, or warty appearance (Fig. 239–1); may have multifocal lesions
- Lesions are usually located on labia majora (Fig. 239–2) but may be seen on the labia minora, clitoris, and perineum.
- The lymph nodes of groin may be palpable.

CAUSE

- The exact etiology is unknown.
- Vulvar intraepithelial neoplasia has been reported in 20% to 30% of invasive squamous cell carcinomas of the vulva, but the malignant potential is unknown.
- Human papillomavirus is found in 30% to 50% of vulvar carcinomas, but its exact role is unclear.
- Chronic pruritus, wetness, industrial wastes, arsenicals, hygienic agents, and vulvar dystrophies have been implicated as causative agents.

DIFFERENTIAL DIAGNOSIS

- Lymphogranuloma inguinale
- Tuberculosis
- Vulvar dystrophies
- Vulvar atrophy
- Paget's disease
- Vulvar sebaceous cysts (Fig. 239–3)
- Vulvar epidermal inclusion cysts (Fig. 239–4)

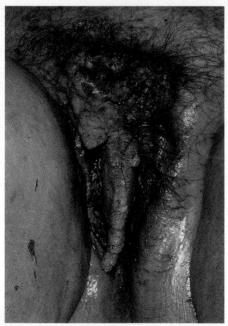

Fig 239–1
Verrucous carcinoma. A relatively small example of verrucous carcinoma showing the smooth pushing edge of the lesion. Excision biopsy was adequate therapy in this patient.
(From Black M, McKay M: Obstetrics and Gynaecological Dermatology, ed 2. St Louis, Mosby, 2002.)

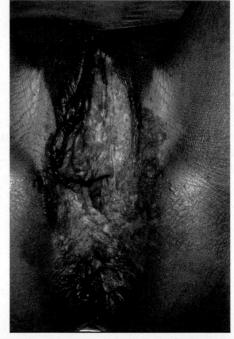

Fig 239–2
Widespread vulvar intraepithelial neoplasia (VIN) was found to hide multiple areas of early invasive cancer of the vulva. The patient also had cervical intraepithelial neoplasia (CIN) 3, and 10 years later she developed a primary invasive vaginal cancer. Multifocal disease of this type is not uncommon and may represent a "field effect" of human papillomavirus (HPV) infection.
(From Black M, McKay M: Obstetrics and Gynaecological Dermatology, ed 2. St Louis, Mosby, 2002.)

WORKUP

- Diagnosis is made histologically by biopsy.
- Thorough examination of the lesion and assessment of spread
- Possible colposcopy of adjacent areas
- Cytologic smear of vagina and cervix
- Cystoscopy and proctosigmoidoscopy may be necessary.

IMAGING STUDIES

- Chest radiography
- Computed tomography (CT) scanning and magnetic resonance imaging (MRI) for assessing local tumor spread

TREATMENT

- Treatment is individualized depending on the stage of the tumor.
- Stage I tumors with <1-mm stromal invasion are treated with complete local excision without groin node dissection.
- Stage I tumors with >1-mm stromal invasion are treated with complete local excision with groin node dissection.
- Stage II tumors require radical vulvectomy with bilateral groin node dissection.
- Advanced-stage disease may require the addition of radiation and chemotherapy to the surgical regimen.

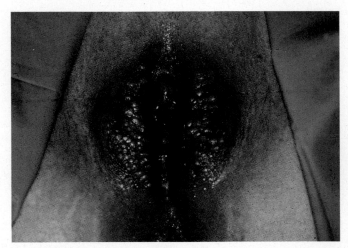

Fig 239–3
Multiple sebaceous cysts on both labia majora. The patient wished removal of the cysts, and a simple excision of both affected areas provided a satisfactory cosmetic result.
(From Black M, McKay M: Obstetrics and Gynaecological Dermatology, ed 2. St Louis, Mosby, 2002.)

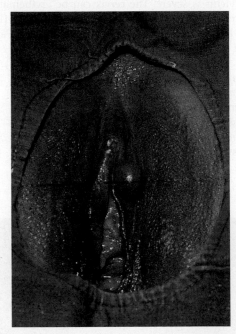

Fig 239–4
Epidermal inclusion cyst, 1 cm in diameter, in the left interlabial fold. Simple excision confirmed the diagnosis and treated the problem. Incision and drainage are not recommended, as the lesion usually recurs unless the cyst wall is removed.
(From Black M, McKay M: Obstetrics and Gynaecological Dermatology, ed 2. St Louis, Mosby, 2002.)

CERVIX

Chapter 240 | Cervicitis

DEFINITION

Cervicitis is an infection of the cervix. It may result from direct infection of the cervix, or it may be secondary to uterine or vaginal infection.

PHYSICAL FINDINGS AND CLINICAL PRESENTATION

Cervicitis is usually asymptomatic or associated with mild symptoms. Copious purulent or mucopurulent vaginal discharge (Fig. 240–1), pelvic pain, and dyspareunia may be present if cervicitis is severe. The cervix can be erythematous and tender on palpation during bimanual examination. The cervix may also bleed easily when obtaining cultures or a Pap smear. May have postcoital bleeding.

CAUSE

- *Chlamydia* (See Fig. 240–2.)
- *Trichomonas*
- *Neisseria gonorrhoeae*
- Herpes simplex
- *Trichomonas vaginalis*
- Human papillomavirus

DIFFERENTIAL DIAGNOSIS

- Carcinoma of the cervix (See Fig. 242–1.)
- Cervical erosion
- Cervical metaplasia

WORKUP

The patient usually presents with a vaginal discharge or history of postcoital bleeding. Otherwise, the patient is diagnosed asymptomatically during routine examination. On examination, there is gross visualization of yellow, mucopurulent material on the cotton swab.

LABORATORY TESTS

On a smear, there will be 10 or more polymorphonuclear leukocytes per microscopic field. Positive Gram stain is found. Cultures should be obtained for *Chlamydia* and *N. gonorrhoeae*. Use a wet mount to look for trichomonads. Obtain a Pap smear.

TREATMENT

Because *Chlamydia* and *N. gonorrhoeae* make up >50% of the cause of infectious cervicitis, if it is suspected, treat without waiting for culture results. Administer ceftriaxone 125 mg IM single dose followed by doxycycline 100 mg PO bid for 7 days. If the patient is pregnant, treat with azithromycin 1 g single dose instead of using doxycycline, which is contraindicated in pregnant or nursing mothers.

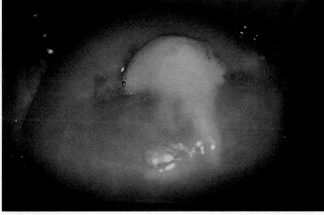

Fig 240–1
Mucopurulent cervicitis caused by *Chlamydia trachomatis*. (Courtesy of Dr. J. Paavonen.)

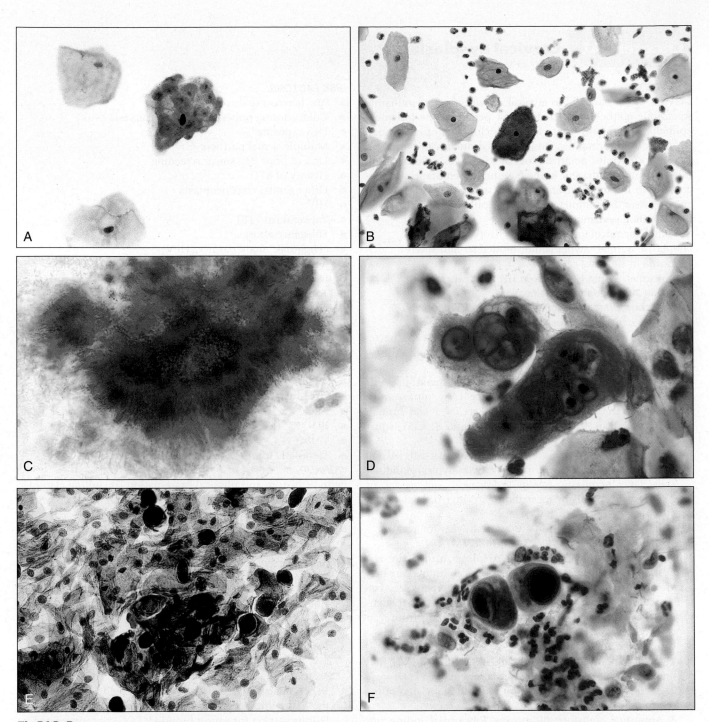

Fig 240-2

Infectious organisms. (**A**) *Trichomonas vaginalis* adherent to a squamous cell in a liquid-based preparation. Liquid preparations tend to have less inflammation and show better preservation of organisms (SurePath). (**B**) Shift in vaginal flora suggestive of bacterial vaginosis in liquid-based preparation. Again the background is cleaner with bacterial adherent to individual cells as well as present in small loose clusters (SurePath). (**C**) *Actinomyces*: loose clumps of bacterial organisms often seen with an eosinophilic center due to inadequate penetration by hematoxylin. The organisms are thin with acute angle branching. (**D**) Herpes: diagnostic herpes consists of multinucleated cells with molded glassy nuclei showing margination of the chromatin. Viral inclusions as seen here may or may not be present. (**E**) *Molluscum contagiosum*: numerous cells with deeply eosinophilic viral inclusions are present. These should be differentiated from the dyskeratotic cells seen in SIL. (**F**) Cytomegalovirus: cytomegalovirus is rarely seen in cervical preparations. The cells are enlarged with a single nucleus containing a prominent nuclear inclusion. Cytoplasmic inclusions, as seen here, may also be present.

(From Silverberg SG: Principles and Practice of Surgical Pathology and Cytopathology, 4th ed. Edinburgh, Churchill Livingstone, 2006.)

Chapter 241 Cervical dysplasia

DEFINITION

Cervical dysplasia refers to atypical development of immature squamous epithelium that does not penetrate the basement epithelial membrane. Characteristics include increased cellularity, nuclear abnormalities, and increased nuclear-to-cytoplasm ratio. A progressive polarized loss of squamous differentiation exists beginning adjacent to the basement membrane and progressing to the most advanced stage (severe dysplasia), which encompasses the complete squamous epithelial layer thickness

Classification systems

Modified Papanicolaou: classes I, II, III, IV, and V

Dysplasia: normal, atypia (mild, moderate, and severe), carcinoma in situ, and cancer

CIN: normal, atypia (CIN I, II, or III), and cancer

Bethesda 2001 Updated Classification

INTERPRETATION/RESULT (INCLUDING SPECIMEN ADEQUACY)

- Negative for intraepithelial lesion or malignancy
- Organisms (i.e., *Trichomonas vaginalis, Candida* sp., bacterial vaginosis), reactive cellular changes (inflammation), atrophy
- Epithelial cell abnormalities: atypical squamous cells (ASC), of undetermined significance (ASC-ultrasound), cannot exclude HSIL (ASC-H), LSIL (CIN 1 and human papillomavirus [HPV]), HSIL (CIN 2 and 3, CIS), squamous cell carcinoma
- Glandular cell abnormalities: atypical glandular cells (AGC): *(specify endocervical, endometrial, or NOS)*, atypical glandular cells, favor neoplastic *(specify endocervical, endometrial, or NOS)* endocervical adenocarcinoma in situ (AIS), adenocarcinoma
- Other: endometrial cells in a woman 40 years of age

PHYSICAL FINDINGS AND CLINICAL PRESENTATION

- Cervical lesions associated with dysplasia usually are not visible to the naked eye; therefore, physical findings are best viewed by colposcopy of a 3% acetic acid–prepared cervix.
- Patients evaluated by colposcopy (see Fig. 232–7) are identified by abnormal cervical cytology screening from Pap smear screening (Fig. 241–1).
- Colposcopic findings
  1. Leukoplakia (white lesion seen by the unaided eye that may represent condyloma, dysplasia, or cancer)
  2. Acetowhite epithelium with or without associated punctation, mosaicism, abnormal vessels
  3. Abnormal transformation zone (abnormal iodine uptake, "cuffed" gland openings)

CAUSE

- May be caused by abnormal reserve cell hyperplasia resulting in atypical metaplasia and dysplastic epithelium
- Strongly associated and initiated by oncogenic HPV infection (high-risk HPV types 16, 18, 31, 33, 35, 45, 51, 52, 56, and 58; low-risk HPV types 6, 11, 42, 43, and 44)

RISK FACTORS

- Any heterosexual coitus
- Coitus during puberty (T-zone metaplasia peak)
- DES exposure
- Multiple sexual partners
- Lack of prior Pap smear screening
- History of STD
- Other genital tract neoplasia
- HIV
- Tuberculosis (TB)
- Substance abuse
- "High-risk" male partner (HPV)
- Low socioeconomic status
- Early first pregnancy
- Tobacco use
- HPV

DIFFERENTIAL DIAGNOSIS

- Metaplasia
- Hyperkeratosis
- Condyloma
- Microinvasive carcinoma
- Glandular epithelial abnormalities
- AIS
- VIN
- VAIN
- Metastatic tumor involvement of the cervix

WORKUP

Periodic history and physical examination (including cytologic screening), depending on age, risk factors, and history of preinvasive cervical lesions

- Consider screening for sexually transmitted disease (Gc, *Chlamydia*, VDRL, HIV, HPV)
- Abnormal cytology (HSIL/LSIL, initial ASC/ASC-ultrasound/ ASC-H in high-risk patients, recurrent in low-risk/post-menopausal patients) and grossly evident suspicious lesions; refer for colposcopy and possible directed biopsy/ ECC (examination should include cervix, vagina, vulva, and anus)
- For glandular cell abnormalities (AGC): refer for colposcopy and possible directed biopsy/ECC, and consider endometrial sampling
- In pregnancy: abnormal cytology followed by colposcopy in the first trimester and at 28 to 32 weeks; only high-grade lesions suspect for cancer biopsied; ECC contraindicated

LABORATORY TESTS

- Gc, *Chlamydia* to rule out STD
- Pap cytology screening (requires appropriate sampling, preparation, cytologist interpretation and reporting) (Fig. 241–2)
- Colposcopy and directed biopsy, ECC for indications (see Workup)
- HPV-DNA typing if identified abnormal cytology

IMAGING STUDIES
- Cervicography
- Computer-enhanced Pap cytology screening (e.g., PAPNET)

TREATMENT
- Superficial ablative techniques (cryosurgery, CO_2 laser, and electrocoagulation diathermy) considered for colposcopy-identified dysplasia (moderate to severe dysplasia or CIS) and negative ECC; mild dysplasia followed conservatively in a compliant patient

- Cone biopsy (LEEP, CO_2 laser, "cold knife" cone biopsy) considered for colposcopy-identified dysplasia (moderate to severe dysplasia or CIS) and positive ECC or if there is a two-grade or more discrepancy between the Pap smear, colposcopy, and biopsy or ECC findings
- Figure 241–3 shows an electrosurgical loop excision
- Hysterectomy if patient has completed childbearing and has persistent or recurrent severe dysplasia or CIS
- Topical 5-fluorouracil (5-FU) is rarely used for recurrent cervicovaginal lesions.

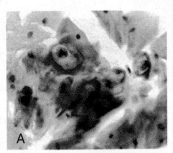

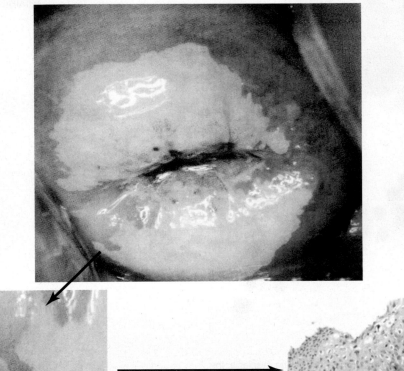

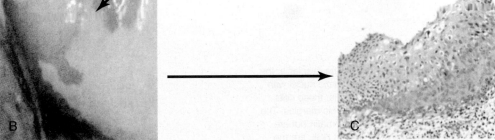

Fig 241–1
A. Cytology reveals a squamous epithelial cell abnormality: low-grade squamous intraepithelial lesion (LSIL) with changes of HPV. In the center is a cell with an enlarged, irregular nucleus; a distinctive perinuclear halo; and clearing of the cytoplasm. Adjacent are several cells with similar findings admixed with superficial and intermediate squamous cells. The background is clean. **B**. Area of biopsy. Acetowhite epithelium with a geographic border and absent vessels. **C**. Histology reveals CIN 1. The epithelium lacks maturation in the lower one third of the epithelium, and the disorderly basal cells exhibit some crowding within the parabasal area. Multinucleated cells are seen near the surface, and koilocytosis is present. There is mild, superficial, chronic inflammation in the stroma.
(From Apgar BS, Brotzman GL, Spitzer M: Colposcopy, Principles and Practice, An Integrated Textbook and Atlas. Philadelphia, WB Saunders, 2002.)

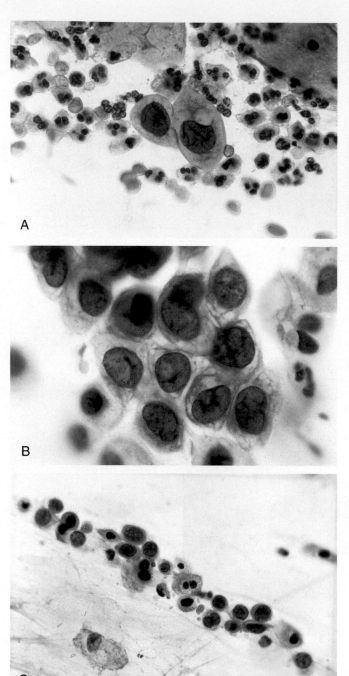

A

B

C

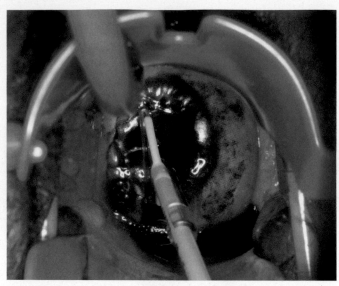

Fig 241–3
An electrosurgical loop excision as the loop is passed under the transformation zone.
(From Apgar BS, Brotzman GL, Spitzer M: Colposcopy, Principles and Practice, An Integrated Textbook and Atlas. Philadelphia, WB Saunders, 2002.)

Fig 241–2
High-grade squamous intraepithelial lesion. (**A**) Moderate dysplasia: the cells show immature cytoplasm and large, hyperchromatic nuclei with a high nuclear to cytoplasmic ratio. (**B**) Severe dysplasia: these cells are arranged in a loose cluster with indistinct cytoplasmic margins. The nuclei demonstrate wrinkled membranes with fine chromatin but are not particularly hyperchromatic. Again, the hallmarks of HSIL are the high N:C ratios and immature cytoplasm to go with the dysplastic nuclei. (**C**) Severe dysplasia: in conventional cytology the dysplastic cells are often found in strings or strands of mucus. The nuclear and cytoplasmic features are similar to those above.
(From Silverberg SG: Principles and Practice of Surgical Pathology and Cytopathology, 4th ed. Edinburgh, Churchill Livingstone, 2006.)

Chapter 242 Cervical cancer

DEFINITION
Cervical cancer is penetration of the basement membrane and infiltration of the stroma of the uterine cervix by malignant cells (Fig. 242–1).

PHYSICAL FINDINGS AND CLINICAL PRESENTATION
- Unusual vaginal bleeding, particularly postcoital
- Vaginal discharge and/or odor
- Advanced cases may present with lower extremity edema or renal failure.
- In early stages, there may be little or no obvious cervical lesion; more advanced cases may present with large, bulky, friable lesions encompassing the majority of the vagina.

CAUSE
- Dysplastic cells progress to invasive carcinoma.
- Thought to be linked to the presence of HPV types 16, 18, 45, and 56 via interaction of E6 oncoproteins on p53 gene product
- There may be an association with past infection with *Chlamydia trachomatis*.

DIFFERENTIAL DIAGNOSIS
- Cervical polyp or prolapsed uterine fibroid
- Preinvasive cervical lesions
- Neoplasia metastatic from a separate primary

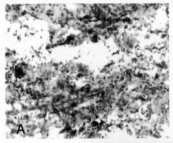

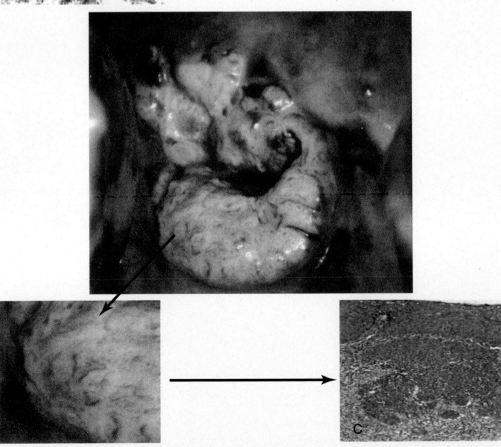

Fig 242–1
(**A**) Cytology reveals only inflammatory changes because of superficial necrosis produced by the cancer. (**B**) Area of biopsy. Dense acetowhite epithelium with atypical blood vessels. (**C**) Histology reveals squamous cell cancer. The basement membrane of the epithelium is breeched, and the abnormal cells extend into the stroma.
(From Apgar BS, Brotzman GL, Spitzer M: Colposcopy, Principles and Practice, An Integrated Textbook and Atlas. Philadelphia, WB Saunders, 2002.)

WORKUP
- Thorough history and physical examination
- Pelvic examination with careful rectovaginal examination
- Colposcopy with directed biopsy and endocervical curettage
- Clinically staged, not surgically staged

LABORATORY TESTS
- Complete blood cell count (CBC), chemistry profile
- Squamous cell carcinoma (SCC) antigen in research setting
- CEA

IMAGING STUDIES
- Chest x-ray
- Depending on stage, may need cystoscopy, colonoscopy, CT scan (Fig. 242–2) or MRI, lymphangiography

TREATMENT
- FIGO stage Ia: cone biopsy or simple hysterectomy
- FIGO stage Ib or IIa: type III radical hysterectomy and pelvic lymphadenectomy *or* pelvic radiation therapy
- Advanced or bulky disease: multimodality therapy (radiation, chemotherapy, and/or surgery); platinum use before radiation therapy

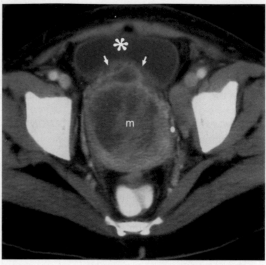

Fig 242–2
CT, cervical cancer. On the axial image, the cervical cancer images as a mass (m). Note the bladder invasion (*arrows*) (bladder).
(From Grainger RG, Allison D: Grainger and Allison's Diagnostic Radiology, A Textbook of Medical Imaging, 4th ed. Edinburgh, Churchill Livingstone, 2001.)

UTERUS

Chapter 243 | Uterine prolapse

DEFINITION

Uterine prolapse refers to the protrusion of the uterus into or out of the vaginal canal (Fig. 243–1). In a *first-degree uterine prolapse*, the cervix is visible when the perineum is depressed. In a *second-degree uterine prolapse*, the uterine cervix has prolapsed through the vaginal introitus, with the fundus remaining within the pelvis proper. In a *third-degree uterine prolapse* (i.e., *complete uterine prolapse, uterine procidentia*), the entire uterus is outside the introitus (Fig. 243–2).

PHYSICAL FINDINGS AND CLINICAL PRESENTATION

- Pelvic pressure
- Bearing-down sensation
- Bilateral groin pain
- Sacral backache
- Coital difficulty
- Protrusion from vagina
- Spotting
- Ulceration of cervix
- Vaginal bleeding
- Examination of patient in lithotomy, sitting, and standing positions and before, during, and after a maximum Valsalva effort
- Erosion or ulceration of the cervix possible in the most dependent area of the protrusion

CAUSE

- Vaginal childbirth and chronic increases in intra-abdominal pressure leading to detachments, lacerations, and denervations of the vaginal support system
- Further weakening of pelvic support system by hypoestrogenic atrophy
- Some cases from congenital or inherited weaknesses within the pelvic support system
- Neonatal uterine prolapse mostly coexistent with congenital spinal defects

DIFFERENTIAL DIAGNOSIS

- Occasionally, elongated cervix; body of the uterus remains undescended.
- Diagnosis is based on history and physical examination. Currently, there is only one genital tract prolapse classification system that has attained international acceptance AND recognition—the pelvic organ prolapse quantification (POPQ).

WORKUP

- If erosion or ulceration of the cervix is present, a Pap smear followed by a cervical biopsy should be performed if indicated.
- If urinary symptoms are significant, further urodynamic workup is indicated, looking for concurrent cystourethrocele, cystocele, enterocele, or rectocele.

LABORATORY TESTS

Urine culture

IMAGING STUDIES

Ultrasound if concurrent fibroids need further evaluation

TREATMENT

- Prophylactic measures
  1. Diagnosis and treatment of chronic respiratory (chronic cough) and metabolic (obesity) disorders
  2. Correction of constipation
  3. Weight control, nutrition, and smoking cessation counseling
  4. Teaching of pelvic muscle exercises

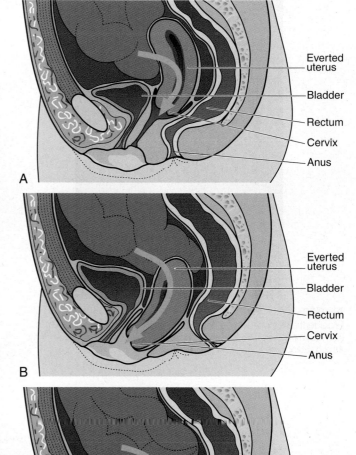

Fig 243–1
Uterine prolapse. (**A**) First-degree, (**B**) second-degree, and (**C**) third-degree prolapse.
(From Drife J, Magowan B: Clinical Obstetrics and Gynaecology. Edinburgh, WB Saunders, 2004.)

- Supportive pessary therapy (Fig. 243–3)
  1. Ring-type pessary (Fig. 243–4) useful for first- or second-degree prolapse
  2. Gellhorn pessary preferred for more advanced prolapse
  3. Use of pessaries in conjunction with continuous hormone replacement therapy, unless contraindicated
  4. Perineorrhaphy under local anesthesia possibly needed to support the pessary if the vaginal outlet is very relaxed
- Hormone replacement therapy at the time of menopause helps preserve tissue strength, maintain elasticity of the vagina, and promote the durability of surgical repairs.
- Gold standard for therapy is vaginal hysterectomy.

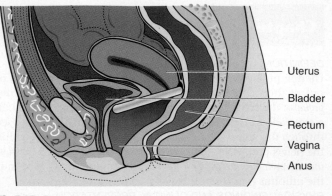

Fig 243–3
Ring pessary in situ. Note that the anterior vaginal wall is elevated to reduce the cystocele and the uterine prolapse has been corrected. (From Drife J, Magowan B: Clinical Obstetrics and Gynaecology, Edinburgh, WB Saunders, 2004)

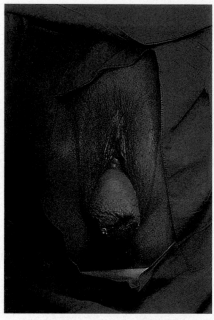

Fig 243–2
Procidentia: a third-degree prolapse of the uterus and vaginal walls. (From Symonds EM, Symonds IM: Essential Obstetrics and Gynaecology, 4th ed. Edinburgh, Churchill Livingstone, 2004.)

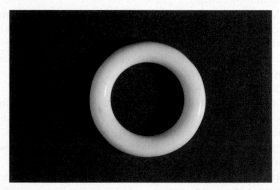

Fig 243–4
A vaginal ring pessary. (From Greer IA, Cameron IT, Kitchener HC, Prentice A: Mosby's Color Atlas and Text of Obstetrics and Gynaecology. London, Harcourt, 2001.)

Chapter 244 Uterine myomas

DEFINITION
Uterine myomas are benign tumors of muscle cell origin (Fig. 244–1). They are discrete nodular tumors that vary in size and number and that may be found subserosal, intramucosal, or submucosal within the uterus or may be found in the cervix or broad ligament or on a pedicle (Fig. 244–2).

PHYSICAL FINDINGS AND CLINICAL PRESENTATION
- Enlarged, irregular uterus on pelvic examination (Fig. 244–3)
- Presenting symptoms:
  1. Menorrhagia (most common)
  2. Chronic pelvic pain (dysmenorrhea, dyspareunia, pelvic pressure)
  3. Acute pain (torsion of pedunculated myoma, infarction, and degeneration)
  4. Urinary symptoms (frequency from bladder pressure, partial ureteral obstruction, complete ureteral obstruction)
  5. Rectosigmoid compression with constipation or intestinal obstruction
  6. Prolapse through cervix of pedunculated submucosal tumor
  7. Venous stasis of lower extremities
  8. Polycythemia
  9. Ascites

CAUSE
Incompletely understood. It is suggested that myomas arise from an original single smooth muscle cell in the myometrium. Each individual myoma is monoclonal. All the cells are derived from one progenitor myocyte. Malignant degeneration of preexisting leiomyoma is extremely uncommon (<0.5%).

DIFFERENTIAL DIAGNOSIS
Leiomyosarcoma, ovarian mass (neoplastic, nonneoplastic, endometrioma), inflammatory mass, pregnancy

WORKUP
- Complete pelvic examination, rectovaginal examination, Pap test
- Estimation of size of mass in centimeters
- Endometrial sampling may be indicated (biopsy or dilation and curettage [D&C]) when abnormal bleeding and pelvic mass are present

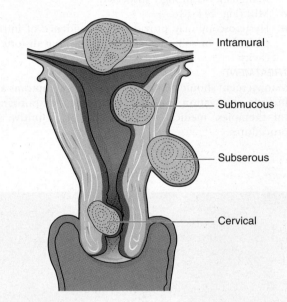

Fig 244–2
Sites of fibroids throughout the uterus.
(From Drife J, Magowan B: Clinical Obstetrics and Gynaecology, Edinburgh, WB Saunders, 2004)

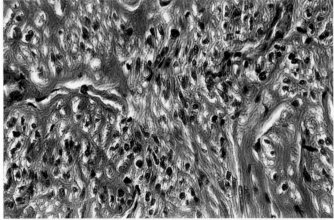

Fig 244–1
Leiomyoma. Uniform ovoid tumor cells in collagenous background.
(From Silverberg SG: Principles and Practice of Surgical Pathology and Cytopathology, 4th ed. Edinburgh, Churchill Livingstone, 2006.)

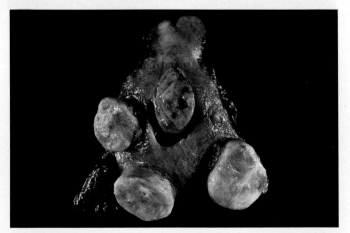

Fig 244–3
Leiomyomatous uterus. Three leiomyomas in this picture demonstrate the typical white, whorled cut surface and the tendency to pop up from the surrounding myometrium when cut. The intraluminal softer structure in the center is an endometrial polyp.
(From Silverberg SG: Principles and Practice of Surgical Pathology and Cytopathology, 4th ed. Edinburgh, Churchill Livingstone, 2006.)

- If urinary symptoms are prominent, cystometry, cystoscopy to rule out bladder lesions, intravenous pyelography (IVP) or urogram to rule out impingement on urinary system

LABORATORY TESTS
- Pregnancy test
- Pap smear
- CBC, erythrocyte sedimentation rate (ESR)
- Fecal occult blood

IMAGING STUDIES
- Pelvic ultrasound (transvaginal may have higher diagnostic accuracy) (Fig. 244–4)
- CT scan (Fig. 244–5) is helpful in planning treatment if malignancy is strongly suspected.
- MRI (Fig. 244–6)
- Hysteroscopy may provide direct evidence of intrauterine pathology or submucosal leiomyoma that distorts uterine cavity.

TREATMENT
Management should be based on primary symptoms and may include observation with close follow-up, temporizing surgical therapies, medical management, or definitive surgical procedures.

NONSURGICAL TREATMENT
- Patient observation and follow-up with periodic repeat pelvic examinations to ensure that tumors are not growing rapidly
- GnRH agonist use results in 40% to 60% reduction in uterine volume. Hypoestrogenism, reversible bone loss, hot flushes associated with use. Limit to short-term use and consider low-dose hormonal replacement to minimize hypoestrogenic effects.
- Regrowth occurs in about 50% of women treated a few months after cessation.
- Indications for GnRH:
  1. Fertility preservation in women with large myomas before attempting conception or preoperative myectomy treatment
  2. Anemia treatment to normalize hemoglobin before surgery
  3. Women approaching menopause to avoid surgery
  4. Preoperative for large myomas to make vaginal hysterectomy, hysteroscopic resection/ablation, or laparoscopic destruction more feasible
  5. Women with medical contraindications for surgery
  6. Personal or medical indications for delaying surgery
- Progestational agents may also result in decrease in uterine size and amenorrhea, allowing iron therapy to treat anemia with limited success.

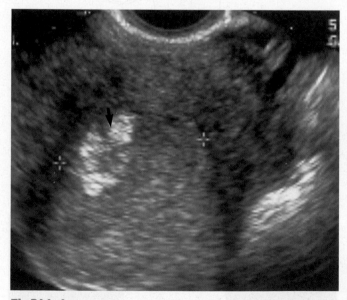

Fig 244–4
Transvaginal ultrasound of leiomyoma with calcifications (*arrow*). (From Grainger RG, Allison D: Grainger and Allison's Diagnostic Radiology, A Textbook of Medical Imaging, 4th ed. Edinburgh, Churchill Livingstone, 2001.)

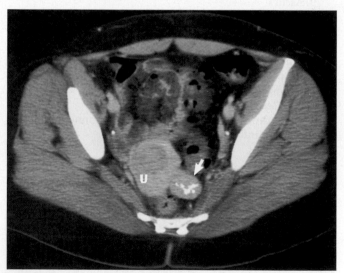

Fig 244–5
CT, calcified leiomyoma. A subserosal leiomyoma with calcifications (*arrow*) is shown on an axial CT scan (U, uterus). (From Grainger RG, Allison D: Grainger and Allison's Diagnostic Radiology, A Textbook of Medical Imaging, 4th ed. Edinburgh, Churchill Livingstone, 2001.)

SURGICAL TREATMENT
- Indications
  1. Abnormal uterine bleeding with anemia, refractory to hormonal therapy
  2. Chronic pain with severe dysmenorrhea, dyspareunia, or lower abdominal pressure/pain
  3. Acute pain, torsion, or prolapsing submucosal fibroid
  4. Urinary symptoms or signs such as hydronephrosis
  5. Rapid uterine enlargement premenopausal or any growth after menopause
  6. Infertility or recurrent pregnancy loss with leiomyoma as only finding
  7. Enlarged uterus with compression symptoms or discomfort
- Procedures
  1. Hysterectomy (definitive procedure)
  2. Abdominal myomectomy (to preserve fertility)
  3. Vaginal myomectomy for prolapsed pedunculated submucous fibroid
  4. Hysteroscopic resection
  5. Laparoscopic myomectomy
  6. Uterine fibroid embolization

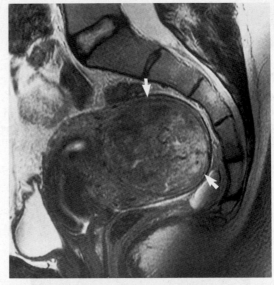

Fig 244–6
MRI of leiomyoma. T2-weighted sagittal MRI. A subserosal leiomyoma (*arrows*) distends the posterior aspect of the uterus, displacing the endometrium.
(From Grainger RG, Allison D: Grainger and Allison's Diagnostic Radiology, A Textbook of Medical Imaging, 4th ed. Edinburgh, Churchill Livingstone, 2001.)

Chapter 245 **Uterine polyps**

A. ENDOMETRIAL POLYPS

DEFINITION

Common benign localized growths of the endometrium consisting of a fibrous tissue core covered by columnar epithelium (Fig. 245–1)

CLINICAL PRESENTATION

Protrusion through the cervical os may be evident (Fig. 245–2). Endometrial polyps may be asymptomatic or may cause menorrhagia. Malignant transformation is rare.

TREATMENT

Surgical removal if symptomatic

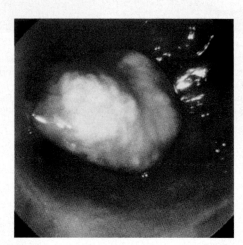

Fig 245–1
Hysteroscopic view of an intrauterine polyp.
Courtesy of Karl Storz Endoscopy (UK) Ltd.

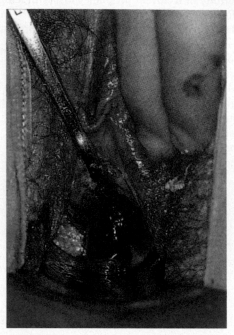

Fig 245–2
Endometrial polyp protruding through the cervical os.
(From Symonds EM, Symonds IM: Essential obstetrics and gynaecology, 4th ed. Edinburgh, Churchill Livingstone, 2004.)

Chapter 246 | Endometrial cancer

DEFINITION

Endometrial cancer is a malignant transformation of endometrial stroma and/or glands typified by irregular nuclear membranes, nuclear atypia, mitotic activity, loss of glandular pattern, irregular cell size (Fig. 246–1)

PHYSICAL FINDINGS AND CLINICAL PRESENTATION

- Abnormal uterine bleeding or postmenopausal bleeding in 90%
- Pyometra or hematometra
- Abnormal Pap smear

CAUSE

Endogenous or exogenous chronic unopposed estrogen stimulation of the endometrium

DIFFERENTIAL DIAGNOSIS

- Atypical hyperplasia
- Other genital tract malignancy (see Fig. 242–1)
- Polyps (see Fig. 245–1)
- Atrophic vaginitis (see Fig. 238–1)
- Granuloma cell tumor
- Fibroid uterus (see Fig. 244–3)

WORKUP

- Complete history and physical examination. Figure 246–2 shows a hysteroscopic view of an endometrial carcinoma.
- Endometrial biopsy or dilation and curettage (Fig. 246–3)

LABORATORY TESTS

- CBC
- Chemistry profile including liver function tests
- Consider CA-125 level

IMAGING STUDIES

- Chest x-ray
- Consider CT scan (Fig. 246–4), MRI (Fig. 246–5), and/or ultrasound (Fig. 246–6)
- Endovaginal ultrasound in postmenopausal women with vaginal bleeding

TREATMENT

- Surgery is the mainstay of treatment, with or without radiation, depending on tumor stage and grade.
- Surgery consists of pelvic washings, total abdominal hysterectomy and bilateral salpingo-oophorectomy, omental biopsy, and selective pelvic and periaortic lymphadenectomy, depending on stage and grade.
- Brachytherapy and/or teletherapy are added in an advanced stage.
- Chemotherapy (cisplatin, Adriamycin) or tamoxifen may also be used.

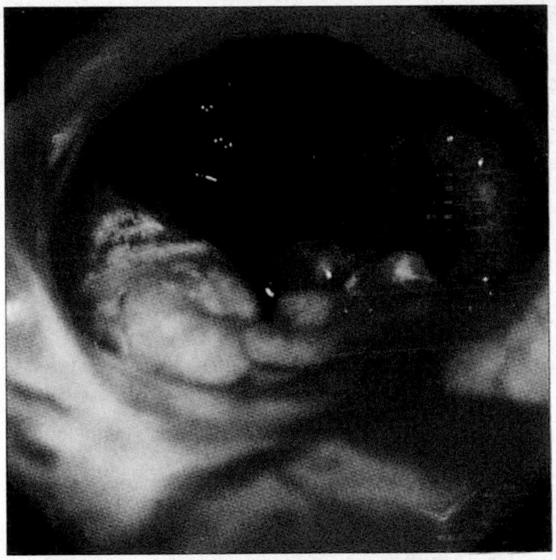

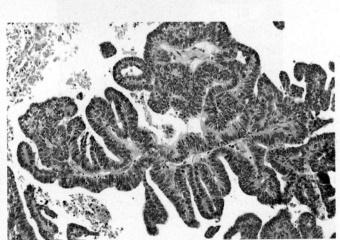

Fig 246–2
A hysteroscopic view of an endometrial carcinoma arising from the posterior uterine wall. [Courtesy of Karl Storz Endoscopy (UK) Ltd.]

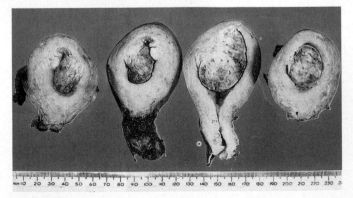

Fig 246–1
Endometrial adenocarcinoma. Multiple sections showing a large endometrial carcinoma invading the substance of the myometrium.
(From Symonds EM, Symonds IM: Essential obstetrics and gynaecology, 4th ed. Edinburgh, Churchill Livingstone, 2004)

Fig 246–3
Endometrioid adenocarcinoma, villoglandular pattern. The papillae in this field are lined by endometrioid-type cells, with ovoid nuclei parallel to one another and perpendicular to the basement membrane.
(From Silverberg SG: Principles and Practice of Surgical Pathology and Cytopathology, 4th ed. Edinburgh, Churchill Livingstone, 2006.)

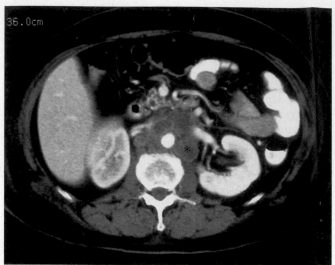

Fig 246-4

Para-aortic lymphadenopathy in a patient with endometrial cancer. Involvement of lymph nodes by tumor relies on size criteria.
(From Grainger RG, Allison D: Grainger and Allison's Diagnostic Radiology, A Textbook of Medical Imaging, 4th ed. Edinburgh, Churchill Livingstone, 2001.)

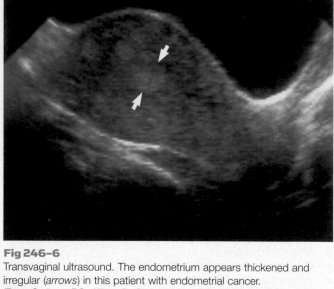

Fig 246-6

Transvaginal ultrasound. The endometrium appears thickened and irregular (*arrows*) in this patient with endometrial cancer.
(From Grainger RG, Allison D: Grainger and Allison's Diagnostic Radiology, A Textbook of Medical Imaging, 4th ed. Edinburgh, Churchill Livingstone, 2001.)

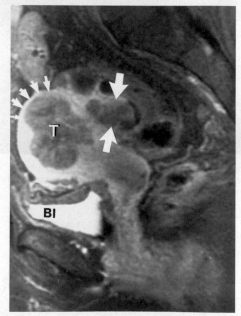

Fig 246-5

Endometrial carcinoma. The sagittal gadolinium-enhanced T1-weighted fat-suppressed spoiled GRE MR image shows an endometrial cancer (T) with deep myometrial invasion. Note the thin rim of normal myometrium (*small arrows*). The disease extends to the adnexae (*large arrows*) (Bl, bladder).
(From Grainger RG, Allison D: Grainger and Allison's Diagnostic Radiology, A Textbook of Medical Imaging, 4th ed. Edinburgh, Churchill Livingstone, 2001.)

OVARIES

Chapter 247 Benign ovarian lesions

DEFINITION
Benign ovarian lesions are clinically indistinguishable from their malignant counterparts. Therefore, all persistent adnexal masses must be considered malignant until proved otherwise.
- Non-neoplastic tumors are as follows:
  - Germinal inclusion cyst
  - Follicle cyst
  - Corpus luteum cyst
  - Pregnancy luteoma
  - Theca lutein cysts
  - Sclerocystic ovaries
  - Endometrioma
- Neoplastic tumors that are derived from coelomic epithelium are as follows:
  - Cystic tumors: serous cystoma, mucinous cystoma, mixed forms
  - Tumors with stromal overgrowth: fibroma, adenofibroma, Brenner tumor
  - Tumors derived from germ cells are dermoids (benign cystic teratomas)

PHYSICAL FINDINGS AND CLINICAL PRESENTATION
- Usually asymptomatic
- Pelvic pain/pressure
- Dyspareunia
- Abdominal pain ranging from mild to severe peritoneal irritation
- Increasing abdominal girth/distention
- Adnexal mass of pelvic examination
- Children: abdominal/rectal mass

CAUSE
- Physiologic
- Endometriosis
- Unknown

DIFFERENTIAL DIAGNOSIS
- Ovarian torsion
- Malignancy: ovary (see Fig. 249–1), fallopian tube, colon
- Uterine fibroid (see Fig. 244–4)
- Diverticular abscess/diverticulitis
- Appendiceal abscess/appendicitis (especially in children)
- Tuboovarian abscess
- Paraovarian cyst
- Distended bladder
- Pelvic kidney
- Ectopic pregnancy (see Fig. 258–2)
- Retroperitoneal cyst/neoplasm

WORKUP
- Complete history and physical examination
- Pelvic examination/rectovaginal examination may reveal firm, irregular, mobile mass
- Laparoscopy/laparotomy to establish diagnosis

LABORATORY TESTS
- Pregnancy test
- Serum tumor markers:
  1. CA–125
  2. α-Fetoprotein (AFP) (endodermal sinus tumor, immature teratoma)
  3. β-Human chorionic gonadotropin (hCG)
  4. Lactic dehydrogenase (LDH) (dysgerminoma)

IMAGING STUDIES
Ultrasound (Fig. 247–1)
- May differentiate adnexal mass from other pelvic masses
- Features that increase risk of malignancy include solid component, papillae, multiple septations/solitary thick septa, ascites, matted bowel, bilaterality, irregular borders
- CT scan with contrast
- Colonoscopy/barium enema, if symptomatic

TREATMENT
Indications for surgery
- Postmenopausal or premenarcheal palpable adnexal mass
- Adnexal mass with suspicious ultrasound features
- Premenopausal woman with persistent cyst >5 cm
- Any adnexal mass >10 cm
- Suspected torsion or rupture

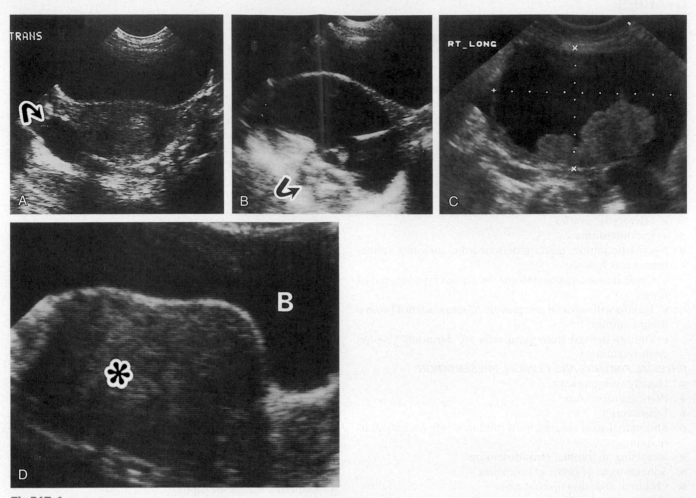

Fig 247–1
Pelvic masses as depicted by TAS. (**A**) Physiologic ovarian cyst arising from the right ovary (*arrow*). (**B**) Dermoid cyst with echogenic component (*arrow*) and a septum. (**C**) Ovarian carcinoma (between *crosses*) containing irregular solid areas. (**D**) Fundal fibroid causing significant enlargement of the uterine outline. B = maternal bladder.
(From Grainger RG, Allison D: Grainger and Allison's Diagnostic Radiology, A Textbook of Medical Imaging, 4th ed. Edinburgh, Churchill Livingstone, 2001.)

Chapter 248 | Polycystic ovary syndrome

DEFINITION

Polycystic ovary syndrome (PCOS) in its complete form associates polycystic ovaries (Figs. 248–1 and 248–2), amenorrhea, hirsutism, and obesity.

PHYSICAL FINDINGS AND CLINICAL PRESENTATION

- Oligomenorrhea or amenorrhea
- Dysfunctional uterine bleeding
- Infertility
- Hirsutism (Fig. 248–3)
- Acne
- Obesity (40% only)
- Insulin resistance (type 2 diabetes mellitus)

CAUSE AND PATHOGENESIS

Elevated serum luteinizing hormone (LH) concentrations and an increased serum LH:FSH ratio result either from an increased GnRH hypothalamic secretion or, less likely, from a primary pituitary abnormality. This results in dysregulation of androgen secretion and increased intraovarian androgen, the effect of which in the ovary is follicular atresia, maturation arrest, polycystic ovaries, and anovulation. Hyperinsulinemia is a contributing factor to ovarian hyperandrogenism, independent of LH excess. A role for insulin growth factor (IGF) receptors has been postulated for the association of PCOS and diabetes.

DIFFERENTIAL DIAGNOSIS

Causes of Amenorrhea

- Primary (unusual in PCOS)
  - Genetic disorder (Turner's syndrome)
  - Anatomic abnormality (e.g., imperforate hymen)
- Secondary
  - Pregnancy
  - Functional (cause unknown, anorexia nervosa, stress, excessive exercise, hyperthyroidism, less commonly hypothyroidism, adrenal dysfunction, pituitary dysfunction, severe systemic illness, drugs such as oral contraceptives, estrogens, or dopamine agonists)

- Abnormalities of the genital tract (uterine tumor, endometrial scarring, ovarian tumor)

LABORATORY TESTS

- Fasting blood glucose to rule out diabetes
- Elevated LH/FSH ratio >2.5
- Prolactin level elevation in 25%
- Elevated androgens (testosterone, DHEA-S)

IMAGING STUDIES

Pelvic ultrasound (Fig. 248–4) reveals the presence of a twofold to fivefold ovarian enlargement with a thickened tunica albuginea, thecal hyperplasia, and 20 or more subcapsular follicles from 1 to 15 mm in diameter.

TREATMENT

The goal is to interrupt the self-perpetuating abnormal hormone cycle:

- Reduction of ovarian androgen secretion by laparoscopic ovarian wedge resection
- Reduction of ovarian androgen secretion by using oral contraceptives or luteinizing hormone–releasing hormone (LH-RH) analogues
- Weight reduction for all obese women with PCOS
- FSH stimulation with clomiphene, or pulsatile LHRH
- Urofollitropin (pure FSH) administration
- Glitazones (e.g., rosiglitazone, pioglitazone) may improve ovulation and hirsutism in the polycystic ovary syndrome
- Metformin is also effective. It reduces insulin secretion and hyperandrogenemia and can restore ovulation in some women.

Choice of Treatment

- The management of hirsutism without risking pregnancy includes oral contraceptives, glucocorticoids, LHRH analogues, or spironolactone (an antiandrogen)

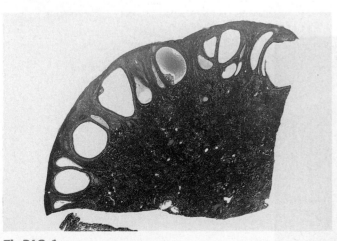

Fig 248–1
Polycystic ovary, showing uniiform cystic follicles in the cortex, prominent stroma, and absence of a corpus luteum or corpora albicantia.
(From Silverberg SG: Principles and Practice of Surgical Pathology and Cytopathology, 4th ed. Edinburgh, Churchill Livingstone, 2006.)

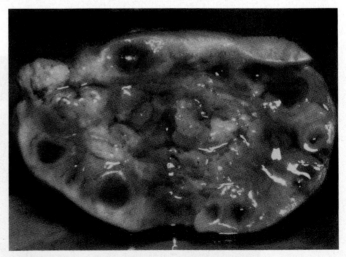

Fig 248–2
Section through a polycystic ovary. The ovary is enlarged and pearly white. The ovarian capsule is thickened.
(From Besser CM, Thorner MO: Comprehensive Clinical Endocrinology, 3rd ed. Mosby, 2002)

- Pregnancy can be achieved with clomiphene (alone or with glucocorticoids, hCG, or bromocriptine), HMG, urofollitropin, pulsatile LHRH, or ovarian wedge resection.
- Laparascopic ovarian diathermy (Fig. 248–5) is a useful alternative to gonadotropin therapy in women resistant to clomiphene and has been shown to be equally effective. It can be usually combined with laparoscopic assessment of the pelvis and tubal insufflation. It is unclear why destroying ovarian tissue, even just unilaterally, can restore ovulatory cycles in these women.

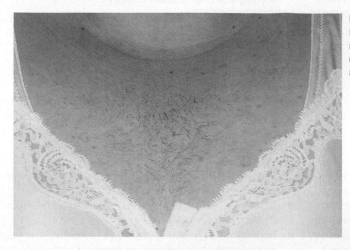

Fig 248–3
Increased hair growth in a patient with polycystic ovary syndrome.
(From Swartz MH: Textbook of Physical Diagnosis, 5th ed, Philadelphia, 2006, WB Saunders)

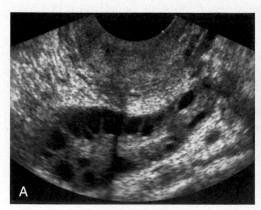
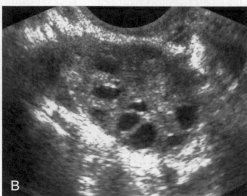

Fig 248–4
Polycystic ovary (PCO) disease. Coronal (**A**) and sagittal (**B**) transvaginal ultrasound shows enlarged ovaries ringed with follicles, the hallmark of PCO. Ovarian volumes of the right and left ovaries are also abnormally increased, 25 μL and 20 μL, respectively.
(Courtesy of Steven C. Horii, MD, Hospital of the University of Pennsylvania.)

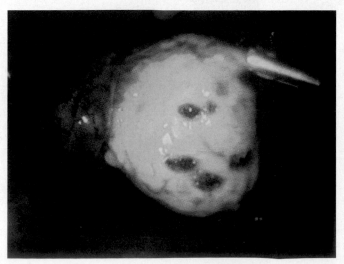

Fig 248–5
Laparoscopic ovarian diathermy.
(From Besser CM, Thorner MO: Comprehensive Clinical Endocrinology, 3rd ed. Mosby, 2002)

Chapter 249 | Ovarian cancer

DEFINITION

Ovarian tumors can be benign, requiring operative intervention but not recurring or metastasizing; malignant, recurring, metastasizing, and having decreased survival; or borderline, having a small risk of recurrence or metastases but generally having a good prognosis.

PHYSICAL FINDINGS AND CLINICAL PRESENTATION

- 60% of patients present with advanced disease
- Abdominal fullness, early satiety, dyspepsia
- Pelvic pain, back pain, constipation
- Pelvic or abdominal mass
- Lymphadenopathy (inguinal)
- Sister Mary Joseph nodule (umbilical mass)

CAUSE

- Can be inherited as site-specific familial ovarian cancer (two or more first-degree relatives have ovarian cancer)
- Breast-ovarian cancer syndrome (clusters of breast and ovarian cancer among first- and second-degree relatives)
- Lynch syndrome
- No family history and unknown etiology in the majority of ovarian cancer cases

DIFFERENTIAL DIAGNOSIS

- Primary peritoneal cancer
- Benign ovarian tumor (see Fig. 247–1B)
- Functional ovarian cyst (see Fig. 247–1A)
- Endometriosis (see Fig. 233–2)
- Ovarian torsion
- Pelvic kidney
- Pedunculated uterine fibroid (see Fig. 244–4)
- Primary cancer from breast, GI tract, or other pelvic organ metastasized to the ovary

LABORATORY TESTS

- CBC
- Chemistry profile
- CA-125 or lysophosphatidic acid level
- Consider: hCG, Inhibin, AFP, neuron-specific enolase (NSE), and LDH in patients at risk for germ cell tumors

IMAGING STUDIES

- Ultrasound (Fig. 249–1)
- Chest x-ray
- Mammogram
- CT scan to help evaluate extent of disease
- Other studies (MRI, BE [barium enema], IVP, etc.) as clinically indicated

TREATMENT

Virtually all cases of ovarian cancer involve surgical exploration. This includes:

- Abdominal cytology
- Total abdominal hysterectomy and bilateral salpingo-oophorectomy (except in early stages where fertility is an issue)
- Omentectomy
- Diaphragm sampling
- Selective lymphadenectomy (pelvis and paraaortic)
- Primary cytoreduction with a goal of residual tumor diameter <2 cm
- Bowel surgery, splenectomy if needed to obtain optimal (<2 cm) cytoreduction
- Optimal cytoreduction is generally followed by chemotherapy (except in some early-stage disease).
- Cisplatin-based combination chemotherapy (cisplatin, paclitaxel) is used for stage II or greater, 6-month treatment.
- Chemotherapy regimens continue to evolve as research continues.
- Consider second-look surgery when chemotherapy is complete.

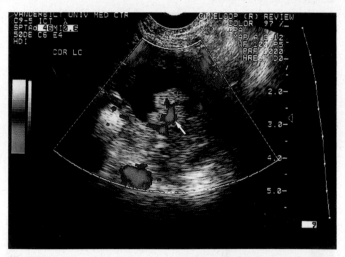

Fig 249–1
Ovarian carcinoma. Coronal transvaginal ultrasound shows a left ovarian cyst with a papillary projection. Central flow within the papillary projection (*arrow*) increases the likelihood of malignancy.
(Courtesy of Dr. Arthur Fleischer, MD, Vanderbilt University Medical Center.)

INFECTIONS

Chapter 250 Pelvic inflammatory disease

DEFINITION

PID is a spectrum of inflammatory disorders of the upper genital tract including a combination of any of the following:
- Endometritis, salpingitis (Fig. 250–1), tuboovarian abscess, or pelvic peritonitis
- Resulting from an ascending lower genital tract infection
- Not related to obstetric or surgical intervention

PHYSICAL FINDINGS AND CLINICAL PRESENTATION
- Lower abdominal pain
- Abnormal vaginal discharge
- Abnormal uterine bleeding
- Dysuria
- Dyspareunia
- Nausea and vomiting (suggestive of peritonitis)
- Fever
- Right upper quandrant (RUQ) tenderness (perihepatitis): 5% of PID cases
- Cervical motion tenderness and adnexal tenderness
- Adnexal mass
- Laparoscopy may reveal adhesions covering the tubes and ovaries in patients with chronic PID (Fig. 250–2)

CAUSE
- *Chlamydia trachomatis*
- *Neisseria gonorrhoeae*
- Polymicrobial infection—*Bacteroides fragilis, Escherichia coli, Gardnerella vaginalis, Haemophilus influenzae, Mycoplasma hominis, U. urealyticum*
- *Mycobacterium tuberculosis* (an important cause in developing countries)
- Cytomegalovirus (CMV)

DIFFERENTIAL DIAGNOSIS
- Ectopic pregnancy (see Fig. 258–2)
- Appendicitis
- Ruptured ovarian cyst
- Endometriosis (see Fig. 233–2)
- Urinary tract infection (cystitis or pyelonephritis)
- Renal calculus
- Adnexal torsion
- Proctocolitis

LABORATORY TESTS
- CBC with differential: leukocytosis
- Elevated acute phase reactants: ESR >15 mm/hr, C-reactive protein
- Gram stain of endocervical exudate: >30 PMNs per high-power field correlates with chlamydial or gonococcal infection
- Endocervical cultures for *N. gonorrhoeae* and *C. trachomatis*
- Fallopian tube aspirate or peritoneal exudate culture if laparoscopy performed
- hCG to rule out ectopic pregnancy

IMAGING STUDIES
- Transvaginal ultrasound to look for adnexal mass has sensitivity for PID of 81%, specificity 78%, accuracy 80%.
- MRI has sensitivity for PID of 95%, specificity 89%, accuracy 93%. It is useful not only for establishing the diagnosis of PID, but also for detecting other processes responsible for the symptoms. Disadvantages are its higher cost and unavailability in certain areas.

TREATMENT
- Antibiotic treatment (e.g., ofloxacin with or without metronidazole as outpatient, cefoxitin plus doxycycline as inpatient). Most patients are treated as outpatients.
- Criteria for hospitalization (2002, Centers for Disease Control and Prevention) as follows:
  1. Surgical emergencies such as appendicitis cannot be excluded.
  2. Tuboovarian abscess
  3. Pregnant patient
  4. Patient is immunodeficient.
  5. Severe illness, nausea, or vomiting precluding outpatient management
  6. Patient unable to follow or tolerate outpatient regimens
  7. No clinical response to outpatient therapy

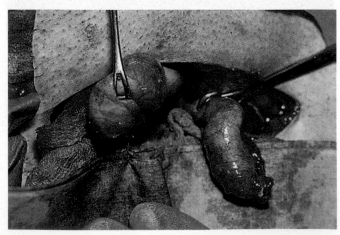

Fig 250–1
Acute salpingitis: the tubes are swollen and engorged.
(From Symonds EM, Symonds IM: Essential Obstetrics and Gynaecology, 4th ed. Edinburgh, Churchill Livingstone, 2004.)

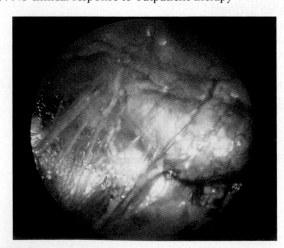

Fig 250–2
Chronic pelvic inflammatory disease: a sheet of fine adhesions covering the tubes and ovary, which is buried beneath the tube.
(From Symonds EM, Symonds IM: Essential Obstetrics and Gynaecology, 4th ed. Edinburgh, Churchill Livingstone, 2004.)

BREASTS

Chapter 251   Fibrocystic breast disease

DEFINITION
Fibrocystic breast disease (FCD) is a "nondisease" that includes nonmalignant breast lesions such as microcystic and macrocystic changes, fibrosis, ductal or lobular hyperplasia, adenosis, apocrine metaplasia, fibroadenoma, papilloma, papillomatosis, and other changes. Atypical ductal or lobular hyperplasia is associated with a moderate increase in breast cancer risk.

PHYSICAL FINDINGS AND CLINICAL PRESENTATION
- Tender breasts
- Nodular areas
- Dominant mass
- Thickening
- Nipple discharge
- Can vary with menstrual cycle

CAUSE
- Although frequently seen and diagnosed, mechanism of development not understood. Figure 251–1 shows a simplified anatomy of the female breast illustrating the major structural components and its corresponding sites of origin of potential lesions.
- Because found in majority of healthy breasts, regarded as nonpathologic process
- With hormone replacement therapy, may be carried into menopausal age

DIFFERENTIAL DIAGNOSIS
- If presenting as dominant mass or masses: exclude possible carcinoma.
- Carcinoma: detection is difficult with FCD, particularly among premenopausal women.
- If presenting with nipple discharge: differentiate from discharge of possible malignant origin (Paget's disease of breast [see Fig. 254–1]).

WORKUP
- Exclude breast carcinoma if breast mass, thickening, discharge, and pain present.
- Perform biopsy of suspected area for histologic confirmation.
- Figure 251–2 shows appearances of benign breast disease.
- An algorithm for the evaluation of a breast lump is shown in Figure 251–3.

IMAGING STUDIES
Mammography and ultrasound studies required:
- For mammographic changes (suspicious densities, microcalcifications, architectural distortion): careful evaluation, including possibly biopsy to exclude breast cancer
- Ultrasound study: to establish cystic nature of clinical or mammographic mass lesion

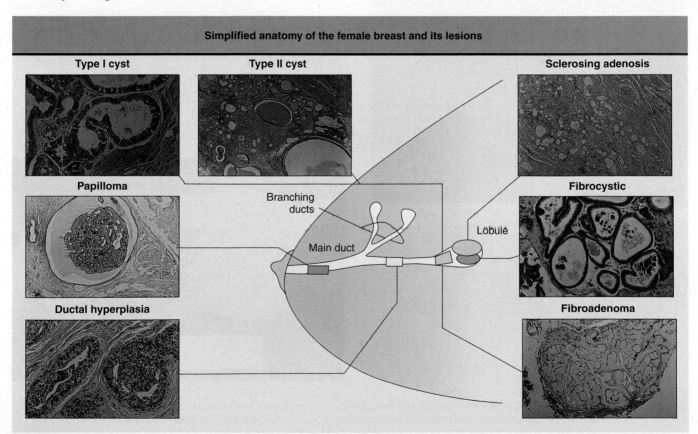

Simplified anatomy of the female breast and its lesions

Type I cyst | Type II cyst | Sclerosing adenosis | Papilloma | Fibrocystic | Ductal hyperplasia | Fibroadenoma

Branching ducts | Main duct | Lobule

Fig 251–1
Simplified anatomy of the female breast illustrating the major structural components and corresponding sites of origin of potential lesions. (From Besser CM, Thorner MO: Comprehensive Clinical Endocrinology, 3rd ed. St Louis, Mosby, 2002.)

TREATMENT

- Not considered a "disease" and does not require treatment
- Surgical intervention diagnostic to eliminate possibility of breast cancer
- Periodic physician examination to follow patients with FCD who have pronounced nodular features
- Aspiration for palpable cysts. (*Note:* Cysts often recur; repeat aspiration is not always required unless pain is a problem.)

For Breast Pain

- Danocrine (Danazol): limited success reported
- Bromocriptine or tamoxifen: used less frequently
- Limited caffeine intake: generally not as successful in controlling pain or nodularity as originally suggested

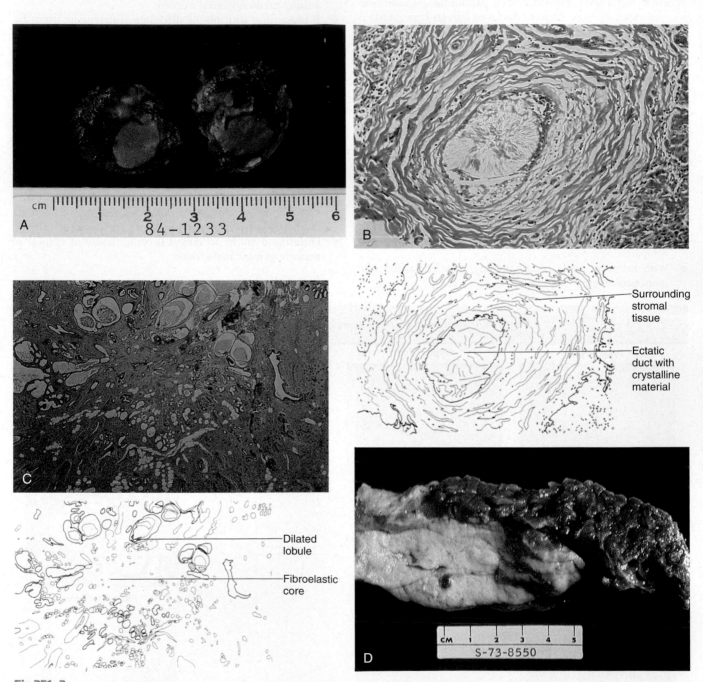

Fig 251–2

Appearances of benign disease. (**A**) Gross appearance of duct ectasia showing a single duct dilated by homogeneous yellow-orange fluid, probably lipid in composition. (**B**) Histologic appearance of duct ectasia showing the characteristic crystalline formation of the intraluminal contents. (**C**) Radial scar demonstrating a central fibroelastic core and peripherally radiating lobules, some of which are typically dilated, as in this example. (**D**) Gross changes with fibrocystic disease showing marked fibrosis and scattered cysts. An area of normal breast tissue is shown in the upper right hand portion of the breast.

(From Besser CM, Thorner MO: Comprehensive Clinical Endocrinology, 3rd ed. St Louis, Mosby, 2002.)

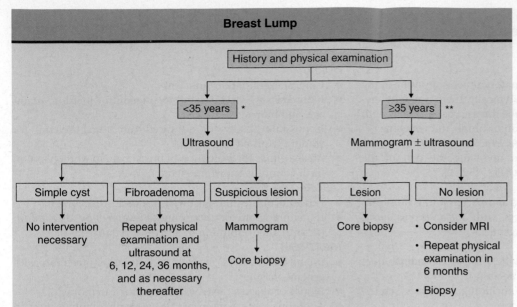

Fig 251–3
Breast lump. Algorithm for evaluation and treatment. With a family history of breast cancer that increases risk, a mammogram ± ultrasound should be performed and biopsy considered even with negative imaging study. Palpable lesions require biopsy even with negative imaging studies. Neoplasms such as invasive lobular carcinoma may be palpable but not seen on mammography or ultrasound. MRI, magnetic resonance imaging.
(From Besser CM, Thorner MO: Comprehensive Clinical Endocrinology, 3rd ed. St Louis, Mosby, 2002.)

Chapter 252 / Breast abscess

DEFINITION
Breast abscess is an acute inflammatory process resulting in the formation of a collection of pus. Typically, there is painful erythematous mass formation in the breast, occasionally with draining through the overlying skin or nipple duct opening.

PHYSICAL FINDINGS AND CLINICAL PRESENTATION
Painful erythematous induration involving the part of the breast leading to fluctuant abscess (Fig. 252–1)

CAUSE
- Lactational abscess: milk stasis and bacterial infection leading to mastitis, then to abscess, with *Staphylococcus aureus* the most common causative agent
- Subareolar abscess:
  1. Central ducts involved, with obstructive nipple duct changes leading to bacterial infection
  2. Cultured organisms mixed, including anaerobes, staphylococci, streptococci, and others

DIFFERENTIAL DIAGNOSIS
- Inflammatory carcinoma (see Fig. 254–1)
- Advanced carcinoma with erythema, edema, and/or ulceration (see Fig. 253–4)
- Rarely, tuberculous abscess
- Hydradenitis of breast skin
- Sebaceous cyst with infection

WORKUP
- Clinical examination sufficient
- If abscess suspected, referral to surgeon for incision, drainage, and biopsy.
- If possible abscess or advanced carcinoma, referral for workup required
- An algorithm for evaluation of breast pain in women not on birth control is shown in Figure 252–2.

LABORATORY TESTS
- Perform culture and sensitivity test of abscess contents.
- If mammogram or ultrasound prevented by discomfort, perform after resolution of abscess if required.

TREATMENT
- Established abscess: incision and drainage, preferably with general anesthesia
- Biopsy of abscess cavity wall to exclude carcinoma
- Antibiotics: the pathogens are generally staphylococci in lactational abscess. Recommended initial antibiotic therapy is nafcillin or oxacillin or cefazolin for 10 to 14 days.
- If acute mastitis is treated early, resolution without drainage is possible.
- Subareolar abscess: broad-spectrum antibiotic treatment (e.g., cephalexin PO or cefazolin IV for 10 to 14 days for more severe infection) and drainage are needed to control acute phase.

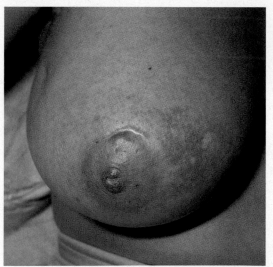

Fig 252–1
Erythema of the breast.
(From Swartz MH: Textbook of Physical Diagnosis, 5th ed, Philadelphia, 2006, WB Saunders.)

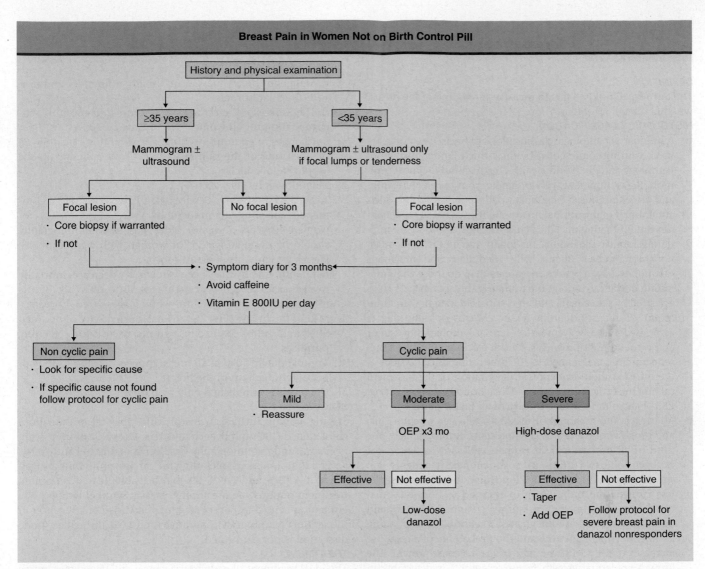

Breast Pain in Women Not on Birth Control Pill

History and physical examination

≥35 years → Mammogram ± ultrasound

<35 years → Mammogram ± ultrasound only if focal lumps or tenderness

Focal lesion
· Core biopsy if warranted
· If not

No focal lesion

Focal lesion
· Core biopsy if warranted
· If not

· Symptom diary for 3 months
· Avoid caffeine
· Vitamin E 800IU per day

Non cyclic pain
· Look for specific cause
· If specific cause not found follow protocol for cyclic pain

Cyclic pain

Mild
· Reassure

Moderate
OEP x3 mo

Effective

Not effective
Low-dose danazol

Severe
High-dose danazol

Effective
· Taper
· Add OEP

Not effective
Follow protocol for severe breast pain in danazol nonresponders

Fig 252–2

Breast pain in women not on birth control pill. Algorithm for evaluation and treatment of breast pain in premenopausal women not on birth control pills. Avoidance of caffeine and use of Vitamin E are suggested even though these strategies have not been proved to be effective. Vitamin E probably acts as a placebo, which is 30% effective in this setting. Avoidance of caffeine may benefit some patients according to anecdotal reports and is not harmful. OEP, oil of evening primrose.

(From Besser CM, Thorner MO: Comprehensive Clinical Endocrinology, 3rd ed. St Louis, Mosby, 2002.)

Chapter 253 | Breast cancer

DEFINITION

The term *breast cancer* refers to invasive carcinoma of the breast, whether ductal or lobular.

HISTOLOGIC CLASSIFICATION

- A number of pathologic classifications of breast carcinoma are used, with those presented by the Armed Forces Institute of Pathology and the World Health Organization the most common. Breast tumors usually originate from breast epithelium and are either ductal or lobular, corresponding to the ducts and lobules of the normal breast. Eighty percent of malignancies are infiltrating ductal carcinomas, less common are infiltrating lobular carcinoma, medullary carcinoma, and mucinous carcinoma. Patients with medullary and mucinous carcinomas have a better survival rate than do those with infiltrating ductal carcinoma. Inflammatory breast cancer is characterized by skin edema and an erysipeloid margin with induration of the surrounding tissue. Microscopically, this is associated with involvement of dermal lymphatics by tumor and carries a poor prognosis. Ductal carcinoma in situ represents carcinoma confined to the preexisting ductal system of the breast without evidence of penetration of the basement membrane by light microscopy. Ductal carcinoma in situ (Fig. 253–1) accounts for 10% to 15% of all breast cancers.

- All breast cancers should be tested for estrogen receptor (ER) and progesterone receptor (PR) proteins. Approximately one third of all premenopausal women will show receptors for estrogen, and two thirds of postmenopausal patients will show receptors to estrogen. ER-positive tumors are usually less virulent and more likely to respond to hormonal manipulation (drug therapy or surgery). Tumors that contain both ERs and PRs have the greatest likelihood of responding to an endocrine maneuver, and the probability of a response increases directly with the titer of the receptor protein. The human epidermal growth factor receptor-2 is detectable in approximately 20% to 30% of breast cancers, and it is now frequently measured in tumor samples from patients with newly diagnosed breast cancer. Human epidermal growth factor receptor-2 is used as a prognostic indicator and may also be predictive of poor response to therapy.

- Fluorescent in situ hybridization (FISH) (Fig. 253–2) is a high-resolution technique that permits the detection of numerous chromosomal alterations in tissue sections or cytologic preparations. This approach is especially suitable in solid tumors and may be performed on metaphase spreads and nuclei in interphase (interphase cytogenetics). A major advantage of FISH over classic cytogenetic techniques is the ability to analyze intact, nondividing tumor cells. FISH is also cheaper and faster than cytogenetics and may be performed on paraffin-embedded tissue.

DIAGNOSIS

1. Breast self-examination and routine physician examination:
   a. Most breast cancers (90%) are discovered first by the woman herself or her sexual partner.
   b. Up to 10% of breast cancers may be clinically evident while mammographically occult

   c. Malignant breast masses are usually nontender and firm with irregular borders.
   d. The American Cancer Society recommends monthly self-examination for all women over the age of 20.
   e. Changes in contour, swelling, any dimpling (Fig. 253–3) or puckering of the skin (Fig. 253–4), or a change in the nipple are of concern.
2. Mammography (Fig. 253–5):
   a. The U.S. Preventive Services Task Force (USPSTF) recommends screening mammography every 1 to 2 years for women 40 years of age or older. Baseline mammography should be done at age 35 for women with significant risk factors for early-onset breast cancer.
   b. Mammography has been shown to decrease mortality from breast cancer for women ages 50 to 69 years, but its role remains controversial for women ages 40 to 49 years.
3. MRI of the breast (Fig. 253–6) has a sensitivity of between 90% and 100%. Its expense limits its use for screening purposes
4. Approximately 50% of all breast cancers develop in the upper outer quadrant of the breast.
5. Diagnosis is established only by biopsy.

STAGING

Staging workup includes a history and physical examination, chest x-ray, a CBC, and liver chemistries. The value of bone scan, liver scan, and mammography has been a matter of controversy. Several tumor markers, including the carcinoembryonic antigen (CEA), CA 15-3, and CA 27-29, may be valuable in determining treatment response and recurrent disease. Sentinel lymph node evaluation is used as part of staging of invasive breast cancer. If the sentinel lymph node is negative for tumor, the axillary node dissection is not performed.

TREATMENT

The ideal treatment of early breast cancer still generates controversy among physicians and patients, with factors such as patient age, cancer stage and prognosis, ER status, type of surgery, role of radiation therapy, need and type of chemotherapy, hormonal therapy, and length of treatment all contributing to the decision-making process.

Some treatment recommendations include the following:
1. Localized DCIS: lumpectomy followed by radiation and tamoxifen
2. Stages I and II: premenopausal (ER negative)
   a. Tumor size <1 cm: lumpectomy and local radiation
   b. Tumor size ≥1 cm: lumpectomy with axillary dissection, six cycles of chemotherapy followed by radiation
3. Stage I: premenopausal (ER positive)
   a. Tumor size <1 cm: lumpectomy, local radiation therapy, and hormonal therapy
   b. Tumor size >1 cm: lumpectomy, six cycles of chemotherapy with radiation and hormonal therapy
4. Stage II: premenopausal (ER negative)
   a. Lumpectomy with dissection and six cycles of chemotherapy and radiation
5. Stages I and II: postmenopausal (ER negative)

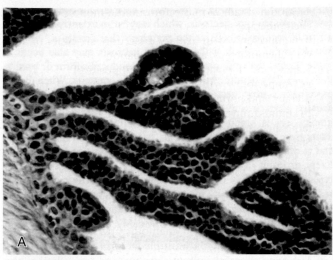

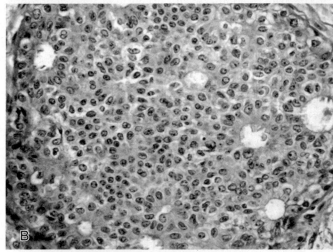

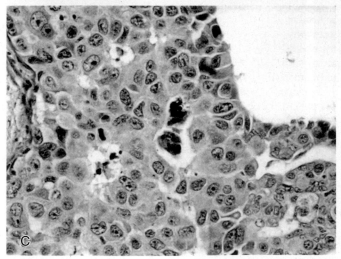

Fig 253–1
Nuclear grading in ductal carcinoma in situ. (**A**) Low nuclear grade.
(**B**) Intermediate nuclear grade. (**C**) High nuclear grade.
(From Silverberg SG: Principles and Practice of Surgical Pathology and
Cytopathology, 4th ed. Edinburgh, Churchill Livingstone, 2006.)

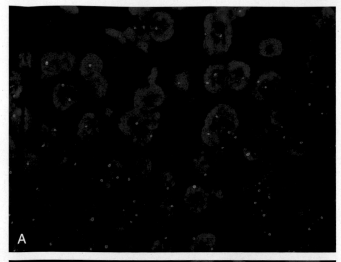

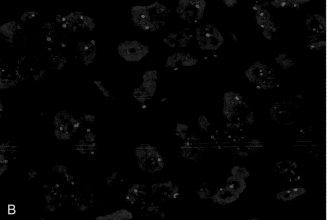

Fig 253–2
FISH. Formalin-fixed paraffin-embedded sections of invasive breast
carcinoma. The green signal represents a centromeric probe for
chromosome 17, whereas the red signal is the gene specific probe
for Her2/neu. (**A**) From a case with no evidence of amplification.
(**B**) Shows Her2/neu amplification.
(Courtesy of Dr. Umadevi Tantravahi, Director of Division of Genetics,
Women and Infants Hospital, Providence, RI.)

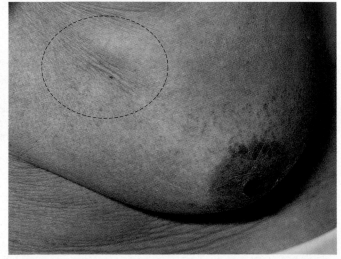

Fig 253–3
Breast carcinoma. Note dimpling of the breast and bloody nipple
discharge.
(From Swartz MH: Textbook of Physical Diagnosis, 5th ed, Philadelphia,
2006, WB Saunders.)

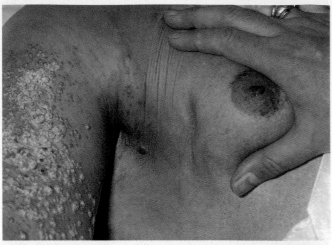

Fig 253–4
Breast dimpling. Note the satellite skin lesions of metastatic breast cancer on the upper arm.
(From Swartz MH: Textbook of Physical Diagnosis, 5th ed, Philadelphia, 2006, WB Saunders.)

   a. Modified radical mastectomy and 6 months of adjuvant chemotherapy, *or*

   b. Lumpectomy with axillary dissection, six cycles of adjuvant chemotherapy, and local radiation

6. Stages I and II: postmenopausal (ER positive)

   a. Lumpectomy with axillary dissection, local radiation therapy, and hormonal therapy *or*

   b. Lumpectomy with axillary dissection, local radiation, and tamoxifen therapy

7. Stage III (locally advanced breast cancer)

   a. Induction chemotherapy followed by modified radical mastectomy followed by 1 to 2 additional years of chemotherapy, *or*

   b. Induction chemotherapy followed by primary radiation followed by 1 to 2 additional years of chemotherapy

8. Stage IV disease: systemic chemotherapy, hormonal therapy, or both, depending on multiple factors

9. The main chemotherapeutic agents used are cyclophosphamide, methotrexate, and 5-fluorouracil (CMF) or doxorubicin substituted for methotrexate (CAF); other useful drugs

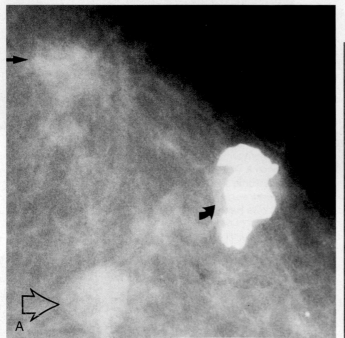
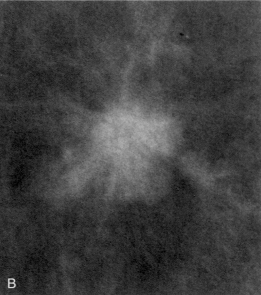

Fig 253–5
Nonmagnified image (**A**) shows lobulated mass (*arrow*) with partially defined borders. Just below this is a circumscribed mass (*open arrow*), most probably a cyst or noncalcified fibroadenoma. Another mass containing coarse calcifications typical of fibroadenoma is present on right (*solid curved arrow*). Magnified image (**B**) of the mass (*straight arrow* in A), which was partially defined on the nonmagnified view shows spiculation indicative of an infiltrating carcinoma.
(From Grainger RG, Allison D: Grainger and Allison's Diagnostic Radiology, A Textbook of Medical Imaging, 4th ed. Edinburgh, Churchill Livingstone, 2001.)

include paclitaxel, docetaxel, vinorelbine, vincristine, vinblastine, mitomycin C, thiotepa, gemcitabine, and cisplatin. Trastuzumab, a monoclonal antibody targeting the extracellular domain of the HER2 protein when combined with paclitaxel after doxorubicin and cyclophosphamide, improves outcomes among women with surgically removed HER2-ositive breast cancer.

10. The main hormonal agents used include tamoxifen, toremifene, megestrol acetate, exemestane, anastrozole, and letrozole. All postmenopausal women with hormone receptor–positive breast cancer benefit from adjuvant tamoxifen therapy regardless of age, tumor stage, or grade. Tamoxifen decreases the risk of cancer recurrence by 47% and risk of death by 26%. If postmenopausal patients who are ER positive develop metastatic disease while on tamoxifen, they should be switched to an aromatase inhibitor. For patients who initially present with metastatic hormone receptor plus breast cancer, aromatase inhibitors are first line of treatment.

11. High-dose chemotherapy (HDCT) and autologous bone marrow transplantation in select patients have produced complete remission rates; duration of the response has not yet been convincingly demonstrated as prolonged, and the median follow-up time is still short. Studies have generally failed to show any significant benefits of bone marrow transplantation over chemotherapy alone.

12. Bisphosphonates (pamidronate) in monthly infusions may decrease the complications and morbidity of skeletal metastases.

13. The use of trastuzumab (Herceptin) in patients whose tumor overexpresses the HER-2 protein has a significant role in treatment of patients with HER2-positive disease. It should however not be used concurrently with anthracyclines because of an increased risk of cardiac toxicity (increased risk of congestive heart failure).

14. Aromatase inhibitors (anastrozole and letrozole) have been shown to be useful in metastatic breast cancer and may also play a role in the treatment of early breast cancer. They function by blocking estrogen synthesis in ER-positive tumors. The aromatase inhibitor letrozole has also been reported to be more effective treatment for metastatic breast cancer and more effective in the neoadjuvant setting than tamoxifen

15. The prophylactic use of tamoxifen may decrease the risk of developing breast cancer by 50%. For postmenopausal women with hormonally responsive tumor using an aromatase inhibitor or switching to an aromatase inhibitor after 2 to 3 years of tamoxifen use improves disease-free survival compared with 5 years of tamoxifen use.

16. Prophylactic bilateral mastectomy reduces the risk of breast cancer development by approximately 90%, and oophorectomy reduces the risk of breast cancer by 50% if performed before menopause in high-risk women (those carrying *BRCA* mutations).

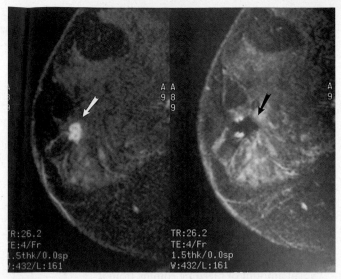

Fig 253–6

MRI-guided wire localization. Images of a patient with malignant axillary adenopathy and unknown primary. Sagittal, fat-expressed contrast-enhanced three-dimensional fast-spin PGR MRI reveals a peripherally enhancing lesion (*arrow* in left image) localized by an MRI-compatible needle (*arrow* in right image). Invasive ductal carcinoma was found at excisional biopsy.
(From Grainger RG, Allison D: Grainger and Allison's Diagnostic Radiology, A Textbook of Medical Imaging, 4th ed. Edinburgh, Churchill Livingstone, 2001.)

a. Factors associated with increased probability of response to treatment
  i. Ambulatory status
  ii. Low number of sites of disease
  iii. High labeling indices
  iv. High thymidine kinase levels
  v. Presence of ERs and PRs

b. Factors associated with decreased probability of response
  i. Prior chemotherapy or radiotherapy
  ii. Presence of bone or liver metastases
  iii. Decreased lymphocyte count (immunocompromise)
  iv. High levels of cathepsin D in node-negative patients
  v. Obesity
  vi. High S phase (DNA synthesis)
  vii. Aneuploidy
  viii. Increased DNA content
  ix. Anaplastic nuclear grade

Chapter 254   Paget's disease of the breast

DEFINITION

Paget's disease of the breast is a malignant disease that presents itself as a scaly, sore, eroding, bleeding ulcer of the nipple. Microscopically, typical large clear cells (Paget's cells) with pale and abundant cytoplasm and hyperchromatic nuclei with prominent nucleoli are found in the epidermal layer. Paget's disease is more often associated with primary invasive or in situ carcinoma of the breast.

PHYSICAL FINDINGS AND CLINICAL PRESENTATION

- Variable
- Itching or burning nipple and/or reported lump
- Very minimal scaly lesion that may bleed when scales are lifted (Fig. 254–1)
- Typical ulcer located on nipple with serous fluid weeping or small amount of bleeding coming from it
- Palpable carcinoma in the breasts of some patients (Fig. 254–2)

CAUSE

- Exact origin unknown
- Possibly migration of either in situ or invasive carcinoma cells in breast to nipple skin to produce Paget's disease

DIFFERENTIAL DIAGNOSIS

- Chronic dermatitis
- Florid papillomatosis of the nipple or nipple adenoma
- Eczema

LABORATORY TESTS

- Biopsy of nipple lesion
- An algorithm foe evaluation and treatment of breast discharge is shown in Figure 254–3.

IMAGING STUDIES

- Mammograms and sonography to search for possible primary carcinoma

TREATMENT

- Fewer patients:
  1. Paget's disease of nipple only finding when mammographically negative breast
  2. Consideration of wide excision of nipple with or without radiation
- Other patients: additional invasive or in situ carcinoma recognized
- Either modified mastectomy or breast conservation treatment
- Presence of underlying in situ or invasive carcinoma in mastectomy specimen of majority of patients
- Systemic adjuvant therapy, depending on extent of invasive carcinoma found

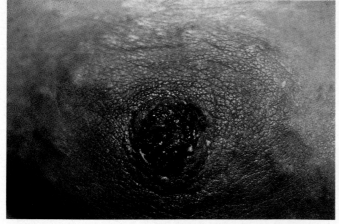

Fig 254–1
Mammary Paget's disease: the nipple shows erythema and erosion.
(Courtesy of the Institute of Dermatology. London, UK.)

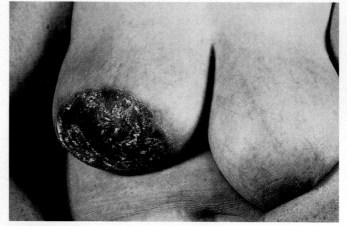

Fig 254–2
Mammary Paget's disease: this patient showed very extensive involvement with crusting of the nipple and areola.
(Courtesy of the Institute of Dermatology. London, UK.)

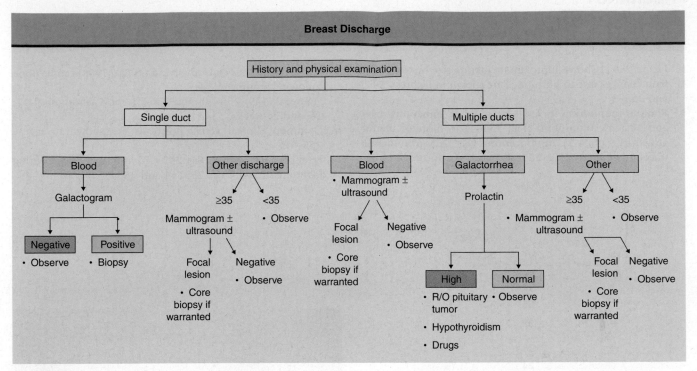

Fig 254–3
Breast discharge. Algorithm for evaluation and treatment. R/O, rule out.
(From Besser CM, Thorner MO: Comprehensive Clinical Endocrinology, 3rd ed. St Louis, Mosby, 2002.)

PREGNANCY

Chapter 255 | **Physiologic changes and prenatal monitoring**

- Figure 255–1 shows approximate uterine size by week.
- Skin changes due to hormones are shown in Figures 255–2 and 255–3.
- Routine monitoring includes periodic examinations, labs, and obstetric ultrasound (Fig. 255–4) to monitor uterine growth (Fig. 255–5). Amniocentesis (Fig. 255–6) under ultrasound guidance (Fig. 255–7) may be performed in high-

risk pregnancies. Fetal karyotyping (Fig. 255–8) can be done following amniocentesis.
- Figures 255–9, 255–10, and 255–11 show gestation at 12, 16, and 24 weeks.
- Common clinical vertex positions are shown in Figure 255–12.
- Fetal blood sampling (Fig. 255–13) and monitoring during labor are shown (Figs. 255–14 and 255–15).

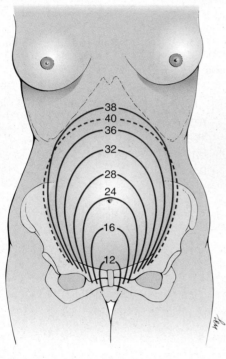

Fig 255–1
Approximate uterine size by week.
(From Swartz MH: Textbook of Physical Diagnosis, 5th ed. Philadelphia, 2006, WB Saunders.)

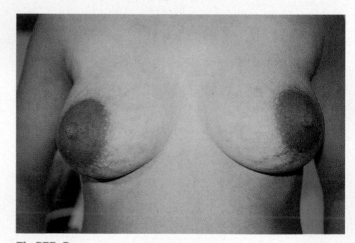

Fig 255–2
Striae gravidarum of the breasts. Note also the marked pigmentation of the areolae.
(From Swartz MH: Textbook of Physical Diagnosis, 5th ed. Philadelphia, 2006, WB Saunders.)

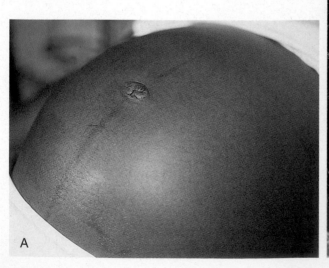

A

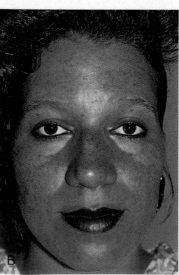

B

Fig 255–3
Skin changes due to high levels of ovarian, placental, and pituitary hormones. **A**, Linea nigra. **B**, Chloasma.
(From Swartz MH: Textbook of Physical Diagnosis, 5th ed. Philadelphia, 2006, WB Saunders.)

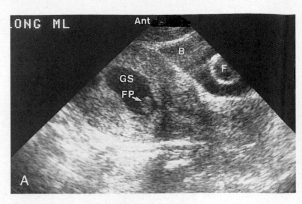
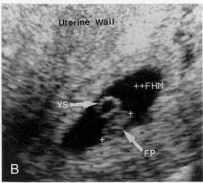

Fig 255-4
Early normal obstetric ultrasound image. A longitudinal transabdominal ultrasound image (**A**) demonstrates the bladder (**B**) and a Foley catheter (F) within it. Superior to and behind the bladder is the uterus with a gestational sac (GS) centrally and a fetal pole (FP) within it. More detail can be obtained using transvaginal ultrasound (**B**) imaging. In this case, the fetal pole (FP) can be measured; a yolk sac (YS) is also seen. The technician has indicated that fetal heart motion was seen (+ + FHM).
(From Mettler FA, Guibertau MJ, Voss CM, Urbina, CE: Primary Care Radiology, Philadelphia, Elsevier, 2000.)

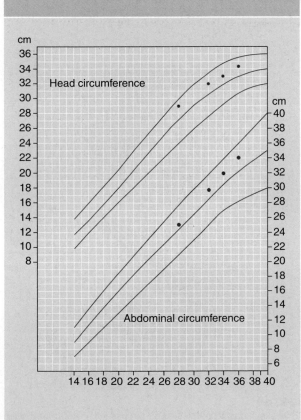

Fig 255-5
Ultrasound growth chart illustrating normal fetal growth in the third trimester on measurement of abdominal circumference and head circumference (lines on the circumference charts indicate mean ± 2 standard deviations).
(From Greer IA, Cameron IT, Kitchener HC, Prentice A: Mosby's Color Atlas and Text of Obstetrics and Gynaecology. London, Harcourt, 2001.)

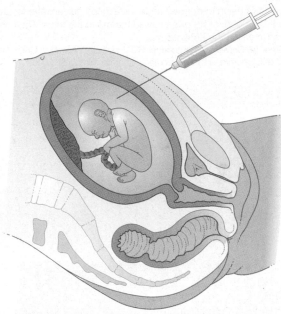

Fig 255-6
Amniotic fluid obtained by the procedure of amniocentesis by inserting a needle into the amniotic sac under ultrasound guidance, avoiding the placenta where possible.
(From Symonds EM, Symonds IM: Essential Obstetrics and Gynaecology, 4th ed. Edinburgh, Churchill Livingstone, 2004.)

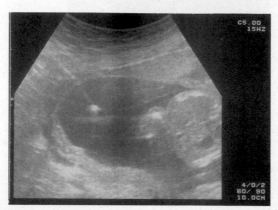

Fig 255–7
Amniocentesis being performed under ultrasound guidance to locate the needle in a pool of liquor and avoid trauma to the fetus. The needle can be seen within the amniotic sac.
(From Greer IA, Cameron IT, Kitchener HC, Prentice A: Mosby's Color Atlas and Text of Obstetrics and Gynaecology. London, Harcourt, 2001.)

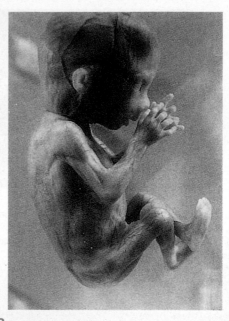

Fig 255–9
At 12 weeks of gestation, the fetus reacts to stimuli. The upper limbs reach their final relative length and the sex of the fetus is distinguishable externally.
(From Symonds EM, Symonds IM: Essential Obstetrics and Gynaecology, 4th ed. Edinburgh, Churchill Livingstone, 2004.)

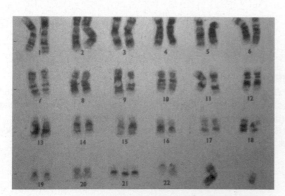

Fig 255–8
Fetal karyotype obtained following amniocentesis precipitated by abnormal "triple test." The karyotype is 47XY with an additional chromosome 21. The fetus has Down syndrome.
(From Greer IA, Cameron IT, Kitchener HC, Prentice A: Mosby's Color Atlas and Text of Obstetrics and Gynaecology. London, Harcourt, 2001.)

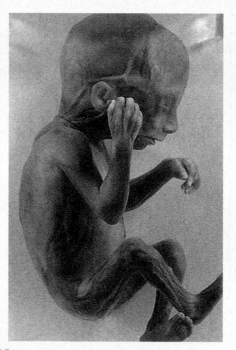

Fig 255–10
At 16 weeks of gestation, the crown–rump length is 122 mm. The lower limbs achieve their final relative length and the eyes face anteriorly.
(From Symonds EM, Symonds IM: Essential Obstetrics and Gynaecology, 4th ed. Edinburgh, Churchill Livingstone, 2004.)

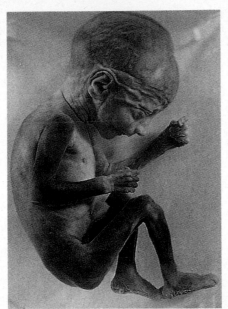

Fig 255–11
At 24 weeks of gestation, the fetal lungs start to secrete surfactant. The eyelids are separated and fine hair covers the body.
(From Symonds EM, Symonds IM: Essential Obstetrics and Gynaecology, 4th ed. Edinburgh, Churchill Livingstone, 2004.)

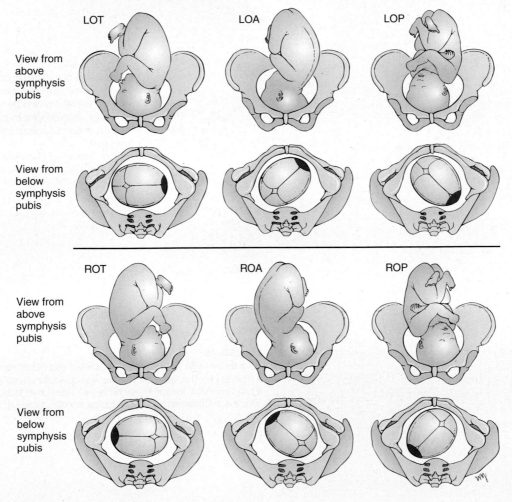

Fig 255–12
Common clinical vertex positions. For each position shown, the top diagram is the view from above the symphysis pubis; the bottom is the view from below the symphysis pubis. "Right" and "left" refer to the mother's side. "Anterior," "posterior," and "transverse" refer to the maternal pelvis. Highlighted area is the fetal occiput. LOA, left occiput anterior; LOP, left occiput posterior; LOT, left occiput transverse; ROA, right occiput anterior; ROP, right occiput posterior; ROT, right occiput transverse.
(From Swartz MH: Textbook of Physical Diagnosis, 5th ed. Philadelphia, 2006, WB Saunders.)

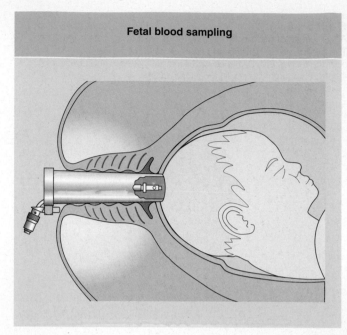

Fetal blood sampling

Fig 255–13
Fetal blood sampling. Amnioscope is inserted into the vagina, guided into the cervix by the examiner's fingers, and pressed against the presenting part. A small 2-mm-deep blade is used to puncture the fetal scalp.
(From Greer IA, Cameron IT, Kitchener HC, Prentice A: Mosby's Color Atlas and Text of Obstetrics and Gynaecology. London, Harcourt, 2001.)

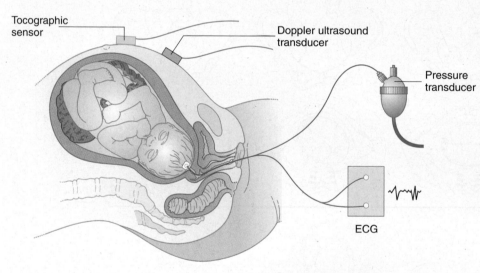

Tocographic sensor

Doppler ultrasound transducer

Pressure transducer

ECG

Fig 255–14
Monitoring during labor: contractions are recorded by intra- and extrauterine tocography; the fetal heart rate is recorded by Doppler ultrasonography or by direct application of an ECG electrode to the presenting part.
(From Symonds EM, Symonds IM: Essential Obstetrics and Gynaecology, 4th ed. Edinburgh, Churchill Livingstone, 2004.)

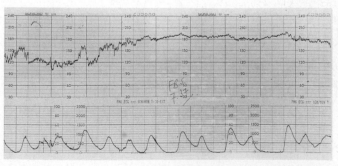

Fig 255–15
Fetal tachycardia and reduced variability. Fetal blood sampling showed a normal pH. The fetal tachycardia was due to maternal pyrexia.
(From Greer IA, Cameron IT, Kitchener HC, Prentice A: Mosby's Color Atlas and Text of Obstetrics and Gynaecology. London, Harcourt, 2001.)

Chapter 256 — Normal labor and delivery

DEFINITION

- Parturition is the process of giving birth. This process incorporates two major events: labor and delivery. Labor is defined as the progressive cervical dilation in response to repetitive uterine contractions. Delivery is the expulsion of the fetus as a result of uterine contractions and cervical dilation.
- The initiation and maintenance of labor are complex. Prostaglandins, cytokines, and sex-steroid hormones appear to play pivotal roles in this process.
- The gestational age is used to classify the type of delivery. Premature labor occurs before 37 weeks of gestation. A delivery before 24 weeks of gestation is referred to as an abortion. Term labor is defined as labor occurring after 37 weeks of gestation.

Initial Evaluation The initial evaluation should determine whether the woman is in labor and identify any conditions that will impact the labor and delivery process. A complete history and physical examination are required. Laboratory tests are also indicated before admission.

Labor See Figure 256–1.
Labor has traditionally been divided into three stages. The first stage is recognized from the onset of labor until complete cervical dilation. The second stage is defined from complete dilation until the delivery of the infant. The interval from delivery of the infant until the delivery of the placenta is known as the third stage. Some have attempted to add a fourth stage, defined as the first hour following the delivery of the placenta, which carries an increased risk of hemorrhage

1. Mechanism of labor
   a. During labor, the fetus undergoes certain movements to maneuver through the pelvis. These movements are known as the seven cardinal movements of labor. They consist of engagement, flexion, descent, internal rotation, extension, external rotation, and expulsion. These movements apply to both vertex and breech presentations. These movements allow the fetus to pass through the pelvis with the least resistance.
   b. Engagement occurs early in labor or before labor. The presenting part reaches the level of the ischial spines. The most common position is occiput anterior. As engagement occurs, the head often rotates transversely. However, the position is usually dictated by the size of the pelvic inlet.
   c. Flexion allows the smallest diameter of the head to pass through the pelvis. Once again, this is dependent on the shape of the pelvis. A platypelloid pelvis may cause some deflexion in some cases and result in a brow or face presentation.
   d. Fetal descent progresses constantly. It is dependent on the uterine contractions and the size of the fetus. The position of the presenting part also plays a role.
   e. As descent takes place, the presenting part undergoes internal rotation. The fetal head rotates from a transverse position to an anterior or a posterior position so as to maneuver through the ischial spines. The rotation is complete by the time the head reaches the perineum.
   f. At the level of the perineum, a combination of uterine contractions and maternal expulsive efforts assist in extension. The extension of the fetal head also allows it to maneuver under the pubic symphysis.
   g. The external rotation occurs after the head is delivered. The rotation restores the fetal head to the initial position it occupied when it became engaged.
   h. The complete expulsion of the infant occurs with the delivery of the shoulders and the rest of the body.

- First stage

The first stage of labor is composed of two phases. The latent phase is the period of gradual cervical effacement and dilation. This period begins with the onset of labor and ends when cervical dilation is approximately 4 to 5 cm. The active phase begins at the conclusion of the latent phase and ends with complete cervical dilation. This period is recognized by rapid cervical dilation. Nulliparous women should dilate at least 1.2 cm/hr and multiparous women at least 1.5 cm/hr during the active phase. The average duration of the entire first stage in nulliparous women is 8 hours; in multiparous women, it averages 5 hours.

- Second stage

The second stage is defined as the period between complete cervical dilation and delivery of the infant. Maternal expulsive efforts are usually spontaneous during this stage if no regional anesthetic is used. These expulsive efforts and the uterine contractions drive the presenting part to the pelvic floor. Delivery is anticipated as the perineum begins to distend.

- Third stage

The period between the delivery of the infant and the delivery of the placenta is termed the third stage of labor. The placenta separates within 5 minutes following the delivery of the infant. This process is often assisted by administering oxytocin into the intravenous (IV) fluid. The separation of the placenta is believed to occur by the rapid reduction of the uterine size resulting in "buckling" of the placental surface area and forming a retroplacental bleed. This bleed eventually propagates and shears off the remaining surface of the placenta.

- Fourth stage

This stage has been recognized as the first hour following the delivery of the placenta. It appears to be a critical period for postpartum hemorrhage. The use of oxytocin and uterine massage will minimize any significant bleeding. The perineal region needs to be frequently noted for any signs of excessive bleeding.

Episiotomy/Lacerations Episiotomy is a surgical incision of the perineum performed during a delivery to provide sufficient area for the delivery of the infant and minimize or avoid lacerations of the perineum and rectum. Episiotomy repair is shown in Figure 256–2.

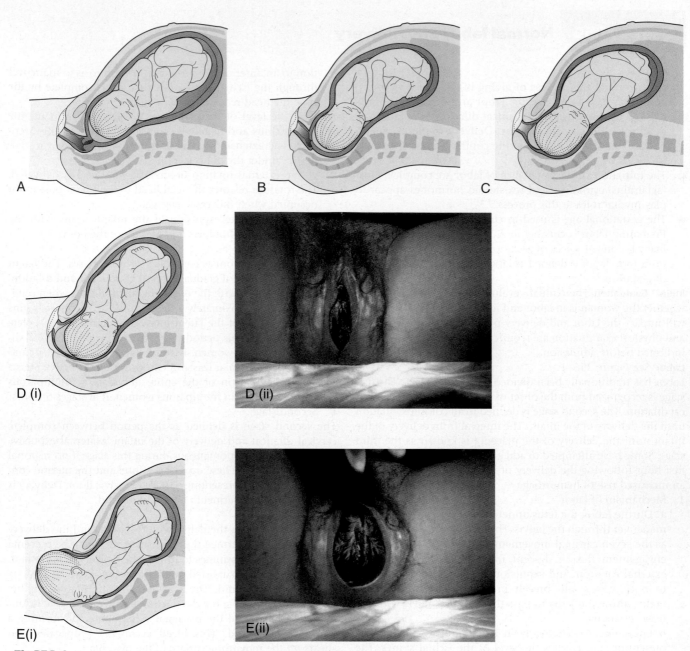

Fig 256-1
Normal labor. See text for details.
(From Drife J, Magowan B: Clinical Obstetrics and Gynaecology. Edinburgh, WB Saunders, 2004.)

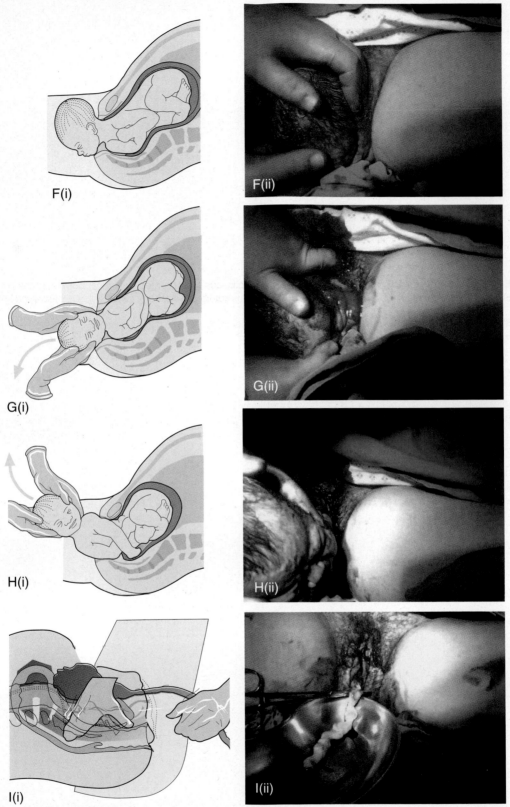

F(i)
F(ii)
G(i)
G(ii)
H(i)
H(ii)
I(i)
I(ii)

Fig 256–1—cont'd
Normal labor. See text for details.
(From Drife J, Magowan B: Clinical Obstetrics and Gynaecology. Edinburgh, WB Saunders, 2004.)

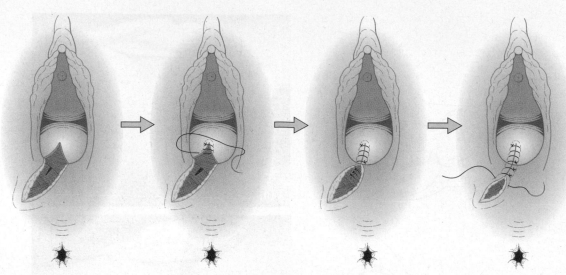

Fig 256-2
Repair of the episiotomy: the posterior vaginal wall may be closed with continuous or interrupted sutures; apposition of the cut levator muscle ensures hemostasis before skin closure. (**A**) Episiotomy wound. (**B**) Continuous suture of posterior vaginal wall. (**C**) Interrupted suture into the perineal skin.
(From Symonds EM, Symonds IM: Essential Obstetrics and Gynaecology, 4th ed. Edinburgh, Churchill Livingstone, 2004.)

Chapter 257　Abnormal labor

Abnormalities of labor are generally described as dystocia. Since 1980, the incidence of cesarean births has increased significantly in the United States. One of the major indications for cesarean births has been dystocia. The exact incidence has been difficult to ascertain because the definition has been vague and generalized. Frequently, generic terms such as cephalopelvic disproportion or failure to progress have been used to describe various dystocias. Every effort should be made to characterize the dystocia encountered precisely so that the correct diagnosis is made.

- Dystocias can be classified into three categories. The categories are a result of problems with uterine contractions, the size of the maternal pelvis, or the size of the fetus. These have been referred to as abnormalities of the power, the passenger, and the passage.

- The most common arrest disorder recognized is an arrest of dilation. This is defined as failure to dilate in the active phase for 2 hours or longer. It is found in approximately 5% of nulliparous labor. An arrest of descent is defined as failure to descend for 1 hour or longer.

- The most common causes of arrest disorders are fetopelvic discrepancy. Many are as a result of positional abnormalities such as occiput transverse or occiput posterior. Uterine dystocia also accounts for a large percentage of arrest disorders. Fetal macrosomia or pelvic contractions account for many of the abnormalities encountered with arrest of descent.

- Dystocia from the fetus is usually caused by a large infant, malposition of the presenting part, or a malpresentation. Treatment for many of these disorders is often an operative delivery by a cesarean section or forceps.

- Malpresentation: Approximately 5% of all labors at term are complicated by malpresentations. These are abnormalities related to the fetal position, or presentation. Malpresentations are the most common cause of fetal dystocia.

1. Breech (Fig. 257–1)

    a. A breech is an abnormal fetal lie in which the head of the infant lies in the uterine fundus. Breeches are described as frank, complete, or footling based on the position of the fetal hips and knees. A frank breech is a fetus who is lying with flexed hips and extended knees. If both the knees and the hips are flexed, it is referred to as a complete breech. When one or both hips are extended, a footling breech is identified. The infants may be designated as single or double footling breeches.

    b. The incidence of breech infants is dependent on the gestational age. Pregnancies less than 28 weeks have an incidence of approximately 25%. This decreases to 7% to 9% by 32 weeks. At term, the incidence of all breeches is 3% to 4%.

    c. Breech presentations have been associated with fetal and uterine anomalies. A careful sonographic evaluation is warranted in persistent breech infants to rule out any anomalies. The perinatal mortality rate of breech presentations varies from 9% to 25%. However, controversy exists because many breeches have anomalies and are premature. The corrected estimates of perinatal mortality at term may not be different from those of infants presenting as vertex.

    d. The mode of delivery remains controversial. A cesarean section should be considered for any breech between 800 and 1500 g. The optimal mode of delivery between 1500 and 2500 g has not clearly been established. A trial of labor may be considered with a breech presentation between 2500 and 3800 g.

- Operative delivery is defined as any delivery requiring an active maneuver. The three most common methods are with forceps, by vacuum, or by a cesarean section.

1. Forceps (Fig. 257–2)

    a. The obstetric forceps is composed of two matched instruments. Each instrument consists of a blade, a shank, a lock, and a handle. The cephalic curve is the area of the blade that is applied to the infant's head. The area of the blade placed on the mother's pelvis is known as the pelvic curve. There is a left and a right blade on all forceps, which correspond to the left and right sides of the mother's pelvis when placed.

    b. There are a variety of classic and modern or special forceps available.

2. Cesarean section (Fig. 257–3)

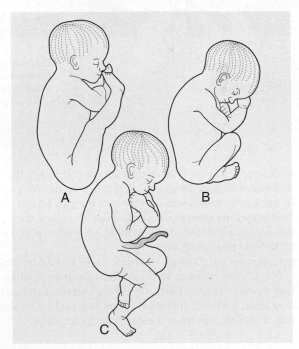

Fig 257–1
Breech presentation. Those presenting by the breech may be (**A**) extended (or frank); (**B**) flexed; or (**C**) footling.
(From Drife J, Magoan B: Clinical Obstetrics and Gynaecology. Edinburgh, WB Saunders, 2004.)

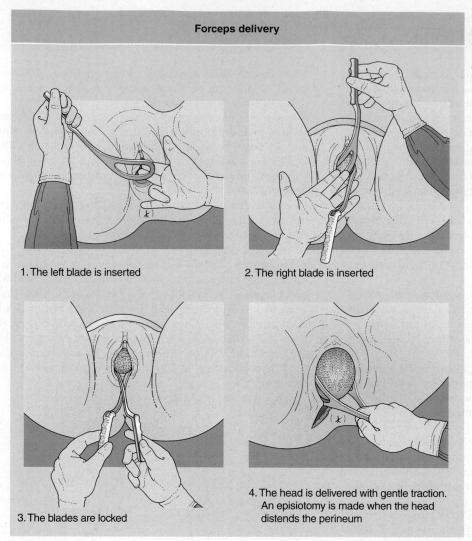

Forceps delivery

1. The left blade is inserted

2. The right blade is inserted

3. The blades are locked

4. The head is delivered with gentle traction. An episiotomy is made when the head distends the perineum

Fig 257–2
Forceps delivery.
(From Greer IA, Cameron IT, Kitchener HC, Prentice A: Mosby's Color Atlas and Text of Obstetrics and Gynaecology. London, Harcourt, 2001.)

a. Cesarean section is a surgical incision through the abdominal wall and the uterus, performed to deliver a fetus. Its use has increased significantly over the past several years, and numerous attempts are under way to reduce the cesarean births in the United States. Most hospitals report a 10% to 35% cesarean birth rate.

b. Cesareans are classified as either classic or low cervical.

(1) Classic cesarean section refers to a delivery of an infant through a vertical incision on the corpus of the uterus. It is associated with increased blood loss and an increased risk of uterine rupture in a subsequent pregnancy.

(2) Low cervical cesarean sections apply to transverse incisions (Kerr incision) performed in the lower, noncontractile portion of the uterus.

(3) Major risks during cesarean sections are infection, anesthetic complications, and hemorrhage. The mortality rate for cesarean section is approximately 5.8 per 100,000 live births.

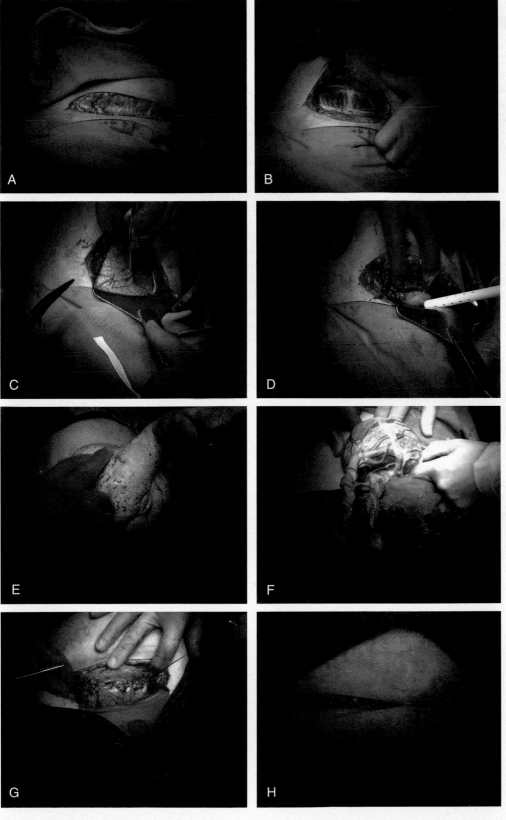

Fig 257-3
Delivery by cesarean section. The table should be tilted 15 degrees to the left side (to reduce aortocaval compression) and a lower abdominal transverse incision made, cutting through the fat (**A**) and the rectus sheath (**B**) to open the peritoneum. The bladder is freed (**C**) and pushed down, and a transverse lower segment incision is made in the uterus (**D**). If the presentation is cephalic the head is then encouraged through the incision with firm fundal pressure from the assistant. Wrigley's forceps are occasionally required. If the baby is presenting by the breech, traction is applied to the baby's pelvis by placing a finger behind each flexed hip to deliver the bottom first (**E**). If transverse, a leg should be identified and pulled to deliver the baby (i.e., internal podalic version). After delivery Syntocinon is given intravenously and after uterine contraction the placenta is delivered (**F**). Hemostasis is obtained with clamps and a check is made to ensure that the uterus is empty and that there are no ovarian cysts. This incision is closed with two layers of dissolving suture to the uterus, one layer to the rectus sheath (**G**) and one layer to the skin (**H**).
(From Drife J, Magowan B: Clinical Obstetrics and Gynaecology. Edinburgh, WB Saunders, 2004.)

Chapter 258 Ectopic pregnancy

DEFINITION

An ectopic pregnancy (EP) is one in which a fertilized ovum implants outside the endometrial lining of the uterus. Figure 258–1 illustrates sites of implantation of EPs.

PHYSICAL FINDINGS AND CLINICAL PRESENTATION

- Abdominal tenderness: 95%
- Adnexal tenderness: 87% to 99%
- Peritoneal signs: 71% to 76%
- Adnexal mass: 33% to 53%
- Enlarged uterus: 6% to 30%
- Shock: 2% to 17%
- Amenorrhea or abnormal vaginal bleeding: 75%
- Shoulder pain: 10%
- Tissue passage: 6% to 7%

CAUSE

- Anatomic obstruction to zygote passage
- Abnormalities in tubal motility
- Transperitoneal migration of the zygote

DIFFERENTIAL DIAGNOSIS

- Corpus luteum cyst
- Rupture or torsion of ovarian cyst
- Threatened or incomplete abortion
- PID (see Figs. 250–1, 250–2)
- Appendicitis
- Gastroenteritis
- Dysfunctional uterine bleeding
- Degenerating uterine fibroids (see Fig. 244–3)
- Endometriosis (see Fig. 233–2)

WORKUP

1. The classic presentation of EP includes the triad of abnormal vaginal bleeding, pelvic pain, and an adnexal mass. Consider in all women with abdominal-pelvic pain and a positive pregnancy test
2. Culdocentesis is clinically useful when other diagnostic modalities are not readily available
   - Positive tap means nonclotting blood with Hct >12%.
   - Negative tap means clear or blood-tinged fluid.
   - Nondiagnostic tap means clotted blood or no fluid.
3. Laparoscopy

LABORATORY TESTS

- hCG: if normal intrauterine pregnancy (IUP), 85% have doubling time of 2 days. If abnormal gestation, will show <66% increase of quantitative human chorionic gonadotropins (QhCG) within 2 days. However, 13% of ectopic pregnancies have a normal doubling time
- Progesterone: decreased production in EP, <5 ng/mL strongly predictive of abnormal pregnancy. If >25 ng/mL, strongly predictive of normal IUP
- Dropping Hct associated with tubal rupture
- Leukocytosis

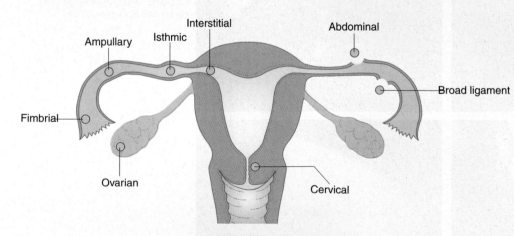

Fig 258–1

Sites of implantation of ectopic pregnancies.
(From Symonds EM, Symonds IM: Essential Obstetrics and Gynaecology, 4th ed. Edinburgh, Churchill Livingstone, 2004.)

IMAGING STUDIES
- Ultrasound (Fig. 258–2): presence of an IUP rules out EP.
- If QhCG > 6000 mIU/mL, should see IUP on abdominal scan, and QhCG > 1500 mIU/mL for transvaginal scan.
- Findings on ultrasound in EP include:
  1. Empty uterus
  2. Adnexal mass
  3. Cul-de-sac fluid
  4. Fetal sac in tube
  5. Fetal cardiac activity in adnexa

TREATMENT

Surgery: can be performed by laparoscopy if patient is stable or by laparotomy if patient is unstable. Salpingiosis: direct injection of chemotherapy into ectopic via laparoscopy, transvaginal ultrasound, or hysteroscopy.
- Conservative surgery-salpingostomy or segmental resection depends on tubal location and size of ectopic.
- Salpingectomy should be considered in the following circumstances:
  1. Ruptured tube
  2. Future fertility not desired
  3. Recurrent ectopic in the same tube
  4. Uncontrolled hemorrhage
- If the patient is stable and compliant the physician may consider medical management with methotrexate. Patient should not have contraindications to methotrexate such as hepatic or renal disease, thrombocytopenia, leukopenia, or significant anemia. There should be no evidence of hemoperitoneum on transvaginal ultrasound. Ectopic should be <4 cm mass with QhCG <30,000 mIU/ml.

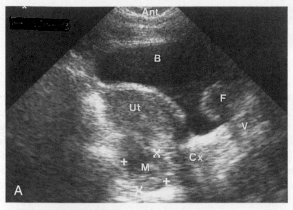
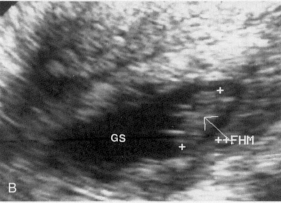

Fig 258–2

Ectopic pregnancy. A longitudinal transabdominal image (**A**) clearly shows the bladder (B), uterus (Ut), and cervix (Cx). There is a Foley ctheter within the bladder. A mass (M) is noted behind the uterus and marked with X and +. A transvaginal ultrasound image (**B**) was performed to get better detail of this abnormality. A gestational sac (GS), a fetal pole, and fetal heart motion (+ +FHM) were identified in this ectopic pregnancy. F = Foley catheter; V = vagina.
(From Mettler FA, Guibertau MJ, Voss CM, Urbina CE: Primary Care Radiology. Philadelphia, Elsevier, 2000.)

Chapter 259   Preeclampsia

DEFINITION
- Preeclampsia involves a triad of hypertension, proteinuria, and edema that develops after the twentieth week of gestation. Mild preeclampsia is defined as a blood pressure of <140/90 mm Hg. Severe preeclampsia is associated with a blood pressure >160/110 mm Hg, proteinuria >5 g in a 24-hour urine collection, oliguria (<400 mL/24 hours), cerebral or visual disturbances, epigastric pain, pulmonary edema, thrombocytopenia, hepatic dysfunction, or severe intrauterine growth retardation.
- HELLP is a serious variant of preeclampsia. HELLP is an acronym for Hemolysis, Elevated Liver function, Low Platelet count

PHYSICAL FINDINGS AND CLINICAL PRESENTATION
- Generalized swelling or nondependent edema (Fig. 259–1), possibly manifested by rapid weight gain (>4 lb/wk) even in the absence of edema
- Auscultation of pulmonary rales
- Right upper quadrant abdominal pain (RUQ) pain (HELLP syndrome or subcapsular liver hematoma)
- Hyperreflexia or clonus
- Vaginal bleeding (placental abruption)
- Acute or chronic fetal compromise manifested by intrauterine growth restriction or fetal tachycardia with late decelerations, respectively
- Wide range of symptoms attributable to multiorgan system dysfunction, involving hepatic, hematologic, renal (Fig. 259–2), pulmonary, and CNS

- Possibility of severe disease despite "normal" blood pressure readings, so a high index of suspicion must be maintained in high-risk situations

DIFFERENTIAL DIAGNOSIS
- Acute fatty liver of pregnancy
- Appendicitis
- Diabetic ketoacidosis
- Gallbladder disease
- Gastroenteritis
- Glomerulonephritis
- Hemolytic-uremic syndrome
- Hepatic encephalopathy
- Hyperemesis gravidarum
- Idiopathic thrombocytopenia
- Thrombotic thrombocytopenic purpura
- Nephrolithiasis
- Pyelonephritis
- Peptic ulcer disease (PUD)
- Systemic lupus erythematosus (SLE)
- Viral hepatitis

WORKUP
- Two blood pressure measurements in lateral recumbent position 6 hours apart, with an absolute pressure >140/90 mm Hg or an increase of 30 mm Hg systolic or 15 mm Hg diastolic from baseline, an increase in the mean arterial pressure (MAP) of 20 mm Hg, or an absolute MAP >105 mm Hg

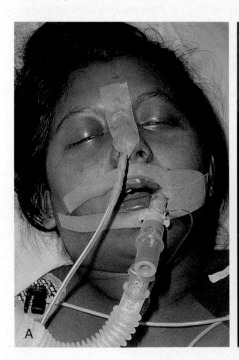 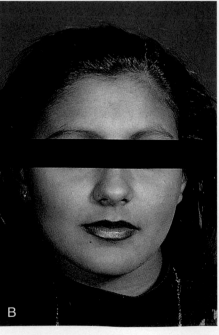

Fig 259–1
Clinical appearance of severe pre-eclampsia. (**A**) Marked facial edema occurs and intubation for treatment of acute pulmonary edema may be required. (**B**) Complete resolution of these features occurs postpartum.
(From Johnson RJ, Feehally J: Comprehensive Clinical Nephrology, 2nd ed. St Louis, Mosby, 2000.)

- Evaluation for proteinuria as defined by >0.1 g/L on urine dipstick or >300 mg protein on a 24-hour urine collection
- Evaluation of fetal status for evidence of intrauterine growth restriction, oligohydramnios, alteration in umbilical or uterine artery Doppler flow, or acute compromise, such as abruption
- Because of the insidious nature of the disease with potential for multiple organ involvement, complete evaluation for preeclampsia in any pregnant patient presenting with CNS derangement or GI complaints after 20 weeks of gestation
- Evaluation for associated conditions such as disseminated intravascular coagulation, hepatic dysfunction, or subcapsular hematoma

LABORATORY TESTS

- High-risk patients: baseline assessment of renal function (24-hour urine collection for protein and creatinine clearance), platelets, blood urea nitrogen (BUN), creatinine, liver function tests (LFTs), and uric acid should be obtained at the first prenatal visit.

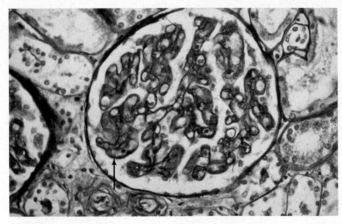

Fig 259–2
Renal changes in preeclampsia include endothelial swelling (E), apparent avascularity of the glomerulus and fibrin deposition (*arrow*) under the basement membrane.
(From Symonds EM, Symonds IM: Essential Obstetrics and Gynaecology. 4th ed. Edinburgh, Churchill Livingstone, 2004.)

- CBC (Hgb, Hct, platelets) may show signs of volume contraction or HELLP syndrome.
- LFTs (AST ALT), LDH are useful in evaluation for HELLP syndrome or to exclude important differentials.
- Hyperuricemia or increased creatinine may indicate decreasing renal function.
- Prothrombin time (PT), partial thromboplastin time (PTT), and fibrinogen should be checked to rule out disseminated intravascular coagulation.
- Peripheral smear may demonstrate microangiopathic hemolytic anemia.
- Complement levels can be used to differentiate from an acute exacerbation of a collagen-vascular disease.
- Increased levels of soluble fms-like tyrosine kinase 1 (SFlT-1) and reduced levels of placental growth factor (PlGF) predict subsequent development of preeclampsia.

IMAGING STUDIES

- CT scan of head if atypical presentation of eclampsia, possibility of intracerebral bleed, or prolonged postictal state
- Sonogram of fetus to evaluate for intrauterine growth retardation (IUGR), amniotic fluid, placenta
- Sonogram of maternal liver if suspect subcapsular hematoma

TREATMENT

- Bed rest in left lateral decubitus position
- Delivery is the treatment of choice and the only cure for the disease. This must be taken in the context of the gestational age of the fetus, severity of the preeclampsia, and the likelihood of a successful induction and reliability of the patient.

Chapter 260 Abruptio placentae

DEFINITION

Abruptio placentae is the separation of placenta from the uterine wall before delivery of the fetus. There are three classes of abruption based on maternal and fetal status, including an assessment of uterine contractions, quantity of bleeding, fetal heart rate monitoring, and abnormal coagulation studies (fibrinogen, PT, PTT) (Fig. 260–1).

- Grade I: mild vaginal bleeding, uterine irritability, stable vital signs, reassuring fetal heart rate, normal coagulation profile (fibrinogen 450 mg%)
- Grade II: moderate vaginal bleeding, hypertonic uterine contractions, orthostatic blood pressure measurements, unfavorable fetal status, fibrinogen 150 mg% to 250 mg%
- Grade III: severe bleeding (may be concealed), hypertonic uterine contractions, overt signs of hypovolemic shock, fetal death, thrombocytopenia, fibrinogen <150 mg%

PHYSICAL FINDINGS AND CLINICAL PRESENTATION

- Triad of uterine bleeding (concealed or per vagina), hypertonic uterine contractions or signs of preterm labor, and evidence of fetal compromise exists.
- More than 80% of cases have external bleeding; 20% of cases have no bleeding but have indirect evidence of abruption, such as failed tocolysis for preterm labor.
- Tetanic uterine contractions are found in only 17% of cases, unless grade II or III abruption.

CAUSE

- Primary etiology: unknown
- Hypertension: found in 40% to 50% of grade III abruptions
- Rapid decompression of uterine cavity, such as is found with polyhydramnios or multifetal gestation
- Blunt external trauma (motor vehicle accident, spousal abuse)

DIFFERENTIAL DIAGNOSIS

- Placenta previa (see Fig. 261–1)
- Cervical or vaginal trauma
- Labor (see Fig. 256–1)
- Cervical cancer (see Fig. 242–1)
- Rupture of membranes

WORKUP

- Initial assessment should evaluate for the source of bleeding, ruling out placenta previa and associated conditions that contraindicate any type of vaginal examination (e.g., pelvic speculum examination).
- Continuous fetal heart monitoring is indicated for all viable gestations (60% incidence of fetal distress in labor); may show early signs of maternal hypovolemia (late decelerations or fetal tachycardia) before overt maternal vital sign changes.
- Actual amount of blood loss is often greater than initially perceived because of the possibility of concealed retroplacental bleeding and the apparent "normal" vital signs. The relative hypervolemia of pregnancy initially protects the gravida until late in the course of bleeding, when abrupt and sudden cardiovascular collapse can occur without warning.

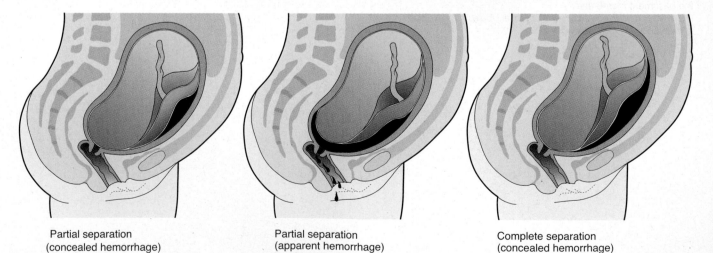

Partial separation
(concealed hemorrhage)

Partial separation
(apparent hemorrhage)

Complete separation
(concealed hemorrhage)

Fig 260–1
Classification of placental abruption.
(From Drife J, Magowan B: Clinical Obstetrics and Gynaecology. Edinburgh, WB Saunders, 2004.)

LABORATORY TESTS
- Baseline Hgb and Hct help quantify blood loss and, even more important, with every four to six determinations can demonstrate significant trends during expectant management.
- Coagulation profile: platelets, fibrinogen, PT, and PTT. Disseminated intravascular coagulopathy (DIC) can develop with severe abruption. If fibrinogen is <150 mg%, estimated blood loss equals 2000 mL, and if fibrinogen is <100 mg%, consider fresh frozen plasma (FFP) to prevent further bleeding.
- Type and antibody screen is important to identify Rh-negative patients who may need Rh immune globulin.

IMAGING STUDIES
Ultrasound should include fetal presentation and status, amniotic fluid volume, placental location, as well as any evidence of hematoma (retroplacental, subchorionic, or preplacental).

TREATMENT
- Stabilization of the mother is the first priority.
- Treatment is dependent on gestational age of the fetus, severity of the abruption, and maternal status.
- Initial assessment for signs of maternal hemodynamic compromise or hemorrhagic shock; large-bore intravenous access, with crystalloid fluid resuscitation using a replacement of 3 mL LR solution for every 1 mL estimated blood loss.

- Indwelling Foley catheter to monitor urine output and maternal volume status, with a goal of 30 mL/hours urine output.
- Assess fetal status and gestational age using sonogram and continuous fetal heart rate monitoring.
- Because of the unpredictable nature of abruptions, cross-matched blood should be made available during the initial resuscitation period.
- In the term fetus or when lung maturity has been documented, delivery is indicated.
- In the preterm fetus or a fetus with an immature lung profile, consider betamethasone 12.5 mg IM q24h for two doses and then delivery, depending on the severity of the abruption and the likelihood of fetal complications from preterm birth.
- C-section should be reserved for cases of fetal distress or for standard obstetric indications.
- In select cases, such as severe prematurity with a stable mother and mild contractions, magnesium sulfate can be used for tocolysis, 6 g IV loading dose then 3 g/hr maintenance, to allow for course of steroids.

Chapter 261   Placenta previa

DEFINITION

Placenta previa is the implantation of the placenta over the internal os. Four degrees of this abnormality have been defined (Fig. 261–1):

- Total placenta previa: the internal os is covered completely.
- Partial placenta previa: the internal os is partially covered.
- Marginal placenta previa: the edge of the placenta is at the margin of the internal os.
- Low-lying placenta: the placenta is implanted in the lower uterine segment, and although its edge does not reach the internal os, it is in close proximity to it.

PHYSICAL FINDINGS AND CLINICAL PRESENTATION

The classic presentation of placenta previa is painless vaginal bleeding, usually in the second or third trimester. Uterine contractions may or may not be present. On physical examination, the uterus is soft and pain free. The fetus is often in breech, transverse lie, or high. Fetal distress is usually not present.

CAUSE

Uncertain

DIFFERENTIAL DIAGNOSIS

- Placenta accreta
- Placenta percreta
- Placenta increta
- Vasa previa
- Abruptio placentae (see Fig. 260–1)
- Vaginal or cervical trauma
- Labor (see Fig. 256–1)
- Local malignancy (see Fig. 242–1)

WORKUP

- Do NOT perform a digital vaginal examination.
- The diagnosis of placenta previa can seldom be firmly established by physical examination alone. A speculum examination in a hospital setting to exclude any local bleeding may be performed.
- This diagnosis should not be dismissed until a thorough evaluation, including sonography, has completely excluded its presence.

LABORATORY TESTS

- A CBC can be used to monitor hemoglobin and hematocrit.
- A Kleihauer-Betke preparation of maternal blood in all Rh-negative women and Rh-immune globulin when indicated

IMAGING STUDIES

- The simplest, most precise, and safest method of placental localization is transabdominal sonography with confirmatory imaging by transvaginal ultrasonography. Transperineal sonography has also proved effective in detection.
- MRI has also been effective in detecting placenta previa, although sonography remains the preferred method.

TREATMENT

- In preterm pregnancies with no active bleeding, close observation and expectant management are indicated. In those with active bleeding, conservative management, including blood transfusions for severe bleeds, is appropriate. The woman should stay in the hospital for at least 48 hours after the bleeding has stopped.

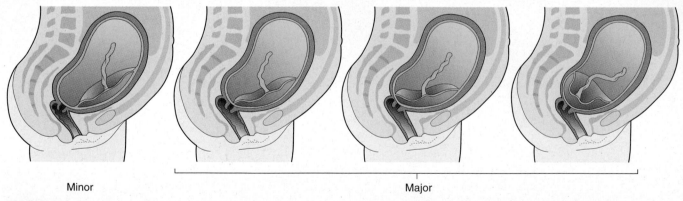

Minor   Major

Fig 261–1
Classification into "major" and "minor" placenta previa depends on the distance of the placenta from the internal os. It is also important to note whether the placenta is anterior or posterior, as cesarean section is more difficult through an anterior placenta.
(From Drife J, Magowan B: Clinical Obstetrics and Gynaecology. Edinburgh, WB Saunders, 2004.)

- Bed rest, preferably in a hospital setting, should be prescribed.
- Initial assessment for signs of maternal hemodynamic compromise or hemorrhagic shock; large-bore intravenous access with crystalloid fluid resuscitation
- Assess fetal status and gestational age using sonogram and continuous fetal heart rate monitoring
- Cross-matched blood should be made available during bleeding episodes; if the hemorrhage is severe, cesarean delivery is indicated despite fetal immaturity
- Tocolytic therapy may be considered in those women in preterm labor, as well as the administration of corticosteroids to enhanced fetal lung maturity

- Cesarean delivery is necessary in nearly all cases of placenta previa.
- Uncontrollable hemorrhage after placental removal should be anticipated secondary to the poorly contractile nature of the lower uterine segment. The need for hysterectomy to control bleeding should be discussed with the patient before delivery, if possible.

Chapter 262 Hydatidiform mole

DEFINITION

Disorder of the placenta with degenerative changes in the stroma or villi combined with neoplastic activity in the chorionic endothelium

CLINICAL PRESENTATION

Vaginal bleeding, severe nausea and vomiting, passage of tissue vaginally. Pathologically, it is characterized by the presence of multiple grapelike vesicles (Fig. 262–1).

DIAGNOSIS

Ultrasound will reveal a "snowstorm" appearance (Fig. 262–2); laboratory evaluation will reveal a very high level of hCG.

TREATMENT

Uterine evacuation, usually by suction curettage

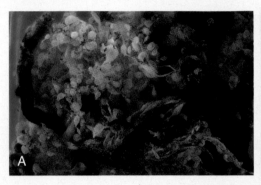 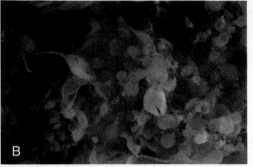

Fig 262–1
(**A**) Pathological appearance of hydatidiform mole following evacuation. (**B**) Note the multiple grapelike vesicles.
(From Greer IA, Cameron IT, Kitchener HC, Prentice A: Mosby's Color Atlas and Text of Obstetrics and Gynaecology. London, Harcourt, 2001.)

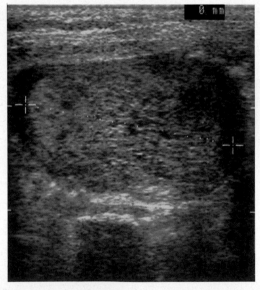

Fig 262–2
Ultrasound showing classic "snowstorm" appearance of hydatidiform mole.

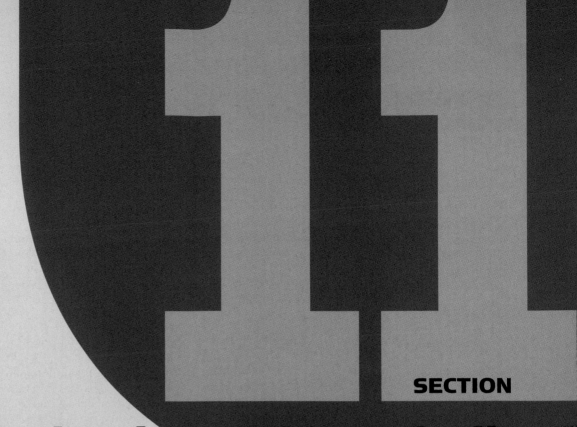

SECTION 11

Endocrine and Metabolic Disorders

Pituitary Disorders
Chapter 263: Hypopituitarism
Chapter 264: Pituitary adenoma
Chapter 265: Diabetes insipidus
Chapter 266: Inappropriate secretion of antidiuretic hormone

Thyroid
Chapter 267: Hypothyroidism
Chapter 268: Hyperthyroidism

Parathyroids
Chapter 269: Hypocalcemia
Chapter 270: Hyperparathyroidism

Adrenal Glands
Chapter 271: Cushing's syndrome
Chapter 272: Addison's disease
Chapter 273: Hypoaldosteronism
Chapter 274: Hyperaldosteronism
Chapter 275: Pheochromocytoma

Reproductive System and Growth
Chapter 276: Normal puberty
Chapter 277: Precocious puberty
Chapter 278: Delayed puberty
Chapter 279: Congenital adrenal hyperplasia
Chapter 280: Klinefelter's syndrome
Chapter 281: Turner's syndrome
Chapter 282: Hypogonadism
Chapter 283: Hirsutism
Chapter 284: Gynecomastia

Disorders of Carbohydrate and Lipid Metabolism
Chapter 285: Diabetes mellitus
Chapter 286: Hypoglycemia and Insulinoma
Chapter 287: Hyperlipidemia
Chapter 288: Multiple endocrine neoplasia (MEN)

PITUITARY DISORDERS

Chapter 263 / Hypopituitarism

DEFINITION

Hypopituitarism is the partial or complete loss of secretion of one or more pituitary hormones resulting from diseases of the hypothalamus or pituitary gland.

PHYSICAL FINDINGS AND CLINICAL PRESENTATION

The onset of hypopituitarism is usually gradual, and symptoms are related to the lack of one or more hormones (Fig. 263–1) and/or mass effect if a pituitary tumor is the cause. Specific symptoms depend on the hormones involved, the severity of the deficiencies, and the patient's age at onset (Fig. 263–2).

- Mass effect of a pituitary tumor can cause headaches and visual disturbances.
- Corticotropin deficiency
  1. Fatigue and weakness, no appetite, abdominal pain, nausea, and vomiting
  2. Hypotension, hair loss, and change in mental status
- Thyrotropin deficiency
  1. Fatigue and weakness, weight gain, cold intolerance, and constipation
  2. Bradycardia, hung-up reflexes, pretibial edema, and hair loss
- Gonadotropin deficiency
  1. Loss of libido, erectile dysfunction, amenorrhea, hot flashes, dyspareunia, infertility
  2. Gynecomastia with lack of hair growth and decreased muscle mass

- Growth hormone deficiency
  1. Growth retardation in children (Fig.263–3)
  2. Easy fatigue, hypoglycemia
  3. Decreased muscle mass and obesity, skeletal maturation delay (Fig.263–4)
- Hyperprolactinemia
  1. Galactorrhea
  2. Hypogonadism
- Vasopressin deficiency
  1. Polyuria, polydipsia and nocturia
  2. Hypotension and dehydration

CAUSE

Hypopituitarism is the result of destruction of pituitary cells caused by the following:

- Pituitary tumors (Fig.263–5)
  1. Macroadenomas >10 mm (Fig. 263–6)
  2. Microadenomas <10 mm
- Pituitary apoplexy caused by hemorrhage or infarction of the pituitary gland
- Pituitary radiation therapy
- Pituitary surgery
- Empty sella: defects in the diaphragma sellae may allow passage of cerebrospinal fluid (CSF) from the suprasellar cistern into the sella turcica. This condition, known as empty sella, is usually an incidental finding, although it may be found in patients with the constellation of headache, endocrine dysfunction, and visual disturbances (Fig. 263–7).

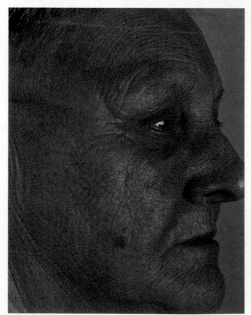

Fig 263–1
A patient with hypopituitarism. Pallor, skin wrinkling, and absence of facial hair can be clearly seen
(From Besser CM, Thorner MO: Comprehensive Clinical Endocrinology, 3rd ed. St. Louis, Mosby, 2002.)

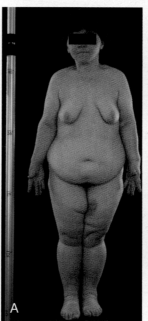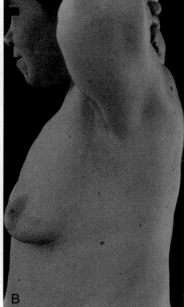

Fig 263–2
A patient with panhypopituitarism. **A,** Short stature, reduced body hair and increased abdominal fat are apparent. **B,** Partial breast development results from estrogen replacement. Failure of adrenal androgen production results in the absence of axillary hair.
(From Besser CM, Thorner MO: Comprehensive Clinical Endocrinology, 3rd ed. St. Louis, Mosby, 2002.)

- Infiltrative disease, including sarcoidosis, hemochromatosis, histiocytosis X, Wegener's granulomatosis, and lymphocytic hypophysitis
- Infection (tuberculosis, mycosis, and syphilis)
- Head trauma
- Internal carotid artery aneurysm

DIFFERENTIAL DIAGNOSIS
- The differential diagnosis is as outlined under "Cause."
- **Postpartum necrosis** *(Sheehan's syndrome):* hypopituitarism secondary to postpartum pituitary hemorrhagic infarction. In the acute phase, magnetic resonance imaging (MRI) may show a high signal intensity within the pituitary gland,

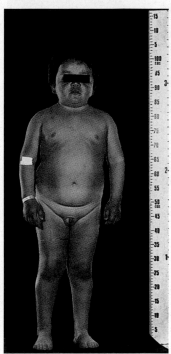

Fig 263–3
A boy with classic growth hormone insufficiency. Such children are very small, tend to be obese, and have underdeveloped genitalia. They have a slow growth rate and usually a retarded bone age. (From Besser CM, Thorner MO: Comprehensive Clinical Endocrinology, 3rd ed. St. Louis, Mosby, 2002.)

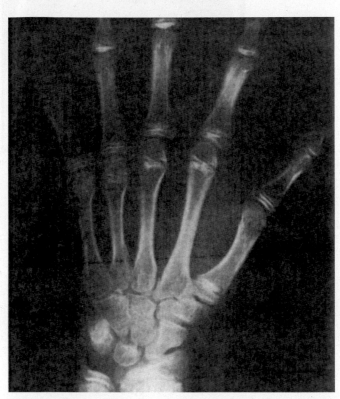

Fig 263–4
Hypopituitarism in a 21-year-old man. Radiograph of the left hand shows marked delay in skeletal maturation, as evidenced by open epiphyses. The bone age is 14 years. (From Grainger RG, Allison DJ, Adam A, Dixon AK [eds]: Grainger & Allison's Diagnostic Radiology, 4th ed. London, Harcourt, 2001.)

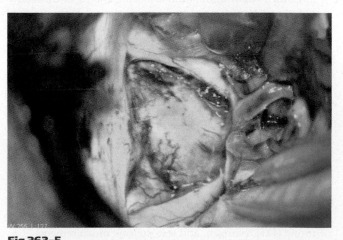

Fig 263–5
Chiasmatic compression. This intraoperative photograph, taken during the transcranial resection of a pituitary adenoma (anterior interhemispheric approach), shows the compression and distortion of the optic chiasm. This patient presented with a progressive bitemporal hemianopic visual field deficit, with progressive loss of visual acuity (20/400). (From Besser CM, Thorner MO: Comprehensive Clinical Endocrinology, 3rd ed. St. Louis, Mosby, 2002.)

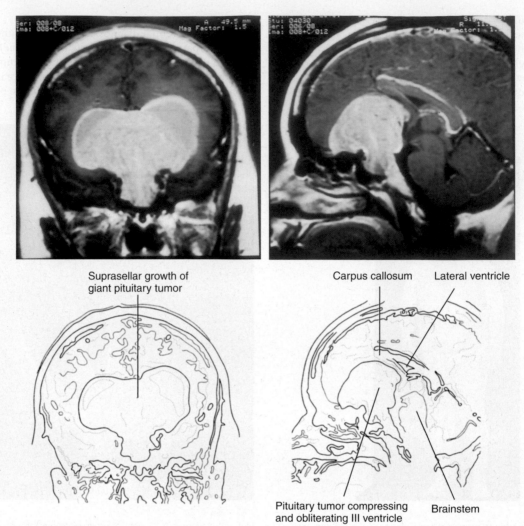

Suprasellar growth of
giant pituitary tumor

Carpus callosum   Lateral ventricle

Pituitary tumor compressing
and obliterating III ventricle   Brainstem

Fig 263–6
Giant pituitary adenoma with extension into the anterior, middle, and posterior cranial fossae, coronal and sagittal views.
(From Besser CM, Thorner MO: Comprehensive Clinical Endocrinology, 3rd ed. St. Louis, Mosby, 2002.)

suggesting the presence of hemorrhage. The gland rapidly diminishes in size until the sella has the appearance of the empty sella. On CT, the pituitary gland in a patient with Sheehan's syndrome may show high density, indicating the presence of clotted blood (Fig. 263–8).

- Pituitary tumors (e.g., craniopharyngiomas and meningioma)
- Metastatic tumors (lung, colon, prostate, melanoma, plasmacytoma) and developmental abnormalities

WORKUP
- Includes basal determination of each anterior pituitary hormone followed by provocative stimulation tests and x-ray imaging.
- Table 263–1 describes dynamic diagnostic tests of hypopituitarism

LABORATORY TESTS
- Corticotropin deficiency:
  1. Serum AM cortisol level usually is low (<3 g/dL).

2. Corticotropin stimulation test using 250 μg of corticotropin given IV and measuring serum cortisol before and 30 and 60 minutes after administration. A normal response is an increase in serum cortisol level more than 20 μg/dL.
3. With pituitary disease, these tests may be indeterminate, and more dynamic testing such as an insulin tolerance (Fig. 263–9) or metyrapone test may be necessary.
- Thyrotropin deficiency
  1. Thyroid-stimulating hormone (TSH) and free thyroxine (T_4) measurements
  2. Primary hypothyroidism shows elevated TSH with low free T_4. Secondary hypothyroidism shows normal or low TSH, with low free T_4 and low triiodothyronine (T_3) resin uptake.
- Gonadotropin deficiency
  1. Follicle-stimulating hormone (FSH), luteinizing hormone (LH), estrogen, and testosterone measurements
  2. In men, hypogonadotropic hypogonadism is seen with low testosterone levels and normal or low FSH and LH levels.

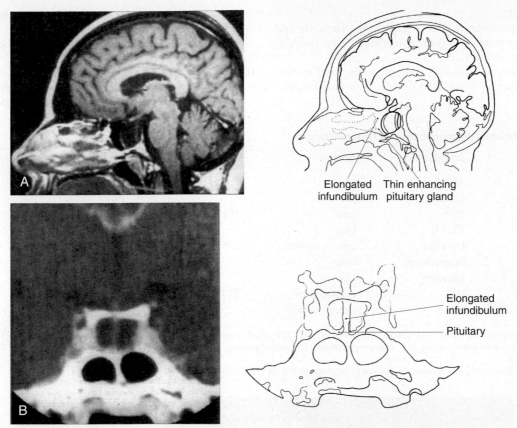

Fig 263–7
Empty sella. **A,** Sagittal T1-weighted postcontrast MRI scan showing a large empty sella with an elongated infundibulum inserting into a thin, enhancing pituitary gland. **B,** Coronal CT scan in a different patient showing insertion of the infundibulum into a thin pituitary.
(From Besser CM, Thorner MO: Comprehensive Clinical Endocrinology, 3rd ed. St. Louis, Mosby, 2002.)

3. In premenopausal women with amenorrhea, low estrogen with normal or low FSH and LH levels is typically seen.
● Growth hormone deficiency
1. Insulin-induced hypoglycemia stimulation test (see Fig. 263–9) using 0.1 to 0.15 U/kg regular insulin given IV and measuring growth hormone 30, 60, and 120 minutes after administration. A normal response is a growth hormone level >10 µg/dL.
2. Serum insulin-like growth factor I can also be measured after provocative testing.
● Vasopressin deficiency
1. Urinalysis shows low specific gravity.
2. Urine osmolality is low.
3. Serum osmolality is high.
4. Fluid deprivation test over 18 hour with inability to concentrate the urine
5. Serum vasopressin level is low.
6. Electrolytes may show hyponatremia and exclude hyperglycemia.

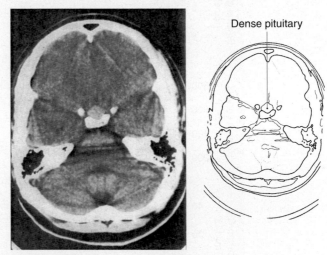

Fig 263–8
Sheehan's syndrome. This axial CT scan shows a dense pituitary caused by hemorrhagic infarction following postpartum uterine hemorrhage.
(From Besser CM, Thorner MO: Comprehensive Clinical Endocrinology, 3rd ed. St. Louis, Mosby, 2002.)

IMAGING STUDIES

- When hypopituitarism has been established clinically and biochemically, imaging of the pituitary gland is necessary to identify the specific lesion.
- MRI is more sensitive than CT scanning of the head in visualizing the pituitary fossa, sella turcica, optic chiasm, pituitary stalk, and cavernous sinuses. It is also more sensitive in detecting pituitary microadenomas.
- CT scanning with coronal cuts through the sella turcica yields better images of bony structures.

TREATMENT

- Hormone replacement therapy and surgery, radiation, or medications in patients with pituitary tumors

---

TABLE 263–1 Dynamic diagnostic tests of hypopituitarism

Pituitary axis	Baseline test	Finding	Dynamic test	Finding
Adrenal	ACTH	Low	ITT	Cortisol peak
	Cortisol	Low		<550 nmol/L
Thyroid	TSH	Low	TRH	Variable
	T3, T4,	Low		
Gonads	LH, FSH	Low to normal	GnRH	Variable
	Testosterone	Low		
	Estradiol	Low		
Growth hormone	GH	Undetectable	IIT	GH peak < 5 ng/mL
	IGF-1	Low to normal		

ACTH, adrenocorticotropic hormone; FSH, follicle-stimulating hormone; GH, growth hormone; GnRH, gonadotropin-releasing hormone; IGF-1; insulin-like growth factor 1; ITT, insulin tolerance test; LH, luteinizing hormone; T3, triiodothyronine; T4, thyroxine; TRH, thyrotropin-releasing hormone; TSH, thyroid-stimulating hormone.
From Besser CM, Thorner MO: Comprehensive Clinical Endocrinology, 3rd ed. St. Louis, Mosby, 2002.

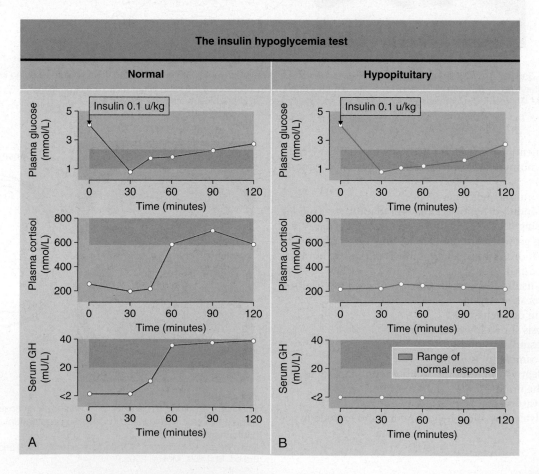

Fig 263–9

Insulin tolerance test. Plasma glucose, plasma cortisol, and serum growth hormone (GH) levels are shown in normal (**A**) and hypopituitary (**B**) subjects. Gonadotropin levels should rise to a minimum of 20 μg/L and cortisol to 550 nmol/L, provided that adequate hypoglycemia is reached with blood glucose concentrations of 2.2 mmol/L or more.
(From Besser CM, Thorner MO: Comprehensive Clinical Endocrinology, 3rd ed. St. Louis, Mosby, 2002.)

Chapter 264   Pituitary adenoma

DEFINITION

Pituitary adenoma is a benign neoplasm of the anterior lobe of the pituitary that causes symptoms by excess secretion of hormones or by a local mass effect as the tumor impinges on other, nearby structures (e.g., optic chiasm, hypothalamus, pituitary stalk). Clinical features of pituitary tumors are noted in Figure 264–1. Pituitary adenomas are classified by their size, function, and features that characterize their appearance.

- Acromegaly is the disease state characterized by a pituitary adenoma that secretes growth hormone (GH).
- A prolactinoma secretes prolactin (PRL). The basic mechanisms in hyperprolactinemia are illustrated in Figure 264–2.
- Cushing's disease is a disease state in which there is hypersecretion of adrenocorticotropic hormone (ACTH).
- Thyrotropin-secreting pituitary adenomas secrete primarily TSH.
- Nonsecretory pituitary adenomas are those in which the neoplasm is a space-occupying lesion whose secretory products do not cause a specific disease state.

PHYSICAL FINDINGS AND CLINICAL PRESENTATION

Prolactinomas See Figure 264–3.

- Females
  - Galactorrhea, prominent Montgomery tubercles (Fig. 264–4)
  - Amenorrhea
  - Oligomenorrhea with anovulation
  - Infertility
  - Estrogen deficiency leading to hirsutism
  - Decreased vaginal lubrication
  - Osteopenia
  - Headaches
- Males
  - Large tumors more common secondary to delayed diagnosis.
  - Possible impotence or decreased libido or hypogonadism
  - Galactorrhea is rare because males lack the estrogen-dependent breast growth and differentiation.

Growth hormone-secreting pituitary adenoma—acromegaly See Figure 264–5.

- Coarse facial features (Fig. 264–6)
- Oily skin
- Prognathism (Fig. 264–7), macroglossia (Fig. 264–8)
- Carpal tunnel syndrome
- Osteoarthritis
- History of increased hat, glove, or shoe size
- Gigantism (Fig. 264–9) in the young before epiphyseal fusion has taken place
- Decreased exercise capacity
- Visual field deficits
- Diabetes mellitus

Corticotropin-secreting pituitary adenoma—Cushing's disease

- Usually present when the tumor is small (1 to 2 mm)
- 50% of the tumors are smaller than 5 mm.
- Other symptoms (see Fig. 264–11)
  1. Truncal obesity
  2. Round facies (moon face)
  3. Dorsocervical fat accumulation (buffalo hump)
  4. Hirsutism

  5. Acne
  6. Menstrual disorders
  7. Hypertension
  8. Striae
  9. Bruising
  10. Thin skin
  11. Hyperglycemia

Thyrotropin-secreting pituitary adenoma

- In males, larger, more invasive, and more rapidly growing tumors that present later in life
- Other symptoms: thyrotoxicosis, goiter, visual impairment

Nonsecretory pituitary adenomas (endocrine inactive pituitary adenoma)

- Usually large at the time of diagnosis
- Symptoms
  1. Bitemporal hemianopia secondary to compression of the optic chiasm
  2. Hypopituitarism secondary to compression of the pituitary gland
  3. Hypogonadism in men and in premenopausal women
  4. Cranial nerve deficits secondary to extension into the cavernous sinus
  5. Hydrocephalus secondary to extension into the third ventricle, compressing the foramen of Monro
  6. Diabetes insipidus secondary to compression of the hypothalamus or pituitary stalk (a rare complication)

CAUSE

- Benign neoplasms of epithelial origin

DIFFERENTIAL DIAGNOSIS

Prolactinoma

- Pregnancy
- Postpartum puerperium
- Primary hypothyroidism
- Breast disease
- Breast stimulation
- Drug ingestion (especially phenothiazines, antidepressants, haloperidol, methyldopa, reserpine, opiates, amphetamines, and cimetidine)
- Chronic renal failure
- Liver disease
- Polycystic ovary disease
- Chest wall disorders
- Spinal cord lesions
- Previous cranial irradiation

Acromegaly

- Ectopic production of GH-releasing hormone from a carcinoid or other neuroendocrine tumor

Cushing's disease

- Diseases that cause ectopic sources of ACTH overproduction (including small cell carcinoma of the lung [see Fig. 271–2], bronchial carcinoid, intestinal carcinoid, pancreatic islet cell tumor, medullary thyroid carcinoma, or pheochromocytoma) resulting in adrenocortical hyperplasia (Fig. 264–10)
- Adrenal adenomas (Cushing's syndrome [Fig. 264–11]), adrenal carcinoma
- Nelson's syndrome (Fig. 264–12)

Clinical features of a pituitary tumor

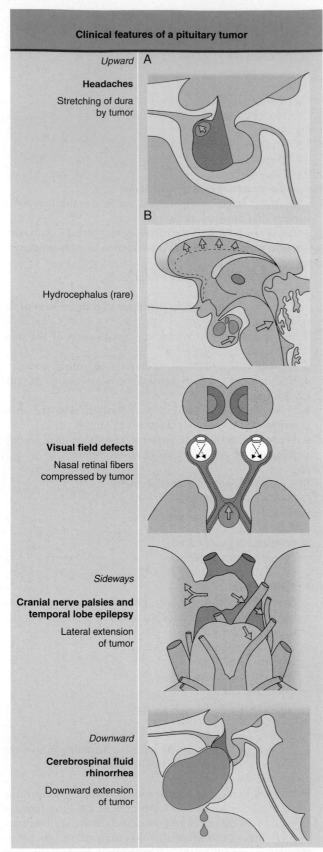

Upward A

Headaches

Stretching of dura
by tumor

B

Hydrocephalus (rare)

Visual field defects

Nasal retinal fibers
compressed by tumor

Sideways

**Cranial nerve palsies and
temporal lobe epilepsy**

Lateral extension
of tumor

Downward

**Cerebrospinal fluid
rhinorrhea**

Downward extension
of tumor

Fig 264–1
Clinical features of a pituitary tumor. The figure illustrates the effects of
local expansion of the tumor (mass effect).
(From Besser CM, Thorner MO: Comprehensive Clinical Endocrinology,
3rd ed. St. Louis, Mosby, 2002.)

Basic mechanisms in hyperprolactinemia

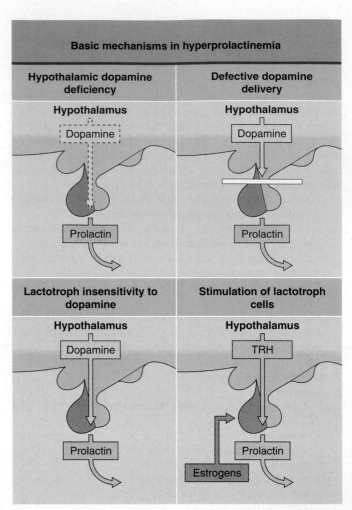

Hypothalamic dopamine deficiency	Defective dopamine delivery
Hypothalamus	**Hypothalamus**
Dopamine	Dopamine
Prolactin	Prolactin

Lactotroph insensitivity to dopamine	Stimulation of lactotroph cells
Hypothalamus	**Hypothalamus**
Dopamine	TRH
Prolactin	Prolactin
	Estrogens

Fig 264–2
Basic mechanisms in hyperprolactinemia. **Top left panel,** Inadequate
synthesis and/or secretion of dopamine from the hypothalamus. **Top
right panel,** Interruption of the hypothalamo-hypophyseal portal circulation. **Bottom left panel,** Decreased sensitivity of the dopamine receptors. (In such cases, lactotropes will be released from dopaminergic inhibition, thereby permitting the release of prolactin.) **Bottom right
panel,** Stimulation of prolactin secretion by estrogens or by excess
thyrotropin-releasing hormone (TRH) in hypothyroidism.
(From Besser CM, Thorner MO: Comprehensive Clinical Endocrinology,
3rd ed. St. Louis, Mosby, 2002.)

Thyrotropin-secreting pituitary adenomas
- Primary hypothyroidism

Nonsecretory pituitary adenoma
- Non-neoplastic mass lesions of various causes (e.g., infectious, granulomatous)

WORKUP

Prolactinoma
- First step: measurement of basal PRL levels
- Elevated PRL levels are correlated with tumor size.
- Levels >200 ng/mL are diagnostic, with levels of 100 to
200 ng/mL being equivocal.
- Basal PRL levels between 20 and 100 ng/mL suggest a
microprolactinoma, as well as other conditions, such as
drug ingestion.
- Basal level lower than 20 ng/mL is normal.

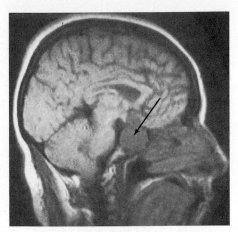

Fig 264–3
Sagittal MRI depicting a large pituitary prolactinoma *(arrow)* in a 13-year-old girl presenting with headaches and galactorrhea. (From Grainger RG, Allison DJ, Adam A, Dixon AK [eds]: Grainger & Allison's Diagnostic Radiology, 4th ed. London, Harcourt, 2001.)

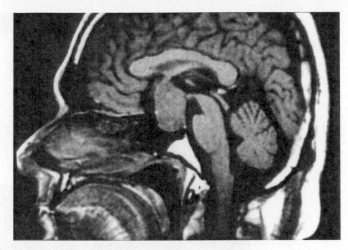

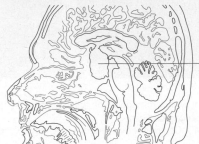

Pituitary tumor with suprasellar extension

Fig 264–5
MRI scan showing a large pituitary tumor with suprasellar extension causing acromegaly.
(From Besser CM, Thorner MO: Comprehensive Clinical Endocrinology, 3rd ed. St. Louis, Mosby, 2002.)

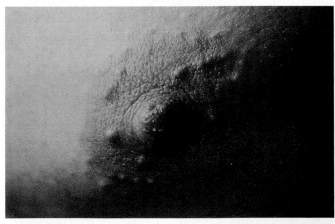

Fig 264–4
Changes in the breast caused by prolactin secretion. Prominent Montgomery tubercles are seen in the breast of a woman with hyperprolactinemia.
(From Besser CM, Thorner MO: Comprehensive Clinical Endocrinology, 3rd ed. St. Louis, Mosby, 2002.)

Acromegaly

- First screening test is the measurement of the serum insulin-like growth factor 1(IGF-1) level, post-serum GH, thyroid-releasing hormone (TRH) stimulation test
- Follow with an oral glucose tolerance test.
- Failure to suppress serum GH to less than 2 ng/mL with an oral load of 100 g glucose is considered conclusive.
- GH–releasing hormone (GH-RH) level >300 ng/mL is indicative of an ectopic source of GH.

Cushing's disease

- Normal or slightly elevated corticotropin level ranging from 20 to 200 pg/mL; normal is 10 to 50 pg/mL.
- Level <10 pg/mL usually indicates an autonomously secreting adrenal tumor.
- Level >200 pg/mL suggests an ectopic corticotropin-secreting neoplasm.

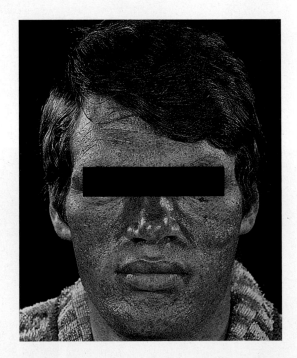

Fig 264–6
Characteristic facial features of a male patient with acromegaly.
(From Besser CM, Thorner MO: Comprehensive Clinical Endocrinology, 3rd ed. St. Louis, Mosby, 2002.)

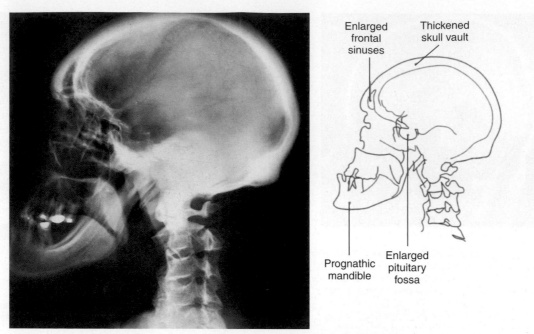

Fig 264-7
Skull radiograph of a patient with acromegaly. The enlarged pituitary fossa and sinuses, thickened skull vault, and prognathism with loss of angle of the mandible can be seen.
(From Besser CM, Thorner MO: Comprehensive Clinical Endocrinology, 3rd ed. St. Louis, Mosby, 2002.)

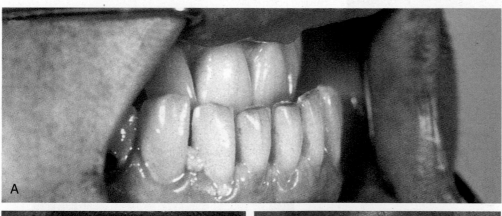

Fig 264-8
Prognathism **(A)** and macroglossia **(B)** in acromegaly. These are shown with a tongue of normal size **(C)** for comparison.
(From Besser CM, Thorner MO: Comprehensive Clinical Endocrinology, 3rd ed. St. Louis, Mosby, 2002.)

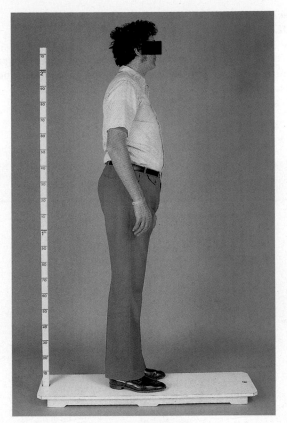

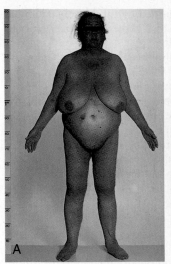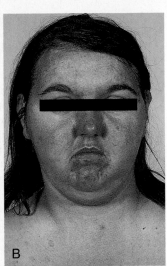

Fig 264-11
Cushing's syndrome. **A,** Typical clinical appearance of a patient with Cushing's syndrome. Central obesity with proximal muscle wasting can be seen. **B,** Typical moon face appearance of a patient with Cushing's syndrome. A plethoric face with acne and hirsutism is characteristic and there is evidence of temporal hair recession.
(From Besser CM, Thorner MO: Comprehensive Clinical Endocrinology, 3rd ed. St. Louis, Mosby, 2002.)

Fig 264-9
Patient 2.3 m (7'6") in height with pituitary gigantism. Gigantism is the rare clinical counterpart of acromegaly and occurs in the young before epiphyseal fusion has taken place.
(From Besser CM, Thorner MO: Comprehensive Clinical Endocrinology, 3rd ed. St. Louis, Mosby, 2002.)

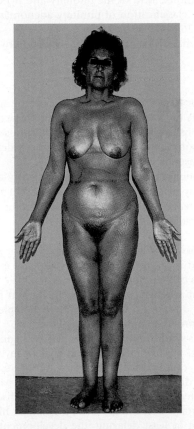

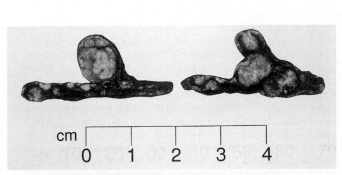

Fig 264-10
Macronodular adrenocortical hyperplasia in a patient with Cushing's disease. Most nodules are 0.5 cm or large in diameter. This patient had multiple endocrine neoplasia (MEN) syndrome type 1.
(From Silverberg SG, Frable WJ, Wick MR, et al [eds]: Principles and Practice of Surgical Pathology and Cytopathology, 4th ed. Philadelphia, Elsevier, 2006.)

Fig 264-12
Appearance of a patient with Nelson's syndrome. The gross pigmentation that occurs in this syndrome is best seen on the flexural surfaces of the body.
(From Besser CM, Thorner MO: Comprehensive Clinical Endocrinology, 3rd ed. St. Louis, Mosby, 2002.)

- Cushing's disease is confirmed by the demonstration of low-dose dexamethasone, which shows the presence of abnormal cortisol suppressibility.
- 24-hour urine collection should demonstrate an increased level of cortisol excretion.

Thyrotropin-secreting pituitary adenoma
- Highly sensitive thyrotropin assays, which evaluate the presence of thyrotoxicosis, are one way to detect a thyrotropin-secreting tumor.
- Free alpha subunit is secreted by more than 80% of tumors; ratio of alpha subunit to thyrotropin <1.
- With central resistance to thyroid hormone, ratio is <1 and the sella is normal.
- Laboratory tests show elevated serum levels of both T_3 and T_4.

Nonsecretory pituitary adenoma
- Visual field testing
- Assessment of pituitary and organ function to determine whether there is hypopituitarism or hypersecretion of hormones (even if the effects of hypersecretion are subclinical)
- TRH to provoke secretion of FSH, LH, and LH–beta subunit; will not elicit response in normal persons
- Exclusion of Klinefelter's syndrome in patients with long-standing primary hypogonadism, elevated gonadotropin levels, and enlargement of the sella

IMAGING STUDIES
- Study of choice: MRI of the pituitary and hypothalamus. A radiologic classification of pituitary adenomas is described in Figure 264–13.
- CT only when MRI is unavailable or is otherwise contraindicated

TREATMENT
Surgery
- Selective trans-sphenoidal resection of the adenoma (Fig. 264–14) is the treatment of choice for prolactinoma, acromegaly, Cushing's disease, and thyrotropin-secreting pituitary adenomas, which all tend to be microadenomas at the time of onset of symptoms.
- Macroadenomas, such as the nonsecretory pituitary adenoma, may also be surgically removed, but risk of recurrence is greater with these tumors and adjunctive therapy such as irradiation may also be necessary.

Radiotherapy
- Radiotherapy (Fig. 264–15) is reserved for patients who have failed surgical treatment and who still experience the symptoms of their adenoma.
- Bilateral adrenalectomy has been done in patients with Cushing's disease on failure of other therapies; complications require lifelong hormone replacement.
- Nelson's syndrome manifests with hyperpigmentation (see Fig. 264–12) following bilateral adrenalectomy for Cushing's syndrome caused by the pituitary tumor responsible for Cushing's disease. It occurs in about 40% of patients undergoing bilateral adrenalectomy for Cushing's disease. Prophylactic pituitary radiotherapy alters the natural history by preventing, or at least delaying, the development of Nelson's syndrome and, if given at the time of adrenalectomy, is believed to reduce the prevalence dramatically.

Medical treatment
PROLACTINOMA
- Bromocriptine
- Other compounds under investigation include pergolide mesylate, a long-acting ergot derivative with dopaminergic properties, as well as other nonergot derivatives.

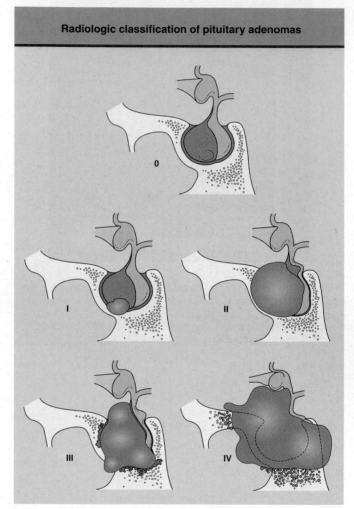

Radiologic classification of pituitary adenomas

Fig 264–13

Radiologic classification of pituitary adenomas. Pituitary tumors are commonly classified on the basis of their size, invasion status, and growth patterns, as proposed by Hardy and Vezina in 1979. Tumors less than or equal to 1 cm in diameter are designated microadenomas, whereas larger tumors are designated macroadenomas—grade 0, intrapituitary microadenoma; normal sellar appearance; grade 1, intrapituitary microadenoma, focal bulging of sellar wall; grade 2, intrasellar macroadenoma, diffusely enlarged sella, no invasion; grade 3, macroadenoma, localized sellar invasion and/or destruction; grade 4, macroadenoma, extensive sellar invasion and/or destruction. Tumors are further subclassified on their basis of their extrasellar extension, whether suprasellar or parasellar.
(From Besser CM, Thorner MO: Comprehensive Clinical Endocrinology, 43rd ed. St. Louis, Mosby, 2002.)

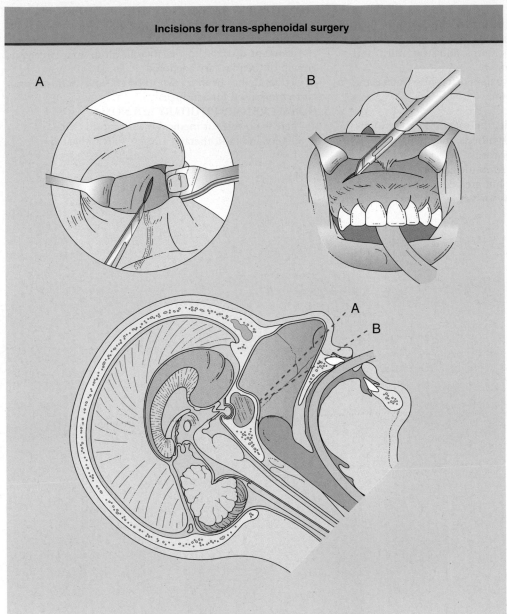

Incisions for trans-sphenoidal surgery

A

B

A

B

Fig 264–14
Incisions for trans-sphenoidal surgery. The endonasal **(A)** and sublabial **(B)** incisions are illustrated, with the direction of approach (bottom panel) afforded by each.
(From Besser CM, Thorner MO: Comprehensive Clinical Endocrinology, 3rd ed. St. Louis, Mosby, 2002.)

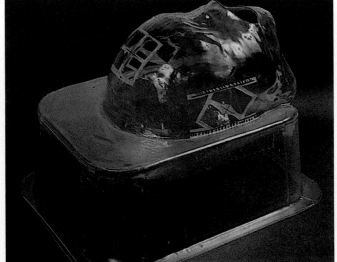

Fig 264–15
An individual head mask used to position the patient accurately during radiotherapy. Three fields are used, and the daily dose of radiation should not exceed 180 cGy.
(From Besser CM, Thorner MO: Comprehensive Clinical Endocrinology, 3rd ed. St. Louis, Mosby, 2002.)

ACROMEGALY

- Octreotide, a somatostatin analogue, is the medical therapy of choice but is limited by side effects, such as biliary sludge and gallstones, nausea, cramps, and steatorrhea, and by its parenteral administration.
- Bromocriptine is less effective than octreotide, but has the advantage of oral administration.

CUSHING'S DISEASE

- Ketoconazole, which inhibits the cytochrome P-450 enzymes involved in steroid biosynthesis, may be effective in managing mild to moderate disease.
- Metyrapone and aminoglutethimide can be used to control hypersecretion of cortisol but are generally used when preparing a patient for surgery or while waiting for a response to radiotherapy.

THYROTROPIN-SECRETING PITUITARY ADENOMA

- Ablative therapy with radioactive iodide or surgery is indicated.
- Treatment directed to the thyroid alone may accelerate growth of the pituitary adenoma.
- Octreotide has been shown to be effective in doses similar to those used for acromegaly.

NONSECRETORY PITUITARY ADENOMA

- There is no role for medical therapy at this time.
- Surgery and radiotherapy are generally indicated.

Chapter 265 Diabetes insipidus

DEFINITION

Diabetes insipidus is a polyuric disorder resulting from insufficient production of antidiuretic hormone (ADH) (pituitary [neurogenic] diabetes insipidus) or unresponsiveness of the renal tubules to ADH (nephrogenic diabetes insipidus). Figure 265–1 describes the various causes of polyuria and polydipsia

PHYSICAL FINDINGS AND CLINICAL PRESENTATION

- Polyuria: urinary volumes ranging from 2.5 to 6 L/day
- Polydipsia (predilection for cold or iced drinks)
- Neurologic manifestations (seizures, headaches, visual field defects)
- Evidence of volume contractions

Note: The previous physical findings and clinical manifestations are generally not evident until vasopressin secretory capacity is reduced to lower than 20% of normal.

CAUSE

Neurogenic diabetes insipidus

- Idiopathic
- Neoplasms of brain or pituitary fossa (craniopharyngiomas, metastatic neoplasms from breast or lung)
- Post-therapeutic neurosurgical procedures (e.g., hypophysectomy)
- Head trauma (e.g., basal skull fracture)
- Granulomatous disorders (sarcoidosis or tuberculosis [TB])
- Histiocytosis (Hand-Schüller-Christian disease, eosinophilic granuloma)
- Familial (autosomal dominant)
- Other: interventricular hemorrhage, aneurysms, meningitis, postencephalitis, multiple sclerosis

Nephrogenic diabetes insipidus

- Drugs: lithium, amphotericin B, demeclocycline, methoxyflurane anesthesia
- Familial: X-linked
- Metabolic: hypercalcemia or hypokalemia
- Other: sarcoidosis, amyloidosis, pyelonephritis, polycystic disease, sickle cell disease, postobstructive

DIFFERENTIAL DIAGNOSIS

- Diabetes mellitus, nephropathies
- Primary polydipsia, medications (e.g., chlorpromazine)
- Osmotic diuresis (e.g., glucose, mannitol, anticholinergics)
- Psychogenic polydipsia, electrolyte disturbances

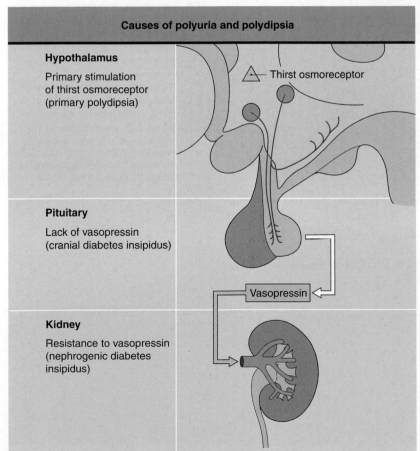

Causes of polyuria and polydipsia

Hypothalamus

Primary stimulation of thirst osmoreceptor (primary polydipsia)

△ — Thirst osmoreceptor

Pituitary

Lack of vasopressin (cranial diabetes insipidus)

Vasopressin

Kidney

Resistance to vasopressin (nephrogenic diabetes insipidus)

Fig 265–1
Causes of polyuria and polydipsia. **Top,** Primary polydipsia is usually related to psychiatric illness. Vasopressin secretion is suppressed by low plasma osmolality induced by the excessive water intake which, if prolonged, may also affect the kidney. **Center,** Cranial diabetes insipidus is caused by a reduction or absence of vasopressin. **Bottom,** In nephrogenic diabetes insipidus, there is resistance to the renal action of vasopressin, with a consequent rise in the plasma vasopressin concentration to a level that is inappropriately high relative to urine osmolality.
(From Besser CM, Thorner MO: Comprehensive Clinical Endocrinology, 3rd ed. St. Louis, Mosby, 2002.)

LABORATORY TESTS

- Decreased urinary specific gravity (≤1.005)
- Decreased urinary osmolarity (usually <200 mOsm/kg), even in the presence of high serum osmolality
- Hypernatremia, increased plasma osmolarity, hypercalcemia, hypokalemia
- The diagnostic workup is aimed at showing that the polyuria is caused by the inability to concentrate urine and determining whether the problem is secondary to decreased ADH or insensitivity to ADH. This is done with the water deprivation test. Figure 265–2 differentiates causes of polyuria.

IMAGING STUDIES

- MRI of the brain if neurogenic diabetes insipidus is confirmed

TREATMENT

- Patient education regarding control of fluid balance and prevention of dehydration with adequate fluid intake
- Daily weight
- Therapy varies with the degree and type of diabetes insipidus.

Neurogenic diabetes insipidus

1. Desmopressin acetate (DDAVP)
2. Vasopressin tannate in oil: useful for long-term management because of its long life
3. In mild cases of neurogenic diabetes insipidus, the polyuria may be controlled with hydrochlorothiazide (HCTZ; decreases urine volume by increasing proximal tubular reabsorption of glomerular infiltrate)

Nephrogenic diabetes insipidus

1. Adequate hydration
2. Low-sodium diet and chlorothiazide to induce mild sodium depletion
3. Polyuria of diabetes insipidus secondary to lithium can be ameliorated by using amiloride.

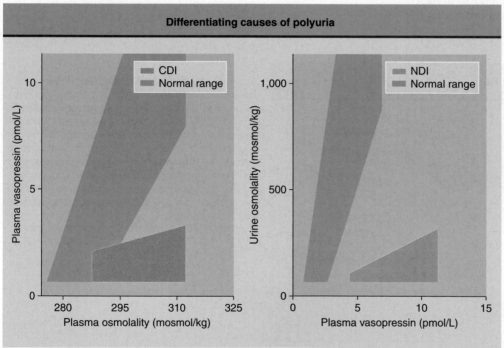

Fig 265–2
Differentiating causes of polyuria.
Left, After osmotic stimulation with 5% hypertonic saline IV, patients with cranial diabetes insipidus (CDI) exhibit values to the right of the normal range, whereas those with nephrogenic diabetes insipidus (NDI) and primary polydipsia will show values within the normal limits.
Right, After overnight dehydration, NDI is usually distinguishable from primary polydipsia by the inappropriately high levels of plasma vasopressin relative to urine osmolality. (From Besser CM, Thorner MO: Comprehensive Clinical Endocrinology, 3rd ed. St. Louis, Mosby, 2002.)

Chapter 266 | Inappropriate secretion of antidiuretic hormone

DEFINITION

The syndrome of inappropriate secretion of antidiuretic hormone (SIADH) is characterized by excessive secretion of ADH in the absence of normal osmotic or physiologic stimuli (increased serum osmolarity, decreased plasma volume, hypotension). Figure 266–1 illustrates the pathophysiology and clinical presentation of inappropriate vasopressin secretion.

PHYSICAL FINDINGS AND CLINICAL PRESENTATION

- The patient is generally normovolemic or slightly hypervolemic; edema is absent.
- Delirium, lethargy, and seizures may be present if the hyponatremia is severe or of rapid onset.
- Manifestations of the underlying disease may be evident (e.g., fever from an infectious process or headaches and visual field defects from an intracranial mass).
- Diminished reflexes and extensor plantar responses may occur with severe hyponatremia.

CAUSE

- Neoplasm: lung, duodenum, pancreas, brain, thymus, bladder, prostate, mesothelioma, lymphoma, Ewing's sarcoma
- Pulmonary disorders: pneumonia, TB, bronchiectasis, emphysema, status asthmaticus
- Intracranial pathology: trauma, neoplasms, infections (meningitis, encephalitis, brain abscess), hemorrhage, hydrocephalus
- Postoperative period: surgical stress, ventilators with positive pressure, anesthetic agents
- Drugs: chlorpropamide, thiazide diuretics, vasopressin, desmopressin, oxytocin, chemotherapeutic agents (vincristine, vinblastine, cyclophosphamide), carbamazepine, phenothiazines, monoamine oxidase (MAO) inhibitors, tricyclic antidepressants, narcotics, nicotine, clofibrate, haloperidol, selective serotonin reuptake inhibitors (SSRIs)
- Other: acute intermittent porphyria, Guillain-Barré syndrome, myxedema, psychosis, delirium tremens, ACTH deficiency (hypopituitarism)

DIFFERENTIAL DIAGNOSIS

- Hyponatremia associated with hypervolemia (congestive heart failure [CHF], cirrhosis, nephrotic syndrome)
- Factitious hyponatremia (hyperglycemia, abnormal proteins, hyperlipidemia)
- Hypovolemia associated with hypovolemia (e.g., burns, GI fluid loss)

LABORATORY TESTS

- Hyponatremia
- Urinary osmolarity > serum osmolarity
- Urinary sodium usually >30 mEq/L
- Normal blood urea nitrogen (BUN), creatinine (indicative of normal renal function and absence of dehydration)
- Decreased uric acid

IMAGING STUDIES

- Chest x-ray to rule out neoplasm or infectious process

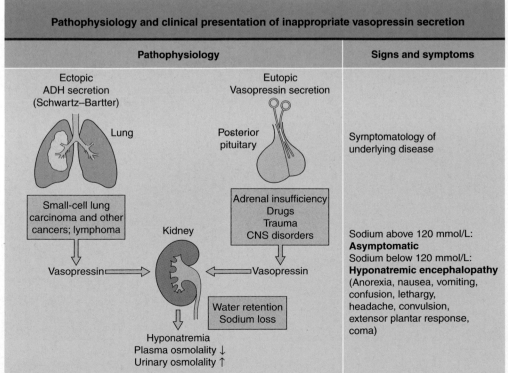

Pathophysiology and clinical presentation of inappropriate vasopressin secretion	
Pathophysiology	**Signs and symptoms**

Ectopic ADH secretion (Schwartz–Bartter)

Eutopic Vasopressin secretion

Lung

Posterior pituitary

Small-cell lung carcinoma and other cancers; lymphoma

Kidney

Adrenal insufficiency
Drugs
Trauma
CNS disorders

Vasopressin → ← Vasopressin

Water retention
Sodium loss

Hyponatremia
Plasma osmolality ↓
Urinary osmolality ↑

Symptomatology of underlying disease

Sodium above 120 mmol/L:
Asymptomatic
Sodium below 120 mmol/L:
Hyponatremic encephalopathy
(Anorexia, nausea, vomiting, confusion, lethargy, headache, convulsion, extensor plantar response, coma)

Fig 266–1
Pathophysiology and clinical presentation of inappropriate vasopressin secretion.
(From Besser CM, Thorner MO: Comprehensive Clinical Endocrinology, 3rd ed. St. Louis, Mosby, 2002.)

TREATMENT

- Fluid restriction to 500 to 800 mL/day
- In emergency situations (seizures, coma), SIADH can be treated with a combination of hypertonic saline solution (slow infusion of 250 mL of 3% NaCl) and furosemide. This increases the serum sodium by causing diuresis of urine that is more dilute than plasma. The rapidity of correction varies depending on the degree of hyponatremia and whether the hyponatremia is acute or chronic. Generally, the serum sodium level should be corrected only halfway to normal in the initial 24 hours and should be increased by <0.5 mEq/L/hr.

- Depending on the underlying cause, fluid restriction may be needed indefinitely. Monthly monitoring of electrolytes is recommended for patients with chronic SIADH.
- Demeclocycline (Declomycin) may be useful in patients with chronic SIADH (e.g., secondary to neoplasm), but use with caution in patients with hepatic disease. Its side effects include nephrogenic DI and photosensitivity.
- Successful treatment of chronic nephrogenic SIADH with urea to induce osmotic diuresis has been reported in children and adults.

THYROID

Chapter 267 Hypothyroidism

DEFINITION

Hypothyroidism is a disorder caused by the inadequate secretion of thyroid hormone.

PHYSICAL FINDINGS AND CLINICAL PRESENTATION

- Hypothyroid patients generally present with the following signs and symptoms: fatigue, dry lethargy, weakness, constipation, weight gain, cold intolerance, muscle weakness, slow speech, slow cerebration with poor memory.
- Skin: dry, coarse, thick, cool, sallow (yellow color caused by carotenemia); nonpitting edema in skin of the eyelids (Fig. 267–1) and hands (myxedema) secondary to infiltration of subcutaneous tissues by a hydrophilic mucopolysaccharide substance
- Hair: brittle and coarse; loss of outer third of eyebrows
- Facies (Fig. 267–2): dulled expression, thickened tongue, thick slow-moving lips.
- Thyroid gland: may or may not be palpable (depending on the cause of the hypothyroidism). A significant enlargement of the thyroid into the chest cavity may impair venous outflow from the head and neck. Elevation of the patient's arms until they touch the sides of the head will result in obstruction and dilation of the cervical veins (*Pemberton's sign* [Fig. 267–3]).
- Heart sounds: distant, possible pericardial effusion (Fig.267–4C, D).
- Pulse: bradycardia. ECG reveals low voltage (see Fig. 267–4A, B).
- Neurologic: delayed relaxation phase of deep tendon reflexes (DTRs), cerebellar ataxia, hearing impairment, poor memory, peripheral neuropathies with paresthesia
- Musculoskeletal: carpal tunnel syndrome, muscular stiffness, weakness.
- Infants with congenital hypothyroidism may reveal periorbital edema, flattened bridge of nose, macroglossia (Fig. 267–5).

CAUSE

Primary hypothyroidism (thyroid gland dysfunction)

- Cause of more than 90% of cases of hypothyroidism
- Hashimoto's thyroiditis is the most common cause of hypothyroidism after 8 years of age.
- Idiopathic myxedema (nongoitrous form of Hashimoto's thyroiditis)
- Previous treatment of hyperthyroidism (radioiodine therapy, subtotal thyroidectomy)
- Subacute thyroiditis
- Radiation therapy to the neck (usually for malignant disease)
- Iodine deficiency or excess
- Drugs (lithium, aminosalicylic acid [PAS], sulfonamides, phenylbutazone, amiodarone, thiourea)
- Congenital (approximately 1 case/4000 live births)
- Prolonged treatment with iodides

Secondary hypothyroidism

- Pituitary dysfunction, postpartum necrosis, neoplasm, infiltrative disease causing deficiency of TSH

Tertiary hypothyroidism

- Hypothalamic disease (granuloma, neoplasm, or irradiation causing deficiency of TRH)

Tissue resistance to thyroid hormone

- Rare

DIFFERENTIAL DIAGNOSIS

- Depression
- Dementia from other causes
- Systemic disorders (e.g., nephrotic syndrome, CHF, amyloidosis)

LABORATORY TESTS

- Increased TSH: TSH may be normal if patient has secondary or tertiary hypothyroidism, is receiving dopamine or corticosteroids, or the level is obtained following severe illness.
- Decreased free T_4
- Other common laboratory abnormalities: hyperlipidemia, hyponatremia, and anemia
- Increased antimicrosomal and antithyroglobulin antibody titers: useful when autoimmune thyroiditis is suspected as the cause of the hypothyroidism

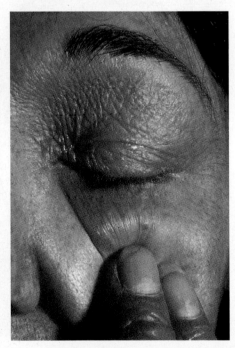

Fig 267–1
Generalized myxedema. Note the waxy infiltrated plaques on the eyelid. (Courtesy of Dr. R. A. Marsden, St. George's Hospital, London.)

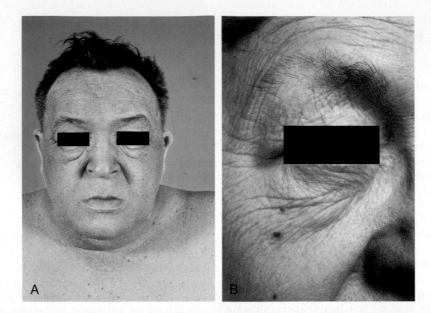

Fig 267-2
A, B, Typical appearance of patients with moderately severe primary hypothyroidism or myxedema. Note the dry skin and sallow complexion, with the absence of scleral pigmentation differentiating the carotenemia from jaundice. Both individuals demonstrate periorbital myxedema. The patient in **B** illustrates the loss of the lateral aspects of the eyebrow, sometimes termed *Queen Anne's sign*. That finding is not unusual in the age group commonly affected by severe hypothyroidism and should not be considered to be a specific sign of the condition.
(From Larsen PR, Kronenberg HM, Melmed S, Polonsky KS: Williams Textbook of Endocrinology, 10th ed. Philadelphia, WB Saunders, 2003.)

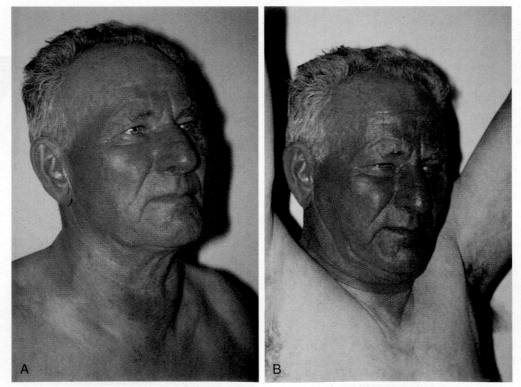

Fig 267-3
A, B, Pemberton's sign.
(From Swartz MH: Textbook of Physical Diagnosis, 5th ed. Philadelphia, WB Saunders, 2006.)

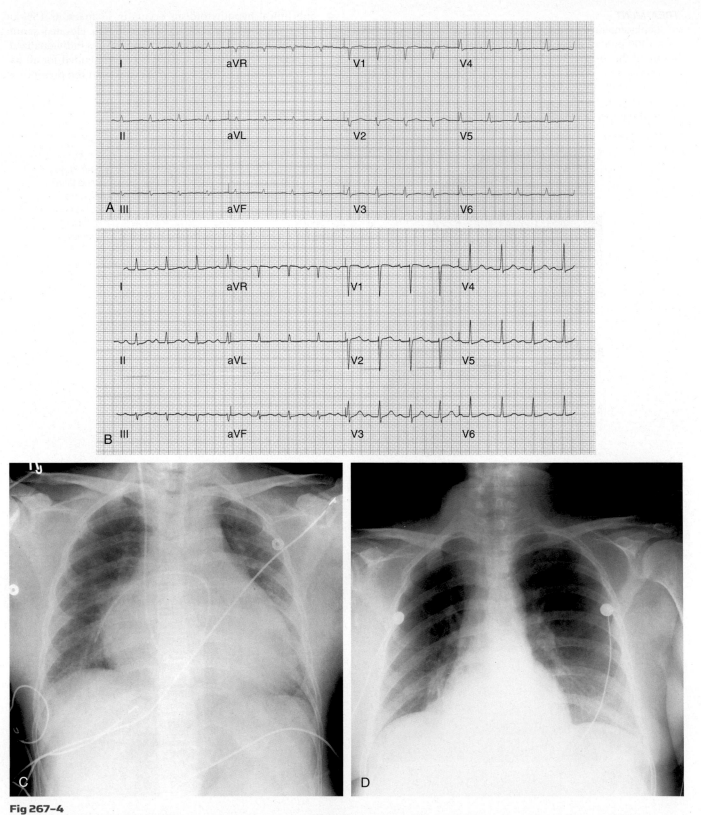

Fig 267–4

Hypothyroidism. **A,** Twelve-lead ECG of a profoundly hypothyroid patient in heart failure. Note the low voltage, widened QRS and flattened T waves. **B,** Twelve-lead ECG from the same patient 5 months later, after thyroid hormone replacement. The ECG is now normal except for first-degree atrioventricular block. **C,** Chest x-ray on admission in heart failure with a pericardial effusion. **D,** Chest x-ray before discharge 3 weeks later with normal cardiac silhouette.

(From Crawford, MH, DiMarco JP, Paulus WJ [eds]: Cardiology, 2nd ed. St. Louis, Mosby, 2004.)

TREATMENT

- Replacement therapy with levothyroxine (L-thyroxine), 25 to 100 μg/day, depending on the patient's age and the severity of the disease. The levothyroxine dose may be increased every 6 to 8 weeks. For monitoring therapy in patients with central hypothyroidism, measurement of serum free thyroxine (free T_4 level) is appropriate and should be maintained in the upper one half of the normal range.

- Subclinical hypothyroidism occurs in as many as 15% of older patients and is characterized by an elevated serum TSH and a normal free T_4 level. Treatment is individualized. Generally, replacement therapy is recommended for all patients with serum TSH >10 mU/L and with the presence of goiter or thyroid autoantibodies.

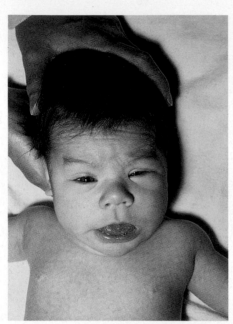

Fig 267–5

Infant with typical stigmata of severe congenital hypothyroidism. Note coarse features, periorbital edema, flattened bridge of nose, and large protruding tongue. Not seen in the picture are umbilical hernia, cutis marmorata, and cold extremities. The infant had a hoarse cry, somnolence, and constipation. Such typical stigmata are rare; most hypothyroid neonates identified in newborn screening programs are not clinically suspected.
(From Besser CM, Thorner MO: Comprehensive Clinical Endocrinology, 3rd ed. St. Louis, Mosby, 2002.)

Chapter 268 Hyperthyroidism

DEFINITION
Hyperthyroidism is a hypermetabolic state resulting from excess thyroid hormone.

PHYSICAL FINDINGS AND CLINICAL PRESENTATION
- Patients with hyperthyroidism generally present with the following clinical manifestations: tachycardia, tremor, hyperreflexia, anxiety, irritability, emotional lability, panic attacks, heat intolerance, sweating, increased appetite, diarrhea, weight loss, menstrual dysfunction (oligomenorrhea, amenorrhea). The presentation may be different in older patients (see below).
- Patients with Graves' disease (Fig. 268–1) may present with exophthalmos, lid retraction lid lag (Graves' ophthalmopathy). The following signs and symptoms of ophthalmopathy may be present: blurring of vision, photophobia, increased lacrimation, double vision, deep orbital pressure, clubbing of fingers associated with periosteal new bone formation in other skeletal areas. Graves' acropachy (Fig. 268–2) and thyroid dermopathy (Fig. 268–3) may be present.
- In older patients, the clinical signs of hyperthyroidism may be masked by manifestations of coexisting disease (e.g., new-onset atrial fibrillation, exacerbation of CHF).
- Older hyperthyroid patients may have only subtle signs (e.g., weight loss, tachycardia, fine skin, brittle nails). This form is known as *apathetic hyperthyroidism* and manifests with lethargy rather than hyperkinetic activity. An enlarged thyroid gland may be absent. Coexisting medical disorders (most commonly cardiac disease) may also mask the symptoms. These patients often have unexplained CHF, worsening of angina, or new-onset atrial fibrillation resistant to treatment.
- Subclinical hyperthyroidism is defined as normal serum free T_4 and T_3 levels with a TSH level suppressed below the normal range and usually undetectable. These patients usually do not present with signs or symptoms of overt hyperthyroidism. Treatment options include observation or a therapeutic trial of low-dose antithyroid agents for 6 months to attempt to induce remission.

CAUSE
- Graves' disease (diffuse toxic goiter): 80% to 90% of all cases of hyperthyroidism
- Toxic multinodular goiter *(Plummer's disease)*
- Toxic adenoma
- Iatrogenic and factitious
- Transient hyperthyroidism (subacute thyroiditis, Hashimoto's thyroiditis)
- Rare causes: hypersecretion of TSH (e.g., pituitary neoplasms), struma ovarii, ingestion of large amount of iodine in a patient with preexisting thyroid hyperplasia or adenoma *(Jod-Basedow phenomenon)*, hydatidiform mole, carcinoma of thyroid, amiodarone therapy

DIFFERENTIAL DIAGNOSIS
- Anxiety disorder
- Pheochromocytoma
- Metastatic neoplasm
- Diabetes mellitus
- Premenopausal state

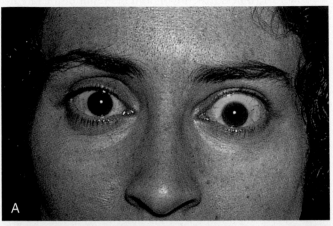
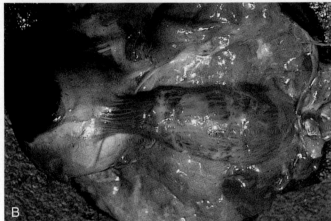
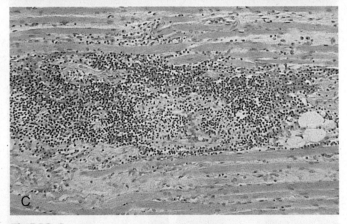

Fig 268–1
Graves' disease. **A,** In Graves' disease, exophthalmos often looks more pronounced than it actually is because of the extreme lid retraction that may occur. This patient, for example, had minimal proptosis of the left eye but marked lid retraction. **B,** Orbital contents obtained postmortem from a patient with Graves' disease. Note the enormously thickened extraocular muscle. **C,** Both fluid and inflammatory cells separating the muscle bundle may be seen. The inflammatory cells are predominantly lymphocytes, plus plasma cells.
(**A,** From Yanoff M, Fine BS: Ocular Pathology, 5th ed. St. Louis, Mosby, 2002; **B, C,** from Hufnagel TJ, Hickey WF, Cobbs WH, et al: Immunohistochemical and ultrastructural studies on the exenterated orbital tissues of a patient with Graves' disease. Ophthalmology. 1984; 91:1411.)

LABORATORY TESTS
- Elevated free T_4
- Elevated free T_3: generally not necessary for diagnosis
- Low TSH (unless hyperthyroidism is a result of the rare hypersecretion of TSH from a pituitary adenoma)
- Thyroid autoantibodies are useful in select cases to differentiate Graves' disease from toxic multinodular goiter (absent thyroid antibodies).

IMAGING STUDIES
- 24-hour radioactive iodine uptake (RAIU) is useful to distinguish suspected hyperthyroidism from iatrogenic thyroid hormone synthesis *(thyrotoxicosis factitia)* and from thyroiditis.
- An overactive thyroid shows increased uptake (Fig.268–4). A normal underactive thyroid (iatrogenic thyroid ingestion, painless or subacute thyroiditis) shows normal or decreased uptake.
- RAIU results also vary with the cause of the hyperthyroidism.
  - Graves' disease: increased homogeneous uptake.
  - Multinodular goiter: increased heterogeneous uptake.

- Hot nodule: single focus of increased uptake (Fig. 268–5)
- RAIU is also generally performed before the therapeutic administration of radioactive iodine to determine the appropriate dose.

TREATMENT

Antithyroid drugs (thionamides)
- Propylthiouracil (PTU) and methimazole (Tapazole) inhibit thyroid hormone synthesis by blocking production of thyroid peroxidase (PTU and methimazole) or inhibiting peripheral conversion of T_4 to T_3 (PTU).
- When antithyroid drugs are used as primary therapy, they are usually given for 6 to 18 months; prolonged therapy may cause hypothyroidism. Monitor thyroid function every 2 months for 6 months, then less frequently.
- The use of antithyroid drugs before radioactive iodine therapy is best reserved for patients in whom exacerbation of hyperthyroidism after radioactive iodine therapy is hazardous (e.g., older patients with coronary artery disease or significant coexisting morbidity). In these patients, the antithyroid drug can be stopped 2 days before radioactive iodine therapy, resumed 2 days later, and continued for 4 to 6 weeks.

Radioactive iodine
- Radioactive iodine (RAI, ^{131}I) is the treatment of choice for patients older than 21 years and younger patients who have not achieved remission after 1 year of antithyroid drug therapy. Radioiodine is also used in hyperthyroidism caused by toxic adenoma or toxic multinodular goiter.
- Contraindicated during pregnancy (can cause fetal hypothyroidism) and lactation. Pregnancy should be excluded in women of childbearing age before radioactive iodine is administered.
- A single dose of radioactive iodine is effective in inducing a euthyroid state in almost 80% of patients.
- There is a high incidence of postradioactive iodine hypothyroidism (more than 50% within first year and 2%/year thereafter); therefore, these patients should be frequently evaluated for the onset of hypothyroidism.

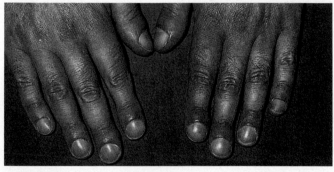

Fig 268–2
Thyroid acropachy. This is marked in the index fingers and thumbs. (From Besser CM, Thorner MO: Comprehensive Clinical Endocrinology, 3rd ed. St. Louis, Mosby, 2002.)

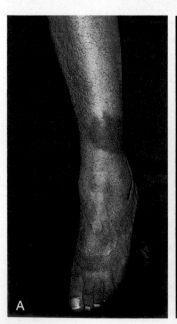
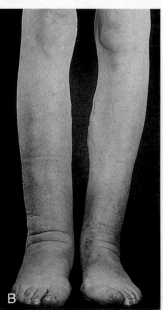
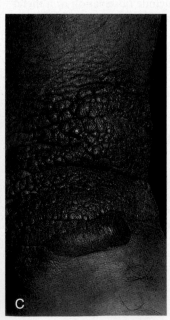

A   B   C

Fig 268–3
Thyroid dermopathy. **A,** Localized plaque on the outer aspect of the skin. **B,** Sheetlike involvement of the lower leg, with coarse skin, thickened hair, and nonpitting edema. **C,** Horny form over shin and dorsum of the foot. (From Besser CM, Thorner MO: Comprehensive Clinical Endocrinology, 3rd ed. St. Louis, Mosby, 2002.)

Surgical therapy (subtotal thyroidectomy)

- Indicated for obstructing goiters, any patient who refuses radioactive iodine and cannot be adequately managed with antithyroid medications (e.g., patients with toxic adenoma or toxic multinodular goiter), and pregnant patients who cannot be adequately managed with antithyroid medication or develop side effects to them
- Patients should be rendered euthyroid with antithyroid drugs before surgery.

- Complications of surgery include hypothyroidism (28% to 43% after 10 years), hypoparathyroidism, and vocal cord paralysis (1%).
- Hyperthyroidism recurs after surgery in 10% to 15% of patients.

Adjunctive therapy

- Propranolol alleviates the beta-adrenergic symptoms of hyperthyroidism.

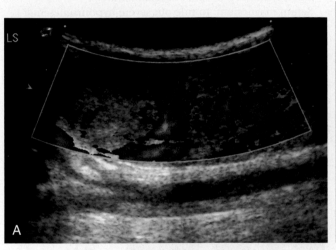

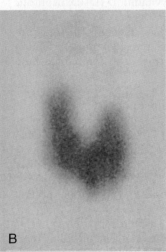

Fig 268–4

Graves' disease. **A,** Longitudinal ultrasound with color Doppler shows diffusely increased vascularity of the thyroid gland. **B,** 99mTc-pertechnetate scan shows a diffusely increased tracer uptake.
(From Grainger RG, Allison DJ, Adam A, Dixon AK [eds]: Grainger & Allison's Diagnostic Radiology, 4th ed. London, Harcourt, 2001.)

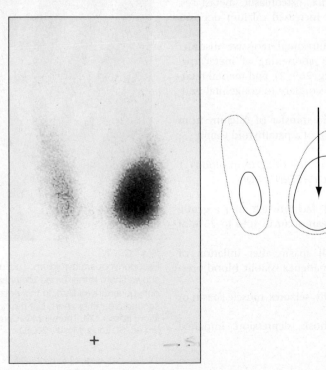

Fig 268–5

Technetium-99m thyroid scan of a toxic adenoma in the left lobe of the thyroid *(arrow).*
(From Besser CM, Thorner MO: Comprehensive Clinical Endocrinology, 3rd ed. St. Louis, Mosby, 2002.)

PARATHYROIDS

Chapter 269 **Hypocalcemia**

CAUSE

- Idiopathic hypoparathyroidism, surgical removal of parathyroids (e.g., neck surgery)
- Renal insufficiency: hypocalcemia caused by the following:
  - Increased calcium deposits in bone and soft tissue secondary to increased serum PO_4^{3-} level
  - Decreased production of 1,25-dihydroxyvitamin D
  - Excessive loss of 25-hydroxyvitamin D (OHD; nephrotic syndrome)
- Hypoalbuminemia: each decrease in serum albumin concentration (g/L) will decrease serum calcium concentration by 0.8 mg/dL but will not change free (ionized) calcium level.
- Vitamin D deficiency:
  - Malabsorption (most common cause)
  - Inadequate intake
  - Decreased production of 1,25-dihydroxyvitamin D (vitamin D–dependent rickets, renal failure)
  - Decreased production of 25-OHD (parenchymal liver disease)
  - Accelerated 25-OHD catabolism (phenytoin, phenobarbital)
  - End-organ resistance to 1,25-dihydroxyvitamin D
- Hypomagnesemia: hypocalcemia caused by the following:
  - Decreased PTH secretion
  - Inhibition of PTH effect on bone
- Pancreatitis, hyperphosphatemia, osteoblastic metastases: hypocalcemia is secondary to increased calcium deposits (bone, abdomen).
- Pseudohypoparathyroidism: autosomal recessive disorder characterized by short stature, shortening of metacarpal bones (Fig. 269–1), obesity (Fig. 269–2), and mental retardation. The hypocalcemia is secondary to congenital end-organ resistance to PTH.
- Hungry bones syndrome: rapid transfer of calcium from plasma into bones after removal of a parathyroid tumor
- Sepsis
- Massive blood transfusion (as a result of EDTA in blood)

PHYSICAL FINDINGS AND CLINICAL PRESENTATION

- Neuromuscular irritability:
  - *Chvostek's sign* (Fig. 269–3): facial twitch after a gentle tapping over the facial nerve (can occur in 10% to 25% of normal adults)
  - *Trousseau's sign:* carpopedal spasm after inflation of blood pressure cuff above the patient's systolic blood pressure for 2 to 3 minutes
  - Tetany, paresthesias, myopathy, seizures, muscle spasm or weakness
- Psychiatric disturbances: psychosis, depression, impaired cognitive function
- Soft tissue calcifications, ocular cataracts
- Cardiovascular manifestations: arrhythmias, CHF (caused by decreased myocardial contractility), increased QT interval, hypotension

LABORATORY TESTS

- Serum albumin: to rule out hypoalbuminemia
- BUN, creatinine: to rule out renal failure
- Serum magnesium: to rule out severe hypomagnesemia
- Serum PO_4^{3-}, alkaline phosphatase: to differentiate hypoparathyroidism from vitamin D deficiency
- Serum PTH level by radioimmunoassay should be ordered only if the diagnosis is uncertain with the preceding tests.
- Markedly increased PTH: pseudohypoparathyroidism
- Increased PTH: vitamin D deficiency
- Decreased PTH: hypoparathyroidism

TREATMENT

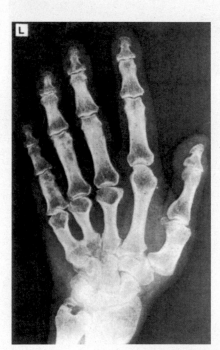
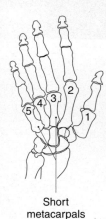

Short metacarpals

Fig 269–1
Pseudohypoparathyroidism. This posteroanterior view of the hand shows short, rather broad metacarpals, an appearance seen in pseudohypoparathyroidism. In this patient, all the metacarpals except the second are rather short, but the number involved may be variable. (From Besser CM, Thorner MO: Comprehensive Clinical Endocrinology, 3rd ed. St. Louis, Mosby, 2002.)

- Acute, severe symptomatic hypocalcemia caused by hypoparathyroidism or vitamin D deficiency: IV calcium gluconate
- Hypoalbuminemia
  - Improve nutritional status.
  - Calcium replacement is not indicated because the free (ionized) calcium level is normal.
- Hypomagnesemia: correct the magnesium deficiency.
  - Severe hypomagnesemia : IV magnesium sulfate
  - Moderate to severe hypomagnesemia: magnesium solution IM
- Chronic hypocalcemia caused by hypoparathyroidism or

vitamin D deficiency
- Calcium supplementation
- Vitamin D replacement
- Chronic hypocalcemia caused by renal failure:
  - Reduction of hyperphosphatemia with sevelamer
  - Vitamin D and oral calcium supplementation

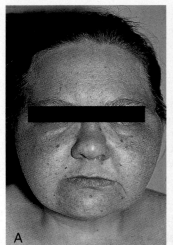
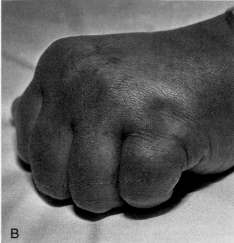

Fig 269–2
Patient with pseudohypoparathyroidism. **A,** Typical round facies characteristic of pseudohypoparathyroidism. **B,** Dimpled knuckle as a result of a shortened fifth metacarpal.
(From Besser CM, Thorner MO: Comprehensive Clinical Endocrinology, 3rd ed. St. Louis, Mosby, 2002.)

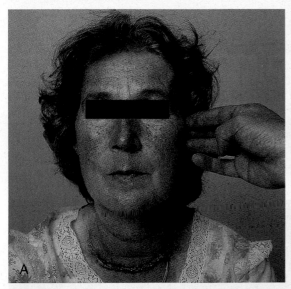
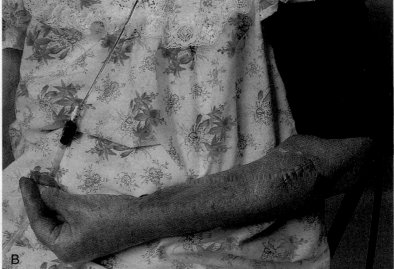

Fig 269–3
Clinical signs of hypocalcemia. **A,** Chvostek's sign is elicited by tapping over the facial nerve, producing a contraction of the upper lip muscle. **B,** Trousseau's sign is produced when a sphygmomanometer cuff is inflated to above systolic pressure for up to 3 minutes. This patient had four-gland hyperplasia and developed transient postoperative hypocalcemia. All four glands were removed, and pieces from one were autotransplanted into the forearm. The site of the transplantation can be seen clearly.
(From Besser CM, Thorner MO: Comprehensive Clinical Endocrinology, 3rd ed. St. Louis, Mosby, 2002.)

Chapter 270 Hyperparathyroidism

DEFINITION
Primary hyperparathyroidism is an endocrine disorder caused by the excessive secretion of PTH from the parathyroid glands.

PHYSICAL FINDINGS AND CLINICAL PRESENTATION
Primary hyperparathyroidism can be classified as asymptomatic (75% to 80%) and symptomatic. Physical examination may be entirely normal. The presence of signs and symptoms varies with the rapidity of development and degree of hypercalcemia. The following abnormalities may be present.

- Gastrointestinal (GI): constipation, anorexia, nausea, vomiting, pancreatitis, ulcers
- Central nervous system (CNS): confusion, obtundation, psychosis, lassitude, depression, coma
- Genitourinary (GU): nephrolithiasis, renal insufficiency, polyuria, decreased urine-concentrating ability, nocturia, nephrocalcinosis (Fig. 270–1)
- Musculoskeletal: myopathy, weakness, osteoporosis, pseudogout, bone pain
- Brown tumors: masses of non-neoplastic reactive tissue that develop as a complication of hyperparathyroidism. The hemorrhage and hemosiderin deposits associated with the massive bone resorption and subsequent microfractures give the lesion its brown color (Fig. 270–2). Clinically, they may produce a mass, which can be painful.
- Other: hypertension, metastatic calcifications, band keratopathy (found in medial and lateral margin of the cornea), pruritus

CAUSE
- Hormonal regulation of calcium homeostasis is noted in Table 270–1. Figure 270–3 illustrates calcium fluxes in a normal adult

- A single adenoma is found in 80% of patients; 90% of the adenomas are found within one of the parathyroid glands (Fig. 270–4) and the other 10% are in ectopic sites (lateral neck, thyroid, mediastinum, retroesophagus).
- Parathyroid gland hyperplasia occurs in 20% of patients.
- Primary hyperthyroidism is associated with multiple endocrine neoplasia (MEN) types I and II.

DIFFERENTIAL DIAGNOSIS
Other causes of hypercalcemia
- Malignancy (Fig. 270–5): neoplasms of the breast, lung, kidney, ovary, pancreas; myeloma, lymphoma
- Granulomatous disorders (e.g., sarcoidosis)
- Paget's disease
- Vitamin D intoxication, milk-alkali syndrome
- Thiazide diuretics
- Other: familial hypocalciuric hypercalcemia, thyrotoxicosis, adrenal insufficiency, prolonged immobilization, vitamin A intoxication, recovery from acute renal failure, lithium administration, pheochromocytoma, disseminated systemic lupus erythematous (SLE)

TABLE 270-1 Hormonal regulation of calcium homeostasis

Hormone	Effect	Control
PTH	Calcium ↑	Calcium ions ↓
	Phosphate ↓	
Calcitonin	Calcium ↓	Calcium ions ↑
	Phosphate ↓	Gastrin
Vitamin D metabolite	Calcium ↑	Phosphate ↓
	Phosphate ↑	PTH ↑

PTH, parathyroid hormone.
From Besser CM, Thorner MO: *Comprehensive Clinical Endocrinology*, 3rd ed. St. Louis, Mosby, 2002.

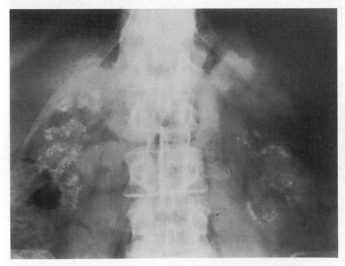

Fig 270–1
Nephrocalcinosis caused by hyperparathyroidism. The patient had passed several small stones.
(From Grainger RG, Allison DJ, Adam A, Dixon AK [eds]: *Grainger & Allison's Diagnostic Radiology*, 4th ed. London, Harcourt, 2001.)

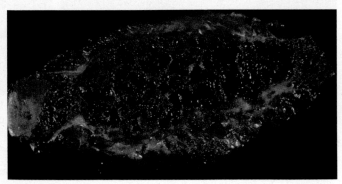

Fig 270–2
Brown tumor of rib. The dark red tumor expands the bone and has a lobular growth pattern.
(From Silverberg SG, Frable WJ, Wick MR, et al [eds]: *Principles and Practice of Surgical Pathology and Cytopathology*, 4th ed. Philadelphia, Elsevier, 2006.)

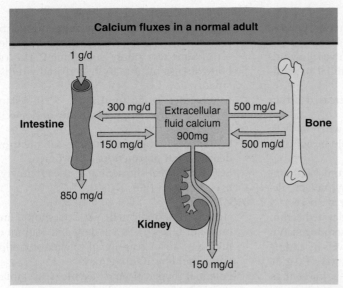

Fig 270-3
Calcium fluxes in a normal adult. As shown here, they appear between the extracellular fluid and gut and between the kidney and bone in a normal adult in zero calcium balance. Note that net calcium absorption (150 mg/day) is equal to calcium losses in the urine.
(From Besser CM, Thorner MO: Comprehensive Clinical Endocrinology, 3rd ed. St. Louis, Mosby, 2002.)

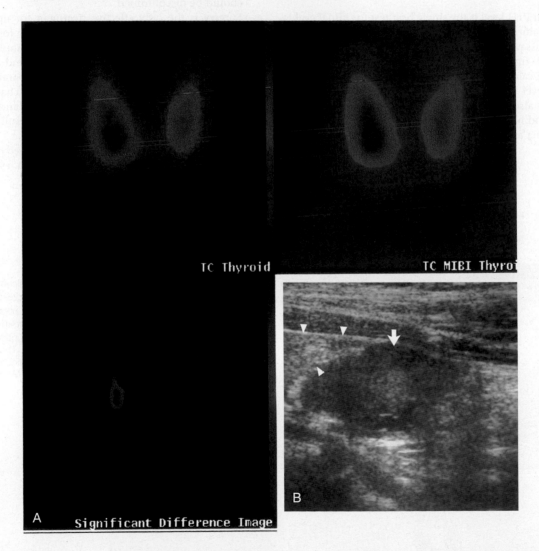

Fig 270-4
Parathyroid adenoma. **A,** ⁹⁹ᵐTc-pertechnetate scintigram (top left) shows uptake by thyroid tissue only; ⁹⁹ᵐTc-MIBI with uptake in both thyroid and parathyroid tissue (top right); subtraction image locating the parathyroid adenoma behind the lower pole of the right lobe of the thyroid gland (bottom left). **B,** Longitudinal ultrasound confirms the parathyroid adenoma *(arrow)* behind the lower pole of the thyroid gland *(arrowheads)*.
(From Grainger RG, Allison DJ, Adam A, Dixon AK [eds]: Grainger & Allison's Diagnostic Radiology, 4th ed. London, Harcourt, 2001.)

LABORATORY TESTS

- Elevated serum ionized calcium, low serum phosphorus, and normal or elevated alkaline phosphatase levels
- Elevated urine calcium level (in contrast with very low urinary calcium levels seen in patients with familial hypocalciuric hypercalcemia)
- Possibly elevated serum chloride levels, decreased serum CO_2, hyperchloremic metabolic acidosis
- A serum albumin level should be determined when measuring serum calcium and the calcium level should be adjusted (see above) in hypoalbuminemic patients.
- Persistent hypercalcemia and an elevated serum PTH confirm the diagnosis of primary hyperparathyroidism. Repeated measurements of serum calcium may be necessary because patients may not have persistently elevated serum calcium level. In malnourished patients, the serum calcium level needs to be corrected for low albumin levels by adding 0.8 mg/dL to the total serum calcium level for every 1.0 g/dL by which the serum albumin concentration is lower than 4 g/dL.
- The serum PTH level is the single best test for initial evaluation of confirmed hypercalcemia. The intact PTH (iPTH) is the best assay. The iPTH distinguishes primary hyperparathyroidism from hypercalcemia caused by malignancy when the serum calcium level is more than 12 mg/dL.
- A high level of urinary cyclic adenosine monophosphate (cAMP) is also suggestive of primary hyperparathyroidism.
- Parathyroid hormone-like protein (PLP) is increased in hypercalcemia associated with solid malignancies.

IMAGING STUDIES

- X-rays of fingers may reveal subperiosteal bone resorption (Fig. 270–6). A bone survey may show evidence of subperiosteal bone resorption (suggesting PTH excess). The classic bone disease of primary hyperparathyroidism is *osteitis fibrosa cystica.*
- Parathyroid localization with ^{99m}Tc-sestamibi has been shown to have a high sensitivity and specificity for single adenomas.
- Screen for osteopenia with measurement of bone mineral density in all postmenopausal women.
- ECG may reveal shortening of the QT interval secondary to hypercalcemia (Fig. 270–7).

TREATMENT

- Unless contraindicated, patients should maintain a high intake of fluids (3 to 5 L/day) and sodium chloride (>400 mEq/day) to increase renal calcium excretion. Calcium intake should be 1000 mg/day.
- Potential hypercalcemic agents (e.g., thiazide diuretics) should be discontinued.
- Surgery is the only effective treatment for primary hyperparathyroidism. It is generally indicated for all patients younger than 50 years and patients with complications from hyperthyroidism, such as nephrolithiasis and osteopenia.
- Percutaneous ethanol injection into the parathyroid gland should be considered in select patients who have undergone a subtotal parathyroidectomy for multigland disease and have recurrent hyperparathyroidism as a result of a remnant gland.
- Asymptomatic older patients can be followed conservatively with periodic monitoring of serum calcium level and review of symptoms.

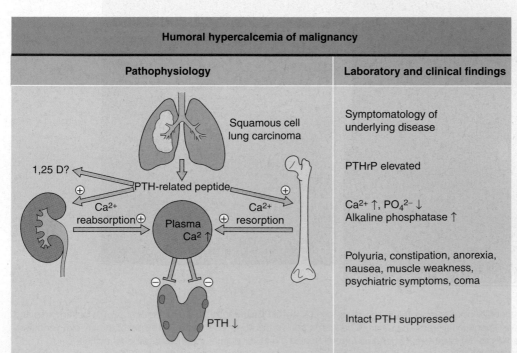

Humoral hypercalcemia of malignancy	
Pathophysiology	**Laboratory and clinical findings**
Squamous cell lung carcinoma	Symptomatology of underlying disease
1,25 D? / PTH-related peptide / Ca^{2+} reabsorption⊕ / Plasma Ca^2 ↑ / Ca^{2+} resorption	PTHrP elevated
	Ca^{2+} ↑, PO_4^{2-} ↓ Alkaline phosphatase ↑
	Polyuria, constipation, anorexia, nausea, muscle weakness, psychiatric symptoms, coma
PTH ↓	Intact PTH suppressed

Fig 270–5

Humoral hypercalcemia of malignancy. 1,25 D, 1,25-dihydroxycholecalciferal; PTH, parathyroid hormone: PTHrP, parathyroid hormone–related peptide. (From Besser CM, Thorner MO: Comprehensive Clinical Endocrinology, 3rd ed. St. Louis, Mosby, 2002.)

- Almost 25% of asymptomatic patients develop indications for surgery during observation.
- Acute severe hypercalcemia (serum calcium > 13 mg/dL) or symptomatic patients can be treated with the following:
- Vigorous IV hydration with normal saline (NS) followed by IV furosemide. Use NS with caution in patients with cardiac or renal insufficiency to avoid fluid overload.

- Bisphosphonates are effective agents. Zoledronate or pamidronate are both effective.
- Cinacalcet is an oral calcimimetic agent that directly lowers PTH levels by increasing the calcium-sensing receptor to extracellular calcium.

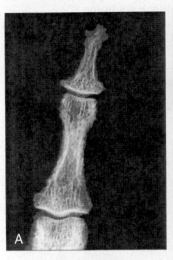
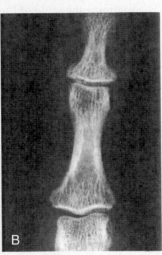

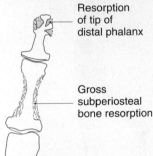

Resorption of tip of distal phalanx

Gross subperiosteal bone resorption

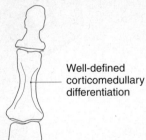

Well-defined corticomedullary differentiation

Fig 270–6

Primary hyperparathyroidism. The phalanges show gross subperiosteal bone resorption, with appearance after healing for comparison. Bony changes are now evident radiologically in a minority of patients with primary hyperparathyroidism. Subperiosteal bone resorption is the earliest radiologic sign and is specific for hyperparathyroidism. Generalized skeletal demineralization is a late finding. **A,** Middle and distal phalanges of the index finger show gross subperiosteal bone resorption of the shafts of the phalanges and also of the tip of the distal phalanx. The bone density is decreased and the texture of the cortex shows a basket weave pattern, with loss of definition of the normal corticomedullary junction. These appearances of gross hyperparathyroidism should be compared with those in **B. B,** Healing has occurred following removal of a parathyroid adenoma. Although subperiosteal bone resorption typically involves the phalanges, it may also occur at many other sites. These include the outer ends and undersurface of the clavicles, the metaphyseal regions of the growing ends of the long bones, the ischial tuberosities, the pubic bones at the symphysis, the sacroiliac joints, and the inner wall of the dorsum sellae.
(From Besser CM, Thorner MO: Comprehensive Clinical Endocrinology, 3rd ed. St. Louis, Mosby, 2002.)

BONE CANCER RESULTING IN HYPERCALCEMIA AND HYPOKALEMIA

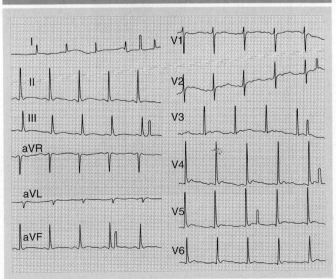

Fig 270–7

Twelve-lead ECG from a patient with bone cancer resulting in hypercalcemia and hypokalemia. Note the short QT interval and prominent U waves.
(From Crawford, MH, DiMarco JP, Paulus WJ [eds]: Cardiology, 2nd ed. St. Louis, Mosby, 2004.)

ADRENAL GLANDS

Chapter 271 | Cushing's syndrome

DEFINITION
Cushing's syndrome is the occurrence of clinical abnormalities associated with glucocorticoid excess secondary to exaggerated adrenal cortisol production or chronic glucocorticoid therapy.

Cushing's disease is Cushing's syndrome caused by pituitary ACTH excess (see later).

PHYSICAL FINDINGS AND CLINICAL PRESENTATION
- Hypertension
- Central obesity (Fig. 271–1) with rounding of the facies (moon facies); thin extremities
- Hirsutism, menstrual irregularities, hypogonadism
- Skin fragility, ecchymoses, red-purple abdominal striae, acne, poor wound healing, hair loss, facial plethora, hyperpigmentation (when there is ACTH excess)
- Psychosis, emotional lability, paranoia
- Muscle wasting with proximal myopathy

Note: The previous characteristics are not commonly present in Cushing's syndrome secondary to ectopic ACTH production. Many of these tumors secrete a biologically inactive ACTH that does not activate adrenal steroid synthesis. These patients may have only weight loss and weakness (Fig. 271–2) .

CAUSE
- Iatrogenic from chronic glucocorticoid therapy (common)
- Pituitary ACTH excess (Cushing's disease; 60%)
- Adrenal neoplasms (30%)
- Ectopic ACTH production (neoplasms of the lung, pancreas, kidney, thyroid, thymus; 10%) (Fig. 271–3)
- Figure 271–4 illustrates the difference between ACTH-dependent and ACTH-independent Cushing's syndrome.

DIFFERENTIAL DIAGNOSIS
- Alcoholic pseudo-Cushing's syndrome (endogenous cortisol overproduction)
- Obesity associated with diabetes mellitus
- Adrenogenital syndrome

LABORATORY TESTS
- Hypokalemia, hypochloremia, metabolic alkalosis, hyperglycemia, hypercholesterolemia
- Increased 24-hour urinary free cortisol (>100 μg/24 hr)
- In patients with a clinical diagnosis of Cushing's syndrome, the initial screening test is the overnight dexamethasone suppression test:
  1. Dexamethasone 1 mg PO given at 11 PM
  2. Plasma cortisol level measured 9 hours later (8 AM)
  3. Plasma cortisol level <5 μg/100 mL excludes Cushing's syndrome.
- Serial measurements (two or three consecutive measurements) of 24-hour urinary free cortisol and creatinine (to ensure adequacy of collection) are undertaken if overnight dexamethasone test is suggestive of Cushing's syndrome. Persistent elevated cortisol excretion (>300 μg/24 hr) indicates Cushing's syndrome.
- The low-dose (2 mg) dexamethasone suppression test is useful to exclude pseudo-Cushing's syndrome if the previous results are equivocal. Corticotropin-releasing hormone (CRH) stimulation after low-dose dexamethasone administration (dexamethasone-CRH test) is also used to distin-

guish patients with suspected Cushing's syndrome from those who have a mildly elevated urinary free cortisol level and equivocal findings.
- The high-dose (8 mg) dexamethasone test and measurement of ACTH by radioimmunoassay (RIA) are useful to determine the cause of Cushing's syndrome.
  1. ACTH undetectable or decreased. Lack of suppression indicates adrenal cause of Cushing's syndrome.

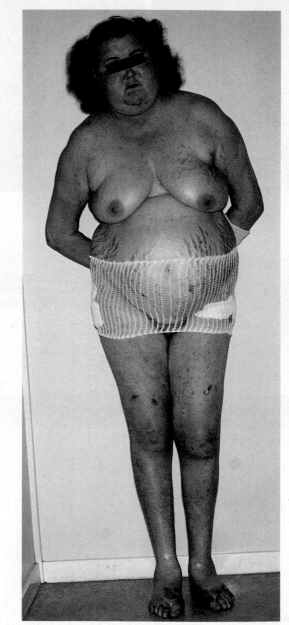

Fig 271–1
This patient has developed gross Cushing's syndrome as a consequence of steroid therapy.
(From McKee PH, Calonje E, Granter SR [eds]: Pathology of the Skin with Clinical Correlations, 3rd ed. St. Louis, Mosby, 2005.)

2. ACTH normal or increased and lack of suppression indicate ectopic ACTH production.

3. ACTH normal or increased and partial suppression suggest pituitary excess (Cushing's disease).

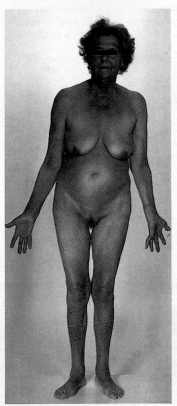

Fig 271-2

Appearance of a patient with classic ectopic adrenocorticotropic hormone syndrome caused by small cell carcinoma of the lung. (From Besser CM, Thorner MO: Comprehensive Clinical Endocrinology, 3rd ed. St. Louis, Mosby, 2002.)

- A single midnight serum cortisol (normal diurnal variation leads to a nadir around midnight) more than 7.5 µg/dL has been reported as 96% sensitive and 100% specific for the diagnosis of Cushing's syndrome.

IMAGING STUDIES

- CT or MRI of adrenal glands in suspected adrenal Cushing's syndrome (Fig. 271–5)
- MRI of pituitary gland with gadolinium in suspected pituitary Cushing's syndrome
- Additional imaging studies to localize neoplasms of the lung, pancreas, kidney, thyroid, or thymus in patients with ectopic ACTH production

TREATMENT

The treatment of Cushing's syndrome varies with its cause.

- Pituitary adenoma: trans-sphenoidal microadenomectomy is the therapy of choice in adults. Pituitary irradiation is reserved for patients not cured by trans-sphenoidal surgery. In children, pituitary irradiation may be considered as initial therapy, because 85% of children are cured by radiation. Stereotactic radiotherapy (photon knife or gamma knife) is effective and exposes the surrounding neuronal tissues to less irradiation than conventional radiotherapy. Total bilateral adrenalectomy is reserved for patients not cured by trans-sphenoidal surgery or pituitary irradiation.
- Adrenal neoplasm
  1. Surgical resection of the affected adrenal
  2. Glucocorticoid replacement for approximately 9 to 12 months after the surgery to allow time for the contralateral adrenal to recover from its prolonged suppression
- Bilateral micronodular or macronodular adrenal hyperplasia: bilateral total adrenalectomy
- Ectopic ACTH
  1. Surgical resection of the ACTH-secreting neoplasm
  2. Control of cortisol excess with metyrapone, aminoglutethimide, mifepristone, or ketoconazole
  3. Control of the mineralocorticoid effects of cortisol and 11-deoxycorticosteroid with spironolactone
  4. Bilateral adrenalectomy: rational approach to patients with indolent, unresectable tumors

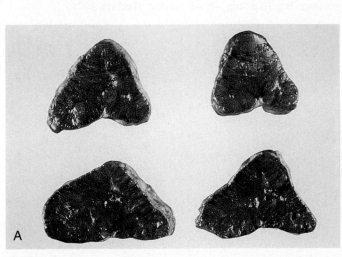

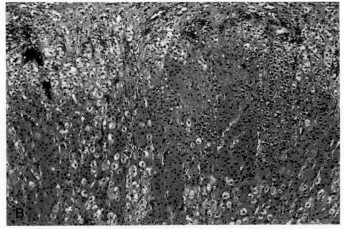

Fig 271-3

A, Ectopic adrenocorticotropic hormone (ACTH) syndrome. Both adrenal glands were enlarged and hyperplastic and, on transverse section, are tan to brown, with radial striations. **B,** Marked diffuse hyperplasia of cortex, with most cells having compact, eosinophilic cytoplasm. Patient had an occult ACTH-producing bronchial carcinoid tumor that was diagnosed several years following bilateral adrenalectomy.

(From Silverberg SG, Frable WJ, Wick MR, et al [eds]: Principles and Practice of Surgical Pathology and Cytopathology, 4th ed. Philadelphia, Elsevier, 2006.)

Cushing's syndrome

ACTH-dependent			ACTH-independent	
Eutopic	Ectopic		Adrenal adenoma/ carcinoma	Ectopic receptor expression (GIP, food-induced Cushing's syndrome)
Cushing's disease	ACTH	CRH/ACTH		

Fig 271–4

Cushing's syndrome. The figure illustrates the difference between adrenocorticotropic hormone (ACTH)–dependent and ACTH-independent Cushing's syndrome. CRH, corticotropin-releasing hormone; GIP, gastric inhibitory peptide.
(From Besser CM, Thorner MO: Comprehensive Clinical Endocrinology, 3rd ed. St. Louis, Mosby, 2002.)

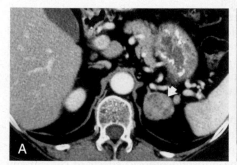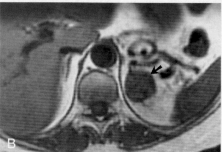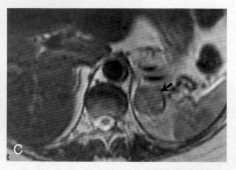

Fig 271–5

Cushing's syndrome caused by adrenocortical adenoma. **A,** Contrast-enhanced CT scan. **B,** T1-weighted spin-echo MR image. **C,** T2-weighted fast spin-echo MR image. All show a 3-cm adenoma *(arrow)* in the left adrenal gland.
(From Grainger RG, Allison DJ, Adam A, Dixon AK [eds]: Grainger & Allison's Diagnostic Radiology, 4th ed. London, Harcourt, 2001.)

DEFINITION

Addison's disease is characterized by inadequate secretion of corticosteroids resulting from partial or complete destruction of the adrenal glands. The hypothalamo–pituitary–adrenal axis in primary and secondary adrenocortical insufficiency is illustrated in Figure 272–1.

PHYSICAL FINDINGS AND CLINICAL PRESENTATION

- Hyperpigmentation (Fig. 272–2): more prominent in palmar creases, buccal mucosa (Fig. 272–3), pressure points (elbows, knees, knuckles), perianal mucosa, and around areolas of nipples
- Hypotension
- Amenorrhea and loss of axillary hair in females

CAUSE

- Autoimmune destruction of the adrenal glands (80% of cases) (Fig. 272–4)
- Tuberculosis (15% of cases)
- Carcinomatous destruction of the adrenal glands
- Adrenal hemorrhage (anticoagulants, trauma, coagulopathies, pregnancy, sepsis)
- Adrenal infarction (arteritis, thrombosis)
- AIDS (adrenal insufficiency develops in 30% of patients with AIDS)
- Other: sarcoidosis, amyloidosis, postoperative, fungal infections

DIFFERENTIAL DIAGNOSIS

- Sepsis
- Hypovolemic shock
- Acute abdomen
- Apathetic hyperthyroidism in older individuals
- Myopathies
- Major depression
- Anorexia nervosa
- Hemochromatosis
- Chronic infection

LABORATORY TESTS

- Increased potassium, decreased sodium and chloride
- Decreased glucose
- Increased BUN-to-creatinine ratio (prerenal azotemia)
- Mild normocytic, normochromic anemia, neutropenia, lymphocytosis, eosinophilia (significant dehydration may mask hyponatremia and anemia)
- Purified protein derivative (PPD) and antiadrenal antibodies
- If the clinical picture is highly suggestive of adrenocortical insufficiency, the diagnosis can be made with the rapid ACTH (Cortrosyn) test:

1. Give 250 mg ACTH by IV push and measure cortisol levels at 0 and 30 minutes.

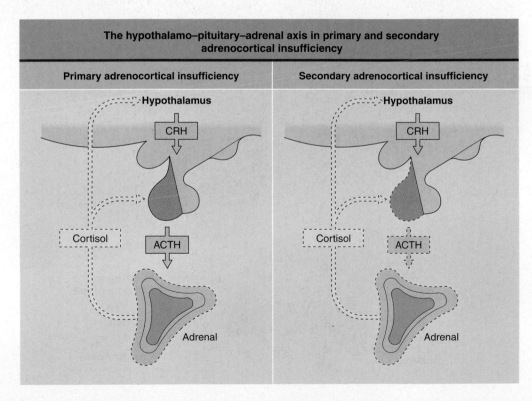

The hypothalamo–pituitary–adrenal axis in primary and secondary adrenocortical insufficiency

Primary adrenocortical insufficiency	Secondary adrenocortical insufficiency
Hypothalamus	Hypothalamus
CRH	CRH
Cortisol	Cortisol
ACTH	ACTH
Adrenal	Adrenal

Fig 272–1

The hypothalamo–pituitary–adrenal axis in primary and secondary adrenocortical insufficiency. In primary adrenocortical insufficiency, circulating adrenocorticotropic hormone (ACTH) levels are elevated because of the negative feedback effects of low circulating cortisol. In secondary adrenocortical insufficiency, low circulating ACTH levels result from hypothalamic or pituitary disease; as a consequence, cortisol levels are low. In secondary adrenocortical failure, aldosterone secretion is maintained because its principal controller is renin.
(From Besser CM, Thorner MO: Comprehensive Clinical Endocrinology, 3rd ed. St. Louis, Mosby, 2002.)

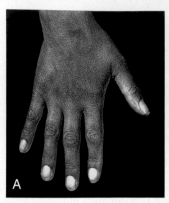 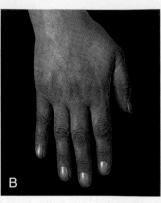

Fig 272–2

Pigmentation of the dorsal surfaces of the hands in a patient with Addison's disease. **A,** Before treatment. **B,** During glucocorticoid therapy. The normal hand color is now restored.
(From Besser CM, Thorner MO: Comprehensive Clinical Endocrinology, 3rd ed. St. Louis, Mosby, 2002.)

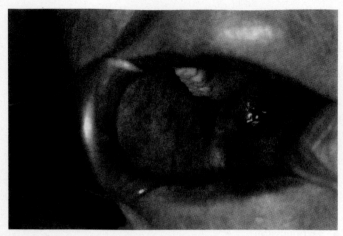

Fig 272–3

Pigmented macules on the gingivae and lips in Addison's disease. (From Callen JP, Jorizzo JL, Piette WW, Zone JJ: Dermatological Signs of Internal Disease, 3rd ed. Philadelphia, WB Saunders, 2003.)

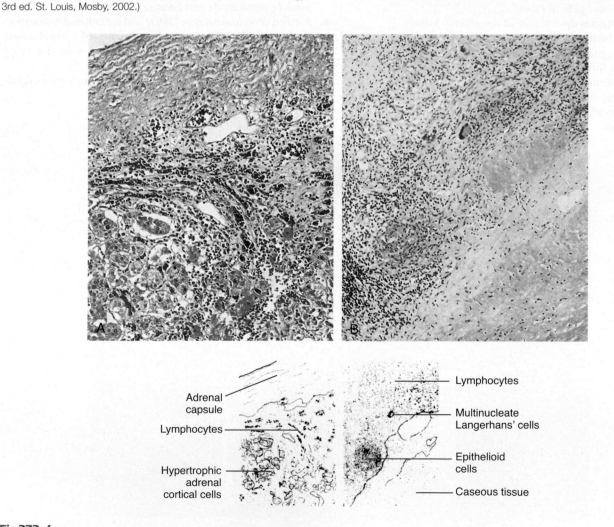

Fig 272–4

Histologic appearance of Addison's disease. The postmortem histology is shown of autoimmune adrenalitis **(A)** and tuberculous adrenalitis **(B)** in patients who died of Addison's disease. **A,** The adrenal capsule is markedly thickened and the surviving cortex consists of scattered hypertrophied adrenocortical cells that are heavily infiltrated with lymphocytes (H&E, ×120). **B,** Pink-staining, amorphous, caseous necrosis can be seen, in addition to tuberculous granulation tissue and a Langerhans' giant cell (H&E, ×80).
(Courtesy of Professor I. Doniach.)

2. Cortisol level <18 mg/dL at 30 or 60 minutes is suggestive of adrenal insufficiency.

3. Measure plasma ACTH. A high ACTH level confirms primary adrenal insufficiency.

- Secondary adrenocortical insufficiency (caused by pituitary dysfunction) can be distinguished from primary adrenal insufficiency by the following:

  1. Normal or low plasma ACTH level following rapid ACTH cosyntropin (Cortrosyn) test

  2. Absence of hyperpigmentation

  3. No significant impairment of aldosterone secretion (because aldosterone secretion is under control of the renin-angiotensin system)

  4. Additional evidence of hypopituitarism (e.g., hypogonadism, hypothyroidism)

IMAGING STUDIES

- Chest x-ray may reveal a small heart.
- Abdominal x-ray film: adrenal calcifications may be noted if the adrenocortical insufficiency is secondary to TB or fungus.
- Abdominal CT scan: small adrenal glands generally indicate idiopathic atrophy or long-standing TB, whereas enlarged glands are suggestive of early TB or potentially treatable diseases.

TREATMENT

- Glucocorticosteroid replacement (Fig. 272–5)
- Addisonian crisis is an acute complication of adrenal insufficiency characterized by circulatory collapse, dehydration, nausea, vomiting, hypoglycemia, and hyperkalemia.

  1. Draw plasma cortisol level; do not delay therapy while waiting for confirming laboratory results.

2. Administer hydrocortisone, 50 to 100 mg IV every 6 hours for 24 hours; if patient shows good clinical response, gradually taper dosage and change to oral maintenance dose (usually prednisone, 7.5 mg/day).

3. Provide adequate volume replacement with D_5 NS solution until hypotension, dehydration, and hypoglycemia are completely corrected. Large volumes (2 to 3 L) may be necessary in the first 2 to 3 hours to correct the volume deficit and hypoglycemia and avoid further hyponatremia.

4. Identify and correct any precipitating factor (e.g., sepsis, hemorrhage).

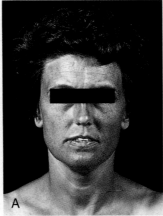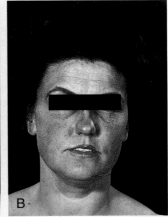

Fig 272–5

Patient with Addison's disease. **A,** Before treatment. Note that the face is thin and pigmented. **B,** During glucocorticoid replacement therapy. (From Besser CM, Thorner MO: Comprehensive Clinical Endocrinology, 3rd ed. St. Louis, Mosby, 2002.)

Chapter 273 Hypoaldosteronism

DEFINITION
Hypoaldosteronism is defined as an aldosterone deficiency or impaired aldosterone function.

PHYSICAL FINDINGS AND CLINICAL PRESENTATION
- Physical examination may be entirely within normal limits.
- Hypertension may be present in some patients.
- Profound muscle weakness and cardiac arrhythmias may be present.

CAUSE
- Hyporeninemic hypoaldosteronism (renin-angiotensin–dependent): decreased aldosterone production secondary to decreased renin production. The typical patient has renal disease secondary to various factors (e.g., diabetes mellitus, interstitial nephritis, multiple myeloma).
- Hyper-reninemic hypoaldosteronism (renin-angiotensin independent): renin production by the kidneys is intact. The defect is in aldosterone biosynthesis or in the action of angiotensin II. Common causes of this form of hypoaldosteronism are medications (e.g., angiotensin-converting enzyme [ACE] inhibitors, heparin), lead poisoning, aldosterone enzyme defects, and severe illness.

DIFFERENTIAL DIAGNOSIS
- Pseudohypoaldosteronism: renal unresponsiveness to aldosterone. In this condition, both renin and aldosterone levels are elevated. Pseudohypoaldosteronism can be caused by medications (spironolactone), chronic interstitial nephritis, systemic disorders (SLE, amyloidosis), or primary mineralocorticoid resistance.

LABORATORY TESTS
- Increased potassium, normal or decreased sodium
- Hyperchloremic metabolic acidosis (caused by the absence of hydrogen-secreting action of aldosterone)
- Increased BUN and creatinine (secondary to renal disease)
- Hyperglycemia (diabetes mellitus is common in these patients)

- Measurement of plasma renin activity following 4 hours of upright posture can differentiate hyporeninemic from hyper-reninemic causes. Renin levels in the normal or low range identify cases that are renin-angiotensin-dependent, whereas high renin levels identify cases that are renin-angiotensin independent. The diagnosis and cause of hypoaldosteronism can be confirmed with the renin-aldosterone–stimulation test:
  - Hyporeninemic hypoaldosteronism: low stimulated renin and aldosterone levels
  - End-organ refractoriness to aldosterone action: high stimulated renin and aldosterone levels
  - Adrenal gland abnormality: high stimulated renin and low aldosterone levels

TREATMENT
- Low-potassium diet with liberal sodium intake (at least 4 g of sodium chloride/day)
- Avoidance of ACE inhibitors and potassium-sparing diuretics
- Judicious use of fludrocortisone in patients with aldosterone deficiency associated with deficiency of adrenal glucocorticoid hormones
- Furosemide to correct hyperkalemia of hyporeninemic hypoaldosteronism
- Treatment of pseudohypoaldosteronism is the same as for hypoaldosteronism; however, the effect is limited because of impaired renal sensitivity.

Chapter 274 — Hyperaldosteronism

DEFINITION

Primary aldosteronism *(Conn's syndrome)* is a clinical syndrome characterized by hypokalemia, hypertension, low plasma renin activity (PRA), and excessive aldosterone secretion. The mechanisms of pathophysiologic changes in primary hyperaldosteronism are shown in Figure 274–1.

PHYSICAL FINDINGS AND CLINICAL PRESENTATION

- Generally asymptomatic
- If significant hypokalemia is present, possible muscle cramping, weakness, paresthesias
- Hypertension
- Polyuria, polydipsia

CAUSE

- Aldosterone-producing adenoma (APA; >60% of cases) (Fig. 274–2)
- Idiopathic hyperaldosteronism (>30% of cases)
- Glucocorticoid-suppressible hyperaldosteronism (<1% of cases)
- Aldosterone-producing carcinoma (<1% of cases)

DIFFERENTIAL DIAGNOSIS

- Diuretic use
- Hypokalemia from vomiting, diarrhea
- Renovascular hypertension
- Other endocrine neoplasms (e.g., pheochromocytoma, deoxycorticosterone-producing tumor, renin-secreting tumor)

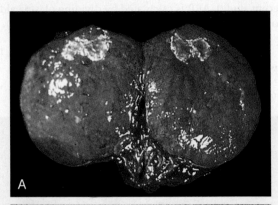

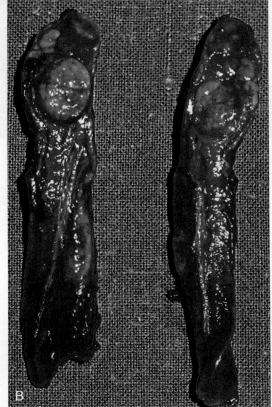

Fig 274–2

Primary hyperaldosteronism. **A,** Adrenal adenoma removed from a patient with primary hyperaldosteronism (Conn's syndrome). The canary yellow color of the adenoma is typical. **B,** Nodular hyperplasia associated with Conn's syndrome. Bilateral hyperplasia occurs in approximately 30% of patients with primary hyperaldosteronism.
(From Besser CM, Thorner MO: Comprehensive Clinical Endocrinology, 3rd ed. St. Louis, Mosby, 2002.)

Mechanism of pathophysiologic changes in primary hyperaldosteronism

Adrenal adenoma

→ ↑ Aldosterone
→ ↑ Sodium retention
→ ↑ Potassium loss
→ ↓ Renin
→ ↓ Angiotensin II

Fig 274–1

Mechanism of pathophysiologic changes in primary hyperaldosteronism. The autonomous production and release of aldosterone from the tumor lead to excessive sodium retention and potassium wasting; these occur largely as a result of the effects of aldosterone on the distal tube of the kidney. Renin release from the kidney is therefore inhibited, which leads to a fall in circulating levels of angiotensin II.
(From Besser CM, Thorner MO: Comprehensive Clinical Endocrinology, 3rd ed. St. Louis, Mosby, 200

LABORATORY TESTS

- Routine laboratory tests can be suggestive but are not diagnostic of primary aldosteronism.
- Common abnormalities include the following:
  - Spontaneous hypokalemia or moderately severe hypokalemia while receiving conventional doses of diuretics
  - Possible alkalosis and hypernatremia
  - As a screening test for primary aldosteronism, an elevated plasma aldosterone-to-renin ratio (ARR), determined randomly from patients on hypertensive drugs, is predictive of primary aldosteronism (positive predictive value, 100% in a recent study). ARR is calculated by dividing plasma aldosterone (mg/dL) by plasma renin activity (mg/mL/hr). ARR >100 is considered elevated.
  - 24-hour urine test for aldosterone and potassium levels (potassium > 40 mEq, aldosterone > 15 µg).

IMAGING STUDIES

- Adrenal CT scans (with 3-mm cuts) may be used to localize neoplasm and identify adrenal hyperplasia (Fig. 274–3).
- Adrenal scanning with ^{75}Se-selenocholesterol (Fig. 274–4), iodocholesterol (NP-59) or 6β-iodomethyl-19-norcholesterol after dexamethasone suppression. The uptake of tracer is increased in those with aldosteronoma and absent in those with idiopathic aldosteronism and adrenal carcinoma.

TREATMENT

- Control of blood pressure and hypokalemia with spironolactone, amiloride, or ACE inhibitors
- Surgery (unilateral adrenalectomy) for APA

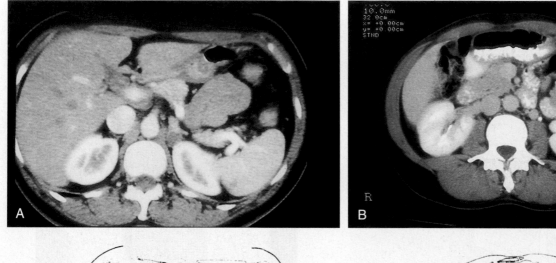

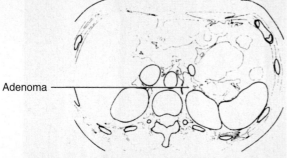

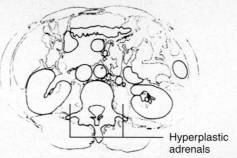

Fig 274–3
Adrenal CT scans in primary aldosteronism demonstrating the presence of a solitary, small, left-sided aldosterone-producing adenoma in a middle-aged woman with hypertension and hypokalemia **(A)** and bilateral hyperplasia in a patient with idiopathic hyperplasia of the adrenal cortex **(B)**. (From Besser CM, Thorner MO: Comprehensive Clinical Endocrinology, 3rd ed. St. Louis, Mosby, 2002.)

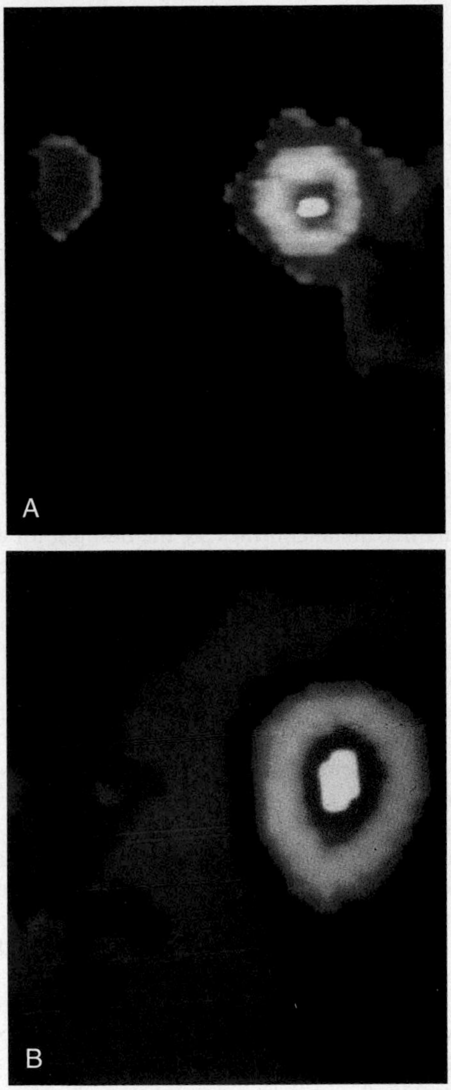

Fig 274–4

^{75}Se-selenocholesterol adrenocortical imaging in Conn's syndrome and Cushing's syndrome. **A,** Posterior view of the abdomen in a patient with Conn's syndrome (primary aldosteronism). It reveals high uptake of ^{75}Se-selenocholesterol in the right adrenal cortex, shown in red and yellow, as compared with the normal uptake in the left adrenal cortex, shown in blue. Production of aldosterone by a Conn's adenoma does not suppress the uptake of ^{75}Se-selenocholesterol by the normal adrenal. The purpose of adrenal cortical imaging is to localize an adenoma or demonstrate bilateral hyperplasia once a positive diagnosis has been made of Conn's or Cushing's syndrome, clinically and biochemically. **B,** A second use is to demonstrate whether an adrenal mass, seen incidentally during CT scanning of the abdomen in a patient with Cushing's syndrome, is caused by a solitary cortisol-secreting adenoma. A high uptake of ^{75}Se-selenocholesterol is seen in the adenoma. In this case, the left adrenal is not visualized because of suppression of adrenocorticotropic hormone by the high cortisol level, thus reducing the normal uptake of ^{75}Se-selenocholesterol.
(From Besser CM, Thorner MO: Comprehensive Clinical Endocrinology, 3rd ed. St. Louis, Mosby, 2002.)

Chapter 275 Pheochromocytoma

DEFINITION

Pheochromocytomas are catecholamine-producing tumors that originate from chromaffin cells of the adrenergic system. They generally secrete both norepinephrine and epinephrine, but norepinephrine is usually the predominant amine.

PHYSICAL FINDINGS AND CLINICAL PRESENTATION

- Hypertension: can be sustained (55%) or paroxysmal (45%)
- Headache (80%): usually paroxysmal in nature; described as pounding and severe
- Palpitations (70%): can be present with or without tachycardia.
- Hyperhidrosis (60%): most evident during paroxysmal attacks of hypertension.
- Physical examination may be entirely normal if done in a symptom-free interval. During a paroxysm, the patient may demonstrate marked increase in systolic and diastolic pressure, profuse sweating, visual disturbances (caused by hypertensive retinopathy), dilated pupils (secondary to catecholamine excess), paresthesias in the lower extremities (caused by severe vasoconstriction), tremor, and tachycardia.

CAUSE

- Catecholamine-producing tumors that are usually located in the adrenal medulla (Fig. 275–1)
- Specific mutations of the RET proto-oncogene cause familial predisposition to pheochromocytoma in MEN-II.

- Mutations in the von Hippel-Lindau tumor suppressor gene (*VHL* gene) cause familial disposition to pheochromocytoma in von Hippel-Lindau disease.
- Recently identified genes for succinate dehydrogenase subunit D (SDHD) and succinate dehydrogenase subunit B (SDHB) predispose carriers to pheochromocytoma and globus tumors.

DIFFERENTIAL DIAGNOSIS

- Anxiety disorder
- Thyrotoxicosis
- Amphetamine or cocaine abuse
- Carcinoid
- Essential hypertension

LABORATORY TESTS

- Plasma-free metanephrines are the best test for excluding or confirming pheochromocytoma and should be the test of first choice for diagnosis of the tumor. Plasma concentrations of normetanephrines higher than 2.5 pmol/mL or metanephrine levels higher than 1.4 pmol/mL indicate a pheochromocytoma with 100% specificity.
- 24-hour urine collection for metanephrines (100% sensitive) will also show increased metanephrines. The accuracy of the 24-hour urinary levels for metanephrines can be improved by indexing urinary metanephrine levels by urine creatinine levels.
- The clonidine suppression test is useful for distinguishing between high levels of plasma norepinephrine caused by release from sympathetic nerves and those caused by release from a pheochromocytoma. A decrease of less than 50% in plasma norepinephrine levels after clonidine administration is normal, whereas persistent elevations are indicative of pheochromocytoma.

IMAGING STUDIES

See Figure 275–2.

- Abdominal CT scanning (88% sensitivity) is useful in locating pheochromocytomas larger than 0.5 inch in diameter (90% to 95% accurate).
- MRI: pheochromocytomas demonstrate a distinctive MRI appearance (100% sensitivity). MRI may become the diagnostic imaging modality of choice.
- Scintigraphy with ^{131}I-MIBG (100% sensitivity): this norepinephrine analogue localizes in adrenergic tissue. It is particularly useful in locating extra-adrenal pheochromocytomas.
- 6-^{18}F-fluorodopamine positron emission tomography is reserved for cases in which clinical symptoms and signs suggest pheochromocytoma and results of biochemical tests are positive but conventional imaging studies cannot locate the tumor. An alternative approach is to use vena caval sampling for plasma catecholamines and metanephrines.

TREATMENT

- Laparoscopic removal of the tumor (surgical resection for both benign and malignant disease)

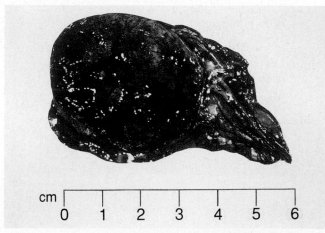

Fig 275–1

Cross section of pheochromocytoma. The tumor is deep brown and faintly nodular and had a positive chromatin reaction.
(From Silverberg SG, Frable WJ, Wick MR, et al [eds]: Principles and Practice of Surgical Pathology and Cytopathology, 4th ed. Philadelphia, Elsevier, 2006.)

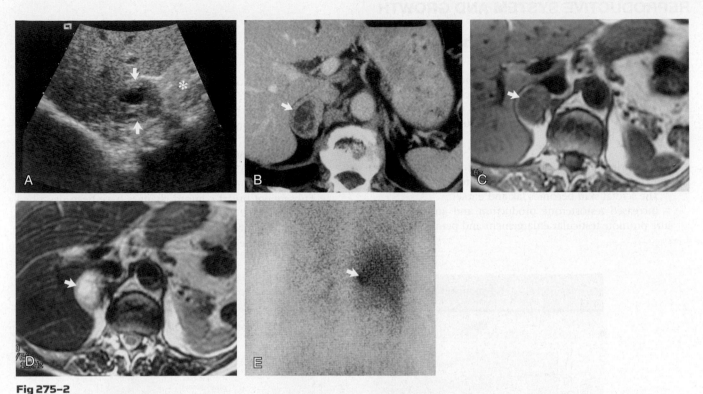

Fig 275–2
Pheochromocytoma with necrosis.
A, Longitudinal ultrasound showing an adrenal mass *(arrows)* lying above the kidney (*) and behind the liver. **B,** Contrast-enhanced CT scan shows a necrotic right adrenal tumor *(arrow)*. Axial **(C)** T1-weighted spin-echo and **(D)** T2-weighted images showing the typical signal intensity pattern of a pheochromocytoma *(arrow)* in the right adrenal gland. **E,** Posterior coronal view from an ^{131}I-MIBG scintigram showing the increased focal uptake in a pheochromocytoma *(arrow)* in the right adrenal gland.
(From Grainger RG, Allison DJ, Adam A, Dixon AK [eds]: Grainger & Allison's Diagnostic Radiology, 4th ed. London, Harcourt, 2001.)

REPRODUCTIVE SYSTEM AND GROWTH

Chapter 276 Normal puberty

- Physical changes during puberty are dependent on exposure of the pituitary to sex steroids. The relationship between growth and other changes in puberty is illustrated in Figure 276–1. The duration of the growth spurt is approximately 6 years for both genders.
- Males
  - The earliest sign is testicular enlargement. An orchidometer (Fig. 276–2) can be used to measure testicular volume.
  - The scrotal skin becomes lax and darker.
  - Increased testosterone production and androgen exposure promote testicular enlargement and penile growth.

- Pubic hair growth (pubarche) usually precedes axillary hair growth. Hair growth follows a typical male pattern (initially at base of penis, then to inner aspects of the thighs, later achieving an inverted triangle distribution).
- Females
  - The earliest sign is the development of a palpable breast bud (thelarche) caused by estrogen secretion from the ovaries.
  - Subsequent breast contour changes have been described by Tanner (Fig. 276–3).
  - Pubic hair development follows breast budding and distributes from the labia to the inner thigh (Fig. 276–4)

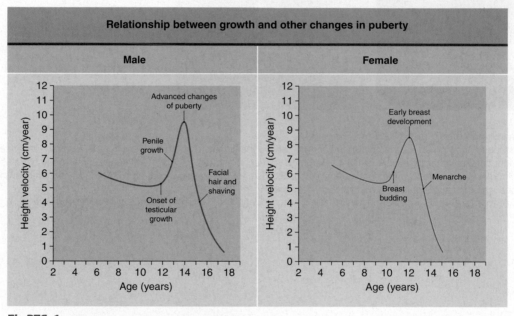

Fig 276–1
Relationship between growth and other changes in puberty.

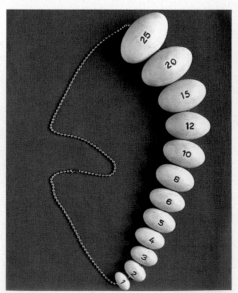

Fig 276–2
Prader's orchidometer. Testicular volume (in milliliters) may be estimated by direct comparison with the ellipsoids. During the assessment of testicular volume, the epididymis should not be included.
(From Besser CM, Thorner MO: Comprehensive Clinical Endocrinology, 3rd ed. St. Louis, Mosby, 2002.)

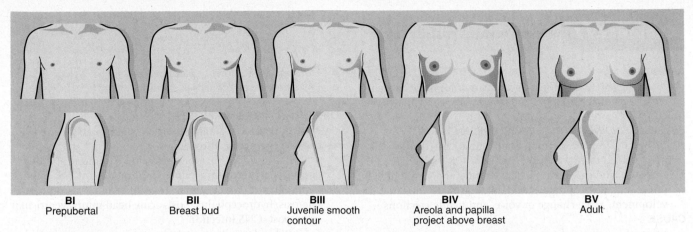

BI	BII	BIII	BIV	BV
Prepubertal	Breast bud	Juvenile smooth contour	Areola and papilla project above breast	Adult

Fig 276–3

Tanner stages of breast development.
(From Drife J, Magowan B: Clinical Obstetrics and Gynaecology. Edinburgh, WD Saunders, 2004.)

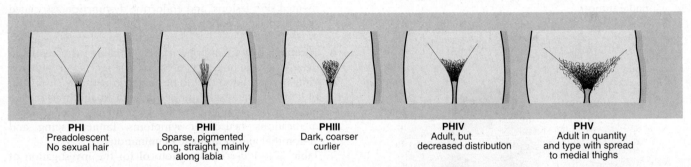

PHI	PHII	PHIII	PHIV	PHV
Preadolescent No sexual hair	Sparse, pigmented Long, straight, mainly along labia	Dark, coarser curlier	Adult, but decreased distribution	Adult in quantity and type with spread to medial thighs

Fig 276–4

Tanner stages of pubic hair development.
(From Drife J, Magowan B: Clinical Obstetrics and Gynaecology. Edinburgh, WD Saunders, 2004.)

Chapter 277 / **Precocious puberty**

DEFINITION
Precocious puberty is defined as sexual development occurring before 8 years of age in males and 9 years of age in females (Fig. 277–1).

PHYSICAL FINDINGS AND CLINICAL PRESENTATION
- In females: breast development, pubic hair development, accelerated growth, and menarche
- In males: increase in testicular volume and penile length, pubic hair development, accelerated growth, muscular development, acne, change in voice, and penile erections

CAUSE
- Idiopathic or true: diagnosis of exclusion
- CNS pathology: tumors, hydrocephalus, ventricular cysts, benign lesions
- Severe hypothyroidism
- Post-traumatic head injury
- Genetic disorders: neurofibromatosis, tuberous sclerosis, McCune-Albright syndrome, congenital adrenal hyperplasia
- Gonadal tumors

- Nongonadal tumors: hepatoblastoma
- Exposure to exogenous sex steroids

DIFFERENTIAL DIAGNOSIS
- Most common diagnoses to consider: premature thelarche and premature adrenarche
- Gonadotropin hormone-releasing hormone (GnRH)–dependent precocious puberty: idiopathic, CNS tumors, hypothalamic hamartomas, neurofibromatosis, tuberous sclerosis, hydrocephalus, post–acute head injury, ventricular cysts, post–CNS infection
- GnRH-independent precocious puberty: congenital adrenal hyperplasia (see Fig. 279–1), adrenocortical tumors (males), gonadal tumors, ectopic human chorionic gonadotropin (hCG)–secreting tumors (chorioblastoma, hepatoblastoma), exposure to exogenous sex steroids, severe hypothyroidism
- *McCune-Albright syndrome:* triad of osteitis fibrosa, pigmented skin lesions, and endocrine dysfunction associated with precocious puberty.

WORKUP
- Thorough history and physical examination are essential to determine whether the patient has true precocious puberty.
- Particular attention should be paid to growth, development, order of appearance of the secondary sexual characteristics, pubertal development in family members (Fig. 277–2), medications, neurologic symptoms, Tanner staging, and abdominal and neurologic examinations.
- Table 277–1 describes a protocol for the investigation of precocious puberty.

LABORATORY TESTS
- GnRH testing will help determine if dependent or independent cause
- Sex hormone studies: LH, FSH, hCG, testosterone (males), estrogen (females)
- T_4, TSH

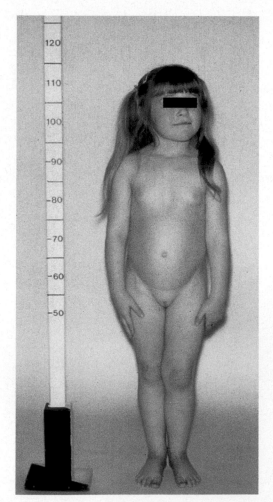

Fig 277–1
Idiopathic central precocious puberty in a 5-year-old girl.
Courtesy of Pharmacia Corporation.)

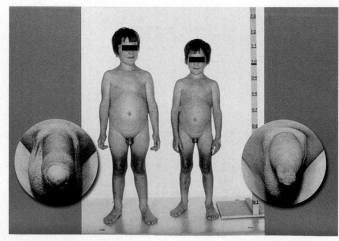

Fig 277–2
Central precocious puberty in 7-year-old boy secondary to neurofibromatosis shown with unaffected twin.
(Courtesy of Pharmacia Corporation.)

IMAGING STUDIES

- CT scanning or MRI of the brain to evaluate for CNS pathology
- Consideration of pelvic ultrasound in female patients to evaluate for cysts, tumors
- Abdominal imaging with CT scanning if intra-abdominal pathology suspected

TREATMENT

Therapy depends on the cause of precocious puberty.

- For true precocious puberty and some CNS lesions, the treatment of choice is leuprolide.
- For other CNS lesions and extragonadal tumors, therapy is dependent on the type of lesion, location of the lesion, and the overall prognosis of the underlying problem.

- For severe hypothyroidism, treatment with thyroid hormone will result in regression of sexual development. The child will subsequently undergo appropriate pubertal development later in life.
- For familial male gonadotropin-independent precocious puberty, ketoconazole or a combination of testolactone and spironolactone can be used.
- Psychological support for the child may be needed with regard to self-image and problems with peer acceptance.

TABLE 277–1 Protocol for investigation of precocious puberty

Workup	Features
History, family history	
Determination of exposure to environmental sex steroids	
Physical examination	Cutaneous lesions (e.g., neurofibromatosis, McCune-Albright syndrome)
	CNS examination
Auxology	Pubertal staging (Tanner)
	Height, weight, height velocity
	Bone age
Hormone measurements	Testosterone/estradiol
	Luteinizing hormone/follicle-stimulating hormone
	Adrenal androgens (DHEA-S, androstenedione)
	17-hydroxyprogesterone ± ACTH stimulation test
	hCG
	Gonadotropin-releasing hormone test
Radiology	Pelvic ultrasound
	Magnetic resonance imaging of the hypothalamic-pituitary region

DNA analysis for known genetic disorders (testotoxicosis, McCune-Albright syndrome)
ACTH, adrenocorticotropic hormone; DHEA-S, dehydroepiandrosterone sulfate; hCG, human chorionic gonadotropin.
From Besser CM, Thorner MO: Comprehensive Clinical Endocrinology, 3rd ed. St. Louis, Mosby, 2002.

Chapter 278 Delayed puberty

CAUSE

- Normal or low serum gonadotropin levels
- Constitutional delay in growth and development
- Hypothalamic and/or pituitary disorders
  - Isolated deficiency of growth hormone
  - Isolated deficiency on Gn-RH
  - Isolated deficiency of LH and/or FSH
  - Multiple anterior pituitary hormone deficiencies
- Associated with congenital anomalies: Kallmann's syndrome, Prader-Willi syndrome (Fig. 278–1), Laurence-Moon-Biedl syndrome, Friedreich's ataxia
- Trauma
- Postinfection
- Hyperprolactinemia
- Postirradiation

- Infiltrative disease (histiocytosis)
- Tumor
- Autoimmune hypophysitis
- Idiopathic
- Functional
- Chronic endocrinologic or systemic disorders
- Emotional disorders
- Drugs: cannabis
- Increased serum gonadotropin levels

Gonadal abnormalities

- Congenital
  - Gonadal dysgenesis
  - Klinefelter's syndrome (Fig.278–2)
  - Turner's syndrome (Fig.278–3)
  - Bilateral anorchism
  - Resistant ovary syndrome
  - Myotonic dystrophy in males
  - 17-Hydroxylase deficiency in females
  - Galactosemia
- Acquired
  - Bilateral gonadal failure resulting from trauma or infection or after surgery, irradiation, or chemotherapy
  - Oophoritis: isolated or with other autoimmune disorders
- Uterine or vaginal disorders

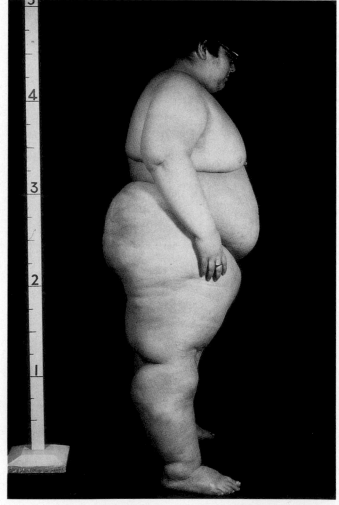

Fig 278–1
Severe obesity in a patient with Prader-Willi syndrome.
(From Besser CM, Thorner MO: Comprehensive Clinical Endocrinology, 3rd ed. St. Louis, Mosby, 2002.)

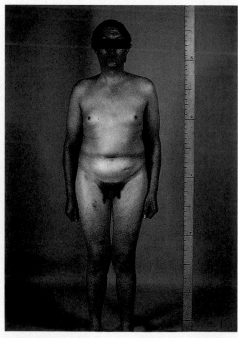

Fig 278–2
Typical appearance of a patient with Klinefelter's syndrome. The patient is hypogonadal, has a female habitus, is poorly virilized with gynecomastia and eunuchoidism, and has a small phallus. The body hair is sparse.
(From Besser CM, Thorner MO: Comprehensive Clinical Endocrinology, 3rd ed. St. Louis, Mosby, 2002.)

- Absence of uterus and/or vagina
- Testicular feminization: complete or incomplete androgen insensitivity

DIFFERENTIAL DIAGNOSIS

- Table 278–1 describes differential diagnostic features of delayed puberty and sexual infantilism
- Evaluation
- Figure 278–4 describes the evaluation of patients with delayed puberty.
- Figure 278–5 illustrates the constitutional delay of growth and puberty.

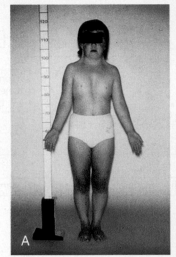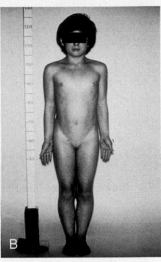

Fig 278–3

Two patients with Turner's syndrome. **A,** Patient has the characteristic dysmorphic features of Turner's syndrome. **B,** Patient has minimal dysmorphic features. In some patients, the only clinical features are short stature and pubertal delay.
(Courtesy of Pharmacia Corporation.)

TABLE 278–1 Differential diagnostic features of delayed puberty and sexual infantilism

Condition	Stature	Plasma gonadotropins	LHRH test, LH response	Plasma gonadal steroids	Plasma DHEA-S	Karyotype	Olfaction
Constitutional delay in growth and adolescence	Short for chronologic age, usually appropriate for bone age	Prepubertal, later pubertal	Prepubertal, later pubertal	Low, later normal	Low for chronologic age, appropriate for bone age	Normal	Normal
Hypogonadotropic hypogonadism							
Isolated gonadotropin deficiency	Normal, absent pubertal growth spurt	Low	Prepubertal or no response	Low	Appropriate for chronologic age	Normal	Normal
Kallmann's syndrome	Normal, absent pubertal growth spurt	Low	Prepubertal or no response	Low	Appropriate for chronologic age	Normal	Anosmia or hyposmia
Idiopathic multiple pituitary hormone deficiencies	Short stature and poor growth since early childhood	Low	Prepubertal or no response	Low	Usually low	Normal	Normal
Hypothalamic-pituitary tumors	Late onset decrease in growth velocity	Low	Prepubertal or no response	Low	Normal or low for chronologic age	Normal	Normal
Primary gonadal failure							
Syndrome of gonadal dysgenesis (Turner's syndrome) and variants	Short stature since childhood	High	Hyper-response for age	Low	Normal for chronologic age	45,X or variant	Normal
Klinefelter's syndrome and variants	Normal to tall	High	Hyper-response at puberty	Low or Normal	Normal for chronologic age	47,XXY or variant	Normal
Familial XX or XY gonadal dysgenesis	Normal	High	Hyper-response for age	Low	Normal for chronologic age	46,XXY or 46,XY	Normal

DHEA-S, dehydroepiandrosterone sulfate; LH, luteinizing hormone; LHRH, luteinizing hormone–releasing hormone.
From Larsen PR, Kronenberg HM, Melmed S, Polonsky KS: Williams Textbook of Endocrinology, 10th ed. Philadelphia, WB Saunders, 2003.

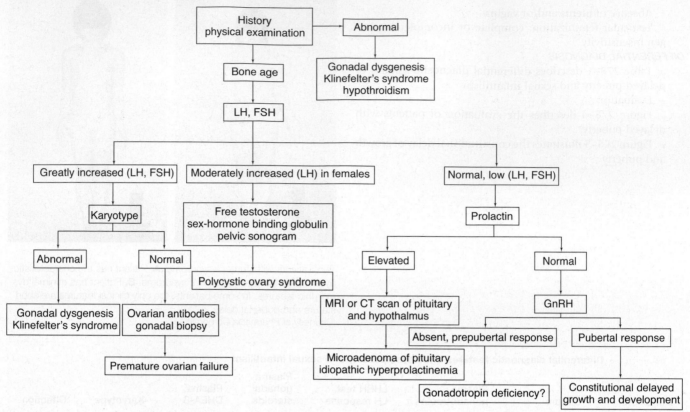

Fig 278-4
Evaluation of patient with delayed puberty. CT, computed tomography; FSH, follicle-stimulating hormone; GnRH, gonadotropin-releasing hormone; LH, luteinizing hormone; MRI, magnetic resonance imaging.
(From Moore WT, Eastman RC: Diagnostic Endocrinology, 2nd ed 2. St Louis, Mosby, 1996.)

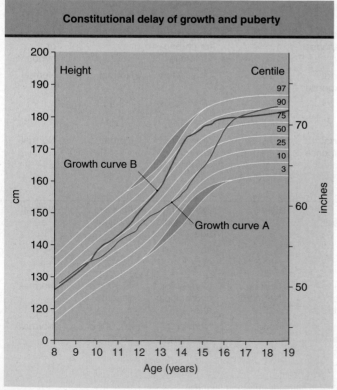

Fig 278-5
Constitutional delay of growth and puberty. Shown are growth curves of two brothers demonstrating the effect of constitutional delay of growth and puberty (growth curve A) in contrast to an unaffected brother (growth curve B).
(Courtesy of Pharmacia Corporation.)

Chapter 279 · Congenital adrenal hyperplasia

DEFINITION

Congenital adrenal hyperplasia (CAH) refers to several different genetic mutations in the enzymes responsible for cortisol synthesis, which are each inherited in an autosomal recessive fashion.

CLINICAL PRESENTATION

- Classic salt-wasting form (impaired cortisol and aldosterone synthesis)
  - Infants are acutely ill with poor weight gain, hypovolemia, hyponatremia, hyperkalemia, and elevated plasma renin.
  - If patients survive infancy, their overall life expectancy is not compromised.
  - Females are born with ambiguous genitalia and may have irregular menses and infertility as adults.
  - Males may have greater penile size and smaller testes than expected during childhood. Males may also develop adrenal rests, or ectopic islands of adrenal cortical tissue in the testes, in childhood and may experience infertility as adults.
  - Both males and females may exhibit rapid growth in childhood (caused by early epiphyseal closure, which then results in short stature in adulthood).
  - Precocious or pseudoprecocious puberty (Fig. 279–1) is common in both males and females.

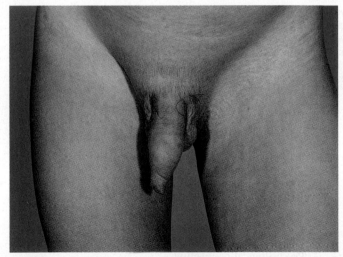

Fig 279–1
Genitalia of a 2-year-old boy with pseudoprecocious puberty secondary to congenital adrenal hyperplasia. Note penile enlargement and pubic hair growth in the presence of prepubertal testes.
(From Besser CM, Thorner MO: Comprehensive Clinical Endocrinology, 3rd ed. St. Louis, Mosby, 2002.)

- Classic non–salt-wasting or simple virilizing form (impaired cortisol synthesis only)
  - Females present with ambiguous genitalia at birth (Fig. 279–2).
  - The normal appearance of male genitalia in the simple virilizing form makes this a difficult diagnosis in male infants.
  - Characterized by precocious puberty, short stature, and testicular adrenal rests, as in the salt-wasting form
- Nonclassic or mild, late-onset form (varying degrees of androgen excess)
  - Usually presents in adolescence or adulthood and is not detected on newborn screening
  - Often asymptomatic, but can be associated with mild virilization
  - Polycystic ovary syndrome (PCOS)–like symptoms occur in women (hirsutism, oligomenorrhea, acne, infertility, insulin resistance, abnormal menses)
  - Associated with infertility in males

CAUSE

In 21-hydroxylase deficiency, the pathways for aldosterone production (from the conversion of progesterone to deoxycorticosterone) and cortisol production (from the conversion of 17-hydroxyprogesterone to 11-deoxycortisol) by the cytochrome P-450 enzyme 21-hydroxylase are interrupted. The production of ACTH is thus stimulated by a negative feedback mechanism, leading to adrenal hyperplasia and mineralocorticoid deficiency as the intermediaries in aldosterone and cortisol synthesis are shunted to the androgen biosynthesis pathway. A recombination event between the active *CYP21A2* gene on chromosome 6p21.3 and the *CYP21A1* pseudogene is thought to create the deficient 21-hydroxylase enzyme.

DIFFERENTIAL DIAGNOSIS

- Precocious puberty (see Figs. 277–1, 272–2)
- PCOS
- Androgen resistance syndromes
- Pseudohermaphroditism
- Mixed gonadal dysgenesis
- Testicular carcinoma
- Leydig cell tumors
- Adrenocortical carcinoma
- Addison's disease
- Pituitary adenoma

LABORATORY TESTS

- For 21-hydroxylase deficiency
  - Prenatal: chorionic villus sampling for genetic testing or measurement of 17-hydroxyprogesterone
  - Neonates, children, and adults: screening for elevated 17-hydroxyprogesterone levels (not done by all states), high-dose cosyntropin stimulation test, and genotyping

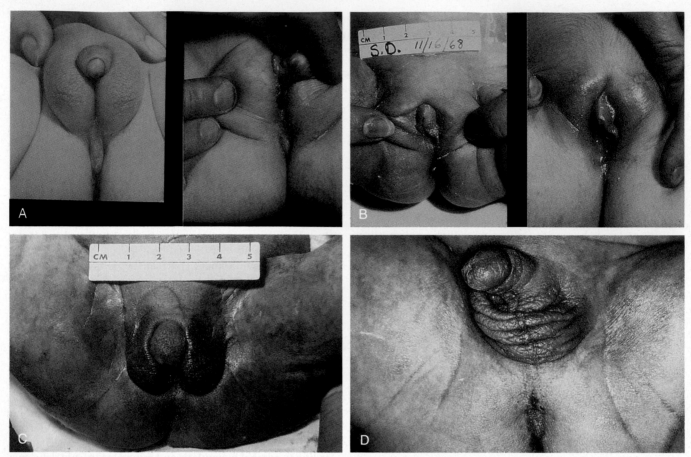

Fig 279-2
Virilization in fetal adrenal steroidogenesis defects. 3β-hydroxysteroid dehydrogenase deficiency is shown in a male **(A)** and female **(B)**. Note the bifid scrotum and third-degree hypospadias in the male and the clitoral hypertrophy with pubic hair development in the female. **C,** Moderately severe virilization in a genetic female infant with 21-hydroxylase deficiency. Clitoral hypertrophy is prominent, with some fusion of the labioscrotal folds. Note the hyperpigmentation of the labia, indicating excessive adrenocorticotropic hormone with its inherent melanocyte-stimulating hormone–like activity. **D,** Complete virilization in a genetic female infant with 21-hydroxylase deficiency. The labia have completely fused to simulate a small phallus, which has undergone circumcision. The infant had vascular collapse, hyponatremia, and hyperkalemia.
(From Besser CM, Thorner MO: Comprehensive Clinical Endocrinology, 3rd ed. St. Louis, Mosby, 2002.)

IMAGING STUDIES
- CT of adrenal glands will reveal adrenal gland enlargement (Fig. 279–3).
- Ultrasound to identify a uterus in cases of ambiguous genitalia
- Ultrasound is preferred to rule out testicular adrenal rest tumors (found in classic and nonclassic forms) and should be done beginning in adolescence. MRI and color flow Doppler may also be used for this purpose.

TREATMENT
- Surgical correction of ambiguous genitalia is recommended by 6 months.
- Bilateral laparoscopic adrenalectomy, with lifelong glucocorticoid and mineralocorticoid replacement (controversial)
- Gene therapy (hypothetical)
- Overall goal is suppression of ACTH.
  - Prenatal: dexamethasone in the first trimester in female fetuses only (controversial because long-term studies are unavailable)
  - Infants: fludrocortisone, NaCl

- Stress states (e.g., major illness) require increased glucocorticoid dosing.

Chronic medical therapy
- Children: hydrocortisone minimizes the risk of iatrogenic short stature found in other corticosteroids with longer half-lives.
- Adolescents and adults: dexamethasone or prednisone
- Fludrocortisone: may decrease glucocorticoid requirement
- Psychological counseling.
- Monitoring of serum 17-hydroxyprogesterone and androstenedione, renin, electrolytes, blood pressure, bone age and density, Tanner staging, growth velocity, weight
- Treatment of simple virilizing form: similar to salt-wasting form, but mineralocorticoid replacement is unnecessary
- Treatment of nonclassic form
1. In adolescent and adult women: oral contraceptives, glucocorticoids, and/ or antiandrogens
2. In children and men, usually no treatment is necessary.

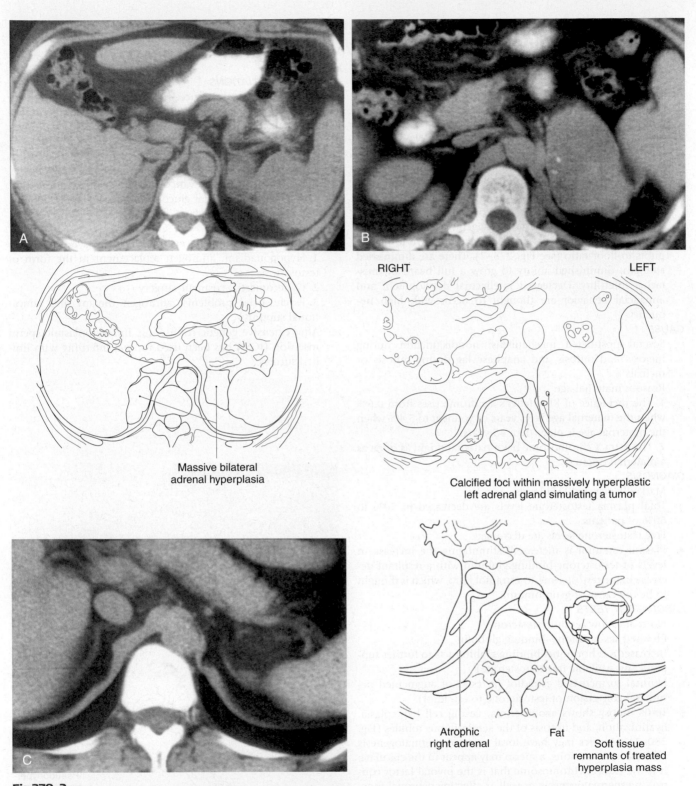

RIGHT LEFT

Massive bilateral
adrenal hyperplasia

Calcified foci within massively hyperplastic
left adrenal gland simulating a tumor

Atrophic
right adrenal

Fat

Soft tissue
remnants of treated
hyperplasia mass

Fig 279–3
Congenital adrenal hyperplasia. **A, B,** Unenhanced axial CT scans in a 50-year-old male patient with previously untreated congenital adrenal hyperplasia show that both adrenal glands are massively enlarged and that the normal contour of the glands has been lost. On the left particularly, an inhomogeneous masslike lesion has resulted and contains foci of calcium. Such severe hyperplasia can, as in this case, simulate the appearance of adrenal carcinomas. **C,** Unenhanced CT scan in the same patient following treatment shows that the right adrenal gland now appears atrophic and that the left adrenal gland cannot be identified. The large mass lesion demonstrated in **B** has been replaced by fat.
(From Besser CM, Thorner MO: Comprehensive Clinical Endocrinology, 3rd ed. St. Louis, Mosby, 2002.)

Chapter 280 Klinefelter's syndrome

DEFINITION

Klinefelter's syndrome is a congenital disorder in which a 47,XXY chromosome complement is associated with hypogonadism and infertility.

PHYSICAL FINDINGS AND CLINICAL PRESENTATION

Classic triad

- Small firm testes, azoospermia, and gynecomastia
- Prepubertal: small testes, gonadal volume <1.5 mL is a result of loss of germ cells before puberty.
- Postpubertal: gynecomastia (periductal fat growth) with small, firm, pea-sized testes. Exaggerated growth of the lower extremities results in a decreased crown-to-pubis–pubis-to-floor ratio (see Fig. 278–2). There are diminished strength, diminished ability to grow a full beard or mustache, infertility. Decreased intellectual development and antisocial behavior are thought to occur with high frequency.

CAUSE

- Several postulated mechanisms: nondisjunction during meiosis and mitosis and anaphase lag during mitosis or meiosis
- Reason: maternal age
  1. The incidence of Klinefelter's syndrome rises from 0.6% when the maternal age is 35 years or younger to 5.4% when the maternal age is older than 45 years.
  2. The extra X chromosome has a paternal origin as often as a maternal origin.

DIAGNOSIS

- Markedly elevated FSH levels
- Total plasma testosterone levels are decreased in 50% to 60% of patients.
- Free testosterone levels are decreased.
- Plasma estradiol is increased, stimulating the increase in levels of testosterone-binding globulin with a resultant decrease in the testosterone-to-estradiol ratio, which is thought to be the cause of gynecomastia.

LABORATORY TESTS

- Normal to low serum testosterone
- Elevated sex hormone–binding globulin
- Increased sex hormone–binding globin (acts to further suppress any available free testosterone)
- Normal to increased estradiol (a result of augmented peripheral conversion of testosterone to estradiol)
- Testis biopsy shows azoospermia, Leydig cell hyperplasia, hyalinization, and fibrosis of the seminiferous tubules (Fig. 280–1). Mosaics may have focal areas of spermatogenesis and, on rare occasions, a sperm may appear in the ejaculate. It is the extra X chromosome that is the pivotal factor controlling spermatogenesis, as well as affecting neuronal function directly, leading to the behavioral abnormalities related to decreased IQ.
- Buccal smear: one sex chromatin body
- Prepubertal male: gonadotropin levels are normal.
- Postpubertal male: gonadotropin levels are elevated, even when the testosterone level is normal.

DISEASE ASSOCIATIONS

- Malignancies: breast cancer (20 times greater than XY men, and 20% the rate of occurrence in women), nonlymphocytic leukemia, lymphomas, marrow dysplastic syndromes, extragonadal germ cell neoplasms
- Autoimmune disorders: chronic lymphocytic thyroiditis, Takayasu's arteritis, taurodontism (enlarged molar teeth), mitral valve prolapse, varicose veins, asthma, bronchitis, osteoporosis, abnormal glucose tolerance testing, diabetes, varicose veins

TREATMENT

- Revolves around three facets of Klinefelter's syndrome:
  1. Hypogonadism: androgen replacement in the form of testosterone
  2. Gynecomastia: cosmetic surgery
  3. Psychosocial problems: androgen therapy and educational support
- After extensive genetic counseling, intracytoplasmic sperm insertion (ICSI) has been used to treat infertility with limited success.

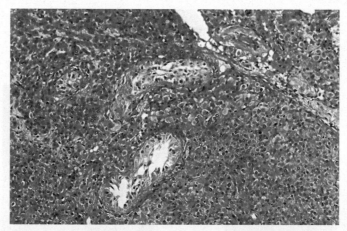

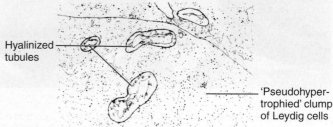

Hyalinized tubules

'Pseudohyper-trophied' clump of Leydig cells

Fig 280–1

Histologic section of a testis of a patient with Klinefelter's syndrome. The dysgenetic seminiferous tubules are evident, and the clumps of Leydig cells give an illusory impression of hyperplasia (H&E). (Courtesy of Professor I. Doniach.)

Chapter 281 **Turner's syndrome**

DEFINITION

Turner's syndrome refers to a pattern of malformation characterized by short stature, ovarian hypofunction, loose nuchal skin, and cubitus valgus.

PHYSICAL FINDINGS AND CLINICAL PRESENTATION

- Turner's phenotype is recognizable at any point on the developmental spectrum (see Fig. 278–3).
- In spontaneous abortions, the most common sex chromosome abnormality detected (45,X chromosome constitution) is found in 75% of affected individuals and accounts for 20% of such cases.
- In fetuses, it is suspected because of ultrasonographic manifestations such as thickening of the nuchal folds, frank nuchal cystic hygromas, or mild shortness of the femora at midtrimester.
- In infants
  1. At birth, may display loose nuchal skin (pterygium colli) and edema on the dorsa of the hands and feet
  2. Canthal folds reflecting midface hypoplasia and redundant skin in the periorbital region
  3. Nipples appearing widely spaced
  4. Heart and cardiovascular system: murmur of aortic stenosis or bicuspid aortic valve or diminished femoral pulses suggestive of aortic coarctation
  5. Renal ultrasonography: renal ectopia, such as pelvic kidney or horseshoe kidneys
- In older children
  1. Slow linear growth
  2. Short stature: may be improved with growth hormone therapy
  3. Delayed or absent menses: secondary sex characteristics possibly normalized with estrogen replacement therapy
  4. Intelligence is often normal, but delays in spatial perception or visual motor integration are commonly observed; frank mental retardation is rare.

CAUSE

- Phenotype caused by absence of the second sex chromosome, whether X or Y
- 45,X chromosome constitution in about 50% of affected individuals
- Other chromosome aberrations (40% of cases): isochromosome Xq (46,X,i[Xq]) or mosaicism (XX/X)
- With deletions involving the short (or p) arm of the X chromosome: short stature but little ovarian hypofunction
- Deletions involving Xq13-q27: ovarian failure
- Usually a deficiency of paternal contribution of sex chromosome, reflecting paternal nondisjunction

DIFFERENTIAL DIAGNOSIS

- *Noonan's syndrome,* an autosomally dominant inherited disorder also characterized by loose nuchal skin, midface hypoplasia, canthal folds, and stenotic cardiac valvular defects and affecting males and females equally; also has normal chromosome constitutions
- Other conditions in the differential diagnosis of loose skin, whether or not associated with edema:
  1. *Fetal hydantoin syndrome* (loose nuchal skin, midface hypoplasia, distal digital hypoplasia)
  2. Disorders of chromosome constitution (trisomy 21, tetrasomy 12p mosaicism)
  3. Congenital lymphedema (Milroy edema)

WORKUP

- Giemsa-banded karyotype to confirm clinical diagnosis
- Once diagnosis is established: cardiologic consultation for evaluation for cardiac valvular abnormalities or aortic coarctation
- Renal ultrasonography
- Endocrine evaluations in older patients with short stature or amenorrhea
- Psychometrics to document known or suspected learning disabilities

LABORATORY TESTS

- As noted, routine Giemsa-banded karyotype on peripheral lymphocytes to confirm the clinical impression in all suspected cases of Turner's syndrome
- Recognition of associated medical problems, such as hypergonadotropic hypogonadism or autoimmune thyroiditis, prompting periodic evaluation of these potential areas

IMAGING STUDIES

- Echocardiography
- Renal ultrasonography
- Abdominal ultrasonography for evaluation of ovarian and uterine size and morphology
- MRI of brain (especially in cases with known or suspected neurologic impairment)
- Radiography (for evaluation of carpal, metacarpal abnormalities, radioulnar synostosis)
- Bone age (for evaluation of short stature)

TREATMENT

- General medical care guided by normal medical standards, with special attention paid to identifying such age-related problems as developmental delays, learning disabilities, slow growth, amenorrhea

Chapter 282 Hypogonadism

CAUSE

Hypergonadotropic hypogonadism

- Hormone resistance (androgen, luteinizing hormone insensitivity)
- Gonadal defects (e.g., Klinefelter's syndrome, myotonic dystrophy)
- Drug induced (e.g., spironolactone, cytotoxins)
- Alcoholism- or radiation-induced
- Mumps orchitis
- Anatomic defects, castration

Hypogonadotropic hypogonadism

- Pituitary lesions (neoplasms, granulomas, infarction, hemochromatosis, vasculitis)
- Drug-induced (e.g., glucocorticoids)
- Hyperprolactinemia
- Genetic disorders

1. *Laurence-Moon-Biedl syndrome:* rare autosomal recessive trait combining retinitis pigmentosa, hypogonadism, developmental delay, and spastic paraplegia

2. *Prader-Willi syndrome:* disorder characterized by severe hypotonia at birth, severe obesity (see Fig. 278–1), short stature (responsive to growth hormone), small hands, and mental retardation. In patients with Prader-Willi syndrome, both hypogonadotropic hypogonadism and hypergonadotropic hypogonadism, perhaps secondary to cryptorchidism, have been reported. More than 50% of children have a chromosomal deletion involving band q11.2 of the long arm of chromosome 15.

3. Delayed puberty

4. Other: chronic disease, nutritional deficiency, Kallmann's syndrome, idiopathic isolated luteinizing hormone or follicle-stimulating hormone deficiency

PHYSICAL FINDINGS AND CLINICAL MANIFESTATIONS

- Nonspecific symptoms associated with testosterone deficiency include depression and irritability.
- Long-standing hypogonadism of all causes can result in characteristic fine facial wrinkling (Fig. 282–1).
- The prepubertal testis measures some 2 cm in length and increases to 4.1 to 5.5 cm in the normal adult. When the seminiferous tubules are damaged before puberty, the testes are small and firm.
- Postpubertal damage characteristically causes small, soft testes. Considerable testicular damage can occur before the overall size is below the lower limits of normal.

- Breast enlargement is a common feature of feminizing states in men and may be an early sign of androgen deficiency.

DIAGNOSTIC EVALUATION

- Figure 282–2 describes the laboratory evaluation of hypogonadism.

TREATMENT

- Variable with cause

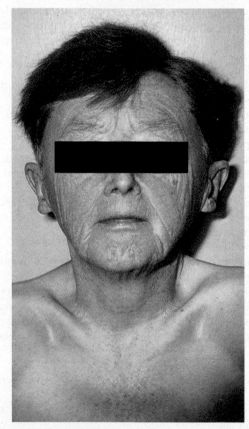

Fig 282–1
Facial appearance in postpubertal hypogonadism. The characteristic perioral wrinkling of the skin can be seen.
(From Besser CM, Thorner MO: Comprehensive Clinical Endocrinology, 3rd ed. St. Louis, Mosby, 2002.)

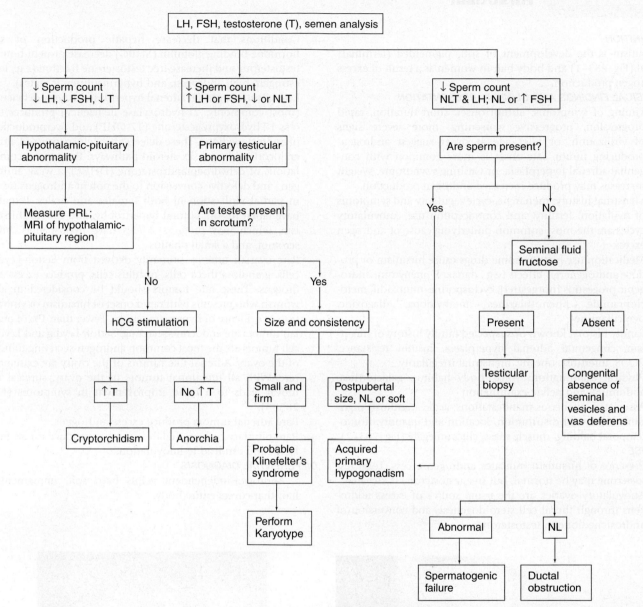

Fig 282–2

Laboratory evaluation of hypogonadism. FSH, follicle-stimulating hormone; hCG, human chorionic gonadotropin; LH, luteinizing hormone; NL, normal; PRL, prolactin; ↑, elevated; ↓, decreased or low.
(From Andreoli TE [ed]: Cecil Essentials of Medicine, 6th ed. Philadelphia, WB Saunders, 2006.)

Chapter 283   Hirsutism

DEFINITION
Hirsutism is the development of stiff, pigmented (terminal) facial (Fig. 283–1) and body hair in women as a result of excess androgen production.

PHYSICAL FINDINGS AND CLINICAL PRESENTATION
- Timing of symptoms: abrupt onset, short duration, rapid progression, progressive worsening, more severe signs of virilization, or later age at onset suggest androgen-producing tumor, late-onset is more common with congenital adrenal hyperplasia, or Cushing's syndrome. Weight increases may produce increased androgen production.
- Menstrual history: menarche, cycle regularity and symptoms of ovulation, fertility, and contraception use. Anovulatory cycles are the most common underlying cause of androgen excess.
- Medication use history: some drugs cause hirsutism or produce androgenergic effects (e.g., danazol, phenytoin, androgenic progestins [norgestrel], cyclosporine, minoxidil, metoclopramide, phenothiazines, methyldopa, diazoxide, penicillamine).
- Family history: known or suspected family history of hirsutism, congenital adrenal hyperplasia, insulin resistance, PCOS, infertility, obesity, menstrual irregularity.
- Physical examination: voice, body habitus, galactorrhea, abdominal and pelvic examination.
- Associated cutaneous manifestations: acne, acanthosis nigricans, striae, hair distribution, location and quantity, frontotemporal balding, muscle mass, clitoromegaly (Fig. 283–2).

CAUSE
- Presence of hirsutism indicates androgen excess. Total testosterone may be normal, but free testosterone is elevated.
- Anovulatory ovaries are the usual source of excess androgens through thecal cell steroidogenesis and conversion of androstenedione to testosterone.
- Conditions that decrease hepatic production of sex hormone-binding globulin (SHBG) decrease protein-bound testosterone and increase free testosterone fraction (e.g., low estrogen, high androgen, and hyperinsulinemic states).
- Late-onset, congenital adrenal hyperplasia enzyme deficiency (most commonly, 21-hydroxylase deficiency) produces excess 17 hydroxyprogesterone (17-OHP) and overproduction of androstenedione. These defects affect glucocorticoid, mineralocorticoid, and sex steroid pathways. Excessive accumulations of dehydroepiandrosterone (DHEA), a weak androgen, and defective conversion to the potent androgens result in partial virilization in both females and males. Females have labial fusion, clitoral hypertrophy, and modest hirsutism, which may progress. Males have hypospadias, bifid scrotum, and a small phallus.
- Rare ovarian tumors, primarily derived from Sertoli-Leydig cells, granulosa theca cells, or hilus cells, produce excess androgens. These rare tumors should be considered in any woman who presents with rapid onset of hirsutism or virilization or evidence of hyperestrogenism. Fewer than 1% of ovarian tumors are endocrine-secreting. Sertoli-Leydig and Leydig cell tumors are the most common androgen-secreting tumors of the ovary. Adrenal-like tumors of the ovary are extremely rare. With all functional tumors of the ovary, surgical removal leads to a rapid improvement in symptoms (Fig. 283–3).
- Rare adrenal tumors produce excess androgens.
- Rare pituitary or hypothalamic tumors produce excess prolactin and can lead to anovulation.

DIFFERENTIAL DIAGNOSIS
- Androgen-independent vellus hair: soft, unpigmented hair that covers entire body.

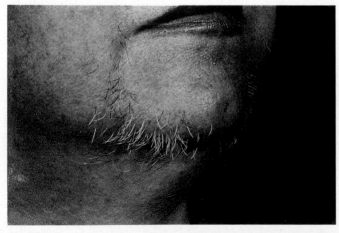

Fig 283–1
Stiff, pigmented (terminal) facial hair in a woman as a result of excess androgen production.
(From Lebwohl MG, Heymann WR, Berth-Jones J, Coulson I [eds]: Treatment of Skin Disease. St. Louis, Mosby, 2002.)

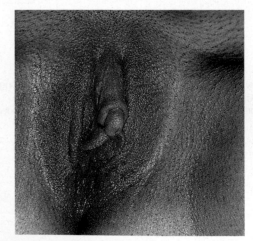

Fig 283–2
Enlarged clitoris in a patient with an androgen-secreting tumor.
(From Besser CM, Thorner MO: Comprehensive Clinical Endocrinology, 3rd ed. St. Louis, Mosby, 2002.)

- Hypertrichosis: diffusely increased total body hair often an adverse response to a medication or systemic illness.
- Polycystic ovary syndrome (PCOS), 75%
- Idiopathic, 5% to 15%
- Congenital adrenal hyperplasia, 1% to 8%
- Insulin resistance syndrome, 3% to 4%
- Drug-induced, <1%
- Ovarian tumor, <1%
- Adrenal tumor, <1%
- Hyperthecosis, <1%
- Hyperprolactinemia, <1%

LABORATORY TESTS

- Total serum testosterone or free testosterone-screen for testosterone secreting tumors. If markedly elevated, may image adrenals and ovaries.
- DHEA-S (DHEA sulfate): screen for adrenal androgen production because this is almost entirely produced by adrenals.
- Prolactin: moderately elevated values should prompt imaging of pituitary-hypothalamic region.
- 17-OHP (17α-hydroxyprogesterone): screen for adrenal enzyme deficiencies.

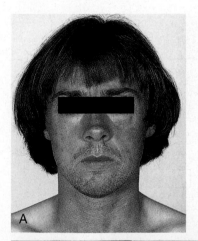

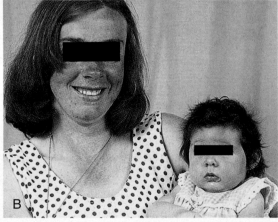

Fig 283–3

Patient with an arrhenoblastoma with associated polycystic ovaries before and after treatment. **A,** Before treatment, the patient had marked facial hirsutism. **B,** The patient is shown successfully treated. The tumor was resected and ovulation ensued after clomiphene and human chorionic gonadotropin therapy.

(From Besser CM, Thorner MO: Comprehensive Clinical Endocrinology, 3rd ed. St. Louis, Mosby, 2002.)

- Other laboratory test considerations, if appropriate:
  - FSH: rule out hypoestrogenic state (perimenopausal).
  - LH: typically elevated in PCOS with low or normal FSH.
  - TSH: rule out hypothyroidism.
  - 24-hour urinary free cortisol: rule out Cushing's syndrome and overproduction of cortisol.
  - Overnight single-dose dexamethasone suppression test: rule out Cushing's syndrome and adrenal hyperfunction.
  - Fasting blood sugar (FBS), 2-hour 75-g oral glucose tolerance test, fasting insulin levels: rule out insulin resistance syndrome.

IMAGING STUDIES

Imaging study considerations, if appropriate:

- Abdominal CT, MRI: rule out adrenal tumor.
- Pituitary-hypothalamic region CT, MRI: rule out pituitary tumor.
- Pelvic ultrasound (high resolution, transvaginal): rule out ovarian tumor.
- Laparoscopy, laparotomy: rule out small ovarian tumor in cases of elevated testosterone levels without radiologic evidence of adrenal or ovarian pathology.

TREATMENT

- Weight reduction: can reduce androgen production, improve menstrual function, and slow hair growth in obese women
- Cosmetic: temporary
  - Shaving: does not stimulate hair growth; lasts days
  - Epilation: electronic plucking
  - Bleaching
  - Mechanical waxing, plucking
  - Depilatories: chemically disrupts sulfide bonds of hair, causing dissolution of hair shaft
  - Pulsed laser: good for pigmented hair; lasts 3 to 6 months
- Cosmetic: permanent
  - Electrolysis: destroys individual hair follicles
  - Combined energies: bipolar radio frequency and pulsed light
- Cosmetic-eflornithine topical 13.9% cream: temporary. Hair growth returns on discontinuation of treatment; slow response over 4 to 8 weeks; applied directly to unwanted facial hair twice daily, with at least 8-hour spaced applications
- Suppress ovarian steroidogenesis and LH through low-dose estrogen and low androgenic progestational agents: slow response to treatment, suppresses new hair growth, established hair unaffected
- Spironolactone (aldosterone-antagonist diuretic inhibits adrenal and ovarian biosynthesis of androgens): when oral contraceptive pills (OCPs) unacceptable, or may be added for disappointing results after 6 months of OCP treatment
- GnRH agonists: inhibits gonadotropin and consequently ovarian androgen and estrogen secretion; may use in combination with low-dose estrogen or progestin or OCP to counter resulting estrogen deficiency
- Dexamethasone: adrenal glucocorticoid suppression is reserved for diagnosis of adrenal enzyme deficiency.
- Metformin-troglitazone therapy reserved for insulin-resistant states.
- Total abdominal hysterectomy or bilateral salpingo-oophorectomy reserved for recalcitrant hirsutism in older woman with hyperthecosis and undesired fertility.

Chapter 284 Gynecomastia

DEFINITION
Excessive breast tissue growth in a male.

CAUSE
- Stimulatory and inhibitory hormones control the growth and differentiation of mammary tissue in the male (Fig. 284-1).
- Estradiol binds to estrogen receptors and stimulates glandular cells, whereas testosterone exerts a generalized inhibitory action on growth and differentiation.
- The balance between stimulatory and inhibitory hormones controls the development and maintenance of breast tissues.
- Table 284-1 describes causes of gynecomastia.

DIAGNOSIS
- The diagnosis between physiologic and pathologic gynecomastia in adult men presents a challenge because of the common presence of breast enlargement in normal men and its association with obesity (Fig. 284-2).

- Important aspects of the history and physical examination in gynecomastia are described in Box 284-1.
- A method of examination for detecting gynecomastia is shown in Figure 284-3.
- Pathologic gynecomastia (Fig. 284-4) is defined as palpable breast tissue larger than 4 cm in diameter, palpable breast tissue larger than 2 cm that is tender, or palpable tissue larger than 2 cm demonstrated to be gradually increasing in diameter on follow-up.
- Mammography may occasionally be necessary to make this distinction, particularly in obese patients (Fig. 284-5).

DIAGNOSIS
- Elimination of contributing factors
- Surgical correction

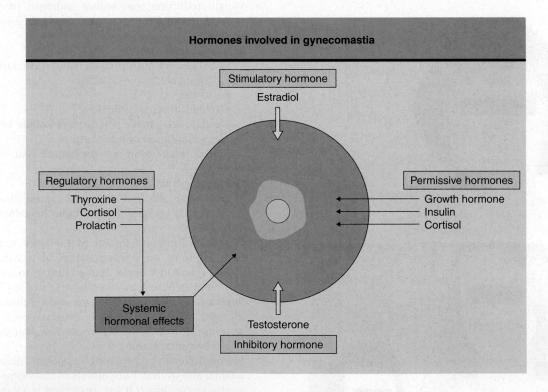

Fig 284-1
Hormones involved in gynecomastia; these affect breast tissue growth and differentiation. The diagram provides a framework for the logical assessment of disorders causing gynecomastia.
(From Besser CM, Thorner MO: Comprehensive Clinical Endocrinology, 3rd ed. St. Louis, Mosby, 2002.)

TABLE 284–1 Causes of pathologic gynecomastia

Feature	Cause(s)
Estradiol excess	Estradiol secretion: adrenal tumors
	Sporadic testicular tumors (sex cord, Sertoli cell, germ cell, Leydig cell)
	Testicular tumors associated with familial syndromes (Peutz-Jeghers, Carney's complex)
	Hepatic tumor with aromatase
	Increased aromatase activity
	Exogenous estrogens or estrogenic substances: drug therapy with estrogens
	Estrogen creams and lotions
	Occupational exposure to various estrogenic substances
	Cannabinoids
	Estrogen analogues: digitoxin
	Elevated estrogen precursors, aromatizable androgens: human chorionic gonadotropin (hCG) excess (eutopic or ectopic); exogenous hormones—testosterone enanthate, testosterone propionate, anabolic steroids, hCG administration
Testosterone deficiency	
Estradiol, testosterone imbalance	Drugs: cytotoxic drug-induced hypogonadism from busulfan, vincristine, nitrosourea, vincristine; combination chemotherapy; steroid synthesis inhibitory drugs
	Androgen resistance: complete testicular feminization
	Partial: Reifenstein's, Lubb's, Rosewater's, and Dreyfus syndromes
	Androgen antagonists: cimetidine, spironolactone, flutamide, bicalutamide, cyproterone acetate
	Blockers of 5_α-reductase
Regulatory hormone excess	Drug therapy with catecholamine antagonists or depleters, sulpiride, metoclopramide; phenothiazines, reserpine, domperidone, tricyclic antidepressants, methyldopa, haloperidol
	Other causes: local trauma, hip spica cast, chest injury, herpes zoster of chest wall, post-thoracotomy, spinal cord injury
	Other chronic illnesses: renal failure, pulmonary tuberculosis, HIV, diabetes mellitus, leprosy, refeeding, gynecomastia
	Drugs associated with gynecomastia with strong relationship of effect: amiodarone, calcium channel blockers, finasteride

From Besser CM, Thorner MO: Comprehensive Clinical Endocrinology, 3rd ed. St. Louis, Mosby, 2002.

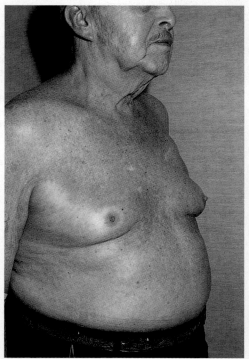

Fig 284–2
Patient with gynecomastia.
(From Swartz MH: Textbook of Physical Diagnosis, 5th ed. Philadelphia, WB Saunders, 2006.)

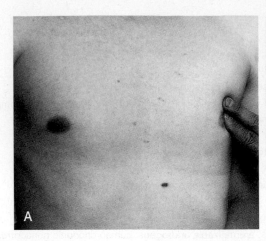
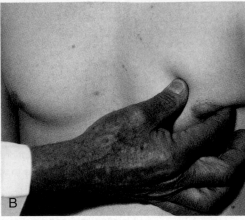

Fig 284–3
Method of examination to detect gynecomastia. **A,** Palpation by pressing down on tissue beneath the nipple in a supine patient is an insensitive method for detecting gynecomastia and is considered incorrect. **B,** Squeezing tissue between the thumb and forefinger in a sitting patient is a more sensitive technique and is considered correct. The examiner should try to flip an edge between normal fat tissue and glandular tissue to distinguish the outer limits of the gynecomastia.
(From Besser CM, Thorner MO: Comprehensive Clinical Endocrinology, 3rd ed. St. Louis, Mosby, 2002.)

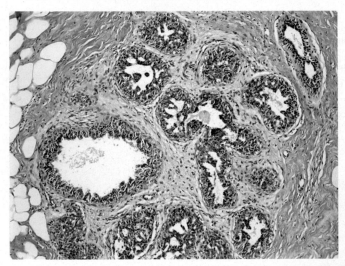

Fig 284–4
Gynecomastia. The stroma is edematous and the ductal proliferation is tufting.
(From Silverberg SG, Frable WJ, Wick MR, et al [eds]: Principles and Practice of Surgical Pathology and Cytopathology, 4th ed. Philadelphia, Elsevier, 2006.)

Box 284–1 Aspects of history and physical examination in gynecomastia

Patient history

Time of onset, rate of progression, degree of pain associated with gynecomastia

Symptoms of androgen deficiency

Use of specific medications

Presence of diabetes, renal, hepatic, cardiac, or pulmonary disease and associated malnutrition

Symptoms of underlying malignancy, especially testicular

Symptoms of estradiol. prolactin, growth hormone, cortisol, or thyroxine excess

History of chest wall trauma

Family history of gynecomastia

Physical examination

Distinguish pseudo- from true gynecomastia.

Determine degree of obesity (calculate body mass index).

Evaluate for signs of hypogonadism.

Quantify testis size and evaluate consistency.

Evaluate for signs of renal or hepatic disease.

Evaluate for evidence of Cushing's syndrome, hyperthyroidism, and hypogonadism.

From Besser CM, Thorner MO: Comprehensive Clinical Endocrinology, 3rd ed. St. Louis, Mosby, 2002.

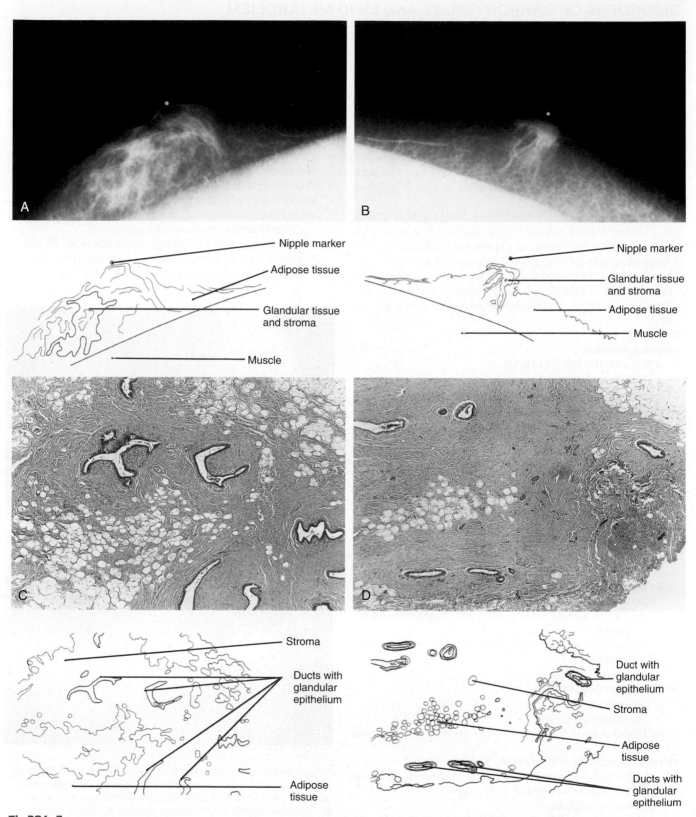

Fig 284–5
Bilateral persistent pubertal gynecomastia. **A, B,** Mammograms of right and left breasts in a 27-year-old male patient with bilateral persistent pubertal gynecomastia. The white circles represent the nipple markers. The glandular elements are apparent as radiopaque areas within bilateral breast tissue. **C, D,** Histologic appearance of the tissue excised from the right and left breasts during reduction mammoplasty. **C,** Ductal tissue interspersed with stroma and a minimal amount of fat tissue. **D,** Ductal tissue contains a predominance of stroma.
(From Besser CM, Thorner MO: Comprehensive Clinical Endocrinology, 3rd ed. St. Louis, Mosby, 2002.)

DISORDERS OF CARBOHYDRATE AND LIPID METABOLISM

Chapter 285 / **Diabetes mellitus**

DEFINITION

Diabetes mellitus (DM) refers to a syndrome of hyperglycemia resulting from many different causes. It can be classified into type 1 (formerly insulin-dependent diabetes mellitus [IDDM]) and type 2 (formerly non–insulin-dependent diabetes mellitus [NIDDM]). Because insulin-dependent and non–insulin-dependent refer to the stage at diagnosis, when a type 2 diabetic needs insulin, he or she remains classified as type 2 and does not revert to type 1.

The American Diabetes Association (ADA) defines DM as (1) a fasting plasma glucose ≥126 mg/dL, (2) a nonfasting plasma glucose ≥200 mg/dL, or (3) glucose ≥200 mg/dL in the 2-hour sample in an oral glucose tolerance test (OGTT). Furthermore, a value of <100 mg/dL of fasting blood sugar is the upper limit of normal for glucose. A fasting glucose between 100 and 126 mg/dL is classified as impaired fasting glucose (IFG).

CAUSE

Idiopathic diabetes

    TYPE 1 DIABETES MELLITUS
- Hereditary factors
1. Islet cell antibodies (found in 90% of patients within the first year of diagnosis)
2. Higher incidence of HLA types DR3, DR4
3. 50% concordance in identical twins
- Environmental factors: viral infection (possibly coxsackie virus, mumps virus)

    TYPE 2 DIABETES MELLITUS
- Hereditary factors: 90% concordance in identical twins
- Environmental factor: obesity

Diabetes secondary to other factors
- Hormonal excess: Cushing's syndrome, acromegaly, glucagonoma, pheochromocytoma
- Drugs: glucocorticoids, diuretics, oral contraceptives
- Insulin receptor unavailability (with or without circulating antibodies)
- Pancreatic disease: pancreatitis, pancreatectomy, hemochromatosis
- Genetic syndromes: hyperlipidemias, myotonic dystrophy, lipoatrophy
- Gestational diabetes

DIFFERENTIAL DIAGNOSIS
- Diabetes insipidus
- Stress hyperglycemia
- Diabetes secondary to hormonal excess, drugs, pancreatic disease

PHYSICAL FINDINGS AND CLINICAL PRESENTATION
- Physical examination varies with the presence of complications and may be normal in early stages.
- Diabetic retinopathy
  - Nonproliferative (background diabetic retinopathy)
  1. Initially: microaneurysms (Fig. 285–1), capillary dilation, waxy or hard exudates, dot and flame hemorrhages (Fig. 285–2), arteriovenous (AV) shunts

2. Advanced stage: microinfarcts with cotton-wool exudates, macular edema
- Proliferative retinopathy: characterized by formation of new vessels (Fig. 285–3), vitreal hemorrhages, fibrous scarring, and retinal detachment
- Cataracts and glaucoma occur with increased frequency in diabetics.
- Peripheral neuropathy: patients often complain of paresthesias of extremities (feet more than hands); the symptoms are symmetrical, bilateral, and associated with intense burning pain (particularly during the night).
- Mononeuropathies involving cranial nerves III, IV, and VI, intercostal nerves, and femoral nerves are also common.
- Physical examination may reveal the following:

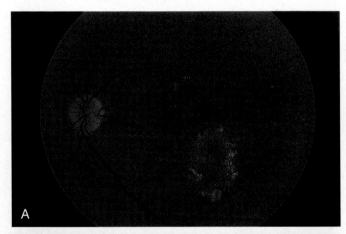

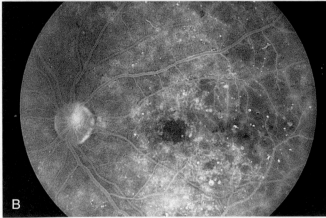

Fig 285–1

Nonproliferative diabetic retinopathy with microaneurysms. **A,** Small dot hemorrhages, microaneurysms, hard (lipid) exudates, circinate retinopathy, an intraretinal microvascular abnormality, and macular edema. **B,** Fluorescein angiography of the eye shown in **A**. Microaneurysms are seen as multiple dots of hyperfluorescence, but the dot hemorrhages do not fluoresce. The foveal avascular zone is minimally enlarged. (From Yanoff M, Duker JS: Ophthalmology, 2nd ed. St. Louis, Mosby, 2004.)

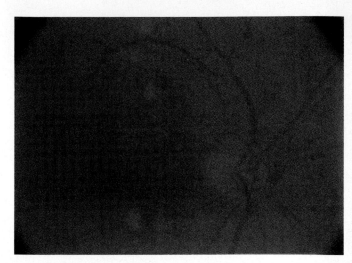

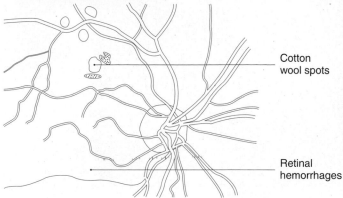

Fig 285-2

Background diabetic retinopathy with cotton-wool spots and retinal hemorrhages.
(Courtesy of Dr. James Tiedeman.)

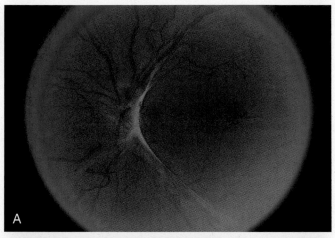

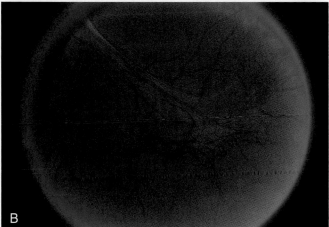

Fig 285-3

Neovascularization. **A,** Neovascularization of the disc with some fibrous proliferation. **B,** Neovascularization elsewhere.
(From Yanoff M, Duker JS: Ophthalmology, 2nd ed. St. Louis, Mosby, 2004.)

1. Decreased pinprick sensation, sensation to light touch, and pain sensation
2. Decreased vibration sense
3. Loss of proprioception (leading to ataxia)
4. Motor disturbances (decreased DTR, weakness and atrophy of interossei muscles). When the hands are affected, the patient has trouble picking up small objects, dressing, and turning pages in a book.
5. Diplopia, abnormalities of visual fields
- Autonomic neuropathy
  - GI disturbances: esophageal motility abnormalities, gastroparesis, diarrhea (usually nocturnal)
  - GU disturbances: neurogenic bladder (hesitancy, weak stream, and dribbling), impotence
  - Orthostatic hypotension: postural syncope, dizziness, light-headedness
- Nephropathy: pedal edema, pallor, weakness, uremic appearance. Diabetic kidney changes are described in Figure 285-4. Early diabetic glomerulopathy is shown in Figure 285-5.
- Foot ulcers (Fig. 285-6): occur in 15% of diabetics (annual incidence, 2%) and are the leading causes of hospitalization. They are usually secondary to peripheral vascu-

lar insufficiency, repeated trauma (unrecognized because of sensory loss), and superimposed infections often leading to gangrene (Fig. 285-7). If a diabetic foot ulcer has been present for weeks and foot pulses are palpable, neuropathy should be considered a major cause. Neuropathy can be detected with a simple examination of the lower extremities using a 10-g monofilament to test sensation. Prevention of foot ulcers in diabetics includes strict glucose control, patient education, prescription foot wear, intensive podiatric care, and evaluation for surgical interventions.
- Neuropathic arthropathy *(Charcot's joints):* bone or joint deformities (Fig. 285-8) from repeated trauma (secondary to peripheral neuropathy).
- *Necrobiosis lipoidica diabeticorum:* plaquelike reddened areas with a central area that fades to white-yellow found on the anterior surfaces of the legs. In these areas, the skin becomes very thin and can ulcerate readily (Fig. 285-9).

LABORATORY TESTS
- Diagnosis is made on the basis of the following tests and should be confirmed by repeated testing on a different day:
  1. Fasting glucose ≥126 mg/dL (ADA criterion)
  2. Nonfasting plasma glucose ≥200 mg/dL

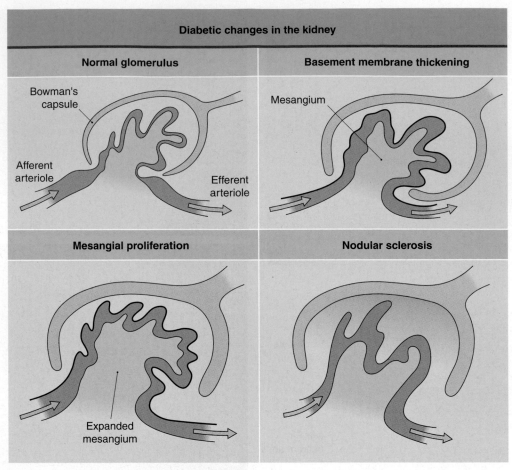

Fig 285–4
Diabetic changes in the kidney. Illustrated here are the progressive changes in the renal glomerular architecture that occur in the diabetic kidney.
(From Besser CM, Thorner MO: Comprehensive Clinical Endocrinology, 3rd ed. St. Louis, Mosby, 2002.)

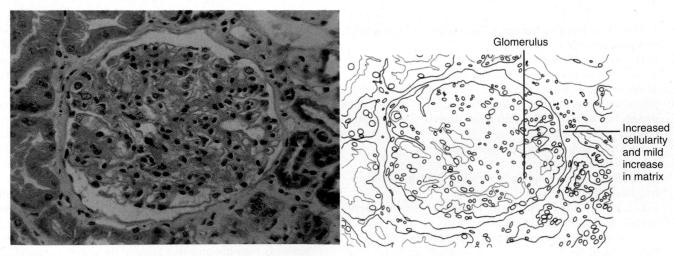

Fig 285–5
Early diabetic glomerulopathy with slight hypercellularity and a mild increase in the mesangial matrix (H&E).
(Courtesy of Dr. Benjamin Sturgill.)

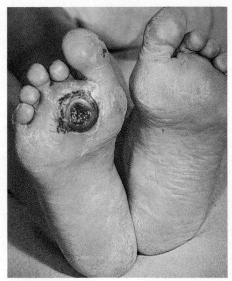

Fig 285-6
Neuropathic plantar ulcer in diabetic osteoarthropathy.
(From Hochberg MC, Silman AJ, Smolen JS, et al [eds]: Rheumatology,
3rd ed. St. Louis, Mosby, 2003.)

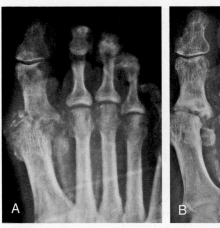

Fig 285-8
Diabetic osteoarthropathy. **A,** Fragmentation and severe osteolysis on
the articular surfaces of the first metatarsophalangeal joint. **B,** The process has healed, with moderate deformation of the articular surfaces.
(From Hochberg MC, Silman AJ, Smolen JS, et al [eds]: Rheumatology,
3rd ed. St Louis, Mosby, 2003.)

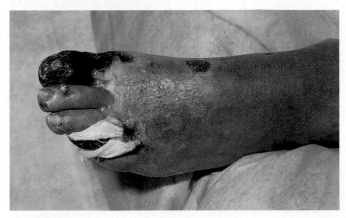

Fig 285-7
Diabetic gangrene.
(From Swartz MH: Textbook of Physical Diagnosis, 5th ed. Philadelphia,
WB Saunders, 2006.)

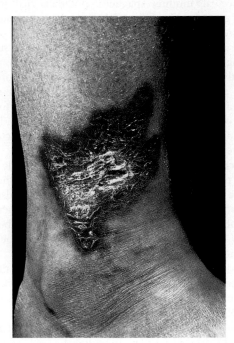

Fig 285-9
Necrobiosis lipoidica. Shown is a chronic lesion with ulceration and
crusting.
(Courtesy of the Institute of Dermatology, London.)

- Use of glycosylated hemoglobin (HbA_{1c}) level is generally
  not recommended for diagnosis because of lack of standard-
  ization of HbA_{1c} values and the imperfect correlation between HbA_{1c} and fasting plasma glucose levels. However,
  some physicians use this test to make the diagnosis of diabetes mellitus if the random plasma glucose is >200 mg/dL
  and the HbA_{1c} level is ≥2 SDs (standard deviations) above
  the laboratory mean.
- Screening for diabetic nephropathy by measuring microalbuminuria is recommended in all patients with diabetes. It can
  be accomplished by any of the following three methods:
  1. Measurement of the albumin-to-creatinine ratio in random spot urine collection. This is the easiest method to
  administer in the office setting because it is an easy assay to
  perform in most laboratories; the physician simply orders
  "Urine for microalbumin level."

  2. Measurement of a 24-hour urine collection for albumin,
  creatinine clearance
  3. Timed (4-hour or overnight) urine collection
- The diagnosis of microalbuminuria should be based on two
  or three elevated levels within a 3- to 6-month period because
  there is a marked variability in daily albumin excretion and
  possible transient elevations in urine albumin from short-
  term hyperglycemia, exercise, severe hypertension, and other
  illnesses, such as sepsis and CHF. Patients with overt nephropathy do not need screening for microalbuminuria

because the level of protein in the urine is high enough to be detected on routine urinalysis.

- A fasting serum lipid panel, serum creatinine, and electrolytes should be obtained annually on all adult diabetic patients.

TREATMENT

- Diet
  - Calories
  1. The diabetic patient can be started on 15 cal/lb of ideal body weight; this can be increased to 20 cal/lb for an active person and 25 cal/lb if the patient does heavy physical labor.
  2. The calories should be distributed as 50% to 60% carbohydrates, less than 30% fat, with saturated fat limited to less than 10% of total calories, and 15% to 20% protein.
  3. The emphasis should be on complex carbohydrates rather than simple and refined starches and on polyunsaturated instead of saturated fats in a ratio of 2:1.
  - Seven food groups
  1. The exchange diet of the ADA includes protein, bread, fruit, milk, and low- and intermediate-carbohydrate vegetables.
  2. The name of each exchange is meant to be all-inclusive (e.g., cereal, muffins, spaghetti, potatoes, rice are in the bread group; meats, fish, eggs, cheese, peanut butter are in the protein group).
  3. The glycemic index compares the rise in blood sugar after the ingestion of simple sugars and complex carbohydrates with the rise that occurs after the absorption of glucose. Equal amounts of starches do not produce the same increase in plasma glucose (pasta equal in calories to a baked potato causes less of an increase than the potato). Thus, it is helpful to know the glycemic index of a particular food product.
  4. Fiber: insoluble fiber (bran, celery) and soluble globular fiber (pectin in fruit) delay glucose absorption and attenuate the postprandial serum glucose peak. They also appear to lower the elevated triglyceride level often present in uncontrolled diabetics. A diet high in fiber should be emphasized (20 to 35 g/day of soluble and insoluble fiber).
  - Other principles
  1. Modest sodium restriction to 2400 to 3000 mg/day. If hypertension is present, restrict to less than 2400 mg/day; if nephropathy and hypertension are present, restrict to less than 2000 mg/day.
  2. Moderation of alcohol intake (two drinks or less/day in men, one drink/day or less in women)
  3. Non-nutritive artificial sweeteners are acceptable in moderate amounts.
- Exercise increases the cellular glucose uptake by increasing the number of cell receptors. The following points must be considered:
  - Exercise program must be individualized and built up slowly.
  - Insulin is more rapidly absorbed when injected into a limb that is then exercised; this can result in hypoglycemia.
- Weight loss: to ideal body weight if the patient is overweight

- Screenings for nephropathy, neuropathy, and retinopathy
- When the previous measures fail to normalize the serum glucose, oral hypoglycemic agents (e.g., metformin, glitazones, or a sulfonylurea) should be added to the regimen in type 2 DM. The sulfonamides and the biguanide metformin are the oldest and most commonly used classes of hypoglycemic drugs.
  - Metformin's primary mechanism is to decrease hepatic glucose output. Because metformin does not produce hypoglycemia when used as a monotherapy, it is preferred for most patients. It is contraindicated for patients with renal insufficiency.
  - Sulfonylureas and repaglinide work best when given before meals because they increase the postprandial output of insulin from the pancreas. All sulfonylureas are contraindicated for patients allergic to sulfa.
  - Acarbose and miglitol work by competitively inhibiting pancreatic amylase. Small intestine glucosidases delay gastrointestinal absorption of carbohydrates, thereby reducing alimentary hyperglycemia. The major side effects are flatulence, diarrhea, and abdominal cramps.
  - Pioglitazone and rosiglitazone increase insulin sensitivity and are useful in addition to other agents in type 2 diabetics whose hyperglycemia is inadequately controlled. Serum transaminase levels should be determined before starting therapy and monitored periodically.
  - Insulin is indicated for the treatment of all type 1 and type 2 DM patients who cannot be adequately controlled with diet and oral agents.
  - Pramlintide (Symlin), a synthetic analogue of human amylin (a hormone synthesized by pancreatic beta cells and cosecreted with insulin in response to food intake), can be used as an adjunctive treatment for patients with type 1 or type 2 DM who inject insulin at mealtime.
  - Exenatide (Byetta), a synthetic peptide that stimulates release of insulin from pancreatic beta cells, can be used as adjunctive therapy for patients with type 2 DM. It is not indicated in type 1 DM and is contraindicated in patients with severe renal impairment.
  - Combination therapy of various hypoglycemic agents is commonly used when monotherapy results in inadequate glycemic control.
  - Continuous subcutaneous insulin infusion (CSII, or insulin pump) provides better glycemic control than conventional therapy and comparable with or slightly better control than multiple daily injections. It should be considered for diabetes presenting in childhood or adolescence and during pregnancy.
  - Low-dose aminosalicylic acid (ASA) to decrease the risk of cerebrovascular disease is beneficial for diabetics older than 30 years with other risk factors (hypertension, dyslipidemia, smoking, obesity).
  - Strict lipid control (low-density lipoprotein [LDL] <70 mg/dL) is indicated for all diabetics. Use of statins is usually necessary to achieve therapeutic goals.

Chapter 286 Hypoglycemia and insulinoma

DEFINITION
- Hypoglycemia can be arbitrarily defined as a plasma glucose level less than 50 mg/dL. To establish the diagnosis, the following three criteria are necessary:
1. Presence of symptoms:
   - Adrenergic: sweating, anxiety, tremors, tachycardia, palpitations
   - Neuroglycopenic: seizures, fatigue, syncope, headache, behavioral changes, visual disturbances, hemiplegia
2. Low plasma glucose level in symptomatic patient
3. Relief of symptoms after ingestion of carbohydrates
- Insulinoma is a pancreatic insulin-secreting tumor that causes symptoms associated with hypoglycemia.

CLASSIFICATION
Reactive hypoglycemia
- Hypoglycemia usually occurs 2 to 4 hours after a meal rich in carbohydrates.
- These patients have no symptoms in the fasting state and rarely experience loss of consciousness secondary to their hypoglycemia because the glucose level rarely goes below 40 mg/dL.
- Patients who have had subtotal gastrectomy rapidly absorb carbohydrates, causing an early and very high plasma glucose level, followed by a late insulin surge that reaches its peak when most of the glucose has been absorbed. This results in hypoglycemia.
- Patients with type 2 (non–insulin-dependent) diabetes can experience hypoglycemia 3 to 4 hours postprandially secondary to a delayed and prolonged second phase of insulin secretion.
- Congenital deficiencies of enzymes necessary for carbohydrate metabolism and functional (idiopathic) hypoglycemia are additional causes of reactive hypoglycemia.

Fasting hypoglycemia
- Symptoms usually appear in the absence of food intake (at night or during early morning).
- Cause: insulinoma, mesenchymal tumors that synthesize insulin-like hormones, adrenal failure, glycogen storage disorders, severe liver or renal disease

Iatrogenic or drug-induced
- Hypoglycemic drugs (e.g., sulfanylureas)
- Excessive insulin replacement
- Factitious
- Ethanol-induced hypoglycemia
- In the hospital setting, a common cause of hypoglycemia is putting noncompliant patients on the regimen that they are supposed to be on at home, not realizing that the patient has been noncompliant.
- Hypoglycemia has also been associated with the use of the antibiotics gatifloxacin and levofloxacin.

DIAGNOSIS
- In a healthy person, when the plasma glucose level is low (e.g., fasting state), the plasma insulin level is also low. The following measurements taken during the hypoglycemic episode are useful in patients presenting with unexplained hypoglycemia:

1. Plasma insulin and proinsulin levels
2. C-peptide (connecting peptide)
3. Plasma and urine sulfonylurea levels
- Factitious hypoglycemia should be considered, especially if the patient has ready access to insulin or sulfonylureas (e.g., medical or paramedical personnel, family members who are diabetic or in the medical profession).
1. To diagnose factitious hypoglycemia secondary to sulfonylureas, screen serum and urine to determine the presence of sulfonylureas.
2. To diagnose factitious hypoglycemia secondary to insulin, the following measurements may be obtained:
   - Insulin level, which is markedly increased following exogenous insulin injection; the proinsulin level, however, is decreased.
   - Insulin antibodies: this test was once considered evidence of factitious hypoglycemia when animal insulin was the only commercial form available. Patients self-administering insulin currently may have no detectable insulin antibodies because of the use of human insulin. Therefore, this test is of limited use in cases of factitious hypoglycemia.
   - C-peptide: insulin is synthesized by the pancreas as a single-chain polypeptide formed of A and B chains joined by the C-peptide. This single-chain polypeptide (proinsulin) is broken down and secreted into the bloodstream as insulin and C-peptide in a 1:1 ratio. Exogenous insulin does not contain C-peptide; thus, C-peptide levels are elevated in patients with insulinoma and sulfonylureas but not after exogenous insulin injection.
3. Pancreatic islet cell neoplasms (insulinomas) are usually small (<3 cm), single, insulin 5–producing adenomas. Insulinomas are almost always solitary. Malignant insulinomas account for 5% of the total; they tend to be larger (6 cm). Metastases are usually to the liver (47%), regional lymph nodes (30%), or both. Measurement of inappropriately elevated serum insulin levels, despite an extremely low plasma glucose level after prolonged fasting (24 to 72 hours), is pathognomonic for these neoplasms.

IMAGING STUDIES
- Abdominal CT scanning or MRI (Fig. 286–1) detects one half to two thirds of insulinomas (abdominal ultrasound is not effective). It should be done only after laboratory tests for insulinoma have confirmed the diagnosis
- The insulinoma can often be located by selective pancreatic arteriography (see Fig. 286–1)

TREATMENT OF INSULINOMA
- Enucleation of single insulinoma
- Partial pancreatectomy for multiple adenomas
- Carbohydrate administration
- Diazoxide directly inhibits insulin release and has an extrapancreatic hyperglycemic effect that enhances glycogenolysis.
- Lanreotide and octreotide (somatostatin analogues)
- Streptozotocin

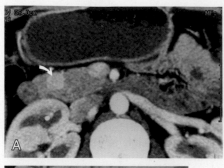
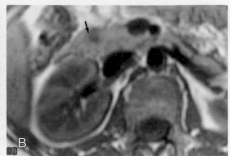
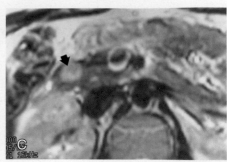

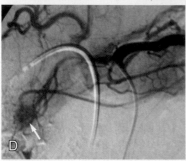

Fig 286–1

Insulinoma. **A,** Contrast-enhanced spiral CT scan demonstrating a small, brightly enhancing insulinoma *(curved arrow)* in the head of the pancreas. Axial T1-weighted spin-echo MRI scan **(B)** and T2-weighted fast spin-echo image **(C)** show the corresponding lesion *(arrow)* on MRI of low signal intensity on the T1- and high signal intensity on the T2-weighted images. **D,** Celiac arteriogram in the same patient shows the vascular blush of the insulinoma *(arrow).*

(From Grainger RG, Allison DJ, Adam A, Dixon AK [eds]: Grainger & Allison's Diagnostic Radiology, 4th ed. London, Harcourt, 2001.)

Chapter 287 **Hyperlipidemia**

DEFINITION

Hyperlipidemia can be defined as an abnormal elevation of plasma cholesterol or triglyceride levels. It is a major contributor to atherosclerosis (Fig. 287–1) and coronary thrombosis (Fig. 287–2). The composition of the major classes of lipoproteins is depicted in Figure 287–3)

PHYSICAL FINDINGS AND CLINICAL PRESENTATION

- Most patients: no physical findings
- Possible findings particularly in the familial forms
  1. Tendon xanthomas (Fig. 287–4)
  2. Xanthelasma (Fig. 287–5)
  3. Arcus corneae (Fig. 287–6)
  4. Eruptive xanthomata on the buttocks (Fig. 287–7)
  5. Lipemia retinalis (Fig. 287–8)
  6. Milky appearance of plasma (Fig. 287–9)

CAUSE

Primary
- Genetics
- Obesity
- Dietary intake

Secondary
- Diabetes mellitus
- Alcohol
- Oral contraceptives
- Hypothyroidism
- Glucocorticoid use
- Most diuretics
- Nephrotic syndrome
- Hepatoma
- Extrahepatic biliary obstruction
- Primary biliary cirrhosis

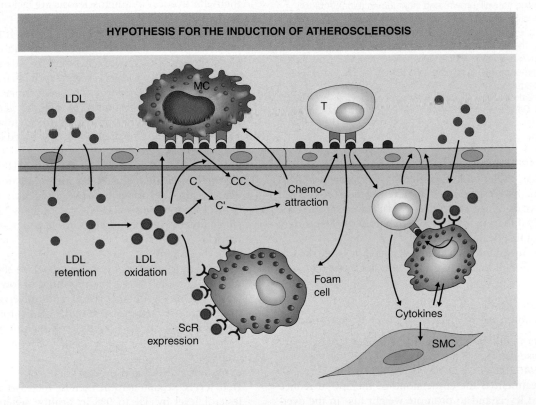

HYPOTHESIS FOR THE INDUCTION OF ATHEROSCLEROSIS

Fig 287–1

Hypothesis for the induction of atherosclerosis. Low-density lipoprotein (LDL) enters the arterial intima through an intact endothelium. In hypercholesterolemia, the influx of LDL exceeds the eliminating capacity and an extracellular pool of LDL with proteoglycans of the extracellular matrix. Intimal LDL is oxidized through the action of free oxygen radicals formed by enzymatic reactions. This generates proinflammatory lipids that induce endothelial expression of the adhesion molecule, vascular cell adhesion molecule-1, activate complement (C), and stimulate chemokine (CC) secretion. All these factors cause adhesion and entry of mononuclear leukocytes, particularly monocytes (MC) and lymphocytes (T). Monocytes differentiate into macrophages, a process promoted by local macrophage colony-stimulating factor secretion in the forming lesion. Macrophages upregulate scavenger receptors (ScR), which internalize oxidized LDL and transform into foam cells. Macrophage uptake of oxidized LDL also leads to presentation of fragments to antigen-specific T cells. This induces an autoimmune reaction that leads to the production of proinflammatory cytokines. Such cytokines include interferongamma, tumor necrosis factor α, and interleukin-1, which act on endothelial cells to stimulate expression of adhesion molecules and procoagulant activity, act on macrophages to activate proteases, endocytosis, nitric oxide (NO), and cytokines, and act on smooth muscle cells (SMCs) to induce NO production and inhibit growth and collagen and actin expression.
(From Crawford, MH, DiMarco JP, Paulus WJ [eds]: Cardiology, 2nd ed. St. Louis, Mosby.)

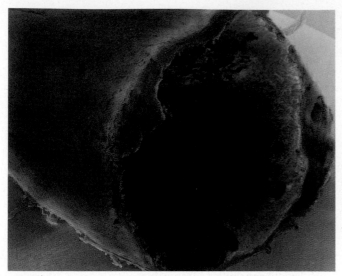

Fig 287–2
Colored scanning electron micrograph of a blood clot of thrombus in-side a coronary artery of the human heart. The artery has been cross-sectioned, showing its wall (brown) and inner lumen (blue). A blood ___ (red) is seen, blocking about 30% of the diameter of the artery. A clot in either of the two coronary arteries that supply blood to the heart lim-its blood flow to the heart, leading to a heart attack. Thrombus forma-tion occurs following disruption of an atherosclerotic plaque, exposing tissue factor on monocytes to flowing blood, which leads to the initia-tion of blood coagulation.
(Courtesy of the Science Photo Gallery), www.sciencephotogallery.co.uk.
From Young NS, Gerson SL, High KA (eds): Clinical Hematology, St. Louis, 2006, Mosby.

DIAGNOSTIC APPROACH

- Serum total cholesterol, high-density lipoprotein (HDL) cholesterol, and triglycerides should be measured in all adults 20 years of age and older at least once every 5 years, particularly if there is a history of premature coronary artery disease in a first degree relative.
- LDL can be measured directly or calculated by using the fol-lowing formula if the triglyceride levels are lower than 400 mg/dL:

  LDL cholesterol =
  total cholesterol − HDL cholesterol − (triglycerides/5)

- All patients should be assessed for the presence of coronary heart disease risk factors and diabetes.

MEDICAL MANAGEMENT OF LIPID DISORDERS

- Dietary treatment is the cornerstone of therapy to reduce blood lipid levels and to promote weight loss in the over-weight patient.
- Drug therapy is initiated when lifestyle changes are insuffi-cient to achieve desired lipid levels. Several medications are now available for treatment.
  - Lipid-lowering agents
1. Statins (3-hydroxy-3-methyglutaryl coenzyme A [HMG-CoA] reductase inhibitors) are effective and generally well tolerated and are agents of choice in patients with elevated LDL cholesterol levels unresponsive to dietary restrictions. They can decrease LDL cholesterol by 20% to 60%, increase

HDL cholesterol by 5% to 15%, and decrease triglycerides by 10% to 40%. All statins necessitate frequent monitoring of liver function tests (alanine aminotransferase [ALT], as-partate transaminase [AST]) for potential toxicity. Concomi-tant use of cyclosporine, fibrates, niacin, or erythromycin can increase the risk of myopathy.
2. Fibrates (fenofibrate, gemfibrozil) are useful in patients with low HDL levels, elevated triglyceride levels, and modest elevations in LDL level. Concomitant use of statins should generally be avoided or used with caution because of in-creased risk of myopathy and rhabdomyolysis.
3. Nicotinic acid (niacin) is useful in patients with low HDL and elevated cholesterol and triglyceride levels. It can result in a 10% to 25% reduction in LDL cholesterol, a 15% to 35% increase in HDL cholesterol, and a 20% to 50% de-crease in triglycerides. Its use, however, is limited by side effects (pruritus, flushing, GI side effects, hepatotoxicity). Some of the newer longer acting preparations are better tolerated.
4. The bile acid sequestrant colesevelam and the cholesterol absorption inhibitors can also be used, but data regarding their effectiveness in atherosclerosis are lacking.
- Hypertriglyceridemia
  - Normal triglyceride levels should be lower than 150 mg/dL. Levels higher than >600 mg/dL may cause pancreatitis.
  - The principal therapy for hypertriglyceridemia is lifestyle changes (weight loss, exercise, avoidance of smoking and al-cohol), and effective control of hyperglycemia in diabetes.
  - Nicotinic acid and fibrates (fenofibrate, gemfibrozil) are effective in reducing severe hyperglyceridemia and may be particularly useful in patients with associated low HDL cho-lesterol levels.
  - Omega-3 polyunsaturated fatty acid (PUFA) lowers tri-glyceride levels by reducing hepatic production of triglycer-ides. It also decreases hepatic production of very low-density lipoproteins (VLDLs) and changes LDL size from small atherosclerotic particles to larger, less atherogenic particles.
- HDL cholesterol
  - Lipid management guidelines recognize the importance of HDL levels by raising the threshold of low HDL choles-terol to <40 mg/dL and award a negative risk factor (re-moves one risk factor from the total count) for HDL choles-terol >60 mg/dL. Each increase in serum HDL level of 1 mg/dL is associated with a 2% to 4 % reduction in cardiac events.
  - Aerobic exercise and modest intake of ethanol will raise HDL levels. Regular aerobic exercise increases the HDL cho-lesterol level by 3% to 9% in healthy sedentary persons. Obesity and cigarette smoking are associated with reduced HDL cholesterol. Diet rich in omega-3 polyunsaturated fatty acids with limited carbohydrates will increase HDL.
  - Therapy with nicotinic acid (20% to 35 % increase), fi-brates (10% to 25% increase), or statins (2% to 15 % in-crease) will increase HDL levels. Use of fibrates or niacin is recommended for persons whose HDL is lower than 40 mg/dL and who have diabetes mellitus or the metabolic syndrome.

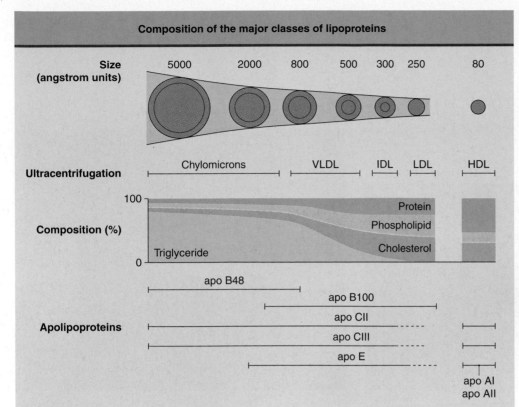

Composition of the major classes of lipoproteins

Fig 287-3
Composition of the major classes of lipoproteins. Although each lipoprotein is distinct with respect to its relative proportions of cholesterol, triglycerides, phospholipids, and apolipoproteins, considerable heterogeneity exists within each lipoprotein class. Lipoproteins are graded according to their density: very low-density lipoprotein (VLDL), low-density lipoprotein (LDL), intermediate-density lipoprotein (IDL), or high-density lipoprotein (HDL). Clinical measures of LDL include both LDL and IDL.
(From Besser CM, Thorner MO: Comprehensive Clinical Endocrinology, 3rd ed. St. Louis, Mosby, 2002.)

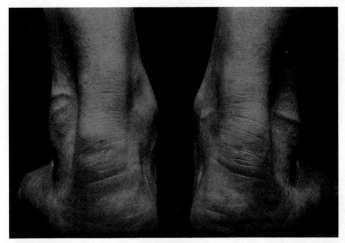

Fig 287-4
Achilles tendon xanthomata.
(From Besser CM, Thorner MO: Comprehensive Clinical Endocrinology, 3rd ed. St. Louis, Mosby, 2002.)

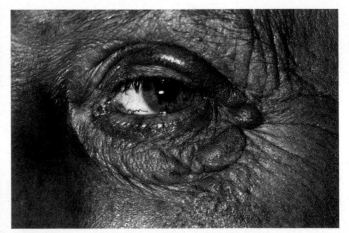

Fig 287-5
Xanthelasmata. Note the yellow periorbital plaques. These are a common manifestation of hypercholesterolemia.
(Courtesy of the Institute of Dermatology, London.)

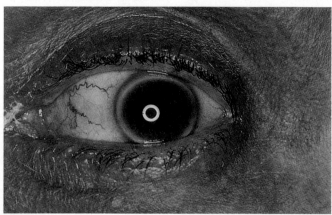

Fig 287–6
Extensive corneal arcus. Early corneal arcus is characterized by depo-
sition of cholesterol at the superior and inferior aspects of the cornea.
With time, the arcus may become totally circumferential, as illustrated.
(From Besser CM, Thorner MO: Comprehensive Clinical Endocrinology,
3rd ed. St. Louis, Mosby, 2002.)

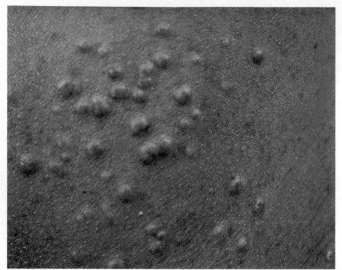

Fig 287–7
Eruptive xanthomata on the buttocks.
(From Besser CM, Thorner MO: Comprehensive Clinical Endocrinology,
3rd ed. St. Louis, Mosby, 2002.)

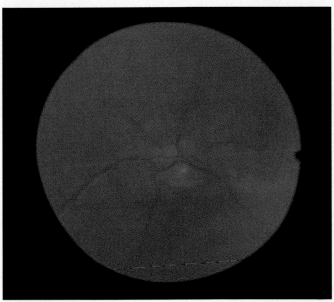

Fig 287-8
Lipemia retinalis seen in association with marked hypertriglyceridemia.
Note the pale color of the retinal vessels (caused by circulating chylo-
microns) against the pink background of the retina.
(From Besser CM, Thorner MO: Comprehensive Clinical Endocrinology,
3rd ed. St. Louis, Mosby, 2002.)

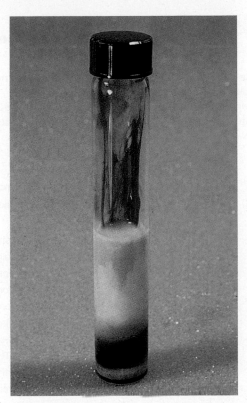

Fig 287-9
Milky appearance of plasma from a patient with marked hypertriglyceridemia.
(From Besser CM, Thorner MO: Comprehensive Clinical Endocrinology,
3rd ed. St. Louis, Mosby, 2002.)

Chapter 288 **Multiple endocrine neoplasia (MEN)**

- Table 288–1 describes the multiple endocrine neoplasia (MEN) syndromes.
- A diagnostic approach to MEN-1 is shown in Figure 288–1.
- Figure 288–2 illustrates a positive nuclear medicine scan in MEN-2B.

TABLE 288–1 Multiple endocrine neoplasia (MEN) syndromes*

Type		Tumors	Biochemical features
MEN-I	Parathyroids (often multiglandular)		Hypercalcemia and ↑ PTH
	Pancreatic islets	Gastrinoma	↑ gastrin and ↑ basal gastric acid output
		Insulinoma	Hypoglycemia and ↑ insulin
		Glucagonoma	Glucose intolerance and ↑ glucagon
		VIPoma	↑ VIP and WDHA
		PPoma	↑ PP
	Pituitary (anterior)	Prolactinoma	Hyperprolactinemia
		GH-secreting	↑ GH
		ACTH-secreting	Hypercortisolemia and ↑ ACTH
		Nonfunctioning	Nil or alpha subunit
	Associated tumors	Adrenocortical	Hypercortisolemia or primary hyperaldosteronism
		Carcinoid	↑ 5-HIAA
		Lipoma	None
MEN-IIA	Medullary thyroid carcinoma		Hypercalcitoninemia*
	Pheochromocytoma		↑ Catecholamines
	Parathyroid		Hypercalcemia and ↑ PTH
MEN-IIB	Medullary thyroid carcinoma		Hypercalcitoninemia
	Pheochromocytoma		↑ Catecholamines
	Associated abnormalities	Mucosal neuromas	
		Marfanoid habitus	
		Medullated corneal nerve fibers	
		Megacolon	

Characteristic tumors and associated biochemical abnormalities are shown. Autosomal dominant inheritance of the MEN syndromes has been established.
*In some patients, basal serum calcitonin concentrations may be normal but show an abnormal rise at 1 and 5 min after stimulation with pentagastrin, 0.5 µg/kg.
ACTH, adrenocorticotropic hormone; GH, growth hormone; 5-HIAA, 5-hydroxyindoleacetic acid; ↑, increased; PR pancreatic polypeptide; PTH, parathyroid hormone; VIP, vasoactive intestinal peptide; WDHA, watery diarrhea, hypokalemia, and achlorhydria.
From Besser CM, Thorner MO: Comprehensive Clinical Endocrinology, 3rd ed. St. Louis, Mosby, 2002.

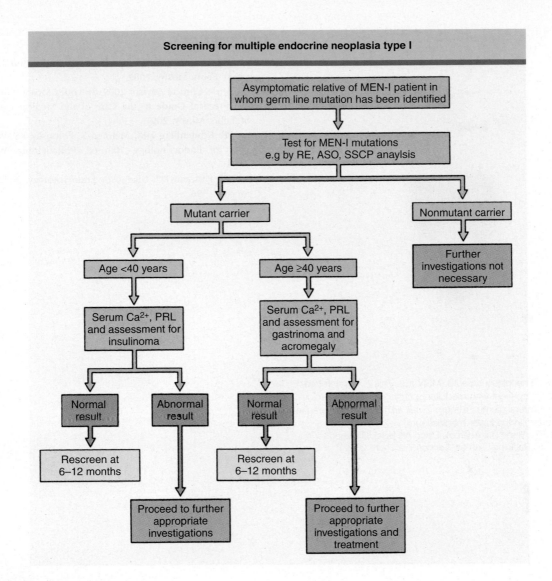

Fig 288–1

Screening for multiple endocrine neoplasia type I (MEN-I). The figure illustrates an approach to screening in an asymptomatic relative of a patient with MEN-I. The relative should first have undergone a clinical evaluation for MEN-I–associated tumors to establish that he or she is asymptomatic. Relatives who are symptomatic, who could also have a test for MEN-I mutations, should proceed to appropriate investigation and management. Mutational analysis for MEN-I is not routinely available at present, and this protocol could instead be adapted for first degree relatives. The MEN-I mutation may be identified directly by DNA sequence analysis or by restriction enzyme (RE), allele-specific oligonucleotide (ASO) hybridization, or another method, such as single-stranded conformational polymorphism (SSCP) analysis. It has been suggested that nonessential genetic testing in a child who is not old enough to make important long-term decisions should be deferred. However, the finding that a child from a family with MEN-I does not have any MEN-I mutations removes the burden of repeated clinical, biochemical, and radiologic investigations and enables health resources to be more effectively directed toward those children who are MEN-I mutant gene carriers. The use of mutational analysis and such screening methods in children is controversial and varies in different countries, as do the approaches to genetic testing and screening for MEN-I.

(Adapted from Thakker RV: Multiple endocrine neoplasia type1. In DeGroot LJ, Jameson JL [eds]: Endocrinology, 4th ed. Philadelphia, WB Saunders, 2001, pp 2503-2517.)

REFERENCES

Besser CM, Thorner MO: Comprehensive Clinical Endocrinology, 3rd ed. St. Louis, Mosby, 2002.

Ferri F: Ferri's Clinical Advisor 2009. St. Louis, Mosby, 2009.

Ferri F: Practical Guide to the Care of the Medical Patient, 7th ed. St. Louis, Mosby, 2007.

Larsen PR, Kronenberg HM, Melmed S, Polonsky KS: Williams Textbook of Endocrinology, 10th ed. Philadelphia, WB Saunders, 2003.

Moore WT, Eastman RC: Diagnostic Endocrinology, 2nd ed. St. Louis, Mosby, 1996.

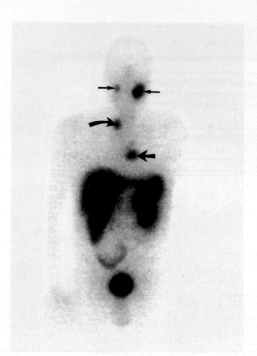

Fig 288–2
Multiple endocrine neoplasia type IIB (MEN-IIB). This ^{111}In-pentetreotide image shows a patient with medullary carcinoma of the thyroid *(curved arrow)*, bilateral glomus tumors *(small arrows)*, and a paraganglioma *(large arrow)* in the lower mediastinum.
(From Grainger RG, Allison DJ, Adam A, Dixon AK [eds]: Grainger & Allison's Diagnostic Radiology, 4th ed. London, Harcourt, 2001.)

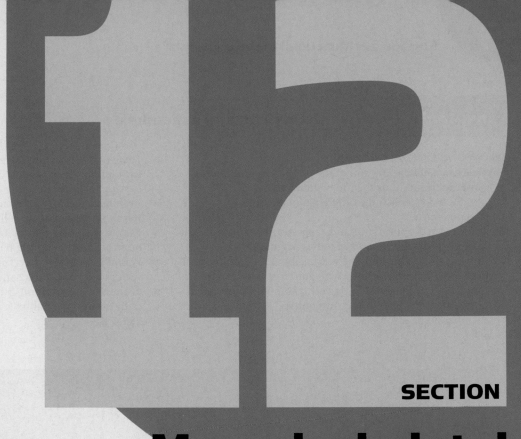

SECTION
Musculoskeletal System

Chapter 289: Diagnostic tests and procedures

Chapter 290: Osteoarthritis

Chapter 291: Rheumatoid arthritis

Chapter 292: Juvenile rheumatoid arthritis

Chapter 293: Systemic lupus erythematosus

Chapter 294: Antiphospholipid antibody syndrome

Chapter 295: Sjögren's syndrome

Chapter 296: Idiopathic inflammatory myopathies
(dermatomyositis, polymyositis)

Chapter 297: Raynaud's syndrome

Chapter 298: Scleroderma

Chapter 299: Mixed connective tissue disease

Chapter 300: Vasculitides

Chapter 301: Spondyloarthropathies

Chapter 302: Crystal-related arthritis

Chapter 303: Fibromyalgia

Chapter 304: Regional rheumatic diseases

Chapter 305: Inherited connective tissue disorders

Chapter 306: Diseases of bone and bone metabolism

Chapter 307: Hypertrophic osteoarthropathy

Chapter 308: Infections

Chapter 309: Bone tumors

Chapter 310: Fractures

Chapter 289 Diagnostic tests and procedures

DIAGNOSTIC EVALUATION

Physical examination The aim of the physical examination is to answer four questions that, in combination with the history, should establish the differential diagnosis.

a. Is it normal?

- The expected appearance and ranges of movement of the musculoskeletal system need to be recognized.
- Abnormalities can be observed as abnormal resting position, swelling, or deformity with abnormal movement. Figures 289-1 through 289-4 reveal commonly observed abnormalities involving the extremities in patients with rheumatologic disorders.

- There may be warmth, crepitus, or tenderness on palpation with instability or weakness and muscle wasting.

b. What is the abnormality?

- An inflamed joint is characterized by pain and tenderness, warmth, redness, and swelling.
- Pain is often apparent by observing movement, and tenderness is elicited by gentle palpation.
- Warmth is mainly detectable in medium and large joints, such as the knee, ankle, and wrist joints (Fig. 289-5).
- Redness is uncommon but is encountered in gout, especially around the hallux (Fig. 289-6) and in infection (Fig. 289-7).

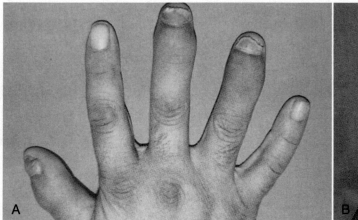
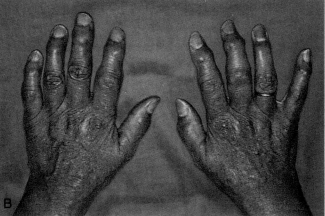

Fig 289-1
Rheumatic disorders affecting the DIP joints. (**A**) Psoriatic arthropathy of two DIP joints and the interphalangeal joint of the thumb, together with nail dystrophy. (**B**) Osteoarthritis is the commonest disorder affecting this segment (Heberden's nodes).
(From Hochberg MC, Silman AJ, Smolen JS, et al [eds]: Rheumatology, 3rd ed. St Louis, Mosby, 2003.)

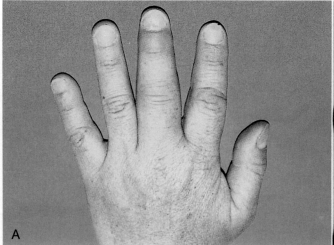
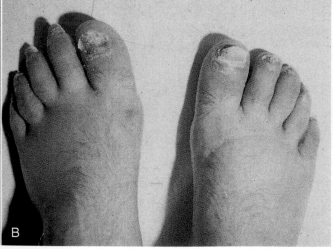

Fig 289-2
Sausage fingers and toes. (**A**) Psoriatic arthropathy—dactylitis at the third finger. (**B**) Reactive arthritis—dactylitis more evident at the second and the third left toes and nail dystrophy
(From Hochberg MC, Silman AJ, Smolen JS, et al [eds]: Rheumatology, 3rd ed. St Louis, Mosby, 2003.)

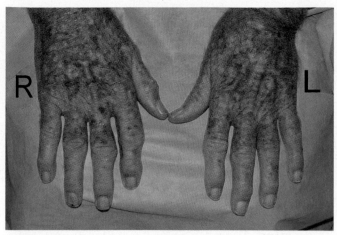

Fig 289-3

Interphalangeal osteoarthritis of the hands. Knobby, hard tissue changes of the DIP joints. Hard and soft tissue changes of the proximal interphalangeal joints, with deformity. The MCP joints and wrists are spared. There is knobby deformity at the base of the left thumb, reflecting at the base of the left thumb, reflecting radial subluxation of the first proximal metacarpal at the first CMC joint.
(From Hochberg MC, Silman AJ, Smolen JS, et al [eds]: Rheumatology, 3rd ed. St Louis, Mosby, 2003.)

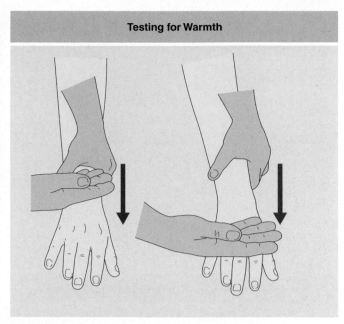

Testing for Warmth

Fig 289-5

Testing for warmth, using the back of the hand.
(From Hochberg MC, Silman AJ, Smolen JS, et al [eds]: Rheumatology, 3rd ed. St Louis, Mosby, 2003.)

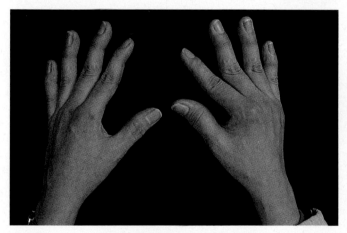

Fig 289-4

Swan-neck deformities in a patient with SLE.
(From Hochberg MC, Silman AJ, Smolen JS, et al [eds]: Rheumatology, 3rd ed. St Louis, Mosby, 2003.)

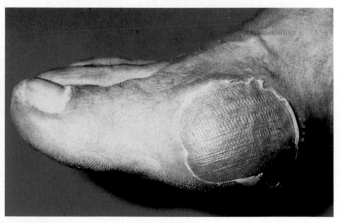

Fig 289-6

Acute gout. The first MTP joint is involved at some time in approximately 75% of patients. Desquamation of the skin often occurs.
(From Hochberg MC, Silman AJ, Smolen JS, et al [eds]: Rheumatology, 3rd ed. St Louis, Mosby, 2003.)

Fig 289-7

Bursitis symptoms are similar to arthritis, but a diagnostic puncture of the bursa containing material in septic bursitis will confirm the diagnosis.
(From Hochberg MC, Silman AJ, Smolen JS, et al [eds]: Rheumatology, 3rd ed. St Louis, Mosby, 2003.)

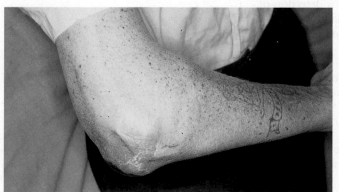

The Bulge Sign in the Knee	The Patellar Tap

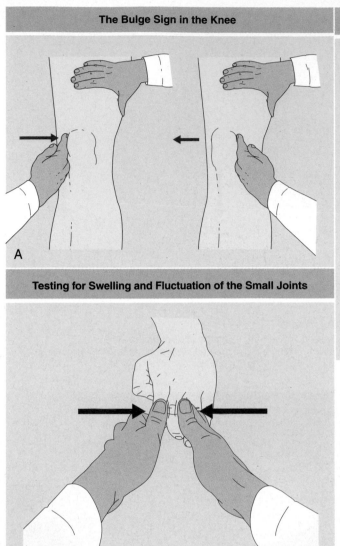

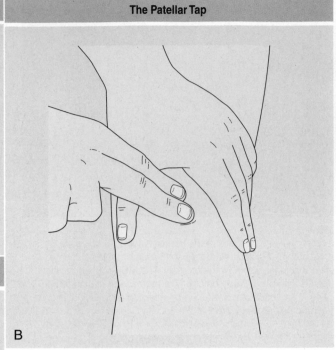

Fig 289–8

Testing for swelling. (**A**) The bulge sign in the knee. The back of the hand gently pushes the fluid from one side of the knee to the other, filling out the 'dimples' on either side of the patella. This is most helpful in detecting small knee effusions. (**B**) The parallel tap. One hand is used to cup the patella and compress the suprapatellar pouch, and the fingers of the other hand press down on the patella to feel for cross-fluctuation. (**C**) Swelling/fluctuation of the small joints of the hand. Detect cross-fluctuation at the joint line with the index fingers and thumbs, with the examiner's fingers squeezing and feeling each side of the joint (as illustrated) or one index finger/thumb squeezing and feeling from side to side and the other from the palmar to the dorsal aspect ('interlocking C')

(From Hochberg MC, Silman AJ, Smolen JS, et al [eds]: Rheumatology, 3rd ed. St Louis, Mosby, 2003.)

- Swelling of an inflamed joint is characterized by its articular origin, is fluctuant because of synovial proliferation or effusion, and is tender, whereas there may be bony swelling along the joint line in osteoarthritis (Fig. 289–8).
- There are a number of specific techniques for detection of synovitis and effusion at different joints. Table 289–1 describes a system for examination of the musculoskeletal system.

  c. What is the pattern of distribution?

- The distribution of involvement of the musculoskeletal structures is of crucial importance in the diagnosis of musculoskeletal conditions.
- Table 289–2 describes characteristic patterns of involvement of the musculoskeletal system.

  d. What other features of clinical importance are there?

- Many musculoskeletal conditions are associated with systemic features.

TABLE 289–1 System for examination of the musculoskeletal system

- Look— at rest, during movement
- Feel
- Move— active, passive, resisted, listen
- Stress
- Special tests

From Hochberg MC, Silman AJ, Smolen JS, et al (eds): Rheumatology, 3rd ed. St Louis, Mosby, 2003.

- Many of them are easily visible as skin signs, such as skin laxity (joint hypermobility syndrome), rashes (Table 289–3), nodules or vasculitis lesions (nodules or vasculitis in rheumatoid arthritis [RA]), gout (tophi), or psoriatic arthritis.

TABLE 289–2 Characteristic patterns of involvement of the musculoskeletal system

Diagnosis	Symmetry	Number of Joints Involved*	Large or Small	Distribution	Upper or Lower Limbs
Rheumatoid arthritis	Symmetrical	Polyarthritis	Large/small	Peripheral	Upper/lower
Ankylosing spondylitis	Asymmetrical	Oligoarthritis	Large	Central and peripheral	Lower
Psoriatic arthritis	Asymmetrical	Oligo/polyarthritis	Large/small	Peripheral	Upper/lower
Reactive arthritis	Asymmetrical	Oligo/polyarthritis	Large/dactylitis	Peripheral	Lower
Gout	Asymmetrical	Mono/oligoarthritis	Large/small	Peripheral	Lower/upper

Oligoarthritis ≤5 joints affected; polyarthritis >5 joints affected.
From Hochberg MC, Silman AJ, Smolen JS, et al (eds): Rheumatology, 3rd ed. St Louis, Mosby, 2003.

TABLE 289–3 Associated skin lesions

Torso and limbs	Livedo reticularis	Systemic lupus erythematosus, antiphospholipid syndrome, vasculitis
	Erythema abigne	Sign of external heat applied to relieve pain
	Erythema migrans	Lyme arthritis
	Palpable purpura	Leukocytoclastic vasculitis
	Psoriasis	Psoriatic arthritis
	Erythema nodosum	Acute sarcoid
	Nodules	Heberden's
		Rheumatoid arthritis
		Gout
		Hyperlipidemia
		Systemic lupus erythematosus
		Rheumatic fever
		Polyarteritis nodosa
		Multicentric histiocytosis
		Sarcoidosis
	Ulcers	Vasculitis, Behçet's disease, Crohn's disease
	Calcinosis cutis	Scleroderma
Face and mouth	Butterfly rash	Systemic lupus erythematosus
	Psoriasis	Psoriatic arthritis
	Heliotrope discoloration	Dermatomyositis
	Oral ulcers	SLE, reactive arthritis, Behçet's disease
	Telangiectasia	Limited cutaneous systemic sclerosis
Nails	Clubbing	Hypertrophic pulmonary osteoarthropathy
	Pitting	Psoriatic arthritis
	Onycholysis	Psoriatic arthritis
	Splinter hemorrhages	Small vessel vasculitis, endocarditis
Hands	Raynaud's phenomenon	Systemic lupus erythematosus, scleroderma, mixed connective tissue disease
	Nail fold capillary abnormalities	Scleroderma, dermatomyositis
	Palmar erythema	Active rheumatoid arthritis, systemic lupus erythematosus
	Gottron's papules	Dermatomyositis
	Telangiectasia	Limited cutaneous systemic sclerosis
	Sclerodactyly	Limited cutaneous systemic sclerosis
	Vasculitic lesions	Rheumatoid arthritis, connective tissue diseases
Feet	Keratoderma blenorrhagica	Reactive arthritis

From Hochberg MC, Silman AJ, Smolen JS, et al (eds): Rheumatology, 3rd ed. St Louis, Mosby, 2003.

- Look at the whole person and his or her posture and movement (Fig. 289–9).
- Examine region by region, comparing one side with the other.
- The key elements of the examination used to identify the clinical signs of musculoskeletal conditions (Table 289–4) are to look, feel, move, and stress (see Table 289–1). Figures 289–10 through 289–12 illustrate diagnostic maneuvers in the examination of a patient's knee. Figure 289–13 illustrates clinical tests for bicipital tendonitis.
- A homunculus (Fig. 289–14) can be used to annotate the examination findings.

TABLE 289–4 Clinical signs of musculoskeletal conditions	
• Attitude	• Movement restricted
• Deformity	• Crepitus
• Swelling	• Warmth
• Skin changes	• Muscle weakness
• Muscle wasting	• Instability
• Tenderness	• Function limited

From Hochberg MC, Silman AJ, Smolen JS, et al (eds): Rheumatology, 3rd ed. St Louis, Mosby, 2003.

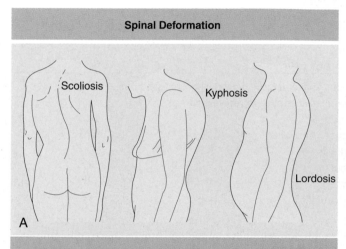

Spinal Deformation

Scoliosis   Kyphosis   Lordosis

A

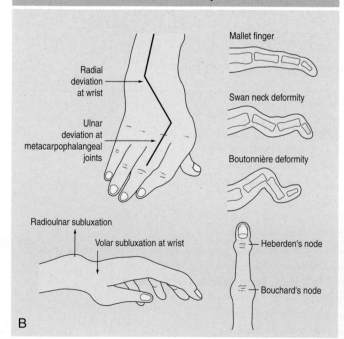

Hand Deformity

Radial deviation at wrist

Ulnar deviation at metacarpophalangeal joints

Radioulnar subluxation

Volar subluxation at wrist

Mallet finger

Swan neck deformity

Boutonnière deformity

Heberden's node

Bouchard's node

B

Fig 289–9
Common deformities of (**A**) the spine and (**B**) the hand. These should be observed during examination. Spinal deformities are best observed from behind and from the side, with the patient in the erect posture.
(From Hochberg MC, Silman AJ, Smolen JS, et al [eds]: Rheumatology, 3rd ed. St Louis, Mosby, 2003.)

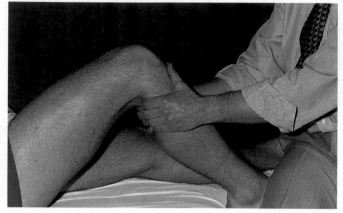

Fig 289–10
The anterior drawer test. The test is performed with the knee in 90° of flexion and should be repeated with the tibia in internal and external rotation.
(From Hochberg MC, Silman AJ, Smolen JS, et al [eds]: Rheumatology, 3rd ed. St Louis, Mosby, 2003.)

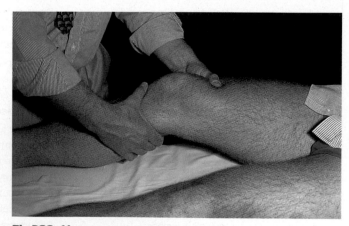

Fig 289–11
Lachman test for tears of the cruciate ligaments.
(From Hochberg MC, Silman AJ, Smolen JS, et al [eds]: Rheumatology, 3rd ed. St Louis, Mosby, 2003.)

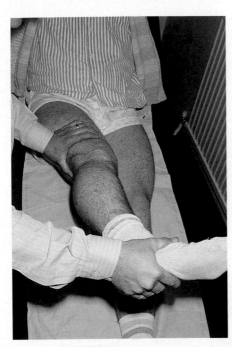

Fig 289–12

The pivot shift test. Anterolateral tibial subluxation is created by applying an internal rotation and valgus force to the tibia while holding the knee in full extension. As the knee is flexed the tibia will suddenly reduce, often accompanied by a click.
(From Hochberg MC, Silman AJ, Smolen JS, et al [eds]: Rheumatology, 3rd ed. St Louis, Mosby, 2003.)

Annotating the Examination Findings

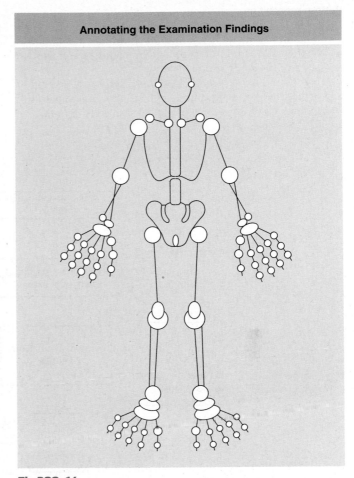

Fig 289–14

Annotating the examination findings. A homunculus can be used to annotate the abnormal findings made during examination.
(From Hochberg MC, Silman AJ, Smolen JS, et al [eds]: Rheumatology, 3rd ed. St Louis, Mosby, 2003.)

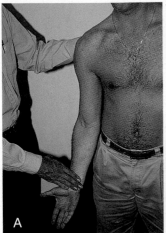
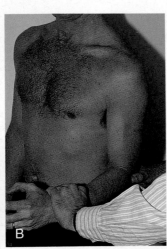
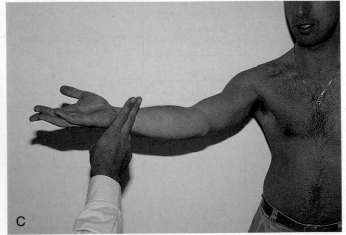

Fig 289–13

Clinical tests for bicipital tendinitis. (**A**) Speed's test. (**B**) Yergason's test. (**C**) Bicipital provocation test.
(From Hochberg MC, Silman AJ, Smolen JS, et al [eds]: Rheumatology, 3rd ed. St Louis, Mosby, 2003.)

Pattern recognition

Pattern recognition is the key to diagnosis of rheumatic disorders—the central questions to be asked are:

- Is there a locomotor problem or a disease of another system?
- Is the condition articular or periarticular?
- Is the condition mechanical (arthrosis) or inflammatory?
- Does it affect appendicular or axial structures or both?

These questions can be answered based on the history (mode of onset, sequence of development, duration of pattern of symptoms) and the physical examination (number, distribution, and pattern of the affected joints or periarticular structures and nature of any systemic involvement). Table 289–5 describes select causes of chronic monoarthritis. An initial approach to acute monoarticular arthritis is described in Figure 298–15. A classification of polyarthritis is described in Table 289–6. A differential diagnosis of a red-hot joint is provided in Table 289–7.

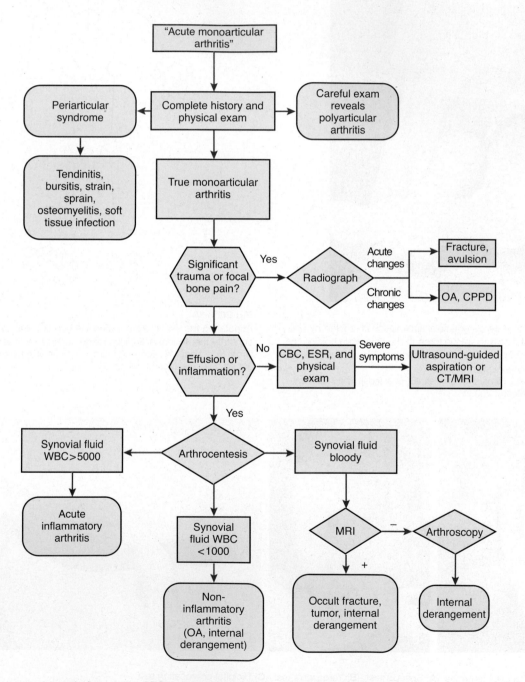

Fig 289–15

Initial approach to acute monoarticular arthritis. CBC, complete blood count; CPPD, calcium pyrophosphate deposition disease; CT, computed tomography; ESR, erythrocyte sedimentation rate; MRI, magnetic resonance imaging; OA, osteoarthritis; WBC, white blood cell count.
(From Harris ED, Budd RC, Genovese MC, Firestein GS, Sargent JS, Sledge CB, Ruddy S: Kelley's Textbook of Rheumatology, ed 7th, Saunders, 2005).

TABLE 289–5 Select causes of chronic monoarthritis

Infectious arthritis	Mycobacterial, fungal, bacterial, viral, Lyme disease
Inflammatory arthritis	Crystal-induced
	Monoarticular rheumatoid arthritis
	EOPA-JCA
	Seronegative spondyloarthopathies (ankylosing spondylitis, reactive arthritis, inflammatory bowel disease arthritis, undifferentiated)
	Psoriatic arthropathy
	Foreign body synovitis (e.g., plant thorn synovitis)
	Sarcoidosis
Noninflammatory arthritis	Osteoarthritis
	Internal derangement
	Osteonecrosis
	Synovial osteochondromatosis
	Reflex sympathetic dystrophy
	Hemarthrosis (e.g., coagulopathy, anticoagulants)
	Neuropathic (Charcot joint)
	Stress fracture
	Transient regional osteoporosis
	Juvenile osteochondroses
Tumors	Pigmented villonodular synovitis
	Lipoma arborescens
	Synovial metastasis from solid tumors
	Synovial sarcoma
Undiagnosed	

From Hochberg MC, Silman AJ, Smolen JS, et al (eds): Rheumatology, 3rd ed. St Louis, Mosby, 2003.

TABLE 289–6 Classification of polyarthritis

Inflammatory
Peripheral polyarticular
    Rheumatoid arthritis
    Systemic lupus erythematosus
    Viral arthritis
    Psoriatic arthritis (occasionally)
Peripheral pauciarticular
    Psoriatic arthritis
    Reiter's syndrome
    Rheumatic fever
    Polyarticular gout
    Enteropathic arthritis
    Behçet's disease
    Bacterial endocarditis
Peripheral with axial involvement
Ankylosing spondylitis (especially juvenile onset)
Reiter's syndrome
Enteropathic arthritis
Psoriatic arthritis
Noninflammatory (osteoarthritis)
Hereditary
    Osteoarthritis of the hands
    Primary generalized osteoarthritis
Traumatic osteoarthritis
    Osteoarthritis following local injury
    Osteoarthritis of the knees in obese people
    Chondromalacia following aggressive exercise programs
    Osteoarthritis in the elderly
Metabolic diseases (may have an unusual pattern)
    Hemochromatosis
    Ochronosis
    Acromegaly
Idiopathic

From Harris ED, Budd RC, Genovese MC, et al: Kelley's Textbook of Rheumatology, 7th ed. Philadelphia, WB Saunders, 2005

TABLE 289–7 The red-hot joint

Infectious	Bacterial	Traumatic
	Neisserial (may be preceded by transient polyarticular disease)	Palindromic rheumatism
	Mycobacterial	Psoriatic arthropathy
	Virus	Reactive arthritis
	Lyme disease	Bacterial endocarditis
Crystal-induced	Gout	
	Calcium pyrophosphate dehydrate (pseudogout type)	
	Hydroxyapatite (acute calcific periarthritis)	

From Hochberg MC, Silman AJ, Smolen JS, et al (eds): Rheumatology, 3rd ed. St Louis, Mosby, 2003.

Imaging studies

a. Conventional radiography is the most commonly used imaging test for evaluating patients with arthritic disorders. Bilateral comparison of joints can help detect subtle alterations in the contours of the articulating bones, subtle joint space narrowing, subluxations, and dislocations and also changes in bone mineral density (Figs. 289–16 and 289–17).

b. Computed tomography (CT), nuclear scintigraphy (bone scan), and magnetic resonance imaging (MRI) (Fig. 289–18) represent useful but much more expensive imaging modalities. These tests are used in diagnosing disorders such as osteomyelitis (Fig. 289–19) and stress fractures (Fig. 289–20) that may not be readily apparent on conventional radiography. Newer techniques involve quantitative analysis of MRI scans to evaluate cartilage loss and monitor response to medical or surgical therapy (Fig. 289–21).

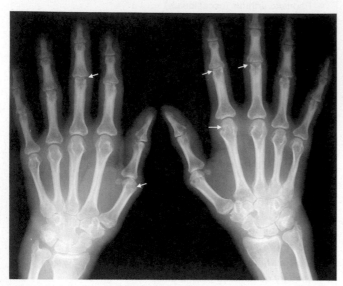

Fig 289–16
Rheumatoid arthritis. Bilateral hand radiographs demonstrate multiple erosions involving predominantly the PIP and MCP joints. Assessment of bilateral involvement and symmetry is helpful in narrowing the differential diagnosis.
(From Hochberg MC, Silman AJ, Smolen JS, et al [eds]: Rheumatology, 3rd ed. St Louis, Mosby, 2003.)

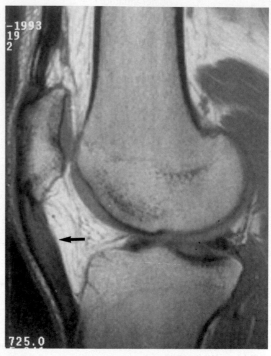

Fig 289–18
MRI appearance of tendinitis. Sagittal T1-weighted image of the knee in a professional basketball player demonstrates abnormal signal and increased size in the patellar tendon, consistent with severe tendinitis (*arrow*). The tendon is normally devoid of signal.
(From Grainger RG, Allison DJ, Adam A, Dixon AK [eds]: Grainger and Allison's Diagnostic Radiology, 4th ed. Philadelphia, Churchill Livingstone, 2001.)

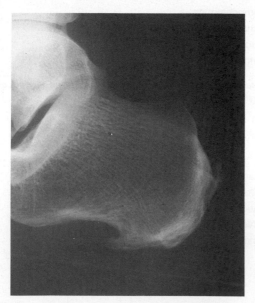

Fig 289–17
Plantar calcaneal spur.
(From Hochberg MC, Silman AJ, Smolen JS, et al [eds]: Rheumatology, 3rd ed. St Louis, Mosby, 2003.)

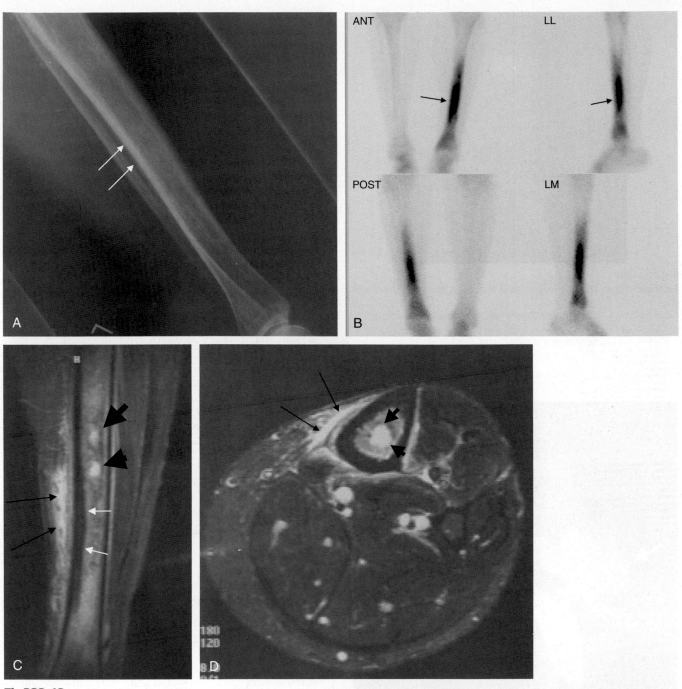

Fig 289–19
Nuclear scintigraphy/bone scan of a patient with clinically suspected osteomyelitis. (**A**) Conventional radiography demonstrates a subtle area of periosteal reaction along the posterior cortex of the tibia (*arrows*). There is also some ill-defined sclerosis in the marrow space. (**B**) Bone scan demonstrates markedly increased radionuclide uptake in the midtibia (*arrow*). (**C, D**). MRI (T2-weighted fat-saturated fast spin-echo) demonstrates soft-tissue edema (*thin black arrows*), periosteal and endosteal thickening (*thin white arrows*) and rounded focal areas of very high signal intensity in the marrow space suggesting liquefaction and Brodie's abscess *(thick black arrows)*.
(From Hochberg MC, Silman AJ, Smolen JS, et al [eds]: Rheumatology, 3rd ed. St Louis, Mosby, 2003.)

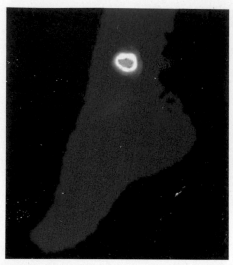

Fig 289–20
Technetium scan showing focal uptake of a stress fracture of the lower tibia.
(From Hochberg MC, Silman AJ, Smolen JS, et al [eds]: Rheumatology, 3rd ed. St Louis, Mosby, 2003.)

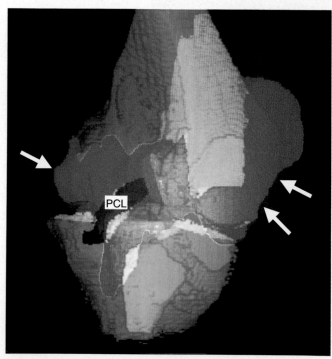

Fig 289–21
Three-dimensional reconstruction of synovial fluid (yellow), femur and tibia (gray) and cruciate ligaments (green, PCL).
(From Hochberg MC, Silman AJ, Smolen JS, et al [eds]: Rheumatology, 3rd ed. St Louis, Mosby, 2003.)

Laboratory tests

a. **Rheumatoid factors (RFs):** autoantibodies directed to the Fc portion of the IgG. A positive RF can be found in rheumatoid arthritis, systemic lupus erythematosus (SLE), and numerous disorders, including sarcoidosis, liver disease, and pulmonary interstitial fibrosis infections, and in normal elderly patients. The sensitivity and specificity of RF are described in Table 289–8. RFs have a physiologic role by enhancing the avidity (and size) of immune complexes, thereby improving immune complex clearance. Some roles for RF in joint pathology are illustrated in Figure 289–22.

b. **Antinuclear antibodies (ANAs):** autoantibodies that can be regarded as probes matching and reflecting basic inflammatory events taking place in affected tissues. The term "ANA" can be used in a very broad sense to indicate all autoantibodies that can potentially be detected by indirect immunofluorescence microscopy on HRp-2 cells, although some of them arguably target cytoplasmic structures. Some ANAs are included as criteria for diagnosis of disease, such as SLE and mixed connective tissue disease (MCTD). Detection of ANAs can strongly support the diagnosis of many other diseases, such as systemic sclerosis, autoimmune Raynaud's syndrome, and primary Sjögren's syndrome (SS). A prominently expressed ANA, as indicated by strong fluorescent staining or a high titer, can antedate the establishment of a clinical diagnosis by many years. ANA patterns related to diagnosis and some common autoantigens targets are described in Table 289–9 and Figures 289–23 and 289–24. An algorithm for use of ANA in the diagnosis of connective tissue disorders is described in Figure 289–25.

TABLE 289–8 Sensitivity and specificity of rheumatoid factor

Diagnosis	≥15 U/mL	≥50 U/mL	≥100 U/mL
Rheumatoid arthritis (RA)	66*	46	26
Sjögren's syndrome	62	52	33
Systemic lupus erythematosus	27	10	3
Mixed connective tissue disease	23	13	6
Scleroderma	44	18	2
Polymyositis	18	0	0
Reactive arthritis	0	0	0
Osteoarthritis	25	4	4
Healthy controls	13	0	0
Sensitivity (%)	66	46	26
Specificity (%)	74	88 (92†)	95 (98†)

*Percentage of positive patients.
†Specificity when a diagnosis of Sjögren's syndrome can be excluded. Rheumatoid factors were determined by nephelometry in 100 patients with RA, in more than 200 patients with other rheumatic diseases, and in 30 healthy control persons.
From Hochberg MC, Silman AJ, Smolen JS, et al (eds): Rheumatology, 3rd ed. St Louis, Mosby, 2003.

TABLE 289–9 Antinuclear antibody patterns related to diagnosis and some common autoantigen targets

Diagnosis	Homogeneous or Fine Grainy Nuclear	Speckled Nuclear	Centromere Kinetochores	Nucleolar Patterns	Cytoplasmic Patterns	Negative
Systemic lupus erythematosus	dsDNA(h) Nucleosomes (h) Ku (g)	Sm/U1RNP (cs) SSA(Ro)/SSB(La) (fs) hnRNPs (l)	Rare	Nucleolin (h) ASE-1 (h)	P-proteins (d) SS-56 (d)	SSA(Ro)
Systemic sclerosis/ Raynaud's syndrome	Topoisomerase I (g) RNA polymerase II, III Ku(g)	U1RNP(cs) U2RNP (cs)	CENP-A, B, C	PM/Scl (h) Th/To (h) Fibrillarin (cl) RNA polymerase 1 (p) NOR-90 (p)	Rare	SSA(Ro
Poly/ dermatomyositis	Ku(g)	Mi-2 (fs) SSA(Ro)-52 (fs) U1RNP(cs)	Rare	PM/Scl (h)	SRP (d) Jo-1 (fs)	Jo-1
Sjögren's syndrome	Rare	SSA(Ro) (fs) SSB(La) (fs) SL	CENP-A, B, C	Nucleolin (h)	SS-56 (d)	SSA(Ro)
Mixed connective tissue disease	Rare	U1RNP (cs) hnRNPs (l) SSA(Ro) (fs)	Rare	Rare	Rare	Rare
APS	*	*	Rare	B23	Rare	Anti-cardiolipin Lupus anti-coagulant

*Depends on primary disease, mostly systemic lupus erythematosus.
cl, clumpy; cs, coarse; d, diffuse; fs, fine speckled; g, grainy; h, homogeneous; l, large; p, punctate
From Hochberg MC, Silman AJ, Smolen JS, et al (eds): Rheumatology, 3rd ed. St Louis, Mosby, 2003.

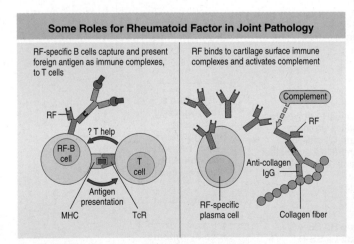

Fig 289–22
Some roles for rheumatoid factor in joint pathology. RF, MHC, TcR (From Hochberg MC, Silman AJ, Smolen JS, et al [eds]: Rheumatology, 3rd ed. St Louis, Mosby, 2003.)

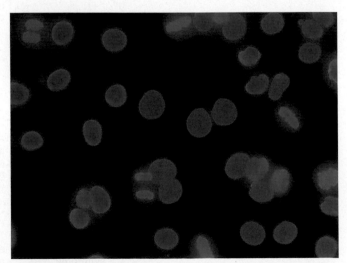

Fig 289–23
Homogeneous nucleoplasmic staining pattern. Note positive staining of chromosomes during mitosis. May appear with peripheral nuclear accentuation.
(From Hochberg MC, Silman AJ, Smolen JS, et al [eds]: Rheumatology, 3rd ed. St Louis, Mosby, 2003.)

Fig 289–24

Large speckled nucleoplasmic staining pattern. Note negative chromosomes in dividing cells.

(From Hochberg MC, Silman AJ, Smolen JS, et al [eds]: Rheumatology, 3rd ed. St Louis, Mosby, 2003.)

c. **Antineutrophil cytoplasmic antibodies (ANCAs):** two different immunofluorescence patterns can be seen.
  • **Cytoplasmic ANCAs (cANCA)** stain the cytoplasm diffusely (Fig. 289–26) and are found primarily in patients with Wegener's granulomatosis.
  • **Perinuclear ANCAS (pANCA)** are directed against myeloperoxidase (MPO) (Fig. 289–27) and can be found in several disorders (Goodpasture's syndrome, Churg-Strauss syndrome, idiopathic necrotizing glomerulonephritis, and microscopic polyarteritis).

d. **Erythrocyte sedimentation rate (ESR):** nonspecific marker of inflammation. May be elevated in infectious, inflammatory, or neoplastic disease. It is most useful for diagnosis and follow-up of giant cell arteritis.

e. **C-reactive protein:** nonspecific marker of inflammation. It changes faster than ESR and may be useful for diagnosis SLE flare-ups and as an indicator of adequate steroid dosage in giant cell arteritis.

f. **Urinalysis and serum creatinine:** useful to monitor renal involvement in rheumatic disease (e.g., SLE glomerulonephritis) and potential toxicity from medications

g. **Uric acid:** useful for diagnosing gout

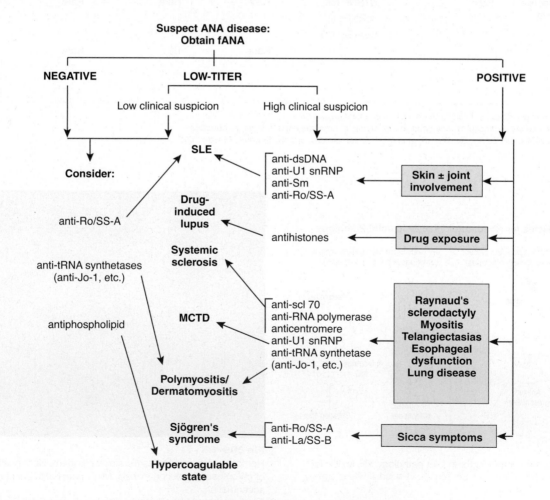

Fig 289–25

Algorithm for the use of antinuclear antibodies (ANAs) in the diagnosis of connective tissue disorders.

(From Harris ED et al (eds): Kelley's Textbook of Rheumatology, 7th ed, Philadelphia, WB Saunders, 2005.)

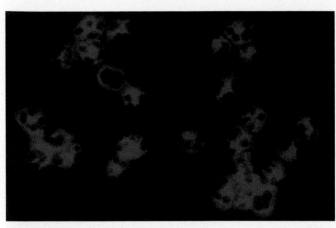

Fig 289–26
cANCA pattern. Demonstration of cytoplasmic antineutrophil cytoplasmic antibodies (cANCAs) by indirect immunofluorescence with normal neutrophils. There is heavy staining in the cytoplasm while the multilobular nuclei (clear zones) are nonreactive. These antibodies are usually directed against proteinase 3 and most patients have Wegener's granulomatosis.
(Courtesy of Dr. Helmut Rennke.).

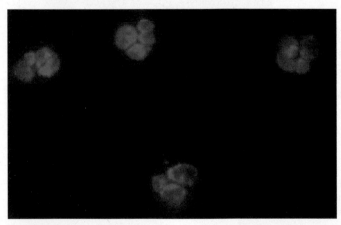

Fig 289–27
pANCA pattern. Demonstration of perinuclear antineutrophil cytoplasmic antibodies (pANCAs) by indirect immunofluorescence with normal neutrophils. Staining is limited to the perinuclear region and the cytoplasm is nonreactive. Among patients with vasculitis, the antibodies are usually directed against myeloperoxidase. However, a pANCA pattern can also be seen with elastase. Non-MPO pANCA can be seen in a variety of nonvasculitic disorders.
(Courtesy of Dr. Helmut Rennke.)

h. **Complete blood cell count (CBC):** a baseline CBC should be obtained in all patients suspected of rheumatic disease and monitored periodically
i. **Others:** ALT, AST, alkaline phosphatase, creatine phosphokinase (CPK), aldolase

Aspiration and injection of joints and synovial fluid analysis
a. Normal synovial fluid is a hypocellular, avascular connective tissue.
b. In disease, the synovial fluid increases in volume and can be aspirated.
c. Changes in synovial fluid composition reflect the pathogenesis of the arthropathy. Synovial fluid analysis is essential for diagnosis in septic arthritis (Fig. 289–28) and crystal-induced synovitides. Table 289–10 describes synovial fluid findings.
d. Elements that change can be either visualized with the light microscope (Fig. 289–29) or measured biochemically.
e. Table 289–11 describes indications for aspirating or injecting joints. Figure 289–30 illustrates the injection of the metacarpophalangeal (MCP) joint.

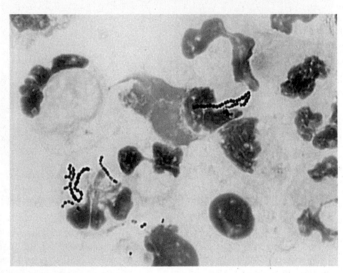

Fig 289–28
Gram-positive cocci (streptococci in this example) within a synovial fluid example. Gram's stain.
(From Hochberg MC, Silman AJ, Smolen JS, et al [eds]: Rheumatology, 3rd ed. St Louis, Mosby, 2003.)

TABLE 289–10 Synovial fluid findings

	Normal	Osteoarthritis	Rheumatoid and Other Inflammatory Arthritis	Septic Arthritis
Gross appearance	Clear	Clear	Opaque	Opaque
Volume (mL)	0–1	1–10	5–50	5–50
Viscosity	High	High	Low	Low
Total white cell count/mm³	<200	200–10,000	500–75,000	>50,000
% Polymorphonuclear cells	<25	<50	>50	>75
Knee joint synovial fluid findings in common forms of arthritis.				

From Hochberg MC, Silman AJ, Smolen JS, et al (eds): Rheumatology, 3rd ed. St Louis, Mosby, 2003.

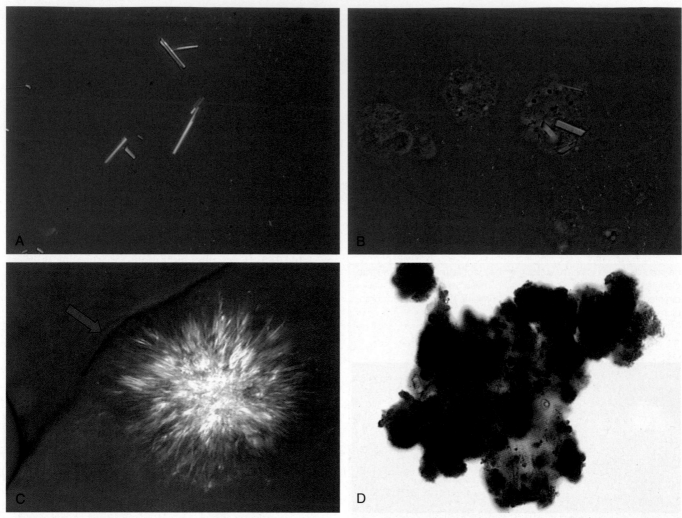

Fig 289–29

A montage of common crystals. (**A**) 'Urate' crystals viewed in polarized light with an interposed quarter-wave plate. (**B**) Pyrophosphate crystals viewed in the same system. Note that the crystals appear duller and that the apparent color of the crystals is the opposite of the urate crystals when related to the long axis of the crystal. (**C**) A lipid droplet (edge arrowed) containing a 'beach ball' of needle-like crystals. (**D**) Hydroxyapatite crystals stained with alizarin red.
(From Hochberg MC, Silman AJ, Smolen JS, et al [eds]: Rheumatology, 3rd ed. St Louis, Mosby, 2003.)

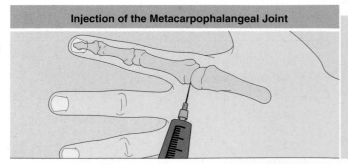

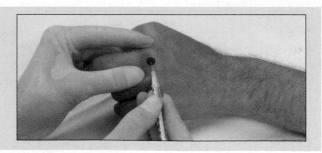

Fig 289–30

Injection of the metacarpophalangeal joint.
(From Hochberg MC, Silman AJ, Smolen JS, et al [eds]: Rheumatology, 3rd ed. St Louis, Mosby, 2003.)

TABLE 289-11 Indications for aspirating or injecting joints

Diagnosis	Mandatory if septic arthritis suspected
	Strongly advised if crystal arthritis or hemarthrosis suspected
	Differentiation of inflammatory from non-inflammatory arthritis
	Imaging studies—arthroscopy and arthrography
	Synovial biopsy
Therapy	To remove tense effusions to relieve pain and improve function
	To remove blood or pus from a joint
	For injection of corticosteroids and other intra-articular therapies
	For tidal lavage of joints

From Hochberg MC, Silman AJ, Smolen JS, et al (eds): Rheumatology, 3rd ed. St Louis, Mosby, 2003.

Percutaneous Muscle Biopsy

Trocar — Subcutaneous fat and fascia — Skin

Quadriceps muscle

Muscle specimen

Cutting trocar moves in

→ Movement of trocar   ← Direction of suction

Minimally invasive procedures

a. Muscle biopsy (Fig. 289–31): useful for suspected inflammatory myopathy
b. Salivary gland biopsy (Fig. 289–32): useful for diagnosing SS, amyloidosis, sarcoidosis
c. Arthroscopy (Fig. 289–33): commonly used for repair of torn meniscus and for decompression of shoulder impingement, it has many other applications, such as obtaining histologic specimens for diagnosis of pigmented villonodular synovitis, fungal arthritis, and tuberculous (TB) arthritis.

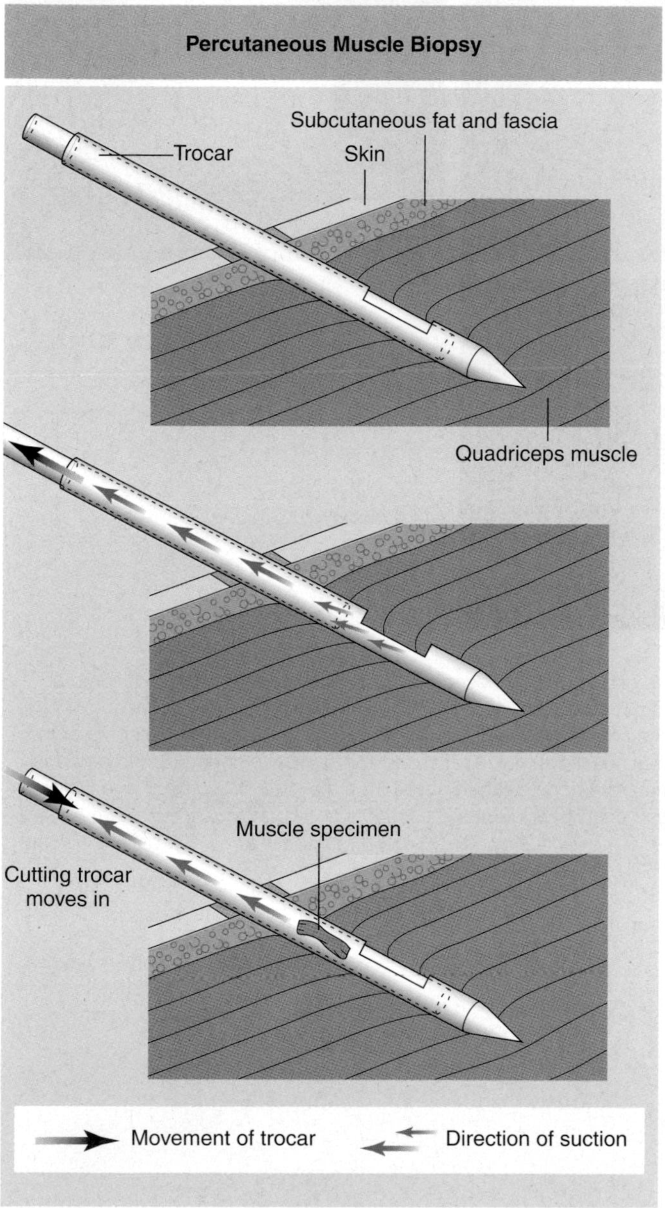

Labial Salivary Gland Biopsy

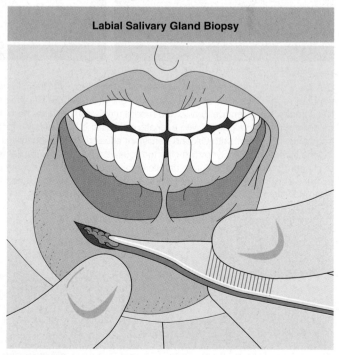

Fig 289–31
Percutaneous muscle biopsy using suction-assisted instrument.
(From Hochberg MC, Silman AJ, Smolen JS, et al [eds]: Rheumatology, 3rd ed. St Louis, Mosby, 2003.)

Fig 289–32
Labial salivary gland biopsy.
(From Hochberg MC, Silman AJ, Smolen JS, et al [eds]: Rheumatology, 3rd ed. St Louis, Mosby, 2003.)

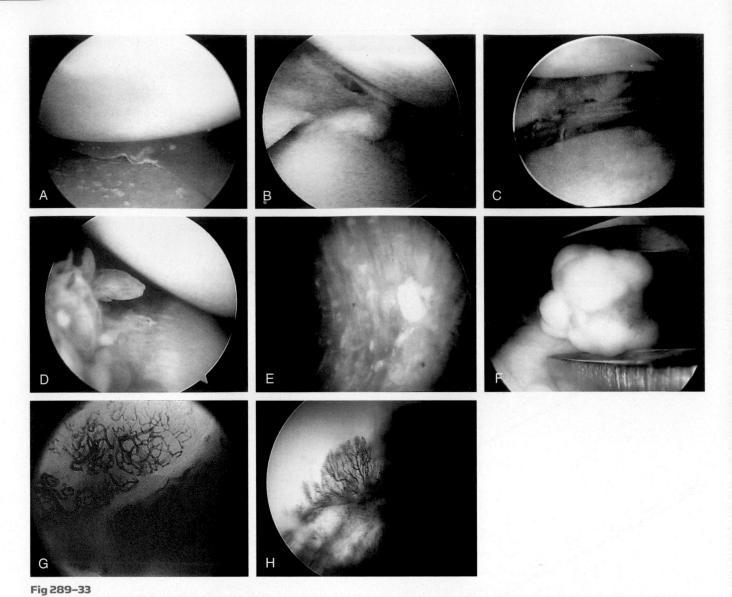

Fig 289–33
Examples of intra-articular pathology seen at arthroscopy. (**A**) Refractile white deposits of monosodium urate on the otherwise normal femoral condyle, meniscus and tibial plateau in a patient with gout. (**B**) Flap tear of the medial meniscus with ulceration of adjacent tibial plateau cartilage. (**C**) Complex (degenerative) tear of the medial meniscus, posterior horn, in a a patient with OA. (**D**) Villous synovitis overlying the outer rim of the medial meniscus in a patient with psoriatic arthritis and knee effusion following minor trauma. (**E**) Hyperemic synovium embedded with cartilage fragments in a patient with OA and persistent effusion. (**F**) Osteocartilaginous loose body being removed from the knee of a patient with OA and locking symptoms. (**G**) Synovium with tortuous vascular pattern (similar to that described for psoriatic arthritis and spondyloarthropathy by Reece et al.) from knee of a patient with undifferentiated arthritis. (**H**) Synovium at edge of pannus invading femoral condyle in knee of a patient with apparent seronegative RA; linear vascular pattern similar to that described for RA by Reece et al.
(From Hochberg MC, Silman AJ, Smolen JS, et al [eds]: Rheumatology, 3rd ed. St Louis, Mosby, 2003.)

Chapter 290 | Osteoarthritis

DEFINITION

Osteoarthritis is a joint condition in which degeneration and loss of articular cartilage occur, leading to pain and deformity. Two forms are usually recognized: primary (idiopathic) and secondary. The primary form may be localized or generalized.

PHYSICAL FINDINGS AND CLINICAL PRESENTATION

- Similar symptoms in most forms: stiffness, pain, and crepitus
- Joint tenderness, swelling
- Decreased range of motion, joint contractures (Fig. 290–1)
- Crepitus with motion
- Bony hypertrophy
- Pain with range of motion
- Distal interphalangeal (DIP) joint involvement possibly leading to development of nodular swellings called Heberden's nodes (Fig. 290–2)
- Proximal interphalangeal (PIP) joint involvement possibly leading to development of nodular swellings called Bouchard's nodes (Fig. 290–2)
- Figures 290–3 and 290–4 illustrate common abnormalities of the hands and feet.

CAUSE

Primary osteoarthritis is of unknown cause. Secondary osteoarthritis may result from a number of disorders including trauma, metabolic conditions, and other forms of arthritis.

DIFFERENTIAL DIAGNOSIS

- Bursitis, tendinitis
- Radicular spine pain
- Inflammatory arthritides
- Infectious arthritis

IMAGING STUDIES

- When the knee is involved with pain, x-rays should always be taken with the patient standing
- X-ray evaluation reveals:
  - Joint space narrowing
  - Subchondral sclerosis
  - New bone formation in the form of osteophytes

TREATMENT

- Rest, restricted use or weight bearing, and moist heat
- Walking aids such as a cane (often helpful for weight-bearing joints)
- Suitable footwear
- Gentle range of motion and strengthening exercise
- Local creams and liniments to provide a counterirritant effect
- Education, reassurance
- Mild analgesics for joint pain
- NSAIDs if inflammation is present
- Occasional local corticosteroid injections
- Viscosupplementation (injection of hyaluronic acid products into the degenerative joint) is of uncertain benefit.
- Nutritional supplements (glucosamine and chondroitin) are unproved.

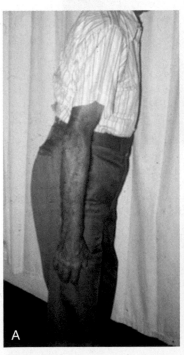
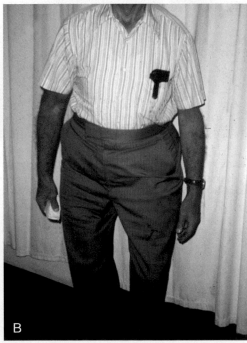

Fig 290–1
Osteoarthritis of the hips. Severe osteoarthritis secondary to pelvic Paget's disease causes medial migration of the femoral heads into the acetabuli, resulting in hip flexion contractures. The patient stands with a bent forward posture apparent from a lateral (**A**) or anterior (**B**) view. (From Hochberg MC, Silman AJ, Smolen JS, et al [eds]: Rheumatology, 3rd ed. St Louis, Mosby, 2003.)

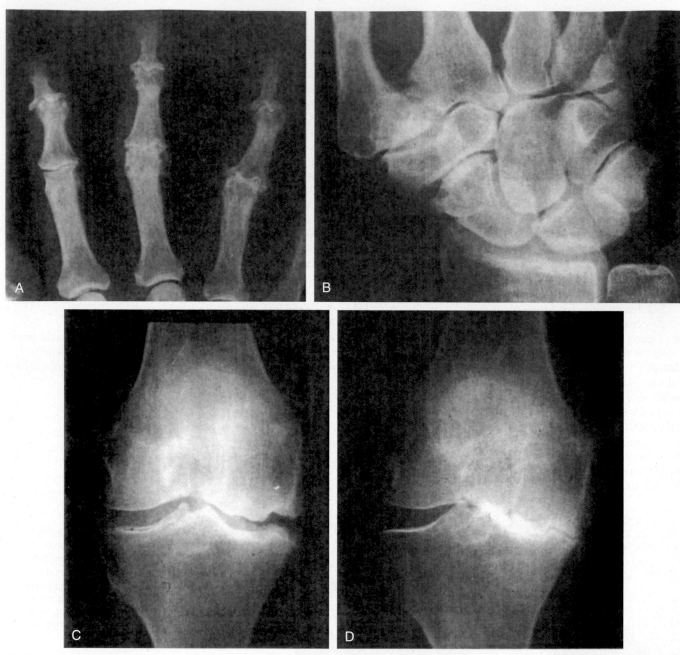

Fig 290-2
Osteoarthritis (degenerative joint disease). (**A**) Primary osteoarthritis of the fingers with characteristic cartilage loss, deviations, and spurs of the proximal (Bouchard's nodes) and distal (Heberden's nodes) interphalangeal joints. (**B**) Primary osteoarthritis of the carpus showing characteristic involvement of the radial side with cartilage loss, subchondral sclerosis, and small spur formation from the base of the first metacarpal to the distal articular surface of the scaphoid. (**C**) Supine film of osteoarthritis of the medial compartment of the femorotibial joint and (**D**) the standing view, more effectively demonstrating the joint space narrowing and varus deformity.
(From Grainger RG, Allison DJ, Adam A, Dixon AK [eds]: Grainger and Allison's Diagnostic Radiology, 4th ed. Philadelphia, Churchill Livingstone, 2001.)

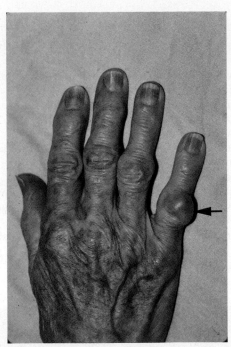

Fig 290-3
Interphalangeal osteoarthritis of the hand, with cystic herniation of the fifth proximal interphalangeal joint.
(From Hochberg MC, Silman AJ, Smolen JS, et al [eds]: Rheumatology, 3rd ed. St Louis, Mosby, 2003.)

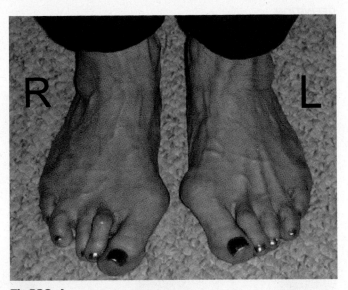

Fig 290-4
MTP and interphalangeal osteoarthritis of the feet. There is bilateral en-largement of the first MTP joint, with medial subluxation of the phalanx. Flexion contraction of toes (particularly of the right second digit) with subluxation of the MTP, has an associated callus over the dorsum of the PIP joint. The right third digit is subluxed under the second digit. There is relaxation of the transtarsal ligament, with medial subluxation of the MTP and bony enlargement of the fifth MTP joints (tailor bunion, bunionette).
(From Hochberg MC, Silman AJ, Smolen JS, et al [eds]: Rheumatology, 3rd ed. St Louis, Mosby, 2003.)

Chapter 291 Rheumatoid arthritis

DEFINITION
Rheumatoid arthritis (RA) is a systemic disorder characterized by chronic joint inflammation that most commonly affects peripheral joints. This process results in the development of pannus, a destructive tissue that damages cartilage.

PHYSICAL FINDINGS AND CLINICAL PRESENTATION
- Usually gradual onset; common prodromal symptoms of weakness, fatigue, and anorexia
- Initial presentation: multiple symmetrical joint involvement, most often in the hands and feet (Fig. 291–1), usually MCP, metatarsophalangeal (MTP), and PIP joints (Fig. 291–2)

- Joint effusions, tenderness, and restricted motion usually present early in the disease
- Eventual characteristic deformities: subluxations, dislocations, and joint contractures (Fig. 291–3)
- Extra-articular findings:
  - Tendon sheaths and bursae frequently affected by chronic inflammation

Possible tendon rupture
  - Rheumatoid nodules (Fig. 291–4) over bony prominences such as the elbow (Fig. 291–5) and shaft of the ulna
  - Splenomegaly, scleritis (Fig. 291–6), peripheral nodules in the lung fields (*Caplan's syndrome*) (Fig. 291–7), pericarditis (Fig. 291–8), and vasculitis (Fig. 291–9)

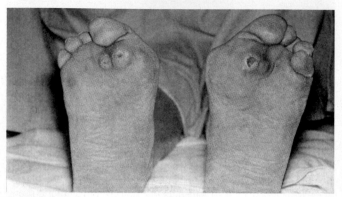

Fig 291–1
Rheumatoid forefoot. Plantar view of the feet in a patient with RA. Hallux valgus, MTP subluxation and bursal swelling under weight-bearing areas are seen. Subluxation of the metatarsal head is associated with clawing of the toes, cock-up digital deformities and over-riding of the toes. The ulcerated burase under the left metatarsal head may become associated with a chronic synovial fistula and secondary infection.
(From Hochberg MC, Silman AJ, Smolen JS, et al [eds]: Rheumatology, 3rd ed. St Louis, Mosby, 2003.)

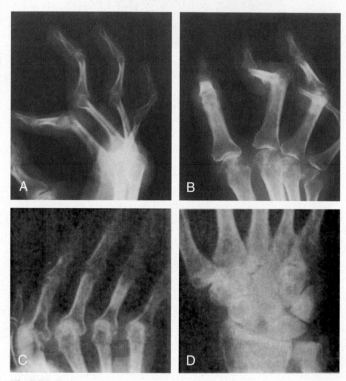

Fig 291–3
Malalignments of the hand and wrist found in rheumatoid arthritis.
(**A**) Swan neck deformities characterized by extension at the proximal interphalangeal joints and flexion at the distal interphalangeal joints are caused by tendon sheath synovitis. Note that there is no bone destruction (**B**) Boutonniére deformities characterized by flexion at the proximal interphalangeal joints and extension at the distal interphalangeal joints and extension at the distal interphalangeal joints are caused by soft-tissue laxity that results in the extensor mechanism of the proximal interphalangeal joint having a flexor function. (**C**) Ulnar deviation of the fingers at the metacarpophalangeal joints is caused by capsular, ligamentous, and muscular laxity. (**D**) Scapholunate ligament rupture results in widening of the scapholunate joint and volar rotation of the scaphoid. The entire carpus drifts in an ulnar direction.
(From Grainger RG, Allison DJ, Adam A, Dixon AK [eds]: Grainger and Allison's Diagnostic Radiology, 4th ed. Philadelphia, Churchill Livingstone, 2001.)

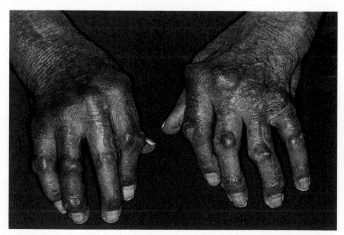

Fig 291–2
Rheumatoid nodules in a patient with long-standing RA treated with low-dose weekly methotrexate
(From Hochberg MC, Silman AJ, Smolen JS, et al [eds]: Rheumatology, 3rd ed. St Louis, Mosby, 2003.)

- Findings of carpal tunnel syndrome resulting from flexor tenosynovitis
- Table 291–1 describes clinical features of RA.

CAUSE

Unknown. There is increasing evidence that the inflammation and destruction of bone and cartilage that occur in many rheumatic diseases are the result of the activation by some unknown mechanism of proinflammatory cells that infiltrate the synovium. These cells, in turn, release various substances, such as cytokines and tumor necrosis factor (TNF) α, which subsequently cause the pathologic changes typical of this group of diseases. Many of the newer therapeutic agents are directed at the suppression of these final mediators of inflammation.

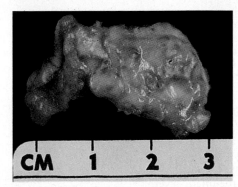

Fig 291–4
Gross anatomic specimen of a rheumatoid nodule. The yellow tissue is caused by fibrinoid necrosis.
(From Hochberg MC, Silman AJ, Smolen JS, et al [eds]: Rheumatology, 3rd ed. St Louis, Mosby, 2003.)

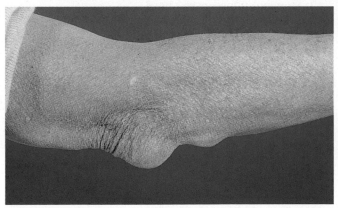

Fig 291–5
A case of olecranon bursitis in later rheumatoid arthritis; a rheumatoid nodule is also shown.
(From Hochberg MC, Silman AJ, Smolen JS, et al [eds]: Rheumatology, 3rd ed. St Louis, Mosby, 2003.)

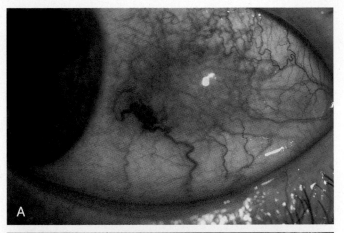

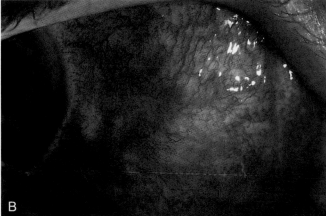

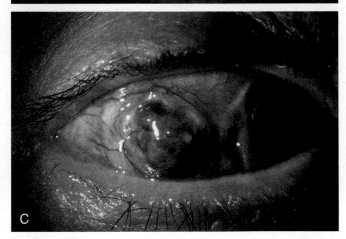

Fig 291–6
Scleritis in RA. (**A**) Nodular episcleritis. (**B**) Anterior scleritis. (**C**) Necrotizing scleritis may expose the underlying uvea. Here it is associated with marginal corneal melting.
(From Hochberg MC, Silman AJ, Smolen JS, et al [eds]: Rheumatology, 3rd ed. St Louis, Mosby, 2003.)

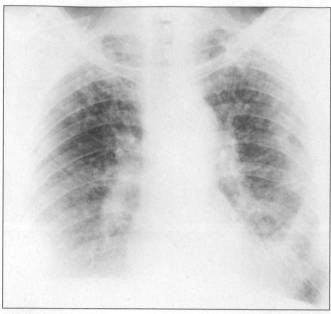

Fig 291–7
Caplan's syndrome.
(From Hochberg MC, Silman AJ, Smolen JS, et al [eds]: Rheumatology, 3rd ed. St Louis, Mosby, 2003.)

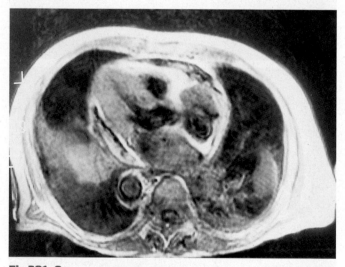

Fig 291–8
MRI of constrictive pericarditis in RA. The dense white infiltrate between the pericardium and gray myocardium is pericardial fluid.
(From Hochberg MC, Silman AJ, Smolen JS, et al [eds]: Rheumatology, 3rd ed. St Louis, Mosby, 2003.)

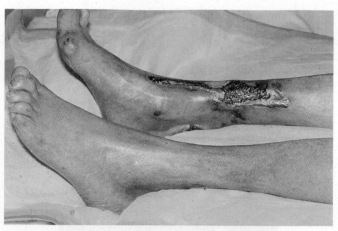

Fig 291–9
Severe ulcers of the lower leg due to necrotizing vasculitis in RA.
(From Hochberg MC, Silman AJ, Smolen JS, et al [eds]: Rheumatology, 3rd ed. St Louis, Mosby, 2003.)

DIFFERENTIAL DIAGNOSIS

- SLE
- Seronegative spondyloarthropathies
- Polymyalgia rheumatica
- Acute rheumatic fever
- Scleroderma

DIAGNOSIS

According to the American College of Rheumatology, RA exists when four of seven criteria are present, with criteria 1 to 4 being present for at least 6 weeks.

1. Morning stiffness over 1 hour
2. Arthritis in three or more joints with swelling
3. Arthritis of hand joints with swelling
4. Symmetrical arthritis
5. Rheumatoid nodules
6. X-ray changes typical of RA
7. Positive serum RF

LABORATORY TESTS

- Increase in RF in 80% of cases (RF also present in the normal population)
- Possible mild anemia
- Usually, elevated acute phase reactants (ESR, C-reactive protein)
- Possible mild leukocytosis
- Usually, turbid joint fluid, which forms a poor mucin clot; elevated cell count, with an increase in polymorphonuclear leukocytes

TABLE 291–1 Clinical features due to manifestations of rheumatoid arthritis (RA), its complications or treatment, or concurrent disease

| Feature | Cause | | | |
	Manifestation of RA	Complication of RA	Side effect of therapy	Concurrent disease
Neuropathy	Vasculitis	Local pressure Entrapment neuropathy Amyloid neuropathy	Chloroquine D-Penicillamine Gold	Diabetes mellitus complication of surgical procedures (hip/knee replacement)
Tendon rupture	Tenosynovitis	Irregular bone edge	Local corticosteroids	Trauma
Ulcers	Vasculitis	Pressure ulcers Perforated nodules Decubitus		Diabetes mellitus Corns, bunions Pyoderma gangrenosa
Anemia/leukopenia	Felty's syndrome	Gastric ulcers Vitamin deficiencies	NSAIDs DMARDs	Multiple myeloma Malignancy
Severe backache	Discitis	Osteoporosis	Corticosteroids	Menopause, aging
Pulmonary insufficiency	Pleuritis Pneumonitis	Cricoarytenoiditis	Methotrexate Gold D-Penicillamine	Congestive heart failure Sarcoidosis Malignancy Uremia/infection
Cardiac insufficiency	Pericarditis Carditis Valve disease Nodules	Conduction abnormalities	NSAIDs	Arteriosclerosis Viral disease Congenital abnormalities
Renal dysfunction	Vasculitis Proliferative glomerulonephritis	Amyloid	NSAIDs DMARDs	Nephrosclerosis Diabetes mellitus Intrinsic renal disease
Gastrointestinal symptoms	Vasculitis	Amyloid	NSAIDs DMARDs	Intestinal disease
Liver and spleen abnormalities	Feltys syndrome Sjögren's syndrome	Amyloid deposition	NSAIDs Azathioprine Methotrexate Other DMARDs	Malignancy Viral infection and other causes
Headache	C1-2 subluxation	Normal pressure hydrocephalus	NSAIDs	Arteriosclerosis Tumors
Eye involvement	Scleromalacia Scleritis (nodules, vasculitis)	Keratoconjunctivitis sicca	Chloroquine Corticosteroids	Eye diseases

From Hochberg MC, Silman AJ, Smolen JS, et al (eds): Rheumatology, 3rd ed. St Louis, Mosby, 2003.

IMAGING STUDIES

Plain radiography

- Usually reveals soft-tissue swelling and osteoporosis early
- Eventually, joint space narrowing, erosion, and deformity visible as a result of continued inflammation and cartilage destruction (Fig. 291–10)

TREATMENT

Proper management requires close cooperation among the primary physician, therapist, rheumatologist, and orthopedist.

- NSAIDs: commonly used as the initial treatment to relieve inflammation (drug of choice for most patients: aspirin, but other NSAIDs also effective)

- Disease-modifying drugs (DMARDs): current recommendations favor early aggressive treatment with DMARDs, seeking to minimize long-term joint damage. Commonly used agents are methotrexate, cyclosporine, hydroxychloroquine, sulfasalazine, leflunomide, and infliximab.
- Oral prednisone
- Intrasynovial steroid injections
- Etanercept, a TNF-α blocker, is indicated in moderately to severely active RA in patients who respond inadequately to DMARDs. The combination of etanercept and methotrexate has been reported to be effective and promising in the treatment of RA.
- Wrist and hand splints (Fig. 291–11) to prevent joint deformities

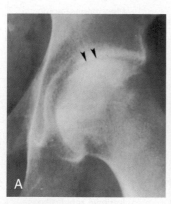 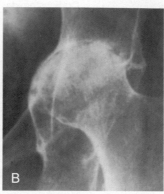

Fig 291–10

Hip involvement in rheumatoid arthritis. (**A**) Early changes of rheumatoid arthritis are focal cartilage loss superiority *(arrowheads)* causing wedge-shaped superolateral joint space. Sclerosis of the opening weight-bearing acetabulum. (**B**) Late changes of rheumatoid arthritis include diffuse cartilage loss, generalized osteopenia, erosion and remodelling of the opposing articular surfaces and resultant surfaces and resultant protrusio acetabuli

(From Grainger RG, Allison DJ, Adam A, Dixon AK [eds]: Grainger and Allison's Diagnostic Radiology, 4th ed. Philadelphia, Churchill Livingstone, 2001.)

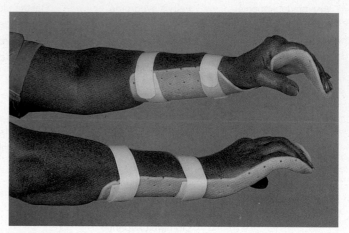

Fig 291–11

Wrist and hand splints.

(From Hochberg MC, Silman AJ, Smolen JS, et al [eds]: Rheumatology, 3rd ed. St Louis, Mosby, 2003.)

Chapter 292 | Juvenile rheumatoid arthritis

DEFINITION

Juvenile rheumatoid arthritis (Still's disease, juvenile chronic arthritis, juvenile idiopathic arthritis) is arthritis beginning before the age of 16 years.

PHYSICAL FINDINGS AND CLINICAL PRESENTATION

Usually one of three types:

Systemic or Acute Febrile Juvenile Rheumatoid Arthritis (20% of Cases):

- Characterized by extra-articular manifestations, especially spiking fevers (Fig. 292–1) and a typical rash (Fig. 292–2) that frequently appears in the evening and may be elicited by gently scratching the skin in susceptible areas (Koebner's phenomenon)
- Possible splenomegaly, generalized lymph adenopathy, pericarditis, and myocarditis
- Often, minimal articular findings overshadowed by systemic symptoms

Pauciarticular or Oligoarticular Form (50% of Cases):

- Involves fewer than five joints
- Usually involves the larger joints, such as the knees, elbows (Fig. 292–3), and ankles
- Systemic features often minimal, and only one to three joints usually involved
- Rarely causes impairment but chronic iridocyclitis develops in approximately 30% of cases with this form, and permanent loss of vision will develop in a high percentage of these patients. Band keratopathy is shown in Figure 292–4.
- Accelerated growth of the affected limb from chronic hyperemia, possibly resulting in a temporary leg length discrepancy (Fig. 292–5) that is eventually equalized in most cases on control of the inflammation

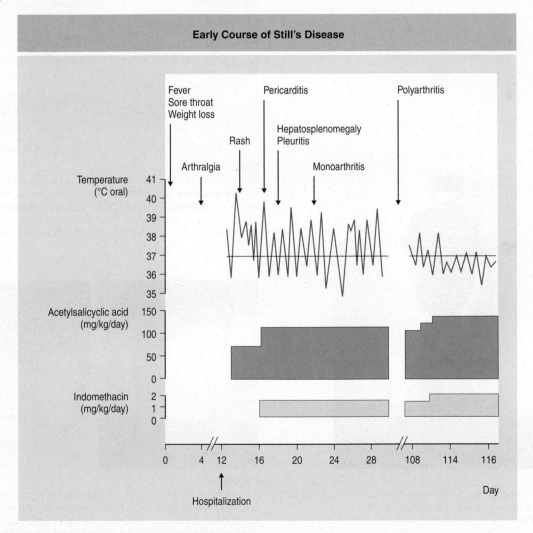

Fig 292-1

Early course of Still's disease. The fever pattern and early evolution of the clinical manifestations in relation to treatment of a typical case of adult Still's disease in a 20-year-old male. The patient was admitted to the hospital on day 12 of the illness. At the time of admission, his hemoglobin was 10.6 g/dL, the white blood cell count was 25,600/mm³, and the erythrocyte sedimentation rate was 32 mm/hr (corrected Wintrobe). From Hochberg MC, Silman AJ, Smolen JS, et al (eds), 3rd ed, St. Louis, Mosby, 2003.

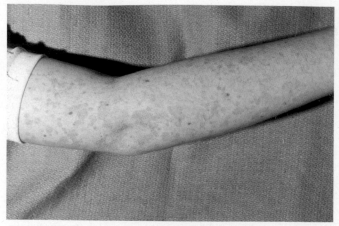

Fig 292-2
The classic erythematous macular rash of systemic juvenile arthritis. This rash is usually nonpruritic and rapidly migratory, most prominent when the child is febrile.
(From Hochberg MC, Silman AJ, Smolen JS, et al [eds]: Rheumatology, 3rd ed. St Louis, Mosby, 2003.)

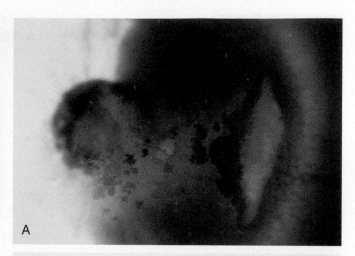

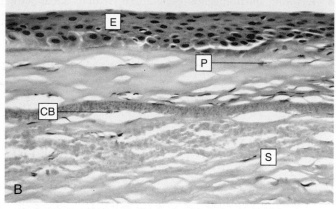

Fig 292-4
Band keratopathy. **A**, Calcium deposits in the cornea of a 13-year-old with juvenile rheumatoid arthritis. **B**, A fibrous pannus (P) is present between the epithelium (E) and a calcified Bowman's membrane (CB). Some deposit is also present in the anterior corneal stroma (S).
(From Yanoff M, Fine BS. Ocular Pathology, 5th ed. St Louis, Mosby, 2002.)

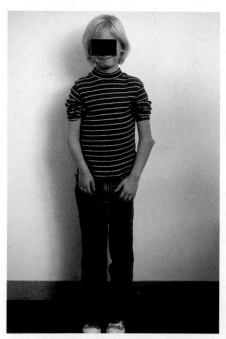

Fig 292-3
Patient with juvenile idiopathic arthritis who has bilateral elbow flexion contractures that prevent straightening of the arms.
(From Yanoff M, Duker JS: Ophthalmology, ed 2, St. Louis, Mosby, 2004)

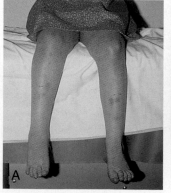
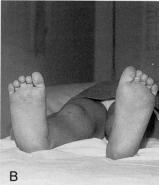

Fig 292-5
Pauciarticular-onset JRA in the right ankle. (**A**) A shorter leg length from the knee to the ankle is demonstrated. (**B**) The right foot is smaller, with underdevelopment of the right forefoot due to disuse.
(From Hochberg MC, Silman AJ, Smolen JS, et al [eds]: Rheumatology, 3rd ed. St Louis, Mosby, 2003.)

Polyarticular Juvenile Rheumatoid Arthritis (30% of Cases):
- Involves five or more joints
- Resembles the adult disease in its symmetrical involvement of the small joints of the hands and feet
- Cervical spine involvement common and may produce marked loss of motion (Fig. 292–6)
- Early closure of the ossification centers of the mandible, often producing a markedly receding chin, a characteristic of this form (Fig. 292–7)
- Systemic manifestations similar to the febrile variety but not as dramatic

CAUSE
Unknown. There is increasing evidence that the inflammation and destruction of bone and cartilage that occur in many rheumatic diseases are the result of the activation, by some unknown mechanism, of proinflammatory cells that infiltrate the synovium. These cells, in turn, release various substances, such as cytokines and TNF-α, which subsequently cause the pathologic changes typical of this group of diseases. Many of the newer therapeutic agents are directed at the suppression of these final mediators of inflammation.

DIFFERENTIAL DIAGNOSIS
- Infectious causes of fever
- SLE
- Rheumatic fever
- Drug reaction
- Serum sickness
- "Viral arthritis"
- Lyme arthritis

LABORATORY TESTS
- Increased ESR
- Low-grade anemia
- High peripheral white blood cell (WBC) count
- RF: rarely demonstrable in the serum of children
- ANAs: often found in children with ocular complications

IMAGING STUDIES
- X-ray findings are similar to those in adult, with soft tissue swelling and osteoporosis early in the disease.
- Joint destruction is less frequent.
- Bony erosion and cyst formation may be present as a result of synovial hypertrophy.

TREATMENT
Proper management requires close cooperation among the primary physician, therapist, rheumatologist, and orthopedist.
- Rest
- Physical and occupational therapy
- NSAIDs
- DMARDs and biologic response modifiers (BRMs)
- Intra-articular steroids
- Systemic corticosteroids

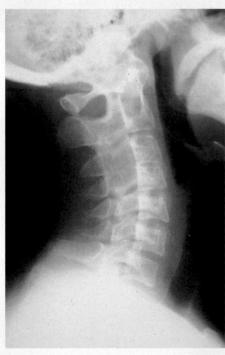

Fig 292–6
Systemic-onset JRA in a child who had a polyarticular course. Her neck shows apophyseal fusion of C2-C4 and undergrowth of adjacent vertebrae.
(From Hochberg MC, Silman AJ, Smolen JS, et al [eds]: Rheumatology, 3rd ed. St Louis, Mosby, 2003.)

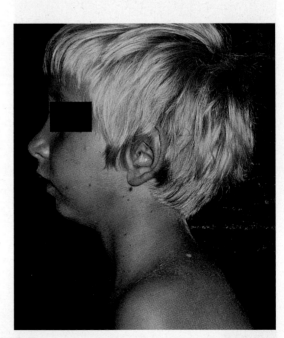

Fig 292–7
Failure of development of the lower jaw some 5 years after systemic onset of disease. The neck is short and slightly flexed.
(From Hochberg MC, Silman AJ, Smolen JS, et al [eds]: Rheumatology, 3rd ed. St Louis, Mosby, 2003.)

Chapter 293 Systemic lupus erythematosus

DEFINITION
SLE is a chronic multisystemic disease characterized by production of autoantibodies and protean clinical manifestations.

PHYSICAL FINDINGS AND CLINICAL PRESENTATION
- Skin: erythematous rash over the malar eminences (Fig. 293–1), generally with sparing of the nasolabial folds (butterfly rash); alopecia; raised erythematous patches with subsequent edematous plaques and adherent scales (discoid lupus) (Fig. 293–2); leg (Fig. 293–3), nasal, or oropharyngeal ulcerations (Fig. 293–4); livedo reticularis; pallor (from anemia); petechiae (from thrombocytopenia)
- Joints: tenderness, swelling, or effusion, generally involving peripheral joints
- Cardiac: pericardial effusion (Fig. 293–5), pericardial rub (in patients with pericarditis), heart murmurs (if endocarditis or valvular thickening or dysfunction)
- Other: fever, conjunctivitis, choroidal vasculitis (Fig. 293–6), dry eyes, dry mouth (sicca syndrome), oral ulcers, abdominal tenderness, decreased breath sounds (pleural effusions [Fig. 293–7])

CAUSE
- Unknown. Autoantibodies are typically present many years before the diagnosis of SLE.

DIFFERENTIAL DIAGNOSIS
- Other connective tissue disorders (e.g., RA, MCTD, progressive systemic sclerosis)
- Metastatic neoplasm
- Infection
- Table 293–1 describes facial lesions that can mimic acute lupus.

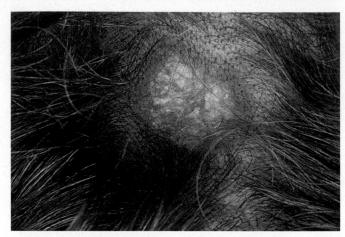

Fig 293–2
Discoid lupus erythematosus: there are considerable scaling and conspicuous background erythema.
(Courtesy of the Institute of Dermatology, London, UK.)

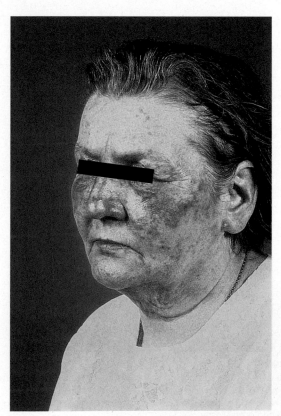

Fig 293–1
Systemic lupus erythematosus: characteristic 'butterfly erythema' on the cheeks and nose.
(Courtesy of R. A. Marsden, MD, St George's Hospital, London, UK)

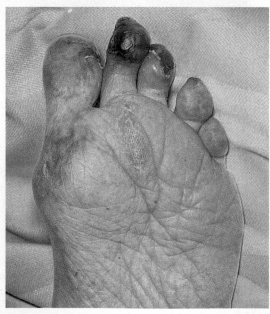

Fig 293–3
Gangrene of the toe in a patient with SLE and vasculitis.
(From Hochberg MC, Silman AJ, Smolen JS, et al [eds]: Rheumatology, 3rd ed. St Louis, Mosby, 2003.)

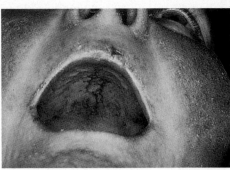

Fig 293–4
Mouth ulcers in a patient with SLE.
(From Hochberg MC, Silman AJ, Smolen JS, et al [eds]: Rheumatology, 3rd ed. St Louis, Mosby, 2003.)

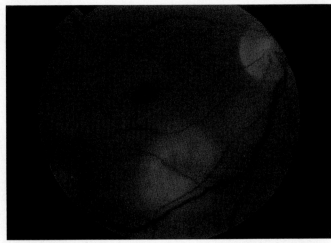

Fig 293–6
Funduscopic examination in a patient with SLE demonstrating choroidal vasculitis.
(From Hochberg MC, Silman AJ, Smolen JS, et al [eds]: Rheumatology, 3rd ed. St Louis, Mosby, 2003.)

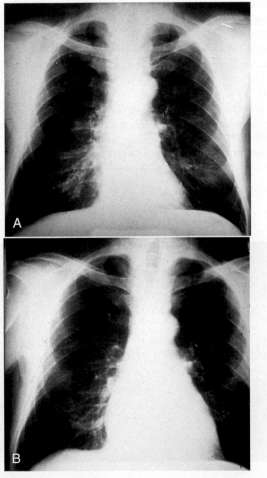

Fig 293–5
Pericardial effusion. Change in cardiac silhouette from (**A**) normal baseline in (**B**) a patient with SLE and acute pericarditis.
(From Hochberg MC, Silman AJ, Smolen JS, et al [eds]: Rheumatology, 3rd ed. St Louis, Mosby, 2003.)

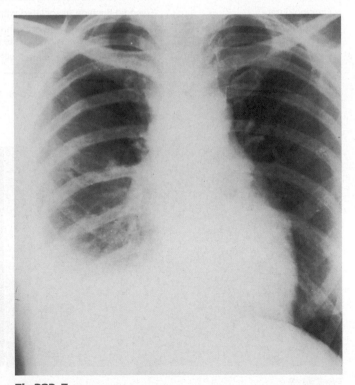

Fig 293–7
Systemic lupus erythematosus causing pleurisy and an associated right pleural effusion.
(From Grainger RG, Allison DJ, Adam A, Dixon AK [eds]: Grainger and Allison's Diagnostic Radiology, 4th ed. Philadelphia, Churchill Livingstone, 2001.)

WORKUP

The diagnosis of SLE can be made by demonstrating the presence of any four or more of the following criteria of the American Rheumatism Association:

1. Butterfly rash
2. Discoid rash
3. Photosensitivity (particularly leg ulcerations)
4. Oral ulcers
5. Arthritis
6. Serositis (pleuritis, pericarditis)
7. Renal disorder (Fig. 293–8) (persistent proteinuria >0.5 g/day or 3+ if quantitation not performed, cellular casts)
8. Neurologic disorder (seizures, microinfarcts [Fig. 293–9], psychosis [in absence of offending drugs or metabolic derangement])
9. Hematologic disorder:
   a. Hemolytic anemia with reticulocytosis
   b. Leukopenia (<4000/mm³ total on two or more occasions)
   c. Lymphopenia (<1500/mm³ on two or more occasions)
   d. Thrombocytopenia (<100,000/mm³ in the absence of offending drugs)
10. Immunologic disorder:
    a. Positive SLE cell preparation (Fig. 293–10)
    b. Anti-DNA (presence of antibody to native DNA in abnormal titer) (Fig. 293–11)
    c. Anti-Sm (presence of antibody to Smith nuclear antigen)
    d. False-positive STS known to be positive for at least 6 months and confirmed by negative TPI or FTA tests

TABLE 293–1 Facial lesions—mimics of acute lupus

Diagnosis	Discriminating features
Dermatomyositis* (occasional)	Heliotrope version more common; rash often involves nasolabial folds; rash has a distinctive pattern at other body locations
Photoallergic/phototoxic drug reactions* (common)	Clinical history of exposure to drugs including sulfa, thiazides, phenothiazines, tetracycline, piroxicam (phototoxic within days of first exposure), naproxen (porphyria-like)
Polymorphous light eruption* (common)	Small papule/papulovesicle variety; occasionally on face and commonly on forearms, chest or thighs, very pruritic, fewer recurrences with further sun exposure over the season
Porphyria* (rare)	Vesicular/bullous lesions and skin fragility in photosensitive distribution; may coexist with SLE
Pellagra* (rare)	Mucosal erythematous patches and ulcers antedate rash; associated with gastrointestinal and psychological disturbances
Early acne rosacea	Malar erythema involving nasolabial folds
Carcinoid (rare)	Episodic flushing associated with other systemic symptoms, including diarrhea
Erysipelas (rare)	Bridge of nose and one or both cheeks involved with raised, rapidly spreading, warm erythematous rash, which may later vesiculate and crust in the febrile patient
Parvovirus infection (occasion)	Episodic flushing associated with other systemic symptoms, including diarrhea

Photosensitive processes.
From Hochberg MC, Silman AJ, Smolen JS, et al (eds): Rheumatology, 3rd ed. St Louis, Mosby, 2003.

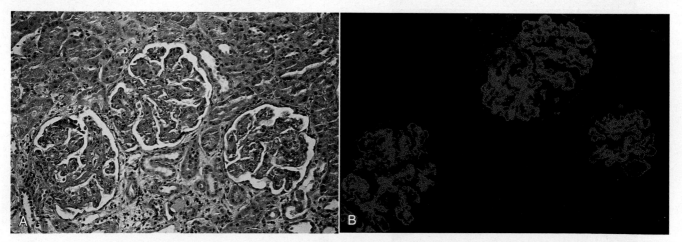

Fig 293–8
Lupus nephritis class iv (diffuse proliferative lupus nephritis). (**A**) Low power view shows the diffuse and global distribution of the endocapillary proliferation. (Hematoxylin and eosin stain.) (**B**) Diffuse and global deposition of IgG throughout the glomerular mesangium and outlining the peripheral capillary walls. (Immunofluorescence, anti-IgG.)
(From Hochberg MC, Silman AJ, Smolen JS, et al [eds]: Rheumatology, 3rd ed. St Louis, Mosby, 2003.)

11. ANA: an abnormal titer of ANA by immunofluorescence or equivalent assay at any time in the absence of drugs known to be associated with "drug-induced lupus" syndrome

LABORATORY TESTS

Suggested initial laboratory evaluation of suspected SLE:

- Immunologic evaluation: ANA, anti-DNA antibody, anti-Sm antibody
- Other laboratory tests: CBC with differential, platelet count (Coombs' test if anemia detected), urinalysis (24-hour urine collection for protein if proteinuria is detected), PTT and anticardiolipin antibodies in patients with thrombotic events, blood urea nitrogen (BUN), creatinine to evaluate renal function

IMAGING STUDIES

- Chest x-ray for evaluation of pulmonary involvement (e.g., pleural effusions, pulmonary infiltrates)
- Echocardiogram to screen for significant valvular heart disease (Fig. 293–12) (present in 18% of patients with SLE); echocardiography can identify a subset of lesions (valvular thickening and dysfunction) other than verrucous (Libman-Sacks) endocarditis that are prone to hemodynamic deterioration

TREATMENT

- Joint pain and mild serositis are generally well controlled with NSAIDs; antimalarials are also effective (e.g., hydroxychloroquine).
- Cutaneous manifestations are treated with the following:
  1. Topical corticosteroids; intradermal corticosteroids are helpful for individual discoid lesions, especially in the scalp
  2. Antimalarials (e.g., hydroxychloroquine and quinacrine)

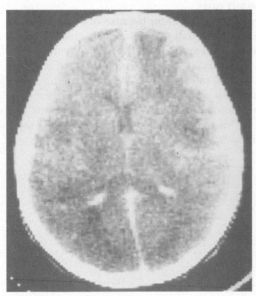

Fig 293–9
CT scan of the brain, demonstrating microinfarcts.
(From Hochberg MC, Silman AJ, Smolen JS, et al [eds]: Rheumatology, 3rd ed. St Louis, Mosby, 2003.)

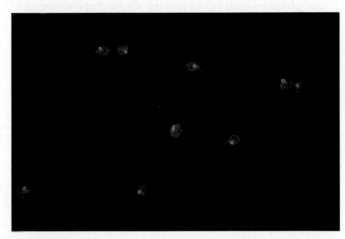

Fig 293–11
Systemic lupus erythematosus: anti-dsDNA (Crithidia luciliae).
(Courtesy of G. Swana, MD, St Thomas' Hospital, London, UK)

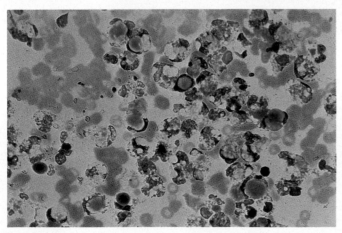

Fig 293–10
Systemic lupus erythematosus: LE cells. The patient's serum is incubated with normal neutrophils. Note the ingested nuclear debris.
(Courtesy of N. Slater, MD, St Thomas' Hospital, London, UK)

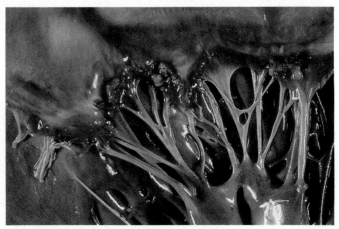

Fig 293–12
Libman-Sacks endocarditis: note the small yellow, glistening vegetations on the cusps of the mitral valve.
(Courtesy of C. Fletcher, MD, Brigham and Women's Hospital and Harvard Medical School, Boston)

3. Sunscreens that block ultraviolet (UV) A and UVB radiation

4. Immunosuppressive drugs (methotrexate or azathioprine) can be used as steroid-sparing drugs.

- Renal disease

1. The use of high-pulsed doses of cyclophosphamide given at monthly intervals is more effective in preserving renal function than is treatment with glucocorticoids alone. The combination of methylprednisolone and cyclophosphamide is superior to bolus therapy with methylprednisolone or cyclophosphamide alone in patients with lupus nephritis. For patients with proliferative lupus nephritis, short-term therapy with IV cyclophosphamide followed by maintenance therapy with mycophenolate mofetil or azathioprine appears to be more efficacious and safer than long-term therapy with IV cyclophosphamide. In the treatment of severe proliferative lupus nephritis, mycophenolate mofetil represents an excellent alternative to cyclophosphamide.

2. The use of plasmapheresis in combination with immunosuppressive agents (to prevent the rebound phenomenon of antibody levels after plasmapheresis) is generally reserved for rapidly progressive renal failure or life-threatening systemic vasculitis.

- Central nervous system (CNS) involvement: treatment generally consists of corticosteroid therapy; however, its efficacy is uncertain, and it is generally reserved for organic brain syndrome. Anticonvulsants and antipsychotics are also indicated in select cases; headaches are treated symptomatically.

- Hemolytic anemia: treatment of Coombs'-positive hemolytic anemia consists of high doses of corticosteroids; nonhemolytic anemia (secondary to chronic disease) does not require specific therapy.

- Thrombocytopenia

1. Initial treatment consists of corticosteroids.

2. In patients with poor response to steroids, encouraging results have been reported with the use of danazol, vincristine, and immunoglobulins. Combination chemotherapy with cyclophosphamide and prednisone combined with vincristine, vincristine and procarbazine, or etoposide may be useful in patients with severe refractory idiopathic thrombocytopenic purpura.

3. Splenectomy generally does not cure the thrombocytopenia of SLE, but it may be necessary as an adjunct in managing select cases.

- Infections are common because of compromised immune function secondary to SLE and the use of corticosteroid, cytotoxic, and antimetabolite drugs; pneumococcal bacteremia is associated with high mortality rate.

- The leading cause of death in SLE is infection (one third of all deaths); active nephritis causes approximately 18% of deaths, and CNS disease causes 7% of deaths; the survival rate is 75% over the first 10 years. Blacks and Hispanics generally have a worse prognosis.

Chapter 294 | Antiphospholipid antibody syndrome

DEFINITION

The antiphospholipid antibody syndrome (APS) is characterized by arterial or venous thrombosis and/or pregnancy loss AND the presence of antiphospholipid antibodies (aPLs). aPLs are antibodies directed against either phospholipids or proteins bound to anionic phospholipids. Four types of aPLs have been characterized:

- False-positive serologic tests for syphilis
- Lupus anticoagulants (LA)
- Anticardiolipin antibodies (ACL)
- Anti–β_2 glycoprotein-1 antibodies

The syndrome is referred to as primary APS when it occurs alone and as secondary APS when in association with SLE, other rheumatic disorders, or certain infections or medications. APS can affect all organ systems and includes venous and arterial thromboses, recurrent fetal losses, and thrombocytopenia.

PHYSICAL FINDINGS AND CLINICAL PRESENTATION

- **Thrombosis:** patients with APS are at risk for both venous and arterial thromboses, although venous thromboses are more common, occurring as the initial manifestation of APS in approximately 30% of APS patients. Of all patients with venous thrombosis, 5% to 20% have aPL. The most common site for deep venous thrombosis is the calf, but thromboses may also occur in the renal, hepatic, axillary, subclavian, vena cava, and retinal veins. The most common site of arterial thrombosis is the cerebral vessels. Other common sites are the coronary, renal, mesenteric arteries, and arterial bypass. Recurrent thrombosis is common with APS.
- **CNS:** stroke, transient ischemic attack (TIA), migraine, multi-infarct dementia, epilepsy, movement disorders, transverse myelopathy, depression, and Guillain-Barré syndrome
- **Pulmonary:** pulmonary embolism and infarction, pulmonary hypertension (HTN), adult respiratory distress disorder (ARDS), intra-alveolar pulmonary hemorrhage, and a postpartum syndrome characterized by fever, pleuritic chest pain, dyspnea, and patchy infiltrates with pleural effusion on chest radiography
- **Cardiology:** Libman-Sacks endocarditis, intracardiac thrombosis, coronary artery disease (CAD), myocardial infarction (MI)
- **Gastrointestinal:** abdominal pain, gastrointestinal (GI) bleed secondary to ischemia, splenic or pancreatic infarction, hepatic vein thrombosis, Budd-Chiari syndrome (second most common cause of BCS)
- **Renal:** proteinuria, acute renal failure, HTN, renal infarct, renal artery or vein thrombosis, postpartum hemolytic-uremic syndrome
- **Hematology:** thrombocytopenia, hemolytic anemia
- **Endocrine:** Addison's disease secondary to adrenal hemorrhage and, less frequently, thrombosis
- **Cutaneous:** livedo reticularis, cutaneous necrosis (Fig. 294–1), skin ulcerations, gangrene of digits
- **Obstetrics:** recurrent spontaneous abortion (secondary to placental vessel thrombosis and ischemia)
- **Catastrophic APS:** widespread thrombotic disease with visceral damage

CAUSE

- aPLs react with negatively charged phospholipids
- Possible mechanisms of thrombosis includes effects of aPL on platelet membranes, endothelial cells, and clotting components such as prothrombin and protein C or S
- Recently shown that prephospholipids are not immunogenic and that a binding protein (β_2-glycoprotein I) may be the key immunogen in the APS

DIFFERENTIAL DIAGNOSIS

Other hypercoagulable states (inherited or acquired)

- Inherited: antithrombin (AT) III, protein C or S deficiency, factor V Leiden, prothrombin gene mutation
- Acquired: heparin-induced thrombopathy, myeloproliferative syndromes, cancer, hyperviscosity
- Hyperhomocysteinemia
- Nephrotic syndrome

WORKUP

Diagnostic criteria of APS include at least one clinical criterion and at least one laboratory criterion:

- Clinical:
  1. Venous, arterial, or small vessel thrombosis OR
  2. Morbidity with pregnancy defined as
  - Fetal death at >10 weeks' gestation OR
  - Premature births before 34 weeks' gestation secondary to eclampsia, preeclampsia, or severe placental insufficiency OR
  - Three or more unexplained consecutive spontaneous abortions at >10 weeks' gestation

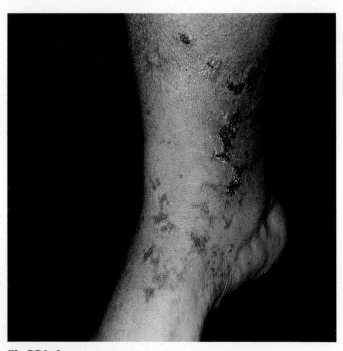

Fig 294–1
Primary antiphospholipid antibody syndrome.
(From Callen JP, Greer KE, Paller AS, Swinyer LJ: Color Atlas of Dermatology, ed 2, Philadelphia, 2000, WB Saunders)

- Laboratory:
  1. IgG and/or IgM anticardiolipin antibody in medium or high titers OR
  2. Lupus anticoagulant activity found on two or more occasions, at least 6 weeks apart

LABORATORY TESTS

Laboratory testing of ACL and LA antibodies indicated in:

- Patient with underlying SLE or collagen-vascular disease with thrombosis
- Patient with recurrent, familial, or juvenile DVT or thrombosis in an unusual location (mesenteric or cerebral)
- Possibly in patients with lupus or lupus-like disorders in high-risk situations (e.g., surgery, prolonged immobilization, pregnancy)

Abnormal tests include:

- False-positive test for syphilis (RPR/VDRL)
- Lupus anticoagulant activity, demonstrated by prolongation of activated partial thromboplastin time (aPTT) that does not correct with 1:1 mixing study
- Presence of anticardiolipin antibodies (ELISA for anticardiolipin is most sensitive and specific test [>80%])
- Presence of anti–β_2-glycoprotein I antibody

TREATMENT

- Treatment of APS: positive aPL and major or recurrent thrombotic events
- Initial anticoagulation with heparin, then lifelong warfarin treatment to maintain INR 3.0 to 4.0

Pregnant Women

- Who are positive for aPL antibodies, without history of non-placental thrombotic event (e.g., DVT), or positive for aPL antibodies with history of <3 spontaneous abortions:
  - Aspirin (ASA) 81 mg at conception and heparin 10,000 IU SQ q12h at time of documented viable intrauterine pregnancy (approximately 7 weeks' gestation) until 6 weeks postpartum
  - A mid-interval PTT should be checked and should be normal or similar to baseline before therapy.
- Who carry a diagnosis of APS and who should already be chronically anticoagulated:
  - Warfarin should be discontinued secondary to its teratogenic effects.
  - ASA 81 mg and heparin SQ to PTT of 1.5 to 2× control value
  - Intravenous immunoglobulins (IVIg) and prednisone have also been used with success if aspirin and heparin fail.

Chapter 295 Sjögren's syndrome

DEFINITION

SS is an autoimmune disorder characterized by lymphocytic and plasma cell infiltration and destruction of salivary and lacrimal glands with subsequent diminished lacrimal and salivary gland secretions.

- *Primary:* Dry mouth (xerostomia) and dry eyes (xerophthalmia) develop as isolated entities.
- *Secondary:* associated with other disorders

PHYSICAL FINDINGS AND CLINICAL PRESENTATION

- Dry mouth with dry lips (cheilosis), erythema of tongue and other mucosal surfaces, carious teeth
- Dry eyes (conjunctival injection, decreased luster, and irregularity of the corneal light reflex)
- Possible salivary gland enlargement (Fig. 295–1) and dysfunction with subsequent difficulty in chewing and swallowing food and in speaking without frequent water intake
- Purpura (nonthrombocytopenic, hyperglobulinemic, vasculitic) may be present (Fig. 295–2).
- Evidence of associated conditions (e.g., RA or other connective disease, lymphoma, hypothyroidism, chronic obstructive pulmonary disease (COPD), trigeminal neuropathy, chronic liver disease, polymyopathy)

CAUSE

Autoimmune disorder

DIFFERENTIAL DIAGNOSIS

- Medication-related dryness (e.g., anticholinergics)
- Age-related exocrine gland dysfunction
- Mouth breathing
- Anxiety
- Other: sarcoidosis, primary salivary hypofunction, radiation injury, amyloidosis

WORKUP

Workup involves ocular and oral examination and laboratory and radiographic testing to demonstrate the following criteria for diagnosis of primary and secondary SS.

PRIMARY

- Symptoms and objective signs of ocular dryness:

1. *Schirmer's test:* <8 mm wetting per 5 minutes (Fig. 295–3)
2. Positive Rose Bengal or fluorescein staining of cornea and conjunctiva to demonstrate keratoconjunctivitis sicca

- Symptoms and objective signs of dry mouth:

1. Decreased parotid flow using Lashley cups or other methods
2. Abnormal biopsy result of minor salivary gland (focus score >2 based on average of four assessable lobules)

- Evidence of systemic autoimmune disorder:

1. Elevated titer of RF >1:320
2. Elevated titer of ANA >1:320
3. Presence of anti–SS A (Ro) or anti–SS B (La) antibodies

SECONDARY

- Characteristic signs and symptoms of SS (described in "Physical Findings")
- Clinical features sufficient to allow a diagnosis of RA, SLE, polymyositis, or scleroderma

LABORATORY TESTS

- Positive ANA (>60% of patients) with autoantibodies anti–SS A and anti–SS B may be present.
- Additional laboratory abnormalities may include elevated ESR, anemia (normochromic, normocytic), abnormal liver function studies, elevated serum β_2-microglobulin levels, and elevated RF.
- A definite diagnosis SS can be made with a salivary gland biopsy.

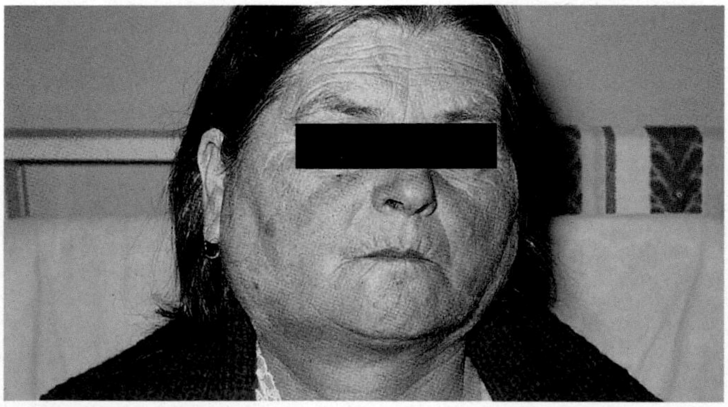

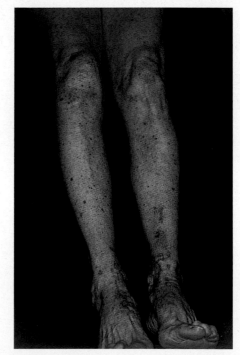

Fig 295–1
Patient with primary Sjögren's syndrome. Parotid gland enlargement. (From Hochberg MC, Silman AJ, Smolen JS, et al [eds]: Rheumatology, 3rd ed. St Louis, Mosby, 2003.)

Fig 295–2
Palpable purpura. Lower extremities of a primary Sjögren's syndrome patient.
(From Hochberg MC, Silman AJ, Smolen JS, et al [eds]: Rheumatology, 3rd ed. St Louis, Mosby, 2003.)

TREATMENT

- Adequate fluid replacement. Ameliorate skin dryness by gently blotting dry after bathing, leaving a small amount of moisture, and then applying a moisturizer.
- Proper oral hygiene to reduce the incidence of caries
- Use artificial tears frequently.
- Pilocarpine is useful to improve dryness. A cyclosporine ophthalmic emulsion may also be useful for dry eyes. Recommended dose is 1 drop bid in both eyes.
- Cevimeline, a cholinergic agent with muscarinic agonist activity, is effective for the treatment of dry mouth in patients with SS.
- Interferon alfa has been shown to significantly improve stimulated whole saliva output and decrease complaints of xerostomia.
- Periodic dental and ophthalmology evaluations to screen for complications

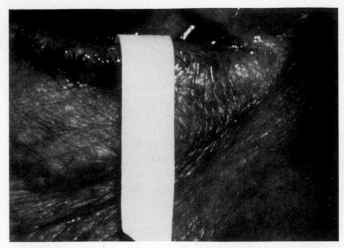

Fig 295–3
Patient with Sjögren's syndrome. Schirmer's test. Wetting of less than 5 mm/5 min of the filter paper strip is shown.
(From Hochberg MC, Silman AJ, Smolen JS, et al [eds]: Rheumatology, 3rd ed. St Louis, Mosby, 2003.)

<table>
<tr><td>**Chapter 296**</td><td>**Idiopathic inflammatory myopathies (dermatomyositis, polymyositis)**</td></tr>
</table>

DEFINITION

Inflammatory myopathies are idiopathic diseases of muscle characterized clinically by muscle weakness and pathologically by inflammation and muscle fiber breakdown. The three most common are dermatomyositis (DM), polymyositis (PM), and inclusion body myositis.

PHYSICAL FINDINGS AND CLINICAL PRESENTATION

DM and PM

- Most patients have a subacute onset, over weeks to months.
- Symmetrical proximal muscle weakness involving the neck flexors, shoulder, and pelvic girdles.
- Difficulty getting up from a chair, climbing stairs, reaching for objects above head, or combing hair.
- Distal muscle and ocular involvement is uncommon.
- Sensation and reflexes are preserved.
- Dysphagia and dysphonia result from pharyngeal muscle involvement.
- Esophageal dysmotility often occurs in DM.
- Respiratory failure from associated pulmonary fibrosis.
- Cardiac conduction abnormalities can be seen with DM.
- Systemic autoimmune disease occurs frequently in PM, and rarely in DM.
- Skin findings in DM:
  1. Heliotrope rash on the upper eyelids (Fig. 296–1)
  2. Erythematous rash on the face
  3. May also involve the back and shoulders (*shawl sign*), neck and chest (V-shape), knees, and elbows
  4. Photosensitivity
  5. *Gottron's papules* (violaceous papules overlying dorsal interphalangeal or MCP areas, elbow or knee joints) (Fig. 296–2)
  6. Nail cracking, thickening, and irregularity with periungual telangiectasia
  7. *Mechanic's hand:* fissured, hyperpigmented, scaly, and hyperkeratotic; also associated with increased risk of interstitial lung disease

CAUSE

- DM: complex, immune-mediated microangiopathy
  1. Adaptive immune response via humorally mediated complement attack.
- PM: unknown
  1. Cell-mediated immune major histocompatibility-I (MHC-1) process directed against muscle fibers is likely, given biopsy features.
  2. A viral etiology has been proposed secondary to the presence of autoantibodies to histidyl transferase antibody, anti–Jo-1 antibody, and signal recognition particle.

DIAGNOSIS

- Characteristic pattern of muscle weakness for each type
- Electromyelography (EMG) and nerve conduction studies should be consistent with myopathic features.
- Laboratory tests listed below.

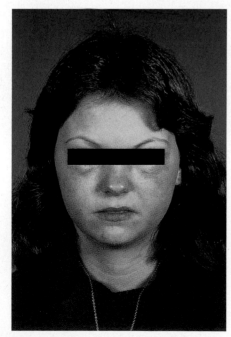

Fig 296–1
Dermatomyositis: note the characteristic red-mauve discoloration around the eyes. There is also spread onto the cheeks.
(Courtesy of R. A. Marsden, MD, St. George's Hospital, London, UK)

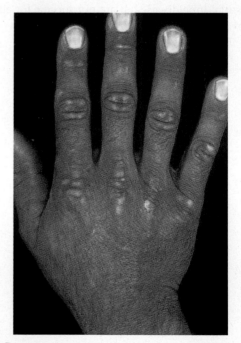

Fig 296–2
Dermatomyositis: characteristic purple papules on the knuckles (Gottron's sign).
(Courtesy of the Institute of Dermatology, London, UK.)

- Biopsy required for diagnosis and should confirm inflammation *before* treatment started: myopathic features (variation in fiber size, fiber splitting, fatty replacement of muscle tissue, and increased endomysial connective tissue) should be seen in addition to the following:

  1. DM: perifascicular atrophy, MAC deposition along capillaries

  2. PM: endomysial infiltrates composed of CD8+ T cells and macrophages invading non-necrotic muscle fibers that express MHC-I antigen

DIFFERENTIAL DIAGNOSIS

- Muscular dystrophies
- Amyloid myoneuropathy
- Amyotrophic lateral sclerosis
- Myasthenia gravis
- Eaton-Lambert syndrome
- Drug-induced myopathies (e.g., quinidine, NSAIDs, penicillamine, HMG-CoA reductase inhibitors)
- Diabetic amyotrophy
- Guillain-Barré syndrome
- Hyperthyroidism or hypothyroidism
- Lichen planus
- Amyopathic DM (rash without weakness)
- SLE (see Fig. 293–1)
- Contact atopic or seborrheic dermatitis
- Psoriasis

LABORATORY TESTS

- Creatine kinase is the most sensitive muscle enzyme test for muscle breakdown and can be elevated as much as 50 times above normal in DM and PM.
- Aldolase, AST, ALT, alkaline phosphatase, and LDH can be elevated.
- Anti–Jo-1 antibodies are seen in myositis with associated interstitial lung disease but are not specific for either DM or PM.

- Electrolytes, thyroid-stimulating hormone (TSH), Ca^{2+}, and Mg^{2+} should be requested to exclude other causes of weakness.
- ECG for cardiac involvement.

IMAGING STUDIES

- Chest radiograph to rule out pulmonary involvement. If suspicious for pulmonary interstitial disease, a high-resolution computed tomography (CT) scan of the chest may be helpful.
- Videofluoroscopy or barium swallow study to look for upper esophageal dysfunction in patients with dysphagia and DM

TREATMENT

- Sun-blocking agents with SPF 15 or greater for skin protection in patients with DM
- Physical therapy is beneficial for gait training and increasing muscle tone and strength.
- Occupational therapy to assist with activities of daily living
- Speech therapy for dysphagia and swallowing problems
- Prednisone
- Use IV immunoglobulin or cyclophosphamide if patient fails to improve on prednisone or muscle enzymes begin rising when tapering off prednisone.
- Hydroxychloroquine can be used to treat the cutaneous lesions of DM.

DEFINITION

Raynaud's phenomenon is a vasospastic disorder usually affecting the digital arteries precipitated by exposure to cold temperatures or emotional distress and manifesting in a triphasic discoloration of the fingers or toes.

PHYSICAL FINDINGS AND CLINICAL PRESENTATION

- The classic manifestation is the triphasic color response to cold exposure (Fig. 297–1), which may or may not be accompanied by pain.
  1. Pallor of the digit resulting from vasospasm
  2. Blue discoloration (cyanosis) secondary to desaturated venous blood
  3. Red (rubor) with or without pain and paresthesia when vasospasm resolves and blood returns to the digit
- Color changes are well delineated, symmetrical, and usually bilateral involving the fingers and toes but sparing the thumbs.
- Fingertips are most often involved, but feet, ears, and nose can be affected.
- Duration of attacks can range from seconds to hours.
- Chronic skin changes resulting from repeated attacks may include skin thickening and brittle nails. Ulcerations and, rarely, gangrene may occur (Fig. 297–2).

- Secondary Raynaud's phenomenon may be associated with typical findings of the underlying disease (e.g., sclerodactyly and telangiectasia in **CREST** [Calcinosis, Raynaud's phenomenon, Esophageal dysmotility, Sclerodactyly, and Telangiectasia] syndrome).

CAUSE

- Primary Raynaud's phenomenon is generally referred to as Raynaud's disease when no cause can be found.
- Primary Raynaud's phenomenon has been shown to have a familial tendency, and five potential chromosomal regions have been identified that may be linked to its pathogenesis.
- Attacks are usually triggered by cold or emotional stimuli but can also be triggered by vibration, caffeine, tobacco, pseudoephedrine, contact with polyvinylchloride (PVC), or frozen foods.
- Proposed mechanisms of pathogenesis include:
  1. Upregulation or sensitization of postsynaptic α_2-receptors in the digits
  2. Increased endothelin-1 (potent endothelium-derived vasoconstrictor), and decreased localized vasodilation medicated by CGRP.
- Secondary Raynaud's phenomenon has many causes:
  1. CREST syndrome
  2. Scleroderma
  3. MCTD, polymyositis, and dermatomyositis
  4. SLE
  5. RA
  6. Thromboangiitis obliterans (Buerger's disease)
  7. Drug induced (beta-blockers, ergotamine, methysergide, vinblastine, bleomycin, oral contraceptives)

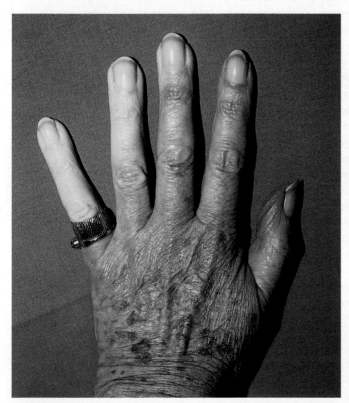

Fig 297–1
Triphasic color response to cold exposure is the classic manifestation of Raynaud's syndrome.
(From Lebwohl MG, Heymann WR, Berth-Jones J, Coulson I [eds]: Treatment of skin disease, St. Louis, 2002, Mosby)

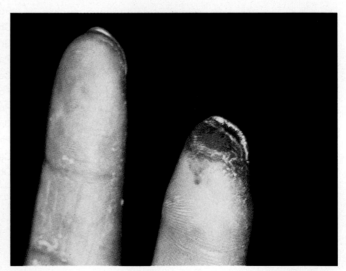

Fig 297–2
Finger necrosis in secondary Raynaud's phenomenon. The second and third fingers of a 42-year-old woman with scleoderma. A typical sclerosis of the skin often leads to a cufflike strangulation of the microcirculation, with concomitant finger tip necrosis.
(From Crawford, MH, DiMarco JP, Paulus WJ [eds]: Cardiology, ed 2, St. Louis, 2004, Mosby)

8. Polycythemia, cryoglobulinemia, and certain vasculitides
9. Carpal tunnel syndrome
10. Tools causing vibration
11. Estrogen replacement therapy without progesterone

DIAGNOSIS

- The diagnosis of Raynaud's phenomenon can be made by a history of well-demarcated digit discoloration induced by cold exposure and a physical examination looking for possible secondary causes.
- Initial pallor is typically necessary for the diagnosis to be made.
- The triphasic color changes can sometimes be induced in the office by placing the hand in an ice bath.

DIFFERENTIAL DIAGNOSIS

Table 297–1 describes the differential diagnosis of Raynaud's phenomenon.

WORKUP

- Once the diagnosis of Raynaud's phenomenon is established, differentiating primary from secondary is helpful in treatment and prognosis. History and physical examination usually make this distinction, whereas certain laboratory studies may predict secondary causes (see "Laboratory Tests").

- One test available but not commonly used is the nailfold microscopy. If positive, it may indicate the presence of underlying collagen-vascular disease and would therefore suggest a diagnosis of secondary Raynaud's phenomenon.

LABORATORY TESTS

- CBC, electrolytes, BUN, creatinine, ESR, ANA, VDRL, RF, and urinalysis should be included in the initial evaluation.
- If the history, physical examination, and initial laboratory tests suggest a possible secondary cause, specific serologic testing (e.g., anticentromere antibodies, anti–Scl 70, cryoglobulins, complement testing, and protein electrophoresis) may be indicated.

IMAGING STUDIES

- Chest x-ray may be helpful if a secondary cause, such as scleroderma, is suggested.
- Barium swallow may be helpful if CREST syndrome is suspected.
- Angiography is rarely needed for Raynaud's phenomenon but may be helpful in diagnosing Buerger's disease as a possible etiology.

TABLE 297–1 Differential diagnosis of Raynaud's phenomenon

Structural vasculopathies	Large and medium arteries	Thoracic outlet syndrome
		Brachiocephalic trunk disease (atherosclerosis, Takayasu's arteritis)
	Small artery and arteriolar	Systemic lupus erythematosus
		Dermatomyositis
		Overlap syndromes
		Cold injury
		Vibration disease
		Arteriosclerosis (thromboangiitis obliterans)
		Chemotherapy (bleomycin, vinblastine)
		Polyvinyl chloride disease
Normal blood vessels	Abnormal blood elements	Cryoglobulinemia
		Cryofibrinogenemia
		Paraproteinemia
		Cold agglutinin disease
		Polycythemias
	Abnormal vasomotion	Primary (idiopathic) Raynaud's phenomenon
		Drug-induced (ergots sympathomimetics)
		Pheochromocytoma
		Carcinoid syndrome
		Other vasospastic disorders (migraine, Prinzmetal's angina)

From Hochberg MC, Silman AJ, Smolen JS, et al (eds): Rheumatology, 3rd ed. St Louis, Mosby, 2003.

TREATMENT

- Avoid medications that may precipitate Raynaud's phenomenon (see "Cause").
- Avoid cold exposure. Use warm gloves, hats, and garments during the winter months or before going into cold environments (e.g., air-conditioned rooms).
- Avoid stressful situations.
- Avoid nicotine, caffeine, and over-the-counter decongestants.
- Typically, patients with Raynaud's phenomenon respond well to nonpharmacologic measures.
- Medications should be used if the above mentioned treatment does not work. Goal is to prevent digital ulcers and gangrene.
- Calcium channel blockers are the most effective treatment for Raynaud's phenomenon.

- Patients who do not tolerate or fail to respond to calcium channel blocker therapy can try other vasodilator drugs alone or in combination. Options include nitroglycerin, nitroprusside, hydralazine, papaverine, minoxidil, prazosin, niacin, and topical nitrates.
- Anticoagulation and thrombolytic therapy can be considered during the acute phase of an ischemic event when embolic or thrombotic complications are suspected. Aspirin (81 mg/day) therapy can be considered in all patients with secondary RP with a history of ischemic ulcers or thrombotic events; however, caution should be exercised, because aspirin can theoretically worsen vasospasm via inhibition of prostacyclin.
- Chemical (lidocaine or bupivacaine) or surgical sympathectomy has been reported to be effective in relief of symptoms for very severe, refractory cases; however, results of this therapy may be short-lived.

Chapter 298 / Scleroderma

DEFINITION

Scleroderma is a connective tissue disorder characterized by thickening and fibrosis of the skin (Fig. 298–1) and variably severe involvement of diverse internal organs.

PHYSICAL FINDINGS AND CLINICAL PRESENTATION

Physical Findings

SKIN

- Begins on hands (Fig. 298-2), then face (Fig. 298–3); skin is shiny, taut, sometimes red with loss of creases and hair
- Later, skin tightening may limit movement.
- Pigmentary changes occur.
- Skin atrophy occurs in late stages.

MUSCULOSKELETAL

- Symmetrical inflammatory arthritis
- Myopathy

GI INVOLVEMENT

- Esophageal dysmotility with heartburn, dysphagia, odynophagia
- Delayed gastric emptying
- Small bowel dysmotility with abdominal cramps and diarrhea
- Colon dysmotility with constipation
- Increased incidence of primary biliary cirrhosis

PULMONARY MANIFESTATIONS

- Pulmonary fibrosis with symptoms of dyspnea and nonproductive cough and fine inspiratory crackles on examination
- Pulmonary hypertension

CARDIAC INVOLVEMENT

- Myocardial fibrosis leading to congestive heart failure

RENAL INVOLVEMENT

- Malignant hypertension
- Rapidly progressive renal failure

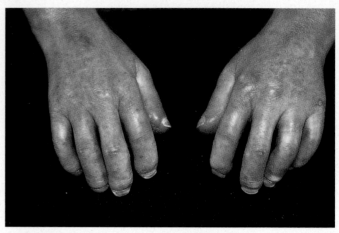

Fig 298–2
Systemic sclerosis: early stage showing characteristic swollen, sausage-shaped fingers.
(Courtesy of the Institute of Dermatology, London, UK.)

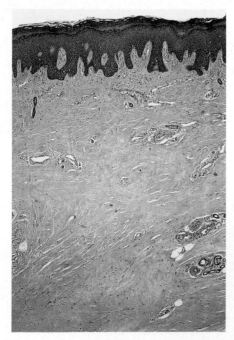

Fig 298–1
Systemic sclerosis: scanning view of acral skin showing dermal fibrosis. The specimen was a foot amputation performed because of severe vascular involvement.
(From Mckee PH, Calonje E, Granter SR [eds]: Pathology of the skin with clinical correlations, ed 3, St. Louis, 2005, Mosby)

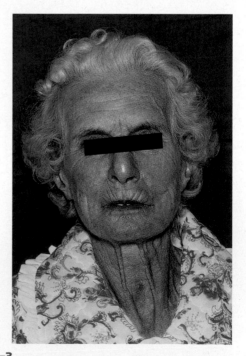

Fig 298–3
Systemic sclerosis: note the thinned lips and characteristic radiating furrows.
(Courtesy of R. A. Marsden, MD, St. George's Hospital, London, UK)

OTHER ORGAN INVOLVEMENT

- Hypothyroidism
- Erectile dysfunction
- Sjögren's syndrome
- Entrapment neuropathies
- Severe vascular involvement may result in intimal fibrosis and obliteration of the lumen (Fig. 298–4)

CREST SYNDROME

- Calcinosis (Fig. 298–5), Raynaud's syndrome, esophageal dysmotility, sclerodactyly, telangiectasias (Fig. 298–6) (in CREST, scleroderma is limited to distal extremities)

CLINICAL PRESENTATION

- Raynaud's phenomenon (Fig. 298–7): initial complaint in 70% (*Note:* The prevalence of Raynaud's syndrome is 5% to 10% of the general population; most do not progress to scleroderma.)

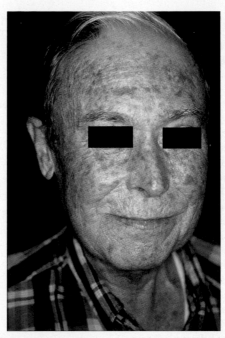

Fig 298–6
Facial telangietasias. Extensive facial telangiectasias in a man with CREST syndrome.
(From Hochberg MC, Silman AJ, Smolen JS, et al [eds]: Rheumatology, 3rd ed. St Louis, Mosby, 2003.)

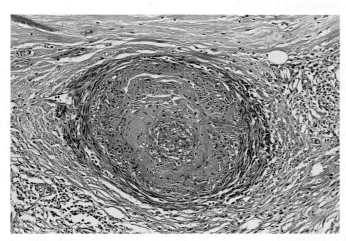

Fig 298–4
Systemic sclerosis: severe vascular involvement characterized by intimal fibrosis and obliteration of the lumen. Note the surrounding chronic inflammation and scarring.
(From McKee PH, Calonje E, Granter SR [eds]: Pathology of the skin with clinical correlations, ed 3, St. Louis, 2005, Mosby)

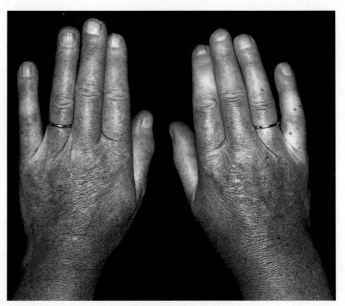

Fig 298–7
Raynaud's phenomenon in a patient with systemic sclerosis. The white discoloration is an essential clinical finding in Raynaud's phenomenon. The asymmetrical involvement and the presence of telangiestasia point to a possibility of a secondary cause for the Raynaud's phenomenon. Digital pitting scarring is one of the main criteria for the diagnosis of the systemic sclerosis.
(From Hochberg MC, Silman AJ, Smolen JS, et al [eds]: Rheumatology, 3rd ed. St Louis, Mosby, 2003.)

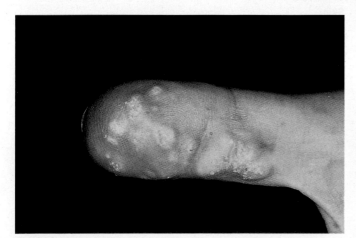

Fig 298–5
Subcutaneous calcinosis. Calcinosis of the finger tip.
(From Hochberg MC, Silman AJ, Smolen JS, et al [eds]: Rheumatology, 3rd ed. St Louis, Mosby, 2003.)

- Finger or hand swelling, sometimes associated with carpal tunnel syndrome. Digital gangrene (Fig. 298–8) may occur with CREST syndrome.
- Arthralgias/arthritis
- Internal organ involvement

CAUSE

Unknown. Unifying features exist despite heterogenous patterns of organ involvement and disease progression:

- Extracellular connective tissue activation
- Frequent immunologic abnormalities
- Inflammation
- Vasoconstriction

DIFFERENTIAL DIAGNOSIS

Dermatologic

- Mycosis fungoides
- Amyloidosis
- Porphyria cutanea tarda
- Eosinophilic fasciitis
- Reflex sympathetic dystrophy (RSD)

Systemic

- Idiopathic pulmonary fibrosis
- Primary pulmonary hypertension
- Primary biliary cirrhosis
- Cardiomyopathies
- GI dysmotility problems
- SLE and overlap syndromes

LABORATORY TESTS

- Antinuclear antibodies (homogeneous, speckled, or nucleolar patterns)
- Negative antibody to native DNA

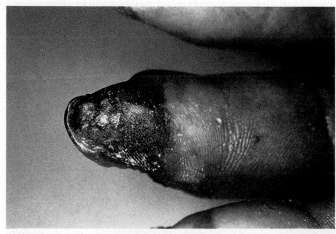

Fig 298–8
Digital gangrene. Sharply demarcated gangrene of several weeks duration of the fingertip of a woman with CREST syndrome.
(From Hochberg MC, Silman AJ, Smolen JS, et al [eds]: Rheumatology, 3rd ed. St Louis, Mosby, 2003.)

- Negative anti-Sm antibody
- Anti-nRNP positive in 20%
- RF positive in 30%
- Anticentromere antibodies in fewer than 10% with systemic illness and in 50% to 95% with limited scleroderma (i.e., good prognosis if positive)
- Positive extractable nuclear antibody to SCL 70 in 30%
- Routine biochemistry tests may indicate specific organ involvement (e.g., liver, kidney, muscle)

IMAGING AND OTHER STUDIES

Arthritis

- Joint radiographs

GI

- Barium swallow
- Cine esophagography
- Endoscopy
- Esophageal manometry

Pulmonary

- Chest radiograph
- Pulmonary function tests (PFTs)
- Chest CT scan
- Bronchoscopy with biopsy
- Gallium lung scan
- Bronchoalveolar lavage

Heart

- ECG
- Ambulatory (Holter) ECG monitoring
- Echocardiography
- Cardiac catheterization

Kidney

- Renal biopsy

Skin

- Skin biopsy

TREATMENT

- D-Penicillamine; recombinant human relaxin; supportive therapies used

Raynaud's syndrome

- Calcium channel blockers
- Peripheral alpha$_1$-adrenergic blockers

Arthralgias

- NSAIDs

Skin

- Moisturizing agents

Esophageal reflux

- H$_2$-receptor blockers
- Proton pump inhibitors

Pulmonary hypertension and fibrosis

- Oxygen
- Lung transplant

Renal involvement

- Angiotensin-converting enzyme inhibitors
- Dialysis
- Renal transplantation

Chapter 299 Mixed connective tissue disease

DEFINITION
The term *mixed connective tissue disease* describes a set of connective tissue symptoms that sometimes overlap with other known connective tissue diseases (SLE, progressive systemic sclerosis, polymyositis) but whose exact significance remains under debate. The disorder is sometimes referred to as an "overlap syndrome," but many prefer the term *undifferentiated connective tissue disease*.

PHYSICAL FINDINGS AND CLINICAL PRESENTATION
- Polyarthritis, polyarthralgia
- Raynaud's phenomenon, hand swelling (Fig. 299–1), or sclerodactyly
- Esophageal hypomotility, myalgia, and muscle weakness
- Other: pericarditis, facial erythema, psychosis

CAUSE
- Autoimmune disorder

DIFFERENTIAL DIAGNOSIS
- Other connective tissue disorders (SLE, progressive systemic sclerosis, polymyositis)

LABORATORY TESTS
- RF is often present in low titers.
- If myositis is present, muscle enzyme (CPK) levels increase.
- Positive ANA is often present with a speckled pattern.
- ESR is elevated.
- Anti-RNP antibodies may be present.

TREATMENT
- Except for pulmonary and scleroderma-like symptoms, response to corticosteroids is excellent in most cases.
- Rheumatoid symptoms may respond to NSAIDs, but other cases may not even respond to gold or penicillamine.
- Immunosuppressive agents are used on occasion, but the best therapeutic options remain uncertain.

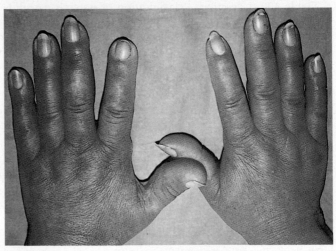

Fig 299–1
Swollen hands in mixed connective tissue disease. The presence of symmetrical puffy hands is a common early finding. Similar changes are often seen in the early stages of scleroderma.
(From Hochberg MC, Silman AJ, Smolen JS, et al [eds]: Rheumatology, 3rd ed. St Louis, Mosby, 2003.)

Chapter 300 **Vasculitides**

- Table 300–1 describes a classification of systemic vasculitis based on the size of the dominant vessel. The major categories of noninfectious vasculitis are noted in Figure 300–1.
- Figure 300–2 illustrates the pathogenesis of vasculitis.
- Vasculitis mimics are described in Table 300–2.
- An investigative approach to vasculitis is described in Table 300–3.

TABLE 300–1 Classification of systemic vasculitis

Dominant vessel	Primary	Secondary
Large arteries	Giant cell arteritis	Aortitis associated with RA
	Takayasu's arteritis	Infection (e.g., syphilis, TB)
Medium arteries	Classic PAN	Hepatitis B–associated PAN
	Kawasaki disease	
Small vessels and medium arteries	Wegener's granulomatosis*	Vasculitis secondary to RA, systemic lupus erythematosus, Sjögren's syndrome
	Churg–Strauss syndrome*	Drugs†
	Microscopic polyangiitis*	Infection (e.g., HIV)
Small vessels (leukocytoclastic)	Henoch–Schönlein purpura	Drugs†
	Cryoglobulinemia	Hepatitis C–associated
	Cutaneous leucocytoclastic angiitis	Infection

*Diseases most commonly associated with ANCA (antimyeloperoxidase and antiproteinase 3 antibodies) and a significant risk of renal involvement, and most responsive to immunosuppression with cydophosphamide.
†For example sulfonamides, penicillins, thiazide diuretics, and many others.
PAN, polyarteritis nodosa; RA, rheumatoid arthritis; TB, tuberculosis.
From Hochberg MC, Silman AJ, Smolen JS, et al (eds): Rheumatology, 3rd ed. St Louis, Mosby, 2003.

TABLE 300–2 Vasculitis mimics

Multisystem disease				
Infection	Subacute bacterial endocarditis		Others	Ergot
	Neisseria			Radiation
	Rickettsiae			Degos syndrome
Malignancy	Metastatic carcinoma			Severe Raynaud's syndrome
	Paraneoplastic			Acute digital loss
Other	Sweet's syndrome			Buerger's disease
Occlusive vasculopathy			**Angiographic**	
Embolic	Cholesterol crystals		Aneurysmal	Fibromuscular dysplasia
	Atrial myxoma			Neurofibromatosis
	Infection		Occlusion	Coarctation
	Calciphylaxis			
Thrombotic	Antiphospholipid syndrome			
	Procoagulant states			
	Cryofibrinogenemia			

From Hochberg MC, Silman AJ, Smolen JS, et al (eds): Rheumatology, 3rd ed. St Louis, Mosby, 2003.

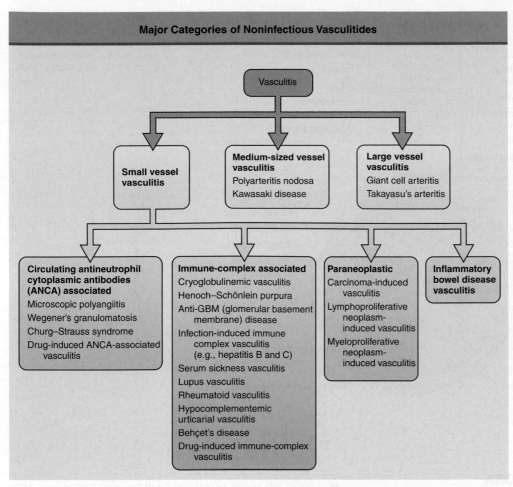

Major Categories of Noninfectious Vasculitides

Vasculitis

Small vessel vasculitis

Medium-sized vessel vasculitis
Polyarteritis nodosa
Kawasaki disease

Large vessel vasculitis
Giant cell arteritis
Takayasu's arteritis

Circulating antineutrophil cytoplasmic antibodies (ANCA) associated
Microscopic polyangiitis
Wegener's granulomatosis
Churg–Strauss syndrome
Drug-induced ANCA-associated vasculitis

Immune-complex associated
Cryoglobulinemic vasculitis
Henoch–Schönlein purpura
Anti-GBM (glomerular basement membrane) disease
Infection-induced immune complex vasculitis (e.g., hepatitis B and C)
Serum sickness vasculitis
Lupus vasculitis
Rheumatoid vasculitis
Hypocomplementemic urticarial vasculitis
Behçet's disease
Drug-induced immune-complex vasculitis

Paraneoplastic
Carcinoma-induced vasculitis
Lymphoproliferative neoplasm-induced vasculitis
Myeloproliferative neoplasm-induced vasculitis

Inflammatory bowel disease vasculitis

Fig 300–1
The major categories of noninfectious vasculitis. Not included are vasculitides that are known to be caused by direct invasion of vessel walls by infectious pathogens, such as rickettsial vasculitis and neisserial vasculitis.
(From Johnson RJ, Feehally J: Comprehensive Clinical Nephrology, 3rd ed, St. Louis, Mosby, 2007)

TABLE 300–3 Investigation of vasculitis

Assessment of Inflammation	Serological Tests
Blood count and differential (total white cell count, eosinophils)	ANCA (including proteinase 3 and myeloperoxidase)
Acute-phase response (ESR and CRP)	Antinuclear antibodies
Liver function	Rheumatoid factor
Assessment of Organ Involvement	Anticardiolipin antibodies
Urine analysis (proteinuria, hematuria, casts)	Complement
Renal function (creatinine clearance, 24-hour protein excretion, biopsy)	Cryoglobulins
	Differential Diagnosis
Chest radiograph	Blood cultures
Liver function	Viral serology (HBV, HCV, HIV, CMV)
Nervous system (nerve conduction studies, biopsy)	Echocardiography (two-dimensional, transesophageal, or both)
Muscle (EMG, creatine kinase, biopsy)	
Cardiac function (ECG, echocardiography)	
Gut (angiography)	
Skin (biopsy)	

CRP, C-reactive protein; ECG, electrocardiogram; EMG, electromyogram; ESR, erythrocyte sedimentation rate; HBV, HCV, hepatitis B and C viruses; CMV, cytomegalovirus.
From Hochberg MC, Silman AJ, Smolen JS, et al (eds): Rheumatology, 3rd ed. St Louis, Mosby, 2003

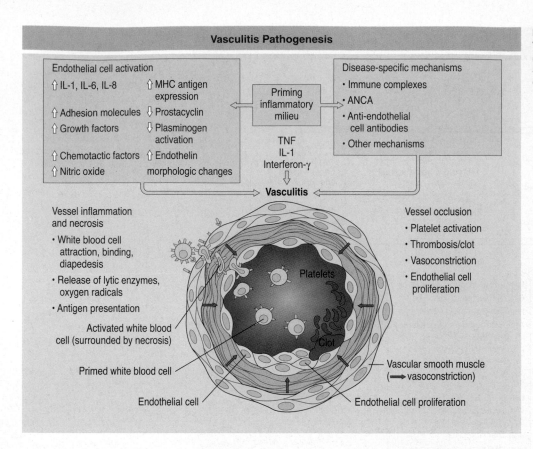

Vasculitis Pathogenesis

Endothelial cell activation
- ⬆ IL-1, IL-6, IL-8
- ⬆ Adhesion molecules
- ⬆ Growth factors
- ⬆ Chemotactic factors
- ⬆ Nitric oxide
- ⬆ MHC antigen expression
- ⬇ Prostacyclin
- ⬇ Plasminogen activation
- ⬆ Endothelin morphologic changes

Priming inflammatory milieu

TNF
IL-1
Interferon-γ

Disease-specific mechanisms
- Immune complexes
- ANCA
- Anti-endothelial cell antibodies
- Other mechanisms

Vasculitis

Vessel inflammation and necrosis
- White blood cell attraction, binding, diapedesis
- Release of lytic enzymes, oxygen radicals
- Antigen presentation

Vessel occlusion
- Platelet activation
- Thrombosis/clot
- Vasoconstriction
- Endothelial cell proliferation

Platelets

Clot

Activated white blood cell (surrounded by necrosis)

Primed white blood cell

Endothelial cell

Vascular smooth muscle (⟶ vasoconstriction)

Endothelial cell proliferation

Fig 300–2
Vasculitis pathogenesis. (From Hochberg MC, Silman AJ, Smolen JS, et al [eds]: Rheumatology, 3rd ed. St Louis, Mosby, 2003.)

A. POLYARTERITIS NODOSA

DEFINITION
- Polyarteritis nodosa is a vasculitic syndrome involving medium-size to small arteries (Fig. 300–3), characterized histologically by necrotizing inflammation of the arterial media and inflammatory cell infiltration (Fig. 300–4). The presence of any three of the following ten items allows the diagnosis of polyarteritis nodosa with a sensitivity of 82% and a specificity of 86%:
  1. Weight loss >4 kg
  2. Livedo reticularis
  3. Testicular pain or tenderness
  4. Myalgias, weakness, or leg tenderness
  5. Neuropathy
  6. Diastolic blood pressure >90 mm Hg
  7. Elevated BUN or creatinine
  8. Positive test for hepatitis B virus
  9. Arteriography revealing small or large aneurysms and focal constrictions between dilated segments (Fig. 300–5)
  10. Biopsy of small or medium-size artery containing WBCs

PHYSICAL FINDINGS AND CLINICAL PRESENTATION
- Typical presentation is subacute, with the onset of constitutional symptoms over weeks to months.
- Weight loss, nausea, vomiting
- Testicular pain or tenderness
- Myalgias, weakness, or leg tenderness
- Neuropathy (mononeuritis multiplex), foot drop

- Livedo reticularis, ulceration of digits, abdominal pain after meals, hematemesis, hematochezia, hypertension, asymmetrical polyarthritis (tending to involve the large joints of lower extremities); true synovitis occurs only in a minority of patients
- Fever may be present (polyarteritis nodosa is often a cause of fever of unknown origin) and can range from intermittent, low-grade fevers to high fevers with chills.
- Tachycardia is common and often striking.

CAUSE
- Unknown
- Hepatitis B virus–associated PAN appears to be an immune complex–mediated disease.

DIFFERENTIAL DIAGNOSIS
- Cryoglobulinemia
- SLE
- Infections (e.g., SBE, trichinosis, *Rickettsia*), lymphoma

LABORATORY TESTS
- Elevated BUN or creatinine, positive test for hepatitis B virus or hepatitis C
- Elevated ESR and C-reactive protein, anemia, elevated platelets, eosinophilia, proteinuria, hematuria
- Biopsy of small or medium-size artery of symptomatic sites (muscle, nerve) is >90% specific. Biopsies of the gastrocnemius muscle and sural nerve are commonly performed.
- Assays for ANA and RF are negative; however, low, nonspecific titers may be detected

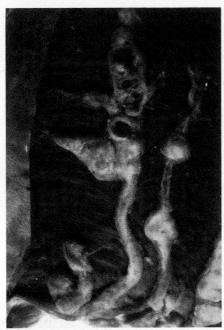

Fig 300-3
Polyarteritis nodosa: coronary arteries showing conspicuous aneurysmal dilatation are now very rarely seen (museum specimen). (Courtesy of the Department of Pathology, St Thomas' Hospital, London, UK.)

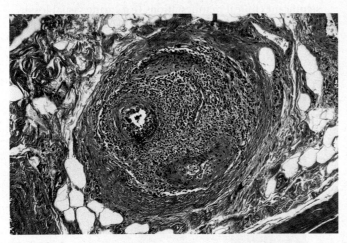

Fig 300-4
Necrotizing vasculitis with fibrinoid necrosis in polyarteritis nodosa. (From Silverberg SG: Principles and Practice of Surgical Pathology and Cytopathology. Churchill Livingstone, ed 4, 2006)

IMAGING STUDIES
Arteriography can be done in patients with negative biopsies or if there are no symptomatic sites. Visceral angiography will reveal aneurysmal dilation of the renal, mesenteric, or hepatic arteries.

TREATMENT
Prednisone 1 to 2 mg/kg/day; cyclophosphamide in refractory cases

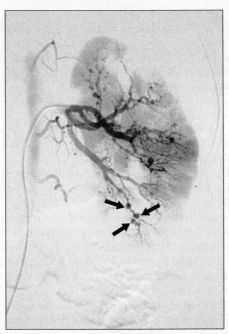

Fig 300-5
Renal angiogram in polyarteritis nodosa. Angiogram shows patchy renal perfusion defects and aneurysms *(arrows)*. (From Johnson RJ, Feehally J: Comprehensive Clinical Nephrology, ed 2, St. Louis, Mosby, 2000)

B. POLYMYALGIA RHEUMATICA

DEFINITION
Polymyalgia rheumatica is a disorder of unknown cause affecting older patients. It is characterized by shoulder and hip stiffness and an elevated ESR.

PHYSICAL FINDINGS AND CLINICAL PRESENTATION
● Symptoms are frequently of sudden onset but are often present for months before the diagnosis is made.
● Neck, shoulder, low back, and thigh pain are common complaints.
● Morning stiffness lasting 2 to 3 hours is typical, and patients often have difficulty getting out of bed.
● Malaise, weight loss, depression, and a low-grade fever are common constitutional symptoms and may suggest systemic inflammation.
● Physical findings are usually limited. Synovitis may be present in peripheral joints and may also be responsible for the proximal girdle symptoms in spite of the fact that they appear to be "muscular" in nature.
● Mild soft tissue tenderness may be present.
● Distal extremity manifestations (knee, wrist, MCP joints) may occur in 25% to 45% of patients.
● The temporal arteries should be carefully examined because of the strong relation of polymyalgia rheumatica with temporal or giant cell arteritis.

CAUSE
Unknown

DIFFERENTIAL DIAGNOSIS
● RA: RF is negative in polymyalgia.
● Polymyositis: enzyme studies are negative in polymyalgia.
● Fibromyalgia

WORKUP

The diagnosis of polymyalgia rheumatica is suggested by the following findings:

- Pain and stiffness of pectoral and pelvic musculature
- Patient >50 years old
- Morning stiffness >1 hour
- Normal motor strength
- Symptoms for at least 4 to 6 weeks
- Elevated ESR (>45)
- Rapid clinical response to low-dose corticosteroid therapy

LABORATORY TESTS

- CBC, ESR, and rheumatoid factor should be performed.
- Mild anemia may be present.

TREATMENT

- Prednisone 10 to 20 mg/day is given. The response is often so dramatic that it can be used to confirm the diagnosis. Improvement is usually noted within 24 to 48 hours. Generally, if the initial prednisone dose is 20 mg/day, reduce by 2.5 mg every weeks to 10 mg/day, then by 1 mg/day every month if tolerated.
- Steroids are gradually tapered over the next few weeks as soon as symptoms permit, but small doses (5 mg/day) may be needed for 2 years or longer.
- NSAIDs may be tried in mild cases.
- Physical therapy is usually unnecessary.

C. GIANT CELL ARTERITIS

DEFINITION

Giant cell arteritis (GCA) is a segmental systemic granulomatous arteritis affecting medium-size and large arteries in individuals >50 years old. Inflammation primarily targets extracranial blood vessels, and although the carotid system is usually affected, pathology in posterior cerebral artery has been reported.

PHYSICAL FINDINGS AND CLINICAL PRESENTATION:

GCA can present with the following clinical manifestations:

- Headache, often associated with marked scalp tenderness
- Constitutional symptoms (fever, weight loss, anorexia, fatigue)
- Polymyalgia syndrome (aching and stiffness of the trunk and proximal muscle groups)
- Visual disturbances (transient or permanent monocular visual loss)
- Intermittent claudication of jaw and tongue on mastication

Important physical findings in GCA:

- Vascular examination: tenderness, decreased pulsation, and nodulation of temporal arteries; diminished or absent pulses in upper extremities

CAUSE

Vasculitis of unknown etiology

DIAGNOSIS

Clinical history and vascular examination are the cornerstones of diagnosis.

The presence of any three of the following five items allows the diagnosis of GCA with a sensitivity of 94% and a specificity of 91%:

- Age at onset >50 years
- New-onset or new type of headache

- Temporal artery tenderness, dilated temporal arteries (Fig. 300–6), decreased pulsation
- Westergren ESR >50 mm/hr
- Temporal artery biopsy with vasculitis and mononuclear cell infiltrate or granulomatous changes (Fig. 300–7)

DIFFERENTIAL DIAGNOSIS

- Other vasculitic syndromes
- Nonarteritic anterior ischemic optic neuropathy (AION)
- Primary amyloidosis
- TIA, stroke
- Infections
- Occult neoplasm, multiple myeloma

LABORATORY TESTS

- ESR >50 mm/hr; however, up to 22.5% patients with GCA have normal ESR in early stages.
- C-reactive protein is typically included in laboratory investigation; it has greater sensitivity than ESR.
- Mild to moderate normochromic normocytic anemia, elevated platelet count

IMAGING STUDIES

- Reliability of color duplex ultrasonography of temporal artery is controversial as it is thought that it does not improve diagnostic accuracy over careful physical examination.
- Fluorescein angiogram of ophthalmic vessels may be warranted to differentiate between arteritic AION (i.e., GCA) and nonarteritic AION.

TREATMENT

- Intravenous methylprednisolone is indicated in those with significant clinical manifestations (e.g., acute visual loss).
- Oral prednisone (1 mg/kg/day) may be used under less urgent circumstances or following the initial period of treat-

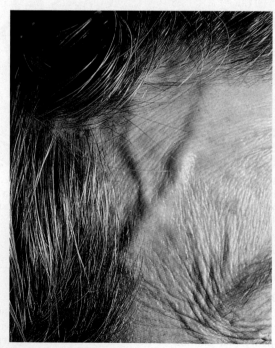

Fig 300–6
Dilated temporal arteries in a patient with giant cell arteritis.
(From Hochberg MC, Silman AJ, Smolen JS, et al [eds]: Rheumatology, 3rd ed. St Louis, Mosby, 2003.)

ment with intravenous methylprednisolone. High-dose oral regimen should be continued at least until symptoms resolve and ESR returns to normal. Prednisone treatment may generally last up to 2 years and is tapered over several months.

D. TAKAYASU'S ARTERITIS

DEFINITION

Takayasu's arteritis refers to a chronic systemic granulomatous vasculitis (Fig. 300–8) primarily affecting large arteries (aorta and its branches).

PHYSICAL FINDINGS AND CLINICAL PRESENTATION

Takayasu's arteritis most frequently involves the aortic arch and its branches and can manifest as:

- Arm claudication, weakness, and numbness
- Amaurosis fugax, diplopia, headache, and postural dizziness
- Systemic symptoms
  - Low-grade fever
  - Malaise
  - Weight loss
  - Fatigue
  - Arthralgia and myalgia

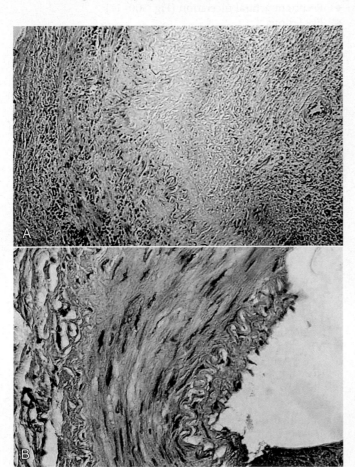

- Vascular bruits of the carotid artery, subclavian artery, and aorta
- Discrepancy of blood pressures between the upper extremities
- Absent pulses
- HTN
- Retinopathy
- Aortic insufficiency murmur

CAUSE

- The cause of Takayasu's arteritis is unknown. A delayed hypersensitivity to mycobacteria and spirochetes is a theory but remains to be substantiated.
- Infiltration of inflammatory cells into the vasa vasorum and media of large elastic arteries leads to thickening and narrowing or obliteration as well as aneurysmal dilation.

DIAGNOSIS

Criteria have been established for the diagnosis of Takayasu's arteritis by the American College of Rheumatology in 1990 and include:

- Age of disease <40 years
- Claudication of extremities
- Decreased brachial artery pulse
- Systolic BP difference >10 mm Hg between left and right arms
- Bruit over subclavian arteries or aorta
- Abnormal arteriogram
- Takayasu's arteritis is diagnosed if at least three of the six criteria are present, giving a sensitivity of 90% and a specificity of 98%.

DIFFERENTIAL DIAGNOSIS

Other causes of inflammatory aortitis must be excluded:

- Giant cell arteritis
- Syphilis
- Tuberculosis
- SLE
- Rheumatoid arthritis
- Buerger's disease
- Behçet's disease
- Cogan's syndrome

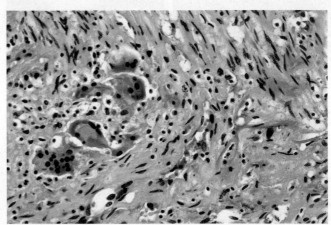

Fig 300–7
A, Temporal artery biopsy positive for giant cell arteritis. Note destruction of elastic lamina and complete luminal occlusion. **B,** Normal temporal artery specimen.
(From Yanoff M, Duker JS: Ophthalmology, ed 2, St. Louis, Mosby, 2004)

Fig 300–8
Takayasu's arteritis: high power showing granulomatous inflammation. The features are indistinguishable from giant cell arteritis.
(From McKee PH, Calonje E, Granter SR [eds]: Pathology of the skin with clinical correlations, ed 3, St. Louis, 2005, Mosby)

- Kawasaki disease
- Spondyloarthropathies

WORKUP

Any young patient with findings of absence pulses and loud bruits merits a workup for Takayasu's arteritis. The workup generally includes blood testing to look for signs of inflammation and imaging studies with the angiogram being the diagnostic gold standard.

LABORATORY TESTS

- CBC may reveal an elevated WBC count.
- ESR is elevated in active disease.

IMAGING STUDIES

- Ultrasound: Carotid, thoracic, and abdominal ultrasound are useful adjunctive imaging studies in diagnosing occlusive disease resulting from Takayasu's arteritis.
- Doppler and noninvasive upper and lower extremity studies are helpful in assessing blood flow and absent pulses.
- CT scan is used to assess the thickness of the aorta.
- Angiogram can show narrowing (Fig. 300–9) of the aorta and/or branches of the aorta, aneurysm formation, and poststenotic dilation. Angiographic findings are classified as four types:
  1. Type I: Lesions involve only the aortic arch and its branches.
  2. Type II: Lesions only involving the abdominal aorta and its branches.
  3. Type III: Lesions involving the aorta above and below the diaphragm.
  4. Type IV: Lesions involving the pulmonary artery.

TREATMENT

- Corticosteroids are the treatment of choice.
- Patients are monitored for symptoms and by following the ESR. If symptoms have resolved and the ESR is normal, attempts to taper prednisone are made.
- Patients who cannot be tapered off the corticosteroids or who have relapse of the disease are given methotrexate
- Cyclophosphamide can be given with glucocorticoids as adjunctive therapy in relapse or treatment-resistant patients.

E. BEHÇET'S SYNDROME

DEFINITION

Behçet's disease is a chronic, relapsing, inflammatory disorder characterized by the presence of recurrent oral aphthous ulcers, genital ulcers, uveitis, and skin lesions (Fig. 300–10). According to the International Study Group for Behçet's disease, the diagnosis of Behçet's disease is established when recurrent oral ulceration is present along with at least two of the following in the absence of other systemic diseases:

- Recurrent genital ulceration (Fig. 300–11)
- Eye lesions
- Skin lesions
- Positive pathergy test

PHYSICAL FINDINGS AND CLINICAL PRESENTATION

- Behçet's disease typically affects individuals in the third to fourth decade of life and primarily presents with painful aphthous oral ulcers. The ulcers occur in crops measuring 2 to 10 mm in size and are found on the mucous membranes of the cheek, gingiva, tongue, pharynx, and soft palate.
- Genital ulcers are similar to the oral ulcers.
- Decreased vision secondary to uveitis, keratitis, or vitreous hemorrhage, or occlusion of the retinal artery or vein may occur.
- Skin findings include nodular lesions, which are histologically equally divided into erythema nodosum–like lesions, superficial thrombophlebitis, and acne-like lesions, which are found at sites uncommon for ordinary acne (arms and legs)
- Arthritis and arthralgias
- CNS meningeal findings including headache, fever, and stiff neck can occur. Cerebellar ataxia and pseudobulbar palsy occur with involvement of the brainstem.
- Vasculitis leading to both arterial and venous inflammation or occlusion can result in signs and symptoms of a myocardial infarction, intermittent claudication, deep venous thrombosis, hemoptysis, and aneurysm formation.

CAUSE

The etiology of Behçet's disease is unknown. An immune-related vasculitis is thought to lead to many of the manifestations of Behçet's disease. What triggers the immune response and activation is not yet known.

DIFFERENTIAL DIAGNOSIS

- Ulcerative colitis
- Crohn's disease
- Lichen planus
- Pemphigoid

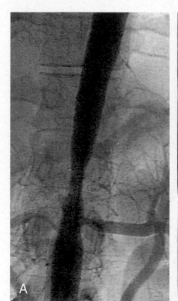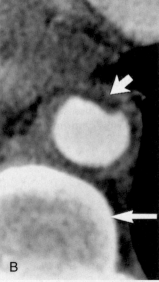

Fig 300–9

Takayasu's arteritis: (**A**) A 19-year-old woman with hyperaorta with narrowing of the lumen, occlusion of the celiac and superior mesenteric arteries, severe stenosis of the right renal artery, and mild stenosis of the left renal artery. There are prominent collaterals via the inferior mesenteric artery. (**B**) CT scan of the lower thoracic aorta (*short thick arrow*) shows that it is much more abnormal than was suspected on the aortogram. The aortic wall is thickened and irregular, and showed some enhancement with IV contrast. The lower dorsal vertebra is indicated by the *long lower arrow*.

(From Grainger RG, Allison DJ, Adam A, Dixon AK [eds]: Grainger and Allison's Diagnostic Radiology, 4th ed. Philadelphia, Churchill Livingstone, 2001.)

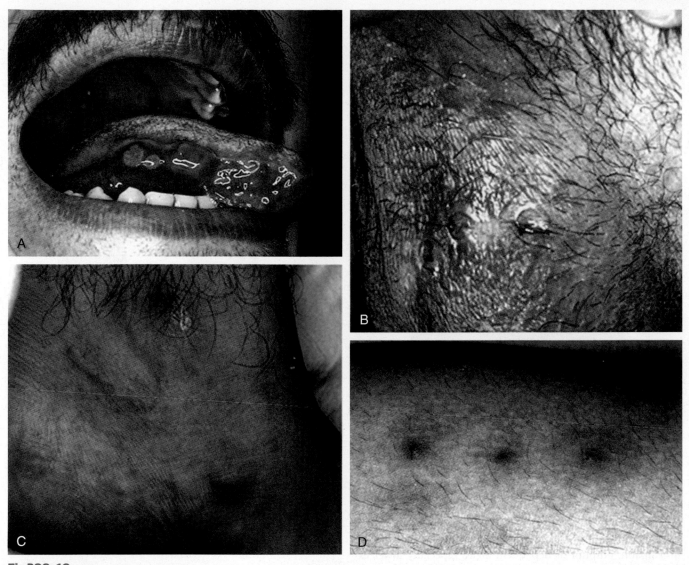

Fig 300–10
Mucocutaneous findings in Behcet's syndrome. (**A**) Oral apthae. (**B**) Genital ulceration. (**C**) Erythema-nodosum–like nodular lesions. (**D**) Multiple
positive pathergy tests.
(From Hochberg MC, Silman AJ, Smolen JS, et al [eds]: Rheumatology, 3rd ed. St Louis, Mosby, 2003.)

- Herpes simplex infection
- Benign aphthous stomatitis
- SLE
- Reiter's syndrome
- Ankylosing spondylitis
- AIDS
- Hypereosinophilic syndrome.
- Sweet's syndrome

LABORATORY TESTS
There are no diagnostic laboratory tests for Behçet's disease.

IMAGING STUDIES
CT scan, MRI, and angiography are useful for detecting CNS
and vascular lesions.

TREATMENT
Treatment is directed at the patient's clinical presentation (e.g.,
mucocutaneous lesions, ocular lesions, arthritis, GI, CNS, or
vascular lesions).

- Oral and genital ulcers: Topical corticosteroids (e.g., triamcinolone acetonide ointment applied tid). Tetracycline tablets 250 mg dissolved in 5 mL water and applied to the ulcer
for 2 to 3 minutes. Colchicine, thalidomide, dapsone, pentoxifylline, azathioprine, methotrexate
- Ocular lesions: anterior uveitis is treated with topical corticosteroids, infliximab
- CNS disease: chlorambucil. Patients not responding to chlorambucil can be tried on cyclosporine. In CNS vasculitis,
cyclophosphamide or prednisone can be used.
- Arthritis: NSAIDs, sulfasalazine
- GI lesions: sulfasalazine, prednisone
- Vascular lesions: prednisone, cytotoxic agents, heparin/
warfarin

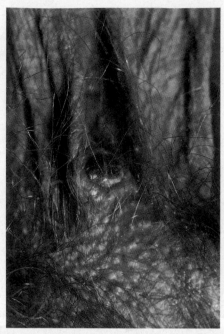

Fig 300–11
Behcet's disease: there is a typical scrotal ulcer with central slough.
(Courtesy of D. A. H. Yates, MD, St Thomas' Hospital, London, UK.)

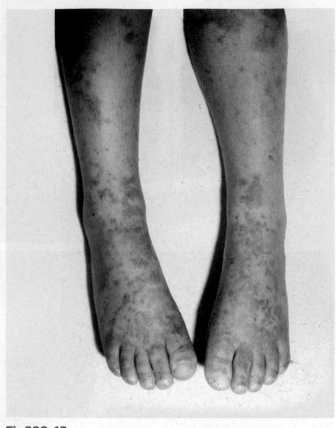

Fig 300–12
Lower extremity vasculitic rash usually found in Henoch-Schönlein purpura. However, it may be seen in other vasculitic disorders such as microscopic polyarteritis or Wegener's granulomatosis.
(From Hochberg MC, Silman AJ, Smolen JS, et al [eds]: Rheumatology, 3rd ed. St Louis, Mosby, 2003.)

F. HENOCH-SCHÖNLEIN PURPURA

DEFINITION
Henoch-Schönlein purpura (HSP) is a systemic small-vessel immune complex–mediated leukocytoclastic vasculitis characterized by a triad of palpable purpura, abdominal pain, and arthritis. It may also present with GI bleeding, arthralgias, and renal involvement.

PHYSICAL FINDINGS AND CLINICAL PRESENTATION
- Palpable purpura of dependent areas, especially lower extremities (Fig. 300–12), and areas subjected to pressure such as the beltline.
- Subcutaneous edema.
- Arthralgias and arthritis in 80%

- GI symptoms are seen in approximately one third of patients. Common findings are nausea, vomiting, diarrhea, cramping, abdominal pain, hematochezia, and melena.
- Anecdotally may follow URI.
- Renal involvement is seen in up to 80% of older children, usually within the first month of illness; <5% progress to end-stage renal failure; major cause of morbidity

CAUSE

- Presumptive etiology is exposure to a trigger antigen that causes antibody formation.
- Antigen-antibody (immune) complex deposition then occurs in arteriole and capillary walls of the skin, renal mesangium, and GI tract. IgA deposition is most common.
- Antigen triggers postulated include drugs, foods, immunization, and upper respiratory and other viral illnesses. Group A streptococcal infection is the most common precipitant in children, seen in up to one third of cases.
- Serologic and pathologic evidence suggests an association between parvovirus B19 and HSP, which may explain observed cases of HSP that do not respond to corticosteroids or other immunosuppressive therapy.

DIAGNOSIS

- Diagnosis is clinical.
- Skin manifestations are most common.
- Palpable purpura is seen in 70% of adult patients, whereas GI complaints are more common in children.
- Skin biopsy will show leukocytoclastic vasculitis.
- The presence of two of the following four American College of Rheumatology criteria yields a diagnostic sensitivity of 87.1% and specificity of 87.7%:
  - Palpable purpura unrelated to thrombocytopenia
  - Age <20 years at onset of first symptoms
  - Bowel angina or ischemia
  - Granulocytic infiltration of arteriole or venule walls on biopsy

DIFFERENTIAL DIAGNOSIS

- Polyarteritis nodosa
- Meningococcemia
- Thrombocytopenic purpura

LABORATORY TESTS

- Electrolytes, BUN, and creatinine
- Urinalysis
- CBC
- Prothrombin time, fibrinogen, and fibrin degradation products
- Blood cultures

Laboratory abnormalities are not specific for HSP. Leukocytosis and eosinophilia may be seen. IgA levels are elevated in approximately 50% of patients. Glomerulonephritis may be present (microscopic hematuria, proteinuria, and red blood cell [RBC] casts).

IMAGING STUDIES

Imaging studies are not useful in diagnosis of HSP. Arteriography or magnetic resonance angiography may be helpful in distinguishing from polyarteritis nodosa.

TREATMENT

- Corticosteroids are given if renal or severe GI disease, although benefits are not clear.
- Corticosteroids and azathioprine may be beneficial if rapidly progressive glomerulonephritis present. Pulse methyl prednisolone therapy has also been proposed in patients with glomerulonephritis, mesenteric vasculitis, or pulmonary involvement.
- NSAIDs for arthritis and arthralgias.

Chapter 301 Spondyloarthropathies

- Spondyloarthropathies or "spondyloarthritides" are seronegative arthritis syndromes characterized clinically by back pain, extra-articular disorders, and peripheral arthritis.
- These disorders show familial aggregation and are typically associated with HLA genes of the major histocompatibility complex, particularly HLA-B27.
- *Enthesitis*, inflammatory lesion at the insertion of tendon into bone, is the hallmark clinical feature of spondyloarthropathies (Fig. 301–1).
- *Dactylitis* or "sausage digit" (Fig. 301–2) is a feature of seronegative spondyloarthropathies in general.
- The principal differences among the seronegative spondyloarthropathies are summarized in Table 301–1.

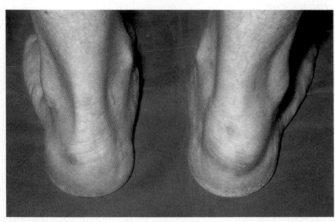

Fig 301–1
Enthesitis involving the insertion of the right Achilles tendon.
(From Hochberg MC, Silman AJ, Smolen JS, et al [eds]: Rheumatology, 3rd ed. St Louis, Mosby, 2003.)

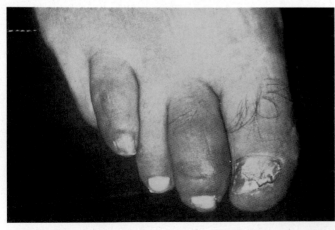

Fig 301–2
Dactylitis of the second toe.
(From Hochberg MC, Silman AJ, Smolen JS, et al [eds]: Rheumatology, 3rd ed. St Louis, Mosby, 2003.)

A. ANKYLOSING SPONDYLITIS

DEFINITION
Ankylosing spondylitis is a chronic inflammatory condition involving the sacroiliac joints and axial skeleton characterized by ankylosis and enthesitis (inflammation at tendon insertions).

PHYSICAL FINDINGS AND CLINICAL PRESENTATION
- Morning stiffness
- Fatigue, weight loss, anorexia, and other systemic complaints in more severe forms
- Bilateral sacroiliac tenderness (sacroiliitis)
- Limited lumbar spine motion
- Loss of chest expansion measured at the nipple line <2.5 cm, reflecting rib cage involvement
- Occasionally, peripheral joint involvement (large joints are more commonly affected)
- Possible extraskeletal manifestations affecting the cardiovascular system (aortic insufficiency, heart block, cardiomegaly), lungs (pulmonary fibrosis), and eye (uveitis)
- Tenderness at tendon insertion sites, especially the Achilles tendons
- Radiation below the knee is rare

CAUSE
Unknown. Genetic factors play an important role. Destructive changes probably due to release of cytokines and tumor necrosis factor.

DIFFERENTIAL DIAGNOSIS
- Diffuse idiopathic skeletal hyperostosis (DISH, Forestier's disease)
- Other spondyloarthropathies

WORKUP
The modified New York criteria are often used for diagnosis:
- Low back pain of at least 3 months' duration improved by exercise and not relieved by rest
- Limitation of lumbar spine movement in sagittal and frontal planes. Evaluation of true lumbar flexion (Fig. 301–3)
- Decreased chest expansion below normal values for age and sex
- Bilateral sacroiliitis of minimal grade or greater
- Unilateral sacroiliitis of moderate grade or greater

LABORATORY TESTS
- Elevated sedimentation rate, C-reactive protein
- Absence of RF and ANA
- Possible mild hyperchromic anemia
- Presence of HLA/B27 antigen in >90% of patients (although this antigen is often present in the general population)

IMAGING STUDIES
- Early radiographic features are those of bilateral sacroiliitis on plain films (Fig. 301–4).
- Vertebral bodies may become demineralized and a typical "squaring off" occurs.
- With progression, calcification of the annulus fibrosus and paravertebral ligaments develops, giving rise to the so-called bamboo spine appearance (Fig. 301–5).
- End result may be a forward protruding cervical spine and fixed dorsal kyphosis (Fig. 301–6).

TABLE 301-1 Seronegative spondyloarthropathies

	Ankylosing Spondylitis	Reiter's Syndrome	Psoriatic Arthritis	Arthritis Associated With Gastrointestinal Disease
Characteristics and presentation	Insidious onset of constant back pain lasting longer than 3 mo in patient younger than 40 yr of age Pain and stiffness are improved by exercise; patients often walk around at night to gain relief from nocturnal back pain Associated with anterior uveitis (25%), aortitis (5%)	Arthritis usually follows episode of urethritis Eye involvement: bilateral conjunctivitis, uveitis, keratitis, retinitis Dermatitis: usually painless mucocutaneous lesions on glans penis and mouth, hyperkeratotic lesions on palms and soles (keratoderma blennorrhagicum)	Arthritis usually involves DIP joints, Often resulting in "sausage" digits Skin lesions usually precede arthritis Nail changes (pitting) often accompany psoriatic arthritis	Occurs with Whipple's disease (up to 90% of patients) and with Crohn's disease (20%) After intestinal bypass With ulcerative colitis (10%) Remission of underlying disorder usually results in complete remission of the arthritis May be associated with erythema nodosum, pyoderma gangrenosum, anterior uveitis
Association with HLA-B27	Strong association	Strong association	No significant association	No significant association except in patients with IBD and sacroiliitis
Characteristic radiographic patterns of spine	Radiographs of spine initially show straightening of lumbar part of spine; in advanced disease diffuse syndesmophyte formation may result in fusion of entire spine (bamboo spine)	Unlike ankylosing spondylitis, distribution of syndesmophytes is asymmetric and nonmarginal	Similar to Reiter's syndrome	Radiographic evaluation may be normal or may reveal sacroiliitis
Peripheral arthritis	Oligoarticular hips, shoulder	Oligoarticular Asymmetrical Lower extremities	DIP joints Usually asymmetrical and oligoarticular but can be variable	Large joints (knees, ankles) Symmetrical
Therapy	NSAIDs, physical therapy	Joint immobilization NSAIDs Topical corticosteroids for conjunctivitis; corticosteroid therapy; physical therapy	Treat skin disease NSAIDs Methotrexate Etanercept	Treat underlying disorder Sulfasalazine for sacroiliitis associated with IBD

DIP, distal interphalangeal: IBD, inflammatory bowel disease: NSAID, nonsteroidal anti-inflammatory drug.
From Ferri F: Practical Guide to the Care of the Medical Patient, 7th ed. St Louis, Mosby, 2007.

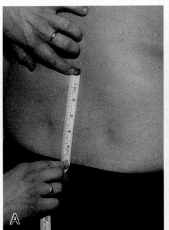
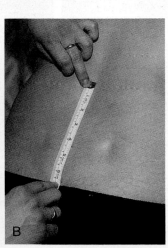

Fig 301-3
Macrae's modification of Schober's test. (**A**) The lumbosacral junction is identified between the dimples of Venus, and measurement made 5 cm below and 10 cm above. (**B**) The distraction of these marks is proportional to true lumbar flexion. In the example shown, the patient has AS and skin distraction is limited.
(From Hochberg MC, Silman AJ, Smolen JS, et al [eds]: Rheumatology, 3rd ed. St Louis, Mosby, 2003.)

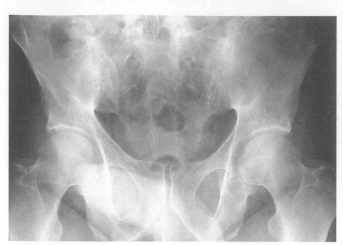

Fig 301–4
Ankylosing spondylitis. Plain radiograph of the pelvis demonstrating bilateral sacroiliitis with fusion of the sacroiliac joints.
(From Hochberg MC, Silman AJ, Smolen JS, et al [eds]: Rheumatology, 3rd ed. St Louis, Mosby, 2003.)

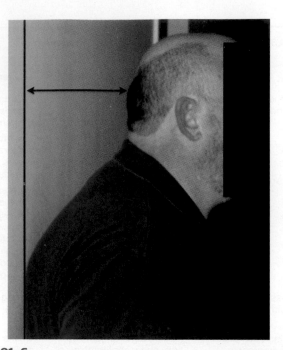

Fig 301–6
Patient with advanced ankylosing spondylitis involving the axial skeleton, demonstrating a characteristic posture with forward stoop of the neck. The *black lines* illustrate the occiput-to-wall measurement, obtained when a patient with black to the wall attempts to touch the wall with his occiput. An unaffected individual performing this test is able to touch the occiput to the wall.
(From Yanoff M, Duker JS: Ophthalmology, ed 2, St. Louis, Mosby, 2004)

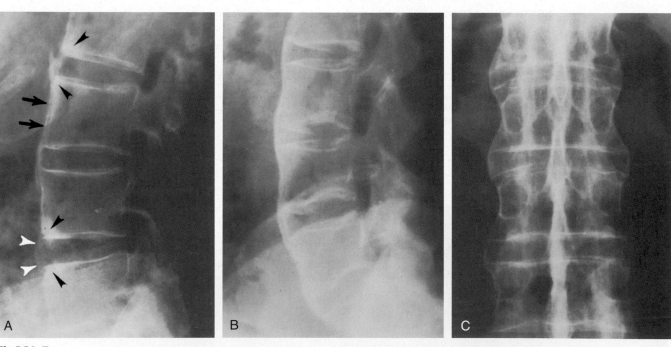

Fig 301–5
Ankylosing spondylitis involving the spine. (**A**) Early manifestations of ankylosing spondylitis in the lumbar spine include the development of an osteitis *(black arrowheads)* at the corners of vertebral body end plates that results in sclerosis and bone resorption. Early syndesmophytes *(white arrowheads)* are gracile, curvilinear calcifications extending from corner to corner. Mineralization of the anterior longitudinal ligament *(black arrows)* may contribute to the squared appearance of a vertebral body. (**B**) Lateral view shows mature appearance of ankylosed invertebral discs and apophyseal joints. These syndesmophytes are fairly thick. (**C**) gracile syndesmophytes at all levels create the 'bamboo spine' appearance.
(From Grainger RG, Allison DJ, Adam A, Dixon AK [eds]: Grainger and Allison's Diagnostic Radiology, 4th ed. Philadelphia, Churchill Livingstone, 2001.)

- MRI may be helpful in detecting early inflammatory lesions and is especially helpful when the history is suggestive but plain films are normal.

TREATMENT
- Exercises primarily to maintain flexibility; general aerobic activity also important
- Postural training
  1. Patients must be instructed to sit in the erect position and to avoid stooping; otherwise, a flexion contracture of the spine may develop, which can become so severe that the patient cannot see forward.
  2. Sleeping should be in the supine position on a firm mattress; pillows should not be placed under the head or knees.
- NSAIDs are often effective in relieving symptoms.
- New research into the use of tumor necrosis factor antagonists such as etanercept appears promising.

B. REITER'S SYNDROME

DEFINITION

Reiter's syndrome is one of the seronegative spondyloarthropathies, so called because serum RF is not present in these forms of inflammatory arthritis. Reiter's syndrome is an asymmetrical polyarthritis that affects mainly the lower extremities and is associated with one or more of the following:
- Urethritis
- Cervicitis
- Dysentery
- Inflammatory eye disease
- Mucocutaneous lesions

PHYSICAL FINDINGS AND CLINICAL PRESENTATION
- Polyarthritis
  1. Affecting the knees and ankles
  2. Commonly asymmetrical
- Heel pain and Achilles tendinitis, especially at the insertion of the Achilles tendon
- Plantar fasciitis
- Large effusions
- Dactylitis or "sausage toe" (Fig. 301–2)
- Urethritis
- Uveitis or conjunctivitis; uveitis can progress to blindness without treatment
- Keratoderma blennorrhagicum, circinate balanitis
  1. Hyperkeratotic lesions on soles of the feet, toes, penis, hands
  2. Closely resembles psoriasis
- Aortic regurgitation similar to that seen in ankylosing spondylitis

CAUSE
- Epidemic Reiter's syndrome following outbreaks of dysentery has been well described.
- Genetically susceptible HLA-B27 individuals are at risk for developing Reiter's syndrome following infection with certain pathogens:
  1. *Salmonella*
  2. *Shigella*
  3. *Yersinia enterocolitica*
  4. *Chlamydia trachomatis*

- Symptom complex indistinguishable from Reiter's syndrome has been described in association with HIV infection.

DIFFERENTIAL DIAGNOSIS
- Ankylosing spondylitis
- Psoriatic arthritis
- RA
- Gonococcal arthritis-tenosynovitis
- Rheumatic fever

LABORATORY TESTS
- Elevated but nonspecific ESR
- No specific laboratory tests to diagnose Reiter's syndrome

IMAGING STUDIES

Plain radiographs
- Juxta-articular osteopenia of affected joints
- Erosions and joint space narrowing in more advanced disease
- Periostitis and reactive new bone formation at the insertions of the Achilles tendon and the plantar fascia (Fig. 301–7)
- Sacroiliitis
  1. Unilateral or bilateral
  2. Indistinguishable from ankylosing spondylitis
- Vertebral bridging osteophytes

TREATMENT
- Enteric or urethral infection should be treated with appropriate antibiotic coverage.
- Uveitis should be treated with steroid eye drops in consultation with an ophthalmologist.
- Achilles tendinitis and plantar fasciitis may be treated with injections of methylprednisolone (40 to 80 mg).
- Sulfasalazine may be effective.
- Persistent and uncontrolled disease may be managed with cytotoxic drugs (methotrexate, azathioprine) in consultation with a rheumatologist.
- Flares treated with NSAIDs
- Physical therapy to maintain range of motion of the back and other joints

C. PSORIATIC ARTHRITIS

DEFINITION

Psoriatic arthritis is an inflammatory spondylarthritis occurring in patients with psoriasis who are usually seronegative for RF.

PHYSICAL FINDINGS AND CLINICAL PRESENTATION
- Usually gradual clinical onset
- Asymmetrical involvement of scattered joints
- Selective involvement of the DIP joints (described in "classic" cases but present in only 5% of patients)
- Symmetrical arthritis similar to RA in 15% of patients
- Possible development of predominant sacroiliitis in a small number of cases
- Advanced form of hand involvement (arthritis mutilans) in some patients
- Dystrophic changes in the nails (pitting, ridging) in many patients with DIP involvement (Fig. 301–8)
- Fingers (see Fig. 289–2) often assume a "sausage" appearance (dactylitis)

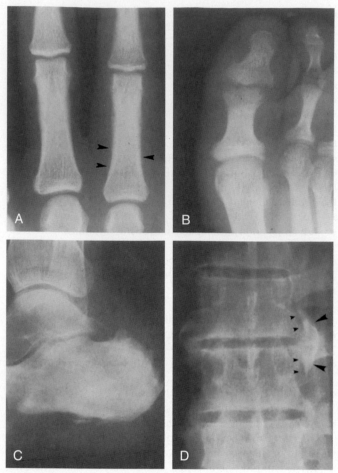

Fig 301–7
Reiter's arthropathy. (**A**) Posteroanterior view shows involvement of the ring finger with soft-tissue swelling, mild dimineralization and early periosteal reaction (arrowheads). (**B**) Anteroposterior view of the foot shows involvement of the great toe with soft-tissue swelling, mild demineralization, cartilage loss of the metatarsophalangeal joint, and erosions of the interphalangeal joint. (**C**) Lateral view of calcaneus shows sclerosis and diffuse enthesitis characterized by shaggy 'whiskered' new bone formation. (**D**) Paravertebral ossification (*large arrowheads*) along the thoracic spine shown as a large bony bar extending from midbody to midbody and in this example is partially separated from the spine by a lucent cleft (*small arrowheads*).
(From Grainger RG, Allison DJ, Adam A, Dixon AK [eds]: Grainger and Allison's Diagnostic Radiology, 4th ed. Philadelphia, Churchill Livingstone, 2001.)

CAUSE
Unknown. Destructive changes probably due to release of cytokines and TNF.

DIFFERENTIAL DIAGNOSIS
- RA
- Erosive osteoarthritis
- Gouty arthritis
- Ankylosing spondylitis

LABORATORY TESTS
- Slight elevation of ESR
- Possible mild anemia
- Possible HLA-B27 antigen (especially in patients with sacroiliitis)

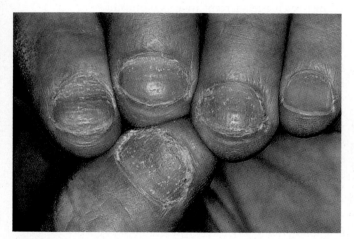

Fig 301–8
Psoriasis: there is conspicuous nail pitting.
(Reproduced with permission from Hordinksy, M.E., Sawaya, M.E., Scher, R.K. (eds) (2000) Atlas of hair and nails. Philadelphia: WB Saunders.)

IMAGING STUDIES

- Peripheral joint findings similar to those in rheumatoid arthritis but erosive changes in the distal phalangeal tufts characteristic of psoriatic arthritis (Fig. 301–9)
- Bony osteolysis; periosteal new bone formation
- Changes in axial skeleton: sacroiliitis, development of vertebral syndesmophytes (osteophytes) that often bridge adjacent vertebral bodies
- Paravertebral ossification
- Spinal changes: do not have same appearance as ankylosing spondylitis; however, spine abnormalities are less common than sacroiliitis

TREATMENT

- Rest
- Splinting
- Joint protection
- Physical therapy
- NSAIDs
- Occasional intra-articular steroid injections
- DMARDs: may be necessary in some patients

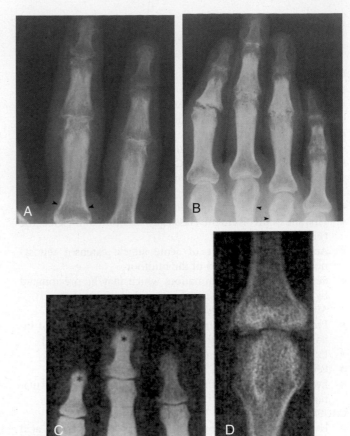

Fig 301–9
Psoriatic arthropathy in the fingers. (**A**) Intermediate stage of psoriatic arthropathy characterized by fusiform soft-tissue swelling (sausage digit), articular cartilage loss, some hypertrophy of proximal phalangeal ligamentous insertions and thin periosteal reaction at the base of the third proximal phalanx *(arrowheads)*. (**B**) Later stage in same patient shows some resolution of soft-tissue swelling, continued maintenance of bone mineral content, spontaneous ankylosis of most interphalangeal joints and destruction of the index finger proximal interphalangeal joint. Note the thin periosteal reaction along the metacarpal necks *(arrowheads)*. (**C**) Productive bone formation involves two distal phalangeal tufts *(asterisk)*. Marginal erosions, present at the bases, are associated with soft-tissue swelling and short thick fingernails. (**D**) Characteristic marginal erosions *(arrowheads)* at a metacarpophalangeal joint.
(From Grainger RG, Allison D- Grainger AND Allison's Diagnostic Radiology, a textbook of Medical Imaging, Churchill Livingstone, ed 4, 2001)

Chapter 302 | **Crystal-related arthritis**

A. GOUT

DEFINITION

Gout is a clinical disorder in which crystals of monosodium urate become deposited in tissue as a result of hyperuricemia. Gout and hyperuricemia can be classified as either primary or secondary if resulting from another disorder.

PHYSICAL FINDINGS AND CLINICAL PRESENTATION

- Usually, initial attack in a single joint or an area of tenosynovium
- Mainly a disease of the lower extremities
- First site of involvement: classically, MP joint of the great toe (Fig. 302–1)
- Another common site of acute attack: extensor tenosynovium on the dorsum of the midfoot
- Severe pain and inflammation, which may be precipitated by exercise, dietary indiscretions, and physical stress
- Attacks following illness or surgery
- Presence of swelling, heat, redness, and other signs of inflammation (the physical findings simulating cellulitis)
- Exquisite soft tissue tenderness
- Fever, tachycardia, and other constitutional symptoms
- Eventually, deposits of urate crystals (tophi) in the subcutaneous tissue (Fig. 302–2)

CAUSE

- Hyperuricemia and gout develop from excessive uric acid production, a decrease in the renal excretion of uric acid, or both.
- Primary gout results from an inborn error of metabolism and may be attributed to several biochemical defects.
- Secondary hyperuricemia may develop as a complication of acquired disorders (e.g., leukemia) or as a result of the use of certain drugs (e.g., diuretics).

DIFFERENTIAL DIAGNOSIS

- Pseudogout
- Rheumatoid arthritis
- Osteoarthritis
- Cellulitis
- Infectious arthritis

LABORATORY TESTS

- Hyperuricemia
- Synovial aspirate: usually cloudy and markedly inflammatory in nature; urate crystals in fluid: needle-shaped and birefringent under polarized light (Fig. 302–3)

IMAGING STUDIES

- Plain radiography to rule out other disorders
- No typical findings in early gouty arthritis but late disease possibly associated with characteristic punched-out lesions and joint destruction (Fig. 302–4)

TREATMENT

- Quick-acting NSAIDs such as ibuprofen
- Colchicine
- Corticosteroids or ACTH for those who are intolerant of NSAIDs or colchicine
- Intra-articular cortisone when oral medication cannot be given
- General measures such as rest, elevation, and analgesics as needed until acute pain subsides
- Modification of diet (avoidance of foods high in purines [e.g., anchovies, organ meat, liver, spinach, mushrooms, asparagus, oatmeal, cocoa, sweetbreads]) and lifestyle
- Moderation in alcohol intake
- HTN and its management requiring careful assessment and possibly nondiuretic drugs

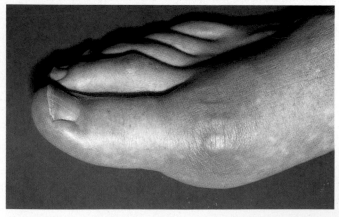

Fig 302–1
Redness as seen in gout. This is a valuable indicator of the intensity of underlying joint inflammation
(From Hochberg MC, Silman AJ, Smolen JS, et al [eds]: Rheumatology, 3rd ed. St Louis, Mosby, 2003.)

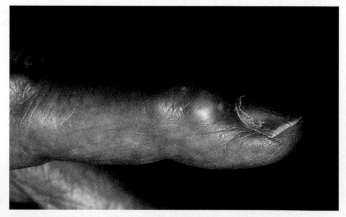

Fig 302–2
Tophus overlying a Heberden's node in a woman on a diuretic.
(From Hochberg MC, Silman AJ, Smolen JS, Weinblatt ME, Weisman MH eds: *Rheumatology*, 3rd ed, St. Louis, Mosby 2004)

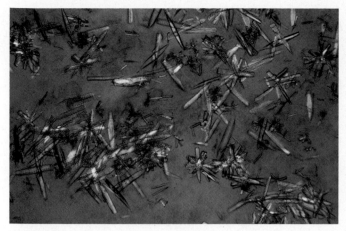

Fig 302-3
Gout: characteristic needle-shaped crystals.
(Courtesy of G.T. McKee, M.D., Massachusetts General Hospital,
Boston)

B. PSEUDOGOUT

DEFINITION
Pseudogout is one of the clinical patterns associated with a crystal-induced synovitis resulting from the deposition of calcium pyrophosphate dehydrate (CPPD) crystals in joint hyaline and fibrocartilage. The cartilage deposition is termed *chondrocalcinosis.* Tissue sites of CPPD deposition are shown in Figure 302-5.

PHYSICAL FINDINGS AND CLINICAL PRESENTATION
- Symptoms are similar to those of gouty arthritis with acute attacks and chronic arthritis.
- Knee joint is most commonly affected (Fig. 302-6).
- Swelling, stiffness, and increased heat in affected joint

CAUSE
- Unknown
- Often associated with various medical conditions, including hyperparathyroidism and amyloidosis

DIFFERENTIAL DIAGNOSIS
- Gouty arthritis
- RA
- Osteoarthritis
- Neuropathic joint

WORKUP
- Diagnosis dependent on the identification of CPPD crystals
- The American Rheumatism Association–revised diagnostic criteria for CPPD crystal deposition disease (pseudogout) are often used:

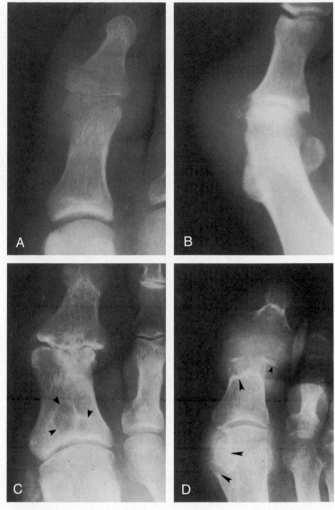

Fig 302-4
Gout of the great toe may have a spectrum of presentation. (**A**) Acute inflammatory gout presented as symmetrical interphalangeal soft-tissue swelling and uniform cartilage loss. This pattern of radiologic presentation is easily confused with rheumatoid arthritis. (**B**) Chronic tophaceous gout presented as a large eccentric periarticular mass with a few small flecks of mineralization giving a lacelike pattern at the periosteal surface. Note that the bone mineral content is normal and that the metatarsophalangeal cartilage is fairly well preserved. (**C**) Chronic articular gout presented with interphalangeal joint cartilage and subchondral cortical destruction. Note that despite the degree of joint involvement, the bone mineral content is maintained. Small intraosseous tophi are present in the base of the proximal phalanx *(arrowheads)* and a small mineralized tophus is located medial to the metatarsal head. (**D**) Chronic tophaceous gout presented with destruction of the interphalangeal joint. The chronicity of the mass has permitted the distal and proximal phalanges to form mineralized margins called 'clasps' around the tophus *(small arrowhead).* Note that other bone erosions of the proximal phalanx and metatarsal head *(large arrowheads)* are more distant from the joint (periarticular) than the marginal erosions of rheumatoid arthritis.
(From Grainger RG, Allison DJ, Adam A, Dixon AK [eds]: Grainger and Allison's Diagnostic Radiology, 4th ed. Philadelphia, Churchill Livingstone, 2001.)

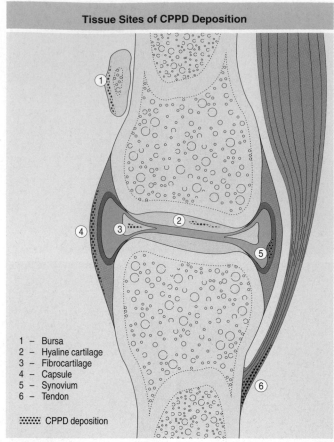

Tissue Sites of CPPD Deposition

1 – Bursa
2 – Hyaline cartilage
3 – Fibrocartilage
4 – Capsule
5 – Synovium
6 – Tendon

:::::: CPPD deposition

Fig 302–5
Tissue sites of CPPD deposition.
(From Hochberg MC, Silman AJ, Smolen JS, et al [eds]: Rheumatology, 3rd ed. St Louis, Mosby, 2003.)

1. Criteria

I. Demonstration of CPPD crystals (obtained by biopsy, necroscopy, or aspirated synovial fluid) by definitive means (e.g., characteristic "fingerprint" by x-ray diffraction powder pattern or by chemical analysis)

II. (a) Identification of monoclinic and/or triclinic crystals showing either no or only a weakly positive birefringence by compensated polarized light microscopy (Fig. 302–7)
    (b) Presence of typical calcifications in x-rays (Fig. 302–8)

III. (a) Acute arthritis, especially of knees or other large joints, with or without concomitant hyperuricemia
    (b) Chronic arthritis, especially of knees, hips, wrists, carpus, elbow, shoulder, and MCP joints, especially if accompanied by acute exacerbations; the following features are helpful in differentiating chronic arthritis from osteoarthritis:

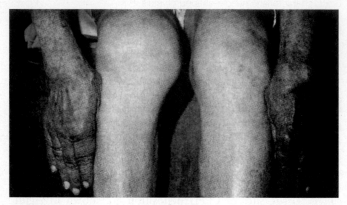

Fig 302–6
Chronic pyrophosphate arthropathy.
(From Hochberg MC, Silman AJ, Smolen JS, et al [eds]: Rheumatology, 3rd ed. St Louis, Mosby, 2003.)

1. Uncommon site—for example, the wrist, MCP, elbow, shoulder
2. Appearance of lesion radiologically—for example, radio-carpal or patellofemoral joint space narrowing, especially if isolated (patella "wrapped around" the femur)
3. Subchondral cyst formation
4. Severity of degeneration—progressive, with subchondral bony collapse (microfractures), and fragmentation, with formation of intra-articular radiodense bodies
5. Osteophyte formation and inconstant
6. Tendon calcifications, especially Achilles, triceps, obturators

2. Categories

Definite—criteria I or II (a) plus (b) must be fulfilled.
Probable—criteria II (a) or II (b) must be fulfilled.
Possible—criteria III (a) or (b) should alert the clinician to the possibility of underlying CPPD deposition.

LABORATORY TESTS

Crystal analysis of the synovial fluid aspirate to reveal rhomboid calcium pyrophosphate crystals

IMAGING STUDIES

Plain radiographs to reveal the following:

- Stippled calcification in bands running parallel to the subchondral bone margins
- Crystal deposition in menisci, synovium, and ligament tissue; triangular wrist cartilage and symphysis pubis are often affected

TREATMENT

- NSAIDs
- Colchicine
- Aspiration/steroid injection
- General measures such as rest and elevation as needed

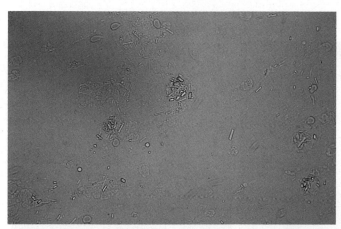

Fig 302–7
Synovial fluid CPPD crystals.
(From Hochberg MC, Silman AJ, Smolen JS, et al [eds]: Rheumatology, 3rd ed. St Louis, Mosby, 2003.)

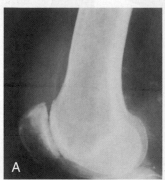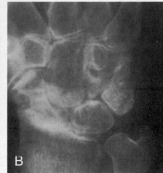

Fig 302–8
Calcium pyrophosphate dehydrate crystal disease. (**A**) Lateral view of knee shows the presence of a large joint effusion indicating the acute inflammatory syndrome–'pseudogout.' Note the irregular articular surfaces of the patellofemoral joint, a manifestation of CPPD arthropathy. (**B**) Posteroanterior view of the wrist shows focal cartilage loss at the radioscaphoid joint with subchrondral sclerosis of the opposing articular surfaces. Other than minor chondrocalcinosis of the ulnar triangular cartilage, the remainder of the wrist is unremarkable.
(From Grainger RG, Allison DJ, Adam A, Dixon AK [eds]: Grainger and Allison's Diagnostic Radiology, 4th ed. Philadelphia, Churchill Livingstone, 2001.)

Chapter 303   Fibromyalgia

DEFINITION
Fibromyalgia is a poorly defined disorder characterized by multiple trigger points and referred pain.

PHYSICAL FINDINGS
- Tender "nodules" and tender points (Fig. 303–1)
- Skin rolling tenderness and reactive hyperemia (Fig. 303–2)

CAUSE
- Unknown

DIFFERENTIAL DIAGNOSIS
- Polymyalgia rheumatica
- Referred discogenic spine pain
- RA
- Localized tendinitis
- Connective tissue disease
- Osteoarthritis
- Thyroid disease
- Spondyloarthropathies

WORKUP
- Subsets of this disorder are often described:
  1. If symptoms develop in conjunction with other conditions (rheumatoid disease or acute stress)
  2. If findings are more regionally distributed, such as those in the neck following motor vehicle accidents
- The primary condition is often suggested by the following criteria from the American College of Rheumatology:
  1. History of widespread pain
  2. Pain in 11 of 18 selected tender spots on digital palpation (mainly in the spine, elbows, and knees)

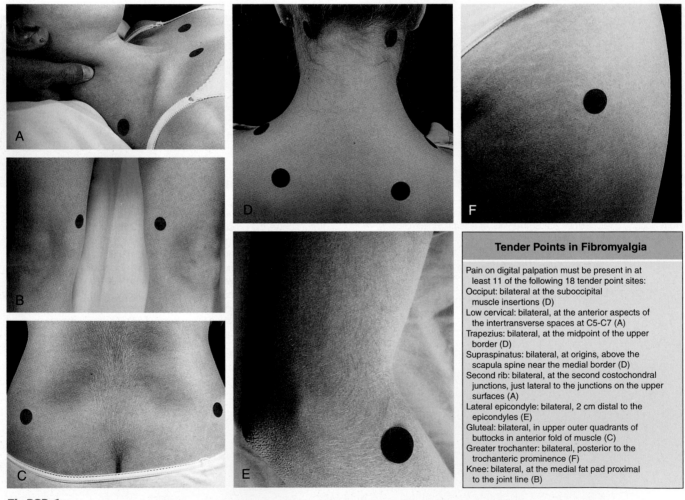

Tender Points in Fibromyalgia

Pain on digital palpation must be present in at least 11 of the following 18 tender point sites:
Occiput: bilateral at the suboccipital muscle insertions (D)
Low cervical: bilateral, at the anterior aspects of the intertransverse spaces at C5-C7 (A)
Trapezius: bilateral, at the midpoint of the upper border (D)
Supraspinatus: bilateral, at origins, above the scapula spine near the medial border (D)
Second rib: bilateral, at the second costochondral junctions, just lateral to the junctions on the upper surfaces (A)
Lateral epicondyle: bilateral, 2 cm distal to the epicondyles (E)
Gluteal: bilateral, in upper outer quadrants of buttocks in anterior fold of muscle (C)
Greater trochanter: bilateral, posterior to the trochanteric prominence (F)
Knee: bilateral, at the medial fat pad proximal to the joint line (B)

Fig 303–1
Locations of the nine pairs of tender points for diagnositc classification of fibromyalgia.
(From Hochberg MC, Silman AJ, Smolen JS, et al [eds]: Rheumatology, 3rd ed. St Louis, Mosby, 2003.)

LABORATORY TESTS

There are no abnormalities in fibromyalgia, but laboratory assessment may be required to rule out other conditions and may include:

- CBC, ESR, rheumatoid factor, ANA
- CPK, T_4, TSH

TREATMENT

- Explanation, reassurance
- Tricyclic antidepressants for sleep disturbance
- Aerobic and stretching exercise, particularly swimming
- Mild analgesics; avoidance of chronic narcotic use
- Trigger point injections
- Physical therapy
- Pregabalin and/or duloxetine may be effective in pain relief

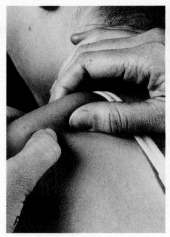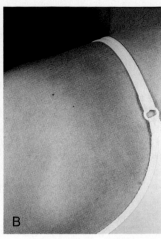

Fig 303–2
Skin rolling tenderness (**A**) and reactive hyperemia (**B**) in fibromyalgia. (From Hochberg MC, Silman AJ, Smolen JS, et al [eds]: Rheumatology, 3rd ed. St Louis, Mosby, 2003.)

Chapter 304 Regional rheumatic diseases

A. JAW

1. Temporomandibular joint syndrome

DEFINITION

Temporomandibular joint (TMJ) syndrome refers to a group of disorders leading to symptoms affecting the TMJ.

PHYSICAL FINDINGS AND CLINICAL PRESENTATION

- Otalgia
- Odontalgia
- Headaches (frontal, temporal, retro orbital)
- Tinnitus
- Dizziness
- Clicking or popping sounds with movement of the TMJ (Fig. 304–1)
- Joint locking
- Tender to palpation
- Limited range of motion of the TMJ (Figs. 304–2 and 304–3)

CAUSE

Causes of TMJ syndrome are multifactorial, encompassing local anatomic anomalies to familiar disease processes that can involve the TMJ.

- Myofascial pain-dysfunction syndrome (MPD): the most common cause of TMJ syndrome and results from teeth grinding and clenching the jaw (bruxism)
- Internal TMJ derangement: abnormal connection of the articular disc to the mandibular condyle
- Degenerative joint disease
- RA
- Gouty arthritis
- Pseudogout
- Ankylosing spondylitis

- Trauma
- Prior surgery (orthodontic, intra-articular steroid injection)
- Tumors

DIFFERENTIAL DIAGNOSIS

The differential diagnosis of TMJ syndrome is thought of in terms of etiology and includes the list as mentioned previously under "Cause." MDS, internal TMJ derangement, and degenerative joint disease represent >90% of all causes of TMJ syndrome.

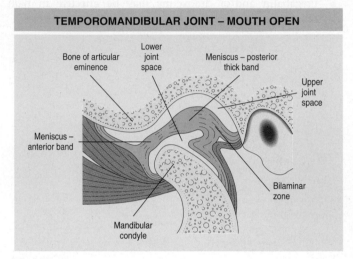

Fig 304–2

The temporomandibular joint in the open position.
(From Hochberg MC, Silman AJ, Smolen JS, et al [eds]: Rheumatology, 3rd ed. St Louis, Mosby, 2003.)

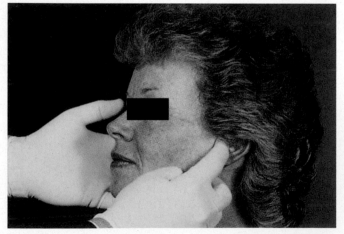

Fig 304–1

Extraoral examination
(From Hochberg MC, Silman AJ, Smolen JS, et al [eds]: Rheumatology, 3rd ed. St Louis, Mosby, 2003.)

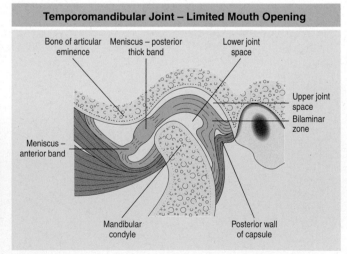

Fig 304–3

Limited opening of the temporomandibular joint showing anterior displacement of the meniscus.
(From Hochberg MC, Silman AJ, Smolen JS, et al [eds]: Rheumatology, 3rd ed. St Louis, Mosby, 2003.)

IMAGING STUDIES
- Plain x-rays: The most common x-rays are the panoramic, transorbital, and transpharyngeal views in both opened and closed positions.
- Arthrography is helpful in looking for meniscus involvement.
- CT scanning is very accurate in diagnosing meniscal and osseous derangements of the TMJ.
- MRI can better visualize soft tissue inflammation, if present.

TREATMENT
- Soft diet to rest the muscles of mastication
- Heat 15 to 20 minutes four to six times per day
- Massage of the masseter and temporalis muscles
- Formed splints or bite appliances (Fig. 304–4)
- Range-of-motion exercises
- NSAIDs, titrated to relieve symptoms
- Muscle relaxants
- In degenerative joint disease of the TMJ, intra-articular steroid injection can be tried

B. HAND AND WRIST
1. Carpal tunnel syndrome

DEFINITION

Carpal tunnel syndrome is an entrapment neuropathy involving the median nerve at the wrist (Fig. 304–5). It is the most common entrapment neuropathy in the upper extremity.

PHYSICAL FINDINGS AND CLINICAL PRESENTATION
- Nocturnal pain
- Occasional median nerve sensory impairment (often only index and long fingers)
- Positive *Tinel's sign* at wrist (tapping over the median nerve on the flexor surface of the wrist produces a tingling sensation radiating from the wrist to the hand) (Fig. 304–6)
- Positive *Phalen's test* (reproduction of symptoms after 1 minute of gentle, unforced wrist flexion) (Fig. 304–7)

- *Carpal compression test:* pressure with the examiner's thumb over the patient's carpal tunnel for 30 seconds elicits symptoms
- Thenar atrophy in long-standing cases (Fig. 304–8)

CAUSE
- Idiopathic in most cases
- Space-occupying lesions in carpal tunnel (tenosynovitis, ganglia, aberrant muscles)
- Often associated with hypothyroidism, hormonal changes of pregnancy
- Job-related mechanical overuse may be a risk factor.
- Traumatic injuries to the wrist

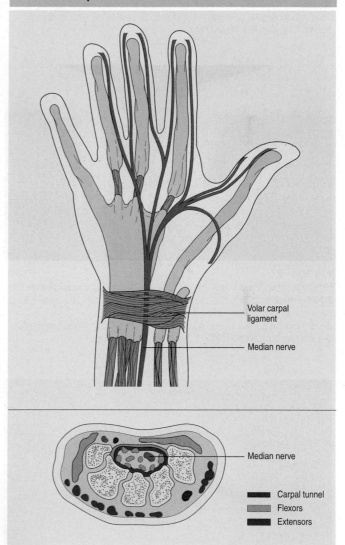

The Carpal Tunnel and Course of the Median Nerve

Volar carpal ligament

Median nerve

Median nerve

Carpal tunnel
Flexors
Extensors

Fig 304–5
The carpal tunnel and course of the median nerve. The space for the median nerve and flexor tendons is very confined. The median nerve courses under the region occupied by the palmaris longus and flexor carpi radialis tendons.
(From Hochberg MC, Silman AJ, Smolen JS, et al [eds]: Rheumatology, 3rd ed. St Louis, Mosby, 2003.)

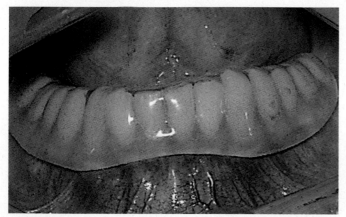

Fig 304–4
Occlusal splint.
(From Hochberg MC, Silman AJ, Smolen JS, et al [eds]: Rheumatology, 3rd ed. St Louis, Mosby, 2003.)

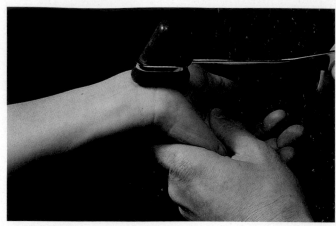

Fig 304-6
Tinel's sign. The wrist is held in extension while gentle percussion is performed over and just proximal to the transverse carpal ligament.
(From Hochberg MC, Silman AJ, Smolen JS, et al [eds]: Rheumatology, 3rd ed. St Louis, Mosby, 2003.)

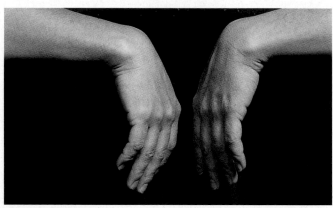

Fig 304-7
Phalen's (wrist flexion) test. With the wrists held in unforced flexion for 30-60 seconds, a positive test reproduces or worsens the patient's symptoms.
(From Hochberg MC, Silman AJ, Smolen JS, et al [eds]: Rheumatology, 3rd ed. St Louis, Mosby, 2003.)

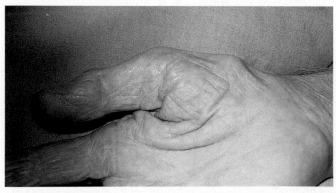

Fig 304-8
Thenar muscle atrophy. Chronic entrapment of the median nerve in the carpal tunnel or more proximally may produce thenar atrophy, as seen in this patient.
(From Hochberg MC, Silman AJ, Smolen JS, et al [eds]: Rheumatology, 3rd ed. St Louis, Mosby, 2003.)

DIFFERENTIAL DIAGNOSIS
- Cervical radiculopathy
- Chronic tendinitis
- Vascular occlusion
- Reflex sympathetic dystrophy (RSD)
- Osteoarthritis
- Other arthritides
- Other entrapment neuropathies

IMAGING STUDIES
Routine x-rays may be helpful in establishing cause or ruling out other conditions.

ELECTRODIAGNOSTIC STUDIES
Nerve conduction velocity tests and EMG are useful in establishing the diagnosis and ruling out other syndromes.

TREATMENT
- Elimination of repetitive trauma
- Occupational splints or braces
- NSAIDs
- Injection of carpal canal on ulnar side of palmaris longus tendon at wrist flexor crease (avoiding median nerve) (Fig. 304-9)
- Low-dose oral corticosteroids are also effective for symptom relief in select patients.
- Stretching exercises
- Surgical referral in cases of failed medical management or signs of motor weakness. Results of surgery usually excellent with return to full activity in 4 to 6 weeks.

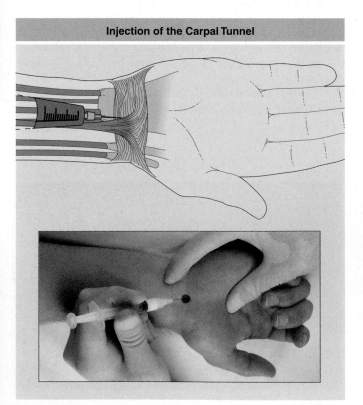

Injection of the Carpal Tunnel

Fig 304-9
Injection of the carpal tunnel.
(From Hochberg MC, Silman AJ, Smolen JS, et al [eds]: Rheumatology, 3rd ed. St Louis, Mosby, 2003.)

2. Pronator syndrome

DEFINITION

A form of compression neuropathy of the median nerve in the proximal forearm caused primarily by the pronator teres muscle. Occasionally, only the anterior interosseus motor branch is affected, sometimes causing a very specific separate clinical presentation.

PHYSICAL FINDINGS AND CLINICAL PRESENTATION

- Forearm discomfort and fatigue, often resulting from repetitive pronation
- Insidious onset
- Nocturnal paresthesias are not typical.
- Vague numbness in the hand, primarily in thumb and index finger, may be present.
- Tenderness and enlargement of the pronator teres may be present.
- Tinel's sign may be positive at the site of compression.
- Although there are no reliable provocative tests, painful paresthesias may occasionally be elicited with forced pronation of the forearm against resistance.
- Motor impairment is rare.

Anterior interosseus nerve syndrome

- Forearm pain and weakness
- Patient may be unable to form a circle when trying to pinch the index finger and thumb because of inability to flex distal phalanges of thumb and index finger.
- Sensation to the hand is not affected.

CAUSE

- Localized anatomic compression (Fig. 304–10)
- Trauma
- Traumatic cut down or phlebotomy

DIFFERENTIAL DIAGNOSIS

- Carpal tunnel syndrome
- Cervical disc syndrome with radiculopathy
- Tendon rupture
- Tendinitis

WORKUP

- Electrodiagnostic studies may be helpful; they are indicated if symptoms persist longer than 4 to 6 weeks or if motor weakness is suspected.
- Plain radiography to rule out bony abnormalities causing compression

TREATMENT

- Rest, bracing of forearm, sling
- Stretching exercises, physical therapy
- NSAIDs

3. Dupuytren's contracture

DEFINITION

Dupuytren's contracture is a disease of the palmar fascia characterized by nodular fibroblastic proliferation that often results in progressive contractures of the fascia and flexion deformity of the fingers.

PHYSICAL FINDINGS AND CLINICAL PRESENTATION

- Usually asymptomatic
- Most common complaints: deformity and interference with the use of the hand by the flexed, contracted fingers
- Process usually begins in the ulnar side of the hand, often starting at the ring finger.
- Isolated painless nodules that eventually harden and mature into a longitudinal cord that extends into the finger

- Lesion often begins in the distal palmar crease.
- Overlying skin adherent to the fascia
- Later stages: fibrous cord begins to contract and pull the finger into flexion (Fig. 304–11)
- Possible involvement of other fingers, particularly the small finger

CAUSE

Unknown. Pathologically, the contracture consists of proliferating vascular tissue that later develops into mature collagen.

DIFFERENTIAL DIAGNOSIS

- Soft tissue tumor
- Tendon cyst

TREATMENT

- Stretching exercises
- Local heat
- Excision of rare nodule that is painful (at any stage)

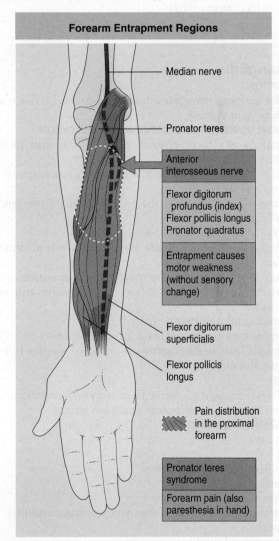

Forearm Entrapment Regions

Median nerve

Pronator teres

Anterior interosseous nerve

Flexor digitorum profundus (index)
Flexor pollicis longus
Pronator quadratus

Entrapment causes motor weakness (without sensory change)

Flexor digitorum superficialis

Flexor pollicis longus

Pain distribution in the proximal forearm

Pronator teres syndrome

Forearm pain (also paresthesia in hand)

Fig 304–10
Forearm entrapment regions. The median nerve may be compressed at several locations in the forearm, most commonly as it traverses the pronator teres muscle. The anterior interosseous branch of the median nerve is solely motor, thus entrapment produces no sensory deficit. (From Hochberg MC, Silman AJ, Smolen JS, et al [eds]: Rheumatology, 3rd ed. St Louis, Mosby, 2003.)

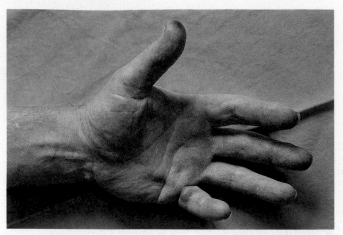

Fig 304–11
Dupuytren's contracture of the palmar fascia.
(From Hochberg MC, Silman AJ, Smolen JS, et al [eds]: Rheumatology, 3rd ed. St Louis, Mosby, 2003.)

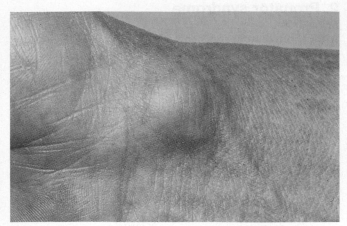

Fig 304–12
A ganglion on the volar aspect of the wrist
(From Hochberg MC, Silman AJ, Smolen JS, et al [eds]: Rheumatology, 3rd ed. St Louis, Mosby, 2003.)

4. Ganglion

DEFINITION
Ganglia are cystic structures thought to derive from a tendon sheath or joint capsule.

PHYSICAL FINDINGS AND CLINICAL PRESENTATION
- Most ganglia occur on the dorsum of the wrist (50% to 70%)
- Volar wrist (18% to 20%) is the next most common site (Fig. 304–12).
- Ganglia can also involve the proximal digital flexor tendons and the DIP joints.
- Left and right hands are equally affected.
- Ganglia are usually solitary, firm, smooth, round, and fluctuant.
- Pain from mass effect or compression up against nearby structure may be present (e.g., median nerve and radial nerve).
- Hand numbness may be present.
- Patient may experience hand muscle weakness.
- Ganglia usually develop over a period of months but may arise suddenly.

CAUSE
Ganglia are thought to derive from synovial herniation or expansion from the joint capsule or tendon sheath.

DIFFERENTIAL DIAGNOSIS
- Lipoma
- Fibroma
- Epidermoid inclusion cyst
- Osteochondroma
- Hemangioma
- Infection (tuberculosis, fungi, and secondary syphilis)
- Gout
- Rheumatoid nodule
- Radial artery aneurysm
- De Quervain's tenosynovitis of the wrist (see Fig. 304–15)

IMAGING STUDIES
- Radiograph of the hand and wrist is done to rule out other bone or joint abnormalities.
- Ultrasound studies are helpful in the diagnosis of ganglia, demonstrating smooth cystic walls that may be septated.
- CT scan can be done if the ultrasound is equivocal.
- MRI (Fig. 304–13) aids in differentiating malignant bone lesions from cystic structures.
- Arthrography may demonstrate a communication between the joint and ganglia (not commonly done).

TREATMENT
Treatment is indicated for pain, muscle weakness, and cosmetic purposes.
- Aspiration with a large-bore needle (18-gauge) followed by injection of 20 to 40 mg of triamcinolone acetonide can be tried.
- This may be repeated if the ganglia recurs (35% to 40%).
- Total ganglionectomy is the surgical procedure of choice.

5. Trigger finger

DEFINITION
Digital stenosing tenosynovitis (trigger finger) refers to an inflammatory process of the digital flexor tendon sheath.

PHYSICAL FINDINGS AND CLINICAL PRESENTATION
- Hand pain
- Painful triggering or snapping with flexion and extension of the affected digit
- Locking or loss of active digital extension is the most common symptom
- The digit possibly fixed in flexion (trapped or incarcerated)
- Usually affects one digit
- If more digits are involved, a systemic cause most likely present (e.g., diabetes, rheumatoid arthritis)
- A palpable tender nodule noted at the MCP joint of the affected digit
- Pain over the flexor tendon with resisted flexion
- Pain with passive stretching

CAUSE
Trigger finger is described as being primary or secondary:
- Primary (idiopathic)

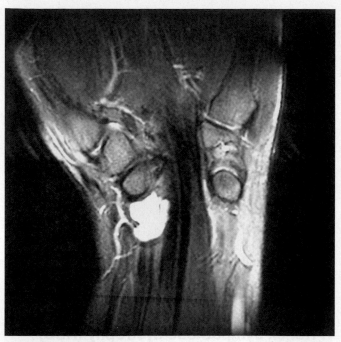

Fig 304–13
Ganglion. A 2-cm ganglion cyst has arisen proximal to the scaphiod on the volar aspect of the wrist. As expected from its fluid content, it returns increased signal on this T2W sequence.
(From Grainger RG, Allison DJ, Adam A, Dixon AK [eds]: Grainger and Allison's Diagnostic Radiology, 4th ed. Philadelphia, Churchill Livingstone, 2001.).

Injection of the Flexor Digital Tendon Sheath in Trigger Finger

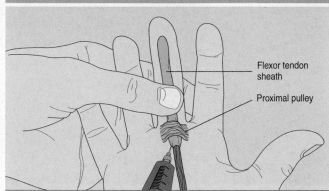

Flexor tendon sheath

Proximal pulley

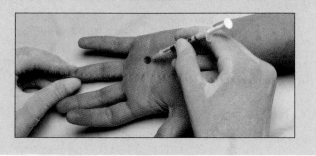

Fig 304–14
Injection of the flexor digital tendon sheath in trigger finger.
(From Hochberg MC, Silman AJ, Smolen JS, et al [eds]: Rheumatology, 3rd ed. St Louis, Mosby, 2003.)

- Secondary
  1. Diabetes
  2. Rheumatoid arthritis
  3. Hypothyroidism
  4. Histiocytosis
  5. Amyloidosis
  6. Gout

DIFFERENTIAL DIAGNOSIS
- Dupuytren's contracture (see Fig. 304–11)
- de Quervain's tenosynovitis
- Acute digital tenosynovitis
- Proliferative tenosynovitis
- Carpal tunnel syndrome
- Flexion tendon rupture
- Trauma

LABORATORY TESTS
- CBC with differential
- Electrolytes, BUN, and creatinine
- Blood glucose
- Thyroid function tests
- Uric acid
- RF

TREATMENT
- In primary idiopathic trigger finger steroid injection, 15 to 20 mg depomethylprednisolone acetate in 1 mL 1% lidocaine has been used with success (Fig. 304–14).
- Triamcinolone 10 mg with 1 mL of 1% lidocaine is an alternative steroid choice to be used in patients who do not respond to the first injection.

- If symptoms do not resolve in 3 weeks, a repeat injection can be tried.
- Surgical release is indicated in patients with refractory symptoms (e.g., locked digits) despite nonpharmacologic and acute treatment.
- Surgery is also indicated in patients with recurrent symptoms despite steroid injection therapy.

6. de Quervain's tenosynovitis
DEFINITION
de Quervain's tenosynovitis refers to a stenosing inflammatory process of the first dorsal retinacular compartment containing the tendons of the abductor pollicis longus (APL) and extensor pollicis brevis (EPB).

PHYSICAL FINDINGS AND CLINICAL PRESENTATION
- Pain over the styloid process of the radius
- Swelling (Fig. 304–15)
- Positive Finkelstein's test (Fig. 304–16)
- Crepitance

CAUSE
- The cause is usually repetitive use or overuse of the hands (e.g., typing, writing, nailing, etc.). Acute trauma can also cause tenosynovitis of the radial styloid.

DIAGNOSIS
- The diagnosis of de Quervain's tenosynovitis is based on the clinical triad of:
  1. Tenderness over the radial styloid
  2. Swelling over the first dorsal retinacular compartment
  3. Positive Finkelstein's test

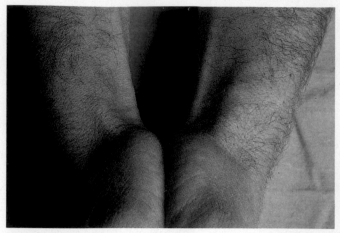

Fig 304–15
de Quervain's tenosynovitis of the wrist.
(From Hochberg MC, Silman AJ, Smolen JS, et al [eds]: Rheumatology, 3rd ed. St Louis, Mosby, 2003.)

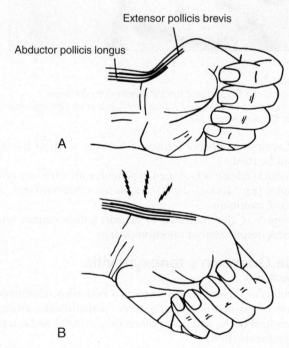

Fig 304–16
Finkelstein's test is positive in de Quervain's stenosing synovitis. Ulnar flexion of the wrist produces pain over the dorsal compartment containing the extensor policis brevis and abductor pollicis longus.
(From Noble J [ed]: *Textbook of primary care medicine*, ed 2, St Louis, 1996, Mosby.)

- Sometimes 1.5 mL of 1% lidocaine can be injected into the tenosynovial sac, and if all three physical signs resolve, the diagnosis is confirmed.

DIFFERENTIAL DIAGNOSIS
- Carpal tunnel syndrome
- Arthritis (e.g., degenerative osteoarthritis or RA)
- Gout
- Infiltrative tenosynovitis

- Radiculopathy
- Wrist ganglion (see Fig. 304–12)
- Compression neuropathy (e.g., superficial branch of the radial nerve "bracelet syndrome")
- Infection (e.g., tuberculosis, bacterial)

LABORATORY TESTS
- ESR is usually normal in patients with de Quervain's tenosynovitis.
- Aspiration to rule out gout
- Gram stain and culture of aspirate

IMAGING STUDIES
- Radiographic studies of the hand

TREATMENT
- Rest
- Splinting
- Physiotherapy
- Corticosteroid injection using 20 to 40 mg triamcinolone acetonide and 1% lidocaine is effective in relieving pain.
- NSAIDs
- Surgical release is generally reserved for patients not responding to NSAIDs and corticosteroid injection therapy.

7. Reflex sympathetic dystrophy (RSD)

DEFINITION
RSD refers to a painful neuropathic symptom complex affecting an extremity following trauma, surgery, or nerve injury to that limb.

PHYSICAL FINDINGS AND CLINICAL PRESENTATION
RSD is divided into three stages:
- Acute stage (occurring within hours to days after the injury)
  1. Burning or aching pain occurring over the injured extremity
  2. Hyperalgesia (exquisitely sensitive to touch)
  3. Edema (Fig. 304–17)
  4. Dysthermia
  5. Increased hair and nail growth
- Dystrophic stage (3 to 6 months after the injury)
  1. Burning pain radiating both distal and proximally from the site of injury
  2. Brawny edema
  3. Hyperhidrosis
  4. Hypothermia and cyanosis
  5. Muscle tremors and spasms
  6. Increased muscle tone and reflexes
- Atrophic stage (6 months after injury)
  1. Spread of pain proximally
  2. Cold, pale cyanotic skin
  3. Trophic skin changes with subcutaneous atrophy
  4. Fixed joints
  5. Contractures

CAUSE
- The cause of RSD is unknown. It is thought to represent dysfunction of the sympathetic nervous system.
- Any injury can precipitate RSD including:
  1. Crush blunt trauma, burns, frostbite
  2. Surgery
  3. Parkinson's disease
  4. Cerebrovascular accident
  5. Myocardial infarction
  6. Osteoarthritis, cervical, and lumbar disc disease

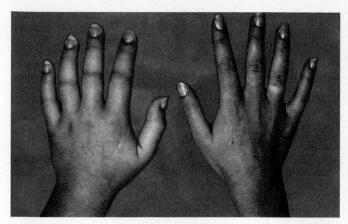

Fig 304–17
Reflex sympathetic dystrophy syndrome. There is diffuse edematous swelling of the entire left hand.
(From Hochberg MC, Silman AJ, Smolen JS, et al [eds]: Rheumatology, 3rd ed. St Louis, Mosby, 2003.)

7. Carpal tunnel and tarsal tunnel syndrome
8. Diabetes
9. Hyperthyroidism
10. Isoniazid therapy

DIFFERENTIAL DIAGNOSIS
The differential diagnosis includes all the causes mentioned under "cause."

IMAGING STUDIES
● No imaging studies are diagnostic of RSD. Three-phase bone imaging may be helpful.
● Autonomic testing, although not commonly done, has been proposed.
  1. Measuring resting sweat output
  2. Measuring resting skin temperature
  3. Quantitative sudomotor axon reflex test
● Radiographic studies of the affected limb may show diffuse soft-tissue swelling, demineralization (Fig. 304–18), and osteoporosis from disuse.

TREATMENT
Treatment is aimed at relieving the pain and improving disuse atrophy with physical therapy.
● Physical therapy
● Transcutaneous nerve stimulation
● The following have been tried for neuropathic pain relief: Amitriptyline, phenytoin, carbamazepine, calcium channel blockers, and prednisone.
  ● Stellate ganglion and lumbar sympathetic blocks can be tried.
  ● Surgical sympathectomy

C. ELBOW
1. Epicondylitis
DEFINITION
Epicondylitis is an inflammation of the musculotendinous origin of the common extensors at the lateral elbow or the flexor pronator group at the medial elbow.

PHYSICAL FINDINGS AND CLINICAL PRESENTATION
● Local tenderness over affected epicondyle
● Reproduction of pain by resistance against wrist extension (lateral) (Fig. 304–19) or flexion (medial) (Fig. 304–20)

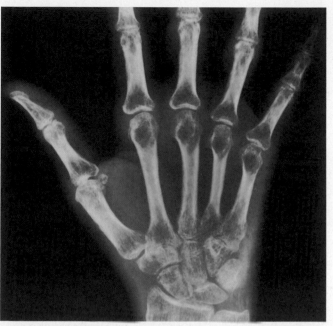

Fig 304–18
Reflex sympathetic dystrophy syndrome involving the right hand. Diffuse soft-tissue swelling with mild periarticular accentuation is evident. Juxta-articular demineralization is also noted, particularly involving the metacarpophalangeal joints and carpus.
(From Grainger RG, Allison DJ, Adam A, Dixon AK [eds]: Grainger and Allison's Diagnostic Radiology, 4th ed. Philadelphia, Churchill Livingstone, 2001.)

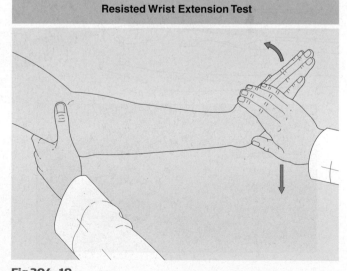

Resisted Wrist Extension Test

Fig 304–19
Resisted wrist extension test.
(From Hochberg MC, Silman AJ, Smolen JS, et al [eds]: Rheumatology, 3rd ed. St Louis, Mosby, 2003.)

CAUSE
- Unknown
- Overuse probably causing minor tendinous tears resulting in inflammation
- Posterior interosseous nerve syndrome: compression of this nerve has occasionally been cited as a possible etiology, es-

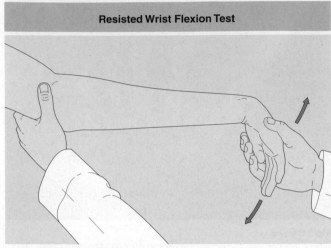

Resisted Wrist Flexion Test

Fig 304-20
Resisted wrist extension test.
(From Hochberg MC, Silman AJ, Smolen JS, et al [eds]: Rheumatology, 3rd ed. St Louis, Mosby, 2003.)

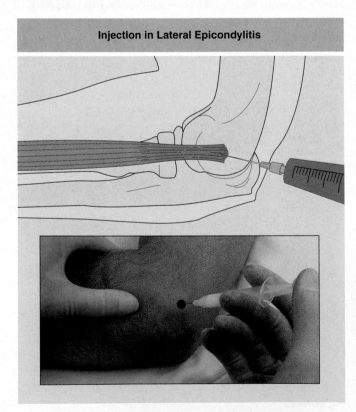

Injection in Lateral Epicondylitis

Fig 304-21
Injection in lateral epicondylitis. Injection of corticosteriod and local anesthetic into the common extensor tendon origin at the lateral humeral epicondyle.
(From Hochberg MC, Silman AJ, Smolen JS, et al [eds]: Rheumatology, 3rd ed. St Louis, Mosby, 2003.)

pecially in cases that have failed traditional medical and surgical treatment. In this disorder, the site of tenderness is 2 to 3 cm distal to the epicondyle.

DIFFERENTIAL DIAGNOSIS
- Cervical radiculopathy
- Intra-articular elbow pathology (osteoarthritis, osteochondritis dissecans, loose body)
- Radial nerve compression
- Ulnar neuropathy
- Medial collateral ligament instability

IMAGING STUDIES
Traction spur or minor soft tissue calcification may be present on plain radiography. Other studies are not usually needed.

TREATMENT
- Rest, restricted activities
- Ice after exercise
- Stretching exercise program
- NSAIDs
- Local corticosteroid/lidocaine injection (Fig. 304–21)
- Counterforce brace
- Proper technique in sports activities
- Intermittent immobilization

2. Cubital tunnel syndrome

DEFINITION
Compression of the ulnar nerve behind the elbow (cubitus) (Fig. 304–22)

PHYSICAL FINDINGS AND CLINICAL PRESENTATION
- Paresthesias and numbness along distribution of ulnar nerve

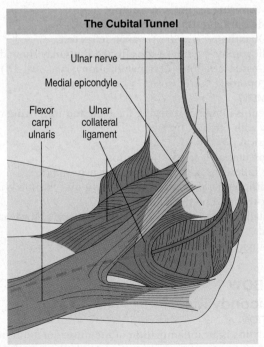

The Cubital Tunnel

Ulnar nerve
Medial epicondyle
Flexor carpi ulnaris
Ulnar collateral ligament

Fig 304-22
The cubital tunnel. The fibro-osseous canal is formed by the medial epicondyle, ulnar collateral ligament, and flexor carpi ulnaris muscle. Elbow flexion decreases the volume of the channel.
(From Hochberg MC, Silman AJ, Smolen JS, et al [eds]: Rheumatology, 3rd ed. St Louis, Mosby, 2003.)

- Positive Tinel's sign at elbow
- Positive elbow flexion test (flexion of elbow with wrist extended for 30 seconds may reproduce symptoms)
- May be diminished sensation to tip of small finger
- Ulnar nerve may be subluxable with elbow motion or by manipulation
- Cubitus valgus may be present if prior bony injury
- Interosseous weakness in long-standing cases with atrophy

CAUSE
- Direct pressure
- Cubitus valgus deformity
- Subluxation of ulnar nerve
- Repeated stretching during throwing motion
- Elbow synovitis
- Local muscular hypertrophy

DIFFERENTIAL DIAGNOSIS
- Medial epicondylitis
- Medial elbow instability
- Carpal tunnel syndrome
- Cervical disc syndrome with radicular arm symptoms
- Ulnar nerve compression at wrist (Guyon's canal)

IMAGING STUDIES
- Routine x-rays may be helpful in establishing cause or ruling out other conditions
- Electrodiagnostic studies: nerve conduction tests and electromyography are useful in establishing diagnosis and ruling out other syndromes.

TREATMENT
- Protect nerve from pressure
- Elbow pads
- Avoid prolonged elbow flexion (talking on the telephone with elbow bent)

D. SHOULDER
1. Rotator cuff syndrome
DEFINITION
Rotator cuff syndrome refers to a spectrum of afflictions involving the tendons of the rotator cuff (primarily the supraspinatus), ranging from simple strains and tendinitis to complete, massive rupture with cuff-tear arthropathy.

PHYSICAL FINDINGS AND CLINICAL PRESENTATION
- Pain, often at night
- Rotator cuff tenderness (Fig. 304–23)
- Referred pain down deltoid, especially with abduction between 70 and 120 degrees ("the painful arc")

- Weakness in abduction or forward flexion
- Increased pain with overhead activities
- Atrophy in long-standing cases of complete tear
- Positive "drop-arm" test (weakness of abduction against downward pressure at 90 degrees)

CAUSE
- Microtrauma from repetitive use (Fig. 304–24)
- Abnormally shaped acromion
- Shoulder instability
- Worsening of process by the overhead throwing motion
- Microcirculatory changes at the musculotendinous junction

DIFFERENTIAL DIAGNOSIS
- Shoulder instability
- Degenerative arthritis
- Cervical radiculopathy
- Avascular necrosis
- Suprascapular nerve entrapment
- Table 304–1 describes the differential diagnosis of shoulder pain.

IMAGING STUDIES
- Plain radiography is generally not helpful for diagnosis
- MRI to evaluate full- or partial-thickness tears (Fig. 304–25), chronic tendinitis, and other causes of shoulder pain
- Since the invention of MRI, arthrography is rarely used.

TREATMENT
- Rest to avoid overhead activity
- Ice or heat for comfort
- Carefully supervised program of stretching and strengthening
- Medication: NSAIDs, subacromial corticosteroid injection (once or twice at 2-week intervals)

2. Milwaukee shoulder
DEFINITION
- Milwaukee shoulder is a complication of shoulder impingement in elderly patients with long-standing supraspinatus tears manifesting with a painful stiff shoulder.
- It is also known as "rotator cuff arthropathy" or "recurrent hemorrhagic shoulder of the elderly."

EPIDEMIOLOGY
- Distinctive type of destructive arthropathy associated with rotator cuff defects and numerous aggregates of basic calcium phosphate (BCP) crystals in the fluid of the affected joint.

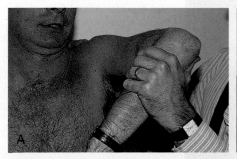 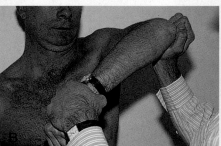 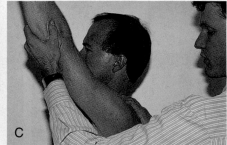

Fig 304–23
Impingement tests. (**A**) Forced passive internal rotation. (**B**) Resisted external rotation. (**C**) Forced passive full forward flexion.
(From Hochberg MC, Silman AJ, Smolen JS, et al [eds]: Rheumatology, 3rd ed. St Louis, Mosby, 2003.)

- Patients are nearly over 70 years old, and approximately 70% are females.

CLINICAL PRESENTATION

- There is usually a history of months or years of increasing pain and loss of function of the affected shoulder.
- The pain may be mild but is usually most apparent at night and on joint use.

- Because motion hurts, most patients keep the shoulder still, causing further deconditioning, muscle atrophy, and contracture. Fibrosis and joint restriction eventually set in.
- Physical examination reveals reduced range of motion, crepitation, and pain.
- The rotator cuff is generally destroyed and a joint effusion is typically present (Fig. 304–26).

DIAGNOSIS

- Aspiration of the affected shoulder joint (Fig. 304–27) yields blood-tinged fluid that has a low-predominantly mononuclear cell count.
- Radiographs in Milwaukee shoulder syndrome (Fig. 304–28) may show upward subluxation of the humeral head or arthroscopic evidence of rotator cuff tear defects.
- MRI can be used to further define the anatomic changes, including loss of cartilage, periarticular bone marrow edema, rupture of the rotator cuff tear, synovial hypertrophy and joint effusion (Fig. 304–29).

TREATMENT

- Physical therapy, NSAIDs, arthroscopy in select cases

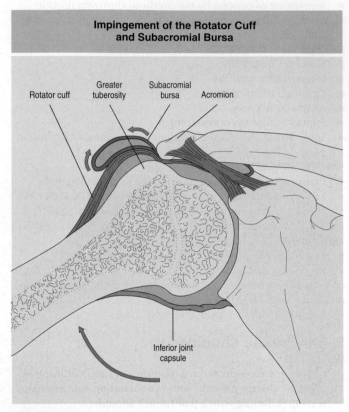

Impingement of the Rotator Cuff and Subacromial Bursa

Rotator cuff · Greater tuberosity · Subacromial bursa · Acromion · Inferior joint capsule

Fig 304–24
Impingement of the rotator cuff and subacromial bursa. Mechanism of impingement of the rotator cuff and subacromial bursa between the humeral head and overlying coracoacromial arch.
(From Hochberg MC, Silman AJ, Smolen JS, et al [eds]: Rheumatology, 3rd ed. St Louis, Mosby, 2003.)

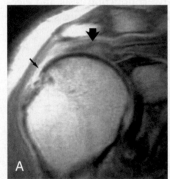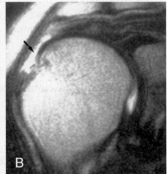

Fig 304–25
Rotator cuff tear. Coronal oblique proton density (**A**) and T2-weighted (**B**) images demonstrate abnormal high signal in the expected region of the distal supraspinatus tendon *(small arrow)*, consistent with a complete tear. The supraspinatus tendon is retracted *(large arrow)*.
(From Grainger RG, Allison DJ, Adam A, Dixon AK [eds]: Grainger and Allison's Diagnostic Radiology, 4th ed. Philadelphia, Churchill Livingstone, 2001.)

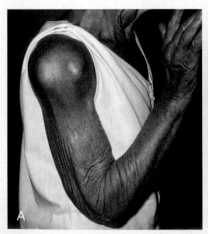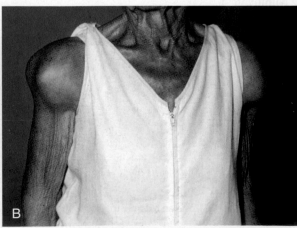

Fig 304–26
Destructive arthropathy (Milwaukee) of the shoulder. A large synovial effusion is apparent (**A**) over the lateral aspect of the humerus or (**B**) anteriorly in front of the glenohumeral joint.
(From Hochberg MC, Silman AJ, Smolen JS, et al [eds]: Rheumatology, 3rd ed. St Louis, Mosby, 2003.)

TABLE 304–1 Differential diagnosis of shoulder pain: clinical and radiographic features of common causes of shoulder pain

Diagnosis	Age	Type of onset	Location of pain	Night pain	Active range of motion	Passive range of motion	Impingement signs	Radiation of pain	Paraesthesia	Weakness	Instability	Radiographic changes	Special features
Rotator cuff tendinitis	Any	Acute or chronic	Deltoid region	+	— guarding	Normal	+++	—	—	Only due to pain	Look for	In chronic cases	Painful arc of abduction
Rotator cuff tears (chronic)	Over 40 years	Often chronic	Deltoid region	++	—	Normal (may _ later)	++	—	—	++	—	+	Wasting of cuff muscles
Bicipital tendinitis	Any	Overuse	Anterior	—	— guarding	Normal	+	Occasionally into biceps	—	Only due to pain	Look for	None	Special examination tests
Calcific tendinitis	30–60 years	Acute	Point of shoulder	++	— guarding	Normal except for pain	+++	—	—	Only due to pain	—	++	Tenderness
Capsulitis "frozen shoulder"	Over 40 years	Insidious	Deep in shoulder	++	—	—	+	—	—	—	—	—	No global range of motion
Acromioclavicular joint	Any	Acute or chronic	Over joint	Lying on side	— full elevation	Normal	—	—	—	—	—	In chronic cases	Local tenderness
Osteoarthrosis of glenohumeral joint	Over 40 years	Insidious	Deep in shoulder	++	—	—	—	—	—	May have mild	—	+++	Crepitus
Glenohumeral instability	Usually <25 years	Episodic	Anterior or posterior	—	Only apprehension	Only apprehension	Possible	—	+ with acute episodes	+ with acute episodes	+++	Often	Stress tests
Cervical spondylosis	Over 40 years	Insidious	Supra-scapular	Often	Normal	Normal	—	++	+++	+	—	In cervical spine	Pain with neck movement
Thoracic outlet syndrome	Any	Usually with activity	Neck shoulder arm	—	Normal	Normal	—	++	++	++	—	—	Special examination tests

From Hochberg MC, Silman AJ, Smolen JS, et al (eds): Rheumatology, 3rd ed. St Louis, Mosby, 2003.

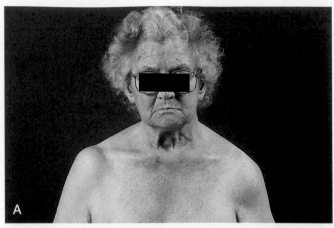

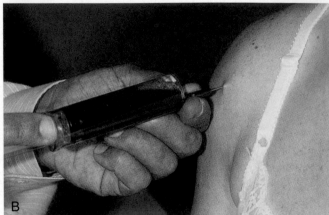

Fig 304–27
BCP crystal-associated destructive arthritis ('Milwaukee shoulder').
(**A**) This elderly patient has visible swellings of both shoulders. (**B**) Aspiration revealed a large amount of bloodstained fluid which contained numerous particles of basic calcium phosphates.
(From Hochberg MC, Silman AJ, Smolen JS, et al [eds]: Rheumatology, 3rd ed. St Louis, Mosby, 2003.)

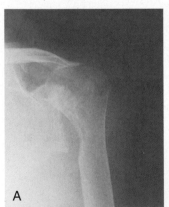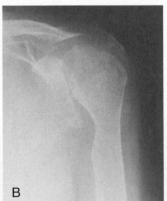

Fig 304–28
Anteroposterior radiographs of a shoulder joint affected by BCP crystal-associated destructive arthritis ('Milwaukee shoulder'). The extensive destruction of periarticular tissues, including the rotator cuff, has led to instability of the shoulder. The upward subluxation (**A**) of the humerus can be overcome by traction on the shoulder (**B**). Note the extensive atrophic destruction and loss of bone of both the acromion and the glenohumeral joint.
(From Hochberg MC, Silman AJ, Smolen JS, et al [eds]: Rheumatology, 3rd ed. St Louis, Mosby, 2003.)

3. Thoracic outlet syndrome
DEFINITION
Thoracic outlet syndrome is the term used to describe a condition producing upper extremity symptoms thought to result from neurovascular compression at the thoracic outlet (Fig. 304–30). Three types are described based on the point of compression: (1) cervical rib and scalenus syndrome, in which abnormal scalene muscles or the presence of a cervical rib may cause compression; (2) costoclavicular syndrome, in which compression may occur under the clavicle; and (3) hyperabduction syndrome, in which compression may occur in the subcoracoid area.

PHYSICAL FINDINGS AND CLINICAL PRESENTATION
- Symptoms and signs are related to the degree of involvement of each of the various structures at the level of the first rib.
- True venous or arterial involvement is rare.
- Diagnosis is most often used in the consideration of neural pain affecting the arm, which would suggest involvement of the brachial plexus (Figs. 304–31 and 304–32).
  1. *Arterial compression:* pallor, paresthesias, diminished pulses, coolness, digital gangrene, and a supraclavicular bruit or mass
  2. *Venous compression:* edema and pain; thrombosis causing superficial venous dilation about the shoulder
  3. *"True" neural compression:* lower trunk (C8, T1) findings with intrinsic weakness and diminished sensation to the finger and small fingers and ulnar aspect of the forearm
  4. Possible supraclavicular tenderness

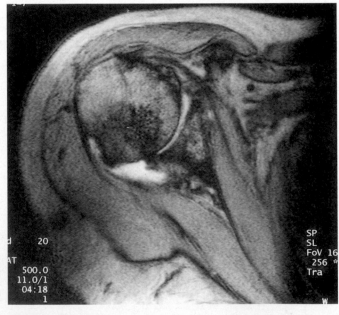

Fig 304–29
Axial T2-weighted MRI scan of a shoulder joint affected by BCP crystal-associated destructive arthritis ('Milwaukee shoulder'). There is advanced glenohumeral joint degeneration with loss of articular cartilage, truncation of the anterior and posterior labrum, narrowing of the joint space, osteophyte formation, muscle atrophy, and joint effusion.
(From Hochberg MC, Silman AJ, Smolen JS, et al [eds]: Rheumatology, 3rd ed. St Louis, Mosby, 2003.)

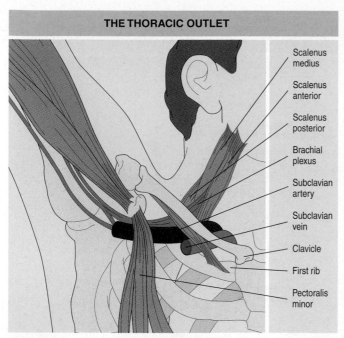

THE THORACIC OUTLET

Scalenus medius
Scalenus anterior
Scalenus posterior
Brachial plexus
Subclavian artery
Subclavian vein
Clavicle
First rib
Pectoralis minor

Fig 304–30
The thoracic outlet. Three narrow channels of the outlet include the scalene triangle, the costoclavicular passage, and the pectoralis minor attachment at the coracoid process.
(From Hochberg MC, Silman AJ, Smolen JS, et al [eds]: Rheumatology, 3rd ed. St Louis, Mosby, 2003.)

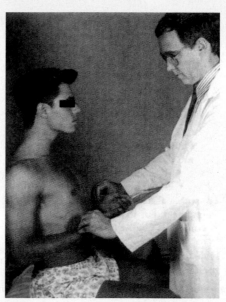

Fig 304–31
The costoclavicular maneuver. The patient takes an exaggerated military position of attention with the shoulders thrust backward and downward. Decreased radial pulse and reproduction of symptoms suggest neurovascular compression between the clavicle and 1st rib.
(From Hochberg MC, Silman AJ, Smolen JS, et al [eds]: Rheumatology, 3rd ed. St Louis, Mosby, 2003.)

5. Provocative tests (*Adson's* [Fig. 304–33], *Wright's*): may reproduce pain but are of disputed usefulness

CAUSE
- Congenital cervical rib or fibrous extension of cervical rib
- Abnormal scalene muscle insertion
- Drooping of shoulder girdle resulting from generalized hypotonia or trauma
- Narrowed costoclavicular interval as a result of downward and backward pressure on shoulder (sometimes seen in individuals who carry heavy backpacks)
- Acute venous thrombosis with exercise (effort thrombosis)
- Bony abnormalities of first rib
- Abnormal fibromuscular bands
- Malunion of clavicle fracture

DIFFERENTIAL DIAGNOSIS
- Carpal tunnel syndrome
- Cervical radiculopathy
- Brachial neuritis
- Ulnar nerve compression
- Reflex sympathetic dystrophy
- Superior sulcus tumor

IMAGING STUDIES
- Arteriography or venography when vascular pathology is strongly suspected clinically
- Cervical spine radiographs to rule out cervical disc disease
- Chest film to rule out lung tumor
- EMG, nerve conduction velocity studies to rule out carpal tunnel syndrome, cervical radiculopathy

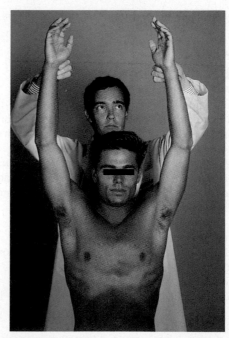

Fig 304–32
The hyperabduction maneuver. The patient lifts his hands above his head with the elbows somewhat flexed and extending out laterally from the body, testing compression by the pectoralis minor at the coracoid process.
(From Hochberg MC, Silman AJ, Smolen JS, et al [eds]: Rheumatology, 3rd ed. St Louis, Mosby, 2003.)

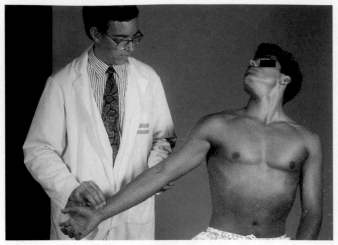

Fig 304–33
The Adson's maneuver. The patient inhales deeply, extends the neck fully, and turns the head to the side being examined. This test for compression in the scalene triangle and is positive if there is a diminution in the radial pulse and reproduction of the patient's symptoms.
(From Hochberg MC, Silman AJ, Smolen JS, et al [eds]: Rheumatology, 3rd ed. St Louis, Mosby, 2003.)

TREATMENT

- Sling for pain relief
- Physical therapy modalities plus shoulder girdle-strengthening exercises
- Postural reeducation
- NSAIDs
- Surgery: generally successful for vascular disorders

E. BACK

1. Lumbar disc syndrome

DEFINITION

Lumbar disc syndromes are diseases resulting from disc disorder, either herniation or degenerative change (spondylosis). Massive disc protrusion may rarely lead to paralysis in the lower extremity, a condition termed *cauda equina syndrome*. Gradual narrowing of the spinal canal (lumbar stenosis), usually from spondylosis, may also cause lower extremity symptoms. Cutaneous innervation of the lower extremities is illustrated in Figures 304–34 and 304–35.

PHYSICAL FINDINGS AND CLINICAL PRESENTATION

- Overlapping clinical syndromes that may result:
  1. Mild herniation without nerve root compression
  2. Herniation with nerve root compression
  3. Cauda equina syndrome
  4. Chronic degenerative disease with or without leg symptoms
  5. Spinal stenosis
- Low back pain, often worsened by activity or coughing and sneezing
- Local lumbar or lumbosacral tenderness
- Paresthesias, usually unilateral
- Restricted low back motion
- Increased pain on bending toward affected side
- Weakness and reflex changes (L4—knee jerk and quadriceps, L5—extensor hallucis longus, S1—ankle jerk and toe walking)

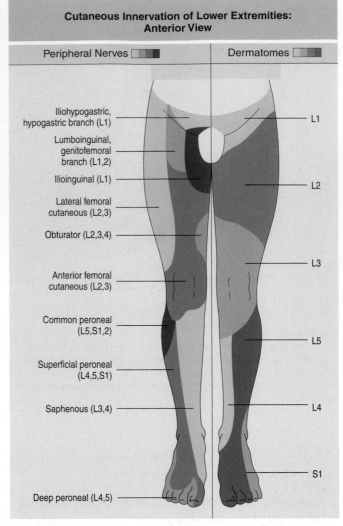

Fig 304–34
Cutaneous sensory innervation. Anterior view of lower extremities illustrating skin areas supplied by nerve roots *(right)* and peripheral nerves *(left)*.
(From Hochberg MC, Silman AJ, Smolen JS, et al [eds]: Rheumatology, 3rd ed. St Louis, Mosby, 2003.)

- Sensory examination usually not helpful
- Lumbar stenosis that possibly produces symptoms (pseudoclaudication), which are often misinterpreted as being vascular. (Pseudoclaudication usually recovers quickly with sitting or spine flexion. Vascular disease is unaffected by spine position and is typically associated with atrophic skin changes and diminished pulses.)
- Positive straight leg raising test if nerve root compression is present

CAUSE

Unknown

DIFFERENTIAL DIAGNOSIS

- Soft-tissue strain/sprain
- Tumor
- Degenerative arthritis of hip
- Insufficiency fracture of hip or pelvis

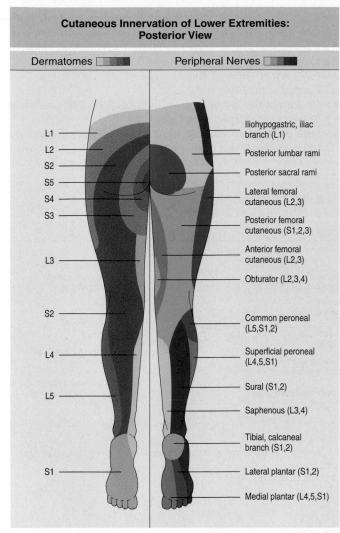

Fig 304–35

Cutaneous sensory innervation. Posterior view of lower extremities illustrating skin areas supplied by nerve roots *(left)* and peripheral nerves *(right)*.

(From Hochberg MC, Silman AJ, Smolen JS, et al [eds]: Rheumatology, 3rd ed. St Louis, Mosby, 2003.)

IMAGING STUDIES

- Plain x-rays may be indicated within the first few weeks; they are usually normal in soft disc herniation, but with chronic degenerative disc disease, loss of height of the disc space and osteophyte formation can occur.
- MRI (Fig. 304–36) may be indicated in patients whose symptoms do not resolve or when other spinal pathology may be suspected.
- Electrodiagnostic studies may confirm the diagnosis or rule out peripheral nerve disorders.

TREATMENT

- Physical therapy for modalities plus a careful gradual exercise program
- NSAIDs
- Muscle relaxants for sedative effect
- Lumbosacral corset brace during rehabilitation process in conjunction with exercise program

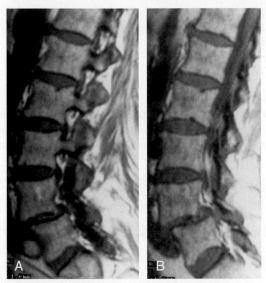

Fig 304–36

Degenerative spondylolisthesis. Parasagittal T1-weighted MRI of the lumbar spine showing anterior slip of L4 on L5 and degeneration in the posterior joints at this level.

(From Grainger RG, Allison DJ, Adam A, Dixon AK [eds]: Grainger and Allison's Diagnostic Radiology, 4th ed. Philadelphia, Churchill Livingstone, 2001.)

- Percutaneous electrical nerve stimulation (PENS) may be beneficial in selected patients with chronic back pain
- Analgesics
- Epidural steroid injection for leg symptoms in selected patients

2. Spinal stenosis

DEFINITION

Spinal stenosis is the pathologic condition compressing or narrowing the spinal canal, nerve root canal, or intervertebral foramina. The lumbar spinal canal in health and disease is shown in Figure 304–37.

PHYSICAL FINDINGS AND CLINICAL PRESENTATION

- Neurogenic claudication: leg, buttock, or back pain precipitated by walking and relieved by sitting
- Radicular leg pain
- Paresthesias
- Difficulty standing or lying in an erect position
- Decreased lumbar extension
- Normal peripheral pulses
- Positive Romberg
- Wide-based gait
- Reduced knee and ankle reflex
- Urine incontinence

CAUSE

Spinal stenosis may be primary or secondary

- Primary stenosis (congenital or developmental narrowing)
  1. Idiopathic
  2. Achondroplasia
  3. Morquio-Ullrich syndrome
- Secondary stenosis (acquired)
  1. Degenerative (hypertrophy of the articular processes, disc degeneration, ligamentum flavum hypertrophy, spondylolisthesis)

2. Fracture/trauma
3. Postoperative (postlaminectomy)
4. Paget's disease
5. Ankylosing spondylitis
6. Tumors
7. Acromegaly

DIFFERENTIAL DIAGNOSIS

Spinal stenosis must be differentiated from other common causes of back and leg pain—osteoarthritis of the knee or hip, osteomyelitis, epidural abscess, metastatic tumors, multiple myeloma, intermittent claudication secondary to peripheral vascular disease, neuropathy, scoliosis, herniated nucleus pulposus, spondylolisthesis, acute cauda equina syndrome, ankylosing spondylitis, Reiter's syndrome, and fibromyalgia.

IMAGING AND OTHER STUDIES

- Lumbar spine film
- CT scan of the lumbosacral spine (Fig. 304–38): sensitivity (75% to 85%), specificity (80%)
- MRI of the lumbosacral spine (Fig. 304–39): sensitivity (80% to 90%), specificity (95%)

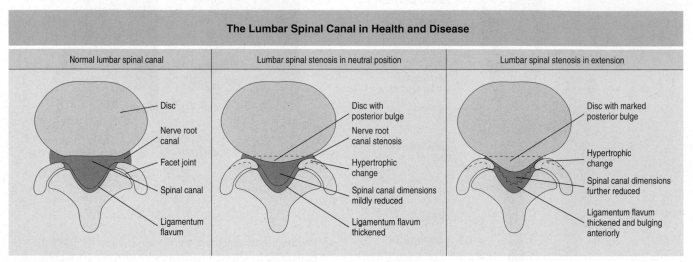

Fig 304–37

The lumbar spinal canal in health and disease. (Left) The normal spinal canal. (Center) The spinal canal in central spinal and nerve root canal stenosis in the neutral position. (Right) The effect of lumbar extension on the spinal canal.
(From Hochberg MC, Silman AJ, Smolen JS, et al [eds]: Rheumatology, 3rd ed. St Louis, Mosby, 2003.)

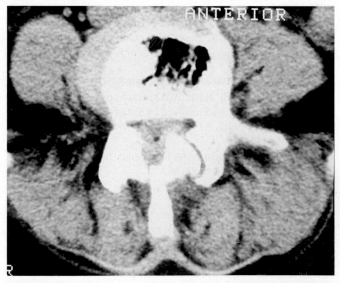

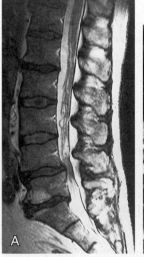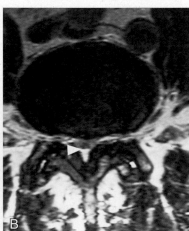

Fig 304–38

Lumbar spine stenosis. CT shows thickened ligamentum flavum, facet joint hypertrophy and posterior disc bulging. Note absence of epidural fat with trefoil deformity of lumbar spinal canal.
(From Hochberg MC, Silman AJ, Smolen JS, et al [eds]: Rheumatology, 3rd ed. St Louis, Mosby, 2003.)

Fig 304–39

Degenerative spinal canal stenosis. Sagittal A, and axial B T2-weighted MRI of the lumbar spine showing a severe spinal canal stenosis at L4-5 with evidence of entrapment of the cauda equina, namely obliteration of the CSF signal from the thecal sac at the site of compression *(white arrowhead)* and redundant coiling of intrathecal spinal roots above.
(From Grainger RG, Allison DJ, Adam A, Dixon AK [eds]: Grainger and Allison's Diagnostic Radiology, 4th ed. Philadelphia, Churchill Livingstone, 2001.)

- Myelogram (rarely performed): sensitivity (77%), specificity (72%). Absolute stenosis is defined as the anteroposterior (AP) diameter of the spinal canal <10 mm. Relative stenosis: 10- to 12-mm AP diameter
- CT and MRI can be used to visualize both the central and lateral canals.
- EMG and nerve conduction velocity are additional studies particularly useful in differentiating peripheral neuropathy from lumbar spinal stenosis.

TREATMENT
- NSAIDs
- Back exercises, abdominal muscle strengthening
- Surgery is indicated in patients with significant compression of nerve roots as determined by MRI or CT and with incapacitating symptoms limiting activities of daily living or with bladder and bowel incontinence.
- Surgical procedures include decompressive laminectomy, arthrodesis, hemilaminectomy, and medial facetectomy.

3. Diffuse idiopathic skeletal hyperostosis (DISH)
DEFINITION
- DISH is a chronic age-related condition with characteristic new bone growth especially at enthuses (region where tendon, ligament, joint capsule, or annulus fibrosis fibers insert into bone).
- Criteria for diagnosis of DISH rely principally on radiologic appearances in the thoracic spine. These typically require the new bone formation to bridge four contiguous vertebral bodies (Fig. 304–40).

CLINICAL FEATURES
- DISH may affect any skeletal structure but is most characteristic in the relatively nonmobile parts of the thoracic spine, where uninterrupted new bone may "flow" from one vertebra to another.

- It is more prominent on the right side of the vertebrae, thought to be a consequence of the pressure effect of the left-sided aorta.
- The deposition of new bone in DISH is usually asymptomatic, apart from increased stiffness in the neck, back, or peripheral joints.
- Important clinical features arise when new bone growth obstructs or impinges on other tissues.
- In the cervical spine, DISH may give rise to dysphagia or cervical myelopathy.

DIAGNOSIS
- DISH cannot be diagnosed without radiologic evaluation.
- Plain films of peripheral areas will show varying degrees of peripheral enthesopathy (Fig. 304–41).
- CT or MRI will provide more detailed images but is not necessary unless the presence of conditions such as spinal stenosis is being sought.

TREATMENT
Physical therapy to maintain range of motion and muscle strength, maintenance of ideal body weight, NSAIDs, surgical intervention (in spinal stenosis or osteophytic dysphagia

4. Scoliosis
DEFINITION
Scoliosis is a lateral curvature of the spine in the upright position, usually 10 degrees or greater. Scoliosis may be classified as either structural (fixed, nonflexible) or nonstructural (flexible, correctable).

PHYSICAL EXAMINATION AND CLINICAL PRESENTATION
- Record patient age (in years plus months) and height.
- Perform neurologic examination to rule out neuromuscular disease.
- Inspect the shoulders and iliac crests to determine if they are level.

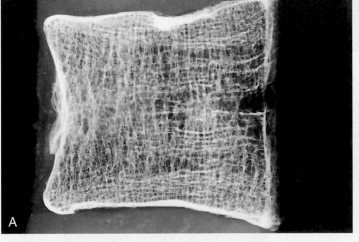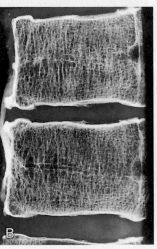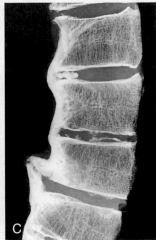

Fig 304–40
Progressive spinal entheseal changes in DISH. The earliest change is shown in (**A**), with ossification at the site of attachment of the anterior longitudinal ligament to the middle of the vertebral body, well away from the annulus. Note the separation of the ossification from the intact cortex, except at the site of attachment. Moderately advanced changes are seen in (**B**), with ossification bridging the disc space, but still firmly attached to cortex at the middle of the vertebral body. Advanced changes are shown in (**C**), with smooth attachment of the new bone to the original cortex. The ossified ligament is much thickened and interrupted at the lower level.
(From Hochberg MC, Silman AJ, Smolen JS, et al [eds]: Rheumatology, 3rd ed. St Louis, Mosby, 2003.)

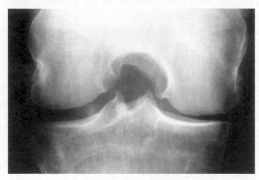

Fig 304-41

Peripheral arthropathy of DISH in the right knee. Ossification of the insertions of the cruciate ligaments reflect thickening and shortening of these structures. There is narrowing of medial compartment space, while lateral compartment space is preserved. Ossification of the margin of the articular cartilage of the medial femoral condyle is seen adjacent to the femoral notch.

(From Hochberg MC, Silman AJ, Smolen JS, et al [eds]: Rheumatology, 3rd ed. St Louis, Mosby, 2003.)

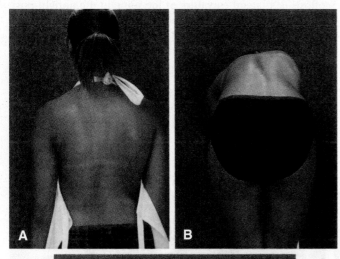

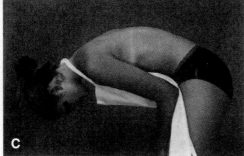

Fig 304-42

Adams Forward Bend test. **A** Scoliosis can be difficult to detect on observation of the standing patient. **B,** With the patient bending forward, and observed from behind, it is much easier to appreciate the asymmetrical trunk rotation seen in scoliosis. **C,** Viewing the patient from the side, one more easily see even subtle degrees of kyphosis note lack of reversal of normal lordosis.

(From Zitelli BJ, Davis HW: Atlas of Pediatric Physical Diagnosis, ed 4th, St. Louis, Mosby 2002)

- Palpate the spinous processes to determine their alignment.
- Have the patient bend forward symmetrically at the waist with the arms hanging free *(Adams' position)*; observe from the back or front to detect abnormal spine rotation (Fig. 304-42).
- Scoliosis may often be associated with kyphosis (kyphoscoliosis), especially in the elderly (Fig. 304-43).

CAUSE
- 90% unknown, usually referred to as idiopathic (genetic)
- Congenital spine deformity
- Neuromuscular disease
- Leg length inequality
- Local inflammation or infection
- Acute pain (disc disease)
- Chronic degenerative disc disease with asymmetrical disc narrowing

Curves of an idiopathic nature or those accompanying congenital deformity or neuromuscular disease are those associated with structural changes. The nonstructural types (leg length discrepancy, inflammation, or acute pain) disappear when the offending disorder is corrected.

IMAGING STUDIES
- Diagnosis of idiopathic scoliosis is confirmed by a standing x-ray of the spine.
- Severity of the curve is measured in degrees, usually by the Cobb method (Fig. 304-44).
- MRI is usually not indicated unless there is (1) pain, (2) a neurologic deficit, or (3) a left thoracic curve (which is often associated with an underlying spinal disorder).

TREATMENT
- Treatment or correction of cause if curve is nonstructural
- Early detection is key in treating genetic curve

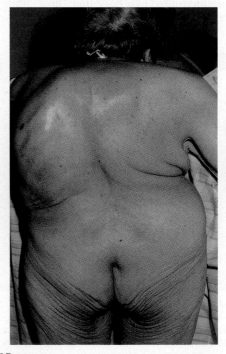

Fig 304-43

Severe kyphoscoliosis.

(From Swartz MH: Textbook of Physical Diagnosis, ed 5, Philadelphia, 2006, WB Saunders)

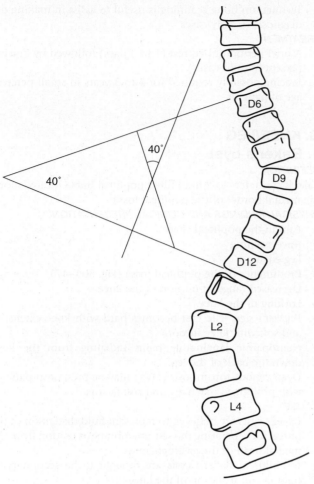

Fig 304–44
Method of measuring the Cobb angle.
(From Grainger RG, Allison DJ, Adam A, Dixon AK [eds]: Grainger and Allison's Diagnostic Radiology, 4th ed. Philadelphia, Churchill Livingstone, 2001.)

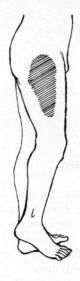

Fig 304–45
Typical location of pain in trochanteric bursitis syndrome. This is also a frequent pain radiation site for lumbar spine lesion, various nerve compression syndromes, and hip disease, particularly in osteonecrosis of the femoral head.
(From Canoso J: Rhematology in primary care, Philadelphia, 1997, WB Saunders.)

- Point tenderness over the greater trochanter is noted.
- Pain is reproduced with resisted hip abduction.

CAUSE

- The specific cause of trochanteric bursitis is not known, although repetitive high-intensity use of the hip joint, trauma, infection (tuberculosis and bacterial), and crystal deposition can precipitate the disease.
- Trochanteric bursitis can occur when other conditions such as osteoarthritis of the knee and hip and bunions of the feet cause changes in the patient's gait, placing varus stress on the hip joint.

DIAGNOSIS

A detailed physical examination and clinical presentation usually make the diagnosis of trochanteric bursitis. Laboratory tests and x-ray images are helpful adjunctive studies used to exclude other conditions either associated with or mimicking trochanteric bursitis.

DIFFERENTIAL DIAGNOSIS

- Osteoarthritis of the hip
- Osteonecrosis of the hip
- Stress fracture of the hip
- Osteoarthritis of the lumbar spine
- Fibromyalgia
- Iliopsoas bursitis
- Trochanteric tendonitis
- Gout
- Pseudogout
- Trauma
- Neuropathy

IMAGING STUDIES

- Plain x-rays of the hip are not very helpful in diagnosing trochanteric bursitis. Sometimes calcifications may be seen around the greater trochanter.
- Bone scan can be done to exclude other disorders but is usually not necessary.
- CT and MRI may show bursitis but are usually not warranted because the results will not alter treatment. They are indicated only when suspecting stress fracture or other disorders.

- Regular observation for curves <20 degrees
- Bracing for idiopathic curves of 20 to 40 degrees to prevent progression
- Surgery for idiopathic curves <40 to 50 degrees in immature patient

F. HIP
1. Trochanteric bursitis

DEFINITION

Trochanteric bursitis is a presumed inflammation or irritation of the gluteus maximus bursa or the bursa separating the greater trochanter from the gluteus medius and gluteus minimus (Fig. 304–45).

PHYSICAL FINDINGS AND CLINICAL PRESENTATION

- Hip pain is the most common complaint. The pain is chronic, intermittent, and located over the lateral thigh.
- Numbness can be present.
- Pain is precipitated with prolonged lying or standing on the affected side.
- Walking, climbing, and running exacerbate the pain.

TREATMENT
- Heat 15 to 20 minutes four to six times per day
- Ultrasound therapy
- Rest
- Partial weight bearing
- Physical therapy to strengthen the back, hip, and knee muscles
- NSAIDs
- Corticosteroid injection

2. Calvé-Legg-Perthes disease

DEFINITION

Calvé-Legg-Perthes disease is a self-limited disorder of unknown etiology caused by ischemia of the immature femoral head that leads to bone necrosis and variable amounts of collapse during the reparative process.

PHYSICAL FINDINGS AND CLINICAL PRESENTATION
- Initial complaint: usually a mildly painful limp
- Pain referred down the inner aspect of the thigh to the knee
- Moderate restriction of motion resulting from hip synovitis (abduction and internal rotation are especially limited)
- Pain at the extremes of movement and tenderness over anterior hip joint

CAUSE

Unknown

DIFFERENTIAL DIAGNOSIS
- Toxic synovitis
- Low-grade septic arthritis
- Juvenile rheumatoid arthritis (JRA) in a young patient

WORKUP

Diagnosis is usually based on the physical findings and eventual radiographic findings.

IMAGING STUDIES
- Plain x-ray to establish the diagnosis (Fig. 304–46)
- AP and frog-leg lateral radiographs

- Technetium bone scanning is useful to assist in making the diagnosis in early cases

TREATMENT
- A brief period of bed rest (1 to 3 days) followed by bracing (except in mild cases)
- Bracing possibly required for 2 to 3 years in small percentage of patients

G. KNEE/LEG
1. Baker's cyst

DEFINITION

Baker's cyst refers to a fluid-filled popliteal bursa located along the medial border of the popliteal fossa.

PHYSICAL FINDINGS AND CLINICAL PRESENTATION
- Pain in the popliteal space
- Knee swelling
- Leg edema
- Prominence of the popliteal fossa (Fig. 304–47)
- Decreased range of motion of the knee
- Locking of the knee
- *Foucher's sign:* The cyst becomes hard with knee extension and soft with knee flexion.
- Neuropathic lancinating pains radiating from the knee down the back of the leg.
- Deep venous thrombosis (DVT) may be present in patients with prolonged inactivity and risk factors.

CAUSE
- Baker's cysts are believed to represent fluid distention of the bursal sac separating the semimembranous tendon from the medial head of the gastrocnemius.
- In children, Baker's cysts are thought to be secondary to trauma and irritation of the knee.
- In adults, Baker's cysts are usually associated with pathologic changes of the knee joint:

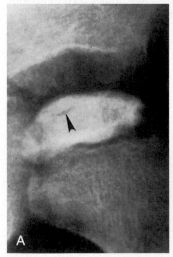
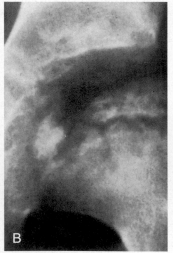
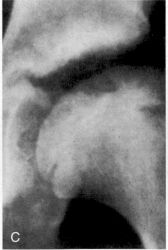
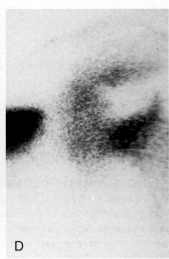

A   B   C   D

Fig 304–46
Calvé-Legg-Perthes' disease. (**A**) Early stage shows a dense femoral capital epiphysis with a small subcortical lucent line *(arrowhead)*. Note that the femoral head is slightly displaced laterally. (**B**) Intermediate stage shows fragmentation of the medial part of the ossification center associated with cystic rarefaction in the proximal metaphysic adjacent to the physis. (**C**) Late stage shows reconstruction of a broad flat deformed femoral head, liable to cause future osteoarthritis. (**D**) Another patient. ^{99}mTc methyl diphophosphonate bone scintigram shows a large cold avascular area *(arrow)* in the lateral portion of the left femoral head. At a later stage, when the femoral head becomes revascularized, the bone scan becomes normal.

(From Grainger RG, Allison DJ, Adam A, Dixon AK [eds]: Grainger and Allison's Diagnostic Radiology, 4th ed. Philadelphia, Churchill Livingstone, 2001.)

- RA
- Osteoarthritis of the knee
- Meniscal tears
- Patellofemoral chondromalacia
- Fracture
- Gout
- Pseudogout
- Infection (tuberculosis)

DIFFERENTIAL DIAGNOSIS
- DVT
- Popliteal aneurysms
- Abscess
- Tumors
- Lymphadenopathy
- Varicosities
- Ganglion

IMAGING STUDIES
- Plain x-ray (AP and lateral views) may show calcification in a solid tumor or in the posterior meniscal area.
- Ultrasound is easy and cost effective and excludes other causes of popliteal fossa pathology.
- MRI of the knee identifies coexisting joint pathology (e.g., osteoarthritis, torn meniscus).

TREATMENT
- NSAIDs, ibuprofen 600 to 800 mg PO tid, or naproxen 500 mg PO bid, can be used to treat Baker's cyst caused by RA, gout, and pseudogout.
- Intra-articular injection or injection of the cyst with corticosteroids.
- Strenuous activity avoidance
- Knee immobilization possibly necessary in some cases

- Surgical procedures addressing the underlying cause or aimed at the cyst include:
  1. Arthroscopic surgery to remove loose cartilaginous fragment
  2. Partial or total meniscectomy
  3. Open excision of the cyst

2. Osgood-Schlatter disease

DEFINITION

Osgood-Schlatter disease is a painful swelling of the tibial tuberosity that occurs in adolescence.

PHYSICAL FINDINGS AND CLINICAL PRESENTATION
- Pain at the tibial tubercle that is aggravated by activity, especially stair-walking and squatting
- Tender swelling and enlargement of the tibial tubercle (Fig. 304–48)
- Increased pain with knee extension against resistance

CAUSE
- Unknown
- May be traumatically induced inflammation

DIFFERENTIAL DIAGNOSIS
- Referred hip pain (any child with hip pain should have a thorough clinical hip examination)
- Patellar tendinitis

IMAGING STUDIES
- Lateral x-ray of the upper portion of the tibia with the leg slightly internally rotated may reveal varying degrees of separation and fragmentation of the upper tibial epiphysis (Fig. 304–49)

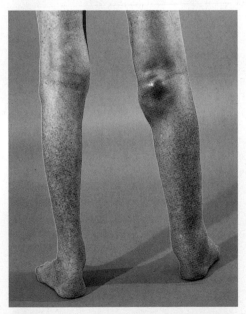

Fig 304–47
Baker's popliteal cyst. Posterior view showing rheumatoid swelling behind the right knee. Swelling of the lower limb was related to venous compression by popliteal synovitis.
(From Hochberg MC, Silman AJ, Smolen JS, et al [eds]: Rheumatology, 3rd ed. St Louis, Mosby, 2003.)

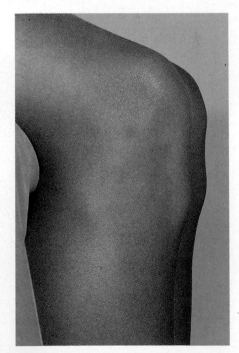

Fig 304–48
Osgood-Schlatter disease. Enlarged tibial tuberosity.
(From Hochberg MC, Silman AJ, Smolen JS, et al [eds]: Rheumatology, 3rd ed. St Louis, Mosby, 2003.)

- Occasionally, fragmented area fails to unite to the tibia and persists into adulthood.

TREATMENT
- Ice, especially after exercise
- NSAIDs
- Gentle hamstring and quadriceps stretching exercises
- Abstinence from physical activity
- Temporary immobilization in a knee splint for 2 to 4 weeks in resistant cases

3. Osteochondritis dissecans

DEFINITION

Osteochondritis dissecans is a disorder in which a portion of cartilage and underlying subchondral bone separates from a joint surface and may even become detached.

The most common joint affected is the knee, with the lateral surface of the medial femoral condyle the most frequent area involved. The capitellum of the humerus, dome of the talus, shoulder, and hip may also be affected.

PHYSICAL FINDINGS AND CLINICAL PRESENTATION
- Pain, stiffness, and swelling
- Intermittent locking if the fragment becomes detached
- Occasionally palpable loose body
- Tenderness at the site of the lesion
- When the knee is involved, positive *Wilson's sign* (pain with knee extension and internal rotation)
- Some asymptomatic cases

CAUSE

Unknown

DIFFERENTIAL DIAGNOSIS
- Fracture
- Neoplasm

IMAGING STUDIES
- Plain x-ray may reveal radiolucent, semilunar line outlining the oval fragment of bone (but findings vary, depending on the amount of healing and stability).
- MRI (Fig. 304–50) or bone scanning is usually not necessary in establishing diagnosis but helpful in determining prognosis and management, especially with regard to the stability of the lesion.

TREATMENT
- Observation every 4 to 6 months for patients in whom the lesion is asymptomatic
- Symptomatic patients who are skeletally immature:
  1. Observation with an initial period of non–weight bearing for 6 to 8 weeks (in knee cases)
  2. When symptoms subside, gradual resumption of activities

H. ANKLE/FOOT
1. Ankle sprain

DEFINITION

An ankle sprain is an injury to the ligamentous support of the ankle. Most (85%) involve the lateral ligament complex. The anterior inferior tibiofibular (AITF) ligament, deltoid ligament, and interosseous membrane may also be injured. Damage to the tibiofibular syndesmosis is sometimes called a *high sprain* because of pain above the ankle.

PHYSICAL FINDINGS AND CLINICAL PRESENTATION
- Often a history of a "pop"
- Varying amounts of tenderness and hemorrhage
- Possible abnormal *anterior drawer test* (pulling the plantar flexed foot forward to determine if there is any abnormal

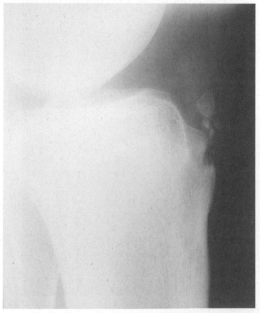

Fig 304–49
Osgood-Schlatter disease. Loose ossicles in the patellar tendon.
(From Hochberg MC, Silman AJ, Smolen JS, et al [eds]: Rheumatology, 3rd ed. St Louis, Mosby, 2003.)

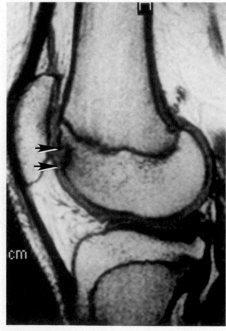

Fig 304–50
Osteochondritis dissecans. Sagittal T1-weighted MRI demonstrating post-traumatic osteochondritis dissecans of the distal femoral epiphysis *(arrows)*.
(From Grainger RG, Allison DJ, Adam A, Dixon AK [eds]: Grainger and Allison's Diagnostic Radiology, 4th ed. Philadelphia, Churchill Livingstone, 2001.)

increase in forward movement of the talus in the ankle mortise) (Fig. 304–51)
- Inversion sprains: tender laterally; syndesmotic injuries: area of tenderness is more anterior and proximal
- Evaluation of motor function

CAUSE
- Lateral injuries usually result from inversion and plantar flexion injuries.
- Eversion and rotational forces may injure the deltoid or AITF ligament or the interosseous membrane.

DIFFERENTIAL DIAGNOSIS
- Fracture of the ankle or foot, particularly involving the distal fibular growth plate in the immature patient
- Avulsion fracture of the fifth metatarsal base

IMAGING STUDIES
X-ray evaluation
1. Usually normal but always performed
2. When done, should include the fifth metatarsal base
3. All minor avulsion fractures should be noted
4. MRI (Fig. 304–52) when diagnosis is uncertain

Varying opinions on the usefulness of arthrograms, tenograms, and stress films

TREATMENT
Ankle sprains are often graded I, II, or III, according to severity, with grade III injury implying complete rupture. The first line of treatment is described by the mnemonic device *RICE:*
- Rest
- Ice
- Compression
- Elevation
- NSAIDs
- In 48 to 72 hours, active range of motion and weight bearing as tolerated

- In 4 to 5 days, exercise against resistance added
- Possible cast immobilization for some patients who require early independent walking; short leg orthoses also available for the same purpose
- Surgery is rarely recommended, even for grade III sprains; reports of equally satisfactory outcomes with nonsurgical treatment

2. Ankle fracture

DEFINITION
Ankle fractures involve the lateral, medial, or posterior malleolus of the ankle and may occur either alone or in some combination. Associated ligamentous injuries are included.

PHYSICAL FINDINGS AND CLINICAL PRESENTATION
- Deformity usually dependent on extent of displacement
- Pain, tenderness, and hemorrhage at the site of injury
- Gentle palpation of ligamentous structures (especially deltoid ligament) to determine the extent of soft tissue injury
- Evaluation of distal neurovascular status; results recorded

CAUSE
- The ankle depends on its ligamentous and bony support for stability. The joint, or *mortise*, is an inverted U with the dome of the talus fitting into the medial and lateral malleoli. The posterior margin of the tibia is often called the *third* or *posterior malleolus*.
- Most common ankle fractures are the result of eversion or lateral rotation forces on the talus (in contrast to common sprains, which are caused usually by inversion).

DIFFERENTIAL DIAGNOSIS
- Ankle sprain
- Avulsion fracture of hindfoot or metatarsal

IMAGING STUDIES
Standard AP and lateral views accompanied by an AP taken 15 degrees internally rotated. The last view is taken to properly visualize the mortise. MRI when diagnosis is uncertain (Fig. 304–53)

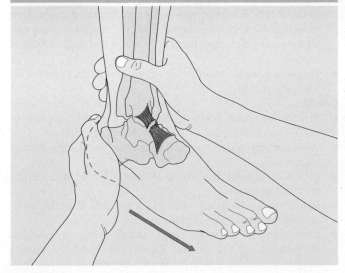

**THE ANKLE JOINT: ANTERIOR DRAW SIGN
(TEAR OF THE ANTERIOR TALOFIBULAR LIGAMENT)**

Fig 304–51
The ankle joint: anterior draw sign (tear of the anterior talofibular ligament).
(From Hochberg MC, Silman AJ, Smolen JS, et al [eds]: Rheumatology, 3rd ed. St Louis, Mosby, 2003.)

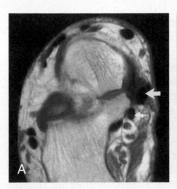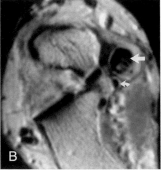

Fig 304–52
Oblique axial T1-weighted MRI of a normal ankle (**A**) demonstrates the normal 2:1 size ratio of the posterior tibialis *(arrow)* and flexor digitorum longus *(small arrow)* tendons. Axial proton density image from a patient who experienced ankle trauma (**B**) shows enlargement of, and abnormal signal within, the posterior tibialis tendon, consistent with a partial tear of that structure *(arrow)*. The flexor digitorum longus tendon is normal *(small arrow)*.
(From Grainger RG, Allison DJ, Adam A, Dixon AK [eds]: Grainger and Allison's Diagnostic Radiology, 4th ed. Philadelphia, Churchill Livingstone, 2001.)

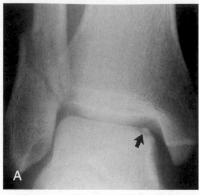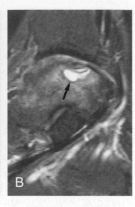

Fig 304–53

Osteochondral fracture of the medial talar dome. Oblique view of the ankle (**A**) demonstrates a lucency separating a small bony fragment from the remainder of the talar dome, consistent with an osteochondral fracture *(arrow)*. There is also a fracture of the lateral malleolus. Sagittal STIR MR image from another patient (**B**) demonstrates an osteochondral fragment of the talar dome separated from the remainder of the talus by high signal fluid *(arrow)*.

(From Grainger RG, Allison DJ, Adam A, Dixon AK [eds]: Grainger and Allison's Diagnostic Radiology, 4th ed. Philadelphia, Churchill Livingstone, 2001.)

TREATMENT

All fractures: elevation and ice to control swelling for 48 to 72 hours

- If there is no widening of the ankle mortise, many injuries can be safely treated with simple casting without reduction:

1. Undisplaced or avulsion fractures of either malleolus below the ankle joint line:
   a. Stability of the joint is not compromised and a short leg walking cast or ankle support is sufficient.
   b. Weight bearing is allowed as tolerated.
   c. In 4 to 6 weeks, protection may be discontinued.
2. Isolated undisplaced fractures of the medial, lateral, or posterior malleolus:
   a. Usually stable and require only the application of a short leg walking cast with the ankle in the neutral position or fracture cast boot.
   b. Immobilization should be continued for 8 weeks.
   c. Fracture line of lateral malleolus may persist roentgenographically for several months, but immobilization beyond 8 weeks is usually unnecessary.
   d. Undisplaced bimalleolar fractures are treated with a long leg cast flexed 30 degrees at the knee to prevent motion and displacement of the fracture fragments. In 4 weeks, a short leg walking cast may be applied for an additional 4 weeks.
3. Isolated fractures of the lateral malleolus that are slightly displaced:
   a. May be treated with casting if no medial injury is present.
   b. A below-knee walking cast is applied with ankle in the neutral position and weight bearing is allowed as tolerated.
   c. Six weeks of immobilization is sufficient.
   d. If medial tenderness is present, suggesting deltoid ligament rupture, a carefully molded cast may suffice if weight bearing is not allowed and the patient is followed closely for signs of instability, especially after swelling recedes. If

significant widening of the medial ankle mortise (increase in the "medial clear space") develops as a result of lateral displacement of the talus, referral for possible reduction is indicated.
   e. If signs of instability are already present at initial examination (widening of the medial clear space with medial tenderness), referral is indicated.
4. Undisplaced fracture of the distal fibular epiphysis:
   a. Often diagnosed clinically
   b. There is tenderness over the epiphyseal plate.
   c. X-ray findings are often negative.
   d. A short leg walking cast is applied for 4 weeks.
   e. Growth disturbance is rare.
5. Isolated posterior malleolar fractures involving less than 25% of the joint surface on the lateral x-ray:
   Safely treated by applying a short leg walking cast or fracture brace. (Fractures involving >25% of the weight-bearing surface should be referred because of the potential for instability and subsequent traumatic arthritis.)

3. Achilles tendon rupture

DEFINITION

Achilles tendon rupture refers to the loss of continuity of the *tendo Achillis,* usually from attrition/trauma.

PHYSICAL FINDINGS AND CLINICAL PRESENTATION

Injury often occurs during an activity that puts great stress on the tendon. Sudden "pop" is often felt followed by weakness and swelling.

- Patient walks flat-footed and is unable to stand on the ball of the foot.
- Tenderness and hemorrhage are present at the site of injury, and a sulcus is usually palpable but may be obscured by an organizing clot if the examination is delayed.
- Although active plantar flexion is usually lost, some plantar flexion occasionally remains because of the activity of the other posterior compartment muscles.
- *Thompson's test* is usually positive. Test measures plantar flexion of the foot when the calf is squeezed with the patient kneeling on a chair; normal foot plantarflexes with calf compression, but movement is absent when *tendo Achillis* is ruptured.
- Excessive passive dorsiflexion of the foot is also present on the injured side

CAUSE

- Relative hypovascularity predisposing to tendon rupture in several tendons (Achilles, biceps, and supraspinatus)
- With advancing age, vascular supply to the tendon further compromised
- Repetitive trauma leading to degeneration of this critical area and weakness
- Rupture of *tendo Achillis* usually 2.5 to 5 cm from the insertion of the tendon into the os calcis
- Most common causative event leading to rupture: sudden dorsiflexion of the plantar flexed foot (landing from a height) or sudden pushing off with the weight on the forefoot

DIFFERENTIAL DIAGNOSIS

- Incomplete (partial) *tendo Achillis* rupture
- Partial rupture of gastrocnemius muscle, often medial head (previously thought to be "plantaris tendon rupture")

DIAGNOSIS

Diagnosis is made on physical examination. MRI (Fig. 304–54) will confirm diagnosis

TREATMENT

- Early referral is necessary for open, end-to-end surgical repair.
- If surgery is contraindicated, a short leg cast applied with the foot in equinus may allow healing.
- In cases of neglected rupture, reconstruction is usually indicated.
- Physical therapy is helpful after repair to restore strength and flexibility.

4. Tarsal tunnel syndrome

DEFINITION

Tarsal tunnel syndrome is a rare entrapment neuropathy that develops as a result of compression of the posterior tibial nerve in the tunnel (Fig. 304–55) formed by the flexor retinaculum behind the medial malleolus of the ankle This retinaculum arises from the medial malleolus and inserts into the medial aspect of the calcaneus.

PHYSICAL FINDINGS AND CLINICAL PRESENTATION

- Symptoms are often vague in contrast to other compression neuropathies such as carpal tunnel syndrome.
- Neuritic symptoms along the course of the posterior tibial nerve in the sole and heel
- The Valleix phenomenon (proximal radiation of the pain) may occur.
- Swelling over tarsal tunnel
- Possible positive Tinel's sign
- Possible reproduction of symptoms with sustained eversion of hindfoot or digital compression of tunnel
- Sensory loss and motor changes unusual

CAUSE

- Space-occupying lesions (ganglia, varicosities, lipomas, synovial hypertrophy) or local tendonitis
- Possibly traction on nerve

DIFFERENTIAL DIAGNOSIS

- Plantar fasciitis
- Peripheral neuropathy
- Proximal radiculopathy
- Local tendinitis
- Peripheral vascular disease
- Morton's neuroma (see Fig. 304–56)

ELECTRICAL STUDIES

Electrodiagnostic testing is often inconclusive. Delayed sensory conduction or increased motor latency may be seen.

TREATMENT

- NSAIDs
- Immobilization for 4 to 6 weeks with ankle orthosis or fracture cast boot
- Medial heel wedge or orthotic to minimize heel eversion
- Local steroid injection into tunnel (avoiding the posterior tibial nerve) if symptoms persist

5. Morton's neuroma

DEFINITION

Morton's neuroma refers to an inflammatory fibrosing process of the plantar digital nerve characterized by pain in the sole of the foot (Fig. 304–56). Morton's neuroma is also described as an interdigital plantar neuropathy with or without plantar neuroma.

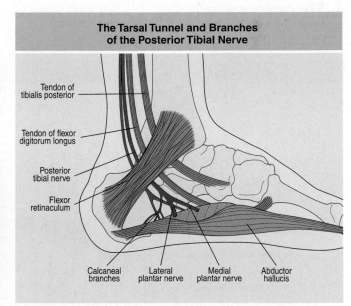

The Tarsal Tunnel and Branches of the Posterior Tibial Nerve

Tendon of tibialis posterior

Tendon of flexor digitorum longus

Posterior tibial nerve

Flexor retinaculum

Calcaneal branches

Lateral plantar nerve

Medial plantar nerve

Abductor hallucis

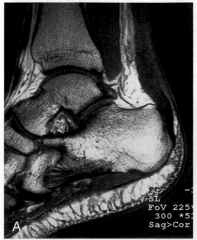
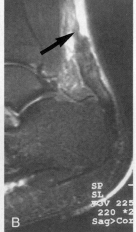

Fig 304–54

Sagittal T1-weighted (**A**) and STIR (**B**) MRI demonstrates discontinuity of the Achilles tendon, with abnormal signal (*arrow*, B) representing hemorrhage and edema. Note how poorly the T1-weighted image demonstrates the disruption; this is because edematous tendon and fluid may look identical with such sequences.
(From Grainger RG, Allison DJ, Adam A, Dixon AK [eds]: Grainger and Allison's Diagnostic Radiology, 4th ed. Philadelphia, Churchill Livingstone, 2001.)

Fig 304–55

The tarsal tunnel and branches of the posterior tibial nerve. Entrapment of branches of the posterior tibial nerve occurs under the flexor retinaculum, which attaches to the medial malleolus. As there are calcaneal as well as medial and lateral plantar branches of the posterior tibial nerve, symptoms of entrapment will depend on which branches are affected.
(From Hochberg MC, Silman AJ, Smolen JS, et al [eds]: Rheumatology, 3rd ed. St Louis, Mosby, 2003.)

PHYSICAL FINDINGS AND CLINICAL PRESENTATION
- Pain is usually located in a specific region, usually in the sole of the foot between the third and fourth metatarsal areas, and is unilateral in the majority of cases.
- Numbness may occur.
- Pain is exacerbated with exercise and relieved with rest and may radiate to the toes and to the ankle.
- Point tenderness is noted on examination, and palpation reveals fullness at the site of discomfort.
- An audible, painful click called *"Murder's click"* is noted in patients with Morton's neuroma after compressing and releasing the forefoot.
- Patients may have neuroma but silent lesions without symptoms.

CAUSE
- Morton's neuroma is thought to be caused by nerve thickening from repeated injury.
- The typical finding is swelling of the plantar digital nerve that pathologically resembles other nerve entrapment syndromes (e.g., median nerve compression in carpal tunnel syndrome).

DIFFERENTIAL DIAGNOSIS
- Diabetic neuropathy
- Alcoholic neuropathy
- Nutritional neuropathy
- Toxic neuropathy
- Osteoarthritis
- Trauma (e.g., fracture)
- Gouty arthritis
- RA

IMAGING STUDIES
- X-ray imaging is primarily done to exclude other causes of foot pain (e.g., fractures, ostearthritis, gouty arthritis).

- MRI can detect and localize a neuroma but is rarely needed to make the diagnosis. MRI can also be performed in patients with recurrent pain after surgical excision of a Morton's neuroma.
- Ultrasound imaging is also being used to locate Morton's neuromas but is rarely needed to make the diagnosis.

TREATMENT
- Changing the type of footwear is the first line of treatment.
- Use open footwear and custom shoe inserts and avoid weight-bearing activities.
- Metatarsal pad with arch support is helpful.
- Participate in ultrasound therapy.
- If conservative measures are unsuccessful, injection of the intermetatarsal bursa with hydrocortisone may help
- NSAIDs
- If nonpharmacologic and acute treatments do not give sufficient relief, surgical excision of the nerve has been successful in 95% of the cases.

6. Bunion deformity and hammer toes

Bunion deformity (hallux abductovalgus) and deformities and flexion contractions of the lower digits (hammer toes) are common in the geriatric population (Fig. 304–57). Patients who have subluxation of MTP joints often develop ulceration over the PIP joints that protrude dorsally. There is an increased incidence in patients with osteoarthritis and RA. Treatment in symptomatic patients is surgical correction.

I. CHEST WALL (COSTOCHONDRITIS)

DEFINITION

Costochondritis is a poorly defined chest wall pain of uncertain cause.

PHYSICAL FINDINGS AND CLINICAL PRESENTATION
- Tenderness of costochondral junctions (second through fifth) and/or sternum (Fig. 304–58)
- Pain with coughing and deep breathing
- Both sides of chest equal in frequency of involvement
- Often associated with anxiety, headache, and hyperventilation

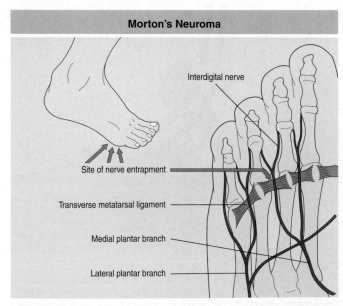

Morton's Neuroma

Interdigital nerve

Site of nerve entrapment

Transverse metatarsal ligament

Medial plantar branch

Lateral plantar branch

Fig 304–56
Morton's neuroma. On the plantar surface of the foot, the interdigital nerve is compressed below the transverse metatarsal ligament and not between the metatarsal heads (plantar view).
(From Hochberg MC, Silman AJ, Smolen JS, et al [eds]: Rheumatology, 3rd ed. St Louis, Mosby, 2003.)

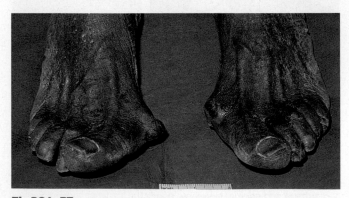

Fig 304–57
Bunion deformity and hammer toes.
(From Swartz MH: Textbook of Physical Diagnosis, ed 5, Philadelphia, 2006, WB Saunders)

CAUSE
- Unknown
- May be a form of regional fibrositis
- May be referred pain from cervical or thoracic spine
- Emotional factors often involved

DIFFERENTIAL DIAGNOSIS
- Cardiovascular disease
- GI disease
- Pulmonary disease
- Osteoarthritis
- Cervical disc syndrome

WORKUP
- There are no laboratory or radiographic abnormalities.
- Testing to rule out or rule in more serious disorders is performed on a case-by-case basis.

TREATMENT
- Explanation, reassurance
- Tricyclic antidepressants for sleep disturbance
- NSAIDs for analgesia

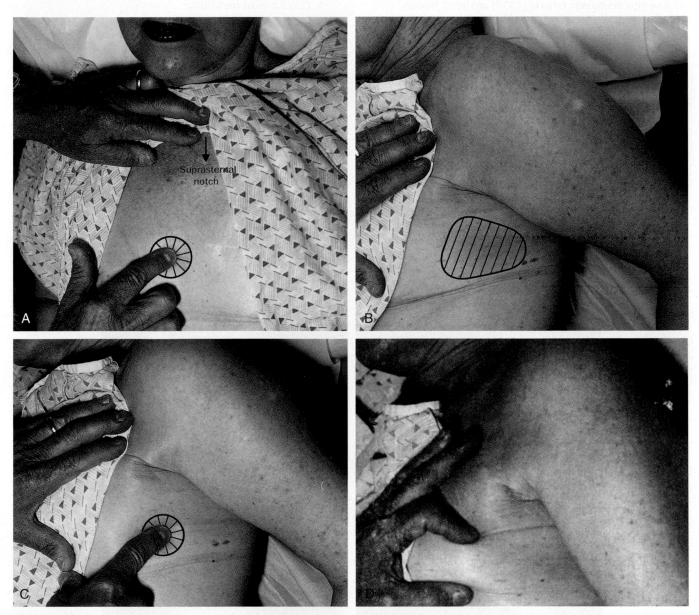

Fig 304–58
Physical examination to detect types of chest wall pain. (**A**) Detection of pain to palpation over the costochondral junctions to elicit the pain of costochondritis and Tietze's syndrome. To provide anatomic orientation, the suprasternal notch is indicated by an *arrow*. (**B**) The area encircled in black indicates an area of diffuse lateral chest wall pain. The patient is examined while lying at 90° on her side. (**C**) Demonstration by palpation of focal lateral chest wall. The area of pain is encircled in black. (**D**). Squeezing of breast tissue between the fingers does not elicit pain in the area where the patient complains of pain. This demonstrates to the patient that her pain is chest-wall in origin (see focal area encircled in black in (**C**) rather than in the breast itself.
(From Besser CM, Thorner MO: Comprehensive Clinical Endocrinology, 3rd ed, St. Louis, Mosby, 2002.)

Chapter 305 — Inherited connective tissue disorders

A. EHLERS-DANLÖS SYNDROME

DEFINITION

Ehlers-Danlos syndrome (EDS) refers to a group of inherited, clinically variable, and genetically heterogeneous connective tissue disorders. EDS is characterized by skin hyperextensibility (Fig. 305–1), skin fragility, joint laxity (Fig. 305–2), and joint hyperextensibility (Fig. 305–3A). The revised classification scheme and diagnostic criteria (1998) are listed below.

CLINICAL PRESENTATION

- Classic (EDS I and II): hyperextensibility ("*Gorlin's sign:*" ability to touch tip of tongue to nose) (see Fig. 305–2), easy scarring and bruising ("cigarette-paper scars") (see Fig. 305–3B), smooth, velvety skin, subcutaneous spheroids (small, firm cystlike nodules) along shins or forearms
- Hypermobility (EDS III): joint hypermobility and some skin hypermobility with or without very smooth skin
- Vascular (EDS IV): thin, translucent skin with visible veins; marked bruising; pinched nose; acrogeria; generalized tissue friability; spontaneous rupture of medium and large arteries and hollow organs, especially the large intestine and uterus
- Kyphoscoliotic (EDS VI): characterized by joint hypermobility, progressive scoliosis; ocular fragility and possible globe rupture, mitral valve prolapse, and aortic dilation
- Arthrochalasia (EDS VII A and B): prominent joint hypermobility with subluxations, congenital hip dislocation, skin hyperextensibility, and tissue fragility

- Dermatosparaxis (EDS VIIC): severe skin fragility with decreased elasticity, bruising, hernias
- Unclassified type:
  1. EDS V: classic characteristics
  2. EDS VIII: classic characteristics and periodontal disease
  3. EDS IX: classic characteristics
  4. EDS X: mild classic characteristics, mitral valve prolapse
  5. EDS XI: joint instability

CAUSE

- Defects of collagen in extracellular matrices of multiple tissues (skin, tendons, blood vessels, and viscera) underlie all forms of EDS.
- EDS I and II are associated with defects in type V collagen, corresponding to mutations of the *COL5A* genes.
- EDS IV involves a deficiency in type III collagen, and several studies suggest that mutations of gene *COL3A1* lead to this deficiency.
- EDS VIIA and VIIB result from a defect in type I collagen, caused by mutations in the *COL1A1* and *COL1A2* genes.

DIFFERENTIAL DIAGNOSIS

- Marfan's syndrome (see Fig. 305–4)
- Osteogenesis imperfecta
- Autosomal dominant cutis laxa
- Familial joint hypermobility

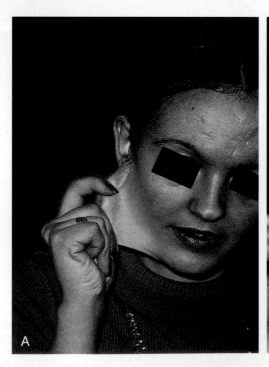
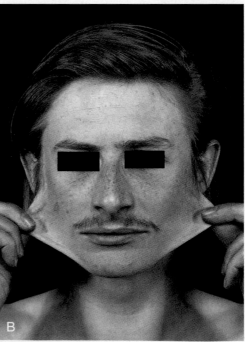

Fig 305–1

(**A, B**) Ehlers-Danlos syndrome: marked hyperelasticity of the skin which, in the younger patient, springs back on release is characteristic. The patient in (**A**) also shows hypertelorism and a widened nasal bridge.

(Courtesy of R. A. Marsden, MD, St George's Hospital, London, UK; [**B**] courtesy of the Institute of Dermatology, London, UK.)

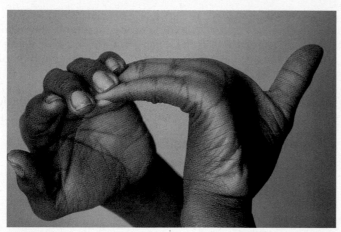

Fig 305-2
(**A, B**) Ehlers-Danlos syndrome: hyperextensible joints are characteristic.
([**A**] Courtesy of F. M. Pope, MD, Northwick Park Hospital, London, UK; [**B**] courtesy of the Institute of Dermatology, London UK.)

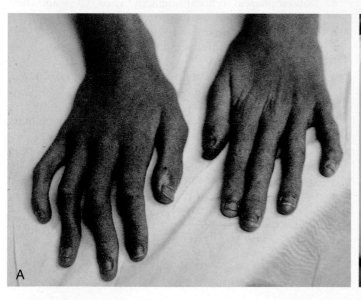

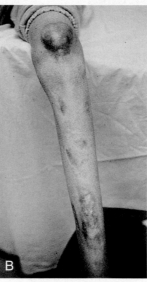

Fig 305-3
Features of Ehlers-Danlos syndrome. (**A**) Hyperextensibility of small joints. (**B**) Cigarette-paper scarring.
(Courtesy of Dr. DK Grange.)

A

B

LABORATORY TESTS

- Limited biochemical assays and gene analyses are performed for known molecular defects.
- Plain radiographs may reveal calcified nodules along the shins or forearms, corresponding to the subcutaneous spheroids.
- Echocardiogram can identify mitral valve prolapsed (MVP) and aortic dilation.

TREATMENT

- All patients should receive genetic counseling about the mode of inheritance of their EDS and the risk of having children with EDS.
- Management of most skin and joint problems should be conservative and preventive. Joint hypermobility and pain in EDS usually does not require surgical intervention. Physical therapy to strengthen muscles is helpful. Surgical repair and tightening of joint ligaments can be performed but ligaments frequently will not hold sutures. Surgical intervention should be considered on an individual basis.
- Vascular type requires special surgical care because of increased tissue friability.
- Patients should be advised to avoid contact sports.
- Elevated blood pressure should be aggressively treated.

B. MARFAN'S SYNDROME

DEFINITION

Marfan's syndrome is an inherited disorder of connective tissue involving skeleton, cardiovascular system, eyes, lungs, and CNS.

PHYSICAL FINDINGS AND CLINICAL PRESENTATION

Diagnostic criteria for Marfan's syndrome

- **Skeleton:** joint hypermobility, tall stature (Fig. 305-4), pectus excavatum, reduced thoracic kyphosis, scoliosis, arachnodactyly, dolichostenomelia, pectus carinatum, and erosion of the lumbosacral vertebrae from dural ectasia†
- **Eye:** myopia, retinal detachment, elongated globe, ectopia lentis†
- **Cardiovascular:** MVP, endocarditis, arrhythmia, dilated mitral annulus, mitral regurgitation, tricuspid valve prolapse, aortic regurgitation, aortic dissection,† dilation of the aortic root†
- **Pulmonary:** apical blebs, spontaneous pneumothorax
- **Skin and integument:** inguinal hernias, incisional hernias, striae atrophicae
- **CNS:** attention-deficit disorder, hyperactivity, verbal-performance discrepancy, dural ectasia, anterior pelvic meningocele†

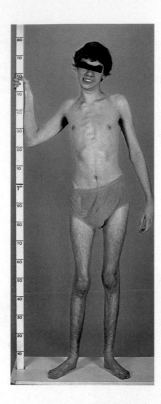

Fig 305–4

A boy with Marfan's syndrome. Arm span is greater than height, and the limbs are long with slender hands and fingers. The cause of death in these patients is usually a dissecting aneurysm in early adult life. (From Besser CM, Thorner MO: Comprehensive Clinical Endocrinology, 3rd ed, St. Louis, Mosby, 2002.)

- If the family history is positive for a close relative clearly affected by Marfan's syndrome, manifestations should be present in the skeleton and one of the other organ systems, and the diagnosis confirmed by linkage analysis or mutation detection.
- If the family history is negative or unknown, the patient should have manifestations in the skeleton, the cardiovascular system, and one other system, and at least one of the manifestations indicated by †.
- Manifestations are listed within each organ system in increasing specificity for Marfan's syndrome; although none is completely specific, those indicated by † are the most specific.

CAUSE

Mutations in the gene that encodes fibrillin-1, the major constituent of microfibrils, which form the frame for elastic fibers. All the manifestations of Marfan's syndrome can be explained by the defective microfibrils.

DIFFERENTIAL DIAGNOSIS

Each of the clinical manifestations of the syndrome may have other causes; however, if the diagnostic criteria are met, the diagnosis is made.

WORKUP

- Echocardiography to establish:
  - MVP
  - Mitral regurgitation
  - Tricuspid valve prolapse
  - Aortic regurgitation
  - Dilation of the aortic root
- Transesophageal echocardiography, chest CT scan, chest MRI, or aortography for suspected aortic dissection
- Chest x-ray for pulmonary apical bullae
- Ophthalmologic examination by ophthalmologist

TREATMENT

- Regular cardiac and aorta monitoring by physical examination and echocardiography
- Endocarditis prophylaxis
- Restriction of contact sports, weight lifting, and overexertion
- Beta-blockers
- Early use of angiotensin-converting enzyme inhibitors in young patients with Marfan's syndrome and valvular regurgitation may lessen the need for mitral valve surgery.
- Genetic counseling
- Monitor aorta during pregnancy (because of increased risk of dissection).

Chapter 306 | Diseases of bone and bone metabolism

A. OSTEOPOROSIS

DEFINITION
Osteoporosis is characterized by a progressive decrease in bone mass that results in increased bone fragility and a higher fracture risk. The various types are as follows:

Primary osteoporosis: 80% of women and 60% of men with osteoporosis
- Idiopathic osteoporosis: unknown pathogenesis; may occur in children and young adults
- Type I osteoporosis: may occur in postmenopausal women (age range: 51 to 75 years); characterized by accelerated and disproportionate trabecular bone loss and associated with vertebral body and distal forearm fractures (estrogen withdrawal effect)
- Type II osteoporosis (involutional): occurs in both men and women >70 years of age; characterized by both trabecular and cortical bone loss, and associated with fractures of the proximal humerus and tibia, femoral neck, and pelvis

Secondary osteoporosis: 20% of women and 40% of men with osteoporosis; osteoporosis that exists as a common feature of another disease process, heritable disorder of connective tissue, or drug side effect (see "Differential Diagnosis")

PHYSICAL FINDINGS AND CLINICAL PRESENTATION
- Most commonly silent with no signs and symptoms
- Insidious and progressive development of dorsal kyphosis ("dowager's hump") (Fig. 306–1), loss of height, and skeletal pain typically associated with fracture, other physical findings related to other conditions with associated increased risk for osteoporosis (see "Risk Factors")

CAUSE
- Primary osteoporosis—multifactorial resulting from a combination of factors including nutrition, peak bone mass, genetics, level of physical activity, age at menopause (spontaneous versus surgical), and estrogen status
- Secondary osteoporosis—associated decrease in bone mass resulting from an identified cause, including endocrinopathies: hypogonadism, hyperthyroidism, hyperparathyroidism, Cushing's syndrome, hyperprolactinemia, acromegaly, diabetes mellitus, gastrointestinal disease, malabsorption, primary biliary cirrhosis, gastrectomy, malnutrition (including anorexia nervosa)

DIFFERENTIAL DIAGNOSIS
- Malignancy (multiple myeloma, lymphoma, leukemia, metastatic carcinoma)
- Primary hyperparathyroidism
- Osteomalacia
- Paget's disease

LABORATORY TESTS
- Biochemical profile to evaluate renal and hepatic function, primary hyperparathyroidism, and malnutrition
- CBC for nutritional status and myeloma
- TSH to rule out the presence of hyperthyroidism
- Consideration of 24-hour urine collection for calcium (excess skeletal loss, vitamin D malabsorption/deficiency), creatinine, sodium, and free cortisol (to detect occult Cushing's disease); no need to measure calcitropic hormones (PTH, calcitriol, calcitonin) unless specifically indicated
- Biochemical markers of bone remodeling; may be useful to predict rate of bone loss and/or follow therapy response; specific biochemical markers followed (e.g., 3-month interval) to document normalization as a response to therapy

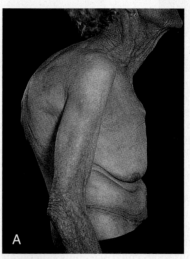

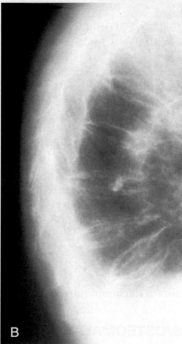

Fig 306–1
Dowager's bump. (**A**) Marked thoracic kyphosis due to multiple osteoporotic fractures in an elderly woman with (**B**) corresponding radiograph.
(From Hochberg MC, Silman AJ, Smolen JS, et al [eds]: Rheumatology, 3rd ed. St Louis, Mosby, 2003.)

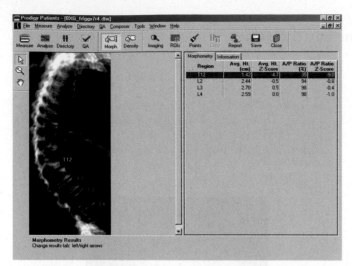

Fig 306–2
Vertebral fracture assessment from a dual x-ray absorptiometry image of the spine. Use of dual energy images facilitates the visualization of the lumbar and thoracic spine in a single image. In this example, a fracture has been identified at T12.
(From Hochberg MC, Silman AJ, Smolen JS, et al [eds]: Rheumatology, 3rd ed. St Louis, Mosby, 2003.)

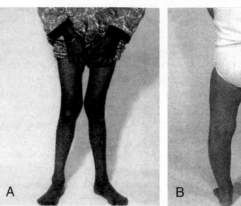
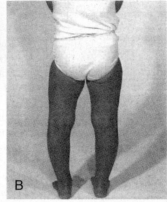

Fig 306–3
Knock knees and bow legs in rickets. (**A**) This boy had simple nutritional vitamin D deficiency. (**B**) This girl had hypophosphatemic rickets.
(From Besser CM, Thorner MO: Comprehensive Clinical Endocrinology, 3rd ed, St. Louis, Mosby, 2002).

IMAGING STUDIES
- BMD determination (dual-energy x-ray absorptiometry [DEXA] scan) (Fig. 306–2) should be performed on all patients with determined risk factors and/or associated secondary causes; accepted screening criteria are currently being investigated.
  1. Normal: BMD <1 SD of the young adult reference mean
  2. Osteopenia: BMD <1 to 2.5 SDs below the young adult reference mean
  3. Osteoporosis: BMD <2.5 SDs below the young adult reference mean
- For patient undergoing treatment: annual BMD to follow response to therapy
- X-ray examination of appropriate part of skeleton to evaluate clinical osteoporotic fracture only (Fig. 306–1)

TREATMENT
- Identification and minimization of risk factors
- Appropriate diagnosis and treatment of secondary causes
- Vitamin D supplement: 400 U/day
- Calcium supplement: 1000 to 1500 mg/day
- Bisphosphonates: alendronate, risedronate, ibandronate, zoledronic acid
- Raloxifene
- Teriparatide
- Synthetic salmon calcitonin intranasally

B. RICKETS/OSTEOMALACIA

DEFINITION
Rickets is a systemic disease of infancy and childhood in which mineralization of growing bone is deficient as a result of abnormal calcium, phosphorus, or vitamin D metabolism. *Osteomalacia* is the same condition in the adult. *Renal osteodystrophy* is a term used to describe a similar condition in patients with chronic kidney disease. Certain forms of the disorder may re-

spond only to high doses of vitamin D and are referred to as vitamin D–resistant rickets (VDRR).

PHYSICAL FINDINGS AND CLINICAL PRESENTATION
The child with classic rickets usually develops a number of specific abnormalities:
- Softening of the skull bones (craniotabes) early in the disorder
- Enlargement of the ribs at the costochondral junctions, producing the "rachitic rosary"
- Limb deformities (Fig. 306–3) and epiphyseal swelling
- Height below normal range
- Irritability and easy fatigability
- Pigeon breast deformity and an indentation of the lower rib cage at the insertion of the diaphragm, sometimes referred to as Harrison's groove; possible decrease in thoracic volume, resulting in diminished pulmonary ventilation

Physical findings in the adult with osteomalacia are more subtle:
- Possible malaise and bone pain
- Many patients presumed to have osteoporosis but may also have osteomalacia

CAUSE
- Deficiency states
  1. True classic VDDR is rare in Western society.
  2. Absorption of vitamin D, however, may be blocked in several GI disorders.
  3. Similar disorders may also prevent absorption of calcium and phosphorus, but in the absence of these other diseases, deficiencies of calcium and phosphorus are also rare.
- Acquired or inherited renal tubular abnormalities that cause resorptive defects and result in rickets and osteomalacia; syndromes include classic VDRR (probably the most common form of rickets seen in general practice)

TABLE 306–1 Serum chemistry in different types of osteomalacia.

Vitamin D deficiency
Calcium ↓
Phosphate ↓ (with normal kidneys)
Secondary hyperparathyroidism
Parathyroid hormone ↑
Serum calcium (normal or abnormal) ↓
Urine calcium ↓
Phosphate ↓ ↓
Chronic renal disease
Glomerular filtration rate ↑
Phosphate ↑
Calcium ↓ (because of impaired formation of 1,25-dihydroxyvitamin D)
Renal phosphorus leak
Serum phosphate ↓
Serum calcium normal

Besser CM, Thorner MO: Comprehensive Clinical Endocrinology, 3rd ed. St Louis, Mosby, 2002.

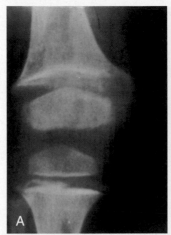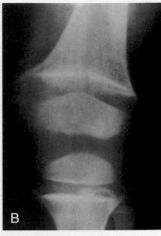

Fig 306–4

Hypophosphatemic rickets. AO radiograph of both knees demonstrates diffuse osteopenia. The growth plates of the distal femora have widened and protrude into the weakened metaphyseal region, causing cupping and widening of the metaphyses. Note also the irregular, indistinct borders of the femoral epiphyses.
(From Grainger RG, Allison DJ, Adam A, Dixon AK [eds]: Grainger and Allison's Diagnostic Radiology, 4th ed. Philadelphia, Churchill Livingstone, 2001.)

- Chronic renal failure:
  1. Can produce renal rickets or renal osteodystrophy
  2. Results in the retention of phosphate

DIFFERENTIAL DIAGNOSIS

- Osteoporosis
- Hyperparathyroidism
- Hyperthyroidism

LABORATORY TESTS

- Requires a high degree of interest because many of the conditions are so similar that only a complicated laboratory evaluation may establish the diagnosis. Serum chemistry in different types of osteomalacia are described in Table 306–1.
- BUN, creatinine, alkaline phosphatase, calcium, and phosphorus levels in any patient suspected of having metabolic bone disease

IMAGING STUDIES

- In rickets:
  1. Characteristic radiographic changes in the ends of growing long bones caused by the lack of calcification of the cartilage matrix (Fig. 306–4)
  2. Widening and irregularity of the epiphyseal plate
- Radiographs in the adult with osteomalacia:
  1. More subtle and often confused with osteoporosis
  2. Bowing of bones (Fig. 306–5). Possible pseudofractures (Looser's zones) where major arteries cross bone
  3. Insufficiency compression deformities in the vertebral bodies (Fig. 306–6)

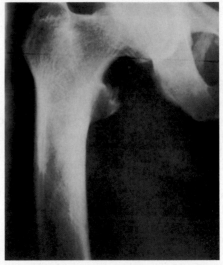

Fig 306–5

Hypophosphatemic osteomalacia. AP radiograph of the femur shows bowing. Notice also the dense bones (typical of this disorder) and ossification at the lesser trochanter and the sacrotuberous ligament.
(From Grainger RG, Allison DJ, Adam A, Dixon AK [eds]: Grainger and Allison's Diagnostic Radiology, 4th ed. Philadelphia, Churchill Livingstone, 2001.)

TREATMENT

- Proper nutrition with replacement of calcium, vitamin D, phosphorus, and other minerals. The need for orthopedic intervention is rare.
- Surgical care is indicated for slipped capital femoral epiphysis, which is fairly common in renal rickets.
- Deformity may require bracing.

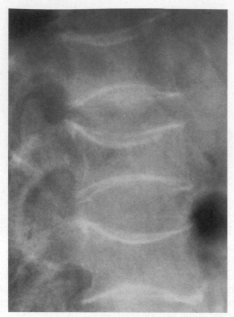

Fig 306–6
Osteomalacia. Lateral view of the lumbar spine in patient with osteomalacia shows moderate osteopenia involving the vertebral bodies. The trabeculae in the vertebral bodies appear indistinct or fuzzy. There is evidence of bone softening with bowing of the end plates. (From Grainger RG, Allison DJ, Adam A, Dixon AK [eds]: Grainger and Allison's Diagnostic Radiology, 4th ed. Philadelphia, Churchill Livingstone, 2001.)

C. OSTEONECROSIS

DEFINITION
Osteonecrosis (avascular necrosis, aseptic necrosis) refers to the death of bone marrow, cortex, and medullary bone caused by interruption of blood supply to the bone.

PHYSICAL FINDINGS AND CLINICAL PRESENTATION
- May be clinically silent
- Pain in the affected bone (hip, knee, or shoulder)
- Pain at rest or with use
- Decreased range of motion of the affected joint
- Joint pain with passive motion

CAUSE
The etiology of osteonecrosis can be divided into:
- Atraumatic
  1. Idiopathic
  2. Alcohol
  3. Hemoglobinopathy (e.g., sickle cell disease)
  4. Connective tissue disorders (SLE, rheumatoid arthritis, vasculitis, antiphospholipid syndrome)
  5. Corticosteroid use
  6. Pregnancy
  7. Estrogen use
  8. Gaucher's disease
  9. Dysbarism
  10. Radiation therapy
- Traumatic
  1. Femoral neck fracture
  2. Septic

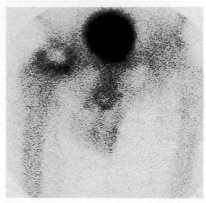

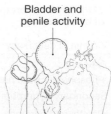

Bladder and penile activity

Increased uptake around focal defect in right femoral head

Fig 306–7
Bone scan in avascular necrosis. There is high uptake around a central defect in the head of the right femur. Activity in the bladder and penis is seen centrally. The result is typical of an avascular necrosis of the head of the femur due to the prolonged corticosteroid therapy. (From Besser CM, Thorner MO: Comprehensive Clinical Endocrinology, 3rd ed, St. Louis, Mosby, 2002.)

DIFFERENTIAL DIAGNOSIS
The differential diagnosis of osteonecrosis is as stated under "Cause" and includes hyperlipidemias, pancreatitis, renal transplantation, chronic liver disease, obesity, and chemotherapy.

LABORATORY TESTS
CBC, electrolytes, BUN, creatinine, LFTs, ESR, ANA, RF, lipid profile, and other serologic tests are used as adjuncts in supporting the diagnosis of avascular necrosis.

IMAGING STUDIES
- Plain films help define and classify the disease course. Staging systems have been developed for osteonecrosis of the femoral head:
  1. Stage I: Initial x-rays are normal, but bone scan is positive.
  2. Stage II: Abnormal radiolucency is noted.
  3. Stage III: deformity with collapse and sclerosis
  4. Stage IV: early osteoarthritis
- Bone scan (Fig. 306–7) reveals decreased uptake at the affected site with a "doughnut sign" and can detect avascular necrosis before the plain x-rays.
- MRI scan is more sensitive and specific than bone scan, especially when looking for osteonecrosis of the femoral head.
- If a MRI is not available, CT scan (Fig. 306–8) of the involved bone is acceptable.

TREATMENT
- Immobilization
- Non–weight bearing with the use of crutches
- Special muscle-strengthening exercise
- NSAIDs can be used for symptom relief.
- For displaced hip fractures, prompt surgical reduction is indicated in attempt to reperfuse the femoral head.
- For patients with stage I or II osteonecrosis (before bone collapse occurs), core decompression treatment is tried to prevent bone collapse.
- In stage III osteonecrosis (after bone collapse), a hemiarthroplasty or total joint replacement is required.
- In stage IV osteonecrosis (arthritis setting in after bone collapse), a total joint replacement is usually required.

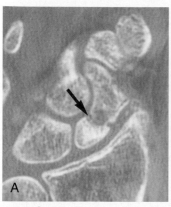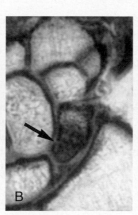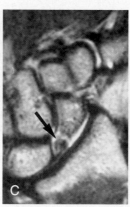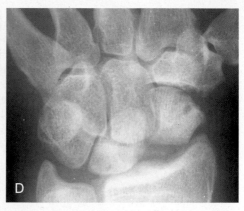

Fig 306–8
Osteonecrosis of the proximal pole of the scaphiod. Direct coronal CT. (**A**) demonstrates the unhealed fracture through the waist of the scaphoid *(arrow)*. The proximal pole is dense, indicating ischemia or osteonecrosis. Coronal T1-weighted (**B**) and T2-weighted (**C**) images demonstrate abnormal low signal in the proximal fragment *(arrows)*. (**D**) An AP radiograph of another patient who suffered AVN of the proximal pole of the scaphoid after a fracture and underwent subsequent resection of the dead bone.
(From Grainger RG, Allison DJ, Adam A, Dixon AK [eds]: Grainger and Allison's Diagnostic Radiology, 4th ed. Philadelphia, Churchill Livingstone, 2001.)

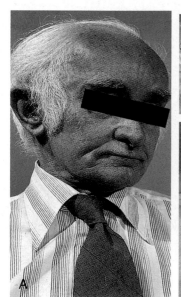
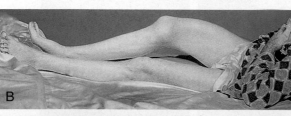
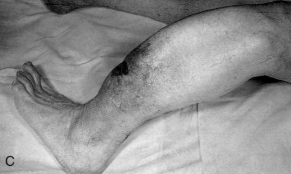

Fig 306–9
Bone deformity in Paget's disease.
(**A**) Marked enlargement of the cranium, with normal facial bones—a hearing aid can be seen. (**B**) Anterior bowing of the femur. (**C**) Marked bowing of the tibia with overlying ulceration.
(From Besser CM, Thorner MO: Comprehensive Clinical Endocrinology, 3rd ed, St. Louis, Mosby, 2002.)

D. PAGET'S DISEASE OF BONE

DEFINITION
Paget's disease of the bone is a disease of bone characterized by repeated episodes of osteolysis and excessive attempts at repair that results in a weakened bone of increased mass. Monostotic (solitary lesion) and polyostotic (numerous lesions) disease are both described.

PHYSICAL FINDINGS AND CLINICAL PRESENTATION
- Many lesions are asymptomatic.
- Onset is variable.
- Symptoms result mainly from the effects of complications:
  1. Skeletal pain, especially hip and pelvis
  2. Bowing of long bones (Fig. 306–9B), sometimes leading to pathologic fracture
  3. Increased heat of extremity (resulting from increased vascularity), overlying ulcerations may be present (see Fig. 306–9C)
  4. Skull enlargement (see Fig. 306–9A) and spinal involvement caused by characteristic bone enlargement, which can produce neurologic complications (vision, hearing loss, radicular pain, and cord compression)
  5. Thoracic kyphoscoliosis
  6. Secondary osteoarthritis, especially of hip
  7. Heart failure as a result of chest and spine deformity and blood shunting

CAUSE
Unknown

DIFFERENTIAL DIAGNOSIS
- Fibrous dysplasia
- Skeletal neoplasm (primary or metastatic)
- Osteomyelitis
- Hyperparathyroidism
- Vertebral hemangioma

LABORATORY TESTS
- Increased serum alkaline phosphatase (SAP)
- Normal serum calcium and phosphorus levels
- Increased urinary excretion of pyridinoline cross-links, although test is expensive and not usually required in routine cases
- Other: bone biopsy only in uncertain cases or if sarcomatous degeneration is suspected (Fig. 306–10)

IMAGING STUDIES
- Appropriate radiographs reflect the characteristic radiolucency and opacity (Fig. 306–11)

- Bone scanning usually reflects the activity and extent of the disease.

TREATMENT
- Bisphosphonates
- Calcitonin
- NSAIDs for pain relief
- General indications for treatment
  1. All symptomatic patients
  2. Asymptomatic patients with high level of metabolic activity or those at risk for deformity
  3. Preoperative, if surgery involves Pagetic site

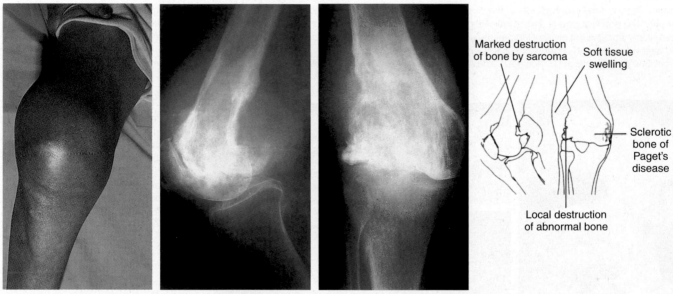

Fig 306–10
Development of osteogenic sarcoma in Paget's disease. Painful swelling developed in the knee of this patient two years after the diagnosis of Paget's disease. Marked bone destruction and soft-tissue swelling can be seen on the radiographs.
(From Besser CM, Thorner MO: Comprehensive Clinical Endocrinology, 3rd ed, St. Louis, Mosby, 2002.)

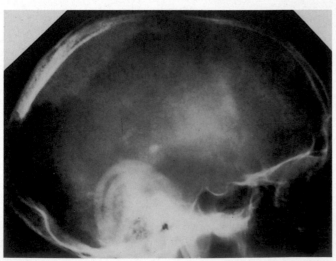

Fig 306–11
Osteoporosis circumscripta (Paget's disease). Extensive loss of bone density affects the lower part of the cranial vault; the margin between abnormal and normal bone is characteristically sharp as seen in the upper posterior parietal region.
(From Grainger RG, Allison DJ, Adam A, Dixon AK [eds]: Grainger and Allison's Diagnostic Radiology, 4th ed. Philadelphia, Churchill Livingstone, 2001.)

Chapter 307 / Hypertrophic osteoarthropathy

DEFINITION

Hypertrophic osteoarthropathy (HOA) is a syndrome of clubbing of the digits, periostitis of long bones, and arthritis. HOA may be primary or secondary to other underlying disease processes.

PHYSICAL FINDINGS AND CLINICAL PRESENTATION

- Primary HOA typically presents with the insidious onset of clubbing of the hands and feet and is described as "spade-like." Other signs and symptoms include:
  1. Joint pain and swelling
  2. Decreased use of the fingers and hands
  3. Facial changes, coarse facial skin grooves
  4. Thickening of the arms and legs
  5. Oily skin, diaphoresis, gynecomastia, and acne
- Secondary HOA patients may present with clinical symptoms before the underlying disorder can be detected. Signs and symptoms are similar to the above mentioned in addition to findings related to the underlying disease (e.g., bronchogenic carcinoma, infective endocarditis).

CAUSE

Unknown; immunologic, endocrine, and vascular etiologies have been suggested.

DIFFERENTIAL DIAGNOSIS

- Other causes of periostitis include Paget's disease, Reiter's syndrome, psoriasis, syphilis, osteoarthritis, RA, and osteomyelitis.
- HOA with the classic finding of clubbing of the digits warrants an investigation into any associated illnesses.

LABORATORY TESTS

- CBC, electrolytes, and urine studies will typically be normal in both primary and secondary HOA.
- ESR will be elevated in secondary HOA.
- LFTs may be abnormal in patients with secondary HOA from GI pathology.
- Alkaline phosphatase may be elevated secondary to periostitis of the long bones.
- Analysis of the synovial fluid from joint effusions reveals a low WBC count with normal viscosity, color, and complement levels.

IMAGING STUDIES

- X-rays of the long bones show periosteal new bone formation (Fig. 307–1).
- A chest x-ray should be obtained to rule out underlying lung cancer.
- Bone scan with technetium-99m commonly reveals uptake along the long bones, phalanxes, and periarticular joint spaces (Fig. 307–1).

TREATMENT

- Treatment of primary HOA is symptomatic. NSAIDs or aspirin will provide bone and joint pain relief.
- For secondary HOA, the treatment of choice is to eradicate the underlying disease (e.g., antibiotics for infective endocarditis, surgery for bronchogenic carcinoma).
- In patients with secondary HOA refractory to NSAIDs and aspirin, vagotomy has been tried with some success. However, the definitive treatment is to treat the underlying disease.

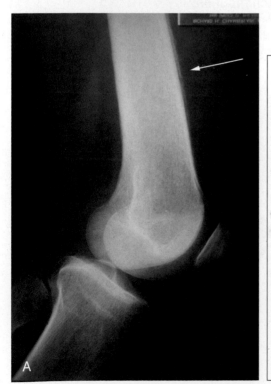
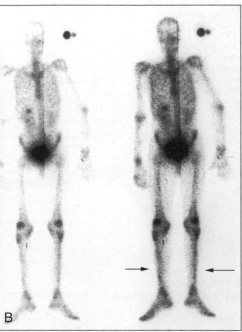

Fig 307–1
Hypertrophic osteoarthropathy. **(A)** Radiograph of knee showing periosteal new bone formation along the shaft of the femur. **(B)** Technetium bone scan with arrows indicating increased uptake in the tibias. (From Hochberg MC, Silman AJ, Smolen JS, et al [eds]: Rheumatology, 3rd ed. St Louis, Mosby, 2003.)

Chapter 308 / Infections

A. INFECTIOUS ARTHRITIS

DEFINITION

Bacterial arthritis is a highly destructive form of joint disease most often caused by hematogenous spread of organisms from a distant site of infection. Direct penetration of the joint as a result of trauma or surgery and spread from adjacent osteomyelitis may also cause bacterial arthritis. Any joint in the body may be affected. Figure 308–1 illustrates routes by which bacteria may reach the joint.

PHYSICAL FINDINGS AND CLINICAL PRESENTATION
- Hallmark: acute onset of a swollen, painful joint (Fig. 308–2)
- Limited range of motion of the joint
- Effusion, with varying degrees of erythema and increased warmth around the joint
- A single joint is affected in 80% to 90% of cases of nongonococcal arthritis
- Gonococcal dermatitis-arthritis syndrome
  1. Typical pattern is a migratory polyarthritis or tenosynovitis
  2. Small pustules on the trunk or extremities
- Generally febrile patient at presentation
- Most commonly affected joints in the adult: knee and hip, but any joint may be involved; in children: hip

CAUSE
- Bacteria spread from another locus of infection.
  1. Highly vascular synovium is invaded by hematogenously spread bacteria.
  2. WBC enzymes cause necrosis of synovium, cartilage, and bone.

3. Extensive joint destruction is rapid if infection is not treated with appropriate IV antibiotics and drainage of necrotic material.
- Predisposing factors: RA, prosthetic joints, advanced age, immunodeficiency
- The most common nongonococcal organisms are *Staphylococcus aureus*, β-hemolytic streptococci, and gram-negative bacilli. Table 308–1 describes bacteriologic findings in bone and joint infections.

DIFFERENTIAL DIAGNOSIS
- Gout
- Pseudogout
- Trauma
- Hemarthrosis
- Rheumatic fever
- Adult or juvenile rheumatoid arthritis
- Spondyloarthropathies such as Reiter's syndrome
- Osteomyelitis
- Viral arthritides
- Septic bursitis

WORKUP
- Joint aspiration, Gram stain, and culture of the synovial fluid (Fig. 308–3)
- Immediate arthrocentesis before other studies are undertaken or antibiotics instituted

LABORATORY TESTS
- Joint fluid analysis
  1. Synovial fluid cell count is usually elevated >50,000 cells/mm^3 with >80% polymorphonuclear cells.

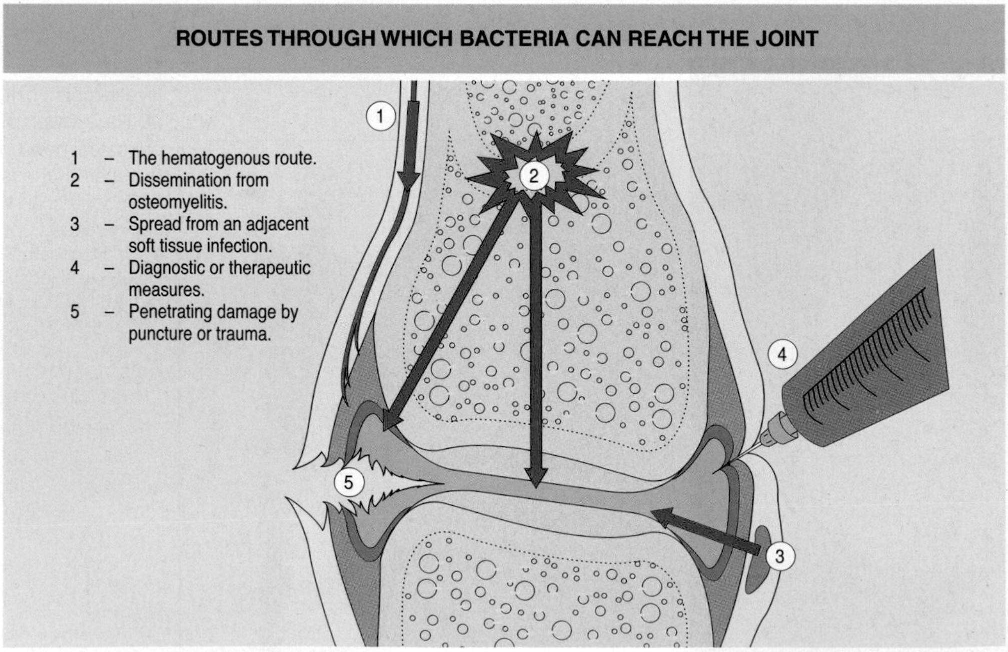

ROUTES THROUGH WHICH BACTERIA CAN REACH THE JOINT

1 – The hematogenous route.
2 – Dissemination from osteomyelitis.
3 – Spread from an adjacent soft tissue infection.
4 – Diagnostic or therapeutic measures.
5 – Penetrating damage by puncture or trauma.

Fig 308–1
Routes through which bacteria can reach the joint.
(From Hochberg MC, Silman AJ, Smolen JS, et al [eds]: Rheumatology, 3rd ed. St Louis, Mosby, 2003.)

TABLE 308–1 Bacteriologic findings in bone and joint infections

	Acute Septic Arthritis	Prosthetic Joint Infection	Bursitis	Acute Hematogenous Osteomyelitis	Chronic Osteomyelitis	Pelvic Osteomyelitis	Spondylitis	Diabetic Osteitis
Staphylococcus aureus	+++	+++	+++	+++	+++	+++	+++	++
Coagulase-negative staphylococci		+++			+			
Hemolytic streptococci	++	++	++	++			++	++
Other streptococci	+	+		+			+	+
Skin anaerobes	+	+++		+	+			++
Gram-negative cocci	+			+				
Haemophilus influenzae	+	+		+				
Gram-negative aerobes	+	++	+	+	+	++	++	++
Pseudomonas aeruginosa	+	+		+	+		+	
Salmonella	+	+		+	+		+	
Intestinal anaerobes		+			+	++		++
Mycobacteria	+	+			+		+	

+ + + = very common (30% or more); + + = common (5%–30%); + = occurs in some circumstances (age, underlying disease, foreign material).
From Hochberg MC, Silman AJ, Smolen JS, et al (eds): Rheumatology, 3rd ed. St Louis, Mosby, 2003.

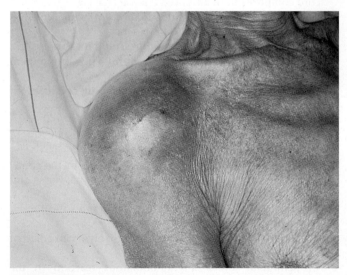

Fig 308–2
Septic arthritis in an elderly patient, here recognized by distention, increased skin temperature and tenderness. The septic arthritis does not always differ from other kinds of arthritis.
(From Hochberg MC, Silman AJ, Smolen JS, et al [eds]: Rheumatology, 3rd ed. St Louis, Mosby, 2003.)

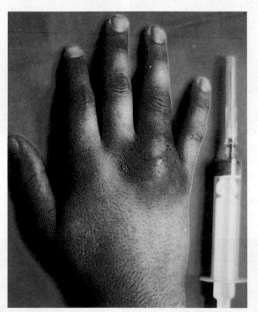

Fig 308–3
The red hot joint. Septic arthritis of the ring finger metacarpophalangeal joint showing swelling and intense redness of the skin.
(From Hochberg MC, Silman AJ, Smolen JS, et al [eds]: Rheumatology, 3rd ed. St Louis, Mosby, 2003.)

2. Counts are highly variable, with similar findings in gout, pseudogout, or RA.
- Blood cultures
- Culture of possible extraarticular sources of infection
- Elevated peripheral WBC count and ESR (nonspecific)

IMAGING STUDIES
- X-ray examination of the affected joint (Fig. 308–4) to rule out osteomyelitis
- CT scan for early diagnosis of infections of the spine, hips, and sternoclavicular and sacroiliac joints.
- Technetium and gallium scintigraphic scans (positive, but do not permit differentiation of infection from inflammation)
- Indium-labeled WBC scans (less sensitive, but more specific)
- MRI (Fig. 308–5)

TREATMENT
- Affected joints aspirated daily to remove necrotic material and to follow serial WBC counts and cultures
- If no resolution with IV antibiotics and closed drainage: open débridement and lavage, particularly in nongonococcal infections
- Prevention of contractures:
  1. After acute stage of inflammation, range-of-motion exercises of the affected joint

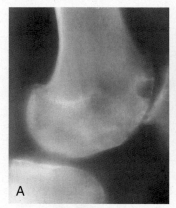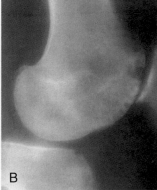

Fig 308–4
Tomogram of right knee of a patient who has *Staphylococcus aureus* septic arthritis and periarticular osteomyelitis. Note the mixed sclerosis and lytic changes suggestive of osteomyelitis.
(From Cohen J, Powderly WG: Infectious Diseases, 2nd ed, St. Louis, 2004, Mosby)

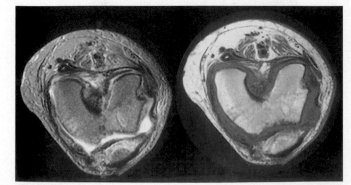

Fig 308–5
MRI scan of right knee of a patient who has *Staphylococcus aureus* septic arthritis. Note the soft tissue inflammation and a joint effusion.
(From Cohen J, Powderly WG: Infectious Diseases, 2nd ed, St. Louis, 2004, Mosby)

2. Physical therapy helpful
- IV antibiotics immediately after joint aspiration and Gram stain of the synovial fluid
- For infections caused by gram-positive cocci: penicillinase-resistant penicillin unless there is clinical suspicion of methicillin-resistant *Staphylococcus aureus*, in which case vancomycin
- Infections caused by gram-negative bacilli: treated with a third-generation cephalosporin or an antipseudomonal penicillin plus an aminoglycoside, pending culture and sensitivity results
- For suspected gonococcal infection, including young adults when the synovial fluid Gram stain is nondiagnostic: ceftriaxone

B. GRANULOMATOUS ARTHRITIS

DEFINITION
The prototype of granulomatous arthritis is tuberculous arthritis. Atypical mycobacteria, sarcoidosis, and sporotrichosis can cause granulomatous involvement of the synovium, but these entities are much less common.

PHYSICAL FINDINGS AND CLINICAL PRESENTATION
- Often no constitutional symptoms (fever and weight loss)
- Possibly no clinical or radiographic evidence of pulmonary tuberculosis
- Spinal infection (Fig. 308–6A, B) most often in the thoracic or upper lumbar area, with back pain as the most common symptom
- Considerable local muscle spasm possible
- Kyphosis and neurologic symptoms resulting from spinal cord compression in advanced disease (see Fig. 308–6C)
- Chronic monoarticular arthritis in the peripheral joints
- Single joint involved in 85% of patients
- Pain, swelling, limitation of motion, and joint stiffness less dramatic than in acute bacterial arthritis; possibly present for months to years
- Seen more often in persons from developing countries, elderly patients, and hemodialysis patients

CAUSE
- Hematogenous spread of organisms from a distant site of infection or by direct spread from bone
- Most commonly affected area: 50% of cases in the spine; next most commonly affected area: large joints (knee and hip)
- Primary infection beginning in the lungs and spreading to the highly vascular synovium
- Tuberculous osteomyelitis commonly involving an adjacent joint
- In peripheral joints, a granulomatous reaction in the synovium causing joint effusion and eventual destruction of underlying bone
- In the spine, infection of the intervertebral disc spreading to adjacent vertebrae
- Osteomyelitis of vertebrae causing collapse, kyphosis, or gibbous deformity, and possibly paraspinal "cold" abscess

DIFFERENTIAL DIAGNOSIS
- Sarcoidosis
- Fungal arthritis
- Metastatic cancer
- Primary or metastatic synovial tumors

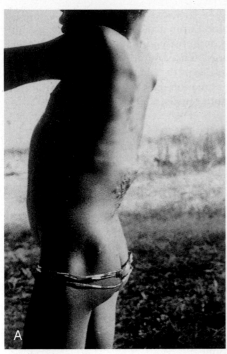
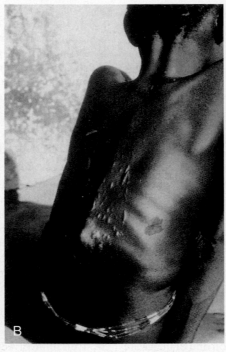
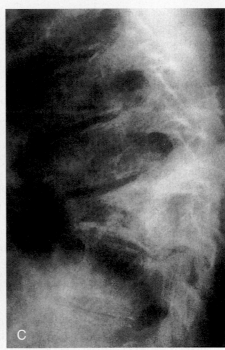

Fig 308–6
Vertebral TB. Tuberculosis of the spine or Pott's disease. Kyphosis is secondary to anterior destruction of vertebral bodies resulting in wedging of adjacent vertebrae and loss of disc space clearly seen by radiography. (Courtesy of Professor J. Cohen, Brighton, UK; © Courtesy of Dr. A. Wightman, with permission from Edmond RTD, Rowland HAK, Welsby PD: A colour atlas of infectious diseases, 3rd ed. London: Mosby; 1995.)

WORKUP

- High index of suspicion needed
- Gold standard: synovial biopsy
- Joint aspiration and culture of the synovial fluid performed while awaiting biopsy
- Positive synovial fluid smear for acid-fast bacilli in 20% of cases; positive culture in 80%
- Elevated synovial fluid protein, low glucose
- Considerable variation in synovial fluid WBC count, but values of 10,000 to 20,000 cells/mm³ typical; may be predominantly polymorphonuclear leukocytes
- Usually positive tuberculin skin test
- Anergy in elderly patients or in advanced disease
- In spinal infections, percutaneous or open biopsy to obtain accurate C&S data

LABORATORY TESTS
Peripheral WBC count and ESR are elevated but nonspecific.

IMAGING STUDIES
- Plain radiographs of the affected joint
  1. Typically demonstrate bony destruction with little new bone formation
  2. Osteopenia and soft tissue swelling in early infections
  3. Later, erosions at the joint margins
  4. In the spine, disc space narrowing with vertebral collapse (wedging) causing characteristic kyphosis
- CT scan: useful in early diagnosis of infections of the spine and to detect paraspinal abscess
- Technetium and gallium scintigraphic scans: may be positive, but do not permit differentiation from inflammation or osteoarthritis

TREATMENT
- Combination chemotherapy
  1. If sensitive TB suspected, give isoniazid plus rifampin for at least 6 months and pyrazinamide for at least the first 2 months plus ethambutol until sensitivity results are available.
  2. Most patients are treated successfully with chemotherapy alone.
  3. Urgent surgical intervention is necessary if spinal cord compression causes neurologic changes.
- Surgical débridement in cases of extensive bone involvement

C. SEPTIC BURSITIS

DEFINITION
Bursitis is an inflammation of a bursa and is usually aseptic. A *bursa* is a closed sac lined with a synovial-like membrane that sometimes contains fluid that is found or that develops in an area subject to pressure or friction.

PHYSICAL FINDINGS AND CLINICAL PRESENTATION
- Swelling, especially if bursa is superficial (olecranon, prepatellar) (Fig. 308–7)
- Local tenderness with pain on pressure against bursa
- Pain with joint movement
- Referred pain
- Palpable occasional fibrocartilaginous bodies (most common in olecranon and prepatellar bursae)

CAUSE
- Acute trauma

- Repetitive trauma
- Sepsis
- Crystalline deposit disease
- RA

DIFFERENTIAL DIAGNOSIS
- Degenerative joint disease
- Tendinitis (sometimes occurs in conjunction with bursitis)
- Cellulitis (if bursitis is septic)
- Infectious arthritis (see Fig. 308–2)

WORKUP
  Aspiration with Gram stain and C&S

IMAGING STUDIES
- Plain radiography to rule out other potential or coexisting bone or joint problems
- MRI

TREATMENT
- Use of relief pads, avoidance of direct pressure
- Rest
- Elevation
- Ice for acute trauma
- Septic:
  1. Appropriate antibiotic coverage and drainage
  2. Aspiration of purulent fluid with a large-bore needle (if there is no rapid clinical response, incision and drainage are indicated)

- Nonseptic:
  1. Aspiration of blood from acute trauma
  2. Application of compression dressing
- Aspiration if excessive fluid volume present, followed by application of compression dressing to prevent fluid reaccumulation (repeat aspiration may be required)
- Steroid injection into bursa
- NSAIDs

D. OSTEOMYELITIS

DEFINITION
Osteomyelitis is an acute or chronic infection of the bone secondary to the hematogenous or contiguous source of infection or direct traumatic inoculation, which is usually bacterial.

PHYSICAL FINDINGS AND CLINICAL PRESENTATION
Hematogenous osteomyelitis Usually occurs in tibia/fibula (children) (Fig. 308–8)
- Localized inflammation: often secondary to trauma with accompanying hematoma or cellulitis
- Abrupt fever
- Lethargy
- Irritability
- Pain in involved bone

Vertebral osteomyelitis Usually hematogenous (Fig. 308–9)
- Fever: 50%
- Localized pain/tenderness
- Neurologic defects: motor/sensory

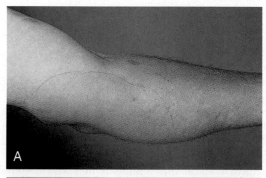
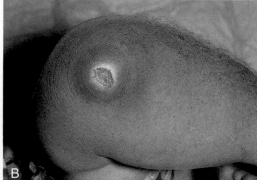

Fig 308–7
Cellulitis at the elbow associated with olecranon bursitis. (**A**) Pale pink erythema on the inner aspect of the elbow. (**B**) Careful inspection demonstrates a focal infection over the point of the elbow. Fluid aspirated from the olecranon bursa yielded a pure culture of *Staphylococcus aureus*. (From Cohen J, Powderly WG: Infectious Diseases, 2nd ed, St. Louis, 2004, Mosby)

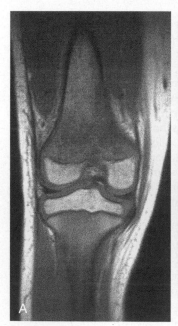
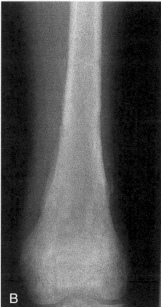

Fig 308–8
Osteomyelitis of the distal femur. The early MR (T1-weighted) (**A**) study shows sparing of the epiphyses. The plain radiograph (**B**) taken some months later shows chronic osteomyelitis with sclerosis from the metaphyses and epiphysis. There are cortical defects and periosteal new bone. (From Grainger RG, Allison DJ, Adam A, Dixon AK [eds]: Grainger and Allison's Diagnostic Radiology, 4th ed. Philadelphia, Churchill Livingstone, 2001.)

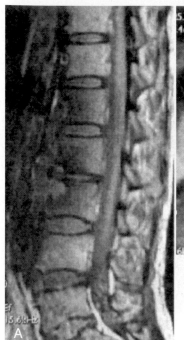

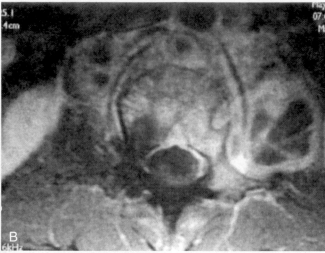

Fig 308-9
(**A,B**) MR images of tuberculous spinal osteomyelitis with scalloping of the vertebrae (tuberculous caries) and paraspinal 'cold' abscesses. (From Grainger RG, Allison DJ, Adam A, Dixon AK [eds]: Grainger and Allison's Diagnostic Radiology, 4th ed. Philadelphia, Churchill Livingstone, 2001.)

Contiguous osteomyelitis: direct inoculation
- Associated with trauma, fractures, surgical fixation
- Chronic infection of skin/soft tissue
- Fever, drainage from surgical site

Chronic osteomyelitis (See Fig. 308–10.)
- Bone pain
- Sinus tract drainage, nonhealing ulcer
- Chronic low-grade fever
- Chronic localized pain

CAUSE
- *Staphylococcus aureus*
- *S. aureus* (methicillin-resistant)
- *Pseudomonas aeruginosa*
- Enterobacteriaceae
- *Streptococcus pyogenes*
- *Enterococcus*
- *Mycobacteria*
- Fungi
- Coagulase-negative staphylococci
- *Salmonella* (in sickle cell disease)

DIFFERENTIAL DIAGNOSIS
- Bone infarction
- Charcot's joint
- Fracture

WORKUP
- CBC with differential, ESR, C-reactive protein
- Blood culturing
- Bone culture
- Pathologic evaluation of bone biopsy for acute/chronic changes consistent with necrosis or acute inflammation

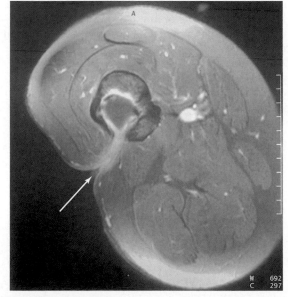

Fig 308-10
Chronic active osteomyelitis in the femur. This case of osteomyelitis was secondary to a fracture and open reduction and internal fixation 30 years before. This axial, contrast-enhanced, fat-suppressed T1-weighted MRI scan shows cortical thickening and a focal intraosseous fluid collection with an enhancing rim, communicating via sinus tract to the surface of the thigh (*arrow*).
(From Cohen J, Powderly WG: Infectious Diseases, 2nd ed, St. Louis, 2004, Mosby)

IMAGING STUDIES
- Bone x-ray examination
- Bone scan
- Gallium scan
- Indium scan
- MRI (most accurate imaging study)

TREATMENT

Surgical débridement in biopsy-positive cases will guide direction for antibiotic therapy. This will vary with type of osteomyelitis. Duration of therapy is usually 6 weeks for acute osteomyelitis; chronic osteomyelitis may need a longer course of medication.

- *S. aureus:* cefazolin IV, nafcillin IV, vancomycin IV (in patient allergic to penicillin)
- *S. aureus* (methicillin resistant): vancomycin IV
- *Streptococcus* spp.: cefazolin or ceftriaxone
- *P. aeruginosa:* piperacillin plus aminoglycoside or ceftazidime plus aminoglycoside
- Enterobacteriaceae: ceftriaxone or fluoroquinolone
- Hyperbaric oxygen therapy: may be useful in chronic osteo myelitis
- Surgical débridement of all devitalized bone and tissue
- Immobilization of affected bone (plaster, traction) if bone is unstable

E. LYME DISEASE

DEFINITION

Lyme disease is a multisystem inflammatory disorder caused by the transmission of a spirochete, *Borrelia burgdorferi*. Lyme disease is spread by the bite of infected *Ixodes* ticks (Fig. 308–11), with it taking 36 to 48 hours for a tick to feed and transmit the infecting organism *B. burgdorferi* to the host.

PHYSICAL FINDINGS AND CLINICAL PRESENTATION

Lyme disease may present in the following stages:
- *Early localized:* early Lyme disease, erythema chronicum migrans (ECM) skin rash (Fig. 308–12), often at site of tick bite; possible fever, myalgias 3 to 32 days after tick bite

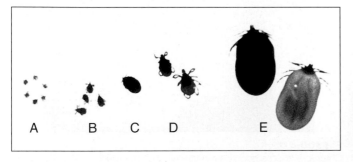

Fig 308–11

The life-cycle stages of *Ixodes scapularis*, the tick that transmits Lyme disease in the northeastern and north central USA. (**A**) Tiny larval ticks, which are <1 mm in diameter. (**B**) Unengorged nymphal ticks, which are only 1–2 mm in diameter. This stage of the tick is primarily responsible for transmission of the spirochete to humans during the late spring and early summer. (**C**) An engorged nymphal tick. (**D**) Unengorged adult male (black) and female (orange) ticks. (**E**) Engorged adult male and female ticks.
(From Hochberg MC, Silman AJ, Smolen JS, et al [eds]: Rheumatology, 3rd ed. St Louis, Mosby, 2003.)

- *Early disseminated:* days to weeks later; multiorgan system involvement, including CNS, joints, cardiac; related to dissemination of spirochete
- *Late persistent:* months to years after tick exposure; affects central and peripheral nervous system, cardiac, joints (Fig. 308–13)
- Common presenting signs and symptoms include:
  - ECM
  - Lymphadenopathy, neck pains, pharyngeal erythema, myalgias, hepatosplenomegaly.
  - Patients will complain of malaise, fatigue, lethargy, headache, fever/chills, neck pain, myalgias, back pain.

CAUSE
- *B. burgdorferi* transmitted from bite of an *Ixodes* tick

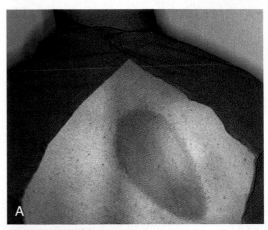

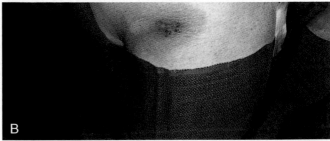

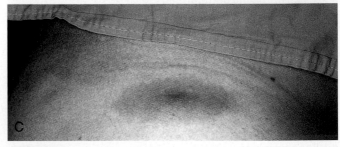

Fig 308–12

Erythema migrans of Lyme disease. Lyme disease usually begins with a slowly expanding skin lesion, erythema migrans, that occurs at the site of a tick bite. (**A**) Classic erythema migrans skin lesion (10 cm in diameter) on the back. The lesion has a redder outer border, with slight central clearing. (**B**) Pale lesion (7 cm in diameter) with several vesicles in the center, near the groin. (**C**) Pale lesion (5 cm in diameter) with a target center over the illiac crest. In each instance, *B. burgdorferi* was isolated from a skin biopsy sample of the lesion.
(Courtesy of Dr. Vijay Sikand, East Lyme, CT, USA.)

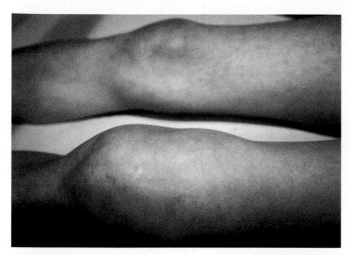

Fig 308–13
The swollen knee of a 9-year-old with Lyme arthritis. In the USA, affected knees may be very swollen and warm, but not particularly painful. In Europe and Asia, the amount of joint swelling is often less. (From Hochberg MC, Silman AJ, Smolen JS, et al [eds]: Rheumatology, 3rd ed. St Louis, Mosby, 2003.)

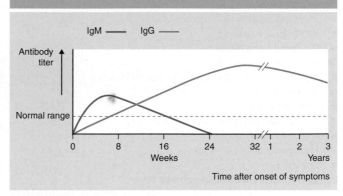

Fig 308–14
The usual serologic response in Lyme disease. Specific IgM becomes detectable 1 to 2 weeks after symptom onset and the appearance of erythema migrans. The later appearance of IgG is frequently concurrent with systemic manifestations. IgG is nearly always elevated with late disease. Typically, and even in untreated patients, IgM falls over 4 to 6 months; persistence for longer than this predicts later manifestations. (From Cohen J, Powderly WG: Infectious Diseases, 2nd ed, St. Louis, 2004, Mosby)

DIAGNOSIS
- Clinical presentation, exposure to ticks in endemic area, and diagnostic testing for antibody response to *B. burgdorferi* (Fig. 308–14)

DIFFERENTIAL DIAGNOSIS
- Chronic fatigue/fibromyalgia
- Acute viral illnesses
- Babesiosis
- Ehrlichiosis

WORKUP
- ELISA testing—Western blot
- Immunofluorescent assay
- Early disease often difficult to diagnose serologically secondary to slow immune response
- Culturing of skin lesions (electron microscopy) and polymerase chain reaction (PCR) of skin biopsy and blood to give definitive diagnosis (available only in reference laboratories)

IMAGING STUDIES
- Echocardiogram if conduction abnormalities are present with cardiac involvement
- CT scan, MRI of head for suspected CNS involvement

TREATMENT
- Early Lyme disease
  - Doxycycline 100 mg bid or amoxicillin 500 mg qid for 10 to 14 days (doxycycline should be avoided in children/pregnant females).
  - Alternative treatments: cefuroxime axetil 500 mg bid for 10 to 14 days, azithromycin 500 mg PO qd for 1 day followed by 250 mg qd for 6 days
- Early disseminated and late persistent infection: 30 days of treatment necessary; doxycycline and ceftriaxone appear equally effective for acute disseminated Lyme disease.
- Arthritis: 30 days of doxycycline or amoxicillin plus probenecid.
- Neurologic involvement requires parenteral antibiotics.

- Ceftriaxone 2 g/day for 21 to 28 days; alternative: cefotaxime 2 g q8h; alternative: penicillin G 5 million U qid
- Cardiac involvement: IV ceftriaxone or penicillin plus cardiac monitoring.
- Prolonged treatment with IV or PO antibiotic therapy for up to 90 days did not improve symptoms more than did placebo.

F. ROCKY MOUNTAIN SPOTTED FEVER

DEFINITION
Rocky Mountain spotted fever (RMSF) is a life-threatening, tick-borne febrile illness caused by infection with *Rickettsia rickettsii*. The infection occurs when *R. rickettsii* in the salivary glands of a vector tick is transmitted into the dermis, spreading and replicating in the cytoplasm of endothelial cells and eliciting widespread vasculitis and end-organ damage.

PHYSICAL FINDINGS AND CLINICAL PRESENTATION
- Incubation: 3 to 12 days
- First symptoms: fever, headache, malaise, and myalgias

Rash
- Appears during first 3 days in 50%; by day 5, 80% have it. No rash in 10%.
- Initial appearance: blanching erythematous macules on wrists and ankles that then spread to the trunk, palms, and soles (Fig. 308–15).
- Lesions may evolve into papules and eventually become nonblanching (petechiae or palpable purpura).

Gastrointestinal symptoms
- Nausea, vomiting, and abdominal pain are common
- Occasionally may mimic an "acute abdomen" (e.g., appendicitis, cholecystitis)
- Mild hepatitis

Cardiopulmonary involvement
- Interstitial pneumonitis
- Myocarditis

Renal problems
- Prerenal azotemia
- Interstitial nephritis
- Glomerulonephritis

Neurologic involvement
- Encephalitis (confusion, lethargy, delirium)
- Ataxia
- Convulsion
- Cranial nerve palsy
- Speech impediment
- Hemiparesis or paraparesis
- Spasticity

Fulminant Rocky Mountain spotted fever
- Early, widespread vascular necrosis leading to multisystem illness and death

CAUSE AND PATHOGENESIS
- Infectious agent: *R. rickettsii* (an intracellular bacterium)
- Vector: dog tick and wood tick (vertical transmission exists in ticks, but horizontal transmission involving rodents represents an important reservoir for the agent). In the United States, *R. rickettsii* is transmitted mainly by the American dog tick *(Dermacentor variabilis)* and the Rocky Mountain wood tick *(D. andersoni)*.
- Pathogenesis: the spread of *R. rickettsii* is hematogenous with attachment to the vascular endothelium, causing a vasculitis. The manifestations of this illness are caused by increased vascular permeability.

DIFFERENTIAL DIAGNOSIS
- Influenza A, enteroviral infection
- Typhoid fever
- Leptospirosis
- Infectious mononucleosis
- Viral hepatitis, sepsis
- Ehrlichiosis
- Meningococcemia, disseminated gonococcal infection
- Secondary syphilis
- Bacterial endocarditis
- Toxic shock syndrome
- Scarlet fever
- Rheumatic fever
- Measles, rubella
- Typhus
- Rickettsialpox
- Lyme disease
- Drug hypersensitivity reaction,
- Idiopathic thrombocytopenic purpura, thrombotic thrombocytopenic purpura
- Kawasaki disease
- Immune complex vasculitis
- Connective tissue disorders

LABORATORY TESTS
- Antibody titers to *R. rickettsii* (by indirect fluorescent antibody test). The diagnosis of RMSF requires a fourfold increase 2 weeks apart and thus is not helpful in the care of the patients despite a sensitivity and specificity of near 100%.
- The only test that can provide a timely diagnosis is the immunohistologic demonstration of *R. rickettsii* in skin biopsy specimens (Fig. 308–16).

TREATMENT
- Oral or intravenous doxycycline

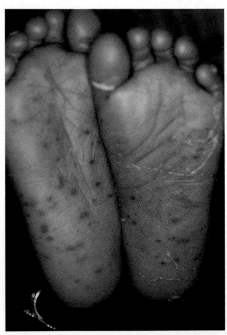

Fig 308–15
Small, purpuric lesion in a patient with Rocky Mountain spotted fever.
(From Callen JP, Jorizzo JL, Bolognia JL, Piette WW, Zone JJ: Dermatological Signs of Internal Disease, 3rd ed, Philadelphia, WB Saunders, 2003)

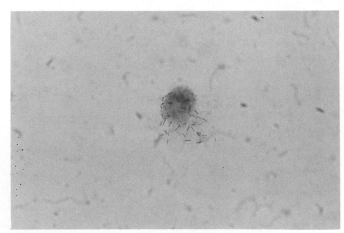

Fig 308–16
Glimenez stain of tissue culture cells infected with spotted fever group rickettsias.
(From Cohen J, Powderly WG: Infectious Diseases, 2nd ed, St. Louis, 2004, Mosby)

Chapter 309 | Bone tumors

DEFINITION

Primary malignant bone tumors are invasive, anaplastic, and have the ability to metastasize. Most arise from the marrow (myeloma), but tumors may develop from bone, cartilage, fat, and fibrous tissues. Leukemia and lymphoma are excluded from this discussion.

1. **Fibrosarcoma and liposarcoma**: Extremely rare. They are similar to those tumors arising in soft tissue.
2. **Osteosarcoma** (Fig. 309–1): A rare primary malignant tumor of bone characterized by malignant tumor cells that produce osteoid or bone. Several variants have been described: parosteal sarcoma, periosteal sarcoma, multicentric, and telangiectatic forms.
3. **Chondrosarcoma**: A malignant cartilage tumor that may develop primarily or secondarily from transformation of a benign osteocartilaginous exostosis or enchondroma.
4. **Ewing's sarcoma** (Figs. 309–2 and 309–3): A malignant tumor of unknown histogenesis.

Benign bone tumors are generally solitary, localized lesions that usually grow slowly and enlarge by pressure and expansion. They generally do not metastasize and threaten life only when they interfere with vital functions (e.g., a benign tumor producing instability at the C1-2 vertebral level).

Common benign bone lesions are:

1. **Chondromas**: These tumors are commonly central in their location in the bone (then referred to as **enchondromas**). They affect the tubular bones of the hands and feet in >50% of cases. Most enchondromas arise in the medulla of the phalanges (Fig. 309–4).
2. **Osteochondromas**: Long bones are commonly affected, especially around the knee where presentation may be related to mechanical interference with movement.

3. **Osteoid osteomas** : Most patients are in the second or third decade of life. The characteristic feature of the lesion is the nidus, a small, circumscribed nodule of osteoid containing vascular, neural elements and mineralized bone. Classically the patient presents with severe pain, often more apparent at rest or at night.
4. **Simple bone cysts** (Fig. 309–5) : They occur predominantly in children and are rarely asymptomatic, although a dull ache may be experienced.
5. **Giant cell tumors** (Fig. 309–6): about 80% occur in patients between ages 18 and 45. They are nearly always found toward the end or margin of a bone, either in the subarticular region or in the subcortical region of a fused apophysis.

PHYSICAL FINDINGS AND CLINICAL PRESENTATION OF MALIGNANT BONE TUMORS

OSTEOSARCOMA

- Most originating in the metaphysis
- 50% to 60% around the knee
- Possible pain and swelling, but otherwise healthy patient
- Osteosarcoma in conjunction with Paget's disease, manifested primarily as a sudden increase in bone pain

CHONDROSARCOMA

- Tumor most commonly involving the pelvis, upper femur, and shoulder girdle
- Painful swelling

EWING'S SARCOMA

- Painful soft tissue mass often present
- Possibly increased local heat
- Midshaft of a long bone usually affected (in contrast to other tumors)
- Weight loss, fever, and lethargy

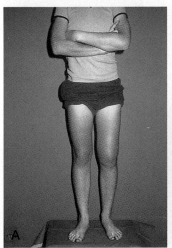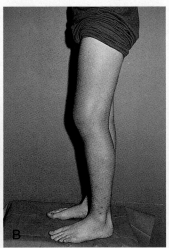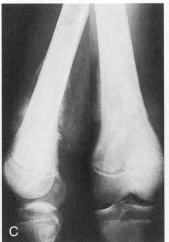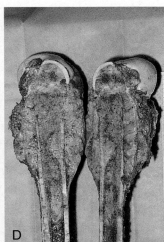

Fig 309–1
Osteosarcoma. (**A,B**) A 16-year-old patient complaining of a painful swelling near the left knee joint. (**C**) Anteroposterior and lateral radiographs of the metaphysis of the femur show patchy increased bone density, extension in the soft tissues and typical Codman's triangle. (**D**) Photograph of the resected specimen, showing the polymorphism of osteosarcoma caused by various stages of differentiation, such as fibroblastic, myxoid, cartilaginous and especially osteoid and reactive processes.
(From Hochberg MC, Silman AJ, Smolen JS, et al [eds]: Rheumatology, 3rd ed. St Louis, Mosby, 2003.)

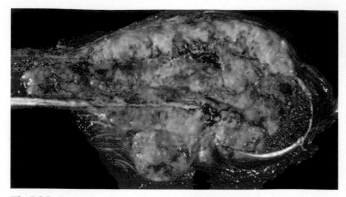

Fig 309–2
Ewing's sarcoma/primitive neuroectodermal tumor. A tan-white tumor destroys the proximal humerus and forms a large soft tissue mass.
(From Silverberg SG: Principles and Practice of Surgical Pathology and Cytopathology. Philadelphia, Churchill Livingstone, 4th ed, 2006)

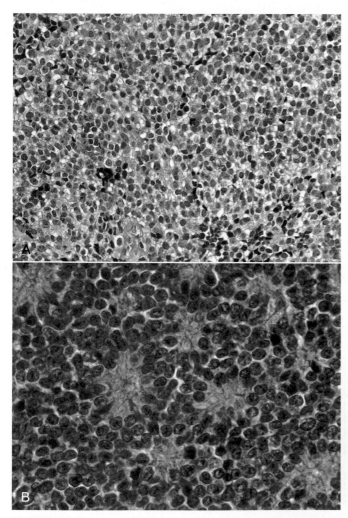

Fig 309–3
Ewing's sarcoma/primitive neuroectodermal tumor. (**A**) Ewing's sarcoma composed of sheets of small round cells. (**B**) Numerous rosettes can be seen in primitive neuroectodermal tumor.
(From Silverberg SG: Principles and Practice of Surgical Pathology and Cytopathology. Philadelphia, Churchill Livingstone, 4th ed, 2006)

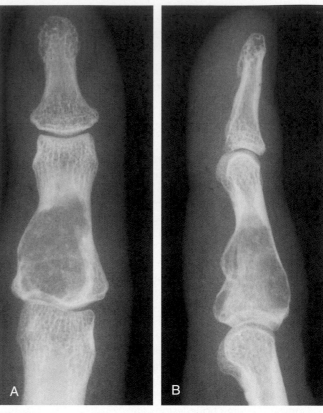

Fig 309–4
Enchondroma of middle phalanx of finger showing expansion and thinning of the cortex. The patient presented as a result of pain associated with infraction of the cortex.
(From Grainger RG, Allison DJ, Adam A, Dixon AK [eds]: Grainger and Allison's Diagnostic Radiology, 4th ed. Philadelphia, Churchill Livingstone, 2001.)

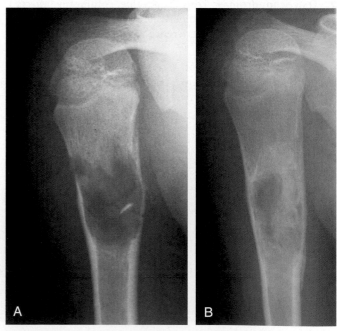

Fig 309–5
Simple bone cyst of the proximal humerus, the commonest site. At presentation (left), pathologic fracture has occurred, giving rise to the 'falling fragment sign.' With healing and metaphyseal growth, the lesion has moved distally into the diaphysis.
(From Grainger RG, Allison DJ, Adam A, Dixon AK [eds]: Grainger and Allison's Diagnostic Radiology, 4th ed. Philadelphia, Churchill Livingstone, 2001.)

DIFFERENTIAL DIAGNOSIS
- Osteomyelitis
- Metastatic bone disease

LABORATORY TESTS
- Slightly elevated alkaline phosphatase in osteosarcoma
- In Ewing's sarcoma: reflective of systemic reaction; include anemia, an increase in WBC count, and an elevated sedimentation rate

- In multiple myeloma:
  1. Bence-Jones protein in the urine
  2. Anemia and elevated sedimentation rate
  3. Characteristic dysproteinemia on serum protein electrophoresis
  4. Diagnostic feature: peak in the electrophoretic pattern suggestive of a monoclonal gammopathy
  5. Rouleaux formation in the peripheral blood smear
  6. Often, presence of hypercalcemia, but alkaline phosphatase levels usually normal

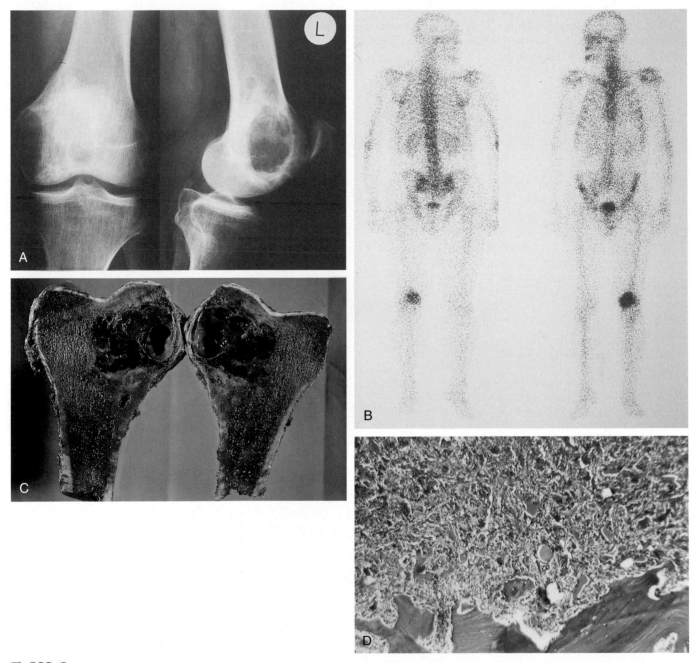

Fig 309–6
Giant cell tumor. (**A**) Anteroposterior and lateral radiographs illustrating a radiolucent lesion located eccentrically in the medial femoral condyle, which expands the thinned cortex. Note the ill-defined borders to the medullary cavity. (**B**) Bone scintigraph revealing increased uptake of the bone-seeking tracer in the tumor. (**C**) Photograph of the resected tumor, showing that some parts of the tumor are grayish white in color or show fleshy and hemorrhagic areas. (**D**) Photomicrograph showing the characteristic histologic pattern of a giant-cell tumor with numerous multinucleated giant cells, uniformaly distributed and separated by mononuclear stromal cells.
(From Hochberg MC, Silman AJ, Smolen JS, et al [eds]: Rheumatology, 3rd ed. St Louis, Mosby, 2003.)

IMAGING STUDIES

- Classic osteogenic sarcoma penetrates the cortex early in many cases.

  1. A blastic (dense), lytic (lucent), or mixed response may be seen in the affected bone.

  2. An aggressive perpendicular sunburst pattern may be present as a result of periosteal reaction, and peripheral Codman's triangles are often noted.

  3. Margins of the tumor are poorly defined.

- Speckled calcifications in a destructive radiolucent lesion are usually suggestive of chondrosarcoma.

- Ewing's sarcoma is characterized radiographically by mottled, irregular destructive changes with periosteal new bone formation. The latter may be multilayered, producing the typical "onion skin" appearance.

- Typical x-ray finding in multiple myeloma is the "punched-out" lesion with sharply demarcated edges.

  1. Multiple lesions are usual.

  2. Diffuse osteoporosis may be the only finding in many cases.

  3. Pathologic fractures are common.

TREATMENT

Combination of chemotherapy, local resection, and radiation therapy. Treatment should be supervised by an orthopedic cancer specialist and oncologist.

Chapter 310 Fractures

CAUSE

- Fractures may occur under a variety of circumstances.
- Most commonly, a fracture is the result of a large force acting acutely on an otherwise normal bone, and disrupting the normal bony architecture.

FRACTURE TYPES

Pathologic fractures

- If the affected bone is already weakened, substantially less force may be required to cause a fracture. Such injuries are referred to as pathologic fractures and are generally associated with primary or secondary tumors in the affected bone.
- Metastatic disease is the most common underlying process, but pathologic fractures through benign tumors such as an enchondroma or solitary bone cyst are not unusual.
- More diffuse processes such as osteoporosis, Paget's disease, renal osteodystrophy, or osteogenesis imperfecta, may result in pathologic fractures.
- A key feature of pathologic fractures is that they tend to be oriented transversely in long bones ("banana fracture"; Fig. 310–1).

Stress fractures

- Stress fractures occur due to chronic repetitive trauma. Such injuries may be difficult to diagnose at initial presentation; subtle periosteal reaction or transverse band of linear sclerosis may develop 1 to 2 weeks after the onset of symptoms. The fracture line is often never identified.
- Skeletal scintigraphy and MRI are very sensitive methods of detection of stress fractures and may be positive at the time of initial presentation.
- Common locations for stress fractures include the metatarsal shafts (first described in military recruits and thus described as "march fractures"), the pubic rami, the femoral neck, the tibial and fibular shafts (Fig. 310–2), and the tuberosity of the calcaneus.

Pelvic fractures

- Pelvic fractures are relatively common in elderly patients and often difficult to visualize on routine radiographs and may require CT for diagnosis (Figs. 310–3 and 310–4).
- In understanding the mechanics of pelvic fractures, it is best to think of the pelvis as a ring; any disruption of one part of the ring necessitates a matching disruption elsewhere in the ring.

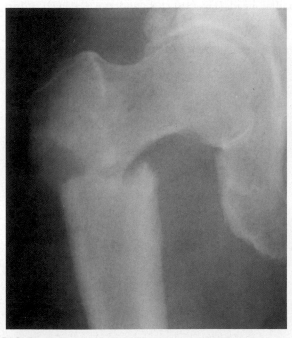

Fig 310–1
Pathologic 'banana fracture'. A transverse subtrochanteric fracture of the right femur with varus angulation is demonstrated. A transverse fracture in a long bone, particularly in the subtrochanteric region of the femur, is almost always due to an underlying abnormality.
(From Grainger RG, Allison DJ, Adam A, Dixon AK [eds]: Grainger and Allison's Diagnostic Radiology, 4th ed. Philadelphia, Churchill Livingstone, 2001.)

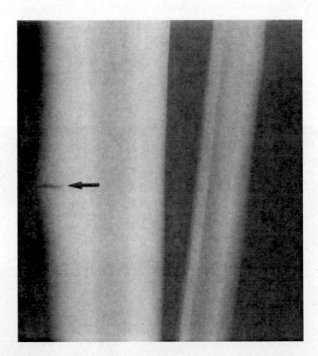

Fig 310–2
Tibial stress fracture. A lateral view of the tibia in a young male basketball player who had had mid-leg pain for 1 month demonstrates anterior cortical thickening and a transverse cortical lucency (arrow). These findings are typical of fatigue fractures that undergo continuing stress.
(From Grainger RG, Allison DJ, Adam A, Dixon AK [eds]: Grainger and Allison's Diagnostic Radiology, 4th ed. Philadelphia, Churchill Livingstone, 2001.)

- Vertical shear forces often result in a particular pattern of injury (*"Malgaigne complex"*) in which a fracture of the medial ileum or sacrum is seen in conjunction with fracture of the superior and inferior rami on the ipsilateral side. Superior displacement of the affected pelvis and hip usually results (Fig. 310–5).

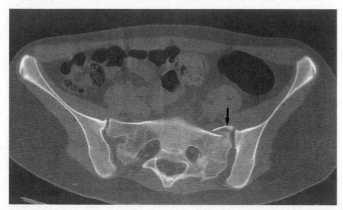

Fig 310–3
CT of a pelvic fracture. Note the fracture fragment arising from the anterior sacrum adjacent to the left sacroiliac joint *(arrow)*. Such fractures can be very difficult to identify and characterize on routine radiographs. (From Grainger RG, Allison DJ, Adam A, Dixon AK [eds]: Grainger and Allison's Diagnostic Radiology, 4th ed. Philadelphia, Churchill Livingstone, 2001.)

Fractures of long bones

- Fractures involving the long bones in adults are described using universally accepted terms.
- Clinically the most important feature is the distinction between **open fractures** (in which the overlying skin is disrupted and the fracture is connected with the outside environment and **closed fractures** (in which the overlying skin is intact).
- Fractures extending right across a bone (i.e., involving "both cortices" radiographically) are called **complete fractures**.
- **Transverse fractures** are those that run at right angles orthogonal to the long axis of the affected bone.
- **Oblique fractures**, as the name implies, cross the shaft at an angle (Fig. 310–6).
- If the inciting injury involves significant torsion, a **spiral fracture** may occur; the fragments created by a spiral fracture are often very sharp and pointed, and may cause soft tissue injury (Fig. 310–7).
- Any fracture that divides the bone into more than two separate fragments is known a **comminuted fracture** (Fig. 310–8).
- An **avulsion fracture** (Fig. 310–9) refers to the separation of a (usually small) bone fragment at the attachment site of a ligament or a tendon.
- In the forearm, the two classic examples of forearm fracture-dislocation complexes are the **Monteggia injury**, which is characterized by an anteriorly angulated fracture of the proximal ulna associated with anterior dislocation of the radial head (Fig. 310–10), and the **Galeazzi injury**, in

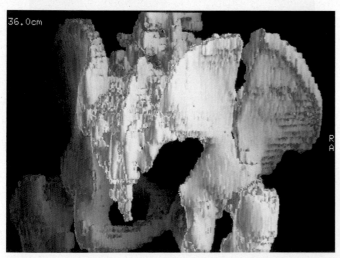

Fig 310–4
Fracture of the right iliac wing. Such fractures are associated with lateral compressive forces, as in this patient involved in a motor vehicle accident. This oblique posterior view from a 3D-reconstructed CT scan demonstrates the lesion, but does not replace the radiographs and axial CT. Extension into the acetabulum is not seen on this 3D reconstruction.
(From Grainger RG, Allison DJ, Adam A, Dixon AK [eds]: Grainger and Allison's Diagnostic Radiology, 4th ed. Philadelphia, Churchill Livingstone, 2001.)

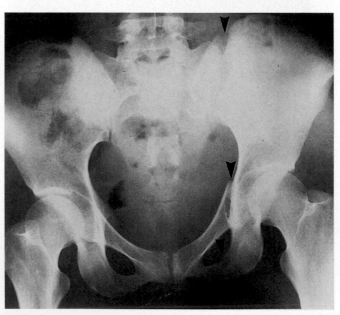

Fig 310-5
A Malgaigne fracture. Note fractures in the left superior and inferior public rami, and in the posterior portion of the left iliac wing adjacent to the sacroiliac joint *(arrowheads)*. There is superior displacement of the left hemipelvis, including the hip.
(From Grainger RG, Allison DJ, Adam A, Dixon AK [eds]: Grainger and z Allison's Diagnostic Radiology, 4th ed. Philadelphia, Churchill Livingstone, 2001.)

which a dorsally angulated distal radial fracture is seen in conjunction with dorsal dislocation of the distal ulna (Fig. 310–11).

- In the wrist, the term **Colles' fracture** is often (inappropriately) used to refer to any fracture of the distal radius resulting from a fall on an outstretched hand; yet Colles specifically described a volarly angulated, impacted fracture of the distal radius with dorsal displacement of the distal fracture segment. Although not in the original description, this fracture is often associated with a separation of the ulnar styloid. The lateral radiograph is generally the most helpful film (Fig. 310–12).

- **Greenstick** (Fig. 310–13) and **torus** (Fig. 310–14) injuries are both incomplete fractures commonly seen in children. In the former, the bone cortex and periosteum break on the convex side of the fracture, whereas the latter occurs when a bone's cortex buckles on the concave side due to a bending force. Buckling may also occur on the concave side of a greenstick fracture.

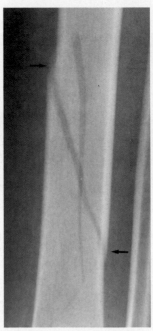

Fig 310–7
Spiral fracture. AP projection of the leg demonstrates a spiral fracture of the tibia. Note the sharp ends of the fracture fragments (arrows), which may cause significant soft-tissue injury.
(From Grainger RG, Allison DJ, Adam A, Dixon AK [eds]: Grainger and Allison's Diagnostic Radiology, 4th ed. Philadelphia, Churchill Livingstone, 2001.)

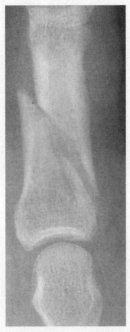

Fig 310–6
An oblique fracture of the proximal phalanx of the fourth digit. There is minimal override of the fracture fragments.
(From Grainger RG, Allison DJ, Adam A, Dixon AK [eds]: Grainger and Allison's Diagnostic Radiology, 4th ed. Philadelphia, Churchill Livingstone, 2001.)

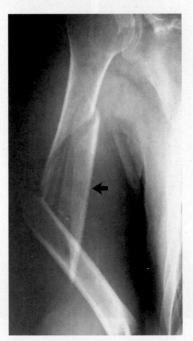

Fig 310–8
A comminuted fracture of the midshaft of the right humerus demonstrates a large medial butterfly fragment (large arrow). There is marked lateral angulation at the fracture line between the major fracture fragments.
(From Grainger RG, Allison DJ, Adam A, Dixon AK [eds]: Grainger and Allison's Diagnostic Radiology, 4th ed. Philadelphia, Churchill Livingstone, 2001.)

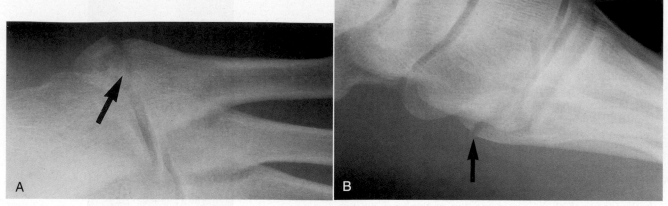

Fig 310–9
Avulsion fracture. AP (**A**) and lateral (**B**) views of the foot demonstrate a horizontal lucency at the base of the fifth metatarsal *(arrow),* representing an avulsion injury at the insertion site of the peroneus brevis tendon. Avulsion fragments are often very small, and can be difficult to detect.
(From Grainger RG, Allison DJ, Adam A, Dixon AK [eds]: Grainger and Allison's Diagnostic Radiology, 4th ed. Philadelphia, Churchill Livingstone, 2001.)

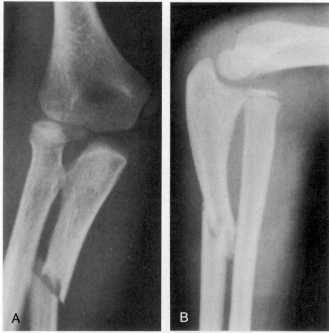

Fig 310–10
Monteggia fracture-dislocation of the proximal forearm. AP (**A**) and lateral (**B**) views demonstrate an anteriorly angulated fracture of the proximal ulna, and anterior of the radius.
(From Grainger RG, Allison DJ, Adam A, Dixon AK [eds]: Grainger and Allison's Diagnostic Radiology, 4th ed. Philadelphia, Churchill Livingstone, 2001.)

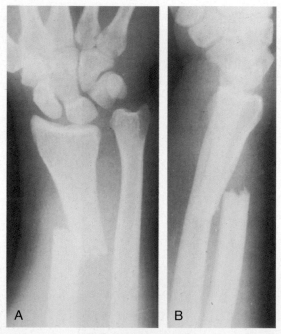

Fig 310–11
Galeazzi fracture-dislocation of the distal forearm. AP (**A**) and lateral (**B**) views of the distal arm demonstrate a displaced fracture of the radius and diastasis of the distal radioulnar joint, with medial ulnar dislocation.
(From Grainger RG, Allison DJ, Adam A, Dixon AK [eds]: Grainger and Allison's Diagnostic Radiology, 4th ed. Philadelphia, Churchill Livingstone, 2001.)

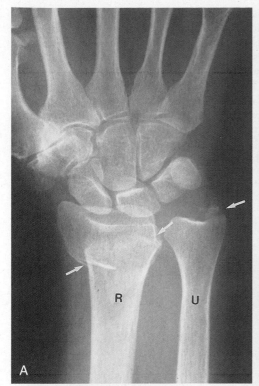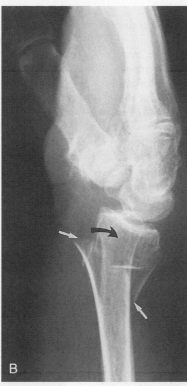

Fig 310–12

Colles' fracture. **A,** An impacted distal radial fracture (R) and a fracture of the ulnar styloid (U) *(white arrows)* are identified on the posteroanterior view in this patient who fell on the outstretched hand.
B, The lateral view of the wrist shows that there is dorsal displacement *(black arrow)* and angulation as well as some impaction of the distal radius. If the fracture of the distal radius extends into the joint, this would be termed a *Barton fracture.*
(From Mettler FA, Guibertau MJ, Voss CM, Urbina CE: Primary Care Radiology, Philadelphia, Elsevier 2000)

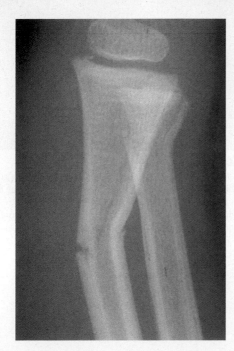

Fig 310–13

Greenstick fractures of the distal radius and ulna.
(From Grainger RG, Allison DJ, Adam A, Dixon AK [eds]: Grainger and Allison's Diagnostic Radiology, 4th ed. Philadelphia, Churchill Livingstone, 2001.)

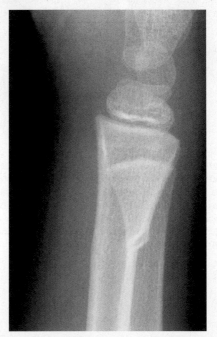

Fig 310–14

Torus fracture of the distal radius.
(From Grainger RG, Allison DJ, Adam A, Dixon AK [eds]: Grainger and Allison's Diagnostic Radiology, 4th ed. Philadelphia, Churchill Livingstone, 2001.)

Cervical spine fractures

- X-ray examination of the cervical spine depends on the patient's clinical condition.
- In severely injured patients (unconscious, major head or neck trauma, spinal cord or root signs, multiple organ system injuries, or multiple fractures), the single most important radiographic examination is the horizontal beam lateral of the cervical spine.
- Care must be taken to ensure that all seven cervical vertebrae are included. If not, a repeat examination should be obtained while pulling down on the patient's arms (Fig. 310–15).

- Failure to visualize the seventh cervical vertebrae and the C7-T1 junction is the most common error made in the radiographic assessment of cervical spine injury.
- A **hangman's fracture** (traumatic spondylolysis of the axis) represent fractures of the neural arch of C2 that are produced by a hyperextension force such as that commonly experienced when the head or face hits the windshield or steering wheel in a motor vehicle accident. This may result in bilateral fractures of the neural arch anterior to the inferior facets. This is the same fracture as caused by a judicial hanging and is therefore often referred to as a hangman's fracture (Fig. 310–16).

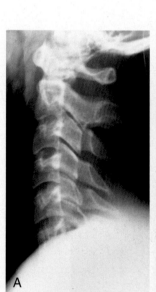 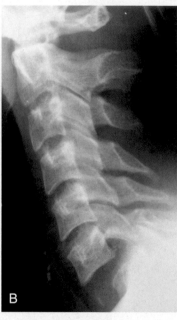

Fig 310–15

We must demonstrate all seven cervical vertebrae. (**A**) Initial cross-table lateral radiographic examination of the spine reveals only six cervical vertebrae. (**B**) A repeat examination was obtained while pulling down on the shoulder, which demonstrates a fracture dislocation at C6-7 not apparent on the initial radiograph.
(From Grainger RG, Allison DJ, Adam A, Dixon AK [eds]: Grainger and Allison's Diagnostic Radiology, 4th ed. Philadelphia, Churchill Livingstone, 2001.)

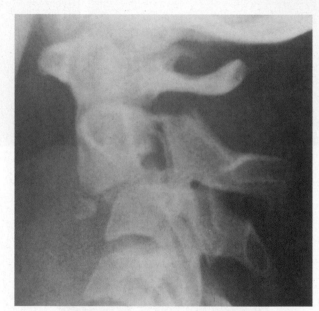

Fig 310–16

Hangman's fracture with wide separation of the fracture fragments and locking of the C2 facets anterior to C3. There is also a small fragment arising from the anterior margin of the vertebral body of C2.
(From Grainger RG, Allison DJ, Adam A, Dixon AK [eds]: Grainger and Allison's Diagnostic Radiology, 4th ed. Philadelphia, Churchill Livingstone, 2001.)

Fractures of thoracic and lumbar vertebrae

- Most fractures of the thoracic and lumbar vertebrae tend to be anterior wedge (compression) fractures, which are usually readily observed in lateral projections (Fig. 310–17). A lesion that may be confused with acute compression fractures is a **Schmorl's nodes** (Fig. 310–18). Schmorl's nodes are usually multiple, are typically located in the end plate, and are characterized by irregular sclerotic margins surrounding an irregular lucent defect.

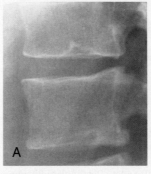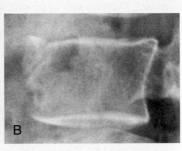

Fig 310–18
Schmorl's nodes. Note the sharply defined domelike densities arising from the end plate in theses two adjacent vertebrae. (**B**) Limbus vertebra. There is a well marginated ossicle at the anterior superior margin of the vertebral body. Note that the underlying vertebral body margin is also well defined. This represents a developmental defect, presumably of the ring apophysis.
(From Grainger RG, Allison DJ, Adam A, Dixon AK [eds]: Grainger and Allison's Diagnostic Radiology, 4th ed. Philadelphia, Churchill Livingstone, 2001.)

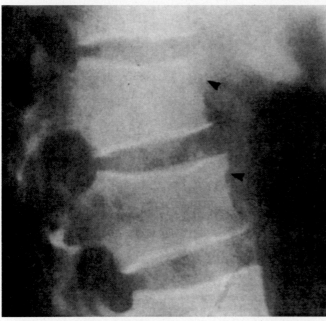

Fig 310–17
Simple wedge (compression) fracture of the bodies of T11 and T12. Note that the posterior walls of the vertebral bodies are maintained and the posterior elements are intact without evidence of dislocation. Fractures of contiguous vertebrae are common in the dorsal spine.
(From Grainger RG, Allison DJ, Adam A, Dixon AK [eds]: Grainger and Allison's Diagnostic Radiology, 4th ed. Philadelphia, Churchill Livingstone, 2001.)

REFERENCES

Canoso J: Rheumatology in primary care. Philadelphia, WB Saunders, 1997.

Cohen J, Powderly WG: Infectious Diseases, 2nd ed. St Louis, Mosby, 2004.

Ferri F: Ferri's Clinical Advisor 2007. St Louis, Mosby, 2007.

Ferri F: Practical Guide to the Care of the Medical Patient, 7th ed. St Louis, Mosby, 2007.

Grainger RG, Allison DJ, Adam A, Dixon AK (eds): Grainger and Allison's Diagnostic Radiology, 4th ed. Philadelphia, Churchill Livingstone, 2001.

Harris ED, Budd RC, Genovese MC, et al: Kelley's Textbook of Rheumatology, 7th ed. Philadelphia, WB Saunders, 2005.

Hochberg MC, Silman AJ, Smolen JS, et al (eds): Rheumatology, 3rd ed. St Louis, Mosby, 2003.

Swartz MH: Textbook of Physical Diagnosis, 5th ed. Philadelphia, WB Saunders, 2006.

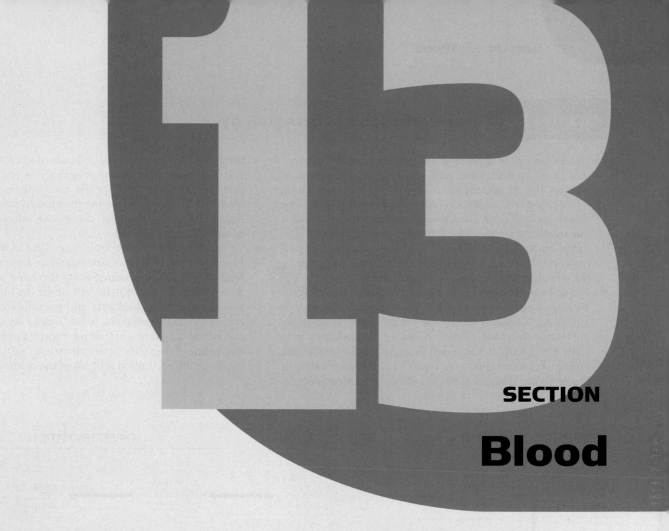

SECTION

Blood

Chapter 311: Basic principles of hematology
Chapter 312: Anemias
Chapter 313: Leukemias
Chapter 314: Myelodysplastic syndrome
Chapter 315: Hodgkin's lymphoma
Chapter 316: Non-Hodgkin's lymphoma
Chapter 317: Hairy cell leukemia
Chapter 318: Plasma cell dyscrasias
Chapter 319: Polycythemia vera
Chapter 320: Thrombocytopenia

Chapter 321: Disseminated intravascular coagulation
Chapter 322: Hypercoagulable state
Chapter 323: Hemophilias
Chapter 324: Von Willebrand's disease
Chapter 325: Felty's syndrome
Chapter 326: Paroxysmal nocturnal hemoglobinuria
Chapter 327: Paroxysmal cold hemoglobinuria
Chapter 328: Histiocytosis X
Chapter 329: Kaposi's sarcoma

Chapter 311   Basic principles of hematology

- Hematopoiesis is defined as the process whereby pluripotent hematopoietic stem cells self-renew and differentiate into all the specialized circulating blood cells, including white blood cells, red blood cells, and platelets (Fig. 311–1). Hematopoiesis occurs in a specialized bone marrow microenvironment, composed of cellular and noncellular elements critical to localization and control of blood cell production. Figure 311–2 illustrates the various stages during the evolution of the mature discocytic red cell.
- Red cell antigens and autoantibodies: blood group antigens are carbohydrate or protein determinants carried on various red blood cell (RBC) membrane components. Blood group autoantibodies have clinical relevance because they may cause hemolysis of transfused antigen-positive RBCs, and during pregnancy they may result in hemolytic disease of the newborn. Testing to detect antibody in a patient's serum

is required before selection of donor blood for transfusion; it is also performed during pregnancy as part of standard prenatal care (Fig. 311–3). The mechanisms of immune-mediated hemolysis following transfusion are illustrated in Figure 311–4. Table 311–1 shows the selection of ABO-compatible donor blood.
- Granulocytopoiesis: neutrophils circulate in the peripheral blood for only 3 to 6 hours, requiring a constitutive high level of neutrophil production by the bone marrow. They arise from pluripotent stem cells under the influence of cytokines, notably granulocyte and granulocyte-macrophage colony-stimulating factors, which induce an intricate transcriptional program that drives morphologic maturation and neutrophil-specific gene expression. Figure 311–5 illustrates the differentiation schema of the neutrophil.

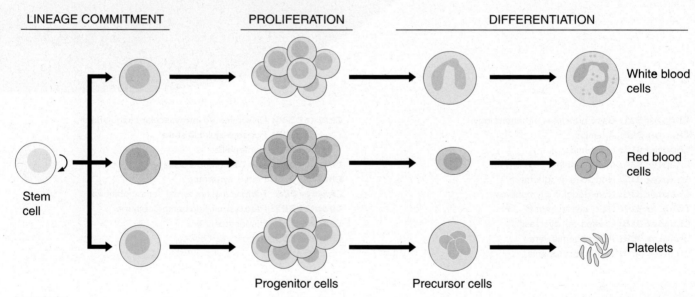

Fig 311–1
Hematopoiesis.
(From Young NS, Gerson SL, High KA [eds]: Clinical Hematology. St. Louis, Mosby, 2006.)

- Immunity can be divided into innate and adaptive immune responses. Major effector cells of the immune response include natural killer (NK) cells, NK T cells, dendritic cells (DCs), macrophages, and granulocytes (Fig. 311–6).
- Megakaryocyte development: in megakaryocyte development, lineage commitment begins when a marrow stem cell gives rise to a bipotent erythromegakaryocytic progenitor cell (see Fig. 311–1). This cell can then further commit to development of either erythrocytes or megakaryocytes. Members of the GATA family of transcription factors, along with obligate cofactor FOG, play a major role in transcriptional regulation of megakaryocytopoiesis (Fig. 311–7).

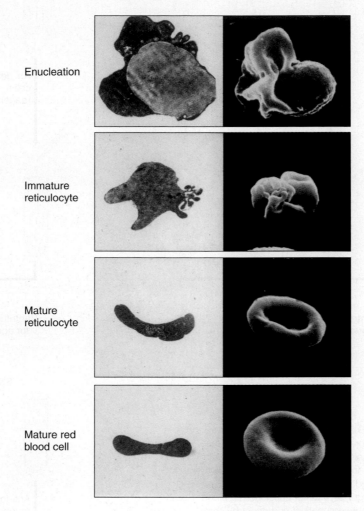

Enucleation

Immature reticulocyte

Mature reticulocyte

Mature red blood cell

Fig 311–2
Transmission (left column) and scanning (right column) electron micrographs showing the various stages during the evolution of the mature discocytic red cell. The non-nucleated immature reticulocyte is produced when the normoblast extrudes its nucleus. The immature reticulocyte is multilobular and motile and contains mitochondria and ribosomes. These motile reticulocytes evolve first to deep cup-shaped nonmotile mature reticulocytes that contain ribosomes and finally to mature, fully hemoglobinized discocytic red blood cells lacking organelles.
(From Young NS, Gerson SL, High KA [eds]: Clinical Hematology. St. Louis, Mosby, 2006.)

ABO AND RH TYPING   SERUM ANTIBODY DETECTION

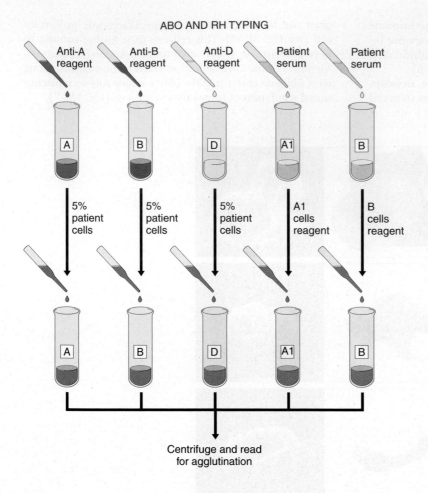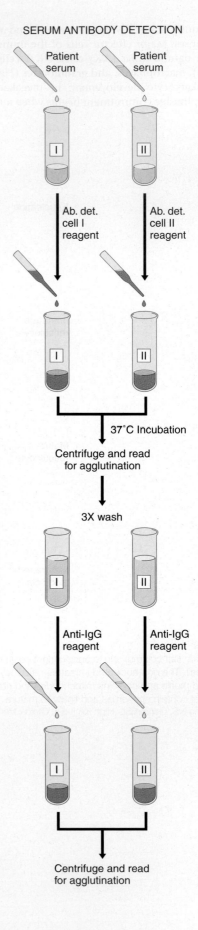

Fig 311–3
Pretransfusion testing of recipient. The protocol includes typing the
recipient's red blood cells (RBCs) for ABO and Rh, and testing of the
recipient's serum (or plasma) for clinically significant blood group antibodies (antibody screen). Because the antibodies involved in ABO and
Rh typing are IgM, the method used is direct agglutination. Because
clinically significant antibodies are IgG, an indirect antiglobulin method
is used. The final step is a match between patient and donor by com-
puter or by physically testing the patient's serum against the selected
donor's RBCs. Ab. det., antibody detection.
(From Young NS, Gerson SL, High KA [eds]: Clinical Hematology. St. Louis,
Mosby, 2006.)

INTRAVASCULAR HEMOLYSIS

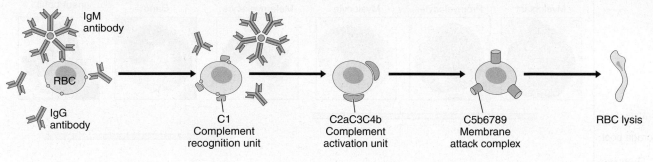

EXTRAVASCULAR HEMOLYSIS

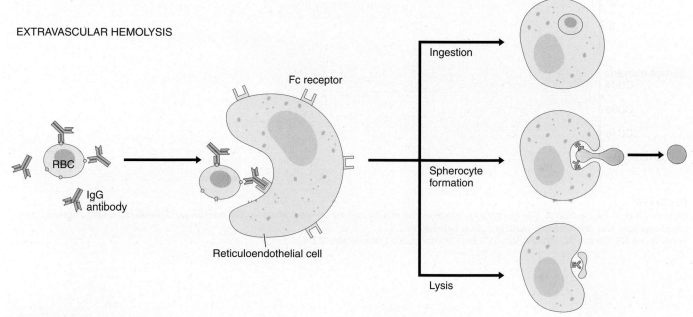

Fig 311–4
Mechanisms of immune-mediated hemolysis following transfusion. RBC, red blood cell.
(From Young NS, Gerson SL, High KA [eds]: Clinical Hematology. St. Louis, Mosby, 2006.)

TABLE 311–1 Selection of ABO-compatible donor blood*

Recipient's type	Donor RBC type				Donor plasma type			
O	—	—	—	O	O	A	B	AB
A	—	A	—	O	—	A	—	AB
B	—	—	B	O	—	—	B	AB
AB	AB	A	B	O	—	—	—	AB

*Group O red blood cell (RBC) donors are called universal donors.
From Young NS, Gerson SL, High KA (eds): Clinical Hematology. St. Louis, 2006, Mosby, 2006.

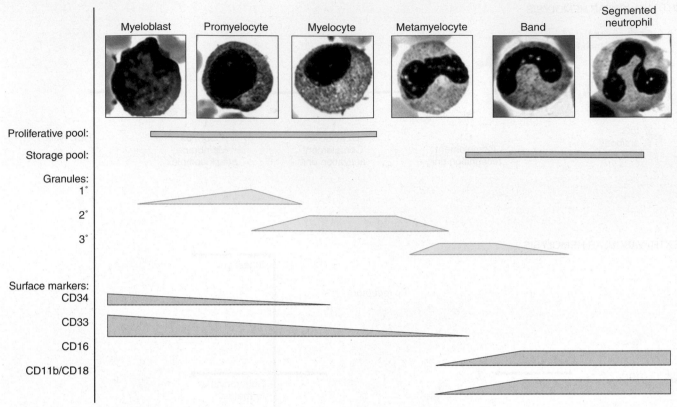

Fig 311–5
Differentiation of the neutrophil. The morphologic stages of neutrophil maturation are correlated with marrow pool distribution, stage-specific granule production, and characteristic surface marker expression.
(From Young NS, Gerson SL, High KA [eds]: Clinical Hematology. St. Louis, Mosby, 2006.)

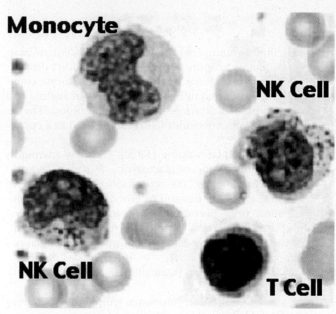

Fig 311–6
Innate immune cells found in the peripheral blood. Shown are a monocyte, two natural killer (NK) cells, and a T lymphocyte. (From Young NS, Gerson SL, High KA [eds]: Clinical Hematology. St. Louis, Mosby, 2006.)

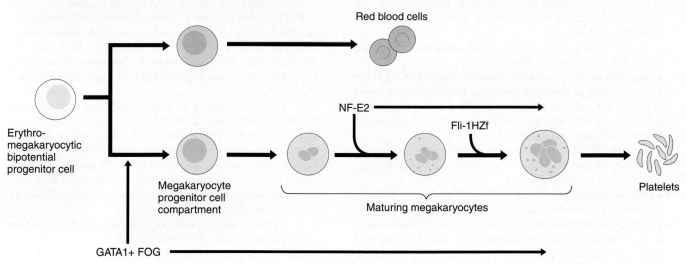

Fig 311–7
Transcriptional regulation of megakaryocytopoiesis.
(From Young NS, Gerson SL, High KA [eds]: Clinical Hematology. St. Louis, Mosby, 2006.)

Chapter 312 Anemias

DEFINITION

Anemia can be defined as a reduction below normal limits in the amount of hemoglobin (Hb) or in the volume of RBCs (hematocrit [Hct]) in a sample of peripheral venous blood.

CAUSE

- Decreased RBC production
  - Deficiency of hematinic agents
  - Bone marrow failure
  - Decreased erythropoietin (renal disease)
- Increased RBC destruction or loss
  - Hemolysis
  - Hemorrhage

DIAGNOSIS

History

- Family and ethnic history: inquire about thalassemia, sickle cell anemia, splenectomy, cholelithiasis at an early age.
- Drug and toxic exposures (e.g., chloramphenicol, methyldopa, quinidine, benzene, alkylating agents)
- Obstetric and menstrual history: excessive menstrual bleeding is a frequent cause of iron deficiency anemia in menstruating women.
- External blood loss: gastrointestinal, genitourinary (inquire about melena, hematochezia, gross hematuria), frequent phlebotomy
- Dietary habits: poor dietary habits and alcohol intake may result in folic acid deficiency.
- Rapidity of onset: gradual onset is suggestive of bone marrow failure or chronic blood loss, whereas sudden onset of symptoms suggests hemolysis or acute hemorrhage.
- History of infection (e.g., sepsis, acquired immunodeficiency syndrome, malaria)
- History of cancer, renal disease, or endocrine disease
- History of diarrhea, abdominal pain, bulky stools (e.g., malabsorption, celiac disease)

Physical examination

- General appearance: evaluate nutritional status.
- Vital signs: hypotension, tachycardia (acute blood loss)
- Skin: pallor of the conjunctiva, lips, oral mucosa, nail beds, and palmar creases; jaundice (hemolysis); petechiae; purpura (thrombocytopenia)
- Mouth: glossitis (pernicious anemia, iron deficiency anemia)
- Heart: listen for flow murmurs, prosthetic valves (increased RBC destruction).
- Abdomen: splenomegaly (hemolysis, neoplasms, infiltrative disorders)
- Rectum: examine stool for occult (or gross) blood.
- Lymph nodes: infiltrative lesions, infections

Laboratory results

- Hb and Hct: provide a guide to diagnosis and severity of anemia. The RBC distribution width (RDW) measures the variability of RBC size and is useful in the diagnostic workup of anemia.
- Reticulocyte count
1. Should be performed before any therapeutic maneuvers and is useful in any diagnostic algorithm (Fig. 312–1)

2. Reticulocyte counts below 1% indicate inadequate marrow production; counts above 4% indicate RBC destruction or acute blood loss. However, the reticulocyte count should be considered in light of the degree of anemia and the shift of reticulocytes to the peripheral blood. The reticulocyte production index (RPI) can be used as a correction method
- Mean corpuscular volume (MCV): classifies anemia as normocytic, microcytic, or macrocytic
1. Normocytic anemia: the reticulocyte count is used to distinguish excess destruction or blood loss (high reticulocyte count) from decreased production (low reticulocyte count). A bone marrow examination is of value in distinguishing the following causes of normocytic anemia and reticulocytopenia:
   a. Marrow hypoplasia (toxic drugs, radiation, infection)
   b. RBC aplasia
   c. Marrow infiltration (myeloma, lymphoma, leukemia)
   d. Myelofibrosis
   e. Renal insufficiency
2. Microcytic anemia (Table 312–1)
   a. Iron deficiency is the most common cause.
   b. Thalassemia, lead poisoning, anemia of chronic disease, and sex-linked sideroblastic anemia are other causes.
   c. The peripheral smear and RBC count may help distinguish iron deficiency from thalassemia minor (relatively high RBC count and basophilic stippling in the latter) (Fig. 312–2).
   d. Assess iron stores by determining the serum ferritin (or marrow iron stain if ferritin is unavailable). If ferritin is low, iron deficiency is proved, but if it is normal or elevated, appropriate workup for thalassemia (Hb electrophoresis), sideroblastic anemia, and anemia of chronic disease (low serum iron, low total iron-binding capacity, increased ferritin, decreased reticulocytes) is warranted. RDW above 15 suggests iron deficiency;
   e. Serum erythropoietin level can be useful in defining and treating anemia of chronic disease.
3. Macrocytic anemia (Fig. 312–3)
   a. Because reticulocytes have a large diameter, an elevated reticulocyte count will read out as an elevated MCV; if the reticulocyte count is elevated, hemolytic studies (haptoglobin, lactate dehydrogenase [LDH], indirect bilirubin) are indicated.
   b. If hemolysis is confirmed, determine the cause with Coombs' test; other studies (as suggested by RBC morphology) may be indicated.
   c. If the reticulocyte count is normal and RBCs are macrocytic, vitamin B_{12} or folate deficiency is possible; therefore RBC folate, serum vitamin B_{12}, and serum folate levels should be determined.
   d. The presence of a megaloblastic bone marrow would enhance the diagnosis of vitamin B_{12} or folate deficiency. If the bone marrow exhibits dyserythropoiesis or white blood cell (WBC) abnormalities, a myelodysplastic anemia is the cause of the macrocytic anemia.

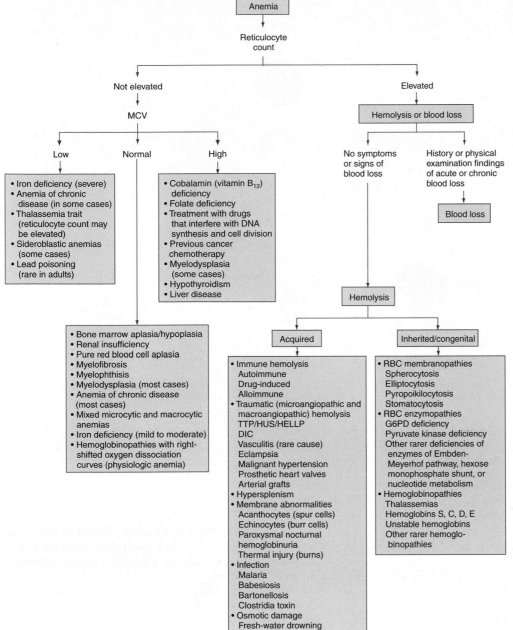

Fig 312–1
Algorithm for the diagnosis of anemias. DIC, disseminated intravascular coagulation; HELLP, hemolysis, elevated liver function, and low platelet count; HUS, hemolytic-uremic syndrome; MCV, mean corpuscular volume; RBC, red blood cell; TTP, thrombotic thrombocytopenic purpura. (From Goldman L, Ausiello D [eds]: Cecil Textbook of Medicine, 22nd ed. Philadelphia, WB Saunders, 2004.)

TABLE 312–1 Differentiating microcytic* anemias using iron studies			
Disorder	**Serum iron**	**Serum TIBC**	**Serum ferritin**
Iron deficiency anemia	Low (<45 μg/dL)	High (>300 μg/dL)	Low (<20 μg/mL)
Anemia of inflammation	Low (<45 μg /dL)	Low or normal (<250 μg/dL)	High (>250 μg/mL)
Anemia of inflammation + iron depletion	Low (<45 μg/dL)	Low or normal (<250 μg/dL)	Normal (<100 μg/mL)
Thalassemia trait	Normal	Normal	Normal
Sideroblastic anemia	High	Normal	Normal

*Mean corpuscular volume < 80 fL.
TIBC, total iron-binding capacity.
From Young NS, Gerson SL, High KA (eds): Clinical Hematology. St. Louis, 2006, Mosby, 2006.

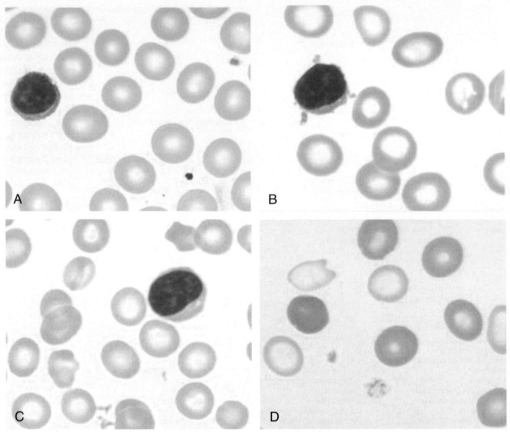

Fig 312–2

Peripheral blood smear photomicrographs (×1000) from patients with microcytic anemias. **A,** Normal red blood cells. **B,** Microcytosis and hypochromia (MCV, 70 fL) caused by iron deficiency. **C,** Microcytosis and hypochromia resulting from β-thalassemia trait (MCV, 67 fL). **D,** Dimorphic red blood cells caused by sideroblastic anemia.
(From Young NS, Gerson SL, High KA [eds]: Clinical Hematology. St. Louis, Mosby, 2006.)

e. A systematic and logical search with avoidance of a "shotgun" diagnostic or therapeutic approach will yield the correct diagnosis (Table 312–2).

• Review peripheral blood smear (Fig. 312–4). RBC morphology should be evaluated for the following:

1. Size

   a. Normal RBCs (see Fig. 312–4A) have a diameter equal to that of the nucleus of a mature lymphocyte.

   b. Microcytosis (see Fig. 312–4B) is seen with iron deficiency, hemoglobinopathies, and sideroblastic anemia.

   c. Macrocytosis (see Fig. 312–4C) indicates megaloblastic anemia, liver disease, or myelodysplasia.

2. Shape

   a. Spherocytes: hereditary spherocytosis, immune, or other hemolytic states

   b. Sickle cell: HbSS (see Fig. 312–4H)

   c. Helmet cells: microangiopathic hemolysis, severe iron deficiency

   d. Teardrop cells (see Fig. 312–4I): myeloproliferative diseases, pernicious anemia, thalassemia

3. Color

   a. Hypochromasia (iron deficiency, sideroblastic anemias)

   b. Hyperchromasia (megaloblastic anemia, spherocytosis)

• Morphology of WBCs and platelets should be noted and any abnormal cells identified; additional abnormalities of diagnostic value that may be present on peripheral smears are noted as follows:

   1. Howell-Jolly bodies (nuclear fragments; see Fig. 312–4K): hemolytic and megaloblastic anemias, splenectomy

   2. Basophilic stippling (see Fig. 312–4L): lead poisoning, thalassemia, hemolytic states

   3. Heinz bodies (denatured Hb; see Fig. 312–4P): unstable hemoglobinopathies, some hemolytic anemias; identification of Heinz bodies requires supravital stain.

   4. Cabot ring (nuclear remnants): megaloblastic anemias

   5. Pappenheimer bodies (see Fig. 312–4Q): postsplenectomy, hemolytic, sideroblastic, and megaloblastic anemias

   6. Rouleaux formation (see Fig. 312–4F): multiple myeloma, Waldenström's macroglobulinemia

   7. Presence of parasites (e.g., *Plasmodium* in malaria [see Fig. 332–5], *Babesia* in babesiosis [see Fig. 332–7])

   8. Nucleated RBCs: extramedullary hematopoiesis, hypoxia, hemolysis

   9. Target cells (see Fig. 312–4D): hemoglobinopathies, iron deficiency, liver disease

   10. Hypersegmented polymorphonuclear neutrophils (PMNs [see Fig. 312–14]): folate–vitamin B_{12} deficiency

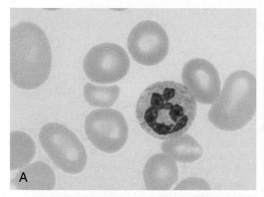
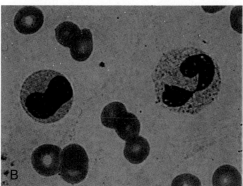
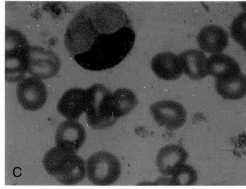
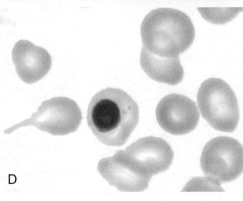

Fig 312–3
Peripheral blood smear photomicrographs (×1000) from patients with macrocytic anemia. **A,** Macrocytes and hypersegmentation resulting from nutritional megaloblastic anemia. **B,** Bilobed neutrophil (Pelger-Huët cell) and a metamyelocyte associated with myelodysplastic syndrome. **C,** Erythrophagocytosis and spurious macrocytosis caused by agglutinated red cells in a patient with *Mycoplasma*-associated cold agglutinin hemolytic anemia. **D,** Nucleated and teardrop red cells associated with myelofibrosis.
(From Young NS, Gerson SL, High KA [eds]: Clinical Hematology. St. Louis, Mosby, 2006.)

TABLE 312–2 Differentiating macrocytic anemias

Disorder	Characteristic findings on initial screening evaluation*
Nutritional megaloblastic anemias	
Cobalamin deficiency	Low serum cobalamin‡; hypersegmented neutrophils
	Increased serum methylmalonic acid and/or homocysteine‡
	Low red cell folate
	High serum iron that falls with specific therapy
	Intrinsic factor antibody is positive in <50% of pernicious anemia patients
Folic acid deficiency	Alcoholism, inadequate diet, or increased requirement (hemolysis, pregnancy)
	Hypersegmented neutrophils; increased serum homocysteine‡
	Low serum and red cell folate†
	Normal serum cobalamin and methylmalonic acid
	High serum iron that falls with specific treatment
Myelodysplastic syndromes	Abnormalities of white blood cells and platelets frequently present
	Hyposegmented neutrophils (Pelger-Huët cells) may be present
	Persistent high serum iron (sideroblastic anemia)
Other marrow disorders	Leukocyte and platelet count abnormalities
	Leukoerythroblastic blood smear: immature white blood cells, nucleated red blood cells
Drugs or substances	Alcohol, cancer chemotherapy, phenytoin, zidovudine, stavudine
Liver disease	Targeted red blood cells, abnormal liver function tests
	Low white blood cell and platelet counts frequently present
Hypothyroidism	High thyroid-stimulating hormone
Spurious macrocytosis	Reticulocytosis; cold agglutinins
	Rouleaux resulting from monoclonal gammopathy

*Reticulocyte count, serum cobalamin, thyroid function test, and peripheral blood smear.
†Serum and red cell folate studies are not recommended. If serum cobalamin is normal and folate deficiency is suspected, it is more cost-effective to treat with folic acid.
‡Tissue cobalamin levels are usually low when serum levels are less than 200 pg/mL, almost always low when levels are below 100 pg/mL, and rarely low when levels are 200-300 pg/mL. Elevated methylmalonic acid levels confirm tissue cobalamin deficiency (if renal function is normal). Both methylmalonic acid and homocysteine are elevated in renal insufficiency.
From Young NS, Gerson SL, High KA (eds): Clinical Hematology. St. Louis, 2006, Mosby, 2006.

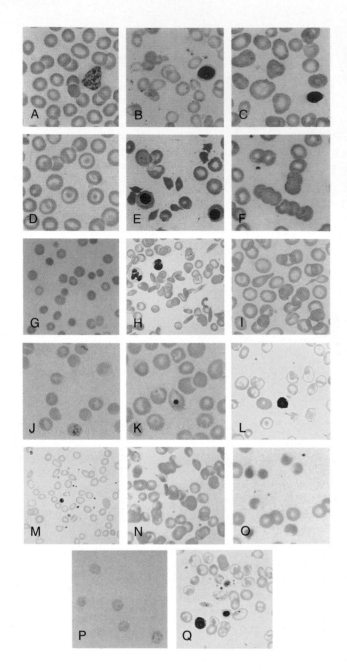

Fig 312–4

Erythrocyte morphology in peripheral blood. **A,** Normal red cells. **B,** Microcytic hypochromic cells typical of iron deficiency. **C,** Macrocytosis typically seen in megaloblastic anemia. **D,** Target cells. **E,** Schistocytes and nucleated red cells. **F,** Rouleaux formation. **G,** Normal red cells and microspherocytes in hereditary spherocytosis. **H,** Sickle cell anemia, showing sickled cells, a Howell-Jolly body, and polychromatophilia. **I,** Teardrop poikilocytes. **J,** Reticulocytes (special stain). **K,** Howell-Jolly body (nuclear remnant). **L,** Homozygous β-thalassemia, showing microcytic and hypochromic erythrocytes, anisocytosis and poikilocytosis, basophilic stippling, a Howell-Jolly body, target cells, and polychromatophilia. **M,** Heterozygous β-thalassemia, showing hypochromia and microcytosis. **N,** Hemoglobin sickle cell disease, showing a hemoglobin C (HbC) crystal, target cells, a folded taco-shaped cell, polychromatophilia, and Pappenheimer bodies. **O,** Eccentrocytes (blister cells) with a lopsided distribution of hemoglobin, typically seen during a hemolytic episode in glucose-6-phosphate dehydrogenase (G6PD) deficiency. **P,** Heinz bodies (supravital stain). **Q,** HbS-β₀–thalassemia, showing a nucleated erythrocyte, Howell-Jolly and Pappenheimer bodies, a sickle cell, target cells, polychromatophilia, and microcytosis (Wright's stain, ×1000). (From Stein JH [ed]: Internal Medicine, 4th ed. St. Louis, Mosby, 1998.)

questration in pulmonary macrophages), paroxysmal nocturnal hemoglobinuria (intravascular hemolysis)

DIFFERENTIAL DIAGNOSIS
- Anemia of chronic disease
- Sideroblastic anemia (see Fig. 312–2D)
- Thalassemia trait (see Fig. 312–2C)

LABORATORY TESTS
- Laboratory results vary with the stage of deficiency.
- Absent iron marrow stores (Fig. 312–5A) and decreased serum ferritin are the initial abnormalities.
- Decreased serum iron and increased total iron-binding capacity (TIBC) are the next abnormalities.
- Hypochromic microcytic anemia is present, with significant iron deficiency (see Fig. 312–5B).
- Peripheral smear in patients with iron deficiency generally reveals microcytic hypochromic RBCs with a wide area of central pallor, anisocytosis, and poikilocytosis when severe.
- Laboratory abnormalities consistent with iron deficiency are low serum ferritin level, elevated RDW, with values generally >15, low MCV, elevated TIBC, and low serum iron.
- The reticulocyte hemoglobin content (CHr) may be a good screening test for iron deficiency. It can be measured using an automated hematology analyzer and represents a relatively inexpensive and fast way to detect iron deficiency.

TREATMENT
- Treatment consists of ferrous sulfate, 325 mg PO daily, for at least 6 months. Calcium supplements can decrease iron absorption; therefore, these two medications should be staggered.
- Parenteral iron therapy is reserved for patients with poor tolerance, noncompliance with oral preparations, or malabsorption.
- Transfusion of packed RBCs is indicated for patients with severe symptomatic anemia (e.g., angina) or life-threatening anemia.

B. SIDEROBLASTIC ANEMIA

DEFINITION

Sideroblastic anemias are blood disorders resulting from defective heme synthesis and are classified as hereditary, acquired, and reversible.

A. IRON DEFICIENCY ANEMIA

DEFINITION

Iron deficiency anemia is anemia secondary to inadequate iron supplementation or excessive blood loss.

PHYSICAL FINDINGS AND CLINICAL PRESENTATION
- Most patients have a normal examination.
- Skin pallor and conjunctival pallor may be present.

CAUSE
- Blood loss from gastrointestinal (GI) or menstrual bleeding (gastrourinary [GU] blood loss less often the cause)
- Dietary iron deficiency (rare in adults)
- Poor iron absorption in patients with gastric or small bowel surgery
- Repeated phlebotomy
- Increased requirements (e.g., during pregnancy)
- Other: traumatic hemolysis (abnormally functioning cardiac valves), idiopathic pulmonary hemosiderosis (iron se-

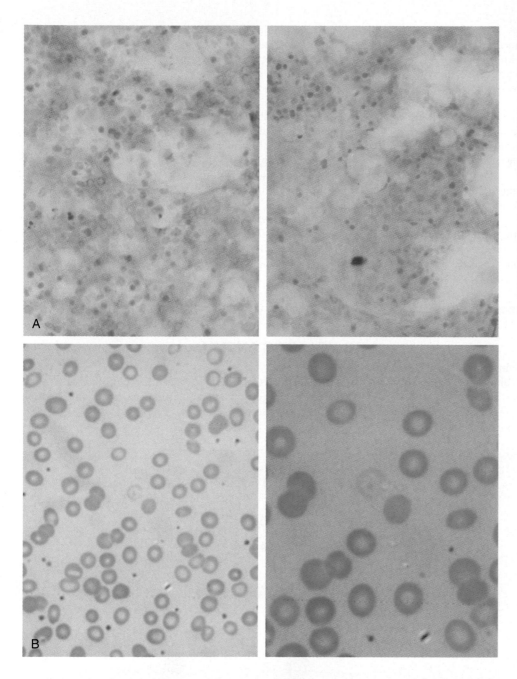

Fig 312–5
Peripheral blood smears in iron deficiency. **A,** Prussian blue staining for iron in the bone marrow of an iron-deficient patient is shown on the left; lack of stainable iron is demonstrated when compared with an iron-replete individual on the right. **B,** Low-power (left) and high-power (right) views. Because of variation in amount of hemoglobin relative to the degree of iron deficiency, hypochromia is variable. Cells are floppy or deformable and appear to have a large degree of size disparity when spread on a glass smear. Automated cell counters more correctly measure the most hypochromic cells as small or microcytic.
(From Young NS, Gerson SL, High KA [eds]: Clinical Hematology. St. Louis, Mosby, 2006.)

PHYSICAL FINDINGS AND CLINICAL PRESENTATION

The symptoms for sideroblastic anemia are the same as for any anemia.

- Symptoms include fatigue, weakness, palpitations, shortness of breath, headaches, irritability, and chest pain.
- Physical findings may include pallor, tachycardia, hepatosplenomegaly, S_3, jugular venous distention (JVD), and rales.

CAUSE

The exact cause in many cases of hereditary and primary acquired sideroblastic anemias remains unknown. However, in some cases, the underlying molecular defect may involve genes encoding the following:

- 5-Aminolevulinate synthase enzyme (ALAS2)
- Mitochondrial iron transporter (ABC7)
- Ferrochelatase
- Cytochrome oxidase
- Mitochondrial proteins (e.g., Pearson marrow-pancrease syndrome)

Primary hereditary sideroblastic anemia may be inherited as a sex-linked recessive disease. Secondary acquired sideroblastic anemia can be caused by alcohol, isoniazid, pyrazinamide, cycloserine, chloramphenicol, and copper deficiency.

DIFFERENTIAL DIAGNOSIS

- Sideroblastic anemia must be differentiated from other causes of microcytic hypochromic anemia: iron deficiency anemia, thalassemia, anemia of chronic disease, lead poisoning, and blood loss.
- Tissue iron overload from sideroblastic anemia may act in a manner similar to hereditary hemochromatosis with liver cirrhosis, diabetes, congestive heart failure, and cardiac arrhythmias.

LABORATORY TESTS

- Sideroblastic anemias are characterized by hypochromic anemia (low Hgb, low Hct, low MCV, high RDW).
- Sideroblastic anemias are characterized by high serum iron levels, low transferrin, and increased transferrin saturation and serum ferritin.
- Free erythrocyte protoporphyrin (FEP) is generally low in hereditary sideroblastic anemia and characteristically increased in acquired sideroblastic anemia.
- Serum copper and zinc levels may assist in the diagnosis of sideroblastic anemias.
- Peripheral smear: dimorphic large and small cells reveal Pappenheimer bodies or siderocytes when stained for iron (Fig. 312–6A).
- Bone marrow shows the classic ringed sideroblasts not seen in normal bone marrow tissue (see Fig. 312–6B,C). The ringed sideroblasts represent iron storage in the mitochondria of normoblasts.

TREATMENT

- Treatment directed at controlling symptoms of anemia and preventing organ damage from iron overload
- Avoid alcohol.
- Hereditary sideroblastic anemia
  1. Almost 35% of patients receiving vitamin B_6 (50 to 200 mg/day) will improve their red blood cell to near-normal values.
  2. The remainder of patients will require blood transfusions to treat symptoms of anemia.
- Primary acquired sideroblastic anemia
  1. Most patients do not respond to vitamin B_6.
  2. Erythropoietin and granulocyte colony-stimulating factor (G-CSF) have shown some success in treating the anemia.
  3. Blood transfusions are indicated for patients with symptomatic anemia.
- Secondary sideroblastic anemia caused by isoniazid, pyrazinamide, and cycloserine can expect a full recovery by withdrawing the medication and by the use of vitamin B_6 (50 to 200 mg/day).
- Hereditary sideroblastic anemia
  1. Organ dysfunction resulting from iron overload will require periodic phlebotomies.
  2. In advanced cases, deferoxamine, is given to maintain serum ferritin levels <500 µg/L.
- Primary acquired sideroblastic anemia: As in the hereditary form, periodic phlebotomies are indicated when serum ferritin levels increase to >500 µg/L and deferoxamine is used in patients refractory to therapeutic phlebotomy and those requiring frequent blood transfusions.

C. APLASTIC ANEMIA

DEFINITION

Aplastic anemia is a bone marrow failure resulting from a variety of causes and characterized by stem cell destruction or suppression leading to pancytopenia.

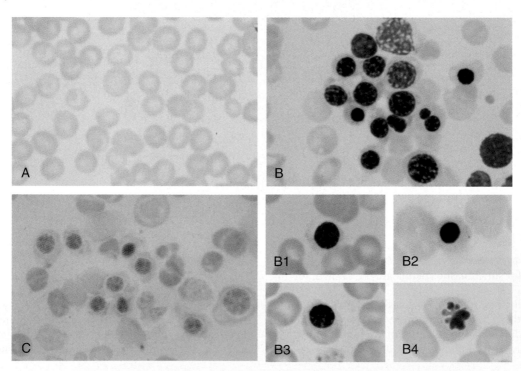

Fig 312–6
Peripheral blood and bone marrow smears from a patient with X-linked sideroblastic anemia. **A,** Peripheral blood smear showing anisopoikilocytosis with hypochromic microcytes and some target cells (May-Grünwald-Giemsa [MGG] stain, ×1250). **B,** Bone marrow smear showing erythroid hyperplasia with predominance of small late erythroblasts. Erythroblasts are small; cytoplasm is often incompletely hemoglobinized with occasional Pappenheimer bodies (MGG, ×1250). **B1-B4,** Bone marrow smear showing erythroid hyperplasia with predominance of small late erythroblasts. Small late dystrophic erythroblasts showing vacuolation, defective hemoglobinization, ill-defined edges, heavily granulated cytoplasm, and nuclear lobulation (MGG, ×1250.) **C,** Bone marrow smear. Most late erythroid cells are ring sideroblasts with numerous (>10) positive granules disposed in a ring surrounding a third or more of the circumference of the nucleus (Perls' reaction, ×1250).
(From Young NS, Gerson SL, High KA [eds]: Clinical Hematology. St. Louis, Mosby, 2006.)

PHYSICAL FINDINGS AND CLINICAL PRESENTATION

- Skin pallor, ecchymosis, petechiae, retinal hemorrhage
- Possible fever, mouth and tongue ulceration, pharyngitis
- Possible short stature or skeletal and nail anomalies in the congenital form
- Possible audible systolic ejection murmur with profound anemia

CAUSE

- In most patients with acquired aplastic anemia, bone marrow failure results from immunologically mediated, active destruction of blood-forming cells by lymphocytes.
- Mutations in *TERT*, the gene for the RNA component of telomerase, cause short telomerases in congenital aplastic anemia and in some cases of apparently acquired hematopoietic failure.

  Common causative factors in aplastic anemia:
  - Toxins (e.g., benzene, insecticides)
  - Drugs (e.g., felbamate, cimetidine, busulfan, and other myelosuppressive drugs, gold salts, chloramphenicol, sulfonamides, trimethadione, quinacrine, phenylbutazone)
  - Ionizing irradiation
  - Infections (e.g., hepatitis C, HIV, EB virus, parvovirus B_{19})
  - Idiopathic
  - Inherited (Fanconi's anemia)
  - Other: immunologic, pregnancy

DIFFERENTIAL DIAGNOSIS

- Bone marrow infiltration from lymphoma, carcinoma, myelofibrosis
- Severe infection
- Hypoplastic acute lymphoblastic leukemia in children
- Hypoplastic myelodysplastic syndrome or hypoplastic acute myeloid leukemia in adults
- Hypersplenism
- Hairy cell leukemia (see Fig. 317–2)

LABORATORY TESTS

- Complete blood cell (CBC) count reveals pancytopenia. Macrocytosis and toxic granulation of neutrophils may also be present. Isolated cytopenias may occur in the early stages.
- Reticulocyte count reveals reticulocytopenia.
- Additional initial laboratory evaluation should include the Ham test to exclude paroxysmal nocturnal hemoglobinuria (PNH) and testing for hepatitis C.
- Diagnostic workup consists primarily of bone marrow aspiration and biopsy and laboratory evaluation (CBC and examination of blood film).
- Bone marrow examination generally reveals paucity or absence of erythropoietic and myelopoietic precursor cells (Fig. 312–7); patients with pure red cell aplasia demonstrate only absence of RBC precursors in the marrow.

IMAGING STUDIES

- Chest x-ray
- Abdominal sonography or CT to evaluate for splenomegaly
- Radiography of hand and forearm in patients with constitutional anemia
- CT of thymus region if thymoma-associated RBC aplasia is suspected

TREATMENT

- Discontinuation of any offending drugs or agents
- Aggressive treatment of neutropenic fevers with parenteral broad-spectrum antibiotics.
- Platelet and RBC transfusions PRN; however, avoid transfusions in patients who are candidates for bone marrow transplantation.
- Immunosuppressive therapy with antithymocyte globulin (ATG) and/or cyclosporine (CSP); ATG in combination with prednisone
- Transplantation of allogeneic marrow or peripheral blood stem cell transplantation from a histocompatible sibling usually cures the underlying bone marrow failure.
- The humanized monoclonal antibody to the interleukin-2 receptor daclizumab has been reported effective in moderate aplastic anemia, producing durable responses in more than 50% of patients.

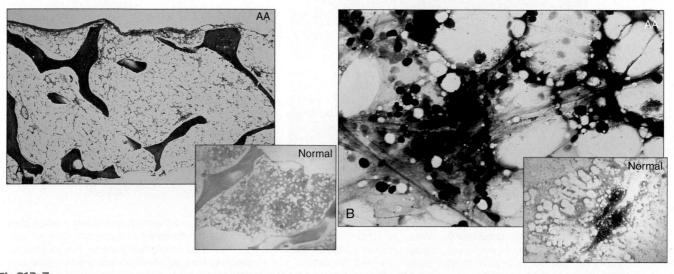

Fig 312–7

Bone marrow morphology in severe aplastic anemia. **A,** Biopsy specimen showing replacement of normal hematopoietic cells with fat. **B,** Aspirate smear, with an overall paucity of cells; myeloid and erythroid precursors and megakaryocytes are absent, and only lymphocytes, plasma cells, and stromal elements are seen.

(From Young NS, Gerson SL, High KA [eds]: Clinical Hematology. St. Louis, Mosby, 2006.)

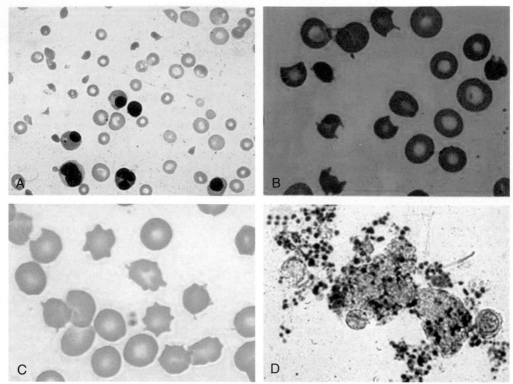

Fig 312–8

Photomicrographs from patients with acquired hemolytic anemias. **A,** Red cell fragmentation and nucleated red blood cells indicating microangio-pathic hemolytic anemia caused by thrombotic thrombocytopenic purpura (×400). **B,** Bite cells caused by severe drug-induced oxidant hemolysis (×1000). **C,** Spur cells from a patient with advanced cirrhosis (×1000). **D,** Urinary hemosiderin stained with Prussian blue (×400) resulting from in-travascular hemolysis in a patient with paroxysmal nocturnal hemoglobinuria.
(From Young NS, Gerson SL, High KA [eds]: Clinical Hematology. St. Louis, Mosby, 2006.)

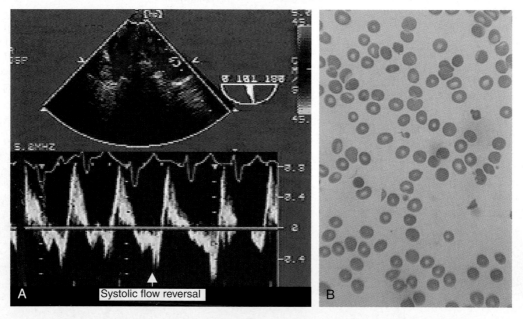

Fig 312–9

Paravalvular leak with hemolytic anemia and heart failure. A 58-year-old woman with a mechanical mitral prosthesis presented with marked ankle edema and shortness of breath worsening over 6 months. The mitral prosthesis had been inserted 9 months earlier for rheumatic mitral valve dis-ease. The patient was in biventricular heart failure, with a murmur of mitral insufficiency and findings of pulmonary hypertension. Transesophageal echocardiography demonstrated a large jet of mitral regurgitation and flow reversal on the pulmonary veins **A,** consistent with a severe paravalvu-lar regurgitation. The hemoglobin concentration was 6.8 g/dL. **B,** Schistocytes were seen on the blood smear, and hemosiderin was recovered in the urinary sediment. The patient underwent successful surgical closure of the paravalvular leak. The markers of hemolysis subsided postopera-tively and the hemoglobin increased to and stayed within the normal range.
(From Crawford MH, DiMarco JP, Paulus WJ [eds]: Cardiology, 2nd ed. St. Louis, Mosby, 2004.)

D. AUTOIMMUNE HEMOLYTIC ANEMIA

DEFINITION

Autoimmune hemolytic anemia (AIHA) is anemia secondary to premature destruction of red blood cells caused by the binding of autoantibodies and/or complement to red blood cells.

PHYSICAL FINDINGS AND CLINICAL PRESENTATION

- Pallor, jaundice
- Tachycardia with a flow murmur may be present if anemia is pronounced.
- Most common presentation is dyspnea, fatigue
- Patients with intravascular hemolysis may present with dark urine and back pain.
- The presence of hepatomegaly and/or lymphadenopathy suggests an underlying lymphoproliferative disorder or malignancy; splenomegaly may indicate hypersplenism as a cause of hemolysis.

CAUSE

- Warm antibody–mediated: IgG (often idiopathic or associated with leukemia, lymphoma, thymoma, myeloma, viral infections, and collagen-vascular disease)
- Cold antibody–mediated: IgM and complement in most cases (often idiopathic, at times associated with infections, lymphoma, or cold agglutinin disease)
- Drug- induced—three major mechanisms
  1. Antibody directed against Rh complex (e.g., methyldopa)
  2. Antibody directed against RBC-drug complex (hapten-induced; e.g., penicillin)
  3. Antibody directed against complex formed by drug and plasma proteins; the drug-plasma protein-antibody complex causes destruction of RBCs (innocent bystander; e.g., quinidine).

DIFFERENTIAL DIAGNOSIS

- Hemolytic anemia caused by membrane defects (paroxysmal nocturnal hemoglobinuria [see Fig. 312–8D], spur cell anemia, Wilson's disease)
- Non–immune-mediated (microangiopathic hemolytic anemia (Fig. 312–8A), hypersplenism (see Fig. 312–8C), cardiac valve prosthesis (Fig. 312–9), giant cavernous hemangiomas, march hemoglobinuria, physical agents, infections, heavy metals, certain drugs [nitrofurantoin, sulfonamides; see Fig. 312–8 B])

LABORATORY TESTS

- Initial laboratory tests: CBC (anemia), reticulocyte count (elevated), liver function studies (elevated indirect bilirubin, LDH), evaluation of peripheral smear; Coombs' test— positive direct Coombs' test (Fig. 312–10) indicates presence of antibodies or complement on the surface of RBC, positive indirect Coombs' test (Fig. 312–11) implies presence of anti-RBC antibodies freely circulating in the patient's serum; haptoglobin level (decreased)

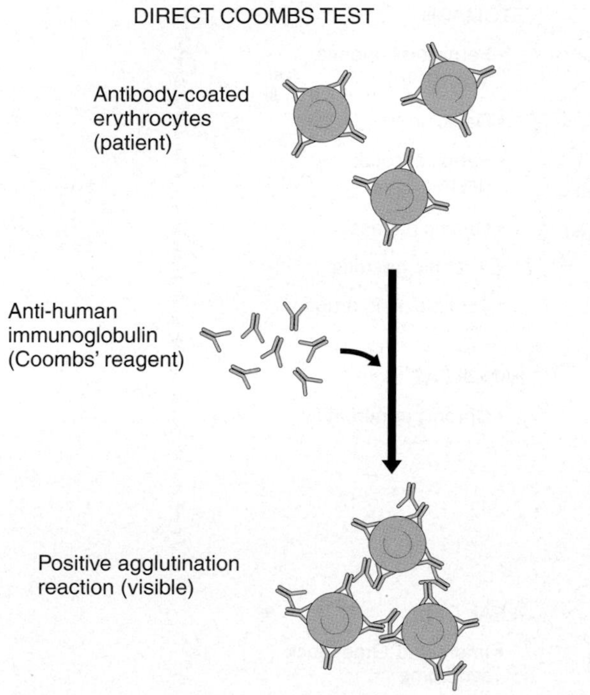

DIRECT COOMBS TEST

Antibody-coated
erythrocytes
(patient)

Anti-human
immunoglobulin
(Coombs' reagent)

Positive agglutination
reaction (visible)

Fig 312–10
Positive direct Coombs' test (direct antiglobulin test). Anti–human immunoglobulin (reagent) is added to the patient's red blood cells, which have been coated with antibody (in vivo). The reagent anti–human immunoglobulin attaches to the antibodies coating the patient's red blood cells, causing visible agglutination.
(From Young NS, Gerson SL, High KA [eds]: Clinical Hematology. St. Louis, Mosby, 2006.)

INDIRECT COOMBS' TEST

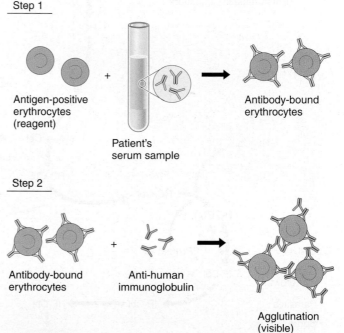

Step 1

Antigen-positive
erythrocytes
(reagent)

+

Patient's
serum sample

Antibody-bound
erythrocytes

Step 2

Antibody-bound
erythrocytes

+

Anti-human
immunoglobulin

Agglutination
(visible)

Fig 312–11
Positive indirect Coombs' test (indirect antiglobulin test). In step 1, reagent red blood cells coated with antigen are added to the patient's serum, which contains antibody. In the presence of antigen-antibody specificity, the antibody from the patient's serum coats the reagent red blood cells (in vitro); this does not result in visible agglutination. In step 2, reagent anti–human immunoglobulin is added to the antibody-bound reagent red blood cells. The reagent anti–human immunoglobulin attaches to the antibodies that are coating the reagent red blood cells, causing visible agglutination.
(From Young NS, Gerson SL, High KA [eds]: Clinical Hematology. St. Louis, Mosby, 2006.)

- IgG antibody and IgM antibody
- Hepatitis serology, antinuclear antibody (ANA)
- Urine tests may reveal hemosiderinuria or hemoglobinuria.

IMAGING STUDIES
- Chest x-ray
- CT of chest and abdomen to rule out lymphoma should also be considered.

TREATMENT
- Discontinuation of any potentially offensive drugs
- Prednisone in warm antibody autoimmune hemolytic anemia. Corticosteroids are generally ineffective in cold antibody autoimmune hemolytic anemia.
- Splenectomy in patients responding inadequately to corticosteroids when RBC sequestration studies indicate splenic sequestration
- Immunosuppressive drugs and/or immunoglobulins only after both corticosteroids and splenectomy (unless surgery

is contraindicated) have failed to produce an adequate remission
- Danazol, usually used in conjunction with corticosteroids (may be useful in warm antibody autoimmune hemolytic anemia)
- Immunosuppressive drugs (azathioprine, cyclophosphamide) may be useful in warm antibody autoimmune hemolytic anemia but are indicated only after both corticosteroids and splenectomy (unless surgery is contraindicated) have failed to produce an adequate remission.

E. PERNICIOUS ANEMIA

DEFINITION
Pernicious anemia is an autoimmune disease resulting from antibodies against intrinsic factor and gastric parietal cells (Fig. 312–12).

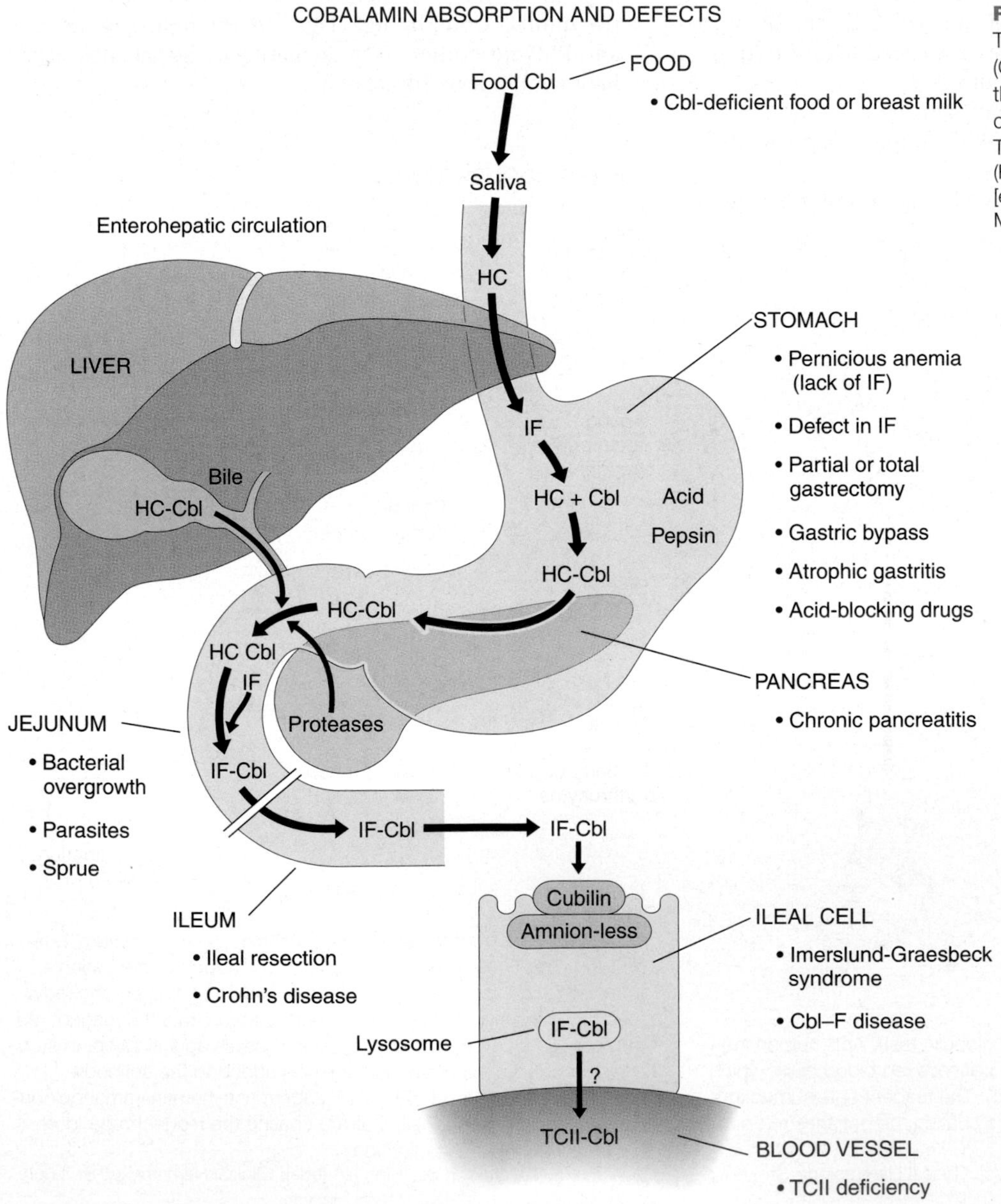

COBALAMIN ABSORPTION AND DEFECTS

Fig 312–12
The normal processes of cobalamin (Cbl) absorption are shown, along with the typical defects causing cobalamin deficiency. IF, intrinsic factor; TCII, transcobalamin II.
(From Young NS, Gerson SL, High KA [eds]: Clinical Hematology. St. Louis, Mosby, 2006.)

PHYSICAL FINDINGS AND CLINICAL PRESENTATION

- Mucosal pallor, glossitis
- Peripheral sensory neuropathy with paresthesias initially and absent reflexes in advanced cases (Fig. 312–13)
- Loss of joint position sense, pyramidal or long track signs
- Possible splenomegaly and mild hepatomegaly
- Generalized weakness and delirium/dementia

CAUSE

- Antigastric parietal cell antibodies in more than 70% of patients, anti-intrinsic factor antibodies in more than 50% of patients
- Atrophic gastric mucosa

DIFFERENTIAL DIAGNOSIS

- Nutritional vitamin B_{12} deficiency
- Malabsorption
- Chronic alcoholism (multifactorial)
- Chronic gastritis related to *Helicobacter pylori* infection
- Folic acid deficiency
- Myelodysplasia

LABORATORY TESTS

- CBC generally reveals macrocytic anemia and leukopenia with hypersegmented neutrophils (Fig. 312–14).
- MCV is generally significantly elevated in the advanced stages.
- Reticulocyte count is low-normal.
- Falsely low serum cobalamin levels can occur in patients with severe folate deficiency, in patients using high doses of ascorbic acid, and when cobalamin levels are measured following nuclear medicine studies (radioactivity interferes with cobalamin radioimmunoassay [RIA] measurement).
- Falsely high-normal levels in patients with cobalamin deficiency can occur in severe liver disease or chronic granulocytic leukemia.
- The absence of anemia or macrocytosis does not exclude the diagnosis of cobalamin deficiency. Anemia is absent in 20% of patients with cobalamin deficiency and macrocytosis is absent in more than 30% of patients at diagnosis. It can be blocked by concurrent iron deficiency or anemia of chronic disease and may be masked by thalassemia trait.
- Schilling test is abnormal in part I; part II corrects to normal after administration of intrinsic factor.
- Laboratory tests used for detecting cobalamin deficiency in patients with normal vitamin B_{12} levels include serum and urinary methylmalonic acid level (elevated), total homocysteine level (elevated), and intrinsic factor antibody (positive).

TREATMENT

- Traditional therapy of a cobalamin deficiency consists of IM injections of vitamin B_{12}, 1000 μg/wk, for the initial 4 to 6 weeks, followed by 1000 μg/month IM indefinitely.
- Oral cobalamin (1000 to 2000 mcg/day) can also be effective in mild cases of pernicious anemia, because about 1% of an oral dose is absorbed by passive diffusion, a pathway that does not require intrinsic factor.

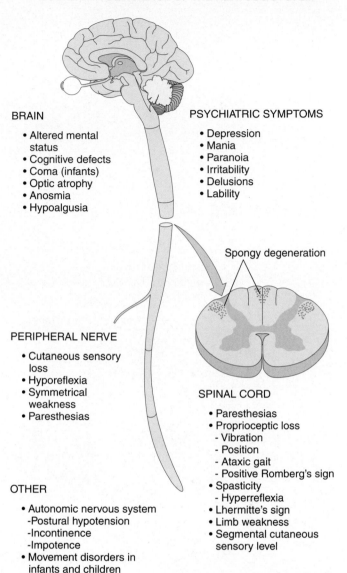

COBALAMIN DEFICIENCY OF THE NERVOUS SYSTEM

BRAIN
- Altered mental status
- Cognitive defects
- Coma (infants)
- Optic atrophy
- Anosmia
- Hypoalgusia

PSYCHIATRIC SYMPTOMS
- Depression
- Mania
- Paranoia
- Irritability
- Delusions
- Lability

Spongy degeneration

PERIPHERAL NERVE
- Cutaneous sensory loss
- Hyporeflexia
- Symmetrical weakness
- Paresthesias

SPINAL CORD
- Paresthesias
- Proprioceptic loss
  - Vibration
  - Position
  - Ataxic gait
  - Positive Romberg's sign
- Spasticity
  - Hyperreflexia
- Lhermitte's sign
- Limb weakness
- Segmental cutaneous sensory level

OTHER
- Autonomic nervous system
  - Postural hypotension
  - Incontinence
  - Impotence
- Movement disorders in infants and children

Fig 312–13
Characteristic symptoms and signs seen in cobalamin deficiency of the nervous system are shown, along with a schematic demonstration of the spongy degeneration seen in the dorsal and sometimes lateral columns of the spinal cord.
(From Young NS, Gerson SL, High KA [eds]: Clinical Hematology. St. Louis, Mosby, 2006.)

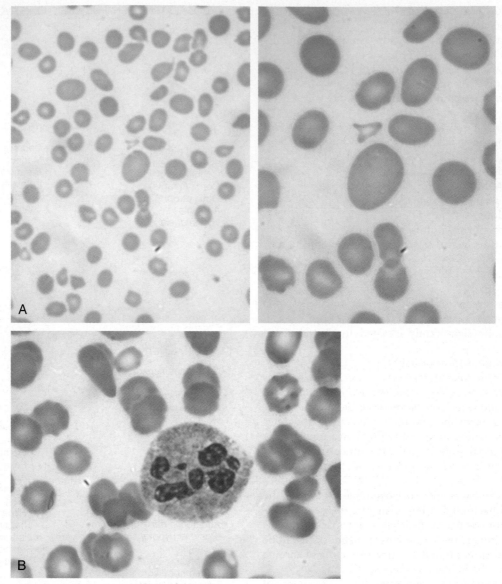

Fig 312–14
Characteristic hematologic abnormalities seen in megaloblastic anemia. **A,** Macro-ovalocytes and marked anisocytosis are seen under low and high power. **B,** A hypersegmented neutrophil with at least six lobes.
(From Young NS, Gerson SL, High KA [eds]: Clinical Hematology. St. Louis, Mosby, 2006.)

F. THALLASEMIA

DEFINITION
Thalassemias are a heterogeneous group of disorders of hemoglobin synthesis that have in common a deficient synthesis of one or more of the polypeptide chains of the normal human hemoglobin, resulting in a quantitative abnormality of the hemoglobin produced. There are no qualitative changes such as those encountered in the hemoglobinopathies (e.g., sickle cell disease).

CLASSIFICATION
β-Thalassemia
- β (+)-Thalassemia (suboptimal β-globin synthesis)
- β (0)-Thalassemia (total absence of β-globin synthesis)
- δ-β–Thalassemia (total absence of both δ-globin and β-globin synthesis)

- Lepore hemoglobin (synthesis of small amounts of fused δ-β–globin and total absence of δ- and β-globin)
- Hereditary persistence of fetal hemoglobin (HPHF) (increased hemoglobin F synthesis and reduced or absence of δ- and β-globin)

α-Thalassemia
- Silent carrier (three α-globin genes present)
- α-Thalassemia trait (two α-globin genes present)
- Hemoglobin H disease (one α-globin gene present)
- Hydrops fetalis (no α-globin gene)
- Hemoglobin constant sprint (elongated α-globin chain)

THALASSEMIC HEMOGLOBINOPATHIES
- Hb Terre Haute
- Hb Quong Sze
- HbE
- Hb Knossos

PHYSICAL FINDINGS AND CLINICAL PRESENTATION

β-Thalassemia

- Heterozygous β-thalassemia (thalassemia minor): no or mild anemia, microcytosis and hypochromia, mild hemolysis manifested by slight reticulocytosis and splenomegaly
- Homozygous β-thalassemia (thalassemia major): intense hemolytic anemia; transfusion dependency; bone deformities (skull [Fig. 312–15] and long bones); hepatomegaly; splenomegaly; iron overload leading to cardiomyopathy, diabetes mellitus, and hypogonadism; growth retardation; pigment gallstones; susceptibility to infection
- Thalassemia intermedia caused by combination of β- and alpha-thalassemia or β- thalassemia and Hb Lepore: resembles thalassemia major but is milder

α-Thalassemia

- Silent carrier: no symptoms.
- α-Thalassemia trait: microcytosis only.
- Hemoglobin H disease: moderately severe hemolysis with microcytosis and splenomegaly.
- The loss of all four α-globin genes is incompatible with life (stillbirth of hydropic fetus).

Note: Pregnancies with hydrops fetalis are associated with a high incidence of toxemia.

CAUSE

- β-Thalassemia: is caused by more than 200 point mutations and rarely, by deletions. The reduction of β-globin synthesis results in redundant α-globin chains (Heinz bodies), which are cytotoxic and cause intramedullary hemolysis and ineffective erythropoiesis. Fetal hemoglobin may be increased.
- α-Thalassemia: several mutations can result in insufficient amounts of α-globin available for combination with non–α-globins.

LABORATORY TESTS

- Hemoblobin electrophoresis.
- See Figure 312–16 (for description of peripheral blood smear abnormalities in thalassemia).

β-Thalassemia

- Microcytosis (MCV, 55 to 80 fL)
- Normal RDW (RBC distribution width)
- Smear: nucleated RBCs, anisocytosis, poikilocytosis, polychromatophilia, Pappenheimer and Howell-Jolly bodies (see Fig. 312–4)
- Hemoglobin electrophoresis: absent or reduced hemoglobin A, increased fetal hemoglobin, variable increase in the amount of hemoglobin A_2
- Markers of hemolysis: elevated indirect bilirubin and LDH, decreased haptoglobin

α-Thalassemia

- Microcytosis in the absence of iron deficiency
- Hemoglobin electrophoresis is normal, except for the presence of hemoglobin H in hemoglobin H disease.

TREATMENT

- Thalassemia minor: no treatment but avoid iron administration for incorrect diagnosis of iron deficiency
- β-Thalassemia major (and hemoglobin H disease)
  1. Transfusion as required, together with chelation of iron with desferrioxamine
  2. Splenectomy for hypersplenism if present.
  3. Bone marrow transplantation. Although hematopoietic stem cell transplantation is the only curative approach for

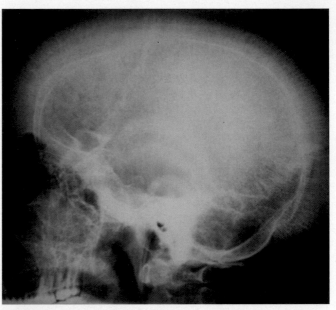

Fig 312–15

Thalassemia. Skull x-ray shows expansion of the diploic marrow and loss of the definition of the outer table. The occipital bone is spared but the frontal sinuses have failed to develop and the maxillary antra contain marrow tissue. A gross hair on end appearance is seen. (From Grainger RG, Allison DJ, Adam A, Dixon AK [eds]: Grainger & Allison's Diagnostic Radiology, 4th ed. London, Harcourt, 2001.)

thalassemia, it has been limited by the high cost and scarcity of HLA-matched donors. Before transplantation, it is necessary to administer myeloablative regimens to eradicate the endogenous thalassemic bone marrow. Commonly used agents are hydroxyurea, azathioprine, fludarabine, busulfan, and cyclophosphamide.

4. Hydroxyurea may increase the level of hemoglobin F.

G. SICKLE CELL ANEMIA

DEFINITION

Sickle cell disease is a hemoglobinopathy characterized by the production of hemoglobin S caused by the substitution of the amino acid valine for glutamic acid in the sixth position of the γ-globin chain. When exposed to lower oxygen tension, RBCs assume a sickle shape, resulting in stasis of RBCs in capillaries. Painful crises are caused by ischemic tissue injury resulting from obstruction of blood flow produced by sickled erythrocytes (Fig. 312–17).

PHYSICAL FINDINGS AND CLINICAL PRESENTATION

See Figure 312–18.

- Physical examination is variable, depending on the degree of anemia and presence of acute vaso-occlusive syndromes or neurologic, cardiovascular, GU, and musculoskeletal complications.
- There is no clinical laboratory finding that is pathognomonic of the painful crisis of sickle cell disease. The diagnosis of a painful episode is made solely on the basis of the medical therapy and physical examination.
- Bones are the most common site of pain. Dactylitis, or hand-foot syndrome (acute, painful swelling of the hands and feet), is the first manifestation of sickle cell disease in

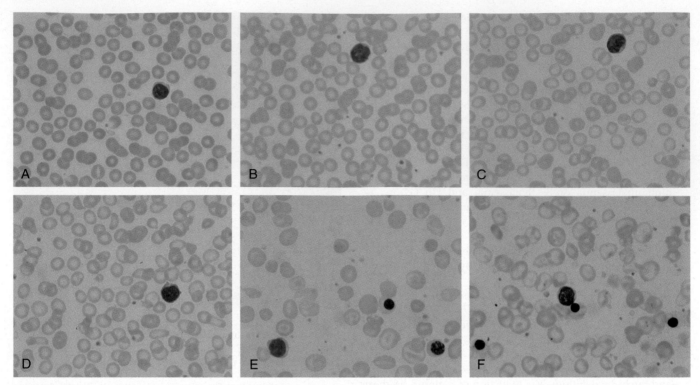

Fig 312–16

Peripheral blood in thalassemia. The blood smears of patients with thalassemia syndromes can demonstrate varying degrees of microcytosis, hypochromia, and basophilic stippling, as well as target cells and elliptocytes, but there is wide variation in red blood cell abnormalities, ranging from normal **A,** to α-thalassemia single-gene deletion **B,** and two-gene deletion **(C),** hemoglobin H disease **(D),** β-thalassemia intermedia **(E),** and β-thalassemia major prior to initiation of transfusion therapy **(F).**
(From Young NS, Gerson SL, High KA [eds]: Clinical Hematology. St. Louis, Mosby, 2006.)

many infants. Irritability and refusal to walk are other common symptoms. After infancy, musculoskeletal pain can be symmetrical, asymmetrical, or migratory, and possibly associated with swelling, low-grade fever, redness, or warmth.
- In children and adults, sickle vaso-occlusive episodes are difficult to distinguish from osteomyelitis, septic arthritis, synovitis, rheumatic fever, or gout.
- When abdominal or visceral pain is present, care should be taken to exclude sequestration syndromes (spleen, liver) or the possibility of an acute condition, such as appendicitis, pancreatitis, cholecystitis, urinary tract infection, pelvic inflammatory disease (PID), or malignancy.
- Pneumonia develops during the course of 20% of painful events and can present as chest and abdominal pain. In adults, chest pain may be a result of vaso-occlusion in the ribs and often precedes a pulmonary event. The lower back is also a frequent site of painful crisis in adults.
- The acute chest syndrome manifests with chest pain, fever, wheezing, tachypnea, and cough. Chest x-ray reveals pulmonary infiltrates. Common causes include infection (mycoplasma, chlamydia, viruses), infarction, and fat embolism.
- Musculoskeletal and skin abnormalities seen in sickle cell anemia include leg ulcers (particularly on the malleoli) and limb-girdle deformities caused by avascular necrosis of the femoral and humeral heads.
- Endocrine abnormalities include delayed sexual maturation and late physical maturation, especially evident in boys.

- Neurologic abnormalities on examination may include seizures and altered mental status.
- Infections, particularly involving *Salmonella*, *Mycoplasma*, and *Streptococcus*, are relatively common.
- Severe splenomegaly secondary to sequestration often occurs in children before splenic atrophy.

DIFFERENTIAL DIAGNOSIS
- Thalassemia (see Fig. 312–16)
- Iron deficiency anemia (see Fig. 312–2)

LABORATORY TESTS
- Anemia (resulting from chronic hemolysis), reticulocytosis, leukocytosis, and thrombocytosis are common. The peripheral smear reveals typical sickle forms and target cells (Fig. 312–19)
- Elevations of bilirubin and LDH are also common.
- Peripheral blood smear may reveal sickle cells, target cells, poikilocytosis, and hypochromia.
- Elevated blood urea nitrogen (BUN) and creatinine may be present in patients with progressive renal insufficiency.
- Urinalysis may reveal hematuria and proteinuria.

IMAGING STUDIES
- Chest x-ray is useful in patients presenting with chest syndrome. Cardiomegaly may be present on chest x-ray examination.
- Bone scanning is useful to rule out osteomyelitis (usually secondary to salmonella). MRI is also effective in diagnosing osteomyelitis.

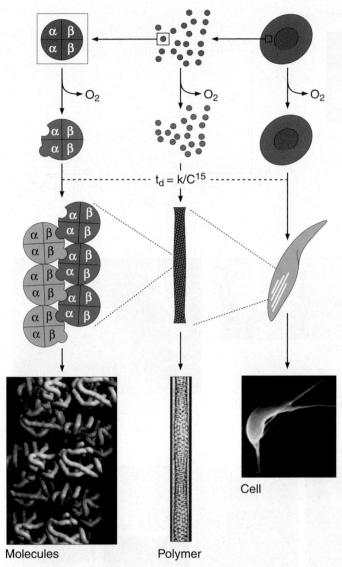

Fig 312-17
Pathophysiology of sickle cell disease. The abnormal sickle hemoglobin polymerizes when deoxygenated, deforming the erythrocyte (red blood cell) and damaging the cell cytoskeleton. The rigid cells can obstruct or slow blood flow.
(From Young NS, Gerson SL, High KA [eds]: Clinical Hematology. St. Louis, Mosby, 2006.)

Molecules   Polymer   Cell

$$t_d = k/C^{15}$$

- CT or MRI of the brain is often needed in patients presenting with neurologic complications such as transient ischemic attack (TIA), cerebrovascular accident (CVA), seizures, or altered mental status.
- Transcranial Doppler is a useful commodity to identify children with sickle cell anemia who are at risk for stroke.
- Doppler echocardiography can be used to diagnose pulmonary hypertension

TREATMENT

- Aggressively diagnose and treat suspected infections (*Salmonella* osteomyelitis and pneumococcal infections occur more often in patients with sickle cell anemia because of splenic infarcts and atrophy). Antibiotics plus incentive spirometry and bronchodilators, are useful in patients with acute chest syndrome.
- Provide pain relief during the vaso-occlusive crisis. Medications should be administered on a fixed time schedule with a dosing interval that does not extend beyond the duration of the desired pharmacologic effect.
- Aggressively diagnose and treat any potential complications (e.g., septic necrosis of the femoral head, priapism, bony infarcts, and acute chest syndrome).
- Avoid routine transfusions but consider early transfusions for patients at high risk for complications. Indications for transfusion include aplastic crises, severe hemolytic crises (particularly during third trimester of pregnancy), acute chest syndrome, and high risk of stroke.
- Hydroxyurea increases hemoglobin F levels and reduces the incidence of vaso-occlusive complications. It is generally well tolerated. Side effects consist primarily of mild reversible neutropenia.
- Replace folic acid.
- Genetic counseling is recommended in all cases.
- Allogeneic stem cell transplantation can be curative in young patients with symptomatic sickle cell disease. However, the death rate from the procedure is almost 10%, the marrow recipients are likely to be infertile, and there is an undefined risk of chemotherapy-induced malignancy.
- Penicillin V, 125 mg PO twice daily, should be administered by age 2 months and increased to 250 mg twice daily by age 3 years. Penicillin prophylaxis can be discontinued after age 5 years, except in children who have had splenectomy.
- Regular immunizations and pneumococcal vaccination are recommended.
- Poloxamer 188, a nonionic surfactant with hemorrheologic and antithrombotic properties, has been reported to produce a significant but relatively small decrease in the duration of painful episodes and an increase in the proportion of patients who achieve resolution of symptoms. A more significant effect was observed in patients who received concomitant hydroxyurea.
- Pulmonary hypertension is a complication of chronic hemolysis and is associated with a high risk of death. It can be detected by Doppler echocardiography in over 30% of adult patients with sickle cell disease. Cardiac catheterization will confirm the diagnosis. It is resistant to hydroxyurea therapy.

SICKLE CELL DISEASE DAMAGES: NONHEMATOLOGIC ORGAN SYSTEMS

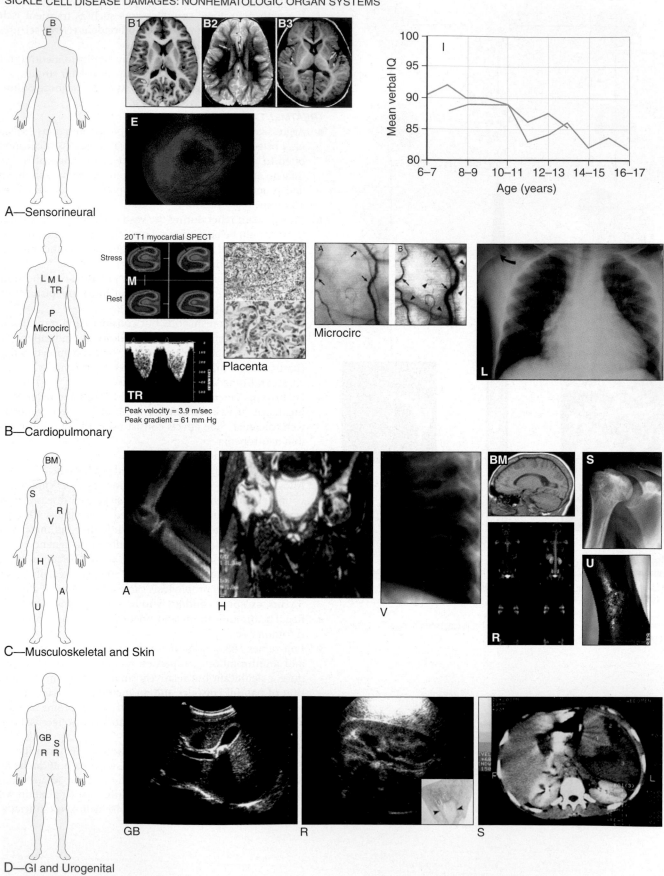

A—Sensorineural

B—Cardiopulmonary

C—Musculoskeletal and Skin

D—GI and Urogenital

Fig 312-18
Legend on opposite page

Fig 312–18

Chronic nonhematologic complications of sickle cell disease. Classic findings on imaging are shown. Several insidious problems can be subclinical until quite severe, but they can be detected by screening tests such as transcranial Doppler ultrasound and echocardiography for tricuspid regurgitant jet. **A,** Sensorineural complications. **B,** Brain complications: **B1,** deep white matter infarct in brain; **B2,** encephalomalacia, extensive in the occipital areas; and **B3,** lacunar infarct. Focal ischemic damage may result from stenotic cerebral arteries and/or microcirculatory abnormalities. Tortuous arteries and collateral vessels may be demonstrated on magnetic resonance angiogram (not shown). **E,** Retinopathy with infarcts and neovascularization can be caused by collateral development around areas of obstruction. Retinopathy can be subclinical until the fragile neovascular tissue bleeds to cause hyphema, or retinal detachment. Annual ophthalmology screening can detect early retinopathy. **I,** Neurocognitive function may decline as shown in the trend of WISC and WISC-R scores of children serially tested during the Cooperative Study of Sickle Cell Disease. This decline is partially attributable to silent infarcts that affect frontal lobes or memory, but also attributable to chronic anemia. However, not every individual with sickle cell disease will have decline in cognitive function. **B,** Cardiopulmonary complications. **L,** Chronic lung disease and cardiac hypertrophy. The chest radiograph shows chronic lung disease as a fine reticular pattern throughout both lungs and cardiomegaly as compensation for increased cardiac output resulting from chronic anemia. Pulmonary function testing often reveals a subclinical mixed obstructive and restrictive respiratory dysfunction. **M,** Myocardial strain. Dilated cardiomegaly is a typical compensation for chronic anemia. Recent studies have indicated a significant incidence of myocardial ischemia, especially with exertion. This single-photon emission CT scan shows abnormal strain on the myocardial wall with stress. **TR,** Tricuspid valve regurgitant jet. Doppler echocardiography detects this indirect measure of pulmonary hypertension. Pulmonary hypertension, indicated by tricuspid regurgitant jet velocity greater than 2.5 m/sec, is associated with high mortality, even though cardiologists may consider this mild pulmonary hypertension in people without chronic anemia. Mitral regurgitation can be caused by distortion of the valve ring. **Microcirc,** Microvascular abnormalities. Abnormally diminished perfusion of the microcirculation, especially during crisis (A) is compared with increased flow at recovery from crisis (B). Abnormal tortuosity of the microvessels are also noted. **Placenta,** Placental abnormalities in a mother with sickle cell disease. Histopathology shows sickled maternal red blood cells in the placental circulation in a primipara with hemoglobin (Hb) SC (sickle cell) at two levels of magnification. In contrast, fetal red blood cells in capillaries are not deformed at the same level of oxygen, in this case because the baby has sickle cell trait. A baby with sickle cell disease would be protected because of high levels of fetal hemoglobin in the newborn period. **C,** Musculoskeletal complications. **BM,** Bone marrow hyperplasia. Increased erythropoietic drive expands the marrow space in many patients with sickle cell disease, here shown as a thickened calvarium. **R,** Rib infarcts. Rib infarcts caused by ischemia can be very painful and associated with acute chest syndrome. Infarcted ribs are highlighted white on the nuclear scan. **V,** Vertebral infarction. Bony collapse of the infarcted vertebral bodies from the normal cylindric shape with rectangular cross-section, into a biconcave shape with a characteristic outline of the letter H on two-dimensional projection (the H sign or fish mouth), seen on radiographs of the thoracolumbar spine. Similar bone infarcts in long bones such as the radius and humerus may appear as sclerotic mottling. **H,** Avascular necrosis of the humeral and femoral heads. Ischemic damage can cause chronic pain, bony collapse, and dislocation of the joint. Avascular necrosis of the femur can be severely disabling. **A,** Arthropathy. The knee displays osteoarthritis with a narrowed joint space, and the long bones have mottled lucencies caused by infarcts. **U,** Leg ulcers. Poor vascular supply of the skin near the malleoli can cause severely painful and disabling ulceration, and healing can take months to years even with appropriate treatment. **D,** Gastrointestinal and genitourinary complications. **GB,** Gallbladder and gallstones. Hemolysis causes increased bilirubin production, and patients with severe hemolysis are chronically jaundiced. Pigmented gallstones form in almost 75% of patients as a result of hemolysis, but can be asymptomatic. **S,** Spleen infarct. Scattered rounded foci of low attenuation in the spleen are noted by CT scan of an adult with Hb SC sickle cell disease. The spleen accumulates infarcts over time and can become a shrunken scar, or a spongy nonfunctional bag that can cause splenic sequestration. Spleen images on the nuclear scan can be speckled with infarcts, or absent because of functional asplenia. **R,** Hyperechoic kidney. This ultrasound finding corresponds to an abnormally heterogeneous texture of the renal cortex as a result of multiple infarcts of the medulla seen in histology (inset with paired *arrowheads* indicating papillary necrosis). Renal ischemic damage to tubules leads to isosthenuria early in childhood. Renal glomerulopathy includes thickened capillaries and proteinuria.
(From Young NS, Gerson SL, High KA [eds]: Clinical Hematology. St. Louis, Mosby, 2006.)

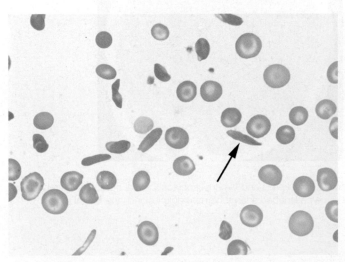

Fig 312–19
Peripheral blood smear of a child with sickle cell anemia (Hb SS). Note the target cells as well as the typical sickle forms (*arrow*).
(From Young NS, Gerson SL, High KA [eds]: Clinical Hematology. St. Louis, Mosby, 2006.)

Chapter 313 Leukemias

A. ACUTE LYMPHOBLASTIC LEUKEMIA

DEFINITION
Acute lymphoblastic leukemia (ALL) is characterized by uncontrolled proliferation of abnormal, immature lymphocytes and their progenitors, ultimately replacing normal bone marrow elements.

PHYSICAL FINDINGS AND CLINICAL PRESENTATION
- Skin pallor, purpura, or easy bruising
- Lymphadenopathy or hepatosplenomegaly
- Fever, bone pain, oliguria, weakness, weight loss, mental status changes due to cerebral leukostasis or stroke (Fig. 313–1)

CAUSE
- Unknown; increased risk in patients with a previous use of antineoplastic agents (e.g., chemotherapy of non-Hodgkin's lymphoma [NHL], Hodgkin's disease, ovarian cancer, myeloma)
- Environmental factors (e.g., ionizing radiation), toxins (e.g., benzene)

DIFFERENTIAL DIAGNOSIS
Acute myeloid leukemia: the distinction between ALL and acute myeloid leukemia and the classification of the various subtypes are based on the following factors:
- Cell morphology
1. Lymphoblasts: a high nucleus-to-cytoplasmic ratio; usually, cytoplasmic granules are not present.
2. Myeloblasts: abundant cytoplasm; often, cytoplasmic granules (Auer rods) are present (see Fig. 313–5).
- Histochemical stains
1. Peroxidase and Sudan black stains: negative in ALL; useful to distinguish nonlymphoid from lymphoid cells

2. Chloroacetate esterase: a pink cytoplasmic reaction identifies granulocytes; useful to distinguish granulocytes from monocytes in patients with acute myeloid leukemia
- Lymphoblastic lymphoma
- Aplastic anemia
- Infectious mononucleosis
- Leukemoid reaction to infection
- Multiple myeloma

LABORATORY TESTS
- CBC reveals normochromic, normocytic anemia, thrombocytopenia.
- Peripheral smear will reveal lymphoblasts.
- Initial blood work should also include BUN, creatinine, serum electrolytes, uric acid, LDH.
- Special diagnostic tests include immunophenotyping, cytogenetics, and cytochemistry.
- The French-American-British (FAB) Cooperative Study Group has classified ALL into three groups (L1 to L3) based on cell size, cytoplasmic appearance, nucleus shape, and chromatin pattern; the most common form is the L2 type.
- Immunologic classification is on the basis of expression of surface antigens by blast cells—T lineage and B lineage.

IMAGING STUDIES
- Chest x-ray, CT to evaluate for the presence of mediastinal mass (Fig. 313–2A) and compression of mediastinal structures (see Fig. 313–2B,C)
- CT or ultrasound of abdomen, pelvis to assess splenomegaly or leukemic infiltration of abdominal organs

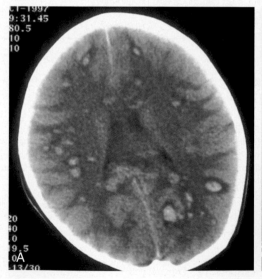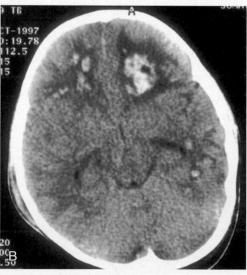

Fig 313–1
A, Axial CT scans of the brain in a child with newly diagnosed acute lymphoblastic leukemia and hyperleukocytosis reveal multiple bilateral hemorrhagic lesions. These lesions typically involve only the white matter. **B,** The same patient had a large hemorrhagic lesion in the frontal region, with associated vasogenic edema.
(From Young NS, Gerson SL, High KA [eds]: Clinical Hematology. St. Louis, Mosby, 2006.)

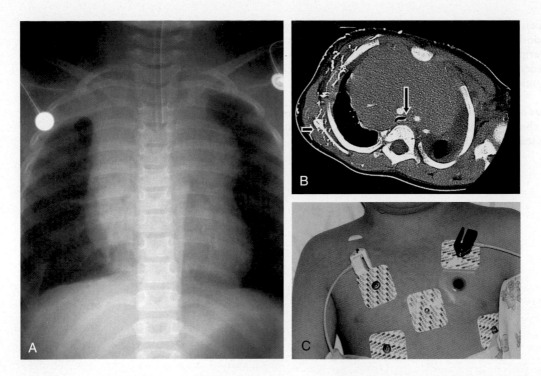

Fig 313-2
A, Chest radiograph of a 10-year-old boy with acute lymphoblastic leukemia shows a large mediastinal mass. **B,** CT scan shows narrowing of the trachea caused by mechanical compression of the mediastinal mass (*long arrow*). **C,** Signs of superior vena cava syndrome include edema of the neck and increased collateral circulation in the chest.
(From Young NS, Gerson SL, High KA [eds]: Clinical Hematology. St. Louis, Mosby, 2006.)

TREATMENT

- Emergency treatment is indicated in patients with intracerebral leukostasis. It consists of one or more of the following:
  1. Cranial irradiation of the whole brain in one- or two-dose fractions
  2. Leukapheresis
  3. Oral hydroxyurea (requires 48 to 72 hours to lower the circulating blast count significantly)
- Urate nephropathy can be prevented by vigorous hydration and lowering the uric acid level with allopurinol and urine alkalization with acetazolamide.
- Infections must be aggressively treated with broad-spectrum antibiotics.
  1. Any febrile or neutropenic patients must have cultures taken and be properly treated with IV antibiotics.
  2. If evidence of infection persists, despite adequate treatment with antibiotics, IV antifungal therapy may be added to provide coverage against fungal infections (*Candida, Aspergillus*).
- Correct significant thrombocytopenia (platelet counts < 20,000/mm³) with platelet transfusion.
- Bleeding secondary to disseminated intravascular coagulation (DIC) is treated with heparin and replacement of clotting factors.
- Induction therapy is intensive chemotherapy to destroy a significant number of leukemic cells and achieve remission.
- Consolidation therapy consists of an aggressive course of chemotherapy, with or without radiotherapy, shortly after complete remission has been attained. Its purpose is to prolong the remission period or cure.
- Meningeal prophylactic therapy with intrathecal chemotherapy, with or without cranial irradiation, is indicated to prevent meningeal sequestration of leukemic cells.
- The goal of maintenance chemotherapy is to maintain a state of remission.
- Bone marrow transplantation: generally patients are candidates for an allograft in the first complete remission if they are between the ages of 20 and 50 years and have matched a sibling donor.

PROGNOSIS
- Generally poorer in adult compared with childhood disease (40% adult cure rate versus 80% cure rate in children)
- Five-year leukemia-free survival is <40%.

B. ACUTE MYELOGENOUS LEUKEMIA

DEFINITION
Acute myelogenous leukemia (AML) is a disorder characterized by uncontrolled proliferation of primitive myeloid cells (blasts), ultimately replacing normal bone marrow elements (Fig. 313-3) and frequently resulting in hematopoietic insufficiency (granulocytopenia, thrombocytopenia, or anemia), with or without leukocytosis.

PHYSICAL FINDINGS AND CLINICAL PRESENTATION
Patients generally come to medical attention because of the effects of the cytopenias.
- Anemia manifests with weakness or fatigue.
- Thrombocytopenia can manifest with bleeding, petechiae, and ecchymosis.
- Neutropenia can result in infections and fever.

- Physical examination may reveal skin pallor, bruises, petechiae; abdominal examination may reveal hepatosplenomegaly; peripheral lymphadenopathy may also be present.
- Hyperleukocytosis can lead to symptoms of leukostasis, such as ocular and cerebrovascular dysfunction or bleeding.

CAUSE
- Risk factors are previous use of antineoplastic agents, chromosomal abnormalities, ionizing radiation, toxins, immunodeficiency states, and chronic myeloproliferative disorders.

DIFFERENTIAL DIAGNOSIS
- Acute lymphocytic leukemia
- Leukemoid reaction
- Myelodysplastic syndrome
- Infiltrative diseases of the bone marrow
- Epstein-Barr virus, other viral infection

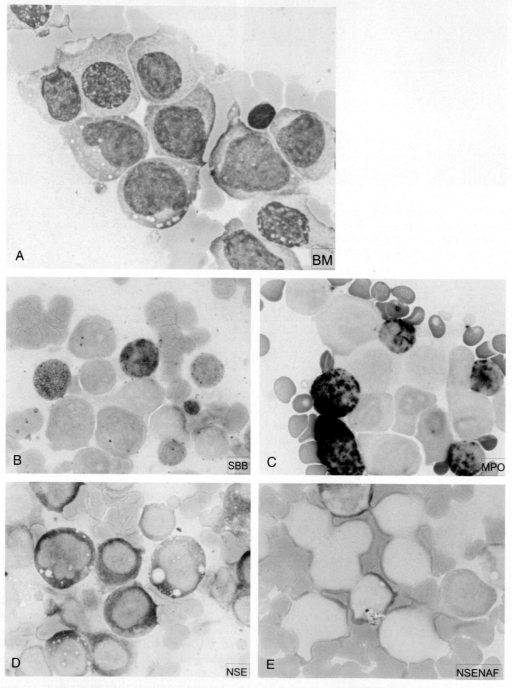

Fig 313–3
Example of diagnostic bone marrow **A,** and immunohistochemical special stains **(B-E)** in case of secondary acute myeloid leukemia with FAB M5 morphology typical of myeloid leukemias with MLL translocations.
(Courtesy of Dr. John Choi.)

LABORATORY TESTS

- CBC reveals anemia, thrombocytopenia. Peripheral WBC count varies from less than 5000/mm³ to more than 100,000/mm³.
- Additional laboratory findings may include elevated LDH and uric acid levels, decreased fibrinogen, and increased fibrin degradation products (FDP) secondary to DIC.
- Cytogenetic abnormalities (Fig. 313–4) are common (chromosome 8 is most frequently involved in AML).
- The distinction between ALL and AML and the classification of the various subtypes are based on the following factors:
  1. Cell morphology: myeloblasts reveal abundant cytoplasm; cytoplasmic granules are often present (Auer rods; Fig. 313–5).
  2. Histochemical stains
  a. Peroxidase and Sudan black stains are negative in ALL.
  b. Chloroacetate esterase: a pink cytoplasmic reaction identifies granulocytes; useful to distinguish granulocytes from monocytes in patients with AML
- AML is diagnosed by the presence of at least 30% blast cells and positive peroxidase or Sudan black histochemical stain in the bone marrow aspirate.
- The FAB Cooperative Study Group has classified AML into seven categories (M1 to M7) based on the type and percentage of immature cells.

IMAGING STUDIES

- Chest x-ray is useful to evaluate for the presence of mediastinal masses.
- CT of the abdomen may reveal hepatosplenomegaly or leukemic involvement of other organs.

TREATMENT

- Emergency treatment consisting of one or more of the following is indicated in patients with intracerebral leukostasis:
  1. Cranial irradiation
  2. Leukapheresis
  3. Oral hydroxyurea
- Urate nephropathy can be prevented by vigorous hydration, lowering uric acid level with allopurinol, and urine alkalinization with acetazolamide.
- Infections must be aggressively treated with broad-spectrum antibiotics.
- Correct significant thrombocytopenia with platelet transfusions.
- Bleeding secondary to DIC is treated with heparin and replacement of clotting factors.
- Intensive induction chemotherapy to destroy a significant number of leukemic cells and achieve remission
- Consolidation therapy consists of an aggressive course of chemotherapy, with or without radiation, shortly after complete remission has been attained, to prolong the remission period or cure. Complications of consolidation therapy are usually secondary to severe bone marrow suppression (anemia, thrombocytopenia, granulocytopenia).
- Autologous bone marrow transplantation should be considered in patients younger than 55 years without a sibling donor. Allogeneic bone marrow transplantation is generally available to less than 20% of patients; usually performed mainly in patients younger than 40 years because of a higher incidence of graft-versus-host disease (GVHD) with advancing age.
- Remission can be achieved in almost 80% of patients younger than 55 years. Remission rates are highest in children.
- Cure for allogeneic bone marrow transplantation approaches 60%; cure rates with autologous transplantation are slightly lower.

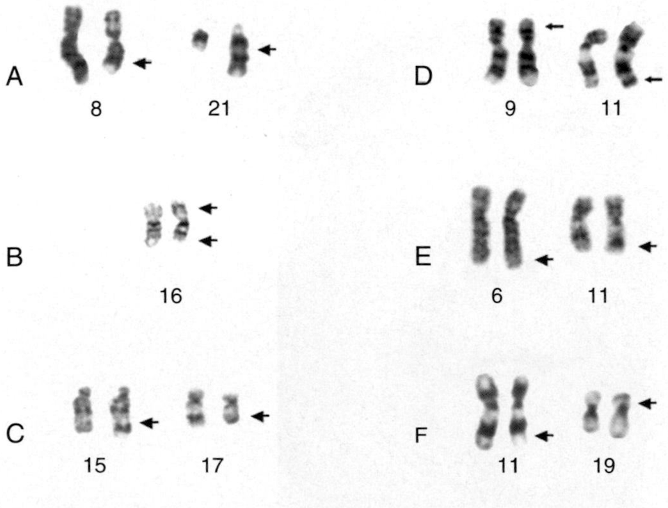

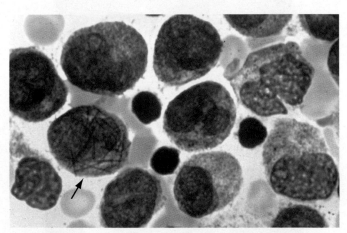

Fig 313–4
G-banded partial karyotypes demonstrating recurrent chromosome abnormalities whose presence is used to classify AML.
A, t(8;21)(q22;q22). **B,** inv(16)(p13q22). **C,** t(15;17)(q22;q12a~21).
D-F, The most frequent among more than 30 recurring translocations involving chromosome band 11q23 in AML: **D,** t(9;11)(p22;q23); **E,** t(6;11)(q27;q23); **F,** t(11;19)(q23;p13.1).
(From Young NS, Gerson SL, High KA [eds]: Clinical Hematology. St. Louis, Mosby, 2006.)

Fig 313–5
Acute promyelocytic leukemia (M3 according to FAB classification). One of the leukemic cells contains bundles of Auer rods (faggot cell) (*arrow*). Leukemic cells may contain one or multiple Auer rods in their cytoplasm. (Romanowsky stain, ×1000).
(From Silverberg SG, Frable WJ, Wick MR, et al [eds]: Principles and Practice of Surgical Pathology and Cytopathology, 4th ed. Philadelphia, Elsevier, 2006.)

C. CHRONIC LYMPHOCYTIC LEUKEMIA

DEFINITION

Chronic lymphocytic leukemia (CLL) is a lymphoproliferative disorder characterized by the proliferation and accumulation of mature-appearing neoplastic lymphocytes.

PHYSICAL FINDINGS AND CLINICAL PRESENTATION

- Lymphadenopathy, splenomegaly, and hepatomegaly in most patients
- Variable clinical presentation according to stage of the disease. Intense facial erythema may be present (Fig. 313–6).
- Abnormal CBC: many cases are diagnosed on the basis of laboratory results obtained after routine physical examination.
- Some patients come to medical attention because of weakness and fatigue (secondary to anemia), lymphadenopathy.
- Viral illnesses (e.g. herpes zoster, varicella) may prove fatal in some patients because of their weakened immune system (Fig. 313–7).

CAUSE

- CLL is a disease derived from antigen-experienced B lymphocytes that differ in the level of immunoglobulin V gene mutations.

DIFFERENTIAL DIAGNOSIS

- Hairy cell leukemia (see Fig. 317–2)
- Lymphoma (see Fig. 313–8B)
- Prolymphocytic leukemia (see Fig. 313–8C)
- Viral infections
- Waldenström's macroglobulinemia

LABORATORY TESTS

- Proliferative lymphocytosis ($\geq$15,000/dL) of well-differentiated lymphocytes is the hallmark of CLL (Fig. 313–8).
- There is monotonous replacement of the bone marrow by small lymphocytes (marrow contains $\geq$30% of well-differentiated lymphocytes).
- Hypogammaglobulinemia and elevated LDH may be present at the time of diagnosis.
- Anemia or thrombocytopenia, if present, indicates a poor prognosis.

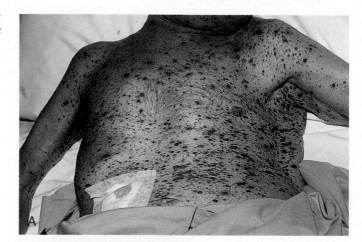

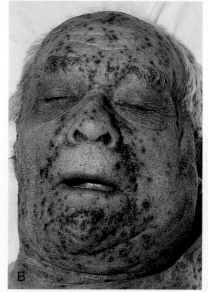

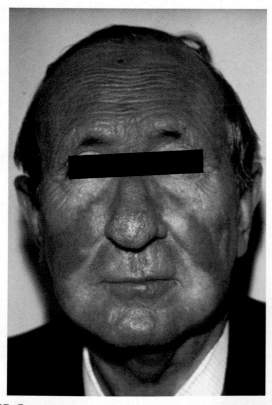

Fig 313–6
Chronic lymphocytic leukemia. There is intense facial erythema. (Courtesy of Dr. R. A. Marsden, St. George's Hospital, London.)

Fig 313–7
A, B, Disseminated cutaneous lesions in a patient with chronic lymphocytic leukemia who developed fatal varicella despite rapid initiation of intravenous acyclovir therapy. Varicella lesions are numerous and hemorrhagic.
(From Cohen J, Powderly WG: Infectious Diseases, 2nd ed. St. Louis, Mosby, 2004.)

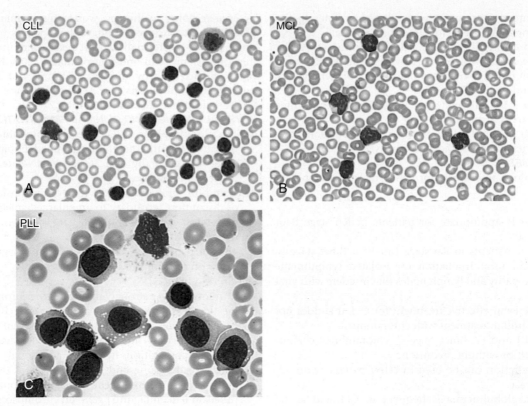

Fig 313–8
Peripheral blood smears distinguishing chronic lymphocytic leukemia (CLL) **A,** from mantle cell lymphoma (MCL) **B,** and prolymphocytic leukemia (PLL) (**C**).
(From Young NS, Gerson SL, High KA [eds]: Clinical Hematology. St. Louis, Mosby, 2006.)

- Trisomy 12 is the most common chromosomal abnormality (Fig. 313–9), followed by 14q+, 13q, and 11q; these all indicate a poor prognosis.
- New laboratory techniques (CD38, fluorescence in situ hybridization [FISH]) can identify patients with early-stage CLL at a higher risk of rapid disease progression. Staining of mononuclear cells by a two-color (fluorescein isothiocyanate–phycoerythrin) flow cytometric assay using antibodies to the chemokine receptors (e.g., CXCR1, CXCR2) can aid in staging and prognosis. An increase in expression of chemokine receptors CXCR4 and CCR7 correlates with advanced Rai stage (stage IV). The presence of V gene mutations, CD38+, or ZAP 70+ cells also has prognostic relevance. Patients with clones having few or no V gene mutations or many CD38+ or ZAP 70+ B cells are associated with an aggressive, usually fatal course.

STAGING
Rai and colleagues have divided CLL into five clinical stages:

Stage 0: characterized by lymphocytosis only ($\geq$15,000/mm^3 on peripheral smear, bone marrow aspirate $\geq$40% lymphocytes). The coexistence of lymphocytosis and other factors increases the clinical stage.

Stage 1: lymphadenopathy

Stage 2: lymphadenopathy/hepatomegaly

Stage 3: anemia (Hgb <11 g/mm^3)

Stage 4: thrombocytopenia (platelets <100,000/mm^3)

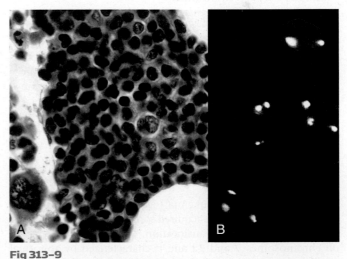

Fig 313–9
Chronic lymphocytic leukemia (CLL). **A,** Note the interstitial pattern of infiltration from a patient with CLL (H&E stain, ×603). **B,** Three of the four leukemic cells from a patient with mixed CLL/PLL (prolymphocytic leukemia) have trisomy 12 (fluorescence in-situ hybridization, ×1000).
(Courtesy of Dr. Russell Brynes.)

Another well-known staging system developed by Binet divides chronic lymphocytic leukemia into three stages:

Stage A: Hgb ≥10 g/dL, platelets ≥100,000/mm³, and fewer than three areas involved (the cervical, axillary, and inguinal lymph nodes [whether unilaterally or bilaterally]; the spleen; and the liver)

Stage B: Hgb ≥10 g/dL, platelets ≥100,000/mm³, and three or more areas involved

Stage C: Hgb <10 g/dL, low platelets (<100,000/mm³), or both (independent of the areas involved)

IMAGING STUDIES

- CT of abdomen to evaluate for hepatomegaly and splenomegaly

TREATMENT

- Observation is appropriate for patients in Rai stage 0 or Binet stage A.
- Symptomatic patients in Rai stage I or II or Binet stage B: chlorambucil; local irradiation for isolated symptomatic lymphadenopathy and lymph nodes that interfere with vital organs
- Fludarabine is an effective treatment for CLL that does not respond to initial treatment with chlorambucil.
- Rai stages III and IV, Binet stage C: chlorambucil chemotherapy, with or without prednisone
- Splenic irradiation can be used in select patients with advanced disease.
- Hypogammaglobulinemia is frequent in CLL and is the chief cause of infections. Immune globulin may prevent infections but has no effect on survival. Infections should be treated with broad-spectrum antibiotics. Patients should be monitored for opportunistic infections.
- Recombinant hematopoietic cofactors (e.g., granulocyte-macrophage colony-stimulating factor and granulocyte colony-stimulating factor) may be useful to overcome neutropenia related to treatment.
- Erythropoietin may be useful to treat anemia unresponsive to other measures.

PROGNOSIS

- Generally directly related to the clinical stage (e.g., the average survival in patients in Rai stage 0 or Binet stage A is more than 120 months, whereas for RAI stage 4 or Binet stage C it is approximately 30 months). Overall 5-year survival is 60%. Measurement of ZAP 70 intracellular protein (where available) is also a useful indicator of prognosis.

D. CHRONIC MYELOGENOUS LEUKEMIA

DEFINITION

Chronic myelogenous leukemia (CML) is a malignant clonal stem disease caused by an acquired somatic mutation that fuses, through chromosomal translocation, the *ABL* and *BCR* genes on chromosomes 9 and 22 and is characterized by abnormal proliferation and accumulation of immature granulocytes. CML manifests with a chronic phase (CP-CML) lasting months to years, followed by an advanced phase (AP-CML) characterized by poor response to therapy, worsening anemia, or decreased platelet count. The second phase then evolves into a terminal phase (acute transformation) that degenerates into acute leukemia (mostly myeloid and approximately 20% lymphoid subtype), characterized by an elevated number of blast cells and numerous complications (e.g., sepsis, bleeding). The phases of CML are described in Table 313–1.

PHYSICAL FINDINGS AND CLINICAL PRESENTATION

- The chronic phase usually reveals splenomegaly; hepatomegaly is not infrequent, but lymphadenopathy is very unusual and generally indicates the accelerated proliferative phase of the disease.
- Common complaints at the time of diagnosis are weakness or discomfort secondary to an enlarged spleen (abdominal discomfort or pain). Splenomegaly is present in up to 40% of patients at diagnosis.
- 40% of patients are asymptomatic and diagnosis is based solely on an abnormal blood count.

CAUSE

- Current evidence strongly implicates the chromosome translocation t(9;22)(q34;q11.2) as the cause of chronic granulocytic leukemia. This translocation is present in more than 95% of patients. The remaining patients have a complex or variant translocation involving additional chromosomes that have the same end result (fusion of the *BCR* [break point cluster region] gene on chromosome 22 to *ABL* [Abelson leukemia virus] gene on chromosome 9).

DIFFERENTIAL DIAGNOSIS

- Lymphoma (see Fig. 313–8B)
- CLL (see Fig. 313–8A)
- Myelodysplastic syndrome (see Fig. 314–3)

LABORATORY TESTS

- Elevated WBC count (generally >100,000/mm³) with a broad spectrum of granulocytic forms (Fig. 313–10A,C).
- Bone marrow demonstrates hypercellularity with granulocytic hyperplasia, increased ratio of myeloid cells to erythroid cells, and increased number of megakaryocytes. Blasts and promyelocytes constitute less than 10% of all cells (see Fig. 313–10B).
- The Philadelphia chromosome, which results from the reciprocal translocation between the long arms of chromosomes 9 and 22, (Fig. 313–11), is present in more than 95% of patients with CML. Its presence (Ph') is a major prognostic factor because the survival rate of patients with Philadelphia chromosome is approximately eight times better than that of those without it. Some believe that Ph⁻ defines CML and that those who are Ph⁻ have another disease.
- Leukocyte alkaline phosphatase (LAP) is markedly decreased (used to distinguish CML from other myeloproliferative disorders).
- Anemia and thrombocytosis are often present.
- Additional laboratory results are elevated vitamin B_{12} levels (caused by increased transcobalamin 1 from granulocytes) and elevated blood histamine levels (because of increased basophils).

TABLE 313–1 Definitions of phases of chronic myelogenous leukemia	
WHO Criteria	**IBMTR Criteria**
Chronic phase	
Ability to reduce spleen size and restore and maintain normal blood count with appropriate therapy	Not specifically denned
Accelerated phase—one or more of the following:	
Blasts 10%-19% of WBCs in peripheral blood and/or nucleated bone marrow cells	Blasts 10%-19% in blood or marrow
Peripheral blood basophils $\geq$ 20%	Peripheral blood basophils $\geq$ 20%
Persistent thrombocytopenia (<100 _ 10^9/L unrelated to therapy, or persistent thrombocytosis (>1000 _ 10^9/L) unresponsive to therapy	Persistent thrombocytopenia (<100 _ 10^9/L) unrelated to therapy
Increasing spleen size and increasing WBC count unresponsive to therapy	Persistent thrombocytosis (>1000 _ 10^9/L) unresponsive to therapy
Cytogenetic evidence of clonal evolution	
Blastic Phase—one or more of the following:	
Blasts >20%	
Extramedullary blast cell proliferation	
Large foci or clusters of blasts in the bone marrow biopsy	

IBMTR, International Bone Marrow Transplant Registry; WBC, white blood cell; WHO, World Health Organization.
From Young NS, Gerson SL, High KA (eds): Clinical Hematology. St. Louis, 2006, Mosby, 2006.

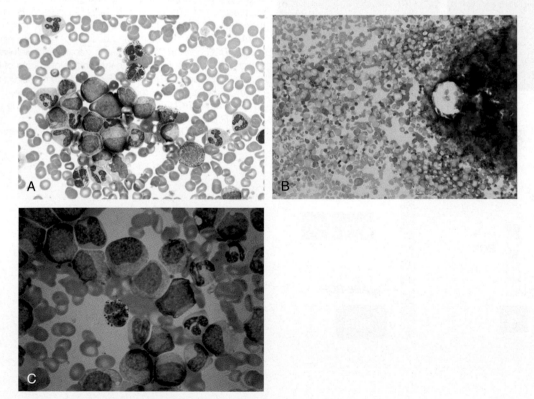

Fig 313–10
Hematologic morphology in chronic myelogenous leukemia (CML). **A,** Peripheral blood in chronic phase disease. **B,** Bone marrow in chronic phase disease. **C,** Peripheral blood in blastic phase disease.
(From Young NS, Gerson SL, High KA [eds]: Clinical Hematology. St. Louis, Mosby, 2006.)

IMAGING STUDIES
- Chest x-ray
- CT of abdomen, pelvis

TREATMENT
- Treatment with a potential to cure CML or prolong survival should be used during the chronic phase of the disease because it is often futile when administered during the advanced phase. Imatinib mesylate, an oral tyrosine kinase inhibitor, is effective and indicated as first-line treatment for CML myeloid blast crisis, accelerated phase, or CML in its chronic phase. More than 60% of patients have a major cytogenetic response (<35% Philadelphia chromosome-positive cells in the marrow) and more than 80% have progression-free survival after 24 months. Complete hematologic response usually occurs in less than 1 month.
- Allogeneic stem cell transplantation (SCT) following intense chemotherapy is the only curative treatment for CML in a chronic phase unresponsive to imatinib. Generally, only 20% of patients are candidates for SCT given the limitations of age or lack of HLA-matched related donors.
- Transplantation of marrow from an HLA-matched unrelated donor is also now recognized as safe and effective therapy for select patients with chronic myelogenous leukemia.

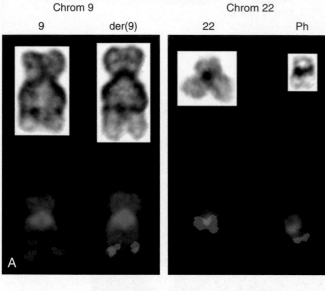

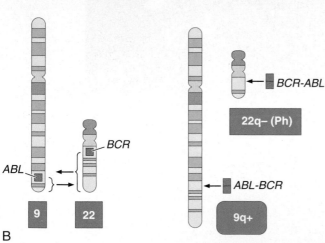

Fig 313–11

A, Chromosomes 9q+ and 22q−. The upper left panel shows a normal chromosome 9 and an abnormal chromosome 9 with extra material on the long arm [9q+ or der(9)]; the upper right panel shows a normal chromosome 22 followed by an abnormal chromosome 22 with loss of material from the long arm (22q− or Ph). The lower panel shows the corresponding chromosomes subjected to fluorescent in situ hybridization to locate the positions of the *ABL* (red) and *BCR* (green) genes, respectively. The normal chromosome 9 shows two red signals and the normal chromosome 22 shows two green signals. The Ph chromosome shows both red and green signals and a yellow signal where the red and green overlap, consistent with the presence of a *BCR-ABL* fusion gene; the 9q+ also shows both red and green signals with a yellow signal where the red and green overlap, consistent with the presence of a reciprocal *ABL-BCR* fusion gene. **B,** The Ph chromosome. *Left,* schematic representation of one normal 9 and one normal 22 chromosome showing position of the *ABL* gene at 9q34 and the *BCR* gene at 22q11. The Ph translocation involves reciprocal balanced exchange of genetic between the long arms of both chromosomes, indicated by the arrows. *Right,* The derivative 9q+ (Ph chromosome) and 22q− resulting from the translocation. Note the positions of the *BCL-ABL* fusion gene on 22q− and the reciprocal *ABL-BCR* fusion gene on 9q+.
(From Young NS, Gerson SL, High KA [eds]: Clinical Hematology. St. Louis, Mosby, 2006.)

Chapter 314 | Myelodysplastic syndrome

DEFINITION

Myelodysplastic syndromes (MDSs) are a group of acquired clonal disorders affecting the hemopoietic stem cells and characterized by cytopenias with hypercellular bone marrow (Fig. 314–1A) and various morphologic abnormalities in the hemopoietic cell lines. MDSs show abnormal (dysplastic) hemopoietic maturation. Marrow cellularity is increased, reflecting an effective hematopoiesis, but inadequate maturation results in peripheral cytopenias.

CLASSIFICATION

- Myelodysplasia encompasses several heterogenous syndromes. The FAB classification of myelodysplastic syndromes is based on the proportion of immature blast cells in the blood and marrow and on the presence or absence of ringed sideroblasts or peripheral monocytosis. It includes the following: refractory anemia, refractory anemia with ringed sideroblasts, refractory anemia with excess blasts, chronic myelomonocytic leukemia, and refractory anemia with excess blasts in transformation.
- The World Health Organization has modified the FAB classification by incorporating newer morphologic insights and cytogenetic findings. It includes the following disease subtypes: refractory anemia, refractory anemia with ringed sideroblasts (Fig. 314–2), refractory cytopenia with multilineage dysplasia, refractory cytopenia with multilineage dysplasia and ringed sideroblasts, refractory anemia with excessive blasts (Fig. 314–3), unclassified myelodysplastic syndrome, and myelodysplastic syndrome associated with isolated del(5q) (see Fig. 314–1).

PHYSICAL FINDINGS AND CLINICAL PRESENTATION

- Splenomegaly, skin pallor, mucosal bleeding, ecchymosis may be present.
- Patients often present with fatigue.
- Fever, infection, and dyspnea are common.

CAUSE

- Unknown. However, exposure to radiation, chemotherapeutic agents, benzene, or other organic compounds is associated with myelodysplasia.

DIFFERENTIAL DIAGNOSIS

- Hereditary dysplasias (e.g., Fanconi's anemia, Diamond-Blackfan syndrome)
- Vitamin B_{12}–folate deficiency
- Exposure to toxins (e.g., drugs, alcohol, chemotherapy)
- Renal failure
- Irradiation
- Autoimmune disease
- Infections (tuberculosis [TB], viral infections)
- Paroxysmal nocturnal hemoglobinuria

TREATMENT

- Results of chemotherapy are generally disappointing. Combination chemotherapy regimens generally induce a complete response in only a minority of patients and the average duration of response is less than 1 year.
- Azacitidine, a pyrimidine nucleoside analogue of cytidine, has been shown to improve the quality of life for patients with myelodysplastic syndrome and probably prolong survival.
- The role of myeloid growth factors (granulocyte colony-stimulating factor, granulocyte-macrophage colony-stimulating factor) and immunotherapy is undefined.
- Lenalidomide, a novel analogue of thalidomide, has demonstrated hematologic activity in patients with low-rise myelodysplastic syndrome who have no response to erythropoietin or who are unlikely to benefit from conventional therapy.
- Allogeneic stem cell transplantation should be considered in patients younger than 60 years because this is the established procedure with cure potential.

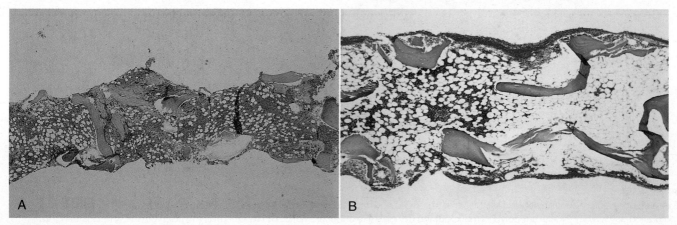

Fig 314–1
Bone marrow biopsies in myelodysplastic syndrome (MDS), low-power views. **A,** Typical hypercellular appearance in a patient with MDS classified as refractory anemia with excessive blasts (RAEB). **B,** Partially hypocellular specimen of a patient with 5q− syndrome.
(From Young NS, Gerson SL, High KA [eds]: Clinical Hematology. St. Louis, Mosby, 2006.)

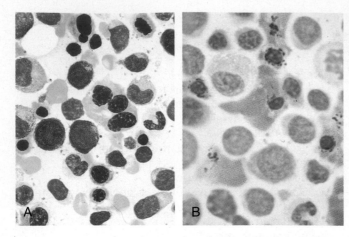

Fig 314-2

A, B, Refractory anemia with ring sideroblasts. Note megaloblastic and megaloblastoid erythropoiesis with erythrons containing multiple nuclei. Ring sideroblasts are evident. (**A,** Romanowsky stain, ×630; **B,** Prussian blue stain, ×1000.).

(From Silverberg SG, Frable WJ, Wick MR, et al [eds]: Principles and Practice of Surgical Pathology and Cytopathology, 4th ed. Philadelphia, Elsevier, 2006.)

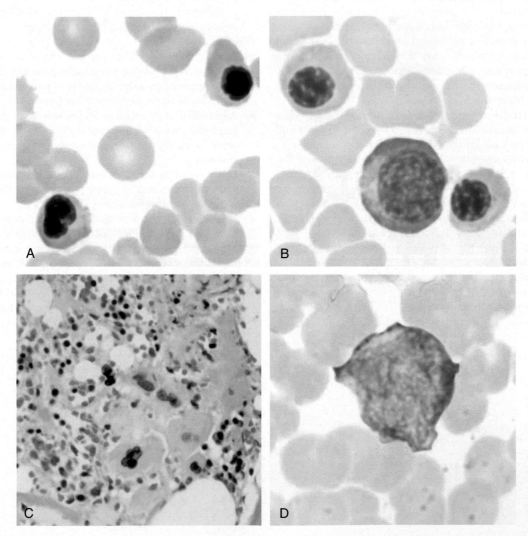

Fig 314-3

Example of refractory anemia with excess blasts in transition. **A,** Orthochromatic normoblasts with nuclear irregularities. **B,** Two normoblasts with maturation asynchrony. Nuclei are polychromatic but the cytoplasm is orthochromatic. **C,** Hypolobated megakaryocytes with clustering. **D,** Increased blasts were seen similar to that shown, approximately 5% to 8% of the marrow cellularity.
(Courtesy of Dr. John Choi.)

| Chapter 315 | **Hodgkin's lymphoma** |

DEFINITION

Hodgkin's disease is a malignant disorder of lymphoreticular origin, characterized histologically by the presence of multinucleated giant cells (*Reed-Sternberg cells*) usually originating from B lymphocytes in germinal centers of lymphoid tissue.

PHYSICAL FINDINGS AND CLINICAL PRESENTATION

- Palpable lymphadenopathy, generally painless
- Most common site of involvement: neck region (Fig. 315–1)
- Symptomatic patients with Hodgkin's disease usually present with the following manifestations:
  - Fever and night sweats: fever in a cyclical pattern (days or weeks of fever alternating with afebrile periods) is known as *Pel-Epstein fever*
  - Weight loss, generalized malaise
  - Persistent, nonproductive cough
  - Pain associated with alcohol ingestion, often secondary to heavy eosinophil infiltration of the tumor sites
  - Pruritus
  - Others: superior vena cava syndrome and spinal cord compression (rare)

LABORATORY TESTS

- Diagnosis can be made with lymph node biopsy. There are four main **histologic subtypes,** based on the number of lymphocytes, Reed-Sternberg cells (Fig. 315–2H), and the presence of fibrous tissue (see Fig. 315–2):
  1. Lymphocyte predominance
  2. Mixed cellularity

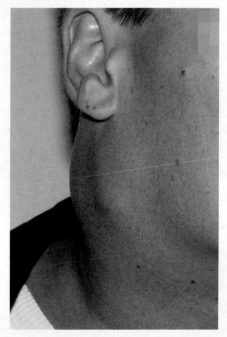

Fig 315–1
Cervical lymph node swelling in a young male with newly diagnosed Hodgkin's lymphoma.
(From Young NS, Gerson SL, High KA [eds]: Clinical Hematology. St. Louis, Mosby, 2006.)

  3. Nodular sclerosis
  4. Lymphocyte depletion
- Nodular sclerosis is the most common type and occurs mainly in young adulthood, whereas the mixed cellularity type is more prevalent after age 50 years.

STAGING

- Ann Arbor staging classification
  Stage I: involvement of a single lymph node region
  Stage II: two or more lymph node regions on the same side of the diaphragm
  Stage III: lymph node involvement on both sides of diaphragm, including spleen
  Stage IV: diffuse involvement of external sites
  Suffix A: no systemic symptoms
  Suffix B: presence of fever, night sweats, or unexplained weight loss of 10% or more body weight over 6 months
  Suffix X: indicates bulky disease more than one third widening of mediastinum or more than 10 cm maximum dimension of nodal mass on a chest film

Proper staging requires the following:

- Detailed history (with documentation of B symptoms and physical examination)
- Surgical biopsy
- Laboratory evaluation (CBC, sedimentation rate, BUN, creatinine, alkaline phosphatase, liver function tests [LFTs], albumin, LDH, uric acid)
- Chest x-ray (posteroanterior [PA] and lateral) (Fig. 315–3)
- Bilateral bone marrow biopsy
- CT scan of the chest (Fig. 315–4) and of the abdomen and pelvis to visualize the mesenteric, hepatic, portal, and splenic hilar nodes
- Positron emission tomography (PET) scan
- Bipedal lymphangiography may be performed only in select patients to define periaortic and iliac lymph node involvement.
- Exploratory laparotomy and splenectomy (select patients)
  1. Decision to perform staging laparotomy depends on the therapeutic plan. It is generally not indicated in patients who have a large mediastinal mass; these patients will generally be treated with combined chemotherapy and radiation. Staging laparotomy may also not be required in patients with clinical stage I or unlikely to have abdominal disease (e.g., women with supradiaphragmatic disease).
  2. Exploratory laparotomy and splenectomy (Fig. 315–5) may be used for patients with clinical stage I to IIA or IIB.
  3. It is useful in identifying patients who can be treated with irradiation alone with curative intent.
  4. Polyvalent pneumococcal vaccine should be given prophylactically to all patients before splenectomy (increased risk of sepsis from encapsulated organisms in splenectomized patients).

CAUSE

- Unknown; evidence implicating Epstein-Barr virus remains controversial.

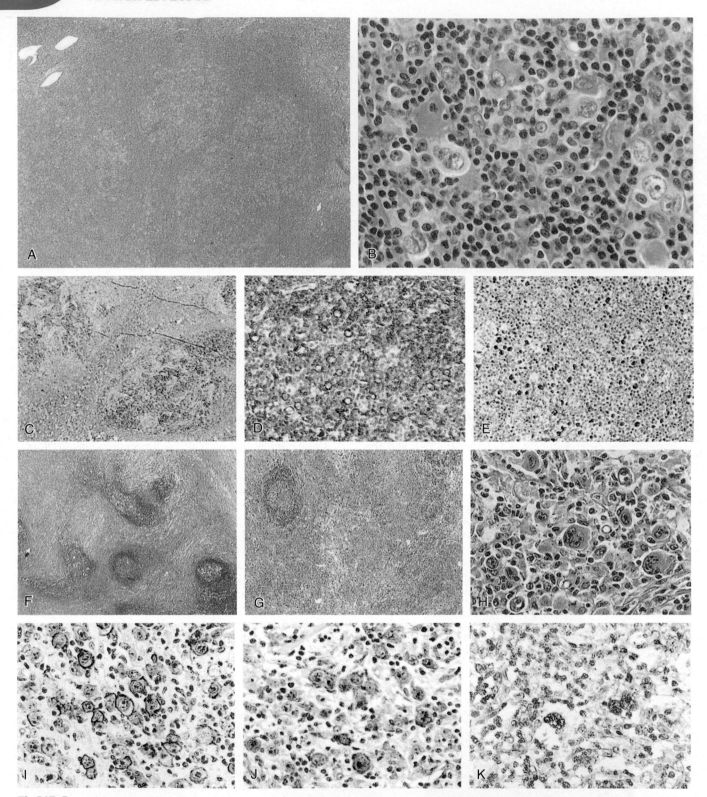

Fig 315–2

Hodgkin's lymphoma. **A-E,** Nodular lymphocyte predominance in Hodgkin's lymphoma. **A,** Low magnification showing large nodules effacing the nodal architecture. **B,** High magnification showing large mononucleated and multilobulated popcorn cells in a background of reactive histiocytes and small lymphocytes. **C,** The nodules are associated with a meshwork of CD21+ follicular dendritic cells. **D,** Immunoperoxidase staining for CD20 showing strong positivity of the large neoplastic cells and small B lymphocytes in the background. **E,** Immunoperoxidase staining for Bcl-6 showing positivity of the neoplastic cells. **F-K,** Classic Hodgkin's lymphoma. **F,** Nodular sclerosis type, showing cellular nodules separated by fibrous bands. G, Mixed cellularity type, showing an interfollicular infiltrate. **H,** Classic Reed-Sternberg cells in a mixed reactive background. **I,** Immunoperoxidase staining for CD30, showing membrane and focally paranuclear Golgi region staining of Reed-Sternberg cells. **J,** Immunoper-oxidase staining for CD15, showing membrane and focally paranuclear Golgi region staining of Reed-Sternberg cells. **K,** In situ hybridization showing positivity of Reed-Sternberg cells for Epstein-Barr virus RNA (EBER).

(From Young NS, Gerson SL, High KA [eds]: Clinical Hematology. St. Louis, Mosby, 2006.)

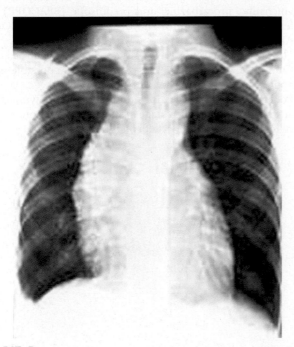

Fig 315–3
Intrathoracic involvement of Hodgkin's lymphoma—a mediastinal mass detected by chest radiograph.
(From Young NS, Gerson SL, High KA [eds]: Clinical Hematology. St. Louis, Mosby, 2006.)

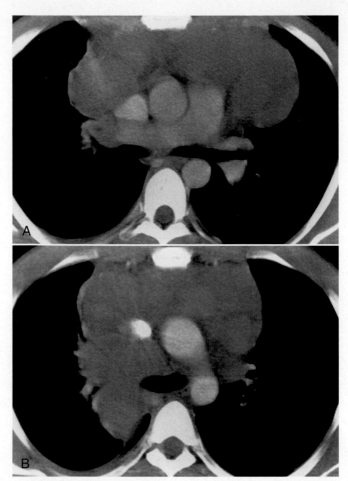

Fig 315–4
Mediastinal masses in lymphoma. **A,** Contrast-enhanced CT scan showing a large anterior mass in a young patient with Hodgkin's disease. No other disease was demonstrated. **B,** Contrast-enhanced CT scan in a patient with mediastinal diffuse large B cell lymphoma (non-Hodgkin's). The mass is involving the anterior and middle mediastinum. This subtype of non-Hodgkin's lymphoma carries a poor prognosis and, as in this patient, often involves the abdominal viscera.
(From Grainger RG, Allison DJ, Adam A, Dixon AK [eds]: Grainger & Allison's Diagnostic Radiology, 4th ed. London, Harcourt, 2001.)

Fig 315–5
Hodgkin's disease. A similar gross pattern of splenic involvement may be seen with large cell lymphoma.
(From Silverberg SG, Frable WJ, Wick MR, et al [eds]: Principles and Practice of Surgical Pathology and Cytopathology, 4th ed. Philadelphia, Elsevier, 2006.)

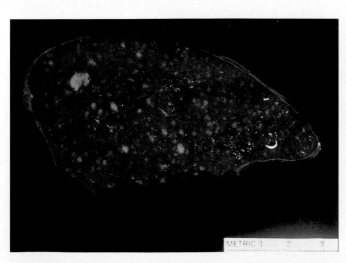

- Non-Hodgkin's lymphoma (see Fig. 316–6)
- Sarcoidosis (see Fig. 137–3)
- Infections (e.g., cytomegalovirus [CMV], Epstein-Barr virus, toxoplasma, HIV)
- Drug reaction

TREATMENT

The main therapeutic modalities are radiotherapy and chemotherapy; the indications for each vary with pathologic stage and other factors.

- Stages I and II: radiation therapy alone unless a large mediastinal mass is present (mediastinal to thoracic ratio ≥ 1.3). In the latter case, a combination of chemotherapy and radiation therapy is indicated.
- Stage IB or IIB: total nodal irradiation is often used, although chemotherapy is performed in many centers.
- Stage IIIA: treatment is controversial. It varies with the anatomic substage after splenectomy.

  1. Stage III$_1$A and minimum splenic involvement: radiation therapy alone may be adequate.

  2. Stage III$_2$ or III$_1$A with extensive splenic involvement: there is disagreement whether chemotherapy alone or a combination of chemotherapy and radiation therapy is the preferred treatment modality.

  3. Stage IIIB and IVB: the treatment of choice is chemotherapy, with or without adjuvant radiotherapy.

- Various regimens can be used for combination of chemotherapy. Most oncologists prefer the combination of doxorubicin plus bleomycin plus vincristine plus dacarbazine (ABVD). Other commonly used regimens are MOPP, MOPP/ABV, MOPP/ABVD, MOPP-BAP.
- In patients with advanced Hodgkin's disease, increased-dose bleomycin, etoposide, doxorubicin, cyclophosphamide, vincristine, procarbazine, and prednisone (BEACOPP) offers better tumor control and overall survival than COPP/ABVD.
- The overall survival at 10 years is approximately 60%.
- Cure rates as high as 75% to 80% are now possible with appropriate initial therapy.
- Poor prognostic features include presence of B symptoms, advanced age, advanced stage at initial presentation, mixed cellularity, and lymphocyte depletion histology.

Chapter 316 Non-Hodgkin's lymphoma

DEFINITION
Non-Hodgkin's lymphoma (NHL) is a heterogeneous group of malignancies of the lymphoreticular system.

PHYSICAL FINDINGS AND CLINICAL PRESENTATION
- Patients often present with asymptomatic lymphadenopathy (Fig. 316–1).
- Approximately one third of NHL originates extranodally. Involvement of extranodal sites can result in unusual presentations (e.g., mouth [Fig. 316–2]). Primary lymphoma accounts for 2% to 5% of gastric tumors. It originates in the submucosa, affecting more frequently the body and the cardia. CT is useful to define extensive gastric wall thickening and the extent of the extraluminal mass. In mucosa-associated lymphoid tissue (MALT) lymphomas, the gastric wall thickening may be minimal and CT is then of limited value in staging and assessment of response (Fig. 316–3)
- NHL cases associated with HIV occur predominantly in the brain (Fig. 316–4).
- Pruritus, fever, night sweats, and weight loss are less common than in Hodgkin's disease.
- Hepatomegaly and splenomegaly may be present.

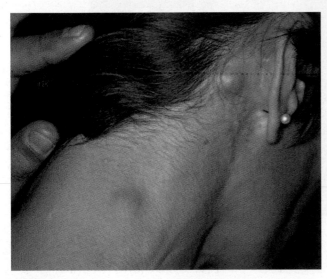

Fig 316–1
Posterior auricular and posterior cervical adenopathy.
(From Swartz MH: Textbook of Physical Diagnosis, 5th ed. Philadelphia, WB Saunders, 2006.)

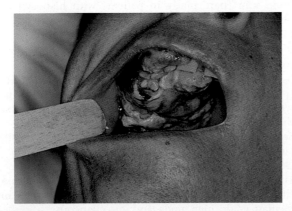

Fig 316–2
Non–Hodgkin's lymphoma. Bulky disease in the gingiva is shown.
(From Cohen J, Powderly WG: Infectious Diseases, 2nd ed. St. Louis, Mosby, 2004.)

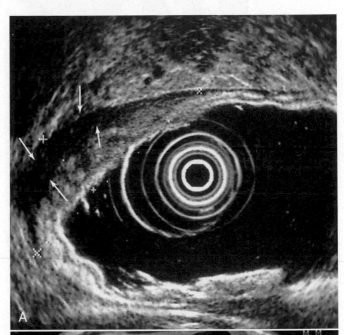
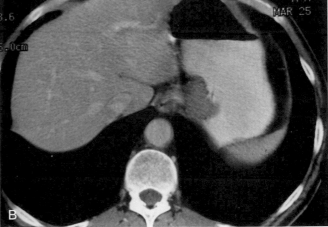

Fig 316–3
MALT lymphoma. **A,** Endoscopic ultrasound showing a narrow sheet of low echogenic tissue in the submucosa (*arrows*). **B,** CT scan in a different patient shows a typical small soft tissue mass in the region of the gastroesophageal junction. The stomach has been fully distended by oral administration of Gastrografin and intravenous injection of hyoscine-*N*-butylbromide.
(Courtesy of Dr. A. McLean, Department of Diagnostic Imaging, St. Bartholomew's Hospital, London.)

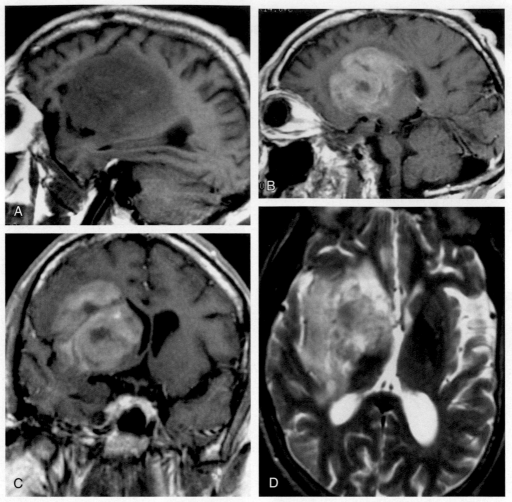

Fig 316–4
Cerebral non-Hodgkin's lymphoma. **A,** T1-weighted (TR = 500, TE = 16) sagittal MRI scan showing a mass of low signal intensity within the right parietal lobe. **B,** This enhances intensely following intravenous administration of gadolinium-DTPA and can be seen to be causing marked mass effect with compression of the right lateral ventricle, both on the contrast-enhanced coronal T1-weighted sequence **(C)** and on an axial T2-weighted (TR = 3800, TE = 95) image **(D)**.
(From Grainger RG, Allison DJ, Adam A, Dixon AK [eds]: Grainger & Allison's Diagnostic Radiology, 4th ed. London, Harcourt, 2001.)

DIFFERENTIAL DIAGNOSIS
- Hodgkin's disease (see Fig. 315–3)
- Viral infections
- Metastatic carcinoma
- Sarcoidosis (see Fig. 137–3)

WORKUP
Initial laboratory evaluation may reveal only mild anemia and elevated LDH and erythrocyte sedimentation rate (ESR). Proper staging of non-Hodgkin's lymphoma requires the following:
- A thorough history, physical examination, and adequate biopsy. Laparoscopic lymph node biopsy can be used on an outpatient basis for most patients with intra-abdominal lymphoma
- Routine laboratory evaluation (CBC, ESR, urinalysis, LDH, BUN, creatinine, serum calcium, uric acid, LFTs, serum protein electrophoresis)
- Chest x-ray (PA and lateral)
- Bone marrow evaluation (aspirate and full bone core biopsy) (Fig. 316–5)
- CT scan of abdomen and pelvis; CT scan of chest (see Fig. 315–4) if chest x-ray films abnormal (Fig. 316–6)
- Bone scan (particularly in patients with histiocytic lymphoma)
- PET scan (Fig. 316–7). Depending on the histopathology, the results of the above studies and the planned therapy, some other tests may be performed.
- β_2-Microglobulin levels should be obtained initially (prognostic value) and serially in patients with low-grade lymphomas (useful to monitor therapeutic response of the tumor).
- Serum interleukin levels have prognostic value in diffuse large cell lymphoma.

CLASSIFICATION
- The Working Formulation of non-Hodgkin's lymphoma for clinical usage subdivides lymphomas into low grade, intermediate grade, high grade, and miscellaneous.

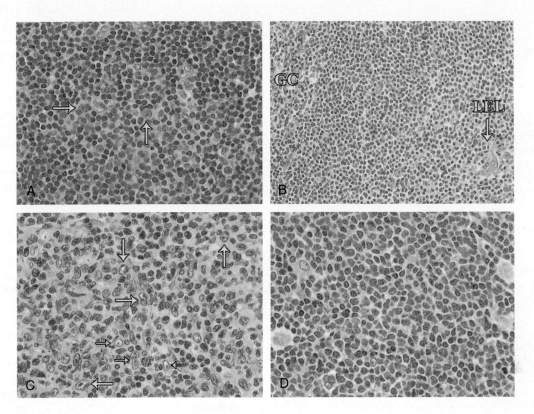

Fig 316–5
Common small B-cell lymphomas. **A,** Small B-cell lymphocytic lymphoma–chronic lymphocytic leukemia, consisting of a diffuse infiltrate of small lymphocytes with scattered prolymphocytes and paraimmunoblasts (*arrows*). **B,** Extranodal marginal zone lymphoma (MALT lymphoma) of the stomach, showing infiltration of the lamina propria by small lymphocytes with irregular nuclei and moderate amounts of clear cytoplasm with destructive infiltration of gastric glands (lymphoepithelial lesion, LEL). A residual germinal center (GC) is seen on the left. **C,** Follicular lymphoma consisting of an admixture of centrocytes (small cleaved cells) and centroblasts (large noncleaved cells) (*long arrows*); nuclei of follicular dendritic cells can also be recognized (*short arrows*). **D,** Mantle cell lymphoma, consisting of an infiltrate of small lymphoid cells with irregular nuclei; scattered histiocytes with abundant eosinophilic cytoplasm are also present.
(From Young NS, Gerson SL, High KA [eds]: Clinical Hematology. St. Louis, Mosby, 2006.)

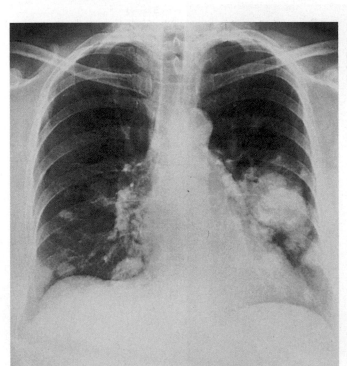

Fig 316–6
Pulmonary involvement by lymphocytic lymphoma showing multiple pulmonary masses.
(From Grainger RG, Allison DJ, Adam A, Dixon AK [eds]: Grainger & Allison's Diagnostic Radiology, 4th ed. London, Harcourt, 2001.)

FDG-PET at diagnosis

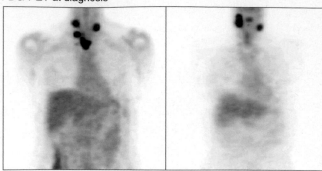

FDG-PET 2 months later after 3 cycles of R-CHOP

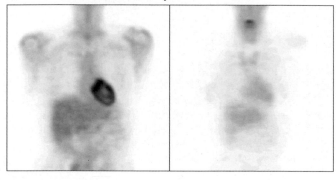

Fig 316–7
Fluorodeoxyglucose–positron emission tomography (FDG-PET) scan before and after treatment with R-CHOP. Resolution of cervical and upper mediastinal disease is shown.
(From Young NS, Gerson SL, High KA [eds]: Clinical Hematology. St. Louis, Mosby, 2006.)

STAGING
- The Ann Arbor classification is used to stage non-Hodgkin's lymphomas. Histopathology has greater therapeutic implications in NHL than in Hodgkin's disease.

TREATMENT
The therapeutic regimen varies with the histologic type and pathologic stage. Following are the commonly used therapeutic modalities.

Low-grade non-Hodgkin's lymphoma (e.g., nodular, poorly differentiated)
- Local radiotherapy for symptomatic obstructive adenopathy
- Deferment of therapy and careful observation in asymptomatic patients
- Chemotherapy

Intermediate- and high-grade lymphomas (e.g., diffuse histiocytic lymphoma)
- Combination chemotherapy regimens

DISPOSITION
- Patients with low-grade lymphoma, despite their long-term survival (6 to 10 years, average), are rarely cured, and the great majority (if not all) eventually die of the lymphoma, whereas patients with a high-grade lymphoma may achieve a cure with aggressive chemotherapy.
- Complete remission occurs in 35% to 50% of patients with intermediate- and high-grade lymphomas. Prognostic factors include the histologic subtype, age of patient, and bulk of disease.

Burkitt's lymphoma

This lymphoma was initially described in African children presenting with jaw tumors and large abdominal tumors (Fig. 316–8) and later found to be associated with the Epstein-Barr virus (EBV). The tumor is composed of medium-sized cells with

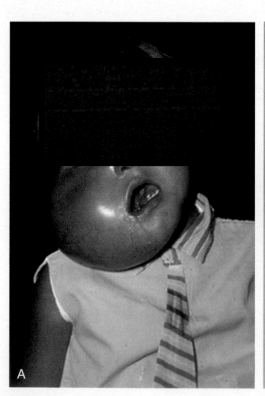

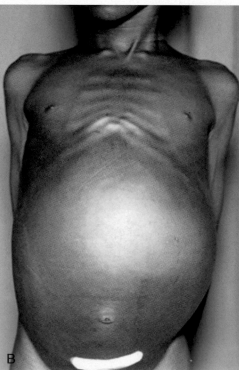

Fig 316–8
Patient with Burkitt's lymphoma involving the jaw **(A)** and the abdomen **(B)**.
(Courtesy of Dr. K. Bathia.)

a high mitotic rate with scattered tangible body macrophages, giving it a starry sky " appearance (Fig. 316–9). This lymphoma can occur sporadically and is found more frequently in immunocompromised hosts (e.g., those with AIDS). It responds well to intensive chemotherapy.

Cutaneous lymphoma (primary cutaneous T cell lymphoma, mycosis fungoides)

- In the skin, primary cutaneous T cell lymphomas (CTCLs; Fig. 316–10) are more common than B cell lymphomas, and mycosis fungoides is the most common form of CTCL.
- Mycosis fungoides refers to a T cell lymphoproliferative disorder with characteristic cutaneous skin lesions and with the potential to disseminate into lymph nodes and viscera.
- Mycosis fungoides characteristically progresses through three phases.
  - Premycotic phase featuring scaly erythematous patches that can last from months to years (Fig. 316–11). During this stage, the diagnosis can only be suspected, because the histopathologic features are not definitive for mycosis fungoides. Lesions are pruritic and can appear anywhere but are usually found in sun-shielded areas.

- Infiltrative plaque phase features raised, indurated, erythematous palpable plaques (Fig. 316–12) that are pruritic and may be associated with alopecia.
  1. Stage IA disease is defined as a patch or plaque skin disease involving less than 10% of the skin surface area.
  2. Stage IB disease is defined as a patch or plaque skin disease involving 10% or more of the skin surface area.
- Tumor phase is characterized by large, lumpy nodules arising from a premycotic patch, plaque, or unaffected skin and represents systemic infiltration and spreading. The tumors can be pruritic and large (more than 10 cm) and ulceration can occur.
  1. Stage II disease is defined by the presence of tumors.
- In approximately 5% of cases of mycosis fungoides, the presentation may be a diffuse, painful, pruritic erythroderma known as *Sézary syndrome* (Fig. 316–13). The peripheral blood smear may reveal Sézary cells (Fig. 316–14)
  1. Stage III disease is defined by the presence of generalized erythroderma.
- Lymphadenopathy can occur during the plaque or tumor stages and may be regional or diffuse.
  1. Stage IVA disease is defined by a lymph node biopsy showing large clusters of atypical cells, more than six cells, or total effacement by atypical cells.
- Infiltration of the liver, spleen, lungs, bone marrow, kidneys, stomach, and brain can occur.
  1. Stage IVB disease is defined by the presence of visceral involvement.

DIAGNOSIS

- Established by skin biopsy. This may be difficult to differentiate from other skin lesions in the early phases of the disease (e.g., premycotic patch or early plaque lesions) and therefore the diagnosis can only be suspected.

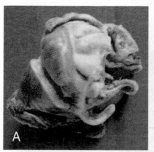
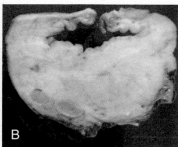
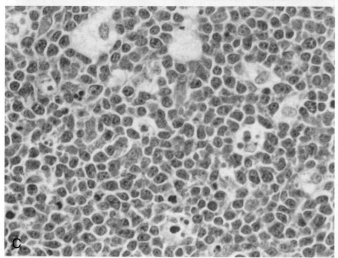

Fig 316–9
Burkitt's lymphoma, sporadic type, in a European child, forming a large ileocecal mass **(A, B)**. The tumor is composed of medium-sized cells with a high mitotic rate, with scattered tingible body macrophages, imparting a so-called starry sky appearance **(C)**.
(From Young NS, Gerson SL, High KA [eds]: Clinical Hematology. St. Louis, Mosby, 2006.)

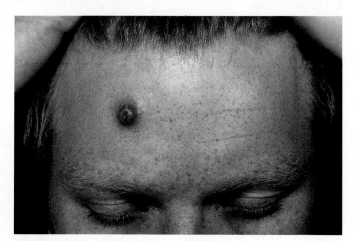

Fig 316–10
Primary cutaneous CD30+ large cell lymphoma—erythematous, ulcerated tumor nodule on the forehead.
(Courtesy of the Institute of Dermatology, London.)

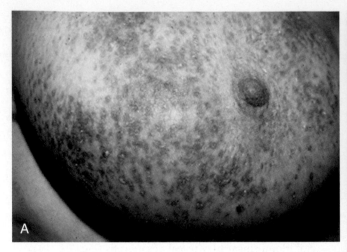

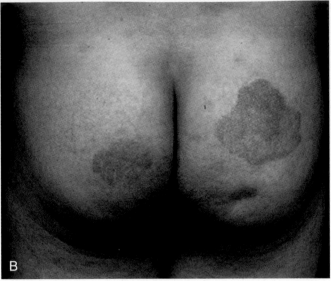

Fig 316–11
Clinical appearance of early mycosis fungoides. **A,** Poikilodermatous patch on the breast showing telangiectasia and epidermal atrophy.
B, Thin plaques of irregular outline on nonexposed sites.
(From Young NS, Gerson SL, High KA [eds]: Clinical Hematology. St. Louis, Mosby, 2006.)

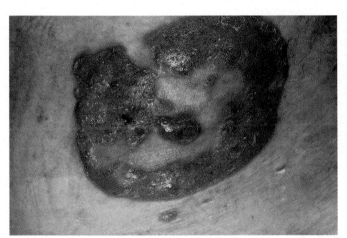

Fig 316–12
Mycosis fungoides, close-up view.
(Courtesy of N. P. Smith, Institute of Dermatology, London.)

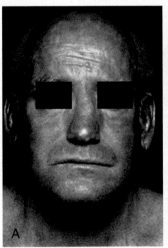

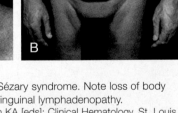

Fig 316–13
A, B, Erythroderma caused by Sézary syndrome. Note loss of body hair, generalized erythema, and inguinal lymphadenopathy.
(From Young NS, Gerson SL, High KA [eds]: Clinical Hematology. St. Louis, Mosby, 2006.)

DIFFERENTIAL DIAGNOSIS

- Contact dermatitis (see Fig. 6–7)
- Atopic dermatitis (see Fig. 6–2)
- Nummular dermatitis (see Fig. 6–5)
- Superficial fungal infections (see Fig. 336–4)
- Drug eruptions (see Fig. 14–1)
- Psoriasis (see Fig. 7–2)
- Photodermatitis (see Fig. 10–2)

TREATMENT

This is guided according to the stage of disease.

- Treatment of patients with Stage IA limited patch or plaque phase include: Topical nitrogen, psoralen plus ultraviolet A (PUVA) light therapy
- Treatment of patients with stage IB or IIA disease is similar to stage IA with topical nitrogen mustard or PUVA.
- Treatment of patients with stage IIB disease with generalized tumor and plaque disease includes skin electron beam therapy followed by adjuvant therapy with topical mustard.

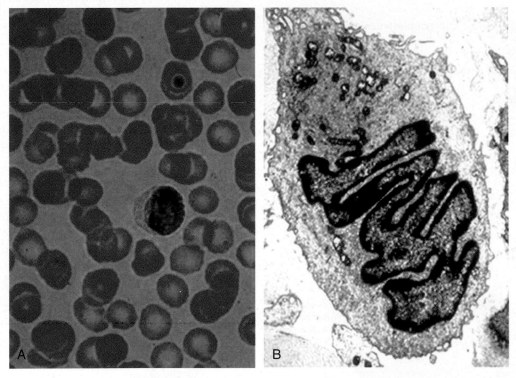

Fig 316–14
Morphology of Sézary cells. **A,** Atypical mononuclear cells on a peripheral blood smear. **B,** Cerebriform nucleus visualized on an ultrathin section. (From Young NS, Gerson SL, High KA [eds]: Clinical Hematology. St. Louis, Mosby, 2006.)

Chapter 317 Hairy cell leukemia

DEFINITION
Hairy cell leukemia is a lymphoid neoplasm characterized by the proliferation of mature B cells with prominent cytoplasmic projections (hairs).

PHYSICAL FINDINGS AND CLINICAL PRESENTATION
See Figure 317–1.
- Usually, splenomegaly (present in more than 90% of cases) secondary to tumor cell infiltration
- Pallor, ecchymosis, and evidence of infection if pancytopenia is severe
- Weakness, lethargy, and fatigue
- Infections (resulting from impaired resistance secondary to neutropenia) and easy bruising (secondary to thrombocytopenia) also common

CAUSE
- Neoplastic disease of the lymphoreticular system of unknown cause

DIFFERENTIAL DIAGNOSIS
  - Other forms of leukemia
  - Lymphoma
  - Viral syndrome

LABORATORY TESTS
- Pancytopenia involving erythrocytes, neutrophils, and platelets is common; anemia is usually present and varies from minimal to severe.
- Hairy cells can account for 5% to 80% of cells in the peripheral blood. The cytoplasmic projections on the cells are redundant plasma membranes (Fig. 317–2).
- Leukemic cells stain positively for tartrate-resistant acid phosphatase (TRAP) stain.
- Bone marrow may result in a dry tap because of increased marrow reticulin.

TREATMENT
- Approximately 8% to 10% of patients are asymptomatic and have minimal splenomegaly and minor cytopenia. They are usually detected on routine laboratory evaluation and do not require initial therapy. They should, however, be frequently monitored for progression of their disease.
- Chemotherapy drugs of choice are the purine analogues 2-chloro-2-deoxyadenosine or 2-deoxycoformycin. They induce complete remissions in up to 85% of patients and partial responses in 5% to 25%.
- The anti-CD 22 recombinant immunotoxin BL 22 can induce complete remission in patients with hairy cell leukemia that is resistant to treatment with purine analogues.

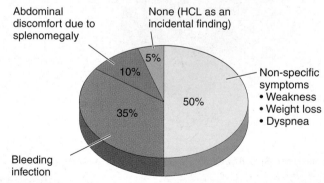

Fig 317–1
Clinical presentations in hairy cell leukemia.
(From Young NS, Gerson SL, High KA [eds]: Clinical Hematology. St. Louis, Mosby, 2006.)

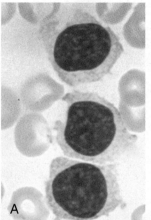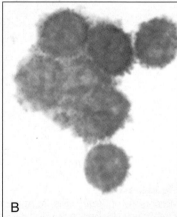

Fig 317–2
Hairy cell leukemia. **A, B,** This composite picture depicts the characteristics of hairy cells. Note the typical evenly distributed nuclear chromatin and hairy cytoplasmic projection. Leukemic cells express CD11c (**A,** Romanowsky stain, ×1000; **B,** immunoalkaline phosphatase stain, ×1000).
(From Silverberg SG, Frable WJ, Wick MR, et al [eds]: Principles and Practice of Surgical Pathology and Cytopathology, 4th ed. Philadelphia, Elsevier, 2006.)

Chapter 318 | **Plasma cell dyscrasias**

A. MULTIPLE MYELOMA

DEFINITION

Multiple myeloma is a malignancy of plasma cells characterized by overproduction of intact monoclonal immunoglobulin or free monoclonal kappa or lambda chains. Diagnostic criteria require the following:

- Presence of more than 10% plasma cells on examination of the bone marrow (or biopsy of a tissue with monoclonal plasma cells)
- Monoclonal protein in the serum or urine. Occasional patients without detectable monoclonal protein are considered to have nonsecretory myeloma.
- Evidence of end-organ damage (calcium elevation, renal insufficiency, anemia, or bone lesions [CRAB])

PHYSICAL FINDINGS AND CLINICAL PRESENTATION

- The median age at diagnosis is 69 years; there is an increased incidence in black men and patients with radiation exposure.
- The patient usually comes to medical attention because of one or more of the following:
  - Bone pain (back, thorax) or pathologic fractures caused by osteolytic lesions or osteoporosis
  - Fatigue or weakness because of anemia resulting from bone marrow infiltration with plasma cells
  - Recurrent infections as a result of multiple factors (e.g., deficiency of normal immunoglobulins, impaired neutrophil function, prolonged physical immobilization); common infecting organisms are *Streptococcus pneumoniae, Staphylococcus aureus, Haemophilus influenzae, Pseudomonas, Escherichia coli,* and *Klebsiella.*
  - Nausea and vomiting caused by constipation and uremia (renal failure resulting from myeloma of kidney [Fig. 318–1], hypercalcemia, amyloidosis, hyperuricemia)
  - Delirium as a result of hypercalcemia from bone resorption resulting from osteoclast-activating factor secreted by myeloma cells (Fig. 318–2) and lysis of bone caused by tumor cell infiltration
  - Neurologic complications, such as spinal cord or nerve root compression, carpal tunnel syndrome secondary to amyloid infiltration, somnolence, blurred vision, or blindness from hyperviscosity
  - Bleeding caused by platelet dysfunction
  - Ecchymoses resulting from amyloid infiltration of capillaries
  - Renal failure

LABORATORY TESTS

- Normochromic, normocytic anemia (60% of patients); rouleaux formation may be seen on peripheral smear (see Fig. 312–4F); thrombocytopenia is observed in 15% of patients at diagnosis.
- Hypercalcemia is present at diagnosis in 20% of cases.
- Elevated BUN, creatinine, uric acid, and total protein levels. Elevated total protein with a normal or low albumin can be a useful diagnostic clue.

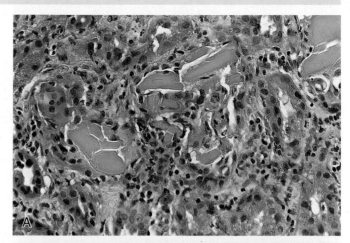
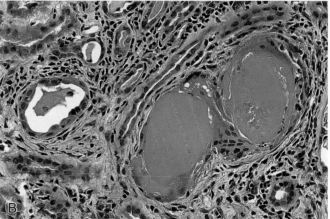
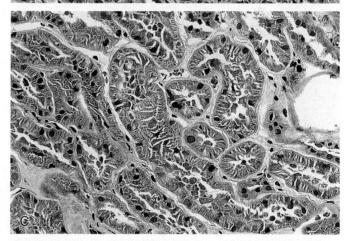

Fig 318–1

Myeloma cast nephropathy. **A,** Numerous hard casts with fracture planes in distal nephrons, typical of myeloma kidney associated with reactive, multinucleated tubular cells **(B)**. **C,** Acute tubulopathy: acute tubular damage (acute tubular necrosis), monoclonal light chain-related (**A,** ×350; **B,** ×500; **C,** ×500).

(From Silverberg SG, Frable WJ, Wick MR, et al [eds]: Principles and Practice of Surgical Pathology and Cytopathology, 4th ed. Philadelphia, Elsevier, 2006.)

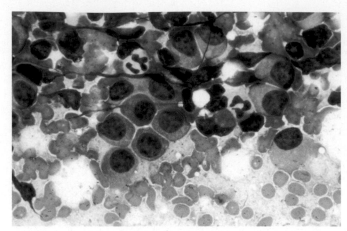

Fig 318–2
The cells of myeloma often have a spoked or cartwheel appearance to the chromatin. The nuclei may be centrally located but are more often placed eccentrically within the cytoplasm (Romanowsky stain).
(From Silverberg SG, Frable WJ, Wick MR, et al [eds]: Principles and Practice of Surgical Pathology and Cytopathology, 4th ed. Philadelphia, Elsevier, 2006.)

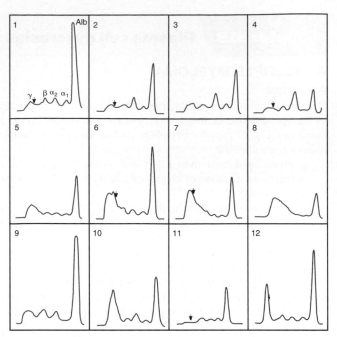

Fig 318–3
Typical serum protein electrophoretic patterns. 1, Normal (*arrow* near gamma region indicates serum application point); 2, acute reaction pattern; 3, acute reaction or nephrotic syndrome; 4, nephrotic syndrome; 5, chronic inflammation, cirrhosis, granulomatous diseases, rheumatoid-collagen group; 6, same as part 5, but gamma elevation is more pronounced, and there is partial (but not complete) beta-gamma fusion; 7, suggestive of cirrhosis but could be found in the granulomatous diseases or the rheumatoid-collagen group; 8, characteristic pattern of cirrhosis; 9, alpha$_1$-antitrypsin deficiency with mild gamma elevation suggesting concurrent chronic disease; 10, same as part 5, but the gamma elevation is marked, the configuration of the gamma peak superficially mimics that of myeloma but is more broad-based, and there are superimposed acute reaction changes; 11, hypogammaglobulinemia or tight-chain myeloma; 12, myeloma, Waldenström's macroglobulinemia, idiopathic or secondary monoclonal gammopathy.
(From Ravel R: Clinical Laboratory Medicine, 6th ed. St. Louis, Mosby, 1995.)

- Proteinuria secondary to overproduction and secretion of free monoclonal kappa or lambda chains (Bence Jones protein)
- Tall homogeneous monoclonal spike (M spike) present on protein immunoelectrophoresis (Fig. 318–3) in approximately 75% of patients; decreased levels of normal immunoglobulins
  - The increased immunoglobulins are generally IgG (75%) or IgA (15%).
  - Approximately 17% of patients have flat level of immunoglobulins but increased light chains in the urine by electrophoresis.
  - A very small percentage (less than 2%) of patients have nonsecreting myeloma (no increase in immunoglobulins and no light chains in the urine) but have other evidence of the disease (e.g., positive bone marrow examination).
- Reduced anion gap resulting from the positive charge of the M proteins and the frequent presence of hyponatremia in myeloma patients.
- Bone marrow examination usually demonstrates nests or sheets of plasma cells; plasma cells usually constitute more than 30% of the bone marrow, and 10% or more are immature.
- Serum hyperviscosity may be present (more common with production of IgA).
- Serum β$_2$-microglobulin has prognostic value because levels greater than 5 mg/L indicate high tumor mass and aggressive disease.
- Elevated serum levels of LDH at the time of diagnosis define a subgroup of myeloma patients with a very poor prognosis.
- Increased interleukin-6 in serum during active stage of myeloma
- The production of DKK1, an inhibitor of osteoblast differentiation, by myeloma cells is associated with the presence of lytic bone lesions in patients with multiple myeloma.

RADIOLOGIC EVALUATION
- X-rays of painful areas usually will demonstrate punched out lytic lesions (70%) (Fig. 318–4).
- Bone scans are not useful because lesions are not blastic.

DIAGNOSTIC CRITERIA
- Presence of 10% or more immature plasma cells in the marrow
- Presence of serum or urinary monoclonal protein
- Osteolytic bone lesions
- Plasmacytomas on tissue biopsy

STAGING
The International Staging System (ISS) divides patients into three distinct stages and prognostic groups solely on the basis of serum β$_2$-microglobulin and albumin level.

Stage I: serum albumin >3.5 g/dL, and serum β$_2$-microglobulin <3.5 μg/mL (median survival, 62 months)

Stage II: neither stage I nor stage III (median survival, 44 months)

Stage III: serum β$_2$-microglobulin >5 μg/mL (median survival, 29 months)

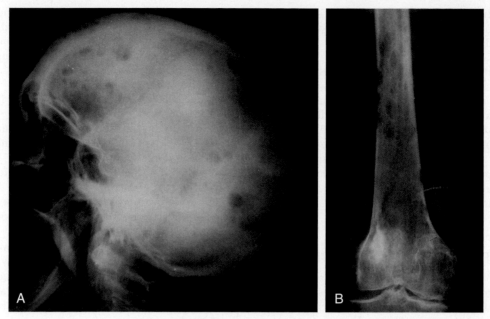

Fig 318–4
Myelomatosis. **A,** Well-defined punched-out lesions are shown in the calvaria. **B,** Discrete round or oval lesions in the femur. The whole marrow is probably infiltrated with myeloma. Visible lesions are those which have eroded the cortex. Similar appearances may occur in carcinomatosis. (From Grainger RG, Alllson DJ, Adam A, Dixon AK [eds]: Grainger & Allison's Diagnostic Radiology, 4th ed. London, Harcourt, 2001.)

TREATMENT
- Newly diagnosed patients with good performance status are best treated with autologous stem cell transplantation (ASCT).
- Induction therapy in patients ineligible for transplantation (old age, coexisting conditions, poor physical conditions) includes the following chemotherapeutic agents:
  1. Thalidomide in combination with melphalan and prednisone.
  2. Melphalan and prednisone: the rates of response to this treatment range from 40% to 60%. Adding continuous low-dose interferon to standard melphalan-prednisone therapy does not improve response rate or survival; however, response duration and plateau phase duration are prolonged by maintenance therapy with interferon.
  3. Vincristine, doxorubicin (Adriamycin), and dexamethasone (VAD) can be used in patients not responding or relapsing after treatment with melphalan and prednisone; methylprednisolone is substituted for dexamethasone (VAMP) in some centers.
- Therapy for relapsed and refractory myeloma
  1. If the relapse occurs more than 6 months after conventional therapy is stopped, the initial chemotherapy regimen can be reinstituted.
  2. Consider autologous stem cell transplantation as salvage therapy in patients who had stem cells cryopreserved early in the course of the disease.
  3. Chemotherapy with vincristine, doxorubicin, and dexamethasone
  4. Thalidomide is also useful to induce responses in patients with multiple myeloma refractory to chemotherapy. Lenalidomide (CC-5013) is an active analogue of thalidomide developed to overcome the toxic effects of thalidomide.

5. Bortezomib is a protease inhibitor that is cytotoxic for multiple myeloma. It is approved for the treatment of refractory multiple myeloma.
- Supportive measures
  1. Control pain with analgesics and radiation therapy to treat painful bone lesions or cord compression. Consider surgical stabilization of pathologic fractures and vertebroplasty or kyphoplasty for select vertebral lesions.
  2. Control hypercalcemia with IV fluids and corticosteroids. The bisphosphonate pamidronate provides significant protection against skeletal complications and improves the quality of life of patients with advanced multiple myeloma. Zoledronic acid has been shown to be as effective as pamidronate in terms of reducing the need for radiation to bone, increasing bone mineral density, and decreasing bone resorption.
  3. Prompt diagnosis and treatment of infections. Common bacterial agents are *S. pneumoniae* and *H. influenzae*. Prophylactic therapy against *Pneumocystis jiroveci* (formerly *P. carinii*) with trimethoprim-sulfamethoxazole must be considered in patients receiving chemotherapy and high-dose corticosteroid regimens.
  4. Prevent renal failure with the following measures:
     a. Adequate hydration
     b. Control hypercalcemia.
     c. Control hyperuricemia (allopurinol and urine alkalinization).
     d. Avoid nephrotoxic agents.(e.g., nonsteroidal anti-inflammatory drugs [NSAIDs]).
     e. Avoid dye contrast studies (e.g., intravenous pyelogram and CT scans with contrast).

5. Erythropoietin therapy or darbepoietin are useful in the treatment of anemia and can decrease the need for transfusion in selected patients.

PROGNOSIS

- The median length of survival after diagnosis is 3 years.
- Prognosis is better in asymptomatic patients with indolent or smoldering myeloma: median survival time is approximately 10 years in persons with no lytic bone lesions and a serum myeloma protein concentration <3 g/dL.
- Adverse outcome is associated with increased levels of β_2-microglobulin, low levels of serum albumin, circulating plasma cells, plasmablastic features in bone marrow, increased plasma cell labeling index, complete deletion of chromosome 13 or its long arm, t(4;14) or t(14;16) translocation, and increased density of bone marrow microvessels.

B. WALDENSTRÖM'S MACROGLOBULINEMIA

DEFINITION

Waldenström's macroglobulinemia (WM) is a plasma cell dyscrasia characterized by the presence of IgM monoclonal macroglobulins.

PHYSICAL FINDINGS AND CLINICAL PRESENTATION

- Fatigue, weight loss, headache, dizziness, vertigo, deafness, and seizures (hyperviscosity syndrome), easy bleeding (e.g., epistaxis)
- Lymphadenopathy (15%), hepatomegaly (20%), splenomegaly (15%)
- Purpura (Fig. 318–5), peripheral neuropathy (5%)

DIAGNOSIS

- The diagnosis of WM is usually established by laboratory blood tests and bone marrow biopsy.
- Symptoms usually occur when the serum viscosity is four times the viscosity of normal serum.

LABORATORY TESTS

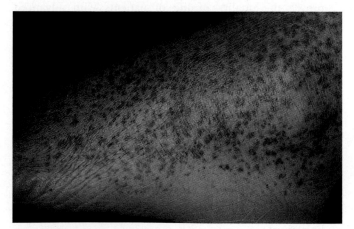

Fig 318–5
Nonpalpable purpura of hyperglobulinemic purpura of Waldenström. (From Hochberg MC, Silman AJ, Smolen JS, et al [eds]: Rheumatology, 3rd ed. St. Louis, Mosby, 2003.)

- CBC with differential: anemia is a common finding, with a median hemoglobin value of approximately 10 g/dL. WBC count is usually normal; thrombocytopenia can occur. Peripheral smear may reveal malignant lymphoid cells in terminal patients.
- Elevated ESR, serum viscosity
- Serum protein immunoelectrophoresis (SPIEP): homogeneous IgM spike
- Urine immunoelectrophoresis: monoclonal light chain usually kappa chains. Bence Jones protein can be seen but is not the typical finding in WM.
- Cryoglobulins, rheumatoid factor, or cold agglutinins may be present.
- Bone marrow biopsy: characteristically reveals lymphoplasmacytoid cells that have infiltrated the bone marrow

TREATMENT

- Asymptomatic patients do not require treatment. These patients should be monitored periodically for the onset of symptoms or changes in blood tests (e.g., worsening anemia, thrombocytopenia, rising IgM, and serum viscosity).
- Symptomatic patients with WM usually receive chemotherapy.

C. MONOCLONAL GAMMOPATHY OF UNDETERMINED SIGNIFICANCE

DEFINITION

Monoclonal gammopathy of undetermined significance (MGUS) is a disorder characterized by a serum M protein concentration less than 3g/dL, less than 10% plasma cells in the bone marrow, absence of anemia, renal insufficiency, hypercalcemia, or bone lesions. M protein may be absent in the urine or present in small amounts.

DEMOGRAPHICS

- Prevalence of MGUS is 1% in patients older than 50 years and 3% in patients older than 70 years.

DIFFERENTIAL DIAGNOSIS

- Multiple myeloma (see Fig. 318–2)
- Macroglobulinemia (see Fig. 318–5)
- Amyloidosis
- Lymphoma (see Fig. 315–2)
- Leukemia (see Fig. 318–8)

CLINICAL APPROACH

- The time interval from the initial diagnosis of MGUS to progression to a more serious disorder ranges from 2 to 29 years (median, 10 years).
- The risk of progression is related to the level of M protein values and to the type of protein (increased risk with higher M protein values and in patients with IgM and IgA M proteins).
- Periodic clinical and laboratory evaluation is recommended.
  - If serum M protein is <2 g/dL, repeat electrophoresis after 6 months; if stable, repeat annually.
  - If serum M protein is >2 g/dL, repeat electrophoresis every 6 months.

Chapter 319   Polycythemia vera

DEFINITION

Polycythemia vera is a chronic myeloproliferative disorder characterized mainly by erythrocytosis (increase in RBC mass). Other clinically important chronic myeloproliferative disorders are chronic myeloid leukemia, *myelofibrosis with myeloid metaplasia* (characterized by massive splenomegaly [Fig. 319–1]), and essential thrombocythemia (Fig. 319–2). Table 319–1 compares important clinical characteristics of chronic myeloproliferative disorders.

DIAGNOSIS

- The JAK_2 mutation is found in >95% of patients with P. Vera. Its presence in patients with polycythemia along with absence of co-existing secondary erythrocytosis is highly suggestive of P. Vera.
- The P. Vera study group requires the following three major criteria or the first two major criteria plus two minor criteria:
  1. Increased RBC mass (>36 mL/kg in men, >32 mL/kg in women)
  2. Normal arterial oxygen saturation (>92%)
  3. Splenomegaly
- Minor criteria
  1. Thrombocytosis (>400,000/mm³)
  2. Leukocytosis (>12,000/mm³)
  3. Elevated leukocyte alkaline phosphatase (>100 U/L)
  4. Elevated serum vitamin B_{12} (>900 pg/mL) or vitamin B_{12} binding protein (>2200 pg/mL)

PHYSICAL FINDINGS AND CLINICAL PRESENTATION

The patient generally comes to medical attention because of symptoms associated with increased blood volume and viscosity or impaired platelet function.

- Impaired cerebral circulation resulting in headache, vertigo, blurred vision, dizziness, TIA, CVA
- Fatigue, poor exercise tolerance
- Pruritus, particularly following bathing (caused by overproduction of histamine)
- Bleeding: epistaxis, upper GI bleeding (increased incidence of peptic ulcer disease [PUD])
- Abdominal discomfort secondary to splenomegaly; hepatomegaly may be present.
- Hyperuricemia may result in nephrolithiasis and gouty arthritis.

  The physical examination may reveal the following:
  - Facial plethora, congestion of oral mucosa, ruddy complexion
  - Enlargement and tortuosity of retinal veins
  - Splenomegaly (found in more than 75% of patients)

DIFFERENTIAL DIAGNOSIS

Smoking

- Laboratory evaluation shows increased Hct, RBC mass, erythropoietin level, and carboxyhemoglobin.
- Splenomegaly is not present on physical examination.

Hypoxemia (secondary polycythemia)

- Living for prolonged periods at high altitudes, pulmonary fibrosis, congenital cardiac lesions with right-to-left shunts

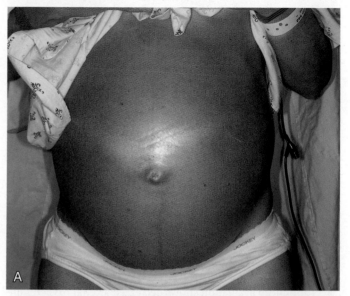
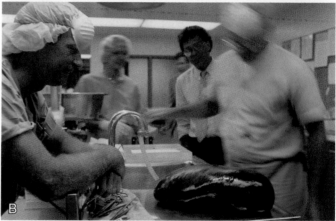
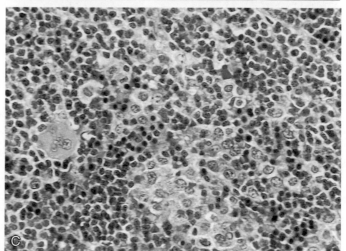

Fig 319–1

A, Massive splenomegaly in a patient with myelofibrosis with myeloid metaplasia. **B,** Surgically removed spleen in myelofibrosis. **C,** Histologic section showing extramedullary hematopoiesis.
(From Young NS, Gerson SL, High KA [eds]: Clinical Hematology. St. Louis, Mosby, 2006.)

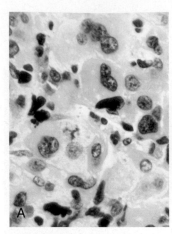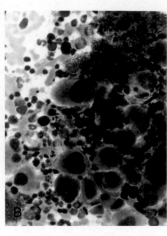

Fig 319-2

A, B, Essential thrombocythemia. Aggregates of megakaryocytes with dysplastic features and clumps of platelets are dominant findings (**A,** H&E stain, ×400; **B,** Romanowsky stain, ×400.).
(From Silverberg SG, Frable WJ, Wick MR, et al [eds]: Principles and Practice of Surgical Pathology and Cytopathology, 4th ed. Philadelphia, Elsevier, 2006.)

- Laboratory evaluation shows decreased arterial oxygen saturation and elevated erythropoietin level.
- Splenomegaly is not present on physical examination.

Erythropoietin-producing states
- Renal cell carcinoma
- Hepatoma
- Cerebral hemangioma
- Uterine fibroids
- Polycystic kidneys

The erythropoietin level is elevated in these patients; the arterial oxygen saturation is normal.
- Splenomegaly may be present with metastatic neoplasms.

Stress polycythemia (Gaisböck's syndrome, relative polycythemia)
- Laboratory evaluation demonstrates normal RBC mass, arterial oxygen saturation, and erythropoietin level; plasma volume is decreased.
- Splenomegaly is not present on physical examination.

Hemoglobinopathies associated with high oxygen affinity
- An abnormal oxyhemoglobin dissociation curve (P50) is present.
- In patients with elevated erythropoietin level, evaluate for secondary erythrocytosis:
- Measure RBC mass by isotope dilution using ^{51}Cr-labeled autologous RBCs (expensive test); a high value eliminates stress polycythemia.
- Measure arterial saturation; a normal value eliminates polycythemia secondary to smoking.
- The diagnosis of hemoglobinopathy with high affinity is ruled out by a normal oxyhemoglobin dissociation curve.

LABORATORY TESTS
- Elevated RBC count (>6 million/mm³), elevated Hgb (>18 g/dL in men, >16 g/dL in women), elevated Hct (>54% in men, >49% in women)
- Increased WBC (often with basophilia); thrombocytosis in the majority of patients
- Elevated leukocyte alkaline phosphatase, serum vitamin B$_{12}$, and uric acid levels
- Low serum erythropoietin level is highly suggestive of polycythemia vera. A normal level does not exclude the diagnosis. If the erythropoietin level is elevated, perform abdominal and pelvic CT to rule out renal cercal carcinoma and other causes of polycythemia.
- Janus kinase 2 mutation (JAK$_2$ VG17F) testing with PCR. Its presence is indicative of P. Vera.
- Bone marrow aspiration revealing RBC hyperplasia and absent iron stores

TREATMENT
- Phlebotomy to keep Hct less than 45% in men and less than 42% in women is the mainstay of therapy.
- Hydroxyurea can be used in conjunction with phlebotomy to decrease the incidence of thrombotic events.
- Interferon alfa-2b is also effective in controlling RBC count without significant side effects.
- Myelosuppressive therapy with chlorambucil is effective but not routinely used because of its leukemogenic potential.

TABLE 319–1 Comparison of important characteristics of chronic myeloproliferative disorders

Characteristic	Polycythemia vera	Chronic myeloid leukemia	Essential thrombocythemia	Chronic idiopathic myelofibrosis
Peripheral blood				
RBC count	↑↑↑	N or ↓	N or ↑	N or ↓
WBC count	N	↑ to ↑↑↑	N	N or ↑
Platelet count	↑↑	N to ↑↑↑	↑↑↑	N or ↑↑
NRBCs	Rare	Occasional	Rare	Many
Anisopoikilocytosis	0 to +	0 to +	0 to +	0 to +++
Bone marrow				
Cellularity	Panhyperplasia, ↓ iron store	Marked myeloid hyperplasia, megakaryocytic hyperplasia	Marked megakaryocytic hyperplasia	Variable; with dysplastic megakaryocytes or dry tap fibrosis
Reticulin fibers				
Early stage	Focal, mild	N to ↑	N	↑ to ↑↑
Late stage	↑↑↑*	↑↑ to ↑↑↑*	N to ↑↑↑*	↑↑↑
Cytogenetic abnormalities	+8, +9, 20q-, or others	Ph chromosome or *BCR-ABL* fusion products	No consistent findings	13q-, 20q-, partial trisomy 1q
Frequency (% of patients)	20-40	>95	5	40-60
Prognosis	Relatively good	Fair to poor	Relatively good	Poor

*Myelofibrosis may develop in 40% of patients with polycythemia vera, 20%-40% with chronic myeloid leukemia, ~5% with essential thrombocythemia.
N, normal; NRBCs, nucleated red blood cells; RBC, red blood cell; WBC, white blood cell.
From Silverberg SG, Frable WJ, Wick MR, et al [eds]: Principles and Practice of Surgical Pathology and Cytopathology, 4th ed. Philadelphia, Elsevier, 2006.

Chapter 320 Thrombocytopenia

DEFINITION
Thrombocytopenia is defined as a platelet count less than 100,000/mm³.

PHYSICAL FINDINGS AND CLINICAL PRESENTATION
- Ecchymoses
- Petechiae (Fig. 320–1)
- Purpura
- Excessive bleeding: menorrhagia, gastrointestinal bleeding, epistaxis

CAUSE
- Increased destruction
- Immunologic
  - Drugs: quinine, quinidine, digitalis, procainamide, thiazide diuretics, sulfonamides, phenytoin, aspirin, penicillin, heparin, gold, meprobamate, sulfa drugs, phenylbutazone, NSAIDs, methyldopa, cimetidine, furosemide, isoniazid, cephalosporins, chlorpropamide, organic arsenicals, chloroquine, platelet glycoprotein IIb/IIIa receptor inhibitors, ranitidine, indomethacin, carboplatin, ticlopidine, clopidogrel
  - Immune thrombocytopenic purpura (ITP): see following discussion.
  - Transfusion reaction: transfusion of platelets with plasminogen activator (PLA) in recipients without PLA-1
  - Fetal-maternal incompatibility
  - Collagen vascular diseases (e.g., systemic lupus erythematosus [SLE])
  - Autoimmune hemolytic anemia
  - Lymphoreticular disorders (e.g., CLL)
- Nonimmunologic
  - Prosthetic heart valves

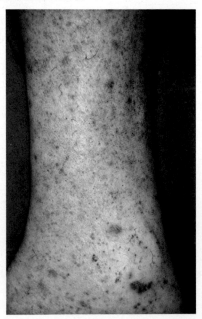

Fig 320–1
Lower extremity petechiae associated with thrombocytopenia.
(From Young NS, Gerson SL, High KA [eds]: Clinical Hematology. St. Louis, Mosby, 2006.)

- Thrombotic thrombocytopenic purpura (TTP)
- Sepsis
- DIC
- Hemolytic-uremic syndrome
- Giant cavernous hemangioma
- Decreased production
  - Abnormal marrow
  - Marrow infiltration (e.g., leukemia, lymphoma, fibrosis)
  - Marrow suppression (e.g., chemotherapy, alcohol, radiation)
  - Hereditary disorders: *Wiskott-Aldrich syndrome*—X-linked disorder characterized by thrombocytopenia, eczema, and repeated infections
  - *May-Hegglin anomaly*: increased megakaryocytes but ineffective thrombopoiesis
  - Vitamin and mineral deficiencies (e.g., vitamin B_{12}, folic acid)
- Splenic sequestration, hypersplenism, chronic liver disease
- Dilutional, as a result of massive transfusion
- A moderate thrombocytopenia (platelet count, 75 to $150 \times 10^3/mm^3$) may be present in healthy women during pregnancy. Such incidental thrombocytopenia during pregnancy generally requires no further investigation other than periodic monitoring of platelet count.

DIAGNOSIS
- Diagnostic approach to undetermined thrombocytopenia (Fig. 320–2)
  - Spurious thrombocytopenia caused by EDTA-induced platelet clumping can be ruled out by repeating the CBC using sodium citrate as an anticoagulant or examining the peripheral blood smear.
  - Thorough history (particularly drug history). The most frequently implicated drugs in pregnancy causing thrombocytopenia are antibiotics (e.g., trimethoprim-sulfamethoxazole), thiazide diuretics, heparin, and NSAIDs.
  - Physical examination: evaluate for presence of splenomegaly (hypersplenism, leukemia, lymphoma).
  - Examine peripheral blood smear. Note platelet size and other abnormalities (e.g., fragmented RBCs may indicate TTP or DIC; increased platelet size suggests accelerated destruction and release of large young platelets into the circulation).
  - Check international normalized ratio (INR), PTT, bleeding time, Coombs' test.
  - LDH (increased in TTP, hemolytic-uremic syndrome [HUS]), haptoglobin (decreased in HUS, TTP)
  - Bone marrow examination: increased megakaryocytes indicate thrombocytopenia resulting from accelerated destruction.

A. Immune thrombocytopenic purpura (ITP)
DEFINITION
ITP is an autoimmune disorder in which antibody-coated or immune complex–coated platelets are destroyed prematurely by the reticuloendothelial system, resulting in peripheral thrombocytopenia.

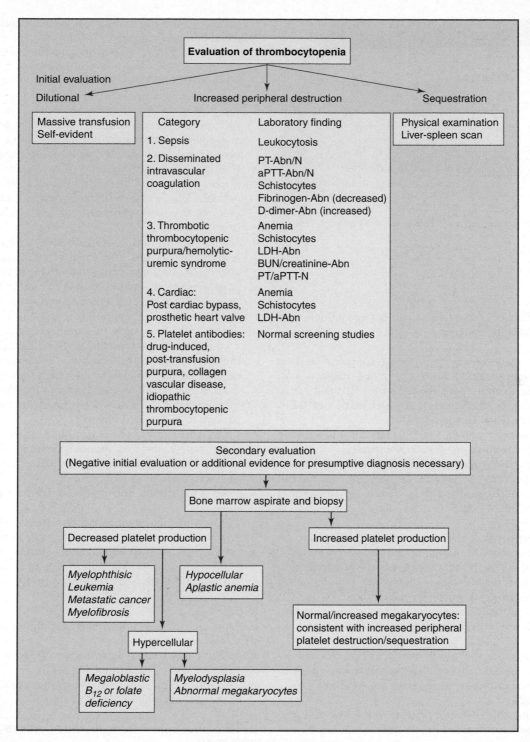

Fig 320–2
Evaluation of thrombocytopenia. Abn, abnormal; aPTT, activated partial thromboplastin time; BUN, blood urea nitrogen; LDH, lactate dehydrogenase; N, normal; PT, prothrombin time.
(From Goldman L, Ausiello D [eds]: Cecil Textbook of Medicine, 22nd ed. Philadelphia, WB Saunders, 2004.)

PHYSICAL FINDINGS AND CLINICAL MANIFESTATIONS
- The physical examination findings may be entirely normal.
- Patients with severe thrombocytopenia may have petechiae, purpura (Fig. 320–3), epistaxis, or heme-positive stool from gastrointestinal bleeding.

- Splenomegaly is unusual; its presence should be a clue to the possibility of other causes of thrombocytopenia.
- The presence of dysmorphic features (e.g., skeletal anomalies, auditory abnormalities) may indicate that a congenital disorder is the cause of the thrombocytopenia.

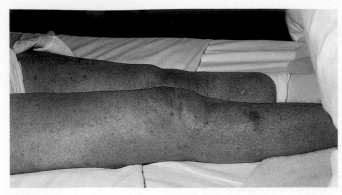

Fig 320-3
Immune thrombocytopenic purpura. These legs show purpura, petechiae and bruising.
(Courtesy of Dr. N. Slater, St. Thomas Hospital, London.)

CAUSE

- Increased platelet destruction caused by autoantibodies to platelet-membrane antigens

DIAGNOSIS

- The history should focus on bleeding symptoms and on excluding other potential causes of thrombocytopenia (e.g., medications, alcohol abuse, risk factors for HIV, family history of hematologic disorders). The presentation of ITP is different in children and adults.
- Children generally present with sudden onset of bruising and petechiae from severe thrombocytopenia.
- In adults, the presentation is insidious; a history of prolonged purpura may be present. In many patients, the disease is diagnosed incidentally by automated laboratories that now routinely include platelet counts.

LABORATORY TESTS

- CBC, platelet count, and peripheral smear: platelets are decreased in number but normal in size or may appear larger than normal. RBCs and WBCs have a normal morphology.
- Additional tests may be ordered to exclude other causes of the thrombocytopenia when clinically indicated (e.g., HIV, antinuclear antibody assessment, thyroid-stimulating hormone [TSH] levels, liver function studies, bone marrow examination).
- The direct assay for the measurement of platelet-bound antibodies has an estimated positive predictive value of 80%. A negative test cannot be used to rule out the diagnosis.

IMAGING STUDIES

- CT of abdomen and pelvis in patients with splenomegaly to exclude other disorders causing thrombocytopenia.

TREATMENT

- Minimize activity to prevent injury or bruising (e.g., contact sports should be avoided).
- Avoid medications that increase the risk of bleeding (e.g., aspirin and other NSAIDs)
- Treatment varies with the platelet count, age of the patient, and bleeding status.
- Observation and frequent monitoring of platelet count in all asymptomatic patients with platelet counts greater than 30,000/mm³
- Methylprednisolone plus IV immunoglobulin and infusion of platelets should be given to patients with neurologic

symptoms, those with internal bleeding, and those undergoing emergency surgery.

- Prednisone, 1 to 1.5 mg/kg daily, continued until the platelet count is normalized, then slowly tapered, is helpful for adults with platelet count below 20,000/mm³ and those who have counts below 50,000/mm³ and significant bleeding. Response rates range from 50% to 75%, and most responses occur within the first 3 weeks. Oral dexamethasone at a dosage of 40 mg/day for 4 consecutive days has also been reported to induce a high response rate (85%)
- High-dose immunoglobulins can be used in children with platelet count below 20,000/mm³ and significant bleeding, or adults with severe thrombocytopenia or bleeding. However, responses are generally transient, lasting no longer than 4 weeks.
- Splenectomy should be considered in adults with platelet count <30,000/ mm³ after 6 weeks of medical treatment or after 6 months if more than 10 to 20 mg of prednisone/day is required to maintain a platelet count >30,000/ mm³. About 75 % of patients who undergo splenectomy achieve complete remission. In children, splenectomy is generally reserved for persistent thrombocytopenia (more than 1 year) and clinically significant bleeding. Appropriate immunizations (pneumococcal, *H. influenzae* vaccine, and meningococcal vaccine) should be administered at least 2 weeks before splenectomy. Splenic irradiation or partial splenic embolization has been used with some success in patients at high risk of surgery
- Rituximab, a monoclonal antibody directed against the CD20 antigen, has been reported useful for ITP patients resistant to conventional treatment and may help prevent serious or fatal bleeding.
- Platelet transfusion only in case of life-threatening hemorrhage
- Chronic: frequent monitoring of platelet count and symptom review in patients with chronic ITP to detect and prevent significant bleeding. Use of danazol, an attenuated androgen, and chemotherapy with cyclophosphamide, vincristine, and prednisone (CVP) has been partially effective in chronic ITP.

PROGNOSIS

- More than 80% of children have a complete remission, usually within a few weeks.
- In adults, the course of the disease is chronic and only 5% of adults have spontaneous remission.
- The principal cause of death from ITP is intracranial hemorrhage (1% of children, 5% of adults).

B. Thrombotic thrombocytopenic purpura

DEFINITION

TTP is a rare disorder characterized by thrombocytopenia and microangiopathic hemolytic anemia. Microthrombi are present and there is extensive purpura (Fig. 320-4).

CAUSE

- In adults, it is usually caused by autoantibody inhibitors of ADAMTS13, a metalloproteinase that cleaves von Willebrand factor multimers.
- It is also caused by severe ADAMTS13 deficiency, thought to lead to the accumulation of unusually large vWF multimers and platelet aggregation.

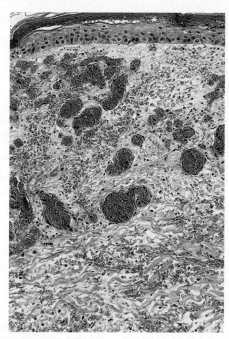

Fig 320-4
Thrombotic thrombocytopenic purpura (TTP). Microthrombi are present and there is extensive purpura.
(From McKee PH, Calonje E, Granter SR [eds]: Pathology of the skin with clinical correlations, 3rd ed. St. Louis, Mosby, 2005.)

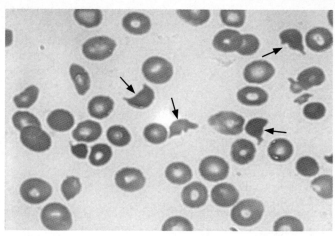

Fig 320-5
Red blood cell fragmentation (schistocytosis). The *arrows* indicate the fragmented red blood cells (schistocytes) in a peripheral blood smear from a 30-year-old man with recurrent thrombotic thrombocytopenic purpura (TTP).
(From Young NS, Gerson SL, High KA [eds]: Clinical Hematology. St. Louis, Mosby, 2006.)

- Many drugs, including clopidogrel, penicillin, antineoplastic agents, oral contraceptives, quinine, and ticlopidine, have been associated with TTP.
- Other precipitating causes include infectious agents, pregnancy, malignancies, allogenic bone marrow transplantation, and neurologic disorders.

PHYSICAL FINDINGS AND CLINICAL PRESENTATION
- Purpura (resulting from thrombocytopenia)
- Jaundice, pallor (resulting from hemolysis)
- Mucosal bleeding
- Fever
- Neurologic symptoms and signs (e.g., fluctuating levels of consciousness)
- Renal failure (resulting from renal cortical infarction and hypertension)
- Hypertension
- There may be clinical overlap with hemolytic-uremic syndrome; however, treatment of this syndrome is similar to treatment of TTP.

LABORATORY TESTS
- Severe anemia and thrombocytopenia
- Elevated BUN and creatinine levels
- Hematuria and proteinuria
- Peripheral blood smear shows severely fragmented RBCs (schistocytes) (Fig. 320-5).
- No laboratory evidence of DIC (normal fibrin degradation product, fibrinogen).

TREATMENT:
- Plasmapheresis with fresh-frozen plasma (FFP) replacement
- Corticosteroids may be effective alone in patients with mild disease or may be administered concomitantly with plasmapheresis plus plasma exchange with FFP.

- Vincristine and cyclosporine can be used in patients whose condition is refractory to plasmapheresis.
- Remission of chronic TTP unresponsive to conventional therapy has been reported after treatment with cyclophosphamide and the monoclonal antibody rituximab.
- Platelet transfusions are contraindicated except in severely thrombocytic patients with documented bleeding.
- Discontinue potential offending agents (e.g., ticlopidine, clopidogrel, penicillin, antineoplastic agents, oral contraceptives).
- Splenectomy in refractory cases. In patients who have had one or more relapses of TTP, splenectomy can also be done during hematologic remission to reduce the frequency of acute relapse and the resulting need for medical therapy.
- Relapse occurs in 20% to 40% of patients who have TTP in remission. Relapsing TTP may be treated with plasma exchange.

C. HELLP syndrome
DEFINITION
The HELLP syndrome is a serious variant of preeclampsia. HELLP is an acronym for **h**emolysis, **e**levated **l**iver function, and **l**ow **p**latelet count. It is the most frequently encountered microangiopathy of pregnancy. There are three classes of the syndrome based on the degree of maternal thrombocytopenia as a primary indicator of disease severity.

Class 1: platelets = 50,000/mm³
Class 2: platelets >50,000 to 100,000/mm³
Class 3: platelets >100,000/mm³

PHYSICAL FINDINGS AND CLINICAL PRESENTATION
- Definitive laboratory criteria remain to be validated prospectively.
- Most commonly used criteria include hemolysis defined by the presence of an abnormal peripheral smear with schistocytes (Fig. 320-6), LDH >600 U/L, and total bilirubin >1.2 mg/dL; elevated liver enzymes—serum aspartate ami-

notransferase (AST) >70 U/L and LDH >600 U/L; low platelet count, less than 100,000/mm³.

- Although many women with HELLP syndrome will be asymptomatic, 80% report right upper quadrant pain and 50% to 60% present with excessive weight gain and worsening edema.

CAUSE

- As with other microangiopathies, endothelial dysfunction, with resultant activation of the intravascular coagulation cascade, has been proposed as the central pathogenesis of HELLP syndrome.

DIFFERENTIAL DIAGNOSIS

- Appendicitis
- Gallbladder disease
- Peptic ulcer disease
- Enteritis
- Hepatitis
- Pyelonephritis
- SLE
- Thrombotic thrombocytopenic purpura–hemolytic-uremic syndrome
- Acute fatty liver of pregnancy

LABORATORY TESTS

- Initial assessment of suspected HELLP syndrome should include CBC to evaluate platelets, urinalysis, serum creatinine, LDH, uric acid, indirect and total bilirubin levels, aspartate transaminase (AST) and alanine aminotransferase (ALT).
- Tests of prothrombin time, partial thromboplastin time, fibrinogen, and fibrin split products are reserved for those women with a platelet count well below 100,000/mm³.

TREATMENT

- Assess gestational age thoroughly. Fetal status should be monitored with nonstress tests, contraction stress tests, and/or biophysical profile.
- Maternal status should be evaluated by history, physical examination, and laboratory testing.
- Magnesium sulfate is administered for seizure prophylaxis regardless of blood pressure.

- Blood pressure control is achieved with agents such as hydralazine or labetalol.
- Indwelling Foley catheter to monitor maternal volume status and urine output

D. Hemolytic-uremic syndrome

DEFINITION

Hemolytic-uremic syndrome (HUS) refers to an acute syndrome characterized by hemolytic anemia, thrombocytopenia, and severe renal failure (Fig. 320–7).

PHYSICAL FINDINGS AND CLINICAL PRESENTATION

- HUS usually preceded by diarrhea in 90% of cases
- Bloody diarrhea (75%)
- Abdominal pain
- Vomiting
- Fever
- Irritability, lethargy, and seizures (10%)
- Hypertension
- Pallor
- Anuria or oliguria

CAUSE

- Pathologically, it is thought that thrombin generation (probably the result of accelerated thrombogenesis) and inhibition of fibrinolysis lead to renal arteriolar and capillary microthrombi preceding renal injury.
- In children
  - E. coli serotype O157:H7 is the leading cause of HUS.
  - The infection is acquired by eating undercooked red meat, especially hamburgers.
- Other causes of HUS in children and adults include the following:
  - Drugs (e.g., cyclosporine, mitomycin, tacrolimus, ticlopidine, clopidogrel, cisplatin, quinine, penicillin, penicillamine, oral contraceptives, quinine used to treat muscle cramps)

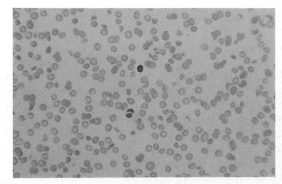

Fig 320–6
Blood film showing microangiopathic hemolytic anemia with fragmentation of red cells.
(From Greer IA, Cameron IT, Kitchner HC, Prentice A: Mosby's Color Atlas and Text of Obstetrics and Gynecology, London, Harcourt, 2001.)

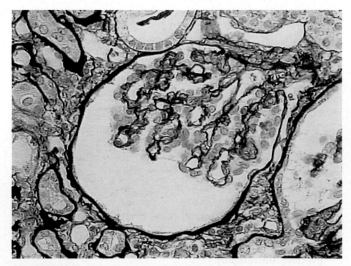

Fig 320–7
Glomerulus from a patient with atypical hemolytic-uremic syndrome with predominant vascular involvement. Severe ischemic changes have occurred. Note the shrinkage of the glomerular tuft and marked thickening and wrinkling of the capillary wall.
(From Johnson RJ, Feehally J: Comprehensive Clinical Nephrology, 2nd ed. St. Louis, Mosby, 2000.)

- Infection (*Salmonella*, *Shigella*, *Yersinia*, group A streptococci, *Clostridium difficile*, *Campylobacter*, coxsackievirus, rubella, influenza virus, EBV)
  - Toxins
  - Pregnancy (usually postpartum) and oral contraceptives
  - HIV-associated thrombotic microangiopathy
  - Pneumococcal infection
- Persons with a relative deficiency in von Willebrand factor–cleaving protease (VMF-CP) are predisposed to nonenteric infection forms of HUS.

DIAGNOSIS
The triad of thrombocytopenia, acute renal failure, and microangiopathic hemolytic anemia establishes the diagnosis of HUS.

DIFFERENTIAL DIAGNOSIS
The differential is vast, including all causes of bloody and nonbloody diarrhea because the GI symptoms usually precede the triad of HUS.
- Thrombotic thrombocytopenic purpura
- Disseminated intravascular coagulation
- Prosthetic valve hemolysis
- Malignant hypertension
- Vasculitis

LABORATORY TESTS
- CBC with hemoglobin <10 g/dL
- Peripheral smear shows the hallmark microangiopathic hemolytic anemia with schistocytes, burr cells, and helmet cells (Fig. 320–8).
- Thrombocytopenia (platelet counts usually <60,000/mm³)
- Reticulocyte count is high.
- LDH level is elevated.
- Haptoglobin is low.
- Indirect bilirubin is elevated.
- BUN and creatinine are elevated.
- Urinalysis reveals proteinuria, microscopic hematuria, and pyuria.
- Stool cultures for *E. coli* O157:H7 are positive in over 90% of cases if obtained during the first week of illness. After the first week, only one third are positive.

TREATMENT
- Blood transfusions for severe anemia
- Antibiotics should be avoided and are not indicated for the treatment of *E. coli* O157:H7.
- Correction of electrolyte abnormalities
- FFP may benefit patients with nonenteric forms of HUS if they are deficient in VMF-CP.

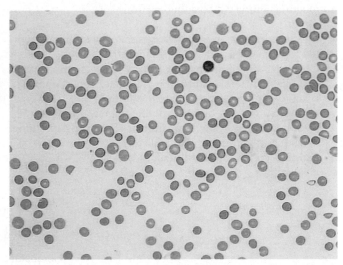

Fig 320–8
Peripheral blood smear from a patient with hemolytic-uremic syndrome. The presence of fragmented red blood cells with the appearance of a helmet is pathognomonic for microangiopathic hemolysis in patients with no evidence of heart valvular disease.
(From Johnson RJ, Feehally J: Comprehensive Clinical Nephrology, 2nd ed. St. Louis, Mosby, 2000.)

Chapter 321   Disseminated intravascular coagulation

DEFINITION
DIC is an acquired thromboembolic disorder characterized by generalized activation of the clotting mechanism, which results in the intravascular formation of fibrin and ultimately thrombotic occlusion of small and midsize vessels. Figure 321–1 describes the mechanisms in DIC.

PHYSICAL FINDINGS AND CLINICAL PRESENTATION
- Wound site bleeding, epistaxis, gingival bleeding, hemorrhagic bullae
- Petechiae, ecchymosis, purpura (Fig. 321–2)
- Dyspnea, localized rales, delirium
- Oliguria, anuria, GI bleeding, metrorrhagia

CAUSE
- Infections (e.g., gram-negative sepsis, Rocky Mountain spotted fever, malaria, viral or fungal infection)
- Obstetric complications (e.g., dead fetus, amniotic fluid embolism, toxemia, abruptio placentae, septic abortion, eclampsia, placenta previa, uterine atony)
- Tissue trauma (e.g., burns, hypothermia rewarming)
- Neoplasms (e.g., adenocarcinomas [GI, prostate, lung, breast], acute promyelocytic leukemia)
- Quinine, cocaine-induced rhabdomyolysis
- Liver failure
- Acute pancreatitis
- Transfusion reactions
- Respiratory distress syndrome
- Toxins (snake bites, amphetamine overdose)
- Other: SLE, vasculitis, aneurysms, polyarteritis, cavernous hemangiomas

DIFFERENTIAL DIAGNOSIS
- Hepatic necrosis: normal or elevated factor VIII concentrations
- Vitamin K deficiency: normal platelet count
- HUS (see Fig. 320–8)
- TTP (see Fig. 320–5)
- Renal failure, SLE, sickle cell crisis, dysfibrinogenemias
- HELLP syndrome (see Fig. 320–6)

LABORATORY TESTS
- Peripheral blood smear generally shows RBC fragments (schistocytes) and low platelet count.
- Coagulation factors are consumed at a rate in excess of the capacity of the liver to synthesize them, and platelets are consumed in excess of the capacity of the bone marrow megakaryocytes to release them. Diagnostic characteristics of DIC are increased prothrombin time (PT), partial throm-

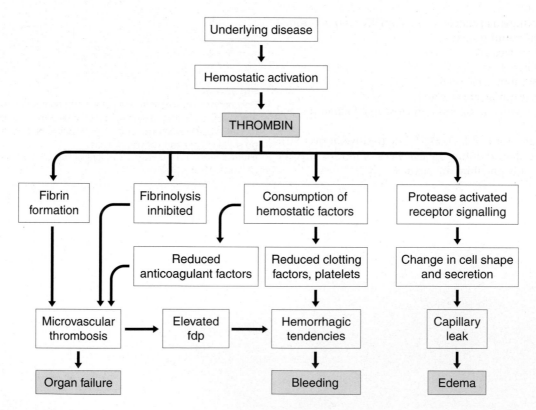

Fig 321–1

Mechanisms in disseminated intravascular coagulation. Systemic activation of hemostatic processes leads to thrombin generation and its consequences, which include intravascular fibrin deposition, depletion of hemostatic factors, and protease-activated receptor-mediated cell signaling responses. As a result, there may be thrombosis of small vessels contributing to organ failure, severe bleeding, capillary leakage, and edema. fdp, fibrin degradation products.

(From Young NS, Gerson SL, High KA [eds]: Clinical Hematology. St. Louis, Mosby, 2006.)

boplastin time (PTT), thrombin time (TT), fibrin split products, D-dimer, decreased fibrinogen level, thrombocytopenia.

- Coagulopathy secondary to DIC must be differentiated from that secondary to liver disease or vitamin K deficiency.

    1. Vitamin K deficiency manifests with prolonged PT and normal PTT, TT, platelet, and fibrinogen level; PTT may be elevated in severe cases.

    2. Patients with liver disease have abnormal PT and PTT; TT and fibrinogen are usually normal unless severe disease is present; platelets are usually normal unless splenomegaly is present.

    3. Factors V and VIII are low in DIC, but normal in liver disease with coagulopathy.

IMAGING STUDIES

Imaging studies are generally not useful. Chest x-ray may be helpful to exclude infectious processes in patients presenting with pulmonary symptoms such as dyspnea, cough, or hemoptysis.

TREATMENT

- Correct and eliminate underlying cause (e.g., antimicrobial therapy for infection, removal of necrotic bowel, evacuation of uterus in obstetric emergencies).
- Give replacement therapy with FFP and platelets in patients with significant hemorrhage:
- Heparin therapy at a dose lower than that used in venous thrombosis (300 to 500 U/hour) may be useful in select cases to increase neutralization of thrombin (e.g., DIC associated with acute promyelocytic leukemia, purpura fulminans, acral ischemia).

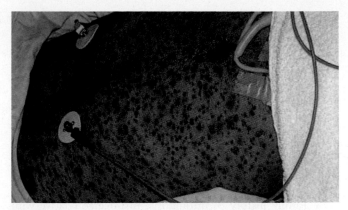

Fig 321–2

Skin lesions in a child with meningococcus sepsis and disseminated intravascular coagulation.

(Courtesy of Dr. Berner, Department for Children and Adolescents, University of Freiburg, Freiburg, Germany.)

Chapter 322   Hypercoagulable state

DEFINITION
A hypercoagulable state is an inherited or acquired condition associated with an increased risk of thrombosis.

HISTORY
A hypercoagulable state is strongly suggested by the following:
- Spontaneous thrombosis (Fig. 322–1): absence of other medical conditions associated with increased risk of thrombosis
- Younger than 50 years at first episode of thrombosis
- Family history of thrombosis: first-degree relative with thrombosis when younger than 50 years
- Recurrent thrombotic events
- Thrombosis in unusual anatomic location (e.g., portal, hepatic, mesenteric, or cerebral vein)
- Thrombosis in pregnancy, postpartum, or associated with oral contraceptive use
- Fetal loss associated with placental infarction, severe or recurrent placental abruption, severe intrauterine growth restriction, severe early-onset preeclampsia
- Warfarin-induced skin necrosis

PHYSICAL FINDINGS AND CLINICAL PRESENTATION
- Inherited thrombophilia is usually associated with venous thrombosis.
- Some acquired thrombophilias are associated with arterial thrombosis.
- Medical conditions associated with increased risk of thrombosis

CAUSE
- Often a multifactorial process with genetic, environmental, and acquired factors
- Multiple genetic factor defects are not uncommon (1% to 2% prevalence); often strong synergistic effect when multiple risk factors are present
- Pregnancy complications may be caused by thrombosis of uteroplacental circulation.

Inherited
FACTOR V LEIDEN (FVL)
- Autosomal dominant mutation with low penetrance
- Causes activated protein C resistance (APCR); 90% of APCR is caused by FVL mutation.
- Most common genetic risk factor for venous thrombosis; accounts for thrombosis in 40% to 50% of inherited cases.
- Oral contraceptive pill (OCP) use in heterozygous carriers is associated with a 35-fold increased risk of thrombosis compared with noncarriers not using OCP.
- May be associated with pregnancy-related complications
- Risk of recurrent thrombotic events not well defined

PROTHROMBIN G20210A MUTATION
- Autosomal dominant mutation with low penetrance
- OCP use in heterozygous carriers is associated with a 16-fold increased risk of thrombosis compared with noncarriers not using OCP
- May be associated with pregnancy-related complications
- Probably low risk of recurrent thrombotic events

PROTEIN C, PROTEIN S, ANTITHROMBIN DEFICIENCY
- Autosomal dominant inheritance.
- Decreased level or abnormal function.
- First episode of thrombosis usually in young adults.
- Increased risk of recurrent thrombosis.
- Associated with an increased risk of venous thrombosis in pregnancy, postpartum (Fig. 322–2) and with OCP use in carriers versus noncarriers
- Associated with adverse pregnancy outcomes

PROTEIN C AND PROTEIN S
- Lifetime risk of thromboembolic event about 50%
- Homozygous condition very rare, usually associated with lethal thrombosis in infancy
- Associated with warfarin-induced skin necrosis, which occurs secondary to depletion of vitamin K–dependent anticoagulant factors sooner than procoagulant factors in the first few days of therapy

ANTITHROMBIN (AT) DEFICIENCY
- Most thrombogenic of the identified inherited factors. The lifetime risk of thromboembolic event is about 70%.
- Homozygous condition very rare, probably not compatible with normal fetal development
- High recurrence risk: about 60% of patients have recurrent thrombosis.
- Can cause heparin resistance

OTHER POSSIBLE CAUSES
- Factor VIII (possibly an important risk factor for thrombosis in blacks)
- Dysfibrinogenemia
- Heparin cofactor II
- Factor XII
- Plasminogen deficiency
- Elevated lipoprotein (a) levels
- Factor IX
- Factor XI

Acquired
ANTIPHOSPHOLIPID ANTIBODY SYNDROME
- Most common cause of acquired thrombophilia
- Can present as arterial or venous thromboembolism or recurrent pregnancy loss
- Thromboembolic events occur in up to 30% of people. There is a high risk of recurrent thrombosis (up to 70% reported).

HYPERHOMOCYSTEINEMIA
- Can be inherited (most commonly an autosomal recessive mutation in methylene tetrahydrofolate reductase gene) but more often secondary to poor dietary intake. Deficiency of folate, vitamin B_6, or vitamin B_{12} accounts for two thirds of cases.
- May be associated with venous and arterial thrombosis, vascular disease, and possibly adverse pregnancy outcomes

MEDICAL CONDITIONS ASSOCIATED WITH INCREASED RISK OF THROMBOSIS
- Trauma
- Chronic medical illness: congestive heart failure (CHF), diabetes mellitus (DM), obesity, nephrotic syndrome, inflammatory bowel disease, paroxysmal nocturnal hemoglobinuria, sickle cell anemia

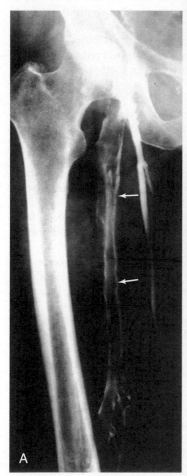

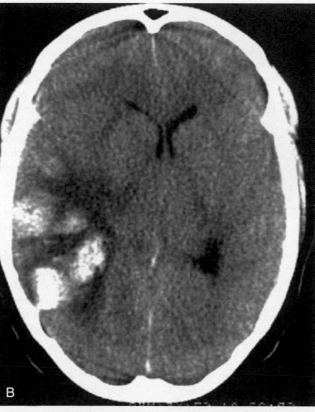

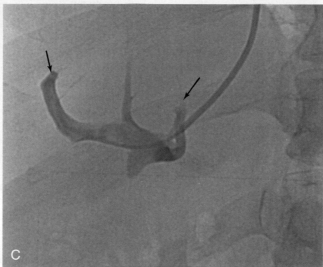

Fig 322–1
Example of venous thrombosis that may occur in patients with inherited thrombophilia. **A,** Deep venous thrombosis of the lower extremity is the most common clinical manifestation of inherited thrombophilia. The *arrows* indicate contrast filling defects in the superficial femoral vein. Thrombosis may also occur at more unusual sites. **B,** Cerebral sinus vein thrombosis, as shown on CT scan of the brain. **C,** Hepatic vein thrombosis in Budd-Chiari syndrome as shown by contrast venography; the *arrows* indicate blockages in the hepatic vein.
(From Young NS, Gerson SL, High KA [eds]: Clinical Hematology. St. Louis, Mosby, 2006.)

- Pregnancy (fivefold increased risk of thrombosis compared with nonpregnant women), postpartum, OCP (fourfold increased risk of thrombosis with OCP use; risk about two times higher with third-generation vs. second-generation OCP), hormone replacement therapy (HRT; twofold increased risk of thrombosis compared with nonusers), tamoxifen
- Immobilization, surgery (especially orthopedic), travel
- Myeloproliferative disorders
- Cancer: disease or treatment related
- Heparin-induced thrombocytopenia and thrombosis
- Cigarette smoking

WORKUP
- History, physical examination, laboratory tests
Note: informed consent should be obtained before genetic testing.
- Timing of workup: ideally 2 weeks after discontinuation of anticoagulation, except for antiphospholipid antibodies, because this will influence duration of anticoagulation.
- Varying recommendations on extent of workup; little cost-effectiveness and outcomes data. It is currently not recommended that individuals with medical conditions associated with increased risk of thrombosis be screened for inherited or acquired defects. A notable exception is made for thrombosis associated with pregnancy, postpartum, or OCP use.

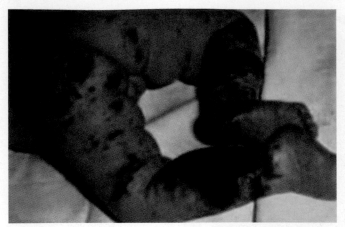

Fig 322–2
Purpura fulminans in a baby with homozygous protein C deficiency.
(From Young NS, Gerson SL, High KA [eds]: Clinical Hematology. St. Louis, Mosby, 2006.)

- Unprovoked venous thrombosis
    - Screen individuals for protein C, protein S, antithrombin deficiency, FVL, prothrombin G20210A mutation, hyperhomocysteinemia, and antiphospholipid antibodies if any of the following are present: younger than 50 years at first episode of thrombosis, family history of thrombosis, recurrent thrombotic events, thrombosis in unusual anatomic location, life-threatening thrombotic event, warfarin-induced skin necrosis, thrombosis in pregnancy, postpartum, with OCP use or characteristic pregnancy complications
    - Screen all white individuals and all women on HRT for FVL, prothrombin G20210A mutation, hyperhomocysteinemia, and antiphospholipid antibodies.
    - Screen all others for hyperhomocysteinemia and antiphospholipid antibodies.
- Arterial thrombosis
    - Screen for antiphospholipid antibody syndromes and hyperhomocysteinemia.

LABORATORY TESTS

- CBC, electrolytes, renal function, liver function tests, PT, PTT, urinalysis

Note: Acute thrombosis, anticoagulation, and many medical conditions can affect the results and must be considered in the interpretation of the workup.

- APCR: screen with second-generation clotting assay (using factor V–deficient plasma); in pregnancy, use genetic test for FVL mutation (polymerase chain reaction [PCR]).
- Prothrombin G20210A mutation: genetic test (PCR)
- Antithrombin deficiency: screen with functional assay (AT heparin cofactor assay). Immunologic assay may be used to differentiate types of AT deficiency.
- Protein C deficiency: functional assay (level and activity) and immunologic assay (level). Functional assay may be false-positive if APCR or elevated factor VIII level is present. Results may be unreliable if lupus anticoagulant (Fig. 322–3) is present.

- Protein S deficiency: screen with measurement of free and total levels; functional assay (level and activity) and immunologic assay (free and total level). Results of functional assay are affected by the presence of APCR and lupus anticoagulant.
- Antiphospholipid antibody syndrome: either of the following found on two occasions at least 6 weeks apart—lupus anticoagulant (clotting assay) or anticardiolipin antibody (IgG and/or IgM).
- Hyperhomocysteinemia: fasting plasma homocysteine level; if normal, but suspicion is high, can proceed with methionine loading test and genotyping for methylene tetrahydrofolate reductase).

IMAGING STUDIES

- As appropriate to diagnose thrombosis and rule out medical conditions associated with increased thrombotic risk

TREATMENT

- OCP, HRT use, smoking should be avoided
- Symptomatic and asymptomatic carriers (identified by family screening) should receive prophylactic anticoagulation in high-risk situations.
- Patients with antithrombin deficiency may benefit from antithrombin concentrates in the perioperative and postoperative periods.
- Patients with hyperhomocysteinemia should receive folic acid supplement (and vitamins B_6 and B_{12} if deficient); this may decrease risk of thrombosis by decreasing plasma homocysteine levels.
- Pregnancy prophylaxis: timing and intensity of therapy are based on the patient's risk (genetic or acquired defect and clinical history).
- Initial therapy is the same as for individuals without thrombophilia.

Venous thrombosis
- Unfractionated heparin or low-molecular-weight heparin (LMWH) followed by warfarin. Continue heparin for at least 5 days or until INR is therapeutic for 48 hours; continue warfarin for 6 months. Aim for an INR of 2 to 3. The intensity of anticoagulation is not affected by the presence of thrombophilia.
- In pregnancy, full heparin anticoagulation for at least 20 weeks, followed by prophylactic heparin for the remainder of the pregnancy. Prophylaxis with heparin or warfarin should be continued for at least 6 weeks postpartum.

Arterial thrombosis
- Anticoagulation and surgical consult for definitive procedure

Protein C deficiency
- Warfarin-induced skin necrosis: after full heparin or LMWH anticoagulation, begin gradual warfarin loading (2 mg/day for 3 days; increase by 2 to 3 mg/day until target INR is reached). Continue heparin for 5 to 7 days until warfarin-induced anticoagulation is achieved.
- Protein C concentrates may be used for deficiency states.

AT deficiency
- AT concentrates may be used if difficulty achieving anticoagulation (heparin resistance), severe thrombosis, or recurrent thrombosis despite adequate anticoagulation
- Lupus anticoagulant (Fig. 322–4)

● LMWH or unfractionated heparin (check heparin levels or antifactor Xa activity) followed by warfarin (INR, 3 to 3.5).

● Duration of therapy

● Must consider risks and benefits: risk of major bleeding 2% to 3%/year in general population on anticoagulation but as high as 7% to 9%/year in older patients.

● Indefinite anticoagulation is suggested if

● One spontaneous thrombosis associated with any of the following:

1. Life-threatening thrombosis
2. More than one genetic defect
3. Presence of antithrombin deficiency or antiphospholipid antibodies

● Two or more spontaneous thromboses

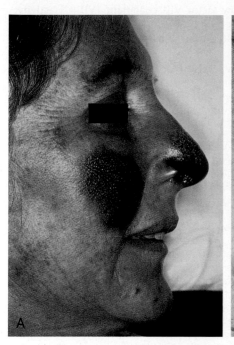
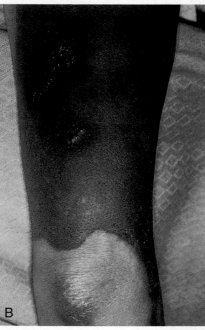

Fig 322–3
Lupus anticoagulant syndrome—extensive gangrene with ulceration affecting the nose **(A)** and cheek, and leg **(B)**.
(Courtesy of Dr. C. Stephens, Poole Hospital, Poole, England.)

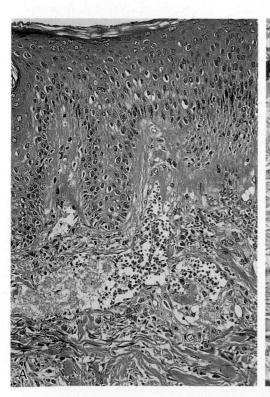
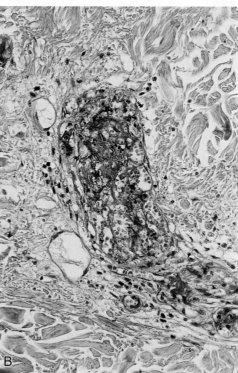

Fig 322–4
Lupus anticoagulant syndrome.
A, Close-up view of occluded vessel. Note the absence of inflammatory changes. **B,** The presence of fibrin is confirmed in this section (phospho-tungstic acid–H&E stain).
(From McKee PH, Calonje E, Granter SR [eds]: Pathology of the skin with clinical correlations, 3rd ed. St. Louis, Mosby, 2005.)

Chapter 323   Hemophilias

DEFINITION
Hemophilia is a hereditary bleeding disorder caused by low factor VIII coagulant activity (hemophilia A) or low levels of factor IX coagulant activity (hemophilia B). Figure 323–1 illustrates the schema of hemostasis and the coagulation cascade.

PHYSICAL FINDINGS AND CLINICAL PRESENTATION
- The clinical features of hemophilias A and B are generally indistinguishable from each other.
- Bleeding is most commonly seen in joints (knees, ankles, elbows) resulting in hot, swollen, painful joints and subsequent crippling joint deformity (Fig. 323–2).
- Bleeding can also occur into the muscles (Fig. 323–3) and the GI tract.
- Compartment syndromes can occur from large hematomas.
- Hematuria may be present.

CAUSE
- Hemophilia A: low factor VIII coagulant (VIII:C) activity; can be classified as mild if factor VIII:C levels are more than 5%, as moderate if levels are 1% to 5%, as severe if levels are less than 1%.
- Hemophilia B: low levels of factor IX coagulant activity

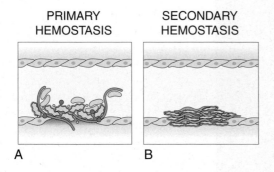

PRIMARY HEMOSTASIS   SECONDARY HEMOSTASIS

A   B

THE COAGULATION SYSTEM

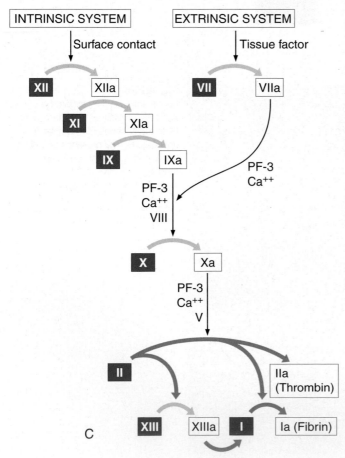

Fig 323–1
A, Schema of primary hemostasis. When vessel injury occurs, von Willebrand factor adheres to the damaged vascular endothelium and serves as a tissue glue to allow platelets to stick to the damaged vessel. Platelets become activated, as small amounts of thrombin (a potent aggregating agent) are formed through activation of the coagulation system through interaction of tissue factor VIIa with damaged vascular endothelium and surface contact (see **C**). Activated platelets adhere to the damaged vascular endothelium, platelet adhesion, and then begin to stick to each other, platelet aggregation. The platelet release reaction occurs, with release of ADP. This series of events serves to allow temporary and early hemostasis through platelet plug formation. The plug becomes stronger and smaller through the action of thrombosthenin, the actin-myosin–like protein, and stops the initial loss of blood. **B,** Schema of secondary hemostasis. The sequence of events following injury and initial formation of the platelet plug and activation of the coagulation cascade include formation of fibrin fibrils on the platelet phospholipid surface, lending strength to the temporary platelet plug structure. Once fibrin becomes cross-linked with factor XIII, or fibrin-stabilizing factor, the clot becomes stronger and secondary hemostasis is achieved. **C,** Coagulation cascade. When vessel injury occurs, as the tissue factor VIIA complex is activated through damaged vascular endothelium, the extrinsic system is activated, with activation of factor X. The intrinsic system is activated through surface contact with factor XI, with subsequent activation of factors IX and VIII, and subsequent activation of the common pathway through factor X. This then activates factors V and II, with subsequent formation of thrombin (IIa) and subsequently fibrin (Ia). This series of linked coagulation reactions, the coagulation cascade, occurs on the platelet-phospholipid surface.
(From Young NS, Gerson SL, High KA [eds]: Clinical Hematology. St. Louis, Mosby, 2006.)

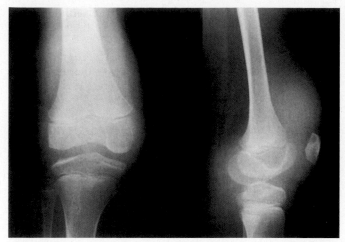

Fig 323–2
Radiograph showing subacute hemophilic arthropathy. There is synovial thickening and radiologic density caused by iron deposition. (From Hochberg MC, Silman AJ, Smolen JS, et al [eds]: Rheumatology, 3rd ed. St. Louis, Mosby, 2003.)

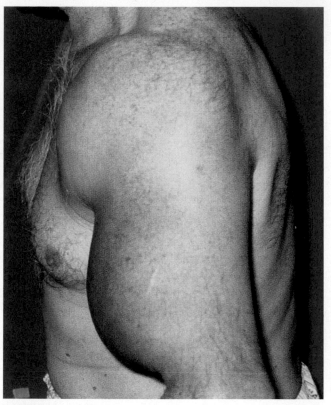

Fig 323–3
Hemocyst, left upper arm.
(From Hochberg MC, Silman AJ, Smolen JS, et al [eds]: Rheumatology, 3rd ed. St. Louis, Mosby, 2003.)

TABLE 323–1 Differential diagnosis of hemophilia

Feature	aPTT	aPTT 1:1 mix	PT	Closure time	Bleeding symptoms
Factor VIII, IX, XI deficiency	↑	nl	nl	nl	Yes
Factor XII deficiency	↑	nl	nl	nl	No
von Willebrand disease	↑	nl	nl	↑	Yes
Lupus anticoagulant	↑	↑	nl	nl	No
Acquired hemophilia (anti–factor VIII)	↑	↑	nl	nl	Yes
Heparin effect	↑	↑	nl	nl	±
Vitamin K deficiency	↑	nl	↑	nl	±
Liver disease	↑	nl	↑	±	±
Disseminated intravascular coagulation	↑	nl	↑	↑	Yes

aPTT, activated partial thromboplastin time; nl, normal; PT, prothrombin time.
From Young NS, Gerson SL, High KA (eds): Clinical Hematology. St. Louis, 2006, Mosby, 2006.

- Both disorders are congenital.
- Spontaneous acquisition of factor VIII inhibitors (acquired hemophilia) is rare.

DIFFERENTIAL DIAGNOSIS
- Other clotting factor deficiencies (Table 323–1)
- Platelet function disorders
- Vitamin K deficiency

LABORATORY TESTS
- PTT is prolonged.
- Reduced factor VIII:C level distinguishes hemophilia A from other causes of prolonged PTT.

- Factor VIII antigen, PT, fibrinogen level, and bleeding time are normal.
- Factor IX coagulant activity levels are reduced in patients with hemophilia B.
- Coagulation factor activity measurement is useful to correlate with disease severity. Normal range is 50 to 150 U/dL, 5 to 20 U/dL indicates mild disease, 2 to 5 U/dL indicates moderate disease, and less than 2 U/dL indicates severe disease with spontaneous bleeding episodes.

TREATMENT
- Avoidance of contact sports
- Patient education regarding the disease, promotion of exercises such as swimming
- Avoidance of aspirin or other NSAIDs
- Orthopedic evaluation and physical therapy evaluation in patients with joint involvement
- Hepatitis vaccination

Hemophilia A
- Reversal and prevention of acute bleeding in hemophilias A and B are based on adequate replacement of deficient or missing factor protein.
- The choice of the product for replacement therapy is guided by availability, capacity, concerns, and cost. Recombinant factors cost two to three times as much as plasma-derived factors, and the limited capacity to produce recombinant factors often results in periods of shortage. In the United States, 60% of patients with severe hemophilia use recombinant products.
- Factor VIII concentrates are effective in controlling spontaneous and traumatic hemorrhage in severe hemophilia.

The new recombinant factor VIII is stable, without added human serum albumin (decreased risk of transmission of infectious agents).
- Recombinant activated factor VII is useful to stop spontaneous hemorrhages and prevent excessive bleeding during surgery in 75% of patients with inhibitors.
- Desmopressin acetate (causes release of factor VIII:C) may be used in preparation for minor surgical procedures in mild hemophiliacs.
- Aminocaproic acid can be given for persistent bleeding that is unresponsive to factor VIII concentrate or desmopressin.

Hemophilia B
- Infuse factor IX concentrates. It is important to remember that factor IX concentrates contain other proteins that may increase the risk of thrombosis with recurrent use. Therefore, factor IX concentrates must be used only when clearly indicated.
- Daily administration of oral cyclophosphamide and prednisone without empirical factor VIII therapy is an effective and well-tolerated treatment for acquired hemophilia.

Chapter 324 / Von Willebrand's disease

DEFINITION

Von Willebrand's disease is a congenital disorder of hemostasis characterized by defective or deficient von Willebrand factor (vWF). There are several subtypes of von Willebrand's disease:

- The most common type (80% of cases) is type I, which is caused by a quantitative decrease in von Willebrand factor;
- Types IIA and IIB are caused by qualitative protein abnormalities.
- Type III is a rare autosomal recessive disorder characterized by an almost complete quantitative deficiency of vWF.

Table 324-1 describes classification of vWD. Acquired von Willebrand's disease (AvWD) is a rare disorder that usually occurs in older patients and generally presents with mucocutaneous bleeding abnormalities and no clinically meaningful family history. It is often accompanied by a hematoproliferative or autoimmune disorder. Successful treatment of the associated illness can reverse the clinical and laboratory manifestations.

PHYSICAL FINDINGS AND CLINICAL PRESENTATION

- Generally normal physical examination
- Mucosal bleeding (gingival bleeding, epistaxis) and GI bleeding may occur.
- Easy bruising (Fig. 324–1)
- Postpartum bleeding, bleeding after surgery or dental extraction, menorrhagia

CAUSE

- Quantitative or qualitative deficiency of vWF

DIFFERENTIAL DIAGNOSIS

- Platelet function disorders
- Clotting factor deficiencies (see Table 323–1)

LABORATORY TESTS

- Normal platelet number and morphology
- Prolonged bleeding time
- Decreased factor VIII coagulant activity
- Decreased von Willebrand factor antigen or ristocetin cofactor
- Normal platelet aggregation studies
- Type II A von Willebrand's disease can be distinguished from type I by absence of ristocetin cofactor activity and abnormal multimer.
- Type IIB von Willebrand's disease is distinguished from type I by abnormal multimer.

TABLE 324–1 Classification of von Willebrand's disease (vWD)

vWD Classification	Description	Inheritance	Laboratory Findings	Multimer Analysis	Prevalence
		Features			
Type 1	Partial quantitative deficiency of VWF; mild to moderate phenotype	Autosomal dominant	Parallel reductions in VWF antigen, VWF activity, and factor VIII	Normal distribution	70%-80%
Type 2A	Qualitative VWF defect caused by missense mutations within the A2 domain; moderate to severe phenotype	Autosomal dominant	Reduced VWF activity to antigen ratio (<0.6)	Loss of midsized and highest molecular weight multimers	10%-15%
Type 2B	Qualitative VWF defect caused by increased binding to platelet GPIb; moderate to severe phenotype	Autosomal dominant	Reduced VWF activity to antigen ratio (<0.6); abnormal RIPA	Loss of highest molecular weight multimers as a result of binding to platelets and clearance	~5%
Type 2M	Qualitative defects in platelet-VWF interaction	Autosomal dominant	Reduced VWF activity to antigen ratio (<0.6)	Normal distribution	Rare
Type 2N	Qualitative defect results in decreased VWF binding of factor VIII; phenotype resembles moderate hemophilia A	Autosomal dominant	Reduced factor VIII level (2%-10%)	Normal distribution	Rare
Type 3	Severe quantitative defect of VWF	Autosomal dominant	Marked reductions or absence in VWF levels; low factor VIII (5%-10%)	Absent	Rare

RIPA, ristocetin-induced platelet aggregation; VWF, von Willebrand factor..
From Young NS, Gerson SL, High KA (eds): Clinical Hematology. St. Louis, 2006, Mosby, 2006.

TREATMENT

- Avoidance of aspirin and other NSAIDs
- Evaluation for likelihood of bleeding (with measurement of bleeding time) before surgical procedures. When a patient undergoes surgery or receives repeated therapeutic doses of concentrates, factor VIII activity should be assayed every 12 hours on the day a dose is administered and every 24 hours thereafter.
- The mainstay of treatment in von Willebrand's disease is the replacement of the deficient protein at the time of spontaneous bleeding, or before invasive procedures are performed.
- Desmopressin acetate (DDAVP) is useful to release stored vWF from endothelial cells. It is used to cover minor procedures and traumatic bleeding in mild type I von Willebrand's disease. DDAVP is not effective in type IIA von Willebrand's disease and is potentially dangerous in type IIB (increased risk of bleeding and thrombocytopenia).
- In patients with severe disease, replacement therapy in the form of cryoprecipitate is the method of choice. The standard dose is one bag of cryoprecipitate/10 kg of body weight.
- Factor VIII concentrate rich in vWF (Humate-P) is useful to correct bleeding abnormalities in types IIA, IIB, and III von Willebrand's disease without alloantibodies. Alloantibodies that inactivate von Willebrand factor and form circulating immune complexes develop in 15% of patients with type III von Willebrand's disease who have received multiple transfusions. In these patients, recombinant factor VIII is preferred because autoantibodies can elicit life-threatening anaphylactic reactions caused by complement activation by immune complexes.
- Life-threatening hemorrhage unresponsive to therapy with cryoprecipitate or factor VIII concentrate may require transfusion of normal platelets.

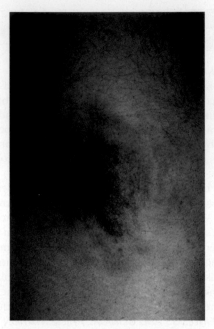

Fig 324–1
Deep hematoma associated with muscular bleed.
(From Young NS, Gerson SL, High KA [eds]: Clinical Hematology. St. Louis, Mosby, 2006.)

Chapter 325 | Felty's syndrome

DEFINITION

Felty's syndrome (FS) is defined as the triad of rheumatoid arthritis (RA), splenomegaly, and granulocytopenia. The hallmark of FS is a persistent idiopathic granulocytopenia, which is defined as a neutrophil count of less than 2000/mm³. Splenomegaly is extremely variable in its extent and varies over time. It is an extra-articular manifestation of seropositive RA in which recurrent local and systemic infections are the major sources of morbidity and mortality.

CLINICAL PRESENTATION

- Rarely, splenomegaly and granulocytopenia are present before the arthritis.
- Articular involvement is usually more severe in patients with FS as compared with other patients with RA; however, one third may have relatively inactive synovitis with an elevated ESR.
- The degree of splenomegaly varies and may be detectable only by imaging studies.
- The degree of splenomegaly has no correlation with the degree of granulocytopenia.
- Patients with FS have a greater frequency of extra-articular manifestations (e.g., nodules, weight loss, Sjögren's syndrome) than other patients with RA.
- Approximately 25% of patients have refractory leg ulcers, often associated with hyperpigmentation of the anterior tibia.
- Mild hepatomegaly is common (up to 68%).
- Patients with FS have a 20-fold increased frequency of infections compared with other RA patients.

CAUSE

- The pathogenesis of FS is probably multifactorial and no clear explanation has been elucidated.

DIFFERENTIAL DIAGNOSIS

- SLE
- Drug reaction
- Myeloproliferative disorders
- Lymphoma, reticuloendothelial malignancies
- Hepatic cirrhosis with portal hypertension
- Sarcoidosis
- Tuberculosis
- Amyloidosis
- Chronic infections

LABORATORY TESTS

- Complete blood count with differential to detect large granular lymphocytes (Fig. 325–1), granulocytopenia, mild to moderate anemia, and mild to moderate thrombocytopenia
- ESR

- Bone marrow biopsy in most patients will show myeloid hyperplasia with an excess of immature granulocyte precursors (maturation arrest).
- Rheumatoid factor: positive in 98%, usually high titer
- ANA: positive in 67%
- Antihistone antibody: positive in 83%
- Antineutrophil cytoplasmic antibodies (77%)
- HLA-DR4: positive in 95%
- Immunoglobulins: level may be higher than in RA patients.
- Complement: level may be lower than in RA patients.

IMAGING STUDIES

- Ultrasonography or CT may be useful in diagnosing splenomegaly.

TREATMENT

- Splenectomy
- Corticosteroids
- Antirheumatic drugs: second-line drugs may improve the granulocytopenia in FS.
- Recombinant G-CSF
- Other immunosuppressants: limited experience with cyclophosphamide, cyclosporine, azathioprine, leflunomide, anti–tumor necrosis factor α antibody.

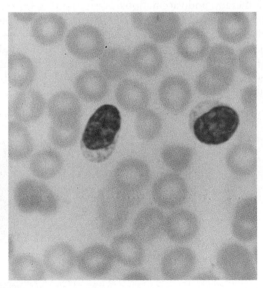

Fig 325–1
Large granular lymphocytes.
(From Hochberg MC, Silman AJ, Smolen JS, et al [eds]: Rheumatology, 3rd ed. St. Louis, Mosby, 2003.)

Chapter 326 Paroxysmal nocturnal hemoglobinuria

DEFINITION

Paroxysmal nocturnal hemoglobinuria (PNH) is a rare disease characterized by episodes of intravascular hemolysis and hemoglobinuria, usually occurring at night. Thrombocytopenia, leukopenia, and recurrent venous thrombosis are also associated with PNH.

PHYSICAL FINDINGS AND CLINICAL PRESENTATION

- Initial manifestations
  - Anemia symptoms (35%)
  - Hemoglobinuria (25%)
  - Bleeding (20%)
  - Aplastic anemia (15%)
  - GI symptoms (10%)
  - Hemolytic anemia (10%)
  - Iron deficiency anemia (5%)
  - Venous thrombosis (5%)
  - Infections (5%)
  - Neurologic symptoms
- Hemoglobinuria: typically, the first morning void reveals dark urine with progressive clearing during the day (Fig. 326–1). The cause for the circadian rhythm is unknown.
- Hemolysis
  - In addition to the circadian hemolysis and resulting hemoglobinuria, episodes of hemolytic exacerbations can accompany infections, menstruation, transfusion, surgery, iron therapy, and vaccinations.
  - Symptoms of severe hemolysis include chest, back, or abdominal pain, headache, fever, malaise, and fatigue.
- Aplastic anemia: may be the presenting manifestation of PNH (therefore, PNH must be in the differential diagnosis of aplastic anemia) or may develop as a later complication of PNH.

- Thrombosis
  - Lower extremity deep venous thrombosis (DVT)
  - Subclavian thrombosis
  - Portal or mesenteric vein thrombosis
  - Hepatic vein thrombosis (Budd-Chiari syndrome)
  - Cerebrovascular thrombosis
- Renal failure
  - Acute renal failure associated with massive hemoglobinuria (acute tubular necrosis)
  - Progressive renal failure associated with thrombosis within renal small veins
- Dysphagia
- Infections (associated with leukopenia or steroid treatment)
- Physical findings include the following:
  - Pallor (anemia)
  - Jaundice (hemolysis)
  - Splenomegaly
  - Unilateral extremity swelling (DVT)
  - Ascites (Budd-Chiari syndrome)

CAUSE AND PATHOGENESIS

- Complement-mediated hemolysis; the erythrocytes are abnormally sensitive to acidified serum.
- Patients have two populations of RBCs, some sensitive to hemolysis (PNH III cells) but not others (PNH I cells) in variable proportions (10% to 75% PNH III cells). About 20% PNH III cells are required for hemoglobinuria to be detectable.
- These protein deficiencies are the result of an acquired mutation located in the X chromosome, which regulates glycosyl phosphatidylinositol (GPI).

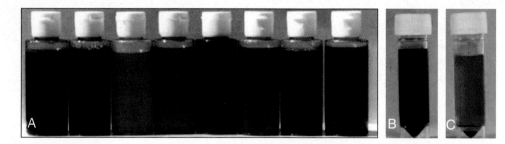

Fig 326–1

A, Urine samples from a patient with paroxysmal nocturnal hemoglobinuria within the short time span of 3 days. Extremely dark urine was first observed in the morning, but this cleared in the course of the day. The term *nocturnal* is a reflection of this finding. Elevated lactate dehydrogenase and a normal creatine phosphokinase in this patient were suggestive of hemolysis and excluded myoglobinuria. Depending on the degree of oxidation of the hemoglobin, the urine can appear red or black. Several weeks later, the urine looked completely normal, suggesting to the eye that the hemoglobinuria is paroxysmal. However, biochemical evidence of hemoglobinuria persists, and hemosiderin was consistently present in the urine sediment. **B,** It is crucial to differentiate hemoglobinuria from hematuria. After centrifugation of the patient's urine, the color—caused by free hemoglobin—remains in the supernatant. **C,** In contrast, after centrifugation of a specimen darkened caused by red cells, a red cell pellet appears, and the supernatant is clear. These simple maneuvers can preempt unnecessary invasive urologic workups.
(From Young NS, Gerson SL, High KA [eds]: Clinical Hematology. St. Louis, Mosby, 2006.)

DIFFERENTIAL DIAGNOSIS
- Other hemolytic anemias

LABORATORY TESTS
- CBC: anemia, leukopenia, thrombocytopenia
- Reticulocytosis
- RBC smear: spherocytes
- Negative Coombs' test
- Low leukocyte alkaline phosphatase
- Elevated LDH
- Low serum haptoglobin
- Low serum iron saturation, low ferritin
- Elevated urine hemoglobin
- Elevated urine urobilinogen
- Elevated urine hemosiderin
- Positive Ham test (acidified serum RBC lysis)
- Normoblastic hyperplasia on bone marrow aspirate or biopsy
- Identification of GPI-anchored protein deficiency on hematopoietic cells using monoclonal antibodies or flow cytometry
- Cytogenetic studies are not diagnostic.

TREATMENT
- Androgenic steroids
- Prednisone
- Eculizumab, a humanized antibody that inhibits the activation of terminal complement components, reduces intravascular hemolysis, hemoglobinuria, and need for transfusion in patients with PNH.
- Iron replacement
- Transfusions
- Treatment and prevention of thrombosis (heparin, warfarin)
- Avoidance of oral contraceptives
- Bone marrow transplantation

Chapter 327   Paroxysmal cold hemoglobinuria

DEFINITION
Paroxysmal cold hemoglobinuria (PCH) is a rare disease characterized by episodic massive intravascular hemolysis after exposure to cold temperatures. Hemolysis may occur in an idiopathic form in adults or, more commonly, after a viral infection in children. It was first described in patients with secondary or tertiary syphilis. Table 327–1 describes a classification system and typical serologic features of the autoimmune hemolytic anemias.

PHYSICAL FINDINGS AND CLINICAL PRESENTATION
- Following cold exposure, red to brown urination begins within minutes to hours.
- Associated symptoms include back, leg, and abdominal pain.
- Headaches, nausea, vomiting, and diarrhea are common.
- May be associated with Raynaud's phenomenon
- Associated with cold urticaria
- Transient splenomegaly and jaundice may occur.
- Symptoms and gross hemoglobinuria usually resolve within hours.
- Symptoms thought to be mediated by smooth muscle dysfunction secondary to nitric oxide toxicity associated with hemoglobinemia.

CAUSE & PATHOGENESIS
- Polyclonal IgG (Donath-Landsteiner antibody) binds to P antigen on RBC membrane when blood is exposed to cold temperatures. As blood warms to body temperature, complement-mediated hemolysis ensues.
- In children, the appearance of the antibody usually follows the onset of a viral respiratory illness by 7 to 10 days. Symptoms may persist for several weeks.
- PCH has been associated with a multiple infectious pathogens, including syphilis, *H. influenzae*, EBV, CMV, influenza A, varicella, measles, mumps, and adenovirus.

DIFFERENTIAL DIAGNOSIS
- Cold agglutinin disease (Fig. 327–1) associated with hemoglobinuria, paroxysmal nocturnal hemoglobinuria, rhabdomyolysis
- Other causes of acute massive intravascular hemolysis

LABORATORY TESTS
- Presence of IgG that reacts with RBCs at reduced temperatures but not at body temperature. In the *Donath-Landsteiner test*, a patient's serum is incubated with donated RBCs and complement at 4°C and then warmed to 37°C. Lysis is observed in a positive test.
- A more sensitive test involves using radiolabelled monoclonal anti-IgG. This is incubated at 4°C with the patient's serum and donor RBCs. The degree of radioactivity on the separated RBCs will be elevated in PCH as compared with a control run at 37°C.
- Elevated bilirubin and LDH
- Abnormal RBC forms such as poikilocytosis, spherocytosis, and anisocytosis
- Erythrophagocytosis by neutrophils and monocytes may be seen.

TREATMENT
- The mainstay of treatment is the avoidance of exposure to cold.
- In children in particular, transfusion may be necessary because the anemia may become life threatening and hemolysis may be ongoing for several weeks.
- Testing and treatment for syphilis if present
- Steroids generally are not found to be helpful.
- Splenectomy is not indicated.

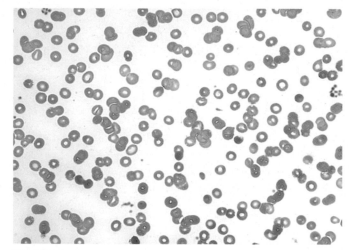

Fig 327–1

In patients with cold agglutinin syndrome, the peripheral blood smear typically reveals red cell agglutination.
(From Young NS, Gerson SL, High KA [eds]: Clinical Hematology. St. Louis, Mosby, 2006.)

TABLE 327–1 **Classification and typical serologic features of the autoimmune hemolytic anemias**

Parameter	Warm autoimmune hemolytic anemia	Cold agglutinin syndrome	Paroxysmal cold hemoglobinuria
Direct antiglobulin test	IgG, IgG, and C3	C3 only	C3 only
Immunoglobulin class	IgG (sometimes IgA)	IgM	IgG
Eluate	IgG	Nonreactive	Nonreactive
Serum	IgG agglutinating red cells at the anti–human globulin phase (panagglutinin)	IgM agglutinating antibody, often with titers >1000, reacting at 30°C in albumin	IgG biphasic hemolysin (Donath-Landsteiner antibody)
Specificity	Rh	I, i	P

From Young NS, Gerson SL, High KA (eds): Clinical Hematology. St. Louis, 2006, Mosby, 2006.

Chapter 328 / Histiocytosis X

DEFINITION

Histiocytosis X is a rare disorder characterized by the abnormal proliferation of pathologic Langerhans cells. These dendritic cells form characteristic infiltrates with eosinophils, lymphocytes, and other histiocytes that may be found in various organs.

PHYSICAL FINDINGS AND CLINICAL PRESENTATION

- A characteristic feature of histiocytosis X is its variable clinical presentation. The clinical spectrum varies.
  1. A benign isolated bony lesion (*eosinophilic granuloma*).
  2. Multiple bone lesions with soft tissue gingival and oral mucosal involvement (*Hand-Schüller-Christian disease*)
  3. An aggressive disseminated disease infiltrating organs and causing organ dysfunction (*Letterer-Siwe disease*)
- Bone lesions (80% to 100%)
  1. May be isolated or multiple
  2. Painful, often worse at night
  3. Skull most often involved, followed by long bones; lesions rarely seen in small bones of the hands and feet
  4. Proptosis
  5. Mastoiditis
  6. Loose teeth
  7. Gingival hypertrophy
- Skin is involved in more than 80% of patients with disseminated disease and in 30% of patients with less extensive disease.
  1. Seborrhea-like scaling of scalp, petechial and purpuric lesions, ulcers, and bronzing of the skin may occur.
  2. Common sites: scalp, neck, trunk, groin, and extremities
- Lymphadenopathy (10%): cervical and inguinal
- Lung involvement may manifest with cough, tachypnea, cyanosis, inspiratory crackles, pleural effusions, or pneumothorax. Diffuse emphysema associated with pulmonary fibrosis is the end stage of a mixed restrictive and obstructive pattern of disease.
- Pulmonary disease is frequent in adults (usually as isolated disease), but can be seen in 23% to 50% of children as well. In children, lung involvement always occurs as part of multisystem disease.
- Liver involvement manifesting as hepatomegaly, with or without jaundice (50% to 60%)
- Involvement of the biliary tree may be seen as biliary fibrosis or sclerosing cholangitis.
- Splenomegaly (5%)
- CNS involvement occurs in 25% to 35% of patients, most often in those with multisystem disease. The most common cerebral site affected is the hypothalamic-neurohypophyseal region, where infiltration and destruction usually result in diabetes insipidus with insatiable thirst and urination. The second most common site of involvement is the cerebellum.
- Involvement of the thymus, parotid glands, and GI tract has been reported in rare cases.

CAUSE

- Unknown
- Initially, histiocytosis was thought to represent an abnormal immune response to a virus or other stimulant, resulting in the proliferation of pathologic Langerhans cells. More recent evidence has suggested histiocytosis X as a monoclonal proliferative neoplastic disorder.
- In adults, pulmonary histiocytosis X appears to be primarily an immune-mediated reactive process and has been linked to cigarette smoking. Cigarette smoke has not been observed as a causative factor in other forms of histiocytosis X.

DIAGNOSIS

- Tissue biopsy revealing pathologic Langerhans cells characterized by the presence of surface nucleoprotein, protein S-100, and CD1a antigen
- Birbeck granules noted on electron microscopy establishes the diagnosis of histiocytosis X.

IMAGING STUDIES

- X-rays of affected areas show lytic lesions, with or without sclerotic margins (Fig. 328–1).
- X-ray bone survey is done, searching for other lesions.

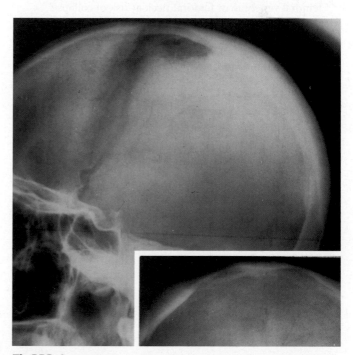

Fig 328–1
Histiocytosis. Shown is a geographic lytic lesion of the skull vault in eosinophilic granuloma. Similar lesions are found in the Hand-Schüller-Christian syndrome. **Insert,** Shown is the beveling so characteristic of the disorder, indicating asymmetrical destruction of the inner and outer tables.
(From Grainger RG, Allison DJ, Adam A, Dixon AK [eds]: Grainger & Allison's Diagnostic Radiology, 4th ed. London, Harcourt, 2001.)

- Bone scan complements the bone survey studies.
- Panoramic dental view of the mandible and maxilla in children with oral involvement
- Chest x-ray can show interstitial reticulonodular infiltrates (Fig. 328–2). This pattern typically progresses toward frank honeycombing fibrosis later in the course of the disease
- High-resolution CT of the chest confirms interstitial lung scarring, nodules, and cysts, and represents an excellent noninvasive means for diagnosis and follow-up of pulmonary histiocytosis X. Pulmonary cysts are bilateral and symmetrical, showing slight upper lobe predominance with relative sparing of the costophrenic angles.
- CT of the temporal bone looking at the mastoid and inner and middle ears.
- Ultrasound of the abdomen may show hepatosplenomegaly.
- Conventional cholangiography or magnetic resonance cholangiopancreatography (MRCP) can confirm the presence of disease in patients suspected to have biliary involvement.
- MRI of the brain visualizing the hypothalamic-hypophyseal region in patients suspected of having diabetes insipidus

TREATMENT

- Isolated bone lesions can be treated by the following:
  - Curettage at the time of diagnosis
  - Intralesional prednisone or vinblastine (Velban) and prednisone injection
  - Radiation therapy is useful only for bone lesions of the femoral vertebrae or femoral neck at risk of collapse.
- Single skin lesions are treated with the following:
  - Topical steroid (e.g., triamcinolone acetonide) applied twice daily
  - Nitrogen mustard in 20% solution
- Solitary lymph node
  - Excision at diagnosis
  - Systemic oral prednisone
- Treatment for multiple bone lesions, skull base lesions, or multisystem disease includes vinblastine plus oral prednisone.

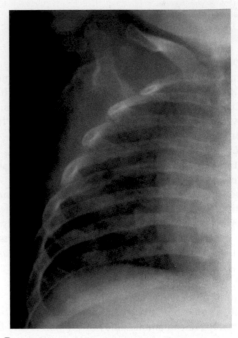

Fig 328–2

Interstitial disease—histiocytosis. There are multiple lytic bone lesions (especially of the right scapula), mediastinal adenopathy, and interstitial infiltrates.
(From Grainger RG, Allison DJ, Adam A, Dixon AK [eds]: Grainger & Allison's Diagnostic Radiology, 4th ed. London, Harcourt, 2001.)

Chapter 329 | Kaposi's sarcoma

DEFINITION

Kaposi's sarcoma (KS) is a vascular neoplasm most frequently occurring in AIDS patients. It can be divided into the following four subsets:

1. Classic Kaposi's sarcoma: most frequently found in older eastern European and Mediterranean men. It consists initially of violaceous macules and papules with subsequent development of plaques and red-purple nodules (Fig. 329–1). Growth is slow, and most patients die of unrelated causes.

2. Epidemic or AIDS-related Kaposi's sarcoma: most frequently occurs in homosexual men. AIDS-related KS affects more than 35% of AIDS patients. Lesions are generally multifocal and widespread. Lymphadenopathy may be associated.

3. Endemic Kaposi's sarcoma: usually affects African children and adults. An aggressive lymphadenopathic form affects African children in particular.

4. Immunosuppression-associated or transplant-associated Kaposi's sarcoma: usually associated with chemotherapy

PHYSICAL FINDINGS AND CLINICAL PRESENTATION

- AIDS-related KS: multifocal and widespread red-purple (Fig. 329–2) or dark plaques and/or nodules on cutaneous or mucosal surfaces
- Generalized lymphadenopathy at diagnosis is present in more than 50% of patients with AIDS-related KS. The initial lesions have a rust-colored appearance, with subsequent progression to red or purple nodules or plaques.
- Most frequently affected areas are the face, trunk, oral cavity, and upper and lower extremities.

CAUSE

- A herpesvirus (HHV-8, Kaposi's sarcoma–associated herpesvirus [KSHV]) has been isolated from patients with most forms of KS and is believed to be the causative agent. It can be transmitted sexually (homosexual, heterosexual activities) and by other forms of nonsexual contact, such as maternal-infant transmission (common in African countries).

DIFFERENTIAL DIAGNOSIS

- Stasis dermatitis (see Fig. 6–17)
- Pyogenic granuloma (see Fig. 25–28)
- Capillary hemangiomas (see Fig. 25–27)
- Granulation tissue
- Postinflammatory hyperpigmentation
- Cutaneous lymphoma (see Fig. 316–10)
- Melanoma (see Fig. 24–1)
- Dermatofibroma
- Hematoma (see Fig. 324–1)
- Prurigo nodularis (see Fig. 6–16)

LABORATORY TESTS

- HIV in patients suspected of AIDS

IMAGING STUDIES

- Chest x-ray (Fig. 329–3)

TREATMENT

- Excisional biopsy often provides adequate treatment for single lesions and resected recurrences in classic Kaposi's sarcoma.
- Liquid nitrogen cryotherapy can result in complete response in 80% of lesions.
- Interlesional chemotherapy with vinblastine is useful for nodular lesions larger than 1 cm in diameter. Intralesional

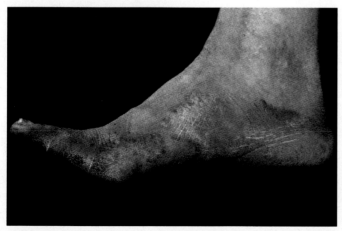

Fig 329–1
Classic Kaposi's sarcoma. The distal extremities are typically involved. (Courtesy of the Institute of Dermatology, London.)

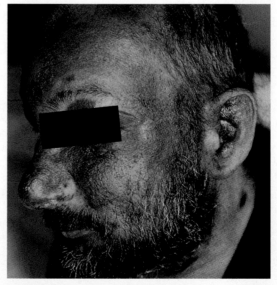

Fig 329–2
Kaposi's sarcoma. There are large confluent hyperpigmented patch stage lesions with lymphedema.
(From Cohen J, Powderly WG: Infectious Diseases, 2nd ed. St. Louis, Mosby, 2004.)

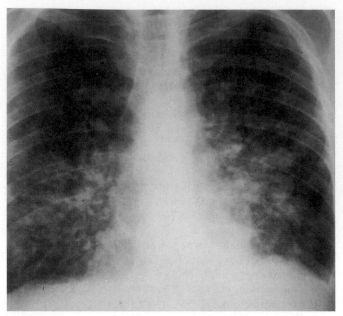

Fig 329-3

Kaposi's sarcoma. A posteroanterior chest film demonstrates coarse linear opacities in the perihilar regions. Some nodular opacities are noted in the right upper lobe. Left pleural fluid is present. This constellation of findings is highly suggestive of Kaposi's sarcoma. (From Grainger RG, Allison DJ, Adam A, Dixon AK [eds]: Grainger & Allison's Diagnostic Radiology, 4th ed. London, Harcourt, 2001.)

injection of interferon alfa-2b has also been reported as effective and well tolerated.

- Radiation therapy is effective for non-AIDS KS and for large tumor masses that interfere with normal function.
- Systemic therapy with interferon is also effective for AIDS-related KS and is often used in combination with azidothymidine (AZT).
- Systemic chemotherapy (vinblastine, bleomycin, doxorubicin, and dacarbazine) can be used for rapidly progressive disease and for classic and African-endemic KS.
- Sirolimus (rapamycin), an immunosuppressive drug, is effective in inhibiting the progression of dermal Kaposi's sarcoma in kidney transplant recipients.
- Oral etoposide is also effective and has less myelosuppression than vinblastine.
- Paclitaxel is also effective in patients with advanced KS and represents an excellent second-line therapy.
- Prognosis is poor in AIDS-related KS. Death is often a result of other AIDS-defining illnesses.
- Prognosis is better in African cutaneous KS and classic sarcoma (patients usually die of unrelated causes).

REFERENCES

Abeloff MD: Clinical Oncology, 3rd ed. Philadelphia, Elsevier, 2004.

Ferri F: Ferri's Clinical Advisor 2007. St. Louis, Mosby, 2007.

Ferri F: Practical Guide to the Care of the Medical Patient, 7th ed. St. Louis, Mosby, 2007.

Young NS, Gerson SL, High KA (eds)]: Clinical Hematology. St. Louis, Mosby, 2006.

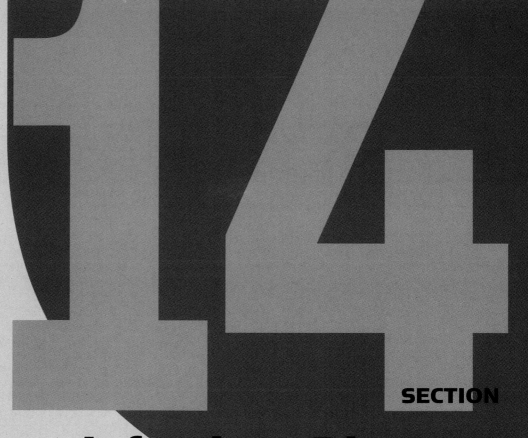

14

SECTION

Infectious Diseases

Chapter 330: Diagnostic tests and procedures
Chapter 331: Human immunodeficiency virus
Chapter 332: Protozoal infections
Chapter 333: Cestode (tapeworm) infestation
Chapter 334: Nematode infestation
Chapter 335: Filariasis
Chapter 336: Fungal infections
Chapter 337: Rheumatic fever
Chapter 338: Infectious mononucleosis
Chapter 339: Thrombophlebitis
Chapter 340: Leprosy
Chapter 341: Tetanus

Chapter 342: Anaerobic infections
Chapter 343: Diphtheria
Chapter 344: Listeriosis
Chapter 345: *Yersinia pestis* (Plague)
Chapter 346: Relapsing fever
Chapter 347: Tularemia
Chapter 348: Brucellosis
Chapter 349: Cat-scratch disease
Chapter 350: Leptospirosis
Chapter 351: Rabies
Chapter 352: Toxic shock syndrome

Chapter 330 | **Diagnostic tests and procedures**

A. GRAM STAIN

Gram staining is used to sort bacteria into two groups based on the composition of their cell wall.

Gm+ organism: bacteria that resist decolorization and appear purple

Gm− organism: bacteria that are decolorized appear red with the counterstain

GRAM-POSITIVE COCCI

1. Streptococci
   a. Lancefield group A streptococci *(Streptococcus pyogenes)*:
      (1) Etiologic agent of acute pharyngitis (group A β-streptococci), wound infections, and localized skin cellulitis
      (2) May be isolated from throat or nasopharyngeal cultures in 15% to 20% of clinically normal children
      (3) Certain strains are associated with acute glomerulonephritis and acute rheumatic fever.
   b. Lancefield group B streptococci *(S. agalactiae):* frequent etiologic agent of neonatal septicemia, neonatal meningitis, and postpartum endometritis
   c. Lancefield group C streptococci *(S. anginosus):* primarily animal pathogens that can occasionally produce pharyngitis and meningitis in humans
   d. Lancefield group D streptococci:
      (1) *S. faecalis* can be associated with subacute bacterial endocarditis (SBE), urinary tract infection (UTI), and biliary tract infections.
      (2) *S. bovis* bacteremia is frequently associated with colon neoplasms.
   e. Lancefield group F streptococci: may be associated with dental abscesses and abscesses in other body tissues
   f. Lancefield group G streptococci: can cause bacteremia in patients with underlying disease (e.g., cancer)
   g. *S. viridans:* most common cause of SBE; may also cause UTI, pneumonia, and wound infections
   h. *S. pneumoniae:* most common cause of bacterial pneumonia (Fig. 330–1)

2. Staphylococci
   a. *Staphylococcus aureus:* most common site of infection is the skin (Fig. 330–2); can also cause pneumonia in debilitated persons or postviral infection, meningitis, and septicemia in immunocompromised hosts, and toxic shock syndrome. MRSA (methicillin-resistant *S. aureus*), a common nosocomial organism and community-acquired MRSA, with a different antibiotic resistance profile than nosocomial MRSA, is an emerging cause of cellulitis and severe lung infections.
   b. *S. epidermidis:* frequent contaminant from cultures from the skin area; infections associated with indwelling catheters, vascular grafts, artificial heart valves, and joint prosthetic devices
   c. *S. saprophyticus:* frequent cause of UTI in young women

GRAM-NEGATIVE DIPLOCOCCI

1. Meningococci: frequent cause of meningitis; can be isolated from the nasopharynx of 5% to 15% of clinically normal persons
2. Gonococci: *Neisseria gonorrhoeae* (Fig. 330–3) causes gonococcal urethritis and salpingitis.

GRAM-NEGATIVE RODS

1. Enteric bacilli: found mostly in the intestinal tract.
   a. *Salmonella* sp.: can cause gastroenteritis, typhoid fever, septicemia; infection is usually transmitted through eggs, undercooked poultry, fecal contamination of food and water
   b. *Shigella* sp.: important cause of bacillary dysentery
   c. *Escherichia coli:* most common cause of UTI and gram-negative bacteremia or septicemia; can also cause diarrhea in adults and children and meningitis in newborns
   d. *Proteus:* responsible for 5% of UTI in hospitalized patients
   e. *Yersinia enterocolitica:* frequent cause of acute enteritis

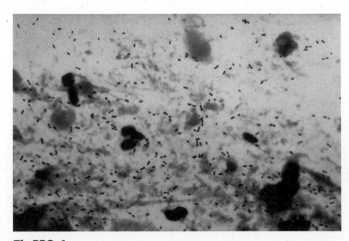

Fig 330–1
Gram stain of a sputum sample infected with *Streptococcus pneumoniae*.
(From Cohen J, Powderly WG: Infectious Diseases, 2nd ed. St Louis, Mosby, 2004.)

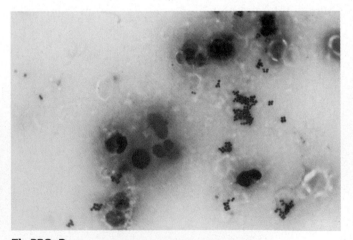

Fig 330–2
Staphylococcus aureus in a Gram stain of pus.
(From Cohen J, Powderly WG: Infectious Diseases, 2nd ed. St Louis, Mosby, 2004.)

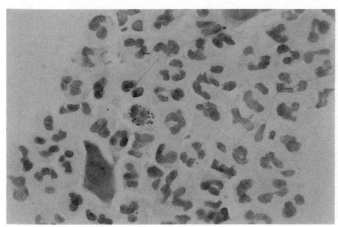

Fig 330-3
Gonorrhea. Gram-stained smear of urethral discharge containing numerous PMNs and Gram-negative intracellular diplococci consistent with *Neisseria gonorrhoeae*.
(From Cohen J, Powderly WG: Infectious Diseases, 2nd ed. St Louis, Mosby, 2004.)

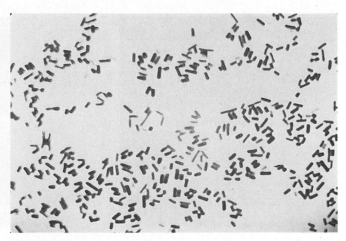

Fig 330-4
Gram stain of *Clostridium perfringens*.
(From Cohen J, Powderly WG: Infectious Diseases, 2nd ed. St Louis, Mosby, 2004.)

2. *Pseudomonas:* found in 10% of nosocomial infections (UTI, extensive burns, pneumonia, malignant otitis media); generally resistant to most antibiotics
3. *Haemophilus influenzae:* a cause of meningitis, acute epiglottitis, otitis media, sinusitis, and pneumonia
4. *Pasteurella multocida:* found in the mouths of cats and dogs; can cause cellulitis and abscess following animal bites
5. *Bordetella pertussis:* etiologic agent of pertussis (whooping cough)
6. *Campylobacter jejuni:* associated with abdominal cramping and bloody diarrhea
7. *Aeromonas:* organism frequently found in water and associated with self-limited diarrhea
8. *Helicobacter pylori:* associated with acute and chronic gastritis, peptic ulcer disease, and possibly gastric carcinoma
9. *Brucella:* infection usually occurs in workers in meat-processing industry, veterinarians, and dairy farmers
10. *Francisella tularensis:* causative agent of tularemia
11. *Vibrio cholerae:* causative agent of epidemic cholera

GRAM-POSITIVE RODS

1. *Listeria monocytogenes:* can cause meningitis in immunocompromised hosts (lymphoma, leukemia, renal transplants)
2. *Clostridia*
   a. *Clostridium perfringens:* etiologic agent of gas gangrene (Fig. 330-4).
   b. *C. tetani:* causative agent for tetanus.
   c. *C. difficile:* most frequent etiologic agent of antibiotic-induced diarrhea (pseudomembranous colitis).
   d. *C. botulinum:* can cause severe food poisoning (botulism)
3. *Bacteroides* sp.: most frequent organisms found in anaerobic infections (e.g., septic abortion, aspiration pneumonia, pelvic abscess) (Fig. 330-5)

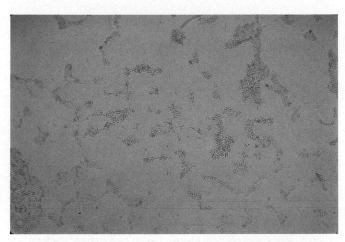

Fig 330-5
Gram stain of *Bacteroides fragilis*.
(Courtesy of Mike Cox.)

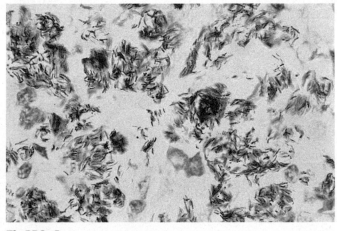

Fig 330-6
Acid-fast stain. The cells are packed with acid-fast bacilli characteristic of *Mycobacterium avium-intracellular* complex (Ziehl-Neelsen stain, ×1000).
(Courtesy of Ann-Marie Nelson, MD.)

B. ACID-FAST BACTERIA (AFB) STAIN

Used to identify mycobacteria (Fig. 330-6), intestinal coccidia (Fig. 330-7), and *Nocardia* species

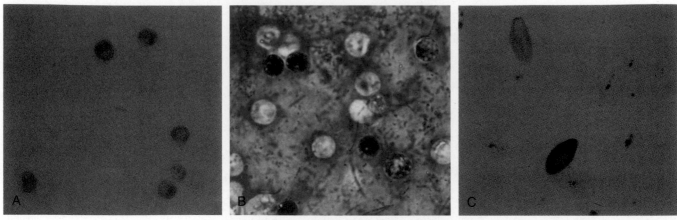

Fig 330–7
Acid-fast–stained smears of fecal specimens showing intestinal coccidia. (**A**) *Cryptosporidium* spp., round, 4 to 6 μm in diameter. (**B**) *Cyclospora* spp., round, 8 to 10 μm in diameter. (**C**) *Isospora belli,* elliptical, 23 to 33 μm long and 10 to 19 μm wide. (Modified Kinyoun stain.) (Courtesy of E. G. Long.)

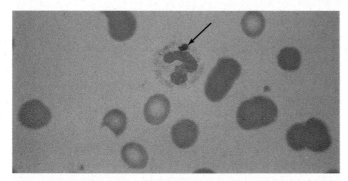

Fig 330–8
Peripheral blood film of a patient with past malaria. The patient had returned 5 days previously from Malawi, having been treated there for malaria. At this stage no parasites were visible on the film. She was confused and delirious on admission and was found to have a profound acidosis (pH 6.98) and acute renal failure, thought to be due to the malaria. She was hypotensive, which suggested a secondary bacterial infection and was found to have a *Salmonella* sepsis. Secondary bacterial infections are not uncommon in severe malaria associated with immunosuppression. The only evidence on blood film for malaria was the presence of malarial pigment (hemozoin) in many of the neutrophils, one of which is demonstrated here (*arrow*).
(From Cohen J, Powderly WG: Infectious Diseases, 2nd ed. St Louis, Mosby, 2004.)

C. PERIPHERAL BLOOD FILM

Examination of the peripheral blood smear can be pivotal in diagnosing several parasitic infections (Fig. 330–8). Table 330–1 describes specific ID diagnosis that can be made from blood film. Giemsa stains and Wright stains of peripheral blood (Fig. 330–9) are commonly used to detect microorganisms.

TABLE 330–1 Specific diagnoses from the blood film—etiologies of acute fever are sometimes established by examination of the blood film

- Malaria
- Babesiosis
- Trypanosomiasis
- Filariasis
- Leptospirosis (dark field)
- Relapsing fever (dark field or staining)
- Bartonellosis
- Ehrlichiosis
- Meningococcemia
- Histoplasmosis, candidemia

From Cohen J, Powderly WG: Infectious Diseases, 2nd 2. St Louis, Mosby, 2004.

D. CULTURES

Cultures of blood, urine, and other potential sites of infection (e.g., cerebrospinal fluid [CSF], sputum, genitalia, stool, skin, wounds, abscesses) should be obtained before therapy whenever possible. Various culturing methods include Agar plating (Figs. 330–10 and 330–11), CAMP test (Fig. 330–12), and culture plating (Fig. 330–13).

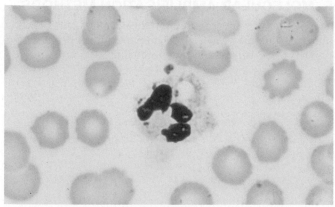

Fig 330–9

Peripheral blood smear of a patient who has pneumococcal sepsis and meningitis. Note polymorphonuclear leukocyte with several bacterial diplococci in the cytoplasm (Wright stain).
(From Cohen J, Powderly WG: Infectious Diseases, 2nd ed. St Louis, Mosby, 2004.)

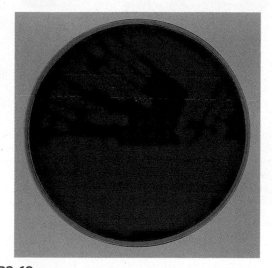

Fig 330–10

β-Hemolytic streptococci group A on a blood agar plate. Note the clear β-hemolytic zone.
(From Cohen J, Powderly WG: Infectious Diseases, 2nd ed. St Louis, Mosby, 2004.)

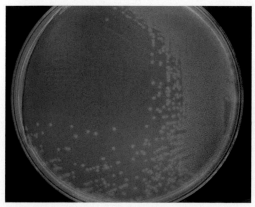

Fig 330–11

Pseudomonas aeruginosa colonies on agar medium.
(Courtesy of Professor E. Bingen)

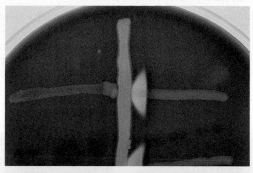

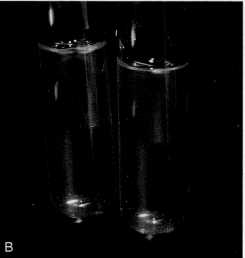

Fig 330–12

Tests for the identification of *Listeria monocytogenes*. (**A**) CAMP test. Enhanced hemolysis patterns for *L. monocytogenes* (*left*) and *Streptococcus agalactiae* (*right*) colonies are shown; these are growing adjacent to a streak of *Staphylococcus aureus* colonies in the center. (**B**) Demonstration of motility of *L. monocytogenes* grown in semisolid agar at room temperature. Note that the migration of the organism from the central stab is more pronounced at the surface of the soft agar, forming the typical umbrella-shaped pattern in both tubes.
(From Cohen J, Powderly WG: Infectious Diseases, 2nd ed. St Louis, Mosby, 2004.)

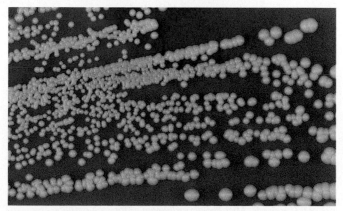

Fig 330–13

Colonies of *Candida albicans* on culture plate.
(From Cohen J, Powderly WG: Infectious Diseases, 2nd ed. St Louis, Mosby, 2004.)

E. DIAGNOSTIC IMMUNOLOGY

Serologic methods in the investigation of infectious diseases include agglutination (antigen-containing particles on a tube or slide together in the presence of antibody) (e.g., Latex agglutination test [Fig. 330–14]), enzyme-linked immunosorbent assay (ELISA), immunoblotting (Western blot [Figs. 330–15 and 330–16]), and fluorescent antibody tests.

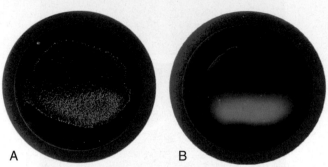

Fig 330–14
Latex agglutination for the identification of β-hemolytic streptococci group A. (**A**) Positive agglutination. (**B**) Negative agglutination.
(From Cohen J, Powderly WG: Infectious Diseases, 2nd ed. St Louis, Mosby, 2004.)

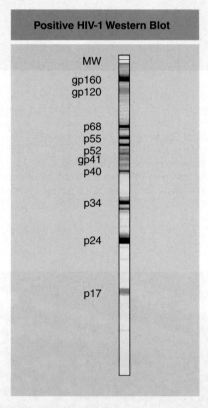

Positive HIV-1 Western Blot

MW
gp160
gp120

p68
p55
p52
gp41
p40

p34

p24

p17

Fig 330–15
Positive HIV-1 Western blot. The binding of the patient's antibodies to viral antigens coated on the strip is revealed by an enzyme-labeled antihuman globulin. gp160, gp120, and gp41 are env gene products. p55, p24, and p17 are gag gene products. p68, p52, and p34 are pol gene products. MW, molecular weight of the viral proteins.
(From Cohen J, Powderly WG: Infectious Diseases, 2nd ed. St Louis, Mosby, 2004.)

F. MOLECULAR AMPLIFICATION METHODS

These techniques are very useful in the diagnosis of hepatitis C, human papilloma virus (HPV), human immunodeficiency virus (HIV), and herpes simplex encephalitis.

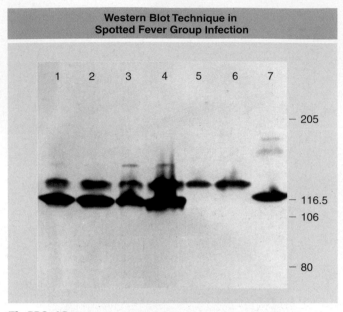

Western Blot Technique in Spotted Fever Group Infection

1 2 3 4 5 6 7

— 205

— 116.5
— 106

— 80

Fig 330–16
Western blot technique in spotted fever group infection. Western blot of pooled mouse antisera to *Rickettsia africae* human isolate (lane 1), *R. africae* tick isolate (lanes 2 through 4), *Rickettsia conorii* Kenyan strain (lane 5), *R. conorii* Moroccan strain (lane 6), and Israeli SFG rickettsia (lane 7). Molecular masses (in thousands) are shown.
(From Cohen J, Powderly WG: Infectious Diseases, 2nd ed. St Louis, Mosby, 2004.)

Chapter 331 | Human immunodeficiency virus

A. THE ASYMPTOMATIC HIV-INFECTED PATIENT

- The human immunodeficiency virus, type 1 (HIV) causes a chronic infection that culminates, usually after several years, in acquired immunodeficiency syndrome (AIDS).
- Acute infection occurs 2 to 6 weeks from the time of viral transmission. Figure 331–1 illustrates the kinetics of viral load and immune response during the phases of HIV-1 infection.

- The acute infection most often is a mild, self-limited mononucleosis-like illness; pharyngitis, mucosal ulcerations (Fig. 331–2), rash (Fig. 331–3), penile ulcer from sexual contact (Fig. 331–4), splenomegaly, and lymphadenopathy commonly occur. Hepatitis and aseptic meningitis are occasionally seen.
- The p24 antigen and the HIV polymerase chain reaction (PCR) will be reactive (Fig. 331–5); positive HIV serology usually first becomes positive 1 month later.

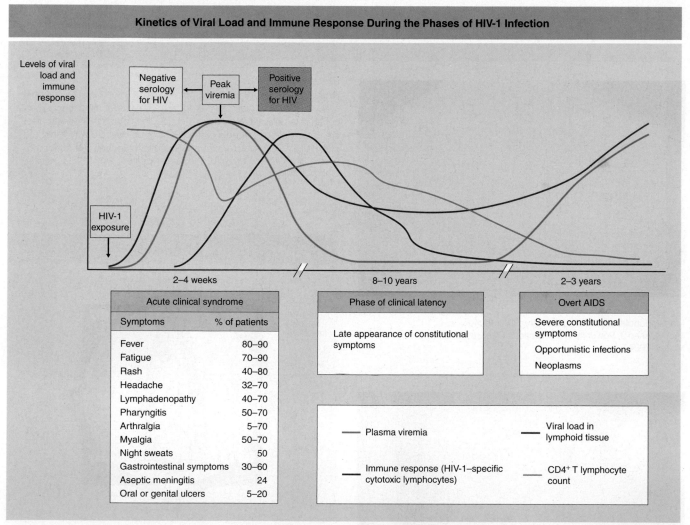

Kinetics of Viral Load and Immune Response During the Phases of HIV-1 Infection

Acute clinical syndrome	
Symptoms	% of patients
Fever	80–90
Fatigue	70–90
Rash	40–80
Headache	32–70
Lymphadenopathy	40–70
Pharyngitis	50–70
Arthralgia	5–70
Myalgia	50–70
Night sweats	50
Gastrointestinal symptoms	30–60
Aseptic meningitis	24
Oral or genital ulcers	5–20

Fig 331–1

Kinetics of viral load and immune response during the phases of HIV-1 infection. After HIV-1 exposure, initial virus replication and spread occur in the lymphoid organs, and systemic dissemination of HIV-1 is reflected by the peak of plasma viremia. A clinical syndrome of varying severity is associated with this phase of primary HIV-1 infection in up to 70% of HIV-1–infected persons. Downregulation of viremia during the transition from the primary to the early chronic phase coincides with the appearance of HIV-1–specific cytotoxic T cells and with the progressive resolution of the clinical syndrome. The long phase of clinical latency is associated with active virus replication, particularly in the lymphoid tissue. During the clinically latent period, CD4+ T cell counts slowly decrease, as does the HIV-1–specific immune response. When CD4+ T cell counts decrease below 200 cells/μL (i.e. when overt AIDS occurs), the clinical picture is characterized by severe constitutional symptoms and by the possible development of opportunistic infections and/or neoplasms.

(From Cohen J, Powderly WG: Infectious Diseases, 2nd ed. St Louis, Mosby, 2004.)

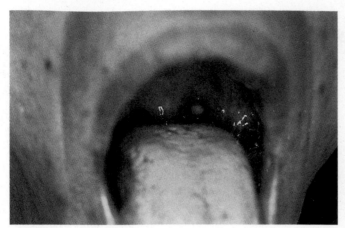

Fig 331–2
Mucosal ulcerations during primary HIV infection.
(From Cohen J, Powderly WG: Infectious Diseases, 2nd ed. St Louis, Mosby, 2004.)

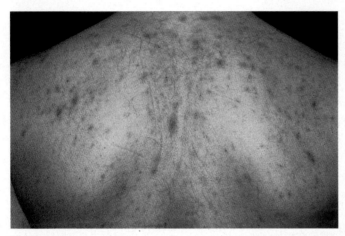

Fig 331–3
Maculopapular rash during primary HIV infection.
(From Cohen J, Powderly WG: Infectious Diseases, 2nd ed. St Louis, Mosby, 2004.)

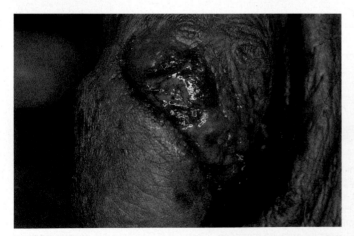

Fig 331–4
Penile ulcer during primary HIV infection.
(From Cohen J, Powderly WG: Infectious Diseases, 2nd ed. St Louis, Mosby, 2004.)

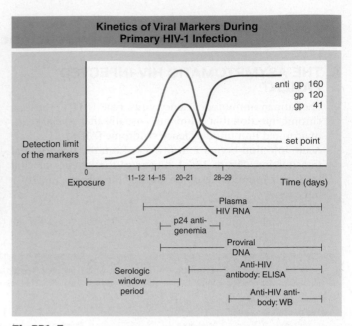

Fig 331–5
Kinetics of viral markers during primary HIV-1 infection. The first positive viral market is plasma RNA 11 to 12 days after infection. p24 antigenemia is detectable on day 14 or 15. The first anti-HIV antibodies are detectable by third-generation ELISAs on days 20–21. (Pink, plasma HIV RNA; purple, p24 antigenemia; blue, anti-HIV antibody.)
(From Cohen J, Powderly WG: Infectious Diseases, 2nd ed. St Louis, Mosby, 2004.)

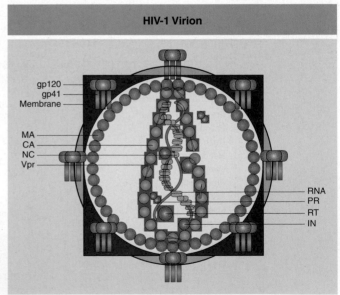

Fig 331–6
HIV-1 virion. The glycoprotein gp120 constitutes the outer envelope of the virus and is noncovalently linked to the transmembrane protein gp41. The matrix protein (p17) bridges the envelope protein with the cone-shaped structure formed by the capsid protein (p24). The viral genomic RNA and processed nucleocapsid (NC; p7) and Pol proteins, reverse transcriptase (RT) and integrase (IN), are located inside the capsid core. PR, protease.
(From Cohen J, Powderly WG: Infectious Diseases, 2nd ed. St Louis, Mosby, 2004.)

- CD4 cells subsequently decline an average of 75/mm^3 per year, but the range is variable. Five percent of infected people are long-term nonprogressors; another 10% progress more rapidly.

CAUSE

- RNA retrovirus HIV-1 (Fig. 331–6) was probably derived from transmission of a simian immunodeficiency virus (SIV) from chimpanzees in Central Africa; a related virus HIV-2 was derived from an SIV found in Sooty Mangebey monkeys from West Africa.
- HIV-1 is the predominant pathogenic retrovirus in human populations; HIV-2 has limited distribution (primarily in West Africa) and tends to be less rapidly immunosuppressive than HIV-1.
- Transmitted by sexual contact, shared needles, blood transfusion, or from mother to child during pregnancy, delivery, or breastfeeding.
- Primary target of infection: CD4 lymphocyte (Fig. 331–7). The HIV-1 life cycle is described in Figure 331–8.
- Direct central nervous system (CNS) involvement: manifested as encephalitis (Fig. 331–9), myelopathy, or neuropathy in advanced cases
- Renal failure (Fig. 331–10), rheumatologic disorders, thrombocytopenia, or cardiac abnormalities

DIFFERENTIAL DIAGNOSIS

- Acute infection: mononucleosis or other respiratory viral infections
- Late symptoms: similar to those produced by other wasting illnesses such as neoplasms, tuberculosis (TB), disseminated fungal infection, malabsorption, or depression
- HIV-related encephalopathy: confused with Alzheimer's disease or other causes of chronic dementia; myelopathy and neuropathy possibly resembling other demyelinating diseases such as multiple sclerosis

Pathogenesis of AIDS

Fig 331–7

Pathogenesis of AIDS. The pathogenesis begins with the binding of HIV to CD4 receptors on the regulatory cells of the immune system. (From Cohen J, Powderly WG: Infectious Diseases, 2nd ed. St Louis, Mosby, 2004.)

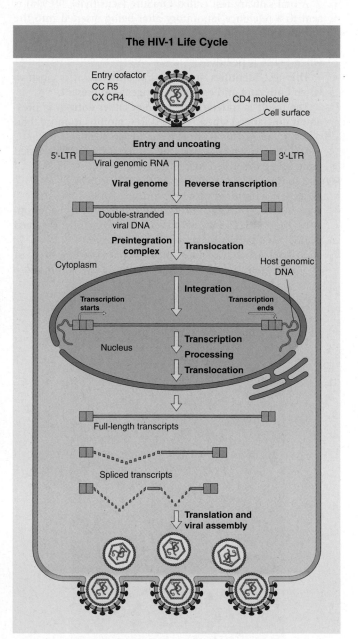

Fig 331–8

The HIV-1 life cycle. The diagram shows the various stages involved, including entry, uncoating, reverse transcription, integration, expression of proviral genome, viral assembly, and particle release. (From Cohen J, Powderly WG: Infectious Diseases, 2nd ed. St Louis, Mosby, 2004.)

LABORATORY TESTS

Three HIV viral antibody screening tests currently are in use:

- ELISA
  - Bound anti-HIV antibody is detected by antihuman antibody labeled with an enzyme. The use of recombinant proteins has reduced false-positive results (specificity, 99.9%).
  - A false-negative finding may result when measured in the acute infection period (sensitivity, 99.9%).
- New rapid serologic-screening assays
  - HIV-antigen–coated gelatin or latex particle agglutination assays. The single-use test can be performed rapidly but may be less sensitive and specific than standard ELISA tests.
  - A oral salivary test called OraSure (sensitivity, 99.9%) is sent to a reference laboratory after being inserted into the mouth for 2 minutes.
- Western blot confirmatory test (Fig. 331–11) is performed when ELISA is positive.
  - This test identifies specific viral antigens; it is positive when both core and envelope antigens are present.
  - The result is indeterminate when either antigen is present; if unchanged when repeated in 6 months in more than one laboratory, this is considered a false-positive result.
  - Laboratory tests for baseline evaluation of HIV-infected patients are described in Table 331–1.

PHYSICAL FINDINGS AND CLINICAL PRESENTATION

Signs and symptoms variable with stage of disease

- Early stage (CD4 cells >400/mm^3): diffuse lymphadenopathy (Fig. 331–12) may be present; the nontender, enlarged glands often persist for more than 3 months.
- High levels of viral replication, 10^9 copies per day, occur at this stage even though the patient remains asymptomatic.

- Quantitative plasma HIV RNA at this stage predicts clinical outcome; those with high viral loads (>55,000 copies/m^2) have a more rapid disease progression to AIDS than those with lower viral loads.
- Middle stage (CD4 cells, 200 to 400/mm^3)

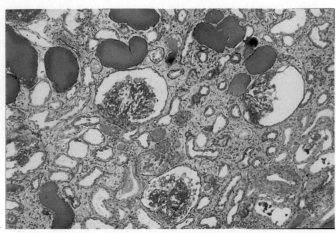

Fig 331–10
HIV-associated nephropathy. Glomerular tufts show varying degrees of collapse, with segmental to global sclerosis. Many tubules show microcystic dilation, with eosinophilic proteinaceous casts. The remaining tubules are lined by simplified epithelium with features suggestive of degeneration and regeneration. Interstitium contains excessive fibrosis and sparse mononuclear infiltrate (periodic acid–Schiff stain, ×130). (From Johnson RJ, Feehally J: Comprehensive Clinical Nephrology, 2nd ed. St Louis, Mosby, 2000)

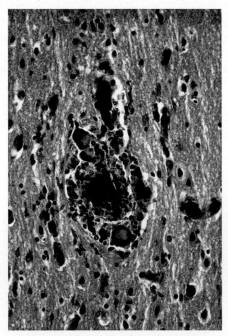

Fig 331–9
HIV encephalitis. The cerebral cortex has perivascular inflammatory infiltrates containing prominent multinucleated cells. (From Silverberg SG: Principles and Practice of Surgical Pathology and Cytopathology, 4th ed. Philadelphia, Churchill Livingstone, 2006.)

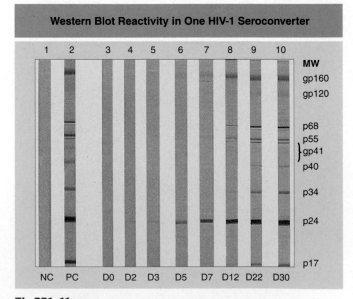

Fig 331–11
Western blot reactivity in one HIV-1 seroconverter. Lanes 1 and 2, negative (NC) and positive controls (PC). Lanes 3–10, serial samples collected on days (D) 0, 2, 3, 5, 7, 12, 22, and 30. Day 0 corresponds to the first collected sample. Anti-p24 was the first antibody detected, rapidly followed by anti-gp160, p55, p40, and gp 120. Later, gp41 and p18 are weakly reactive. (From Cohen J, Powderly WG: Infectious Diseases, 2nd ed. St Louis, Mosby, 2004.)

- *Mycobacterium tuberculosis* infections (Fig. 331–13), recurrent herpes zoster (Fig. 331–14), persistent mucocutaneous herpes simplex infections, and recurrent bacteremias caused by *S. pneumoniae* and *Salmonella* spp. occur.

- Kaposi's sarcoma (Figs. 331–15 and 331–16) and the oral manifestations of HIV infection—candidiasis (Fig. 331–17) and hairy leukoplakia, the latter appearing as painless, raised, grayish lesions—appear.

- AIDS: advanced HIV infection (CD4 cell count <200/mm³): the classic opportunistic infections

- Pneumocystis jirovecii pneumonia (PJP) (Fig. 331–18), cerebral toxoplasmosis (Fig. 331–19), cryptococcosis occurs when CD4 cell count <200/mm³ ; infections due to cytomegalovirus (Fig. 331–20), and MAC (Fig. 331–21) occur at the most advanced stage, usually with CD4 cell count below 50/mm³.

- HIV lipodystrophy may develop (Fig. 331–22).

TABLE 331–1 Laboratory tests for baseline evaluation of HIV-infected patients

- Plasma HIV RNA viral load
- CD4+ lymphocyte count, absolute and percentage
- Complete blood count and differential and platelet count
- Liver (aspartate aminotransferase, lactate dehydrogenase, alkaline phosphatase, bilirubin) and renal (blood urea nitrogen, creatinine) profiles
- Creatine phosphokinase, amylase, uric acid, and triglycerides
- Hepatitis B, hepatitis C, syphilis, cytomegalovirus, and toxoplasmosis serologies
- Tuberculin skin test
- Cultures and smears for sexually transmitted diseases, as indicated by the history and physical examination
- Sputum cultures and smears for mycobacteriae, as indicated by history and physical examination
- Chest radiograph
- Urinalysis
- Pregnancy test (if appropriate)
- Papanicolaou's smear test (if appropriate)
- Eye fundoscopy if the CD4+count is <100/mL

From Cohen J, Powderly WG: Infectious Diseases, 2nd ed. St Louis, Mosby, 2004.

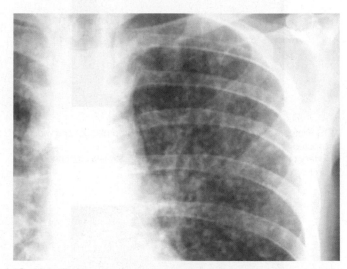

Fig 331–13
Chest radiograph of HIV-infected patient who has miliary tuberculosis. (From Cohen J, Powderly WG: Infectious Diseases, 2nd ed. St Louis, Mosby, 2004.)

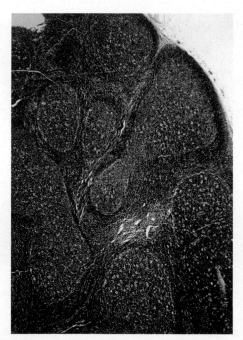

Fig 331–12
HIV-associated lymphadenopathy. "Explosive" reactive follicular hyperplasia is seen.
(From Silverberg SG: Principles and Practice of Surgical Pathology and Cytopathology, 4th ed. Philadelphia, Churchill Livingstone, 2006.)

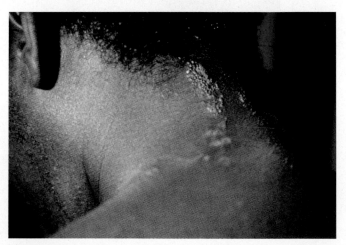

Fig 331–14
Herpes zoster. A painful linear-zosteriform eruption of vesicles on an erythematous base is characteristic of herpes zoster. The eruption may be persistent, and verrucous lesions are not uncommon.
(From Cohen J, Powderly WG: Infectious Diseases, 2nd ed. St Louis, Mosby, 2004.)

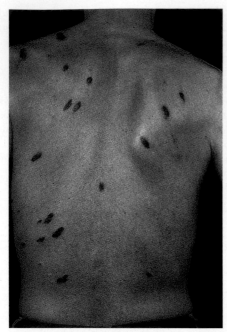

Fig 331–15
AIDS-related Kaposi's sarcoma: darkly pigmented plaques are widely distributed on this young man's back.
(Courtesy of the late N. P. Smith, MD, Institute of Dermatology, London, UK.)

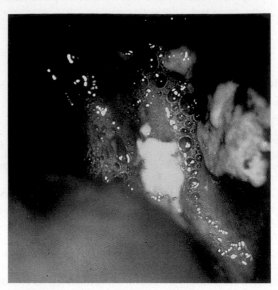

Fig 331–17
Pseudomembranous oral candidiasis ("thrush").
(From Cohen J, Powderly WG: Infectious Diseases, 2nd ed. St Louis, Mosby, 2004.)

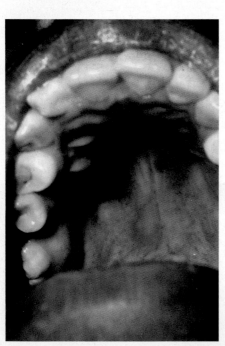

Fig 331–16
AIDS-related Kaposi's sarcoma: oral mucosal lesions are common.
(Courtesy of the Institute of Dermatology, London, UK.)

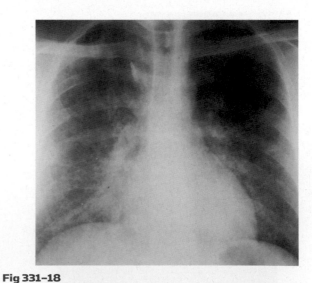

Fig 331–18
P. jirovecii (carinii) pneumonia. A posteroanterior chest film demonstrates the typical bilateral distribution of fine to medium reticular interstitial densities.
(From Grainger RG, Allison DJ, Adam A, Dixon AK [eds]: Grainger and Allison's Diagnostic Radiology, 4th ed. Philadelphia, Churchill Livingstone, 2001.)

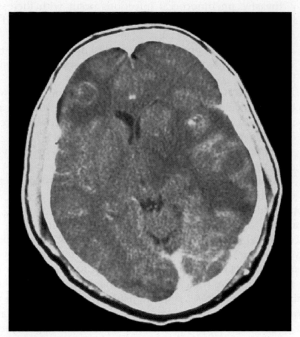

Fig 331–19
Toxoplasmic encephalitis in person who has AIDS. A cranial CT scan shows bilateral contrast-enhanced ring lesions with peripheral edema and mass effect.
(From Cohen J, Powderly WG: Infectious Diseases, 2nd ed. St Louis, Mosby, 2004.)

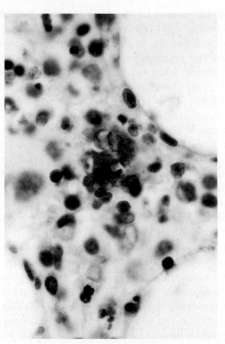

Fig 331–21
Immunoperoxidase stain of *Mycobacterium avium* complex (MAC) in the bone marrow of a patient who has HIV infection and disseminated disease. The presence of mycobacteria in the bone marrow and blood of a patient is the microbiologic hallmark of disseminated MAC disease. The presence of mycobacteria in bone marrow sections using either an immunoperoxidase stain or a conventional acid-fast stain requires the presence of approximately 1.5×10^4 bacilli/g of bone marrow.
(From Cohen J, Powderly WG: Infectious Diseases, 2nd ed. St Louis, Mosby, 2004.)

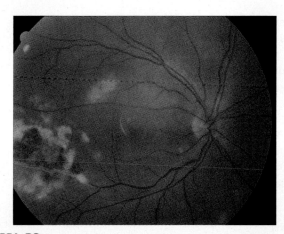

Fig 331–20
Cytomegalovirus retinitis, with characteristic perivascular hemorrhages and exudates.
(From Cohen J, Powderly WG: Infectious Diseases, 2nd ed. St Louis, Mosby, 2004.)

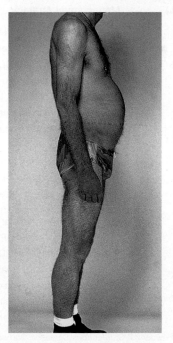

Fig 331–22
Lipodystrophy associated with HIV infection: there is loss of the fat of the extremities. Note the deposition of fat around the abdomen.
(Courtesy of D. McGibbon, MD., Institute of Dermatology, London, UK.)

Management Strategies for the Asymptomatic Patient

- Initial testing: CD4 cell count and HIV viral load measured every 3 to 6 months to guide decisions regarding antiretroviral use and prophylaxis against PCP and MAC infection
- Other testing: identifies previously acquired latent infections that may become reactivated because of loss of T cell function but can be prevented by the use of specific agents
- Serology to *Toxoplasma gondii* (IgG):
  - Clinical infection may be prevented by trimethoprim-sulfamethoxazole (TMP-SMZ) used as prophylaxis for PCP.
- Venereal Disease Research Laboratories (VDRL) test:
  - Lumbar puncture should be performed in patients with a confirmatory specific test (FTA).
  - Treatment with intramuscular benzathine penicillin if the CSF fluid is normal, and intravenous penicillin for 10 days if the CSF VDRL test is reactive or CSF pleocytosis, protein elevation, or hypoglycorrhachia is present.
- PPD skin test showing induration of 5 mm or greater, or patients with exposure to someone with active tuberculosis
  - Treatment with isoniazid 300 mg/day for 9 months or, in case of isoniazid-induced hepatitis, rifampin 600 mg PO qd (only for those not receiving protease inhibitors or nucleoside reverse transcriptase inhibitor agents) for 4 months
- Immunizations:
  - Patients should receive the annual influenza vaccine each fall.
  - Pneumococcal polysaccharide vaccine (Pneumovax) is recommended for all people with HIV infection and is most effective in those with CD4 counts greater than 200.

- Invasive pneumococcal infections occur with increased frequency in HIV-infected people; these people should be revaccinated every 5 years.
- Hib vaccine is not usually recommended for adult use, since the incidence of invasive *H. influenzae* infection is low.
- Hepatitis B vaccination is recommended for people who have no evidence of prior infection with hepatitis B and who are at risk for acquiring it. They should also receive hepatitis A vaccine.
- Tetanus-diphtheria vaccine boosters should be given every 10 years.
- Mumps and rubella vaccines are recommended for susceptible adults.

Prophylactic Agents

Treatment for several opportunistic infections can be discontinued if there has been a sustained CD4 cell count elevation above 200 associated with highly active antiretroviral therapy (HAART) (PCP, toxoplasmosis, cryptococcosis) and 100 for MAC for more than 3 to 6 months. Primary prophylaxis against each of these opportunistic infections should be reintroduced if the CD4 count falls below this range. Table 331–2 describes prophylaxis and treatment for opportunistic infections.

- PJP prophylaxis if CD4 cell level is less than 200/mm^3.
- TMP-SMZ: most effective agent, also provides protection against infections due to *T. gondii*, *Nocardia* spp., and enteric pathogens

---

TABLE 331–2 Prophylaxis and treatment for opportunistic infections

CD4$^+$ lymphocyte count (No./mL)	Management strategy
500	General counseling (safer sex, nutrition, etc.)
	History and physical examination every 3–6 months
	Plasma viral load and CD4 count every 5–6 months
	Pneumovax, annual influenza vaccinations
	Tuberculin skin lest and INH prophylaxis if indicated
	Update diphtheria–pertussis–tetanus (tetanus toxoid for adults) and inactivated polio vaccinations
	Hepatitis B vaccine if at risk
	Syphilis serology
<500	Antiretroviral therapy followed by plasma viral load 1 month later
	Plasma viral load and CD4+ count every 3–4 months
	Herpes suppression if frequent recurrences (more than 4–6 outbreaks/year)
	Relevant history, physical and laboratory investigations at least monthly if symptomatic, diagnosed with AIDS, or on antiretroviral therapy
200	Start prophylaxis for PJP
100	Plasma viral load and CD4+ count every 3–4 months
	Start prophylaxis for toxoplasmosis if seropositive and not on trimethoprim–sulfamethoxazole
<75	Consider MAC prophylaxis
<50	Screening by an ophthalmologist for cytomegalovirus (CMV) retinitis, to be repeated at 3- to 6-monthly intervals; consider CMV prophylaxis

From Cohen J, Powderly WG: Infectious Diseases, 2nd ed. St Louis, Mosby, 2004.

- Dapsone: indicated for those with TMP-SMZ toxicity or who fail TMP-SMZ desensitization; 30% of people with TMP-SMZ rash develop a reaction to dapsone.
- Aerosolized pentamidine is less effective than TMP-SMZ or dapsone in reducing the incidence of PCP in persons with CD4 cell counts less than 100.
- Atovaquone may be considered if the patient is unable to tolerate other prophylactic regimens.
- Prophylaxis against MAC in patients with CD4 cell counts less than 75.
- Azithromycin weekly is the most effective agent in preventing MAC. Emergence of resistant strains may occur with azithromycin (11%).
- Mycobacterial blood culture for MAC should be drawn and returned negative before prophylaxis against MAC is initiated.
- Prophylaxis against *Cryptococcus* (oral fluconazole) and cytomegalovirus (oral ganciclovir) is not indicated because neither drug reduces mortality, both are costly, and they may cause the emergence of resistant strains.

Highly Active Antiretroviral Therapy

- Treatment goals are maximal and durable suppression of viral loads (<50 copies/mL), restoration of immunologic function (CD4 cell count), and prevention of HIV disease progression. Figure 331–23 illustrates possible sites of intervention in the inhibition of HIV replication, and Figure 331–24 describes an approach to antiretroviral therapy.

- The standard regimen is two nucleoside reverse transcriptase inhibitor (NRTI) (AZT/3TC, TNF/3TC, or ABAC/3TC) plus a non-nucleoside reverse transcriptase inhibitor (NNRTI) (Sustiva is the standard agent, although nevirapine has similar virologic activity) or a ritonavir-boosted protease inhibitor (PI) agent (Lopinavir, Atazanavir, Fosamprenavir). Both NNRTI agents and PI agents may be given on a once daily basis to treatment naïve patients.
- Treatment should be offered to all symptomatic patients and those with acute infection. For asymptomatic patients with chronic HIV infection, therapy should be initiated sometime after the CD4 cell count declines below 350 but before it reaches 200. Before treatment is started, CD4 and HIV viral load values should be repeated because of variations in laboratory values.
- After initiating HAART, measure CD4 counts and viral loads at 1 and 4 months. The criteria used to assess initial HAART efficacy are as follows:
- Greater than 1.0 log reduction in HIV viral load within 4 weeks and undetectable viral load (HIV RNA <50 copies/mL) within 4 months.
- CD4 boost >25 cells increase above pretreatment value or >200 absolute value within 6 months after initiating therapy
- An ideal regimen should include preferably three but at least two agents from separate drug classes to which the virus retains susceptibility.

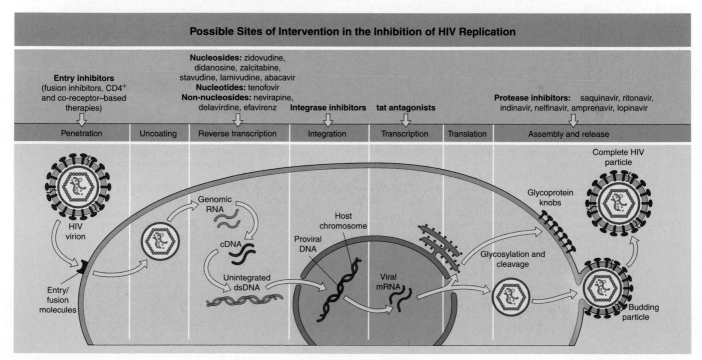

Possible Sites of Intervention in the Inhibition of HIV Replication

Entry inhibitors (fusion inhibitors, CD4+ and co-receptor–based therapies)

Nucleosides: zidovudine, didanosine, zalcitabine, stavudine, lamivudine, abacavir
Nucleotides: tenofovir
Non-nucleosides: nevirapine, delavirdine, efavirenz

Integrase inhibitors

tat antagonists

Protease inhibitors: saquinavir, ritonavir, indinavir, nelfinavir, amprenavir, lopinavir

| Penetration | Uncoating | Reverse transcription | Integration | Transcription | Translation | Assembly and release |

Fig 331–23
Possible sites of intervention in the inhibition of HIV replication.
(From Cohen J, Powderly WG: Infectious Diseases, 2nd ed. St Louis, Mosby, 2004.)

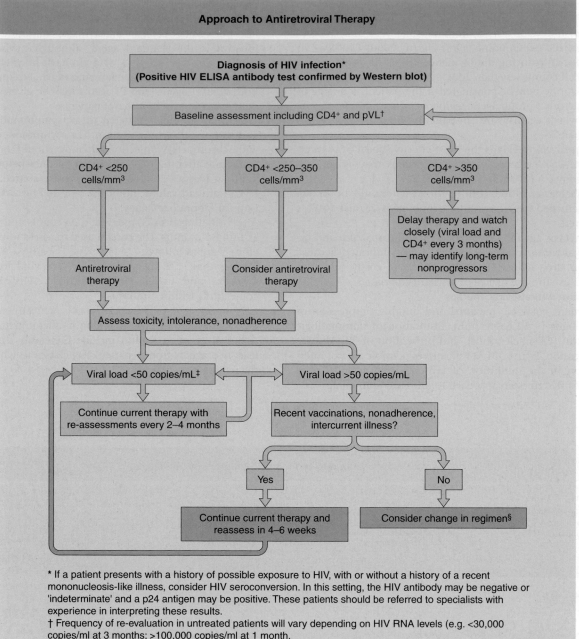

Fig 331-24
Approach to antiretroviral therapy. PI, protease inhibitors.
(From Cohen J, Powderly WG: Infectious Diseases, 2nd ed. St Louis, Mosby, 2004.)

B. SYMPTOMATIC PATIENT WITH AIDS-DEFINING ILLNESS

Infections and Therapy

- <u>Fungal disorders</u>
- *Candida* infection (thrush)
  - Oropharyngeal thrush involving mucous membranes of the mouth (see Fig. 331–17): if severe, consider esophageal involvement, especially with accompanying wasting
  - Diagnosis: usually by clinical appearance—whitish patches with erythematous base; potassium hydroxide preparation may demonstrate budding yeast and pseudohyphae
  - Differential diagnosis: herpes simplex and aphthous ulcers (painful), oral hairy leukoplakia (as a result of Epstein-Barr virus)
  - Treatment: clotrimazole troches or oral fluconazole
- Esophagitis/oropharyngeal candidiasis
  - Oropharyngeal candidiasis is usually present; patient presents with odynophagia or dysphagia.
  - Differential diagnosis: Epstein-Barr virus, cytomegalovirus, giant esophageal ulcers, and cancer, which should be considered in those patients not responding to antifungal therapy; antifungal prophylaxis
  - Treatment: fluconazole
- Cryptococcus (neoformans) infection
  - Patients may have headache, fever, mental status changes, meningismus (only 30%) with cranial nerve palsies; *Cryptococcus* may disseminate to lungs (Fig. 331–25), skin (Fig. 331–26), blood, liver, and prostate. Nuchal rigidity may be absent. Diagnosis is made by spinal fluid analysis; head CT scan should be performed first. Spinal white blood cell, glucose, and protein levels may all be normal. Cryptococcal antigen is the most sensitive (>1:16 in 95% cases). Serum cryptococcal antigen is reactive in more than 90% of patients with CNS involvement.
  - Initial therapy is with amphotericin B for 2 weeks with adjunctive flucytosine, unless preexisting cytopenias prohibit its use. Serum flucytosine levels must be monitored. Maintenance oral fluconazole therapy prevents relapse and

may be withdrawn when HAART-restored CD4 is >200.
- Coccidioidomycosis (Fig. 331–27)
  - Patients should avoid activities associated with increased risk (disturbed native soil, dust storms) in endemic areas.
  - After initial therapy for coccidioidomycosis, lifelong suppressive therapy is recommended with fluconazole or itraconazole.
  - Recommendations for discontinuation of secondary prophylaxis (chronic maintenance therapy) in a patient with a CD4 count greater than 100 on HAART are not available.
  - Fluconazole and itraconazole have potential teratogenicity in pregnant women. Consider amphotericin B (preferred), especially during the first trimester. All HIV-positive women on azole therapy for coccidioidomycosis should maintain birth control precautions.
- Histoplasmosis (Figs. 331–28 and 331–29)

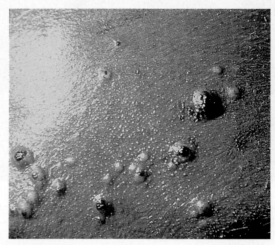

Fig 331–26
Cutaneous cryptococcosis. This lesion is typical of the skin lesions of most endemic mycoses that occur in patients who have AIDS, and such a lesion may therefore also be seen in an AIDS patient who has disseminated histoplasmosis or penicilliosis.
(From Cohen J, Powderly WG: Infectious Diseases, 2nd ed. St Louis, Mosby, 2004.)

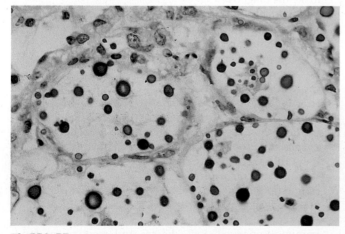

Fig 331–25
Histology of pulmonary cryptococcosis.
(From Cohen J, Powderly WG: Infectious Diseases, 2nd ed. St Louis, Mosby, 2004.)

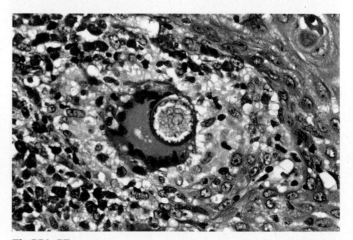

Fig 331–27
Coccidioidomycosis: high-power view of spherule.
(Courtesy of J. Cohen, MD, Dermatopathology Laboratory, Tucson, AZ.)

• HIV-infected people living in or visiting areas endemic for histoplasmosis who have CD4 counts below 200 should avoid activities with increased risks (surface soil dust, contact with chicken droppings, cave exposure).

• Initial therapy for histoplasmosis may include itraconazole rather than amphotericin in non–fulminantly ill patients; chronic maintenance therapy with itraconazole

• Discontinuation of chronic maintenance may be considered if the HAART-restored CD4 count is greater than 200.

• Itraconazole has teratogenicity and embryotoxicity and should not be offered during pregnancy. Treatment with amphotericin B is preferred during the first trimester. HIV-

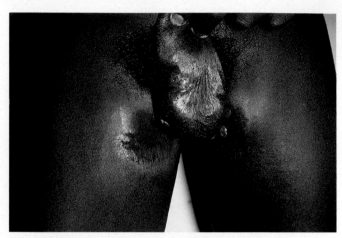

Fig 331–28
Histoplasma capsulatum: note the ulcerated lesions on the scrotum and thigh. This patient was HIV positive.
(Courtesy of C. Furlonge, MD, Port of Spain, Trinidad.)

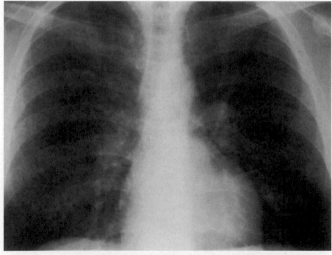

Fig 331–29
Histoplasmosis. A posteroanterior chest film demonstrates the typical findings of histoplasmosis in AIDS patients. A pattern composed of small nodules 2 to 4 mm in diameter is seen in both lungs.
(From Grainger RG, Allison DJ, Adam A, Dixon AK [eds]: Grainger and Allison's Diagnostic Radiology, 4th ed. Philadelphia, Churchill Livingstone, 2001.)

infected women on azole therapy should maintain effective birth control measures.

• *Pneumocystis jirovecii (carinii)* infection
  • Patients have shortness of breath and nonproductive cough with few findings on examination; chest x-ray usually reveals an interstitial infiltrate (see Fig. 331–18), but may be normal.
  • Diagnosis is usually made by sputum induction or by bronchoalveolar lavage, with visualization by monoclonal antibody, methenamine silver stain, or PCR.
  • Oral regimens: treatment in mild cases can be given orally (PO_2 >70 mm Hg; A-a gradient <35 mm Hg) for a 3-week course: TMP-SMZ, TMP-dapsone: trimethoprim, primaquine and clindamycin: primaquine, atovaquone
  • Intravenous regimens: for individuals with moderate-to-severe infections (PO_2 <70 mm Hg or A-a gradient >35 mm Hg) or individuals intolerant to oral formulations: TMP-SMZ, pentamidine, trimetrexate
  • Adjunctive corticosteroid therapy: indicated when PO_2 is less than 70 mm Hg or A-a gradient is greater than 35 mm Hg to prevent early deterioration of oxygenation by decreasing inflammation. Must exclude other opportunistic infections (TB, fungal); 40 mg of prednisone bid days 1 to 5, 40 mg/day for 6 to 10 days; taper over 21-day course of therapy. There is a risk of reactivation of latent infection (cytomegalovirus, histoplasmosis, TB).

• **Mycobacterial infections**
  • *Mycobacterium tuberculosis* may cause pulmonary involvement (see Fig. 331–13), extrapulmonary involvement, or both. Extrapulmonary tuberculosis may involve meningitis, lymphadenitis, or peritonitis. With more advanced disease (CD4 <200), there may be atypical chest x-ray findings, possibly involving the lower lobes.
  • *Mycobacterium avium* complex (MAC) (Fig. 331–30)
  • Symptoms are fever, night sweats, and wasting. Dissemination may involve lymph nodes, liver, and bone marrow, causing marrow suppression, diarrhea with abdominal pain, gastroenteritis, and, rarely, pulmonary involvement. Diagnosis is made by blood culture (special lysis-centrifugation technique), which takes an average of 3 weeks to isolate; cultures of tissue or bone marrow are rarely necessary to make the diagnosis.
  • Combination therapy with at least two agents: clarithromycin and ethambutol. Addition of a third agent (rifabutin) may be considered.

• **Bacterial infections:** patients with HIV may develop infections from *S. pneumoniae, H. influenzae,* or *P. aeruginosa.* Fever with productive cough and lobar infiltrates may occur. Functional humoral response to *S. pneumoniae* may be impaired, leading to recurrent infections caused by these pathogens. Other pathogens include the following:
  • *Salmonella* spp,: recurrent bacteremia; treat with ampicillin, TMP-SMZ, ciprofloxacin, or third-generation cephalosporin, based on sensitivities and clinical presentation; gastrointestinal symptoms may not be present. Avoid raw or undercooked eggs, poultry, meat, and seafood.
  • Listeriosis: in HIV-infected individuals who are severely immunosuppressed. Soft cheeses and ready-to-eat foods (hot dogs, cold cuts) should be avoided or heated until steaming hot.

- Sinusitis: may be routine bacterial infection or involve *P. aeruginosa* or fungi
- Bacillary angiomatosis: an infection involving skin, with red lesions (Fig. 331–31) that can be mistaken for Kaposi's sarcoma; can involve viscera (liver, spleen, bone); caused by *Rochalimaea henselae* or *R. quintana*; treat with erythromycin or doxycycline; other potential bacterial pathogens in HIV are *Rhodococcus equi*, which may cause cavitating pneumonia, and *Nocardia*.
- Viral infections
  - Herpes simplex viral infections
  - May involve mucous membranes, cause genital herpes, or cause rectal or perirectal infection, resulting in proctitis
  - Initial therapy: acyclovir 200 mg PO five times per day for 7 to 10 days; recurrent episodes may need treatment with 400 mg PO three to five times a day for 5 to 7 days or until

clinically resolved; severe disease involving lung, bronchi, and esophagus may require intravenous acyclovir. Intravenous foscarnet or cidofovir can be used to treat infection caused by acyclovir-resistant isolates of herpes simplex virus (HSV).
- Hepatitis C virus (HCV)
  - Patients with HIV infection should be tested for HCV by enzyme immunoassay. If this test result is positive, confirm with recombinant immunoblot assay or PCR for HCV RNA.
  - Patients with HCV and HIV should receive vaccination for hepatitis A if they are negative for hepatitis A antibodies.
  - Patients with HIV-HCV coinfection are at high risk for chronic liver disease and should be evaluated for treatment by providers with experience in treating both HIV and HCV.
- Cytomegalovirus: infection from this virus may cause illness involving the retina (see Fig. 331–20), gastrointestinal tract (including esophagus, colon), and CNS
- Chorioretinitis may develop in 25% of AIDS patients and also may be unilateral, with viremia involving other organs; the patient usually reports decreased vision or "floaters"; ophthalmologic evaluation may be necessary to confirm diagnosis.
- Esophagitis: deep ulcerations are seen, confirmed by the presence of inclusion bodies by biopsy
- Colitis: usually associated with diarrhea, weight loss, and fever; occurs in approximately 10% of AIDS patients
- Retinitis: ganciclovir implant is effective in delaying progression of disease; oral valganciclovir is used to prevent systemic manifestations of disease
- Progressive multifocal leukoencephalopathy (PML): demyelinating disease most often involving posterior cortex of brain (Fig. 331–32), resulting in slowly progressive cognitive impairments. Clinical and radiologic improvement or, in some cases, complete resolution may occur with HAART-associated restoration of CD4 cell counts.
- Parasitic infections
  - Toxoplasmosis
  - Symptoms of *Toxoplasma* encephalitis symptoms: headache, fever, encephalopathy, focal neurologic deficits. Pneumonia, myocarditis, and retinal involvement occur less often.

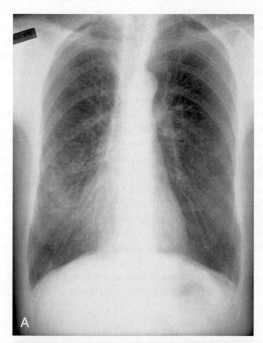

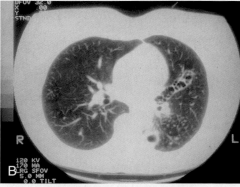

Fig 331–30

Mycobacterium avium complex (MAC) lung disease. (**A**) Interstitial nodular midlung field infiltrates (right > left) in a 64-year-old woman with MAC lung disease. (**B**) Chest CT scan from a 52-year-old woman with MAC lung disease demonstrating three abnormalities that are common in MAC lung disease: bronchiectasis, a cavity and small (<5 mm) nodules. (From Cohen J, Powderly WG: Infectious Diseases, 2nd ed. St Louis, Mosby, 2004.)

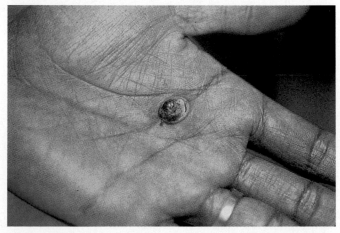

Fig 331–31

Typical appearance of bacillary angiomatosis. (Courtesy of Ciro Martins, MD)

- Diagnosis is usually presumptive, based on multifocal ring enhancing and hypodense mass lesions on CT (see Fig. 331–19), positive toxoplasmic IgG serology, and a clinical and radiologic response to antitoxoplasmic therapy. Other causes of CNS mass lesions in AIDS patients include CNS lymphoma, fungal infection (*Aspergillus, Cryptococcus*), tuberculoma, bacterial abscess.
- Treatment
  (a) Pyrimethamine plus sulfadiazine
  (b) Clindamycin
  (c) Atovaquone, TMP-SMZ, and macrolides may have anti-*Toxoplasma* properties and can be considered as alternative treatments.
- Cryptosporidiosis: Protozoal infection causing watery diarrhea, abdominal pain, and dehydration, particularly worse in patients with CD4 counts less than 50. Diagnosis is made by a modified acid-fast bacilli stain of stool. There is no effective therapy for HIV-infected patients, although nitazoxanide has been used in immunocompetent patients. Azithromycin, when taken for MAC prophylaxis, may reduce the risk for cryptosporidiosis.
- Isosporiasis: Another protozoal infection with a presentation similar to that of *Cryptosporidium* infection, with oocysts found in routine stain of stool; treatment with TMP-SMZ.
- Microsporidiosis (see Fig. 330–7): Also similar to *Cryptosporidium* infection, with oocysts found in special modified trichrome stain of stool; treatment with albendazole (400 mg bid) is only effective against certain species; atovaquone is effective against others.
- Malignancies and HIV and AIDS: Malignancies may be occurring more frequently, as prognosis has been improved with HAART and prevention of opportunistic infections with prophylactic therapies. The following have been listed as AIDS-defining malignancies:
- Kaposi's sarcoma (see Fig. 331–15): found most often in HIV-infected homosexual men and less frequently (<5%) in patients in other HIV risk groups. The lesions from Kaposi's sarcoma may be multifocal, involving skin (79%),

lymph nodes (70%), gastrointestinal tract (45%), and lungs (10%). Treatment is based on extent of involvement; therapy with intralesional vinblastine and with radiation therapy is recommended for localized or small numbers of lesions and chemotherapy with vincristine and vinblastine, etoposide, or bleomycin for aggressive and disseminated disease. Use of many interleukins (e.g., interleukin 4), tumor necrosis factor, and pentoxifylline is investigational.

- Non-Hodgkin's lymphoma: a B cell tumor associated with Epstein-Barr virus; most often extranodal; 30% may occur in patients with CD4 cell counts greater than 200; gastrointestinal tract, CNS, bone marrow, or liver (or other viscera in smaller percentages) are also affected. Chemotherapy regimens have approximately 50% response. Dose-limiting multiagent therapy is myelosuppression.
- Primary CNS lymphoma: most occur in patients with CD4 counts less than 200, but one third occur with CD4 counts greater than 200. Most are unifocal ring-enhancing mass lesions that cause focal neurologic deficits or seizures. Brain biopsy establishes diagnosis.
- AIDS-related cervical cancer: associated with human papillomavirus (Fig. 331–33); often in patients with multiple sexual partners and possibly related to primary association of HIV to cancer development.
- Other cancers associated with HIV infection:
  - Hodgkin's lymphoma: may occur in a patient who is an intravenous drug user or who has sexually acquired disease. Epstein-Barr virus may be linked to both Hodgkin's disease and non-Hodgkin's lymphoma; patients usually present with disseminated stage III or stage IV disease involving bone marrow (50%) or liver and lungs.
  - Anal carcinoma: associated with human papillomavirus and impaired immunity; increased risk in homosexual men
  - AIDS-related cachexia: Megestrol acetate can stimulate appetite and food intake in patients with AIDS-related weight loss. It can result in a statistically significant weight gain and in patient-reported improvement in overall sense of well-being.

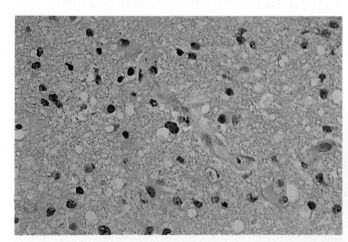

Fig 331–32
Progressive multifocal leukoencephalopathy. Enlarged oligodendroglial cell nuclei are characteristic of this disorder.
(From Silverberg SG: Principles and Practice of Surgical Pathology and Cytopathology, 4th ed. Philadelphia, Churchill Livingstone, 2006.)

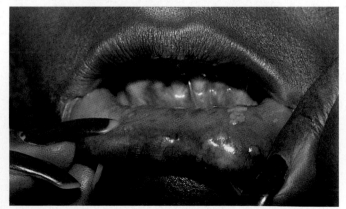

Fig 331–33
Human papillomavirus infection. Human papillomavirus infections are common in HIV-infected patients. They may have unusual features, as demonstrated here, and may be refractory to therapy.
(From Cohen J, Powderly WG: Infectious Diseases, 2nd ed. St Louis, Mosby, 2004.)

Chapter 332 Protozoal infections

A. MALARIA

DEFINITION

Malaria is a protozoan disease caused by the genus *Plasmodium* and transmitted by female *Anopheles* spp. mosquitoes. It is characterized by fever and often presents with classic malarial paroxysm. Four species of genus *plasmodium* usually infect humans:

- *P. falciparum*
- *P. vivax*
- *P. malariae*
- *P. ovale*

PHYSICAL FINDINGS AND CLINICAL PRESENTATION

- Fever is the hallmark of malaria (Fig. 332–1), known as malarial paroxysm, initially daily until synchronization of infection after several weeks, when fever may occur every other day (tertian) in *P. vivax*, *P. ovale*, or *P. falciparum* malaria or every third day (quartan) in *P. malariae* malaria.
- Classic malarial paroxysm characterized by
  1. Cold stage: abrupt onset of cold feeling associated with rigors, shakes
  2. Hot stage: high fever ($\cong 40°$ C) associated with restlessness
  3. Sweating stage: patient defervesces
- Nonspecific symptoms are
  1. Headache
  2. Cough
  3. Myalgia
  4. Vomiting
  5. Diarrhea
  6. Jaundice

P. falciparum

- Most pathogenic of the four species
- Rapidly progresses to high-level parasitemia
- Important cause of the fatal malaria
- Classic malarial paroxysm usually absent
- Incubation period after exposure is 12 days (range: 9 to 60 days)
- Cytoadherence and resetting of red blood cells (RBCs) play central roles in pathogenesis.
- The sequestration of RBC in vital organs (Fig. 332–2) leads to fatal complications.
- Cerebral malaria is a feared complication.
- Retinal hemorrhages (Fig. 332–3) may occur.
- Invades erythrocytes of all ages
- Lacks hypnozoites (intrahepatic stage), does not relapse
- Blood smear usually shows ring form only.
- Pigment color is black.
- Banana-shaped gametocytes; if seen in blood, smear is diagnostic.
- Chloroquine resistance widely present

P. vivax

- Known as tertian malaria: fever occurs every other day
- Duffy blood-group antigen FYA- or FYB-related receptor needed for attachment to RBCs
- FyFy phenotype (most West African) individuals are resistant to *P. vivax* malaria.
- Incubation period after exposure is 14 days (range: 8 to 27 days).
- Hypnozoites may cause relapse of infection after years.
- Infects mainly reticulocytes. Figure 332–4 illustrates the *P. vivax* life cycle.

Tertian and Quartan Malarial Fever Patterns

	Day 1		Day 2		Day 3		Day 4	
	☀	☽	☀	☽	☀	☽	☀	☽

Temperature (°F): 104, 102, 100, 98.6, 98

——— Plasmodium vivax, Plasmodium ovale, Plasmodium falciparum

·····○····· Plasmodium malariae

☀ Daytime

☽ Nighttime

Fig 332–1
Tertian and quartan malarial fever patterns.
(From Cohen J, Powderly WG: Infectious Diseases, 2nd ed. St Louis, Mosby, 2004.)

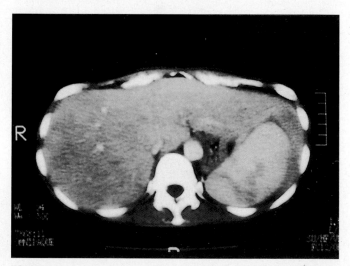

Fig 332–2
Massive hepatosplenomegaly in a patient with severe malarial anemia due to *P. falciparum*. This CT scan of the abdomen was taken of a traveler from West Africa who, after a prolonged history of fevers, presented with a hemoglobin concentration of less than 50 g/L. The scan shows a massively enlarged liver, the left lobe of which is encircling an equally enlarged spleen.
(From Cohen J, Powderly WG: Infectious Diseases, 2nd ed. St Louis, Mosby, 2004.)

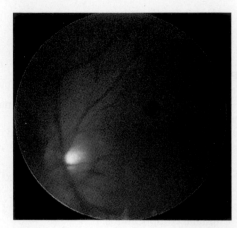

Fig 332-3
Retinal hemorrhage in severe falciparum malaria. Examination of the fundus is important in the physical examination of a patient with severe falciparum malaria as it can give some indication as to prognosis. In this case, the hemorrhage is near the macula. Such hemorrhages have been found in as many as 18% to 30% of patients with cerebral malaria. In children, additional changes of extramacular whitening and changes in which the vessels turn white in isolated segments, often at branch points, occur.
(From Cohen J, Powderly WG: Infectious Diseases, 2nd ed. St Louis, Mosby, 2004.)

Plasmodium Vivax Life Cycle

Human liver stages

Liver cell

② Infected liver cell

⑫ Ruptured oocyst   *Mosquito stages*

a

Exo-erythrocytic cycle

④ Ruptured schizont

③ Schizont

① Mosquito takes a blood meal (injects sporozoites)

⑪ Oocyst

ⅰ Release of sporozoites

Human blood stages

Immature trophozoite (ring stage)

c

Sporogonic cycle

⑧ Mosquito takes a blood meal (ingests gametocytes)

b

Erythrocytic cycle

⑩ Oakinete

Mature trophozoite

Macrogametocyte

⑨ Microgamete entering macrogamete

Exflagellated microgametocyte

P. falciparum

⑥ Ruptured schizont

Schizont

♀ *P. vivax*
P. ovale
P. malariae   ⑦ Gametocytes ♂

⑦ Gametocytes

ⅰ Infective stage

▲ Diagnostic stage

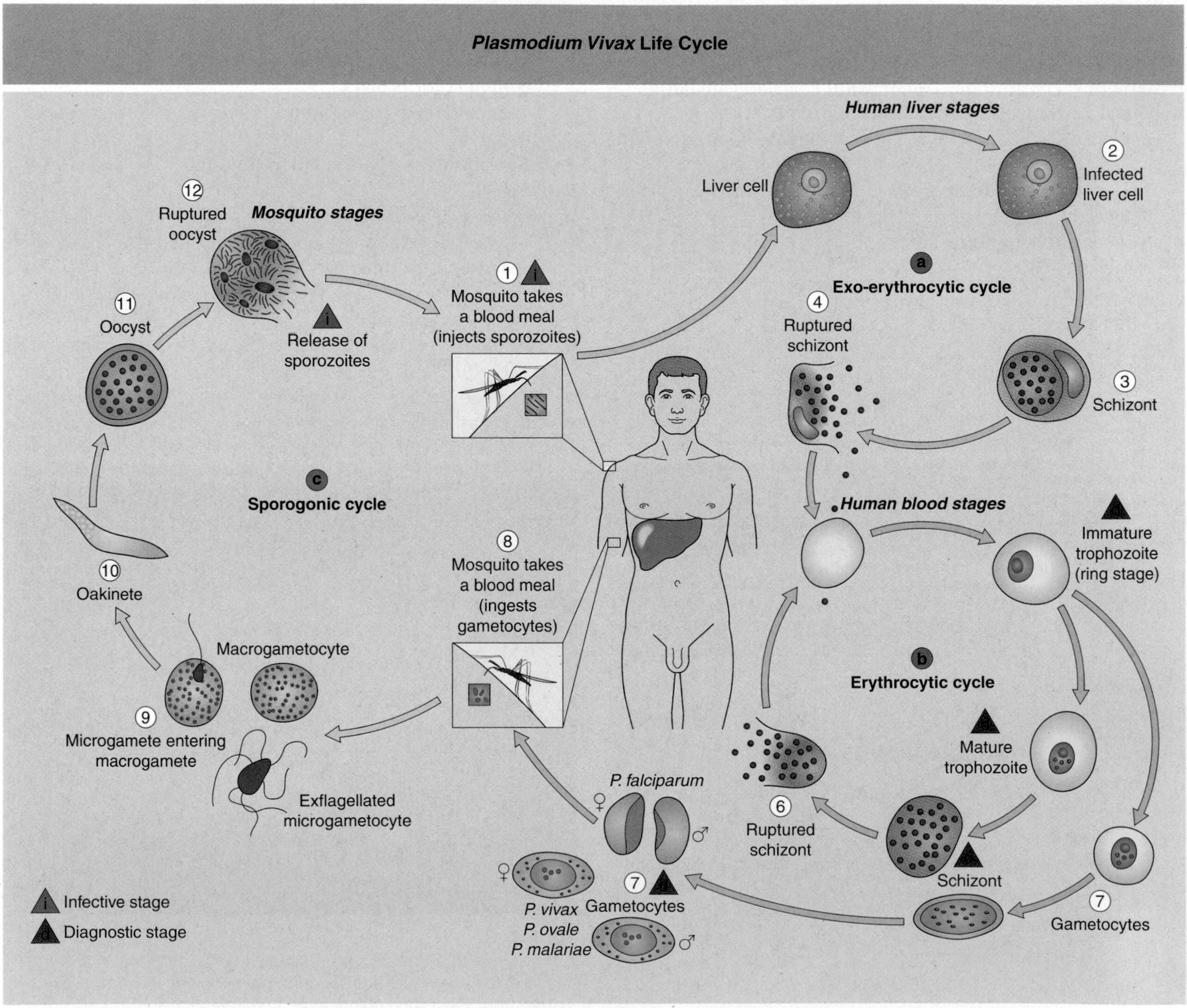

Fig 332-4
Plasmodium vivax life cycle. The life cycle starts when an infected mosquito feeds, inoculating the sporozoite form of the parasite, which infects the hepatocytes. The parasite cells then multiply (liver schizonts) and are liberated into the circulation to invade red cells where they grow (trophozoites) and divide (schizonts). Some trophozoites differentiate into gametocytes infective for mosquitoes.
(From Cohen J, Powderly WG: Infectious Diseases, 2nd ed. St Louis, Mosby, 2004.)

- Irregularly shaped large rings and trophozoites, enlarged RBCs, and Schüffner's dot are seen in peripheral blood smear.
- Pigment color is yellow-brown.
- *P. vivax* from Papua New Guinea have reduced sensitivity to chloroquine.
- Primaquine needed to eradicate the hypnozoites

P. ovale
- Also known as tertian malaria; fever occurs every other day
- Occurs mainly in tropical Africa
- Incubation period after exposure is 14 days (range: 8 to 27 days)
- Hypnozoites may cause relapse of infection.
- Infects mainly reticulocytes
- Infected RBCs seen as enlarged, oval shape containing large ring or trophozoites with Schüffner's dot
- Pigment color is dark brown.
- Primaquine needed to eradicate the hypnozoites
- No chloroquine resistance encountered

P. malariae
- Known as quartan malaria; fever occurs every third day
- Common cause of chronic malarial infection
- May persist 20 to 30 years after leaving the endemic area
- Worldwide distribution
- Incubation period after exposure is 30 days (range: 16 to 60 days)
- Lacks hypnozoites (intrahepatic stage)
- May persist in blood for many years if treated inadequately
- Chronic infection may cause soluble immune-complex, resulting in nephritic syndrome.
- Infects mainly mature RBCs
- Band or rectangular forms of trophozoites are commonly seen in peripheral blood smear.
- Pigment color is brown-black.

Cerebral malaria
- Feared complication of *P. falciparum* infection
- Mortality ~20%
- Pathogenesis is poorly understood.
- Ischemia as a result of sequestration of parasites or cytokines induced by parasite toxin(s) is the key debate.
- Seizure and altered mental status leading to coma are cardinal manifestations.
- Hypoglycemia, lactic acidosis, and elevated circulating tumor necrosis factor (TNF) a may present.
- Cerebrospinal fluid (CSF) studies: no increase in WBC count or protein, raised lactate concentrate, and increased opening pressure, especially in children, may present

DIFFERENTIAL DIAGNOSIS
- Typhoid fever
- Dengue fever
- Yellow fever
- Viral hepatitis
- Influenza
- Brucellosis
- UTI
- Leishmaniasis
- Trypanosomiasis
- Rickettsial diseases
- Leptospirosis

LABORATORY TESTS
- The thick and thin blood films are required to identify malarial parasites (Fig. 332–5).
- The thick smears are more sensitive and primarily used to detect the presence of parasites.
- The thin smears are used for species differentiation and parasite density estimation.
- Persons suspected of having malaria but with no parasite seen in blood smears should have blood smears repeated every 12 to 24 hours for 3 consecutive days.
- Urinalysis: urine specimen may reveal dark urine (Fig. 332–6)
- PCR
  1. It is useful in accurate species diagnosis.
  2. It can detect the low-level parasitemias.
- Quantitative buffy cost (QBC)
  1. This test detects nuclear material of parasites using acridine orange stain.
  2. It is unable to speciate the parasites accurately.
  3. It cannot quantitate parasitemias.
- Para Sight F and Malaria PF test
  1. This test uses a monoclonal antibody to detect *P. falciparum*–specific, histidine-rich protein (HRP)-2
  2. It can detect *P. falciparum* only.
  3. Past infection may confuse diagnosis.
- OptiMal test
  1. This test detects lactate dehydrogenase (LDH) of parasites.
  2. It can differentiate *P. falciparum* from non–*P. falciparum* malaria.

TREATMENT

NON–*P. FALCIPARUM* MALARIA
- Chloroquine
- In the case of *P. vivax* and *P. ovale*, treatment with primaquine is needed to eradicate the exoerythrocytic forms, especially the hypnozoites responsible for relapses.

P. FALCIPARUM MALARIA
- Chloroquine can be used cautiously for *P. falciparum* malaria acquired in chloroquine-sensitive areas (chloroquine is more rapidly effective than quinine)
- Mainstay of treatment is oral quinine sulfate, followed by pyrimethamine with sulfadoxine (Fansider) or doxycycline to eradicate asexual forms of the parasite.

MULTIDRUG-RESISTANT MALARIA:
- Mefloquine, or halofantrine. Combination therapy usually preferred

B. BABESIOSIS

DEFINITION

Babesiosis is a tick-transmitted protozoan disease of animals, caused by intraerythrocytic parasites of the genus *Babesia*. Humans are incidentally infected, resulting in a nonspecific febrile illness.

PHYSICAL FINDINGS AND CLINICAL PRESENTATION
- Incubation period 1 to 4 weeks, or 6 to 9 weeks in transfusion-associated disease
- Gradual onset of irregular fever, chills, diaphoresis, headache, myalgia, arthralgia, fatigue, and dark urine

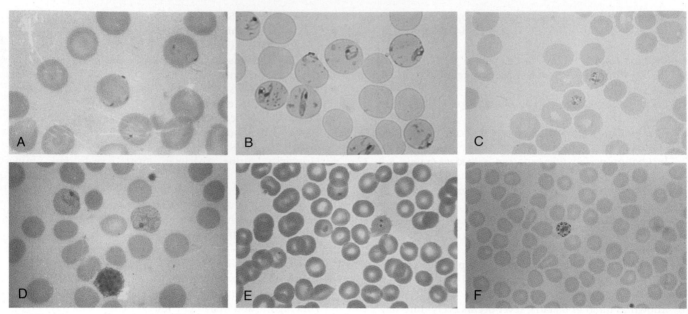

Fig 332–5

Thin blood films from patients with malaria. (**A**) Delicate small ring forms of *Plasmodium falciparum* showing multiply infected red cells and a characteristic "appliqué" form in the uppermost parasite in the central red cell, where the parasite appears as if it is applied to the surface rather than within the red cell. (**B**) Ring forms of *P. falciparum* in a heavy infection and where the pH of the stain is 7.2 rather than 6.7, showing the irregular, basophilic Maurer's clefts in the cytoplasm of infected cells characteristic of *P. falciparum*. (**C**) Very early trophozoites of *P. falciparum* in the peripheral blood film of a patient with severe disease. The relative size and presence of pigment indicate the greater maturity of the parasite and may indicate a poorer prognosis. (**D**) Peripheral blood film from a patient with vivax malaria showing mixed ring and schizont forms. The ring forms are far more fleshy and ameboid and the cytoplasm of the infected cell shows the characteristic regular and eosinophilic Schüffner's dots, which help in diagnosis. (**E**) Peripheral blood film from a patient with ovale malaria showing a small ring form on the left, which could quite easily be mistaken for *P. falciparum*. The larger central parasite has enlarged the cell into an oval shape and has also formed a fimbriated fringe at the upper pole of the cell. (**F**) Peripheral blood film from a patient with malariae malaria showing the characteristic rosette schizont with daughter merozoites (usually eight) around a central piece of pigment (hemazoin). The ring forms of this species characteristically form a band stretching across the width of the red cell.

(From Cohen J, Powderly WG: Infectious Diseases, 2nd ed. St Louis, Mosby, 2004.)

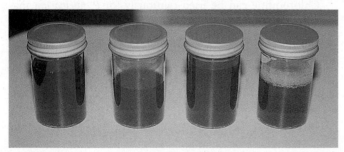

Fig 332–6

Blackwater fever. Urine specimen on admission (*left*) and days 2, 3, and 4 in a cross-Africa traveler with falciparum malaria on quinine treatment, showing the characteristic dark urine of blackwater fever, which showed gradual clearing. The same patient presented with a fever 1 week later and, when treated presumptively for malaria with quinine, developed dark urine once again. Renal function was only mildly impaired.

(From Cohen J, Powderly WG: Infectious Diseases, 2nd ed. St Louis, Mosby, 2004.)

- On physical examination: petechiae, frank or mild hepatosplenomegaly, and jaundice
- Infection with *B. divergens* producing a more severe illness with a rapid onset of symptoms and increasing parasitemia progressing to massive intravascular hemolysis and renal failure

CAUSE

- Vector: Deer tick, *Ixodes scapularis* (also known as *I. dammini*)

  1. Feeds on rodents during the spring and summer while in its larval and nymphal stages and on deer as an adult

  2. During the warmer months in endemic areas, humans are readily infected while engaging in outdoor activities.

- *B. microti*, along with *B. divergens* and *B. bovis*, account for most human infections.

- In the United States, cases caused by *B. microti* are acquired on offshore islands of the northeastern coast, including Nantucket Island, Cape Cod, and Martha's Vineyard in Massachusetts; Block Island in Rhode Island; and Long Island, Fire Island, and Shelter Island in New York; as well as the nearby mainland including Connecticut and New Jersey.

- Sporadic cases reported from California, Georgia, Maryland, Minnesota, Virginia, Wisconsin, and, most recently, the WA-1 strain from Washington State and the MO-1 strain from Missouri.
- *B. divergens* and *B. bovis* are implicated in human disease in Europe, where the disease remains rare and predominantly associated with asplenia.
- Majority of cases are symptomatic
- May be transmissible by transfusion, through platelets and erythrocytes
- Mixed infections (*B. microti* and *Borrelia burgdorferi*) are estimated to occur in 10% (Rhode Island and Connecticut) to 60% (New York) of cases.

DIFFERENTIAL DIAGNOSIS
- Amebiasis (see Fig. 332–11)
- Ehrlichiosis (see Fig. 332–8)
- Hepatic abscess (see Fig. 183–2)
- Leptospirosis
- Malaria (see Fig. 332–5)
- Salmonellosis, including typhoid fever
- Acute viral hepatitis
- Hemorrhagic fevers

LABORATORY TESTS
- CBC to reveal mild to moderate pancytopenia
- Abnormally elevated serum chemistries, including creatinine, liver function profile, lactate dehydrogenase, and direct and total bilirubin levels
- Urinalysis to reveal proteinuria and hemoglobinuria
- Examination of Giemsa- or Wright-stained thick and thin blood films for intraerythrocytic parasites
  1. In its classic, although infrequently seen, form, a "tetrad" or "Maltese Cross" composed of four daughter cells attached by cytoplasmic strands is observed (Fig. 332–7).
  2. More commonly, smaller forms composed of a single chromatin dot are eccentrically located within bluish cytoplasm.

3. Parasitized erythrocytes may be multiply infected but not enlarged, or they may show evidence of pigment deposition, seen with *Plasmodium* species.
- Diagnosis achieved serologically by indirect immunofluorescence assay (IFA) is specific for *B. microti*.
  1. Titer of ≥1:64 is indicative of seropositivity, whereas a titer ≥1:256 is considered diagnostic of acute infection.
  2. Assay is hampered by the inability to distinguish between exposed patients and those who are actively infected.
  3. Immunoglobulin M indirect immunofluorescent antibody test may be highly sensitive and specific for diagnosis.
  4. Babesial DNA by PCR has comparable sensitivity and specificity to microscopic analysis of thin blood smears.

TREATMENT
- In patients with intact spleens: predominantly asymptomatic or, if symptomatic, generally self-limited
- Therapy reserved for the severely ill patient, especially if asplenic, elderly, or immunosuppressed
- Combination of quinine sulfate plus clindamycin
- Combination of atovaquone and azithromycin appears to be as effective as a regimen of clindamycin and quinine with fewer adverse reactions
- Exchange transfusions in addition to antimicrobial therapy: successful treatment for severe infections in asplenic patients associated with high levels of *B. microti* or *B. divergens* parasitemia

C. HUMAN GRANULOCYTIC EHRLICHIOSIS

DEFINITION
Human granulocytic ehrlichiosis (HGE) is a zoonotic infection of granulocytes, caused by an *Ehrlichia* species closely related to *E. phagocytophila, E. equi,* and *E. ewingii,* with multisystem manifestations. The etiologic agent is now known as *Anaplasma phagocytophilum.* The characteristic structures of ehrlichias are the morulas that lie within the vacuoles in host cells (Fig. 332–8). Genogroups of ehrlichias are described in Table 332–1.

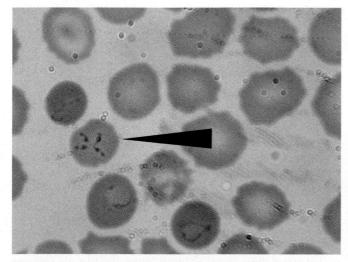

Fig 332–7
Babesia spp. Single and multiple intraerythrocytic parasites can be seen. The *arrow* marks a typical Maltese cross.
(From Cohen J, Powderly WG: Infectious Diseases, 2nd ed. St Louis, Mosby, 2004.)

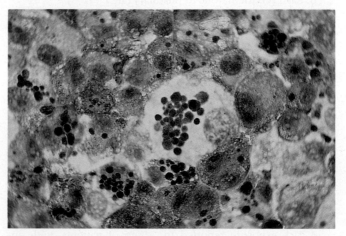

Fig 332–8
Multiple morulas of *Ehrlichia canis* in culture DH82 cells.
(From Cohen J, Powderly WG: Infectious Diseases, 2nd ed. St Louis, Mosby, 2004.)

TABLE 332–1 Genogroups of *Ehrlichia*

Group	Human infection	Animal infection	Vector	Host cell
Group 1: *Ehrlichia* Group				
Ehrlichia caffeenis	Yes	Deer	*Amblyomma*	Monocyte/macrophage
Ehrlichia canis	Possibly	Dogs	*Rhipicephalus*	Monocyte/macrophage
Ehrlichia ewinqii	Yes	Dogs	*Amblyomma*	Neutrophil
Ehrlichia muris	Possibly	Vole	?	Monocyte/macrophage
Ehrlichia ruminantium	No	Cattle, sheep, goats	*Amblyomma*	Endothelium
Group II: *Anaplasma* Group				
Anaplasma bovis	No	Cattle	*Boophilus*	Endothelium
Anaplasma platys	No	Dogs	*Rhipicephalus*	Neutrophil
Anaplasma phagocytophila (incl. *Ehrlichia phagocytophila*, *E. equi*, and "HE" agent)	Yes	Horses, cattle, sheep, deer	*Ixodes*	Neutrophil
Group III: *Neorickettsia* Group				
Neorickettsia helminthoeca	No	Dogs	Fish	Macrophage
Neorickettsia sennetsu	Yes	No	Possibly fish	Monocyte/macrophage
Neorickettsia risticii	No	Horses	Trematode larvae	Monocyte/enterocyte

From Cohen J, Powderly WG: Infectious Diseases, 2nd ed. St Louis, Mosby, 2004.

PHYSICAL FINDINGS AND CLINICAL PRESENTATION
- Most common initial symptoms
  1. Fever
  2. Chills, rigor
  3. Headache
  4. Myalgia
- Subsequent symptoms
  1. Anorexia, nausea
  2. Arthralgia
  3. Cough
  4. Confusion
  5. Abdominal pain
  6. Rash (erythematous to pustular) rare (>11%)
- Complications
  1. Hepatitis
  2. Interstitial pneumonitis
  3. Renal and respiratory failure
  4. Meningitis

CAUSE
- Obligate intracellular gram-negative bacterium (family Rickettsiaceae, genus *Ehrlichia*), now renamed *A. phagocytophilum*
- Vector
  1. Almost certainly tick borne, recently confirmed to be rarely transmitted by infected blood
  2. Transmitted by *Ixodes scapularis* in the northeastern and upper Midwestern states and *Ixodes pacificus* in the Pacific Western states
  3. Tick exposure reported in >90% of patients, with approximately 60% reporting tick bite

- Mammalian host: deer, horses, dogs, white-footed mice, cattle, sheep, goats, bison
- Host inflammatory and immune responses define final spectrum of disease beyond granulocytes, including hepatitis, interstitial pneumonitis, and nephritis with mild azotemia
- Between 6% and 21% of patients with HGE also have serologic evidence of other infection, both transmitted by *Ixodes* spp. tick bites
- Recovery is usual outcome; fatality rate of HGE is <1%

DIFFERENTIAL DIAGNOSIS
- Human monocytic ehrlichiosis (HME)
  1. Caused by *E. chaffeensis* (vector: tick *Amblyomma americanum*)
  2. Rash more common, sometimes petechial
  3. Morulae in monocytes
- Rocky Mountain spotted fever, Colorado tick fever, Q fever, relapsing fever
- Babesiosis
- Leptospirosis
- Lyme disease
- Tularemia
- Typhoid fever, paratyphoid fever
- Brucellosis
- Viral hepatitis
- Meningococcemia
- Infectious mononucleosis
- Hematologic malignancy

LABORATORY TESTS
- Giemsa-stained smear demonstrating morulae of *Ehrlichia* within granulocytes

- CBC progressive leukopenia and thrombocytopenia with nadir near day 7
- C-reactive protein concentration is generally elevated
- Liver function tests (LFTs): increase in hepatic transaminases, LDH, and alkaline phosphatase
- Elevated plasma creatinine concentration may be seen
- Serologic titer (IFA) >80 or fourfold increase in titer to *E. equi* antigen
- PCR to facilitate early diagnosis
- Culture on the first 7 days of illness; not readily available in most clinical laboratories

IMAGING STUDIES
- Chest x-ray examination may show interstitial pneumonitis (unusual)
- MRI of the brain

TREATMENT
- Immediate therapy to limit extent of acute illness and complication
- Tetracycline and doxycycline have activity against the HGE; doxycycline preferred because of a better pharmacokinetic profile
- Rifampin is an alternative drug of choice.

D. AMEBIASIS

DEFINITION
Amebiasis is an infection caused by the protozoal parasite *Entamoeba histolytica*. Although primarily an infection of the colon, amebiasis may cause extraintestinal disease, particularly liver abscess (Fig. 332–9).

PHYSICAL FINDINGS AND CLINICAL PRESENTATION
- Often nonspecific
- Approximately 20% of cases symptomatic
  1. Diarrhea, which may be bloody
  2. Abdominal and back pain
  3. Abdominal tenderness in 83% of severe cases

- Fever in 38% of severe cases
- Hepatomegaly, right upper quadrant (RUQ) tenderness, and fever in almost all patients with liver abscess (may be absent in fulminant cases)

CAUSE
- Caused by the protozoal parasite *E. histolytica*
- Transmission by the fecal-oral route
- Infection usually localized to the large bowel, particularly the cecum where a localized mass lesion (ameboma) may form
- Extraintestinal infection in which the organism invades the bowel mucosa (Fig. 332–10) and gains access to the portal circulation

DIFFERENTIAL DIAGNOSIS
- Severe intestinal infection possibly confused with ulcerative colitis or other infectious enterocolitis syndromes, such as those caused by *Shigella, Salmonella, Campylobacter*, or invasive *Escherichia coli*
- In elderly patients: ischemic bowel possibly producing a similar picture
- Table 332–2 describes common gastrointestinal (GI) parasites.

WORKUP
- Three stool specimens over a period of 7 to 10 days to exclude the diagnosis (sensitivity, 50% to 80%)
- Concentration and staining the specimen with Lugol's iodine or methylene blue to increase the diagnostic yield
- Available culture (rarely necessary in routine cases)

LABORATORY TESTS
- Stool examination is generally reliable (Fig. 332–11).
- Mucosal biopsy is occasionally necessary (Fig. 332–12).
- Serum antibody may be detected and is particularly sensitive and specific for extraintestinal infection or severe intestinal disease.
- Aspiration of abscess fluid is used to distinguish amebic from bacterial abscesses.

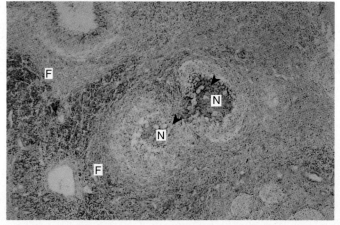

Fig 332–9
Experimental amebic liver abscess. Two characteristic granulomas can be observed with several trophozoites (*arrowheads*) around its necrotic center (N) and epithelioid cells limiting the lesion, surrounded by an area of fibrosis (F).
(From Cohen J, Powderly WG: Infectious Diseases, 2nd ed. St Louis, Mosby, 2004.)

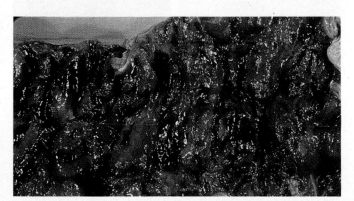

Fig 332–10
Pathology specimen from a fatal case of human amebic colitis. Deep ulcerations into the submucosa have produced abundant hemorrhages.
(Courtesy of Dr. Jesús Aguirre García, Hospital General de México, Secretaria de Salud, Mexico)

TABLE 332–2   Gastrointestinal parasites

Intestinal protozoa	Amebae	Entamoeba *histolytica; Entamoeba dispar* Commensals: *Entamoeba coli* *Entamoeba hartmanni* *Endolimax nana* *Iodamoeba butschlii* *Blastocystis hominis*
	Flagellates	*Giardia lamblia* *Dientamoeba iragilis*
	Ciliate	*Balantidium coli*
	Coccidia	*Cryptosporidium parvum* *Cyclospora cayetanensis* *Isospora belli*
	Microsporidia	*Enterocytozoon bieneusi* *Encephalitozoon intestinalis* (formerly *Septato intestin*)
Intestinal helminths	Nematodes (roundworms)	*Ascaris lumbricoides* *Enterobius vermicularis* Hookworms: *Ancylostoma duodenale* *Necator americanus* *Trichuris trichiura* *Strongyloides stercoralis*
	Trematodes (flukes)	*Fasciolopsis buski* *Heterophyes heterophyes*
	Cestodes (tapeworms)	*Taenia solium* *Taenia saginata* *Hymenolepis nana* *Diphyllobothrium latum*

From Cohen J, Powderly WG: Infectious Diseases, 2nd ed. St Louis, Mosby, 2004.

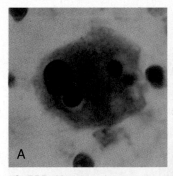 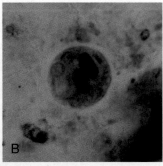

Fig 332–11

Entamoeba histolytica. (**A**) Trophozoite containing ingested red blood cells (the presence of red blood cells confirms the organism is the true pathogen, *E. histolytica*). (**B**) *E. histolytica/E. dispar*, cyst containing four nuclei and chromatoidal bars with smooth, rounded edges (trichrome stain). Note: from the cyst morphology, it is not possible to differentiate pathogenic *E. histolytica* from nonpathogenic *E. dispar*. (From Cohen J, Powderly WG: Infectious Diseases, 2nd ed. St Louis, Mosby, 2004.)

IMAGING STUDIES

Abdominal imaging studies (sonography or CT scan) to diagnose liver abscess

TREATMENT

- Metronidazole is used in the treatment of mild to severe intestinal infection and amebic liver abscess; it may be administered intravenously when necessary.
- Follow-up treatment with iodoquinol should eradicate persistent cysts.
- For asymptomatic patients with amebic cysts on stool examination, use iodoquinol or paromomycin.
- Avoid antiperistaltic agents in severe intestinal infections to avoid risk of toxic megacolon.
- Liver abscess is generally responsive to medical management but surgical intervention indicated for extension of liver abscess into pericardium or, occasionally, for toxic megacolon.

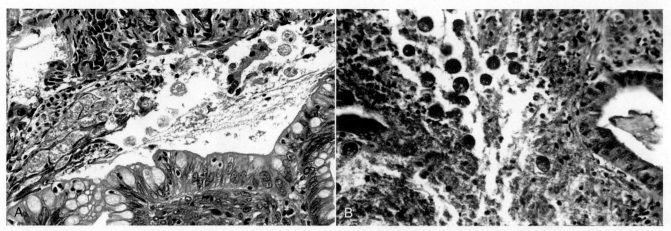

Fig 332–12

Biopsy of a colonic ulcer revealing *Entamoeba histolytica*. (**A**) The large, round trophozoites are present within the necrotic debris at the center of the biopsy. (**B**) A periodic acid–Schiff stain highlights the organisms.
(From Silverberg SG: Principles and Practice of Surgical Pathology and Cytopathology, 4th ed. Philadelphia, Churchill Livingstone, 2006.)

E. GIARDIASIS

DEFINITION

Giardiasis is an intestinal and/or biliary tract infection caused by the protozoal parasite *Giardia lamblia* (Fig. 332–13). The organism is a widespread zoonotic parasite and frequently contaminates fresh water sources worldwide.

PHYSICAL FINDINGS AND CLINICAL PRESENTATION

- More than 70% with one or more intestinal symptoms (diarrhea, flatulence, cramps, bloating, nausea)
- Fever in <20%
- Chronic diarrhea, malabsorption, and weight loss
- GI bleeding is unusual.
- Continuous or intermittent symptoms, lasting for weeks
- Of infected patients, 20% to 25% are asymptomatic.

CAUSE

Infection is acquired by ingestion of viable cysts of the organism, typically in contaminated water or by fecal–oral contact.

DIFFERENTIAL DIAGNOSIS

- Other agents of infective diarrhea (amebae, *Salmonella* sp., *Shigella* sp., *Staphylococcus aureus, Cryptosporidium*, etc.)
- Noninfectious causes of malabsorption

WORKUP

- Stool specimen (three specimens yield 90% sensitivity) or duodenal aspirate for microscopic examination to establish diagnosis and exclude other pathogens.
- Immunoassays for *Giardia* sp. Antigens in stool samples are now routinely used to in most clinical laboratories.

LABORATORY TESTS

- Serum albumin, vitamin B_{12} levels, and stool fat test to exclude malabsorption

IMAGING STUDIES

- Not necessary unless biliary obstruction is suspected
- In detection of organism, possible interference by barium in stool from radiographic studies

TREATMENT

- Adults: metronidazole *or* paromomycin

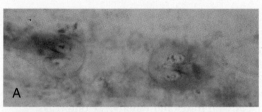

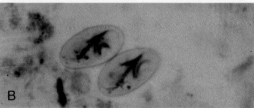

Fig 332–13

Giardia lamblia. (**A**) Trophozoites in mucus; note the sucking disc area, linear axonemes, curved median bodies, and two nuclei (trichrome stain). (**B**) Cysts containing multiple nuclei, linear axonemes, and curved median bodies (iron-hematoxylin stain).
(From Cohen J, Powderly WG: Infectious Diseases, 2nd ed. St Louis, Mosby, 2004.)

F. CRYPTOSPORIDIOSIS

DEFINITION

The intracellular protozoan parasite *Cryptosporidium parvum* is associated with GI disease (Fig. 332–14) and diarrhea, especially in AIDS patients or immunocompromised hosts. It is also associated with waterborne outbreak in immunocompetent hosts.

Other species, including *C. felis, C. muris,* and *C. meleagridis,* are now described to be pathogens as well.

PHYSICAL FINDINGS AND CLINICAL PRESENTATION

- Usually limited to GI tract
- Diarrhea, severe abdominal pain (2 to 28 days)
- Impaired digestion, dehydration
- Fever, malaise, fatigue, nausea, vomiting
- Pneumonia if aspirated

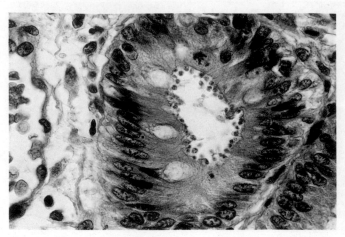

Fig 332–14

Cryptosporidiosis of the colon. Numerous small organisms are evident at the luminal surface of the crypt.

(From Silverberg SG: Principles and Practice of Surgical Pathology and Cytopathology, 4th ed. Philadelphia, Churchill Livingstone, 2006.)

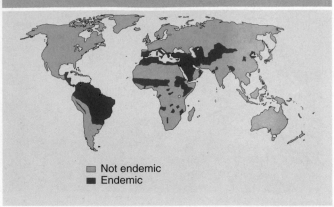

Fig 332–15

Geographic distribution of leishmaniasis. Visceral leishmaniasis (VL): 90% of cases occur in India, Bangladesh, Sudan, and Brazil. Mucocutaneous leishmaniasis (MCL): 90% of cases occur in Bolivia, Brazil, and Peru. Cutaneous leishmaniasis (CL): 90% of cases occur in Afghanistan, Brazil, Iran, Peru, Saudi Arabia, and Syria.

(From Cohen J, Powderly WG: Infectious Diseases, 2nd ed. St Louis, Mosby, 2004.)

CAUSE

Cryptosporidium hominis, Cryptosporidium parvum, C. felis, C. muris, C. meleagridis

DIAGNOSIS

Clinical presentation of acute GI illness, especially associated with HIV or with travel and waterborne outbreaks.

DIFFERENTIAL DIAGNOSIS

- *Campylobacter*
- *Clostridium difficile*
- *Entamoeba histolytica*
- *Giardia lamblia*
- *Salmonella*
- *Shigella*
- *Microsporida*
- Cytomegalovirus
- *Mycobacterium avium*

Disease may cause cholecystitis, reactive arthritis, hepatitis, pancreatitis, pneumonia in immunocompromised or HIV-infected patients

WORKUP

- Stool evaluation looking for characteristic oocyst by modified acid-fast stain
- Serologic testing investigational

TREATMENT

- May be self-limited in normal host, often requiring hydration. Antidiarrhea agents Pepto-Bismol, Kaopectate, or loperamide may give symptomatic relief.
- Pharmacologic treatment with antibiotics has to date varying and usually poor response. Oocyst excretion reduction has been shown with paromomycin/azithromycin and nitazoxanide therapy along with decreasing stool frequency.
- Nitazoxanide elixir has been approved for the treatment of cryptosporidiosis in children ages 1 to 11 years.
- Biliary cryptosporidiosis can be treated with antiretroviral therapy in the HIV setting.

G. LEISHMANIASIS

DEFINITION

Leishmaniasis is an infectious disease caused by a heterogeneous group of protozoan parasites belonging to the genus *Leishmania* and resulting in a variety of different clinical syndromes. Figure 332–15 illustrates the geographic distribution of leishmaniasis.

PHYSICAL FINDINGS AND CLINICAL PRESENTATION

Cutaneous Syndrome

- Localized cutaneous leishmaniasis (Fig. 332–16)
- Mucosal leishmaniasis
- Leishmania recidivans
- Diffuse cutaneous leishmaniasis (Fig. 332–17)

Visceral Syndrome

- Viscerotrophic leishmaniasis: fever, chronic fatigue, malaise, cough, intermittent diarrhea, and abdominal pain. Signs include adenopathy, hepatosplenomegaly (Fig. 332–18), hyperpigmentation of skin, petechiae, jaundice, edema, and ascites.
- Post kala-azar dermal leishmaniasis: generalized cutaneous rash that is often papular or nodular; severe forms with desquamation of skin and mucosa

CAUSE

- Old World parasite: *Leishmania tropica, L. major, L. aethiopica, L. donovani, L. infantum*
- New World parasite: *L. braziliensis* and *L. mexicana* complex, *L. chagasi, L. b. guyanensis, L. b. panamensis*

DIFFERENTIAL DIAGNOSIS

- Malaria
- African trypanosomiasis
- Brucellosis
- Enteric fever
- Bacterial endocarditis

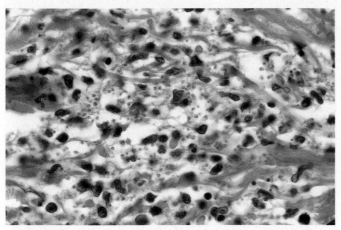

Fig 332-16
Cutaneous leishmaniasis. Numerous amastigote forms of Leishmania are contained in macrophages. Other areas of the biopsy contained a neutrophilic inflammatory response. Despite the numerous organisms, the etiology was not recognized at the time of the initial interpretation (HANDE, ×500).
(From Silverberg SG: Principles and Practice of Surgical Pathology and Cytopathology, 4th ed. Philadelphia, Churchill Livingstone, 2006.)

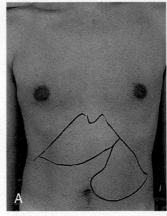
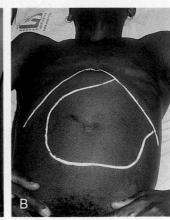

Fig 332-18
Visceral leishmaniasis. (**A**) Hepatosplenomegaly and pallor in a 29-year-old Italian man. (**B**) Splenomegaly and pallor in a 23-year-old Angolan. Both complained of weight loss, fatigue, and fever of several weeks' duration.
(From Cohen J, Powderly WG: Infectious Diseases, 2nd ed. St Louis, Mosby, 2004.)

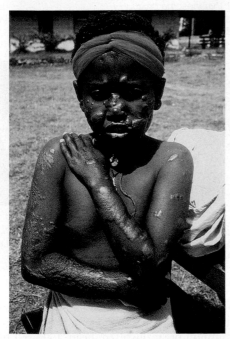

Fig 332-17
Diffuse cutaneous leishmaniasis: note the widespread lesions, many of which appear keloidal.
(Courtesy of the late M. S. R. Hutt, MD, St Thomas' Hospital, London, UK.)

- Generalized histoplasmosis
- Chronic myelocytic leukemia
- Hodgkin's disease and other lymphomas
- Sarcoidosis
- Hepatic cirrhosis
- Tuberculosis

LABORATORY TESTS
- CBC: anemia, neutropenia, thrombocytopenia, and eosinophilia
- LFTs: hypergammaglobulinemia, hypoalbuminemia, and hyperbilirubinemia
- Elevated BUN and creatinine
- Specific diagnosis confirmed by intracellular amastigote in Giemsa-stained impression smears (Fig. 332-19) or sectioned tissue or culture performed in NMN (Novy, MacNeal, Nicolle) or Schneider's medium
- Serologic diagnosis: ELISA, direct agglutination tests, K39 ELISA, PCR, and monoclonal antibody staining of tissue smears
- Montenegro skin test

TREATMENT
- Nonspecific or supportive care
  1. Nutritional diet
  2. Antimicrobial agents for concurrent infections
  3. Blood transfusions
  4. Iron and vitamins
- Specific antileishmanial therapy
  1. Pentavalent antimonials: sodium stibogluconate and sodium antimonygluconate
  2. Miltefosine
  3. Amphotericin B
  4. Pentamidine
  5. Aminosidine
  6. Other agents: allopurinol, ketoconazole, paromomycin (combined with other regimens)
  7. Immunotherapy: IFN-g
  8. Local or tropical treatments and physical therapy, including thermal treatments
  9. Plastic surgery

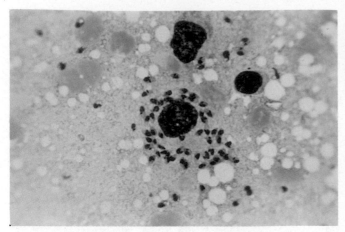

Fig 332–19
Amastigotes (Leishman-Donovan bodies) in bone marrow aspirate from a patient who had *Leishmania infantum* visceral leishmaniasis and AIDS. The nucleus and kinetoplast stain deeply with Giemsa and give the organism its characteristic appearance. *Histoplasma* spp. are the main source of mistaken identification in bone marrow smears but lack these structures. Amastigotes measure 2 to 3 μm in length and are found within macrophages in tissue sections, but usually lie free in smears, because infected macrophages burst as they are smeared.
(From Cohen J, Powderly WG: Infectious Diseases, 2nd ed. St Louis, Mosby, 2004.)

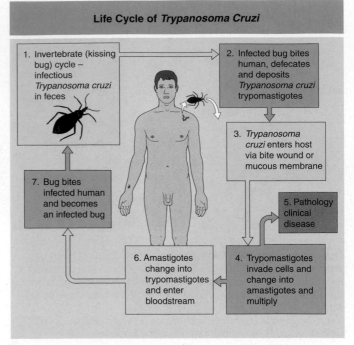

Fig 332–20
Life cycle of *Trypanosoma cruzi*.
(From Cohen J, Powderly WG: Infectious Diseases, 2nd ed. St Louis, Mosby, 2004.)

H. TRYPANOSOMIASIS

DEFINITION

Trypanosomiasis (*Chagas' disease*) is an infection caused by the protozoan parasite *Trypanosoma cruzi*. This is a vector-borne disease transmitted by reduviid ("kissing") insects from multiple wild and domesticated animal reservoirs. Figure 332–20 illustrates the life cycle of this parasite. The disease is characterized by an acute nonspecific febrile illness that may be followed, after a variable latency period, by chronic cardiac, GI, and neurologic sequelae.

PHYSICAL FINDINGS AND CLINICAL PRESENTATION

- Inflammatory lesion that develops about 1 weeks after contamination of a break in the skin with infected insect feces (chagoma)
  1. Area of induration and erythema
  2. Usually accompanied by local lymphadenopathy
- Presence of *Romaña's sign* (Fig. 332–21), which consists of unilateral painless palpebral and periocular edema, when conjunctiva is portal of entry
- Constitutional symptoms of fever, fatigue, and anorexia, along with edema of the face and lower extremities, generalized lymphadenopathy, and mild hepatosplenomegaly after the appearance of local signs of disease
- Myocarditis in a small portion of patients, sometimes with resultant congestive heart failure (CHF)
- Uncommonly, CNS disease, such as meningoencephalitis, which carries a poor prognosis
- Symptoms and signs of disease persisting for weeks to months, followed by spontaneous resolution of the acute illness; patient then in the indeterminate phase of the disease (asymptomatic with attendant subpatent parasitemia and reactive antibodies to *T. cruzi* antigens)

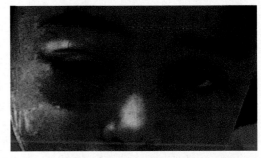

Fig 332–21
Romaña's sign.
(From Cohen J, Powderly WG: Infectious Diseases, 2nd ed. St Louis, Mosby, 2004.)

- Chronic disease may become manifest years to decades after the initial infection:
1. Most common organ involved: heart, followed by GI tract and, to a much lesser extent, the CNS
   a. Cardiac involvement takes the form of arrhythmias or cardiomyopathy, but rarely both.
   b. Cardiomyopathy (Fig. 332–22) is generally bilateral but may affect either ventricle and is often accompanied by apical aneurysms (Fig. 332–23) and mural thrombi.
   c. Arrhythmias are a consequence of involvement of the bundle of His and have been implicated as the leading cause of sudden death in adults in highly endemic areas.
   d. Right-sided heart failure, thromboembolization, and rhythm disturbances associated with symptoms of dizziness and syncope are characteristic.

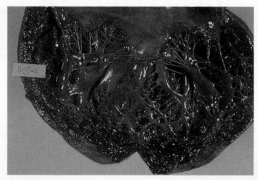

Fig 332–22
A dilated heart from a fatal case of chagasic cardiomyopathy. Chronic heart disease is the commonest cause of death in Chagas' disease. (Courtesy of Dr. J. Cohen, Cordoba, Argentina.)

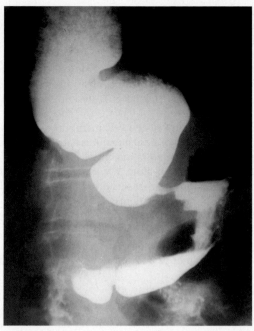

Fig 332–24
Mega-esophagus on radiograph.
(Courtesy of Dr. J. S. Oliveira.)

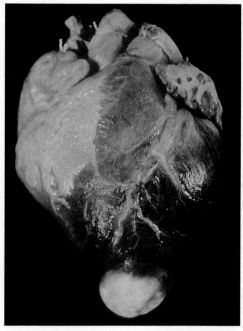

Fig 332–23
Apical aneurysm of the left ventricle in chronic Chagas' disease.
(Courtesy of Dr. J.S. Oliveira)

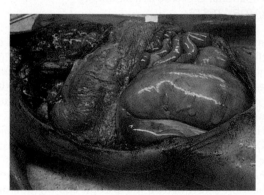

Fig 332–25
Chagasic megacolon at autopsy. Grossly enlarged colon as shown here or other duct dilation is characteristic of chronic Chagas' disease.
(Courtesy of Dr. J. Cohen, Cordoba, Argentina.)

2. Patients with megaesophagus (Fig. 332–24): dysphasia, odynophagia, chronic cough, and regurgitation, frequently resulting in aspiration pneumonitis
3. Megacolon (Fig. 332–25): abdominal pain and chronic constipation, which, when severe, may lead to obstruction and perforation
4. CNS symptoms: most often secondary to embolization from the heart or varying degrees of peripheral neuropathy

CAUSE
● T. cruzi
  1. Found only in the Americas, ranging from the southern half of the United States to southern Argentina
  2. Transmitted to humans by various species of bloodsucking reduviid insects, primarily those of the genera *Triatoma, Panstrongylus,* and *Rhodnius*

3. Usually found in burrows and trees, where infected insects transmit the parasite to nonhuman mammals (e.g., opossums and armadillos), which constitute the natural reservoir
4. Intrusion into enzootic areas for farmland, allowing insects to take up residence in rural dwellings, thus including humans and domestic animals in the cycle of transmission
5. Initial infection of insects by ingesting blood from animals or humans that have circulating flagellated trypanosomes (trypomastigotes)
6. Multiplication of ingested parasites in the insect midgut as epimastigotes, then differentiation into infective metacyclic trypomastigotes in the hindgut whereby the parasites are discharged with the feces during subsequent blood meals

7. Transmission to the second mammalian host through contamination of mucous membranes, conjunctivae, or wounds with insect feces containing infected forms
- In the vertebrate host
  1. Movement of parasites into various cell types, intracellular transformation and multiplication in the cytoplasm as amastigotes, and thereafter differentiation into trypomastigotes
  2. Following rupture of the cell membrane, parasitic invasion of local tissues or hematogenous spread to distant sites, maintaining a parasitemia infective for vectors
- In addition to insect vectors, *T. cruzi* is transmitted through blood transfusions, transplacentally, and, occasionally, secondary to laboratory accidents

DIFFERENTIAL DIAGNOSIS

Acute disease
- Early African trypanosomiasis
- New World cutaneous and mucocutaneous leishmaniasis

Chronic disease
- Idiopathic cardiomyopathy
- Idiopathic achalasia
- Congenital or acquired megacolon

WORKUP

Principal considerations in diagnosis:
- A history of residence where transmission is known to occur
- Recent receipt of a blood product while in an endemic area
- Occupational exposure in a laboratory

LABORATORY TESTS

For acute diagnosis:
- Demonstration of *T. cruzi* in wet preparations of blood, buffy coat, or Giemsa-stained smears (Fig. 332–26)
- Xenodiagnosis, a technique involving laboratory-reared insect vectors fed on subjects with suspected infection thereafter examined for parasites, and culture of body fluids in liquid media to establish diagnosis
  1. Hampered by the length of time required for completion
  2. Of limited use in clinical decision making with regard to drug therapy
  3. Although xenodiagnosis and broth culture are considered to be more sensitive than microscopic examination of body fluids, sensitivities may not exceed 50%.
- Recent advances in serologic testing include immunoblot assay, in situ indirect fluorescent antibody, PCR-based techniques, and an immunochromatographic assay (Chagas Stat Pak).

For chronic *T. cruzi* infection:
- Traditional serologic tests including: complement fixation (CF), indirect immunofluorescence (IIF), indirect hemagglutination, enzyme-linked immunosorbent assay (ELISA), and radioimmune precipitation assay
- Persistent problem with these tests: in addition to sensitivity and specificity, false-positive results
- Saliva ELISA may be useful as a screening diagnostic test in epidemiologic studies of chronic trypanosomiasis infection in endemic areas.

TREATMENT
- Chronic chagasic heart disease: mainly supportive
- Megaesophagus: symptoms usually amenable to dietary measures or pneumonic dilation of the esophagogastric junction

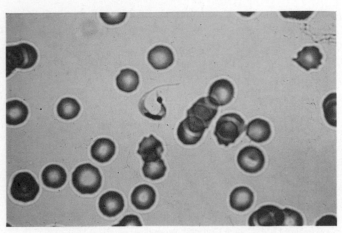

Fig 332–26
Trypanosoma cruzi C-shaped trypomastigote in Giemsa-stained thin blood film.
(From Cohen J, Powderly WG: Infectious Diseases, 2nd ed. St Louis, Mosby, 2004.)

- Chagasic megacolon: in its early stages responsive to a high-fiber diet, laxatives, and enemas
- Nifurtimox: only drug available in the United States for the treatment of acute, congenital, or laboratory-acquired infection. Parasitologic cure in approximately 50% of those treated; should be begun as early as possible

I. SCHISTOSOMIASIS

DEFINITION

Schistosomiasis is caused by infection with parasite blood flukes known as schistosomes.

CAUSE AND PATHOGENESIS
- Human infections are caused by *S. mansoni, S. haematobium, S. japonicum, S. mekongi, and S. intercalatum.* Table 332–3 describes the geographic distribution of human schistosomes.
- Acquisition of disease via contact with fresh water containing infectious free-living cercarial larvae (Fig. 332–27)
- In the United States, most cases are acquired during foreign travel.
- Human disease is primarily associated with the host's granulomatous response to eggs retained in the tissue.

PHYSICAL FINDINGS AND CLINICAL PRESENTATION

ACUTE SYMPTOMS
- Swimmer's itch
- Katayama fever

CHRONIC SYMPTOMS
- Intestinal schistosomiasis
  1. Abdominal pain
  2. Bloody diarrhea
  3. Iron deficiency anemia
  4. Intestinal polyp
  5. Bowel ulcer and strictures
- Hepatic schistosomiasis
  1. Hepatomegaly
  2. Splenomegaly
  3. Portal hypertension, ascites (Fig. 332–28)
  4. Esophageal varices

Life Cycle of Schistosomes

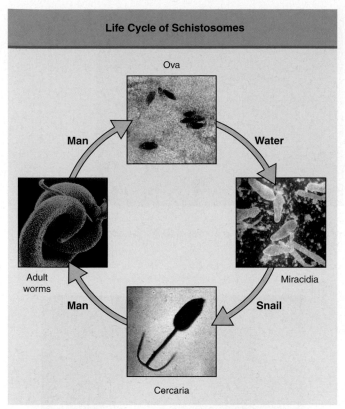

Man — Ova — Water

Adult worms — Miracidia

Man — Cercaria — Snail

Fig 332–27
Life cycle of schistosomes.
(From Johnson RJ, Feehally J: Comprehensive Clinical Nephrology, 2nd ed. St Louis, Mosby, 2000)

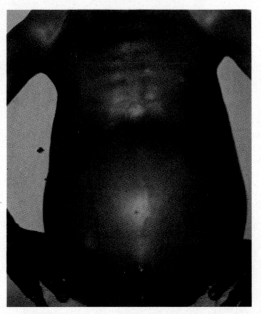

Fig 332–28
Late manifestations of disease caused by *Schistosoma mansoni* infection. Note marked ascites and collateral circulation on anterior abdominal wall.
(Courtesy of Prof. M. A. Madwar.)

TABLE 332–3 Geographic distribution of human schistosomes

Species	Africa	Middle East	Asia	Americas	Caribbean
S. haematobium	+	+	+	+	+
S. mansoni	+	+	+	−	−
S. japonicum	−	−	+	−	−
S. mekongl	−	−	+	−	−
S. intercalatum	+	−	−	−	−

From Cohen J, Powderly WG: Infectious Diseases, 2nd ed. St Louis, Mosby, 2004.

- Urinary schistosomiasis (Fig. 332–29)
  1. Hematuria
  2. Dysuria
  3. Urinary frequency
  4. Fibrosis of bladder and ureters
  5. Squamous cell cancer of bladder
  6. Proteinuria
  7. Nephrotic syndrome

COMPLICATIONS
- Neurologic complication
  1. Granuloma of spinal cord (Fig. 332–30) or brain
  2. Transverse myelitis
  3. Epilepsy or focal neurologic deficit

- Pulmonary complication
  1. Granulomatous pulmonary endarteritis
  2. Pulmonary hypertension (Fig. 332–31)
  3. Cor pulmonale
- Other complications include tubal obstruction and infertility
- Recurrent bacteremia and recurrent UTI

DIFFERENTIAL DIAGNOSIS
- Amebiasis
- Bacillary dysentery
- Bowel polyp
- Prostatic disease
- Genitourinary tract cancer
- Bacterial infections of the urinary tract

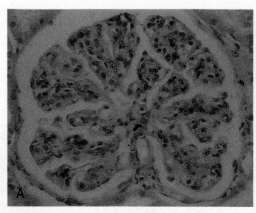
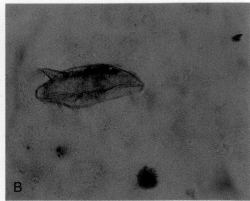

Fig 332–29
Schistosomiasis. (**A**) Membranoproliferative glomerulonephritis in a patient with hepatosplenic schistosomiasis. (**B**) *Schistosoma mansoni* eggs identified in a fecal specimen.
(Courtesy of L. de Moura, São Pablo, Brazil.)

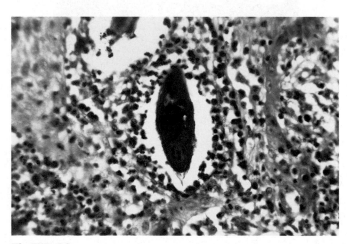

Fig 332–30
Schistosoma hematobium: the terminal spine is characteristic of this species.
(From McKee PH, Calonje E, Granter SR [eds]: Pathology of the Skin With Clinical Correlations, ed 3, St Louis, 2005, Mosby)

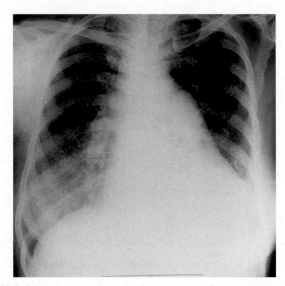

Fig 332–31
Schistosomiasis. A 35-year-old man who presented in gross right heart failure. The heart is enlarged and the main and proximal right and left pulmonary arteries are enlarged, indicating marked pulmonary arterial hypertension. There is fine military nodulation throughout the lungs.
(From Grainger RG, Allison DJ, Adam A, Dixon AK [eds]: Grainger and Allison's Diagnostic Radiology, 4th ed. Philadelphia, Churchill Livingstone, 2001.)

LABORATORY TESTS
- CBC shows eosinophilia, anemia, thrombocytopenia
- LFT with mild increase in alkaline phosphatase and GGT
- Microscopy: stool and urine
- Serology: ELISA for detecting both schistosomal antibodies and antigen
- Rectal biopsy or bladder mucosal biopsy

IMAGING STUDIES
- X-ray of abdomen shows "fetal head" calcification.
- Sonography also documents a thickened bladder wall, hydronephrosis and hydroureter, and bladder polyps or calcification. It also demonstrates the thickened fibrosed portal tracts.
- Esophagoscopy documents esophageal varices.
- Liver biopsy may also demonstrate granuloma (Fig. 332–32) and clay pipestem fibrosis.

TREATMENT
- Praziquantel
- Oxamniquine for recalcitrant infections

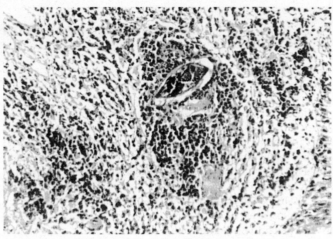

Fig 332–32
Schistosomiasis of the liver. A refractile schistosome ova is located in a portal tract and is associated with an eosinophil-rich granulomatous inflammatory reaction.
(From Cohen J, Powderly WG: Infectious Diseases, 2nd ed. St Louis, Mosby, 2004.)

Chapter 333 Cestode (tapeworm) infestation

DEFINITION
Four species of adult tapeworm may infect humans as the definitive host: *Taenia saginata* (beef tapeworm) (Fig. 333–1), *Taenia solium* (pork tapeworm), *Diphyllobothrium latum* (fish tapeworm), and *Hymenolepis nana*. In addition, *T. solium* may infect humans in its larval form (cysticercosis), and several animal tapeworms may cause infection in an analogous manner. Figure 333–2 illustrates the life cycle of important human tapeworms.

PHYSICAL FINDINGS AND CLINICAL PRESENTATION
- Adult worms
  1. Attach to bowel mucosa
  2. Feed and grow
  3. Cause minimal or no symptoms or sequelae
- Cysticercosis
  1. Mass lesions of brain (neurocysticercosis), soft tissue (Fig. 333–3), viscera
  2. Neurocysticercosis (Fig. 333–4) may cause seizures, hydrocephalus
- Prolonged infection with *D. latum*
  1. Vitamin B$_{12}$ deficiency
  2. Megaloblastic anemia

Fig 333–1
Taenia saginata. A mature worm may be over 33 feet (10 m) long. (From Cohen J, Powderly WG: Infectious Diseases, 2nd ed. St Louis, Mosby, 2004.)

CAUSE
TAPEWORM
- Adult worm resides in small or large bowel; proglottids and eggs passed in stool
- Eggs are ingested by the animal intermediate host.
- Eggs hatch into larvae.
- Larvae disseminate largely in skeletal muscle, brain, viscera.
- Humans eat infected beef (*T. saginata*), infected pork (*T. solium*), or infected fish (*D. latum*).
- Larvae mature into adults within the GI lumen (Fig. 333–5).
- *H. nana* infection is acquired by ingesting eggs in human or rodent feces.

CYSTICERCOSIS
- Humans ingest eggs of *T. solium* in food contaminated with human feces that contain the eggs.
- Eggs hatch into larvae in gut.
- Larvae disseminate widely through tissues (Fig. 333–6) (particularly soft tissue and CNS) forming cystic lesions (Fig. 333–7) containing either viable or nonviable larvae.

WORKUP
- Stool examination for eggs or proglottids (tapeworm)
- Cerebral CT scan (neurocysticercosis)
- Serum antibody (neurocysticercosis)

IMAGING STUDIES
- Tapeworm: incidental finding on upper GI series
- Neurocysticercosis:
  1. Cerebral cysts are readily demonstrated by CT scan or MRI.
  2. Calcified lesions are an incidental finding.

TREATMENT
- All patients with intestinal tapeworm infections should be treated with a single oral dose of praziquantel.
- An alternative therapy to praziquantel for tapeworm infections is niclosamide,
- Therapy that may be considered for symptomatic cysticercosis:
  1. May regress spontaneously
  2. Surgery
  3. Albendazole or praziquantel

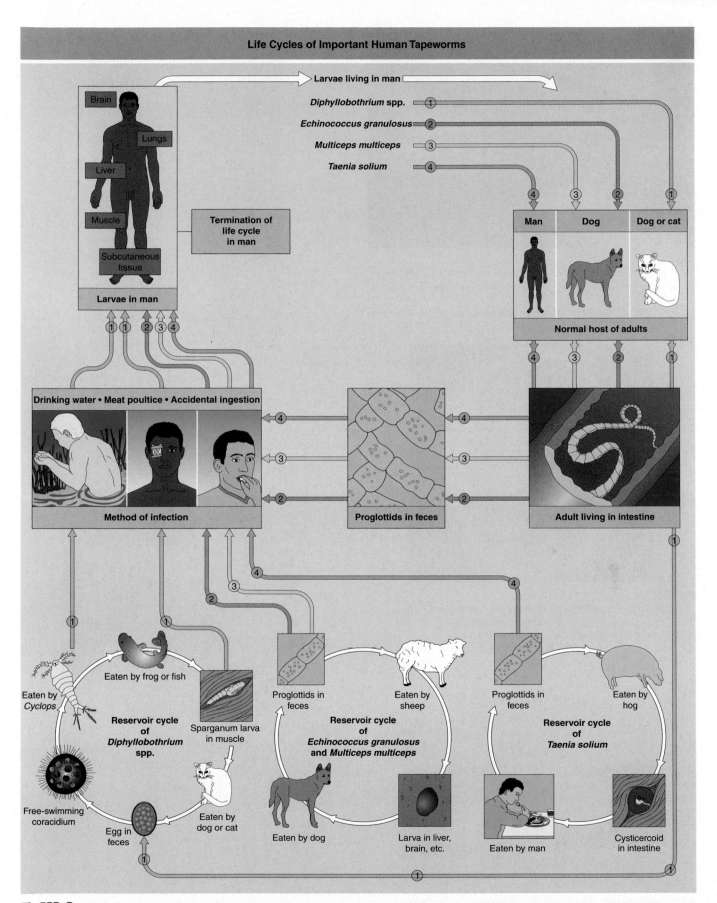

Life Cycles of Important Human Tapeworms

Larvae living in man

Diphyllobothrium spp. ①

Echinococcus granulosus ②

Multiceps multiceps ③

Taenia solium ④

Brain

Lungs

Liver

Muscle

Subcutaneous tissue

Larvae in man

Termination of life cycle in man

Man | Dog | Dog or cat

Normal host of adults

Drinking water • Meat poultice • Accidental ingestion

Method of infection

Proglottids in feces

Adult living in intestine

Eaten by frog or fish

Eaten by *Cyclops*

Reservoir cycle of *Diphyllobothrium* spp.

Sparganum larva in muscle

Proglottids in feces

Eaten by sheep

Reservoir cycle of *Echinococcus granulosus* and *Multiceps multiceps*

Proglottids in feces

Eaten by hog

Reservoir cycle of *Taenia solium*

Free-swimming coracidium

Egg in feces

Eaten by dog or cat

Eaten by dog

Larva in liver, brain, etc.

Eaten by man

Cysticercoid in intestine

Fig 333–2

Life cycles of important human tapeworms. Adults live in tissues, intestines, and blood; humans are accidental hosts.
(From Cohen J, Powderly WG: Infectious Diseases, 2nd ed. St Louis, Mosby, 2004.)

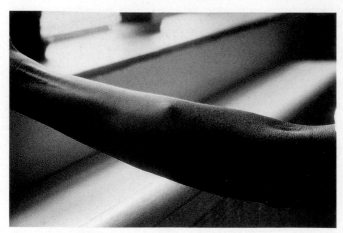

Fig 333-3
Cysticercosis: a solitary nodule is present on the ventral aspect of the forearm. Cysticercosis develops when humans are harboring the larval (cysticercus) stage of the tapeworm.
(Courtesy of S. Lucas, MD, St Thomas' Hospital, London, UK.)

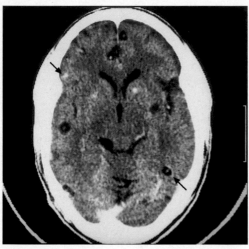

Fig 333-4
Computed tomography appearances in neurocysticercosis. Viable cysts appear as radiolucent defects (*arrowhead*). The central protoscolex appears as a radiodense spot in about 50% (*small arrow*). Cysts that show ring enhancement are probably degenerating. Calcified cysts (*large arrow*) are dead and will not benefit from specific therapy.
(From Cohen J, Powderly WG: Infectious Diseases, 2nd ed. St Louis, Mosby, 2004.)

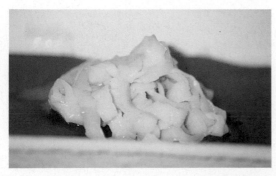

Fig 333-5
Adult beef tapeworm (*Taenia saginata*) passed in a patient's feces.
(From Cohen J, Powderly WG: Infectious Diseases, 2nd ed. St Louis, Mosby, 2004.)

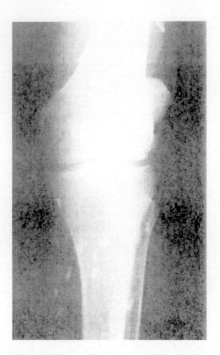

Fig 333-6
Cysticercosis. Anteroposterior radiograph of the knee showing multiple calcified oval cysts aligned along muscle planes.
(From Grainger RG, Allison DJ, Adam A, Dixon AK [eds]: Grainger and Allison's Diagnostic Radiology, 4th ed. Philadelphia, Churchill Livingstone, 2001.)

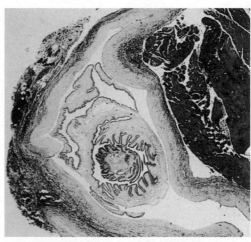

Fig 333-7
Cysticercosis: the worm lies within a cystic cavity surrounded by a dense fibrous capsule.
(Courtesy of S. Lucas, MD, St Thomas' Hospital, London, UK.)

Chapter 334 Nematode infestation

A. HOOKWORM

DEFINITION

Hookworm is a parasitic infection of the intestine caused by helminths.

PHYSICAL FINDINGS AND CLINICAL PRESENTATION

- Nonspecific abdominal complaints
- Because these organisms consume host RBCs, symptoms related to iron deficiency anemia, depending on the amount of iron in the diet and the worm burden
- Fatigue, tachycardia, dyspnea, and high-output failure
- Hypoproteinemia and edema from loss of proteins into the intestinal tract
- Unusual for pulmonary manifestations to occur when the larvae migrate through the lungs
- Skin rash at sites of larval penetration in some individuals without prior exposure

CAUSE

Two species can cause this disease: *Necator americanus* and *Ancylostoma duodenale*. *N. americanus* is the predominant cause of hookworm in the United States. They are soil nematodes (geohelminthic infections) that are acquired by skin contact (i.e., bare feet) with contaminated soils in moist, warm climate.

- Infection occurs via penetration of the skin by the larval form, with subsequent migration via the bloodstream to the alveoli, up the respiratory tract, then into the GI tract. Figure 334–1 illustrates the life cycles of important human roundworms.
- *Ancylostoma* spp. infection can also occur via the oral route through ingestion of contaminated water supplies.
- Sharp mouth parts allow for attachment to intestinal mucosa.
- *Ancylostoma* spp. are more likely to cause iron deficiency anemia because they are larger and remove more blood daily from the bowel wall than the other hookworm species, *Necator americanus*.

DIFFERENTIAL DIAGNOSIS

- Strongyloidiasis
- Ascariasis
- Other causes of iron deficiency, anemia and malabsorption

LABORATORY TESTS

- CBC to show hypochromic, microcytic anemia; possible mild eosinophilia and hypoalbuminemia
- Examine stool for hookworm eggs.

IMAGING STUDIES

Chest x-ray: occasionally shows opacities

TREATMENT

- Albendazole or mebendazole

B. ASCARIASIS

DEFINITION

Ascariasis is a parasitic infection caused by the nematode *Ascaris lumbricoides*. The majority of those infected are asymptomatic;

however, clinical disease may arise from pulmonary hypersensitivity, intestinal obstruction, and secondary complications.

PHYSICAL FINDINGS AND CLINICAL PRESENTATION

- Occurs approximately 9 to 12 days after ingestion of eggs (corresponding to the larva migration through the lungs)
- Nonproductive cough
- Substernal chest discomfort
- Fever
- In patients with large worm burdens, especially children, intestinal obstruction associated with perforation, volvulus, and intussusception
- Migration of worms into the biliary tree, giving clinical appearance of biliary colic and pancreatitis as well as acute appendicitis with movement into that appendage
- Rarely, infection with *A. lumbricoides* producing interstitial nephritis and acute renal failure
- In endemic areas in Asia and Africa, malabsorption of dietary proteins and vitamins as a consequence of chronic worm intestinal carriage

CAUSE

- Transmission is usually hand to mouth, but eggs may be ingested via transported vegetables grown in contaminated soil.
- Eggs are hatched in the small intestine, with larvae penetrating intestinal mucosa and migrating via the circulation to the lungs.
- Larval forms proceed through the alveoli, ascend the bronchial tree, and return to the intestines after swallowing, where they mature into adult worms.
- Estimated time until the female adult worm to begin producing eggs is 2 to 3 months.
- Eggs are passed out of the intestines with feces.
- Within human host, adult worm life span is 1 to 2 years.

DIFFERENTIAL DIAGNOSIS

- Radiologic manifestations and eosinophilia to be distinguished from drug hypersensitivity and Löffler's syndrome

LABORATORY TESTS

- Examination of the stool for *Ascaris* ova (Fig. 334–2)
- Expectoration or fecal passage of adult worm
- Eosinophilia: most prominent early in the infection and subsides as the adult worm infestation established in the intestines
- Anti-ascaris IgG4 blood levels by ELISA is a sensitive and specific marker of infection and may be useful in the evaluation of treatment
- Malondialdehyde levels clearly increase in patients infected with *A. lumbricoides*

IMAGING STUDIES

- Chest x-ray may reveal bilateral oval or round infiltrates of varying size (Löffler's syndrome). NOTE: Infiltrates are transient and eventually resolve.
- Plain films of the abdomen and contrast studies may reveal worm masses in loops of bowel

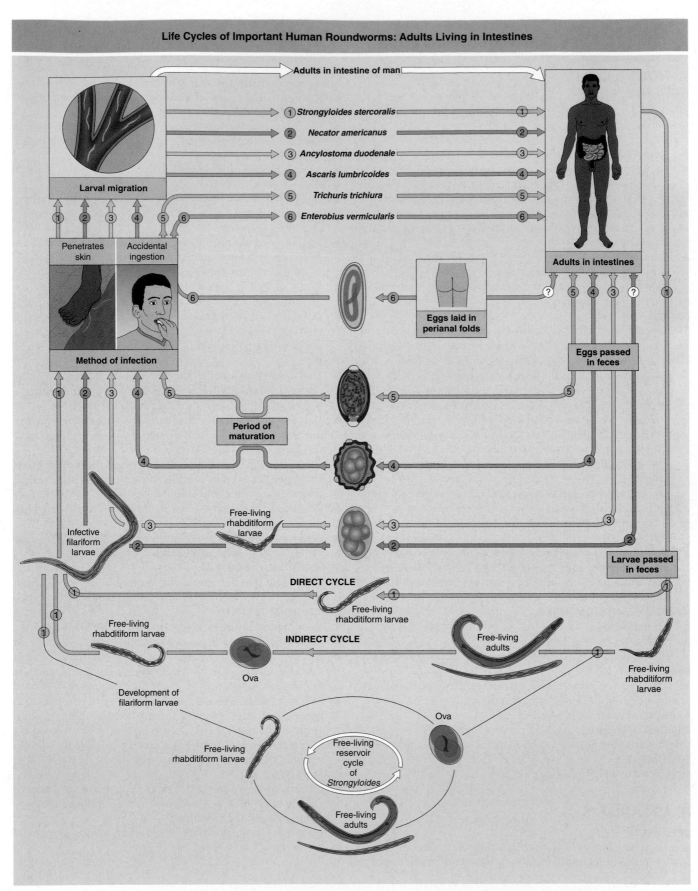

Life Cycles of Important Human Roundworms: Adults Living in Intestines

Adults in intestine of man

① *Strongyloides stercoralis*
② *Necator americanus*
③ *Ancylostoma duodenale*
④ *Ascaris lumbricoides*
⑤ *Trichuris trichiura*
⑥ *Enterobius vermicularis*

Larval migration

Penetrates skin

Accidental ingestion

Method of infection

Adults in intestines

Eggs laid in perianal folds

Eggs passed in feces

Period of maturation

Infective filariform larvae

Free-living rhabditiform larvae

Larvae passed in feces

DIRECT CYCLE

Free-living rhabditiform larvae

Free-living rhabditiform larvae

INDIRECT CYCLE

Free-living adults

Free-living rhabditiform larvae

Ova

Development of filariform larvae

Ova

Free-living reservoir cycle of *Strongyloides*

Free-living rhabditiform larvae

Free-living adults

Fig 334–1
Life cycles of important human roundworms: adult living in the intestines.
(From Cohen J, Powderly WG: Infectious Diseases, 2nd ed. St Louis, Mosby, 2004.)

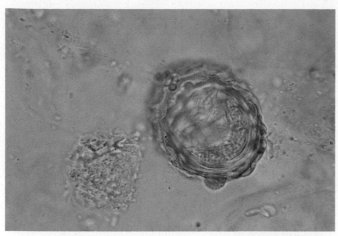

Fig 334–2
Ascaris lumbricoides ovum in feces. The ovum measures 50 to 70 mm × 40 to 50 mm and is elliptical. The rough albuminous coat gives it a mammillated appearance.
(From Cohen J, Powderly WG: Infectious Diseases, 2nd ed. St Louis, Mosby, 2004.)

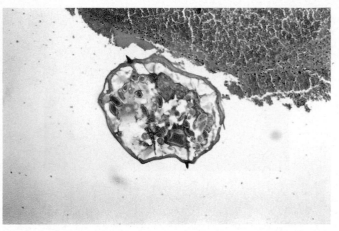

Fig 334–3
Enterobius vermicularis in the lumen of an appendix is an incidental finding. Symptoms occur when the gravid females migrates to the perianal area to lay her eggs. The worm is identified as a nematode by the characteristic "tube within a tube" morphology combined with the prominent lateral alae. In this case, a specific identification can be made because the characteristic pinworm eggs can also be seen within the section (HANDE, ×250).
(From Silverberg SG: Principles and Practice of Surgical Pathology and Cytopathology, 4th ed. Philadelphia, Churchill Livingstone, 2006.)

- Ultrasonography and endoscopic retrograde cholangiopancreatography (ERCP) to identify worms in the pancreaticobiliary tract

TREATMENT
- Mebendazole: drug of choice for intestinal infection with *A. lumbricoides*
- Albendazole
- Pyrantel pamoate
- Piperazine citrate
- Complete obstruction should be managed surgically.
- Aggressive IV hydration, especially in children with fever, severe vomiting, and resultant dehydration

C. ENTEROBIASIS (PINWORMS)

DEFINITION
Pinworms are a noninvasive infestation of the intestinal tract by *Enterobius vermicularis*, a helminth of the nematode family.

PHYSICAL FINDINGS AND CLINICAL PRESENTATION
- Most infested persons are asymptomatic.
- Perianal itching is the most common reported symptom, with scratching leading to excoriation and sometimes secondary infection.
- Rarely insomnia, irritability, anorexia, and weight loss are described.
- Granulomas have been described in various organs resulting from worms wandering outside the intestines and dying there.

CAUSE AND PATHOGENESIS
- *Enterobius vermicularis* is highly prevalent throughout the world, particularly in countries of the temperate zone. Humans are the only host for this worm. Infestation is by fecal-oral route; ingested eggs hatch in the stomach and the larvae migrate to the colon where they mature. Gravid female worms containing an average of 10,000 ova migrate to the perianal skin at night, lay their eggs there, and die. The eggs

embryonate within 6 hours and cause itching; scratching causes egg deposition under fingernails, from which they can contaminate food or lead to autoreinfection.
- *Enterobius vermicularis* may be transmitted between sexual partners, especially those engaging in oral–anal sex.

DIFFERENTIAL DIAGNOSIS
- Perianal itching related to poor hygiene
- Hemorrhoidal disease and anal fissures
- Perineal yeast/fungal infections

WORKUP
Identification of adult worms or eggs. *Enterobius vermicularis* ova are ovoid but flattened on one side and measure approximately 56 × 27 mm (Fig. 334–3). The eggs can be identified on transparent tape placed on the perianal skin on awakening (note: five consecutive negative tests rule out the diagnosis). A single examination detects 50% of infections, three examinations detect 90%, and five examinations detect 99%.

TREATMENT
- Single dose of mebendazole (100 mg) with a repeat dose given after 2 weeks
- Single dose of albendazole (400 mg) with a second dose given 2 weeks later is also highly effective.
- Pyrantel pamoate (11 mg/kg up to 1 g) can prevent against *Enterobius vermicularis*. It is available as a suspension and has minimal toxicity (mild transient GI symptoms, headache, drowsiness). A repeat dose after 2 weeks is recommended because of the frequency of reinfection and autoinfection.
- Other infected family members, classmates, or residents of long-term care facilities should be treated at the same time as the index case.

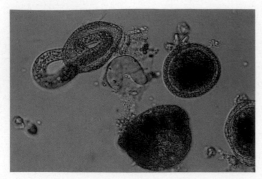

Fig 334-4
Fully embryonated egg of *Toxocara canis* hatching. To the *right* are two unfertilized eggs.
(From Cohen J, Powderly WG: Infectious Diseases, 2nd ed. St Louis, Mosby, 2004.)

D. TOXOCARIASIS (ROUNDWORMS)

Toxocariasis (visceral larva migrans, roundworms)

DEFINITION

Infestation by the canine ascarid *Toxocara canis* (Fig. 334–4). The life cycle of *Toxocara canis* is described in Figure 334–5.

CLINICAL PRESENTATION

- Visceral larva migrans:
    - In humans, *T. canis* eggs hatch and larvae invade but are not able to develop beyond the L2 stage and continue to migrate through the body for a prolonged period.
    - The larvae of *T. canis* excrete a complex mixture of glycoproteins from the larval surface resulting in an intense systemic response consisting of fever cough, wheeze, hepatosplenomegaly, and eosinophilia.
    - Failure to thrive, abdominal pain, and urticaria are also common.
- Ocular infection:
    - If the larva is trapped in the retina, the inflammatory response is localized, leading to ocular complications and endophtlamitis or uveitis.

DIAGNOSIS

- In humans, adult worms do not develop and eggs cannot be found in the stool.
- Diagnosis is made serologically with an antibody capture enzyme immunoassay based on *Toxocara* excretory secretory (TES) antigens.

TREATMENT

Albendazole or diethylcarbamazine

E. TRICHINOSIS

DEFINITION

Trichinosis is an infection by one of various species of *Trichinella*.

PHYSICAL FINDINGS AND CLINICAL PRESENTATION

- Symptoms
    1. May vary widely depending on the time from ingestion of contaminated meat and on worm burden
    2. Most persons are asymptomatic

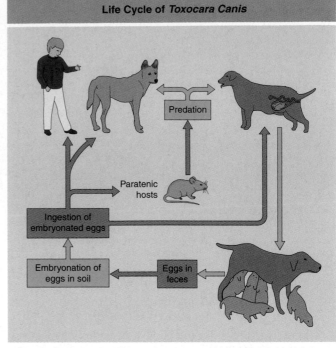

Life Cycle of *Toxocara Canis*

Fig 334-5
Life cycle of *Toxocara canis*. This demonstrates the importance of transplacental transmission in maintaining canine infection and the role of young dogs in transmitting infection to humans.
(From Cohen J, Powderly WG: Infectious Diseases, 2nd ed. St Louis, Mosby, 2004.)

- Enteral phase
    1. Correlates with penetration of ingested larvae into the intestinal mucosa
    2. May last from 2 to 6 weeks
    3. Mild, transient diarrhea and nausea
    4. Abdominal pain
    5. Diarrhea or constipation
    6. Vomiting
    7. Malaise
    8. Low-grade fevers
- Migratory or parenteral phase
    1. In the intestine, maturation and mating
    2. Newborn larvae
        a. Penetrate into lymphatic and blood vessels
        b. Migrate to muscles where they penetrate into muscle cells, enlarge, coil, and develop a cyst wall (Fig. 334–6)
    3. Patients may present with
        a. Fever
        b. Myalgias
        c. Periorbital or facial edema
        d. Headache
        e. Skin rash
        f. Other symptoms caused by the penetration of tissues by the newborn migrating larvae
    4. Peak in symptoms 2 to 3 weeks after infection, then symptoms slowly subside

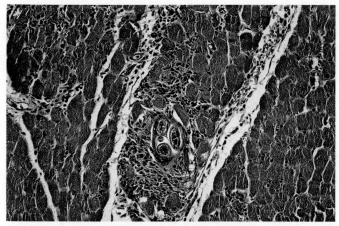

Fig 334–6
Trichinella spiralis associated with a localized inflammatory response.
(From Silverberg SG: Principles and Practice of Surgical Pathology and
Cytopathology, 4th ed. Philadelphia, Churchill Livingstone, 2006.)

- Severe complications
  1. Brain damage by granulomatous inflammation or occlusion of arteries
  2. Cardiac involvement
  3. Can lead to death

CAUSE
- The nematode responsible for this illness is an obligate intracellular parasite belonging to the genus *Trichinella*.
- It is one of the most ubiquitous parasites in the world and may be found in virtually all warm-blooded animals.
- Infection in humans occurs by the ingestion of contaminated animal meat that is raw or partially cooked and contains viable cysts.
- Most cases are now related to the consumption of poorly processed pork or wild game (bear, wild boar, cougar, and walrus).

DIFFERENTIAL DIAGNOSIS
- Different presentations have different differential diagnoses.
- Early illness may resemble gastroenteritis.
- Later symptoms may be confused with:
  1. Measles
  2. Dermatomyositis
  3. Glomerulonephritis

WORKUP
- Antibody assay of serum is usually positive by approximately 2 weeks after infection.
- Muscle biopsy is used to detect the larvae in muscle tissue if diagnosis unclear; best done by placing the tissue between two slides.

LABORATORY TESTS
- CBC: leukocytosis with prominent eosinophilia
- ESR: usually normal
- Elevation of muscle enzymes common (i.e., CPK, aldolase)

IMAGING STUDIES
Soft-tissue radiographs may show calcified cyst walls.

TREATMENT
- Albendazole
- Salicylates to decrease muscle discomfort
- Steroids in critically ill patients
- Mebendazole is an alternative to albendazole.

F. STRONGYLOIDIASIS

DEFINITION
Infection with the parasite *Strongyloides stercoralis* (southern United States) or *Strongyloides fulleborni* (Africa, New Guinea). Humans acquire the infection through penetration of the skin by filariform larvae. The larva subsequently migrates to the lungs and then to the intestines. There the females produce eggs, which release first-stage larvae. The life cycle of *Strongyloides stercoralis* is described in Figure 334–7.

PHYSICAL FINDINGS AND CLINICAL PRESENTATION
- The vast majority of patients are asymptomatic.
- GI symptoms: nausea, anorexia, abdominal pain and bloating, diarrhea
- Cutaneous manifestations: pruritus. urticarial, serpiginous, migratory lesions on buttocks, groin, trunk
- Pulmonary symptoms: cough, wheezing, hemoptysis, pleuritic pain
- Immunocompromised patients may develop Gram-negative sepsis, meningitis, intestinal obstruction

DIFFERENTIAL DIAGNOSIS
- *Entamoeba histolytica* infection
- Cutaneous larva migrans
- Trichinosis
- Cutaneous leishmaniasis

LABORATORY TESTS
- Eosinophilia
- Presence of larvae in stool, duodenal aspirate (Fig. 334–8), respiratory secretions (Fig. 334–9), CSF fluid, ascetic fluid, or urine establishes the diagnosis.

IMAGING STUDIES
- Chest x-ray may demonstrate infiltrates (Fig. 334–9).
- Abdominal x-rays may reveal small bowel obstruction in immunocompromised hosts.

TREATMENT
- Thiabendazole or ivermectin

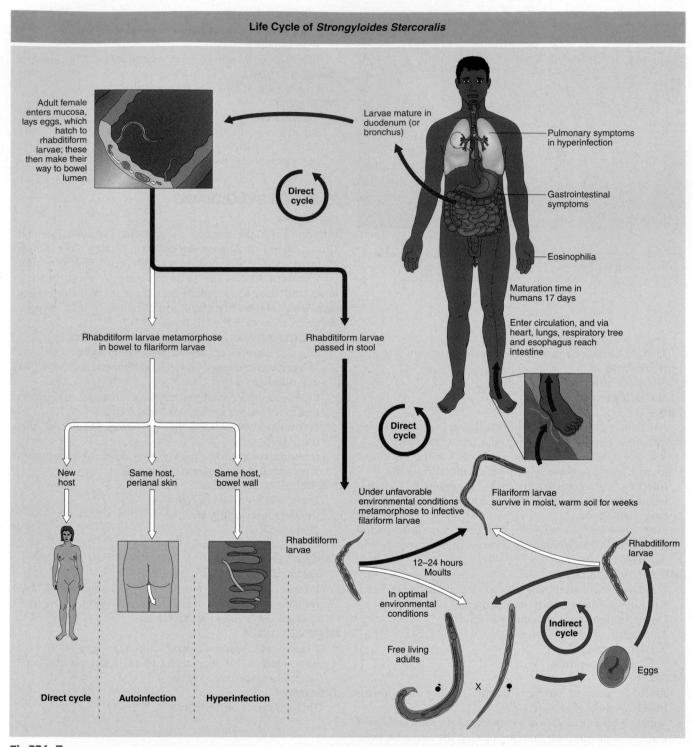

Fig 334–7
Life cycle of *Strongyloides stercoralis*.
(From Cohen J, Powderly WG: Infectious Diseases, 2nd ed. St Louis, Mosby, 2004.)

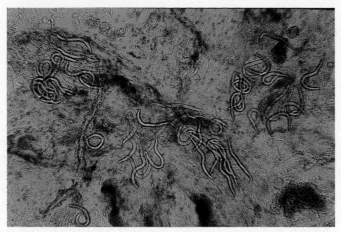

Fig 334–8
Numerous rhabditiform larvae of *Strongyloides* in a duodenal juice
specimen.
(From Cohen J, Powderly WG: Infectious Diseases, 2nd ed. St Louis,
Mosby, 2004.)

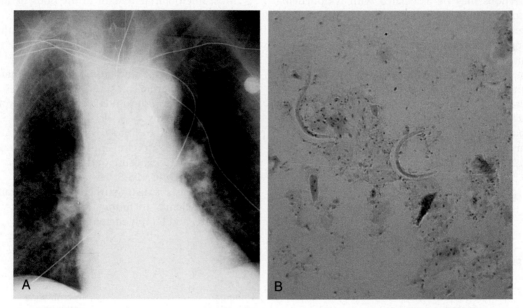

Fig 334–9
Disseminated strongyloidiasis in an immunocompromised patient. (**A**) Chest radiograph showing a diffuse bilateral interstitial process.
(**B**) Gram stain of sputum from the same patient shows filariform larvae of *Strongyloides stercoralis*.
(Courtesy of R. Johnson.)

Chapter 335 Filariasis

DEFINITION

Filariasis is a general term for an infection caused by subcutaneous nematodes (roundworms) of the genera *Wuchereria* and *Brugia,* found in the tropical and subtropical regions of the world. The disease is variably characterized by acute lymphatic inflammation or chronic lymphatic obstruction associated with intermittent fevers or recurrent episodes of dyspnea and bronchospasm. Principal filarial diseases are described in Table 335–1.

PHYSICAL FINDINGS AND CLINICAL PRESENTATION

- Clinical manifestations result from acute lymphatic inflammation or chronic lymphatic obstruction.
- Many patients are asymptomatic despite the presence of microfilaremia.
- Episodes of lymphangitis and lymphadenitis are associated with fever, headache, and back pain.
- Acute funiculitis and epididymitis or orchitis may also be present; all usually resolve within days to weeks but tend to recur.
- Chronic infections may be associated with lymphedema, most commonly manifested by hydrocele.
- It is a progressive disease, leading to nonpitting edema and brawny changes that may involve a whole limb
- Elephantiasis occurs in about 10% of patients, with skin of the scrotum (Fig. 335–1) or leg (Fig. 335–1) becoming thickened and fissured; patient is thereafter plagued by recurrent ulceration and infection.
- Chyluria, a condition that develops when lymphatic vessels rupture into the urinary tract, may occur.
- Onchocerciasis can result in severe pruritus (Fig. 335–2).
- Loiasis (Fig. 335–3) can manifest with angioedema.

CAUSE

Caused by one of three types of nematode parasites, all of which are transmitted to humans by *Culex* spp. mosquitoes:

- *W. bancrofti:* distributed in Africa, areas of Central and South America, the Pacific Islands, and the Caribbean Basin
- *B. malayi:* restricted to Southeast Asia
- *B. timori:* confined to the Indonesian archipelago

After bite of an infected mosquito:

- Filarial larvae move into lymphatic vessels and nodes, settling and maturing over 3 to 15 months into adult male and female worms.
- After fertilization, the female nematode produces large numbers of larvae or microfilariae that enter into the bloodstream via the lymphatics.
- Nocturnal periodicity, characteristic of *B. malayi,* is an increased presence of microfilariae in the circulation during the night.
- Microfilariae of *W. bancrofti* are maximal during late afternoon.
- Most microfilariae remain in the body as immature forms for 6 months to 2 years.
- Infected larvae are ingested by mosquitoes, then transmitted to humans where the microfilariae mature into new adult worms.

Acute and chronic inflammatory and granulomatous changes in the lymphatic channels:

- Result from complex interaction of adult worms and host's immune systems
- Eventually lead to fibrosis and obstruction
- Most likely to develop into obstructive lymphatic disease with recurrent exposure over many years

DIFFERENTIAL DIAGNOSIS

- Elephantiasis is distinguished from other causes of chronic lymph edema, including Milroy's disease, postoperative scarring, and lymph edema of malignancy.

TABLE 335–1 Principal filarial diseases

Disease	Number of people infected worldwide	Parasite	Vector	Principal clinical manifestations	Distribution	Location of microfilariae within the body	Periodicity
Lymphatic filariasis	120 million	*Wuchereria*	Mosquitoes	Lymphedema, elephantiasis, genital pathology (hydrocele)	Tropics worldwide	Blood	Nocturnal (95%), "subperiodic" (5%)
		Brugio malayi	Mosquitoes	Lymphedema, elephantiasis	Asia, India, Philippines	Blood	Nocturnal (75%), "subperiodic" (25%)
Onchocerciasis	17 million	*Onchocerca volvulus*	Black flies	Dermatitis, blindness	Africa (95%), Americas, Yemen	Skin	Minimal
Loiasis	12 million	*Loa loa*	Deer flies	Angioedema, "eyeworm"	Africa	Blood	Diumal

From Cohen J, Powderly WG: Infectious Diseases, 2nd ed. St Louis, Mosby, 2004.

WORKUP

Diagnosis is suspected in individuals who have resided in endemic areas for at least 3 to 6 months or longer and complain of recurrent episodes of lymph angitis, lymphadenitis, scrotal edema, or thrombophlebitis, with or without fever.

LABORATORY TESTS

- Demonstration of microfilariae on a blood smear for definitive diagnosis
- For patients from southeastern Asia: blood sample drawn at night, especially between midnight and 2 AM.
- Occasionally, microfilaremia in chylous urine or hydrocele fluid

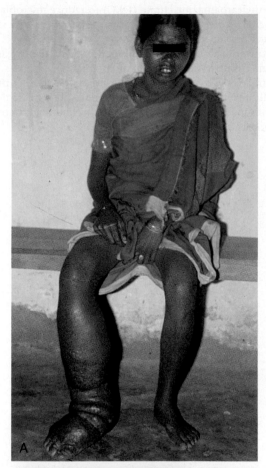

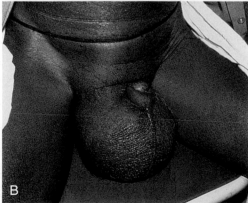

Fig 335–1
Elephantiasis. (**A**) Already advanced elephantiasis in a 14-year-old Indian girl who has bancroftian filariasis. Although such clinical expression of filarial disease is more commonly seen in adults, infection in endemic areas is usually established in early childhood. (**B**) Scrotal elephantiasis in an adult man who has bancroftian filariasis.
(From Cohen J, Powderly WG: Infectious Diseases, 2nd ed. St Louis, Mosby, 2004.)

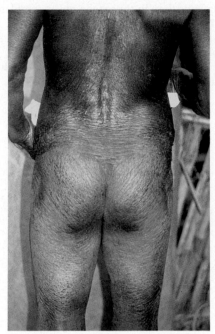

Fig 335–2
Onchocerciasis. Evidence of excoriation caused by the patient's trying to relieve the maddening pruritus caused by onchocerciasis. Note also the marked dermal atrophy associated with chronic infection.
(From Cohen J, Powderly WG: Infectious Diseases, 2nd ed. St Louis, Mosby, 2004.)

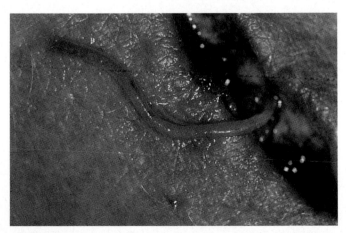

Fig 335–3
Loa loa adult worm. The worm has been teased from the subcutaneous tissue after an incision was made through a small pruritic papule (0.5 cm in diameter) in an expatriate patient who had loiasis. Such papules can occur spontaneously or after treatment with DEC.
(From Cohen J, Powderly WG: Infectious Diseases, 2nd ed. St Louis, Mosby, 2004.)

- Prominent eosinophilia only during periods of acute lymphangitis or lymphadenitis
- Serologic tests for antibody, including ELISA and indirect fluorescent antibody (often unable to distinguish among the various forms of filariasis or between acute and remote infection)
- Immunoassays (such as circulating filaria antigen [CFA]): more successful in antigen detection in patients who are microfilaremic than in those who are amicrofilaremic

IMAGING STUDIES
- Chest x-ray: reticular nodular infiltrates (tropical pulmonary eosinophilia syndrome)
- In men proved to be microfilaremic, scrotal ultrasonography to aid in the detection of adult worms

TREATMENT
- Standard of care for elephantiasis:
  1. Elevation of the affected limb
  2. Use of elastic stockings
  3. Local foot care
- General wound care for chronic ulcers and prevention of secondary infection
- Diethylcarbamazine citrate (DEC) to reduce microfilaremia by 90%. Effect on adult worms, especially those of the *Wuchereria* species, less certain
- Ivermectin alone or in combination with diethylcarbamazine citrate to decrease microfilaremia
- Antibacterial agents (a penicillin or cephalsporin) may be indicated to treat coexisting bacterial soft tissue infection (cellulitis or lymphangiitis), which frequently complicates filariasis of the lower extremities.

Chapter 336 | Fungal infections

A. CANDIDIASIS

DEFINITION
Infection by the fungal organism *Candida* (*C. albicans*, *C. tropicalis*, *C. glabrata*). Most frequently seen in immunocompromised hosts (diabetes, HIV, cancer, chemotherapy) or following use of antibiotics or corticosteroids.

PHYSICAL FINDINGS AND CLINICAL PRESENTATION
- Disseminated candidiasis (Fig. 336–1) is most frequently seen in immunocompromised hosts.
- Thrush, atrophic glossitis (Fig. 336–2)

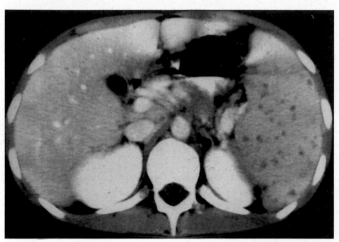

Fig 336–1
Hepatosplenic candidiasis. Multiple abscesses can be seen.
(From Cohen J, Powderly WG: Infectious Diseases, 2nd ed. St Louis, Mosby, 2004.)

- Candida esophagitis (Fig. 336–3), meningitis (seen usually in HIV disease or cancer)
- Vulvovaginal, perirectal candidiasis (Fig. 336–4)
- Intertrigo (skin folds, under breasts, perineum, abdominal wall), interdigital (Fig. 336–5)
- Balanitis (begins with vesicles on penis, can involve scrotum, perineum, buttocks)
- Mucocutaneous candidiasis (diaper rash, perianal area [may cause pruritus ani])
- Candiduria (Fig. 336–6)
- Candida uveitis, retinitis (Fig. 336–7), keratitis

DIFFERENTIAL DIAGNOSIS
- Mucormycosis (see Fig. 336–45)
- Aspergillosis (see Fig. 336–14)
- Tinea infections (corporis, cruris, pedis, capitis)
- Cryptococcosis (see Fig. 336–22)

LABORATORY TESTS
- *Candida* spp. can be identified microscopically (KOH preparation, Gram stain) and by culture.
- Scraping of the affected area will demonstrate the organism.
- *Candida* isolates can also be found in the urine (Fig. 336–8) in hospitalized patients with candiduria.
- Ophthalmoscopic examination may reveal retinal lesions in patients with disseminated candidiasis and *candida* endophthalmititis.
- Blood cultures are usually sterile even in the presence of disseminated infection.

TREATMENT
- Antifungal creams for skin infections
- Fluconazole, itraconazole
- Intravenous amphotericin B for life-threatening infections

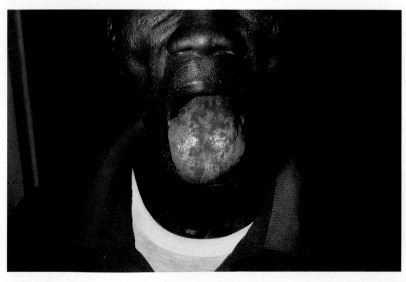

Fig 336–2
Candidial atrophic glossitis with HIV infection: infection with *Candida* is a very common manifestation. In addition to the oral cavity, intertriginous and nail infections may be present. (Courtesy of C. Furlonge, MD, Port of Spain, Trinidad.)

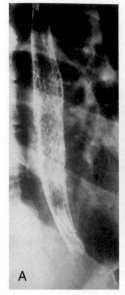
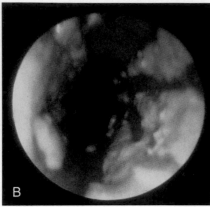

A   B

Fig 336–3
Candidal esophagitis. (**A**) Double-contrast radiography in candidal
esophagitis. (**B**) Endoscopy of same patient.
(From Cohen J, Powderly WG: Infectious Diseases, 2nd ed. St Louis,
Mosby, 2004.)

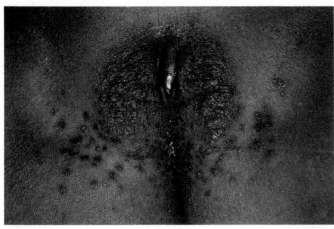

Fig 336–4
Vulvovaginal perirectal candidiasis.
(From Lebwohl MG, Heymann WR, Berth-Jones J, Coulson I [eds]: Treat-
ment of Skin Disease. St Louis, Mosby, 2002.)

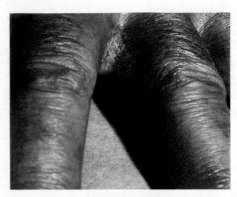

Fig 336–5
Interdigital candidiasis.
(From Cohen J, Powderly WG: Infectious Diseases, 2nd ed. St Louis,
Mosby, 2004.)

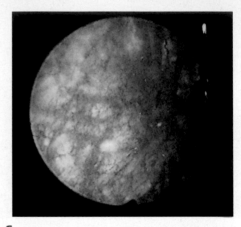

Fig 336–6
Macroscopic appearance of extensive cystitis caused by *C. krusei* as
visualized on cystoscopy. Note the extensive hyperemia, exudative re-
action resembling a "snow storm."
(From Johnson RJ, Feehally J: Comprehensive Clinical Nephrology, 2nd ed.
St Louis, Mosby, 2000.)

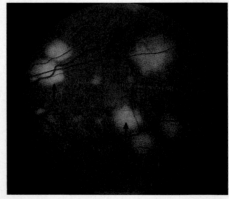

Fig 336–7
Retina of a patient who has lesions (*arrows*) due to disseminated
candidiasis.
(From Cohen J, Powderly WG: Infectious Diseases, 2nd ed. St Louis,
Mosby, 2004.)

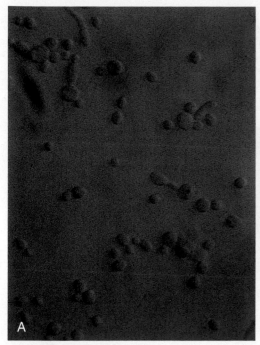

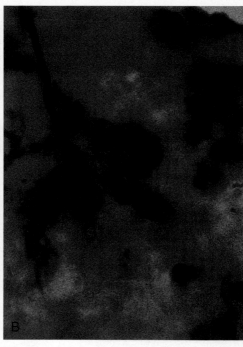

Fig 336–8
Photomicrograph of urine specimen containing *Candida*. (**A**) A high-power (×100) examination of urine demonstrates singlets and yeast (blastospores), budding yeast, and pseudohyphae in a patient with *C. albicans* infection. (**B**) A Gram stain of urine obtained from the same patient, showing pseudo-hyphae.
(From Johnson RJ, Feehally J: Comprehensive Clinical Nephrology, 2nd ed. St Louis, Mosby, 2000.)

B. ASPERGILLOSIS

DEFINITION
Aspergillosis refers to several forms of a broad range of illnesses caused by infection with *Aspergillus* sp.

CAUSE
- *Aspergillus fumigatus* is the usual cause.
- *A. flavus* is the second most important species, particularly in invasive disease of immunosuppressed patients and in lesions beginning in the nose and paranasal sinuses. *A. niger* can also cause invasive human infection.

ALLERGIC ASPERGILLOSIS
- Is a hypersensitivity pneumonitis
- Presents as cough, dyspnea, fever, chills, malaise typically 4 to 8 hours after exposure
- Repeated attacks can lead to granulomatous disease and pulmonary fibrosis.

ALLERGIC BRONCHOPULMONARY ASPERGILLOSIS (ABPA)
- Symptoms occur most commonly in atopic individuals during the third and fourth decades of life.
- Hypersensitivity reaction to *Aspergillus* fungal antigens present in the bronchial tree
- Results from an initial type I (immediate hypersensitivity) and type III reaction (immune complexes)
- Underdiagnosed pulmonary disorder in patients with asthma and cystic fibrosis

ASPERGILLOMAS ("FUNGUS BALLS")
- In the absence of invasion or significant immune response, *Aspergillus* can colonize a preexisting cavity, causing pulmonary aspergilloma.
- Forms masses of tangled hyphal elements, fibrin, and mucus
- Patients typically have a history of chronic lung disease, tuberculosis, sarcoidosis, or emphysema.
- Manifests commonly as hemoptysis
- Many are asymptomatic.

INVASIVE ASPERGILLOSIS
- Patients with prolonged and profound granulocytopenia or impaired phagocytic function are predisposed to rapidly progressive *Aspergillus* pneumonia (Fig. 336–9).
- Typically a necrotizing bronchopneumonia, ranging from small areas of infiltrate to intensive bilateral hemorrhagic infarction
- Most common presentation: unremitting fever and a new pulmonary infiltrate despite broad-spectrum antibiotic therapy in an immunosuppressed patient. Bronchial obstruction may be present (Fig. 336–10).
- Dyspnea and nonproductive cough are common; sudden pleuritic pain and tachycardia, sometimes with a pleural rub, may mimic pulmonary embolism; hemoptysis is uncommon.
- Chest x-ray (Fig. 336–11) may reveal patchy bronchopneumonic, nodular densities, consolidation or cavitation (Fig. 336–12).
- Immunocompromised patients: invasive pulmonary *Aspergillus* (IPA) generally is acute and evolves over days to weeks; less commonly, patients with normal or only mild abnormalities of their immune systems may develop a more chronic, slowly progressive form of IPA.

EXTRAPULMONARY DISSEMINATION
- Cerebral infarction from hematogenous dissemination may occur in immunosuppressed individuals.
- Abscess formation from direct extension or invasive disease in the sinuses (Fig. 336–13)
- Esophageal or gastrointestinal ulcerations may occur in the immunosuppressed host.
- Fatal perforation of the viscus or bowel infarction may occur.
- Necrotizing skin ulcers involving the extremities (Fig. 336–14)
- Osteomyelitis

- Endocarditis in patients who have recently undergone open heart surgery
- Infection of an implantable cardioverter-defibrillator has been reported.

DIFFERENTIAL DIAGNOSIS

- Tuberculosis (see Fig. 102–9)
- Cystic fibrosis (see Fig. 139–31)

- Carcinoma of the lung (see Fig. 132–5)
- Eosinophilic pneumonia
- Bronchiectasis (see Fig. 139–28)
- Sarcoidosis (see Fig. 102–8)
- Lung abscess (see Fig. 139–11)

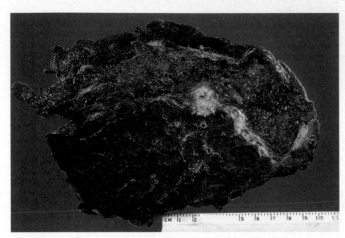

Fig 336–9

Aspergillus niger mycetoma of lung. A large, thick-walled cavity contains brown grumous material due to masses of hyphae.
(From Silverberg SG: Principles and Practice of Surgical Pathology and Cytopathology, 4th ed. Philadelphia, Churchill Livingstone, 2006.)

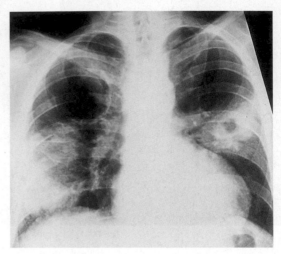

Fig 336–11

Aspergillus pneumonia.
(From Cohen J, Powderly WG: Infectious Diseases, 2nd ed. St Louis, Mosby, 2004.)

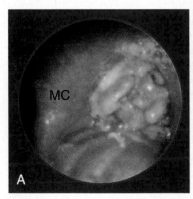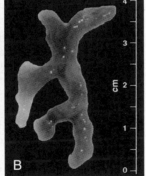

Fig 336–10

A, Endobronchial aspergillosis obstructing the right main-stem bronchus. **B**, Extracted bronchial cast cultured *Aspergillus fumigatus.* Bronchoscopic identification of fungal organisms responsible for histoplasmosis, coccidioidomycois, blastomycosis, cryptococcosis, and mucormycosis is highly indicative of respiratory infection. However, growth of *Aspergillus* and *Candida* species from bronchoscopic washings does not establish the diagnosis of respiratory aspergillosis or candidiasis because these organisms frequently colonize the respiratory tract. In invasis aspergillosis, bronchoscopic specimens are positive for *Aspergillus* species in only 23% of patients. In pulmonary histoplasmosis, bronchoscopy helps in documenting the diagnosis in patients with cavitated lesions, localized infiltrates, and miliary disease caused by histoplasmosis. In 11% of patients with histoplasmosis, bronchoscopy is the only text to document the diagnosis.[33]
(From Gold WM, Murray JF, Nadel JA: Atlas of Procedures in Respiratory Medicine, Philadelphia, WB Saunders, 2002.)

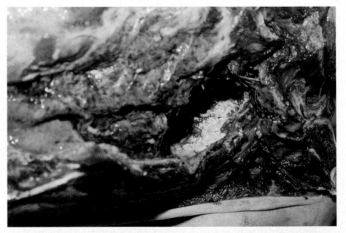

Fig 336–12

Aspergillus fumigatus invasive disease with cavitation. The necrotizing infection has produced cavities in which masses of white mold are growing. The clinical implication of the "mycetomas" is that of the underlying invasive infection.
(From Silverberg SG: Principles and Practice of Surgical Pathology and Cytopathology, 4th ed. Philadelphia, Churchill Livingstone, 2006.)

LABORATORY TESTS

ABPA

- Peripheral blood eosinophilia and an elevated total serum IgE level
- Skin test with *Aspergillus* antigenic extract is usually positive but nonspecific.
- *Aspergillus* serum precipitating antibody is present in 70% to 100% of cases.
- Sputum cultures may be positive for *Aspergillus* spp. but are nonspecific.

ASPERGILLOMAS

- Sputum culture
- Serum precipitating antibody

INVASIVE ASPERGILLOSIS

Definitive diagnosis requires the demonstration of tissue invasion (i.e., septate, acute branching hyphae) (Fig. 336–15) or a positive culture from the tissue obtained by an invasive procedure such as transbronchial biopsy.

- Sputum and nasal cultures: In high-risk patients, a positive culture is strongly suggestive of invasive aspergillosis.
- Serology not helpful, rarely elevated in invasive disease
- Blood cultures: usually negative
- Lung biopsy is necessary for definitive diagnosis.
- Biopsy and culture of extrapulmonary lesions

IMAGING STUDIES

ABPA

- Chest x-ray show a variety of abnormalities from small, patchy, fleeting infiltrates (commonly in the upper lobes) to lobar consolidation or cavitation.
- A majority of patients eventually develop central bronchiectasis.

ASPERGILLOMAS

Chest x-ray or CT scans usually show the characteristic intracavity mass partially surrounded by a crescent of air).

INVASIVE ASPERGILLOSIS

Chest x-ray and CT scanning may reveal cavity formation.

TREATMENT

- **ABPA**
  - Prednisone (0.5 to 1 mg/kg PO) until the chest x-ray has cleared, followed by alternate-day therapy at 0.5 mg/kg PO (3 to 6 months)
  - If a patient is corticosteroid dependent, prophylaxis for the prevention of *Pneumocystis jiroveci* infection and maintenance of bone mineralization should be considered.
  - Bronchodilators and physiotherapy
  - Serial chest x-ray and serum IgE are useful in guiding treatment
  - Itraconazole 200 mg PO bid for 4 to 6 months, then taper over 4 to 6 months may be considered as a steroid-sparing agent or if steroids are ineffective.
- **ASPERGILLOMAS**
  - Controversial and problematic; the optimal treatment strategy is unknown.
  - Up to 10% of aspergillomas may resolve clinically without overt pharmacologic or surgical intervention.
  - Observation for asymptomatic patients
  - Surgical resection/arterial embolization for those patients with severe hemoptysis or life-threatening hemorrhage
  - For those patients at risk for marked hemoptysis with inadequate pulmonary reserve, consider itraconazole 200 to 400 mg/day PO.
- **INVASIVE ASPERGILLOSIS**
  - Amphotericin B
  - Itraconazole
  - Voriconazole
  - Posaconazole and ravuconazole are new azoles currently under investigation.

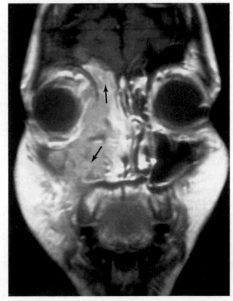

Fig 336–13
Aspergillus sinusitis. Involvement of right maxillary sinus with extension to adjacent structures and the brain (*arrows*). Coronal section. (From Cohen J, Powderly WG: Infectious Diseases, 2nd ed. St Louis, Mosby, 2004.)

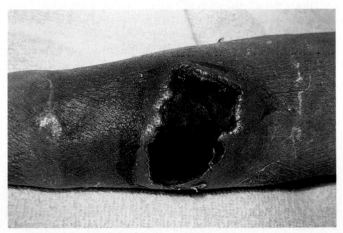

Fig 336–14
Aspergillosis: there is extensive ulceration with characteristic black crusting. Primary cutaneous aspergillosis most often follows trauma, or it may develop in the immunosuppressed. (From Mckee PH, Calonje E, Granter SR [eds]: Pathology of the Skin With Clinical Correlations, 3rd ed. St Louis, Mosby, 2005.)

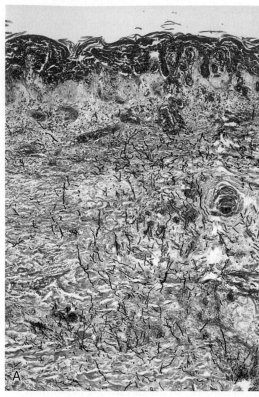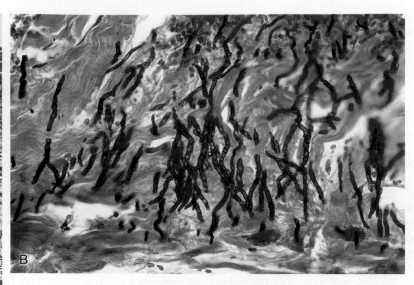

Fig 336–15
Aspergillosis: (**A**) low-power view showing the arboreal growth pattern; (**B**) the hyphae are septate and branch at 45 degrees (methanamine silver). (From McKee PH, Calonje E, Granter SR [eds]: Pathology of the Skin With Clinical Correlations, 3rd ed. St Louis, Mosby, 2005.)

- Caspofungins (Candigas) is the first of a new class of antifungals, the echinocandins approved for the treatment of invasive aspergillosis in patients who fail or are unable to tolerate other antifungal drugs.
- Because azoles and echinocandins target different cellular sites, combination therapy may have additive activity against *Aspergillus sp.* Although still under investigation, some bone marrow transplant units use caspofungin and voriconazole as the preferred initial treatment.
- Cytokine therapy may offer future treatment options in conjunction with the currently available antifungals.

C. HISTOPLASMOSIS

DEFINITION
Histoplasmosis is caused by the fungus *Histoplasma capsulatum* and characterized by a primary pulmonary focus with occasional progression to **chronic pulmonary histoplasmosis (CPH)** or various forms of dissemination. **Progressive disseminated histoplasmosis (PDH)** may present with a diverse clinical spectrum, including adrenal necrosis, pulmonary and mediastinal fibrosis, and ulcerations of the oropharynx and GI tract. In those patients coinfected with the HIV, it is a defining disease for AIDS. Figure 336–16 illustrates the endemic distribution of histoplasmosis in the Americas.

PHYSICAL FINDINGS AND CLINICAL PRESENTATION
- Conidia are deposited in alveoli and then converted to a yeast, where they spread to regional lymph nodes and other organs, particularly the liver and spleen.
- One to 2 weeks later, a granulomatous inflammatory response begins to contain the yeast in the form of discrete granulomas.
- Delayed-type cutaneous hypersensitivity to *Histoplasma* antigens usually occurs 3 to 6 weeks after exposure.
- Clinical disease manifests in various forms, depending on host cellular immunity and inoculum size:
1. Acute primary pulmonary histoplasmosis
   a. Overwhelming number of patients are asymptomatic.
   b. Most clinically apparent infections manifest by complaints of fever, headache, malaise, pleuritic chest pain, nonproductive cough, and weight loss.
   c. Less than 10%, mainly women, complain of arthralgias, myalgias, and skin manifestations such as erythema multiforme or erythema nodosum.
   d. Acute pericarditis presents in smaller percentage of patients.
   e. Hepatosplenomegaly is most commonly observed in children.
   f. With particularly heavy exposure, there is severe dyspnea, marked hypoxemia, impending respiratory failure.
   g. Most patients are asymptomatic within 6 weeks.
2. CPH
   a. Presents insidiously with low-grade fever, malaise, weight loss, cough, sometimes with blood-streaked sputum or frank hemoptysis
   b. Most patients with cavitary lesions present with associated COPD or chronic bronchitis, masking underlying fungal disease.

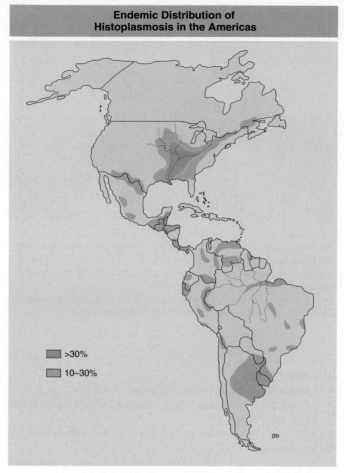

Endemic Distribution of Histoplasmosis in the Americas

■ >30%
□ 10–30%

Fig 336–16
Endemic distribution of histoplasmosis in the Americas. This is based on skin testing surveys.
(From Cohen J, Powderly WG: Infectious Diseases, 2nd ed. St Louis, Mosby, 2004.)

c. Tends to worsen preexisting pulmonary disease and further contribute to eventual respiratory insufficiency
3. PDH
  a. In both acute and subacute forms, constitutional symptoms of fever, fatigue, malaise, and weight loss are common.
  b. Acute form (seen in infants and children) presents with respiratory symptoms, fevers consistently 10° F (38.3° C), generalized lymphadenopathy, marked hepamegaly to splenomegaly, and fulminant course resembling septic shock associated with a high fatality rate.
  c. Subacute form is more common in adults and associated with lower temperatures, hepatosplenomegaly, oropharyngeal ulceration, focal organ involvement (including adrenal destruction, endocarditis, chronic meningitis, and intracerebral mass lesions).
  d. Course of subacute form is relentless, with untreated patient dying within 2 years.
  e. Chronic PDH is found in adults and marked by gradual symptoms of weight loss, weakness, easy fatigability; low-grade fever when present; oropharyngeal ulcerations and hepatomegaly and/or splenomegaly in one third of patients.

  f. Less clinical evidence of focal organ involvement in chronic form than in subacute form.
  g. Natural history of chronic form protracted and intermittent, spanning months to years.
● Histoplasmoma
  1. A healed area of caseation necrosis surrounded by a fibrous capsule
  2. Usually asymptomatic
● Mediastinal fibrosis
  1. A rare consequence of a fibroblastic process that encases caseating mediastinal lymph nodes after primary histoplasma bronchopneumonia; progressive fibrosis producing severe retraction, compression, and distortion of mediastinal structures
  2. Constriction of the bronchi resulting in bronchiectasis, also esophageal stenosis associated with dysphagia, and superior vena cava syndrome
● Presumed ocular histoplasmosis syndrome (POHS)
  1. Diagnosis characterized by distinct clinical features, including atrophic choroidal scars and maculopathy in patient with a history suggestive of exposure to the fungus (e.g., residence in an endemic area)
  2. Patient complains of distortion or loss of central vision without pain, redness, or photophobia
  3. Usually no evidence of systemic infection except for a positive skin reaction to histoplasmin
● In patients with AIDS
  1. Possible presentation as overwhelming infection similar to acute PDH seen in children
  2. Constitutional symptoms: fever, weight loss, malaise, cough, dyspnea
  3. About 10% with cutaneous maculopapular, erythematous eruptions or purpuric lesions on the face, trunk, and extremities
  4. Up to 20% with CNS involvement, manifesting as intracerebral mass lesions, chronic meningitis, or encephalopathy

CAUSE
● *H. capsulatum* is a dimorphic fungus present in temperate zones and river valleys around the world.
● In the United States, it is highly endemic in southeastern, mid-Atlantic, and central states.
● Exists as mold at ambient temperature and favors surface soil enriched with bird or bat droppings

DIFFERENTIAL DIAGNOSIS
● Acute pulmonary histoplasmosis
  1. Mycobacterium tuberculosis
  2. Community-acquired pneumonias caused by *Mycoplasma* and *Chlamydia*
  3. Other fungal diseases, such as *Blastomyces dermatitidis* and *Coccidioides immitis*
● Chronic cavitary pulmonary histoplasmosis: *M. tuberculosis*
● Histoplasmomas: true neoplasms

LABORATORY TESTS
● Demonstration of organism on culture from body fluid (Fig. 336–17) or tissues (Fig. 336–18) to make definitive diagnosis
  1. Especially high yield in patients with AIDS
  2. Characteristic oval yeast cells in neutrophils stained with Wright-Giemsa on peripheral smear (Fig. 336–19)
  3. Preparations of infected tissue with Gomori's silver methenamine for revealing yeast forms, especially in areas of caseation necrosis

1195

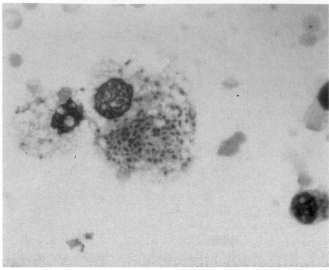

Fig 336–17
Cytologic specimen from bronchoalveolar lavage fluid showing intracellular *Histoplasma capsulatum*.
(From Cohen J, Powderly WG: Infectious Diseases, 2nd ed. St Louis, Mosby, 2004.)

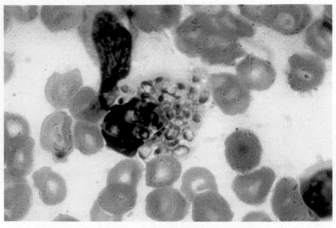

Fig 336–19
This Wright-stain smear of a patient with disseminated histoplasmosis shows the morphology that is most difficult to differentiate from leishmaniasis. Each organism has only one nuclear body that is pushed to the edge of the cell wall (Wright, ×1000).
(From Silverberg SG: Principles and Practice of Surgical Pathology and Cytopathology, 4th ed. Philadelphia, Churchill Livingstone, 2006.)

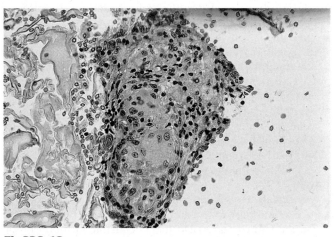

Fig 336–18
Histoplasmosis of lung. Small granulomas are present with multinucleated giant cells. Organisms of histoplasmosis were easily demonstrated with special stains (HANDE, ×400).
(From Silverberg SG: Principles and Practice of Surgical Pathology and Cytopathology, 4th ed. Philadelphia, Churchill Livingstone, 2006.)

- Serologic tests, including complement-fixing (CF) antibodies and immunodiffusion assays
- Detection of *Histoplasma* antigen in urine: may be influenced by infections with *Blastomyces* and *Coccidioides*
- In PDH
  1. Pancytopenia
  2. Marked elevations in alkaline phosphatase and alanine aminotransferase common
- In chronic meningitis (majority of cases)
  1. CSF pleocytosis with either lymphocytes or neutrophils predominating
  2. Elevated CSF protein levels
  3. Hypoglycorrhachia

IMAGING STUDIES
- Chest x-ray in acute pulmonary histoplasmosis
  1. Singular or multiple patchy infiltrates, especially in the lower lung fields
  2. Hilar or mediastinal lymph adenopathy with or without pneumonitis
  3. Diffuse nodular or confluent bilateral miliary infiltrates (Fig. 336–20) characteristic of heavier exposure
  4. Infrequent pleural effusions, except when associated with pericarditis
- Chest x-ray in histoplasmoma: coin lesion displaying central calcification, ranging from 1 to 4 cm in diameter, predominantly located in the subpleural regions
- Chest x-ray in CPH:
  1. Upper lobe disease frequently associated with cavities
  2. Preexisting calcifications in the hilum associated with peribronchial streaking extending to the parenchyma
- Chest x-ray in acute PDH: hilar adenopathy and/or diffuse nodular infiltrates
- CT scan of adrenals to reveal bilateral enlargement and low-attenu ation centers

TREATMENT
- No drug therapy is required for asymptomatic pulmonary disease.
- Brief course of therapy with ketoconazole or itraconazole may be beneficial in some patients with acute pulmonary distress.
- Same therapy appropriate for immunocompetent, mild to moderately symptomatic patients with CPH and subacute and chronic forms of PDH, but duration for 6 to 12 months
- Use amphotericin B in patients hypersensitive to or intolerant of azole therapy.
- Give amphotericin B for life-threatening disease or continued illness as a result of primary failure or relapse of adequate azole therapy.

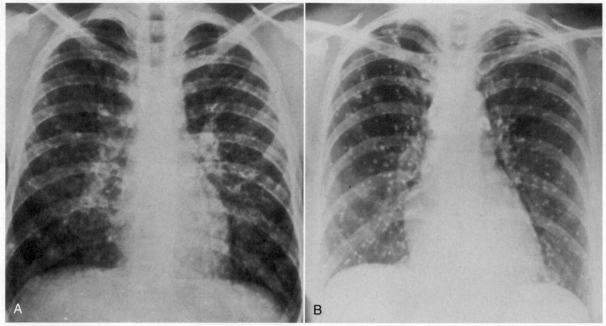

Fig 336–20
Histoplasmosis. (**A**) Acute inhalational histoplasmosis in a 15-year-old boy. The lungs show widespread small areas of consolidation, which may eventually calcify. (**B**) Appearance of such calcification in another patient.
(From Grainger RG, Allison DJ, Adam A, Dixon AK [eds]: Grainger and Allison's Diagnostic Radiology, 4th ed. Philadelphia, Churchill Livingstone, 2001.)

1. For acute pulmonary histoplasmosis associated with acute respiratory distress syndrome (ARDS), acute PDH, and histoplasma meningitis
2. Prednisone 60 to 80 mg/day beneficial for severe fungal hypersensitivity complicating acute pulmonary disease
- Endocarditis: surgical treatment with excision of infected valve or graft combined with amphotericin
- For pericardial disease:
  1. Antifungal therapy: no apparent benefit
  2. Best managed with NSAIDs
- For POHS:
  1. Antifungal therapy: no apparent benefit
  2. May respond to laser therapy

D. CRYPTOCOCCOSIS

DEFINITION
Cryptococcosis is an infection caused by the fungal organism *Cryptococcus neoformans*.

PHYSICAL FINDINGS AND CLINICAL PRESENTATION
- More than 90% present with meningitis; almost all have fever and headache.
- Meningismus, photophobia, mental status changes are seen in approximately 25%.
- Increased intracranial pressure.
- Most common infections outside the CNS:
  1. In the lungs (fever, cough, dyspnea) (Fig. 336–21)
  2. In the skin (cellulitis, papular eruption, erythematous nodules) (Fig. 336–22)
  3. In the lymph nodes (lymphadenitis)
  4. Potential involvement of virtually any organ

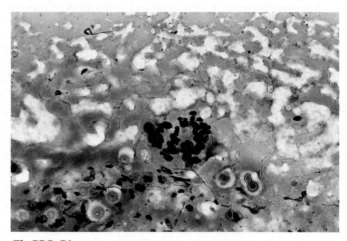

Fig 336–21
Cryptococcus neoformans infection of lung. Patient with acquired immunodeficiency syndrome and pulmonary infiltrates. Many round yeast are present and show thick capsules and narrow-based budding (Diff-Quik stain, ×600).
(From Silverberg SG: Principles and Practice of Surgical Pathology and Cytopathology, 4th ed. Philadelphia, Churchill Livingstone, 2006.)

CAUSE
- Caused by the fungal organism *C. neoformans*
  There are three varieties of *Cryptococcus* spp. and four serotypes based on the capsular polysaccharide: Serotype A is *Cryptococcus neoformans* var. *grubii* and serotype D is known as *Cryptococcus neoformans* var. *neoformans*. Both are ubiquitous in nature and cause disease primarily in immunocompromised patients. Serotypes B and C are known as *C.*

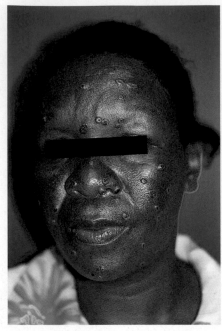

Fig 336-22
Cryptococcosis: multiple erythematous nodules are present.
(Courtesy of N. C. Dlova, MD, Nelson R. Mandela School of Medicine, University of Kwa Zulu-Natal, South Africa.)

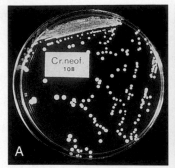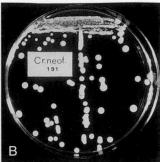

Fig 336-23
Cryptococcus neoformans. (**A**) Thinly encapsuiated. (**B**) With a thick capsule.
(From Cohen J, Powderly WG: Infectious Diseases, 2nd ed. St Louis, Mosby, 2004.)

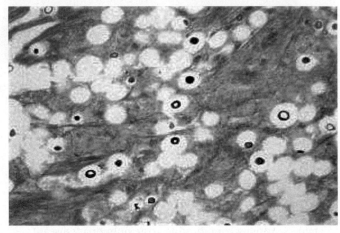

Fig 336-24
Cryptococcosis: the organisms are positive with methenamine silver.
(From McKee PH, Calonje E, Granter SR [eds]: Pathology of the Skin With Clinical Correlations, 3rd ed. St Louis, Mosby, 2005.)

neoformans var. *gatti*. This organism is found primarily in subtropical areas in association with Eucalyptus trees and causes disease in normal hosts.
- Transmission by the respiratory route
- Disseminates to the CNS in most cases, usually without recognizable lung involvement
- Almost always in the setting of AIDS or other disorders of cellular immune function
- Neutropenia alone poses a much lower risk of significant cryptococcal infection.

DIFFERENTIAL DIAGNOSIS
- Subacute meningitis (caused by *Listeria monocytogenes, Mycobacterium tuberculosis, Histoplasma capsulatum*, viruses)
- Intracranial mass lesion (neoplasms, toxoplasmosis, TB)
- Pulmonary involvement confused with *P. jiroveci* pneumonia when diffuse or confused with TB or bacterial pneumonia when focal or involving the pleura
- Skin lesions confused with bacterial cellulitis or molluscum contagiosum

WORKUP
- Lumbar puncture to exclude cryptococcal meningitis
- CT scan of the head when focal lesion or increased intracranial pressure is suspected.
- Biopsy of enlarged lymph nodes and skin lesions if feasible

LABORATORY TESTS
- Culture (Fig. 336-23) and India ink stain (60% to 80% sensitive in culture-proved cases) examination of the CSF in all cases when CNS involvement is suspected
- Blood and serum cryptococcal antigen assay (90% sensitivity and specificity)
- Culture and histologic examination of biopsy material (Fig. 336-24)

IMAGING STUDIES
- CT scan or MRI of the head if focal neurologic involvement is suspected
- Chest x-ray to exclude pulmonary involvement (Fig. 336-25)

TREATMENT
- Therapy is initiated with IV amphotericin B with or without flucytosine.
- After stabilization (usually several weeks), consider fluconazole or voriconazole
- Alternative: IV fluconazole for initial therapy in patients unable to tolerate amphotericin B

E. COCCIDIODOMYCOSIS

DEFINITION
Coccidioidomycosis is an infectious disease caused by the fungus *Coccidioides immitis*. It is usually asymptomatic and characterized by a primary pulmonary focus with infrequent progression to chronic pulmonary disease and dissemination to other organs.

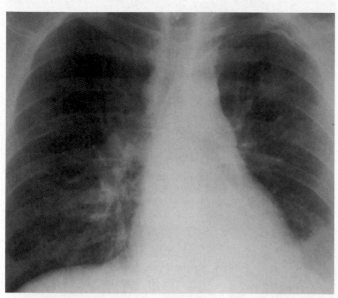

Fig 336–25

Cryptococcosis. An anteroposterior chest film demonstrates a fine reticular interstitial pattern, right paratracheal and hilar adenopathy, and left pleural fluid. Although the interstitial pattern may simulate that seen with pneumocystis pneumonia, the presence of adenopathy and pleural fluid should direct attention toward another diagnosis. (From Grainger RG, Allison DJ, Adam A, Dixon AK [eds]: Grainger and Allison's Diagnostic Radiology, 4th ed. Philadelphia, Churchill Livingstone, 2001.)

PHYSICAL FINDINGS AND CLINICAL PRESENTATION

- Asymptomatic infections or illness consistent with a non-specific upper respiratory tract infection in at least 60%
- Symptoms of primary infection—cough, malaise, fever, chills, night sweats, anorexia, weakness, and arthralgias (desert rheumatism)—in remaining 40% within 3 weeks of exposure
- Erythema nodosum and erythema multiforme more common in women
- Scattered rales and dullness on percussion
- Spontaneous improvement within 2 weeks of illness, with complete recovery usual
- Pulmonary nodules and cavities in <10% of those patients with primary infection; one half of these patients asymptomatic
- In a small portion of these patients: a progressive pneumonitis, often with a fatal outcome
- Immunocompromised or diabetic patients may progress to chronic pulmonary disease
- Over many years, granulomas rupture, leading to new cavity formation and continued fibrosis, often accompanied by hemoptysis
- Disseminated or extrapulmonary disease in approximately 0.5% of acutely infected patients
  1. Early signs of probable dissemination: fever, malaise, hilar adenopathy, and elevated ethrymatosus sedimentation rate (ESR) persisting in the setting of primary infection
  2. Most organs are susceptible to dissemination, with heart and GI tract generally spared.

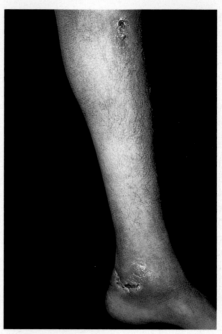

Fig 336–26

Coccidioidomycosis: ulcerated nodules are present on the knee and ankle. (Courtesy of R. Arenas, MD, and J. C. Salas, MD, Monterrey, Mexico.)

- Musculoskeletal involvement: bone lesions often unifocal, ribs, long bones, and vertebral lesions are common.
  1. Joint lesions predominantly unifocal, most commonly involving the ankle and knee, and often accompanying adjacent sites of osteomyelitis.
- Meningeal involvement: headache, fever, weakness, confusion, lethargy, cranial nerve defects, seizures; meningeal signs often minimal or absent.
- Cutaneous involvement: variable lesions—pustules, papules, plaques, nodules (Fig. 336–26), ulcers, abscesses, or verrucous proliferative lesions
  1. Dissemination and fatal outcomes most common in men, pregnant women, neonates, immunocompromised hosts, and individuals of dark-skinned races, especially those of African, Filipino, Mexican, and Native American ancestries

CAUSE

- *Coccidioides immitis* is endemic to North and South America.
- In the United States, endemic areas coincide with the Lower Sonoran Life Zone, with semiarid climate, sparse flora, and alkaline soil in Arizona, California, New Mexico, and Texas.
- Fungus exists in the mycelial phase in soil, having barrel-shaped hyphae (arthroconidia). Arthrospores are aerosolized and deposit in the alveoli, then fungus converts to thick-walled spherule.
- Internal spherical spores (endospores) are released through spherule rupture and mature into new spherules (parasitic cycle).
- Fungus incites a granulomatous reaction in host tissue, usually with caseation necrosis.

DIFFERENTIAL DIAGNOSIS
- Acute pulmonary coccidioidomycoses:
  1. Community-acquired pneumonias caused by *Mycoplasma* and *Chlamydia*
  2. Granulomatous diseases, such as *Mycobacterium tuberculosis* and sarcoidosis
  3. Other fungal diseases, such as *Blastomyces dermatitidis* and *Histoplasma capsulatum*
- Coccidioidomas: true neoplasms

WORKUP
- Suspected in patients with a history of residence or travel in an endemic area, especially during periods favorable to spore dispersion (e.g., dust storms and drought followed by heavy rains)

LABORATORY TESTS
- CBC may reveal eosinophilia, especially with erythema nodosum
- Routine chemistries: usually normal but may reveal hyponatremia
- Elevated serum levels of IgE; associated with progressive disease
- CSF cell counts and chemistry: pleocytosis with mononuclear cell predominance associated with hypoglycorrhachia and elevated protein level
- Definitive diagnosis based on demonstration of the organism by culture from body fluids (Fig. 336–27) or tissues (Fig. 336–28)
  1. Greatest yield with pus, sputum, synovial fluid, and soft tissue aspirations, varying with the degree of dissemination
  2. Possible positive cultures of blood, gastric aspirate, pleural effusion, peritoneal fluid, and CSF, but less frequently obtained
- Serologic evaluations
  1. Latex agglutination and complement fixation
  2. Elevated serum CFA titers ≥1:32 strongly correlated with disseminated disease, except with meningitis where lower titers seen
  3. In meningeal disease: CFA detected in CSF except with high serum CFA titers secondary to concurrent extraneural disease
  4. ELISA against a 33-kDa spherule antigen to detect and monitor CNS disease
- Skin test: coccidioidin, the mycelial phase antigen, and spherulin, the parasitic phase antigen
  1. Positive (>5 mm) 1 month following onset of symptomatic primary infection
  2. Useful in assessing prior infection
  3. Negative skin test with primary infection: latent or future dissemination

IMAGING STUDIES
Chest X-ray Examination
- Reveals unilateral infiltrates, hilar adenopathy (Fig. 336–29), or pleural effusion in primary infection
- Shows areas of fibrosis containing usually solitary, thin-walled cavities that persist as residua of primary infection
- Possible coccidioidoma, a coinlike lesion representing a healed area of previous pneumonitis

TREATMENT
- Supportive care in mild symptomatic disease

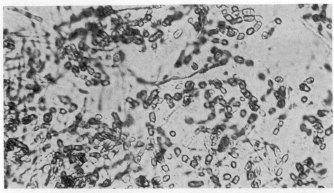

Fig 336–27
Coccidioides immitis, mycelial form in culture at 86° F. This shows hyaline, septate, branching hyphae and chains of arthroconidia, often in alternating cells.
(From Cohen J, Powderly WG: Infectious Diseases, 2nd ed. St Louis, Mosby, 2004.)

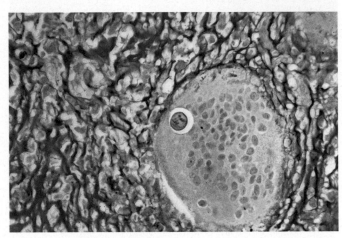

Fig 336–28
Coccidioidomycosis. A developing spherule of *Coccidioides immitis* is located within a multinucleated giant cell. The primary differential at this stage of development is with *Cryptococcus neoformans* and *Blastomyces dermatitidis* (periodic acid × Schiff stain, ×250).
(From Silverberg SG: Principles and Practice of Surgical Pathology and Cytopathology, 4th ed. Philadelphia, Churchill Livingstone, 2006.)

- In general, drug therapy is not required for patients with asymptomatic pulmonary disease and most patients with mild symptomatic primary infection.
- Chemotherapy is indicated under the following circumstances:
  1. Severe symptomatic primary infection
  2. High serum CFA titers
  3. Persistent symptoms >6 weeks
  4. Prostration
  5. Progressive pulmonary involvement
  6. Pregnancy
  7. Infancy
  8. Debilitation
  9. Concurrent illness (e.g., diabetes, asthma, COPD, malignancy)
  10. Acquired or induced immunosuppression
  11. Racial group with known predisposition for disseminated disease

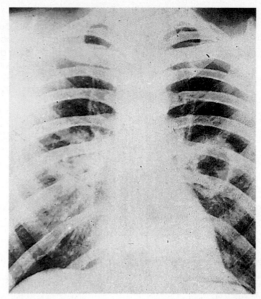

Fig 336–29
Coccidioidomycosis, showing hilar lymphadenopathy and a cavity in the left lung.
(From Cohen J, Powderly WG: Infectious Diseases, 2nd ed. St Louis, Mosby, 2004.)

- Fluconazole
- Itraconazole
- Amphotericin B is the classic therapy for disseminated extra-neural disease.

With meningeal disease: Intrathecal amphotericin B remains the traditional treatment modality, given alone or preceding the use of oral agents.

- For osteomyelitis, soft tissue closed-space infections, and pulmonary fibrocavitary disease: surgical débridement, drainage, or resection, respectively, in addition to oral azole therapy or parenteral administration of amphotericin B

F. NOCARDIOSIS

DEFINITION
Nocardiosis is an infection caused by aerobic actinomycetes found in soil (Fig. 336–30) and characterized by lung, soft tissue, or CNS involvement.

PHYSICAL FINDINGS AND CLINICAL PRESENTATION
- Inhalation of *Nocardia* organisms is the most common mode of entry, and pneumonia is the most common presentation, with 75% manifesting with fever, chills, dyspnea, and a productive cough
  1. Presentation can be acute, subacute, or chronic.
  2. Nocardiosis should be suspected if soft tissue abscesses or CNS tumors or abscesses form in conjunction with the pulmonary infection.
  3. Pulmonary infection may spread into the pericardium, mediastinum, and superior vena cava.
- Cutaneous disease usually occurs via direct inoculation of the organism as a result of skin puncture by a thorn or splinter (Fig. 336–31), surgery, IV catheter use, or animal scratches or bites manifesting in:
  1. Cellulitis

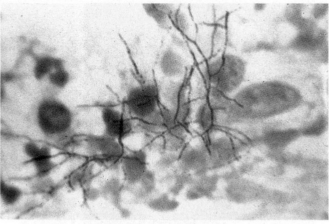

Fig 336–30
Nocardia: the organisms appear mainly as irregular staining filaments in this specimen, but a variety of forms, including rods and cocci, is often seen.
(Courtesy of A. E. Prevost, MD, and H. P. Lambert, MD, St George's Hospital, London, UK.)

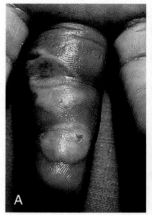 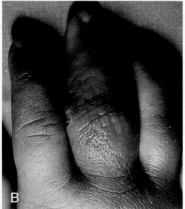

Fig 336–31
Primary cutaneous nocardial infection is characteristically painless, localized, and slowly progressive. (**A**) There are marked swelling and erythema in this child's finger. (**B**) However, because the finger was painless, the child was not brought to medical attention until the infection had progressed to involve the entire finger.
(From Cohen J, Powderly WG: Infectious Diseases, 2nd ed. St Louis, Mosby, 2004.)

  2. Lymphocutaneous nodules appearing along lymphatic sites draining the infected puncture wound (Fig. 336–32)
  3. *Mycetoma (Madura foot)*, a chronic deep nodular infection usually involving the hands or feet that can cause skin breakdown, fistula formation, and spread along the fascial planes to infect surrounding skin, subcutaneous tissue, and bone
- The CNS system is infected in approximately one third of all cases. Brain abscesses is the most common pathologic finding.
- Dissemination of nocardiosis may infect other tissues and organs including the kidneys, heart, skin, and bone.

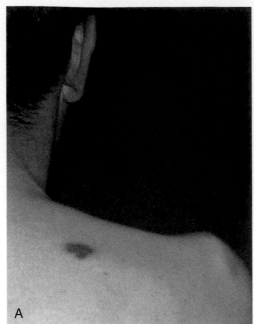

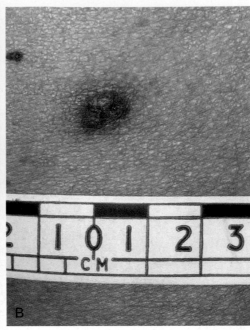

A

B

Fig 336–32
Nocardiosis: (**A**) this cutaneous nodule developed in an immunocompromised young male; (**B**) a different
lesion is shown in close-up view.
(Courtesy of R. A. Marsden, St
George's Hospital, London, UK.)

CAUSE

- The most common *Nocardia* species leading to infection in humans are:
  1. *N. asteroides* (causing more than 80% of the cases of pulmonary nocardiosis)
  2. *N. brasiliensis* (most common cause of mycetoma)
  3. *N. otitidiscaviarum*
- *N. asteroides* has two subgroups
  1. *N. farcinica*
  2. *N. nova*

DIFFERENTIAL DIAGNOSIS

- There are no pathognomonic findings separating nocardiosis pneumonia from other infectious etiologies of the lung. Diagnoses presenting in a similar manner and often confused for nocardiosis are:
  1. Tuberculosis
  2. Lung abscess
  3. Lung tumor
  4. Other causes of pneumonia
  5. Actinomycosis
  6. Mycosis
  7. Cellulitis
  8. Coccidioidomycosis
  9. Histoplasmosis
  10. Aspergillosis
  11. Kaposi's sarcoma

WORKUP

All patients with suspected nocardiosis need laboratory identification of the microorganism by obtaining sputum in the case of pneumonia, cultures of the infected skin lesions in mycetoma or lymphocutaneous disease, or the sampling of any purulent material (e.g., brain abscess, lung abscess, and pleural effusion).

LABORATORY TESTS

- Blood tests are not very sensitive in the diagnosis of nocardiosis.

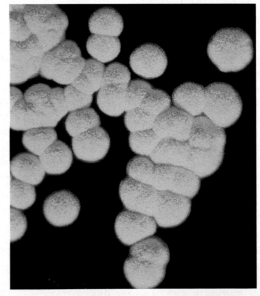

Fig 336–33
Colonies of *Nocardia asteroides*, showing a smooth, chalky-white
appearance.
(From Cohen J, Powderly WG: Infectious Diseases, 2nd ed. St Louis,
Mosby, 2004.)

- Gram stain shows gram-positive beaded filaments with multiple branches
- Gomori methenamine silver staining may detect the organism.
- *Nocardia* species are acid-fast on a modified Ziehl-Neelsen stain.
- *Nocardia* are slow-growing organisms, and colony growth in cultures (Fig. 336–33) may take up to 2 to 3 weeks.

IMAGING STUDIES
- Chest x-ray may demonstrate infiltrates, densities, nodules, cavitary masses, or multiple abscesses.
- CT scan of the brain is indicated in the appropriate clinical setting to exclude CNS brain abscesses.

TREATMENT
- Supportive therapy with oxygen in patients with pneumonia
- Chest physiotherapy
- For any abscess formation, surgical drainage indicated (e.g., skin, lung, or brain)
- There are no prospective randomized trials to date highlighting the most effective treatment of nocardiosis. Nevertheless, sulfonamides are generally considered the treatment of choice.
- Trimethoprim-sulfamethoxazole
- Amikacin has been the IV antibiotic of choice.
- Alternative drug treatment includes minocycline, erythromycin, ampicillin, ofloxacin, clarithromycin

G. ACTINOMYCOSIS

DEFINITION
Actinomycosis is an indolent, slowly progressive infection caused by both anaerobic or microaerophilic bacteria that normally colonize the mouth, vagina, and colon. Actinomycosis is characterized by the formation of painful abscesses, soft tissue infiltration, and draining sinuses.

PHYSICAL FINDINGS AND CLINICAL PRESENTATION
Actinomycosis can affect any organ. Although not typically considered as opportunistic pathogens, *Actinomyces* species capitalize on tissue injury or mucosal breach to invade adjacent structures in the head and neck regions. As a result, dental infections and oromaxillofacial trauma are common antecedent events. Characteristic manifestations include:
- Cervicofacial disease (most common site):
  1. Occurs in the setting of poor dental hygiene, recent dental surgery, or minor oral trauma
  2. Painful soft tissue swelling commonly seen at the angle of the mandible
  3. Fever, chills, and weight loss
  4. Trismus
  5. Soft tissue facial infection with sinus tract or fistula formation
- Thoracic disease:
  1. Can involve the lungs, pleura, mediastinum, or chest wall (Fig. 336–34)
  2. Presumed secondary to aspiration of *Actinomyces* organisms in patients with poor oral hygiene
  3. Fever, cough, weight loss, and pleuritic chest pains are common symptoms.
  4. Signs of pneumonia or pleural effusion may be present.
  5. With extension beyond the lungs to mediastinal structures and the chest wall, signs and symptoms of pericarditis, empyema, chest wall sinus drainage, and tracheoesophageal fistula can all occur.
- Abdominal disease:
  1. Occurs most commonly after appendectomy, perforated bowel, diverticulitis, or surgery to the GI tract

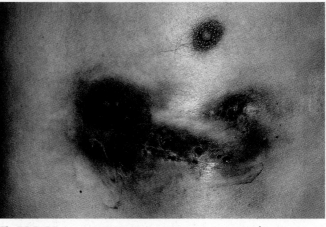

Fig 336–34
Actinomycosis: extensive intrathoracic disease has resulted in involvement of the anterior chest wall. Numerous sinuses are evident. (Courtesy of P. Duhra, MD, Coventry and Warwickshire Hospital, Coventry, UK.)

  2. Lesions develop most commonly in the ileocecal valve, causing abdominal pain, fever, weight loss, and a palpable mass.
  3. Extension may occur to the liver, causing jaundice and abscess formation.
  4. Sinus tracts to the abdominal wall can occur.
- Pelvic disease:
  1. Commonly occurs by extension from abdominal disease of the ileocecal valve to the right adnexa (80% of cases)
  2. Endometritis

CAUSE
- Actinomycosis is most commonly caused by *Actinomyces israelii*. Other causes are *A. naeslundii*, *A. odontolyticus*, *A. viscosus*, *A. meyeri*, and *A. gerencseriae*.
- *Actinomyces* are gram-positive, non–spore-forming, filamentous, anaerobic or microaerophilic rods.
- Actinomycosis infections are polymicrobial, usually associated with *Streptococcus*, *Bacteroides*, *Eikenella corrodens*, *Enterococcus*, and *Fusobacterium*.
- Infects individuals only after entry into disrupted mucosa or tissue injury

DIFFERENTIAL DIAGNOSIS
- Cervicofacial disease: odontogenic abscesses, brachial cleft cyste
- Pulmonary disease: nocardiosis, botryomycosis, chromomycosis, fungal disease of the lung, tuberculosis
- Intestinal disease: intestinal tuberculosis, ameboma, Crohn's disease, colon cancer
- Pelvic disease: chronic pelvic inflammatory disease, Crohn's disease
- CNS disease: other forms of brain abscess, brain tumors, toxoplasmosis, intracranial hematoma

LABORATORY TESTS
- Isolating *"sulfur granules"* from tissue specimens or draining sinuses confirms the diagnosis of actinomycosis. *Actinomyces* are noted for forming characteristic sulfur granules in infected tissue but not in vitro. The term *sulfur granule* is a misnomer, reflecting only the yellow color of the granule in pus, because the granules are not composed of any sulfur at all.

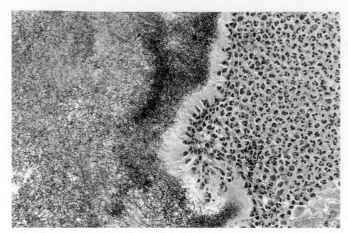

Fig 336-35
Sulfur granule of actinomycosis with well-demonstrated sulfur granule composed of thin, delicate branching bacilli visible on HANDE. The bulk of the granule is composed of amorphous material (HANDE, ×450).
(From Silverberg SG: Principles and Practice of Surgical Pathology and Cytopathology, 4th ed. Philadelphia, Churchill Livingstone, 2006.)

1. Sulfur granules are nests of *Actinomyces* species (Fig. 336-35). Sulfur granules may be macroscopic or microscopic.
2. Sulfur granules are crushed and stained for identification of *Actinomyces* organisms and may take up to 3 weeks to grow in culture media.

IMAGING STUDIES
● Imaging studies are useful adjunctive tests in localizing the site and spread of infection.
   1. Chest x-ray
   2. CT scans of the head, chest, abdomen, and pelvic areas are useful.

TREATMENT
● Incision and drainage of abscesses
● Excision of sinus tract
● Penicillin 10 to 20 million units per day in 4 divided doses for 4 to 6 weeks
● In penicillin-allergic patients, erythromycin, tetracycline, clindamycin, or cephalosporins (depending on the type of penicillin allergy) are reasonable alternatives.
● Chloramphenicol has been used for CNS actinomycosis.

H. BLASTOMYCOSIS

DEFINITION
Blastomycosis is a systemic pyogranulomatous disease caused by a dimorphic fungus, *Blastomyces dermatitidis*

PHYSICAL FINDINGS AND CLINICAL PRESENTATION
● Acute infection: 50% symptomatic, median incubation 30 to 45 days, symptoms are nonspecific: mimic influenza or bacterial infection with abrupt onset of myalgias, arthralgias, chills and fever; transient pleuritic pain, cough that is initially nonproductive; resolution within 4 weeks is usual
● Chronic or recurrent infection: indolent, progressive; includes pulmonary or extrapulmonary disease

● *Pulmonary manifestations:* symptoms and signs of chronic pneumonia—productive cough, hemoptysis, pleuritic chest pain, weight loss, low-grade pyrexia
● Extrapulmonary manifestations:
   1. *Cutaneous:* most common; may occur with or without pulmonary disease. Two different lesions:
   Verrucous: beginning as a small papulopustular lesion on exposed body areas that may develop into an eschar with peripheral microabscesses
   Ulcerative: Subcutaneous nodules (cold abscesses) (Fig. 336-36), and rarely cutaneous inoculation blastomycosis may occur.
   2. Bone and joint: 10% to 50% have osteolytic lesions; affects long bones, vertebrae, and ribs; lesions may present with contiguous soft-tissue abscess or draining sinus that spreads to a joint, resulting in pyarthrosis
   3. Genitourinary: 10% to 30%; prostatic involvement is most common and may present as obstruction; epididymis and testes may also be affected
   4. CNS: 5% normal host; 40% AIDS patients; meningitis and abscess formation

CAUSE
Blastomyces dermatitidis exists in warm, moist soil that is rich in organic material. When these microfoci are disturbed, the aerosolized spores or conidia are inhaled into the lungs. Disease at other sites is a result of dissemination from the initial pulmonary infection; the latter may be acute or chronic.

DIFFERENTIAL DIAGNOSIS
PULMONARY INFECTION:
● Tuberculosis
● Bronchogenic carcinoma
● Histoplasmosis
● Bacterial pneumonia
CUTANEOUS INFECTION:
● Bromoderma
● Pyoderma gangrenosum
● *Mycobacterium marinum* infection
● Squamous cell carcinoma
● Giant keratoacanthoma
LABORATORY TESTS
● Presumptive diagnosis can be made by visualizing the distinctive yeast forms in clinical specimens (Fig. 336-37).
● Culture: on Sabouraud's or more enriched media
   1. Aspirated material from abscesses (Fig. 336-38)
   2. Skin scrapings
   3. Prostatic secretions (urine culture with prostatic massage)
● Direct examination of specimens (Fig. 336-39)
   1. Wet preparation with 10% KOH
   2. Histopathology: typically demonstrates pyogranulomas; yeast identification requires special stains
● Serologic tests: a negative test cannot exclude blastomycosis, nor should a positive titer be an indication to start treatment

IMAGING STUDIES
In chronic disease, chest radiographic findings are nonspecific, but lobar or segmental alveolar infiltrates (Fig. 336-40), especially of the upper lobes, are most common and may progress to cavitation.

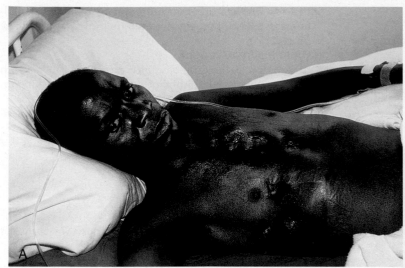

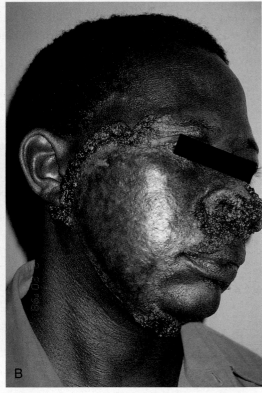

Fig 336–36
Blastomycosis: (**A**) numerous ulcerated and crusted nodules are visible on the chest; the patient had systemic involvement. (**B**) There is severe facial involvement. Note the sepiginous border.
(**A,** Courtesy of W. Weir, MD, Coppetts Wood Hospital, London, UK. **B,** Courtesy of N. C. Dlova, MD, Nelson R. Mandela School of Medicine, University of Kwa Zulu-Natal, South Africa.)

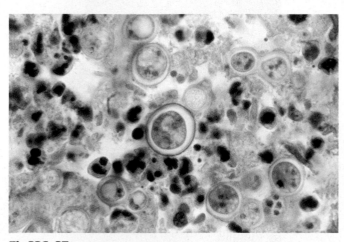

Fig 336–37
Localized blastomycosis was an incidental finding in an autopsy. Yeast cells of *Blastomyces dermatitidis* demonstrate multiple nuclei, thick cell walls, broad-based budding, and an artifactual separation of the cytoplasm from the cell wall (HANDE, ×1000).
(From Silverberg SG: Principles and Practice of Surgical Pathology and Cytopathology, 4th ed. Philadelphia, Churchill Livingstone, 2006.)

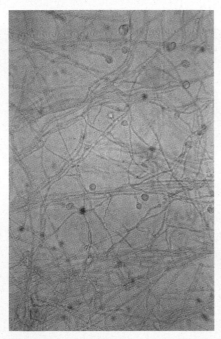

Fig 336–38
Blastomyces dermatitidis, mucelial form in culture at 86° F. This shows hyaline, septate, branching hyphae and short conidiophores bearing colitary oval-to-piriform conidia.
(From Cohen J, Powderly WG: Infectious Diseases, 2nd ed. St Louis, Mosby, 2004.)

TREATMENT
ACUTE BLASTOMYCOSIS
- Treatment remains controversial for acute pulmonary blastomycosis.
- Because the acute form may be benign and self-limited, patients may be closely observed.
- Some patients progress to chronic infection with significant morbidity and therefore may require treatment.

- Patients who are immunocompromised or have extrapulmonary disease or progressive pulmonary disease should be treated.

CHRONIC BLASTOMYCOSIS
- Itraconazole is the drug of choice except for patients with CNS disease or with fulminant illness who require amphotericin B.
- Fluconazole if unable to tolerate itraconazole or amphotericin B
- Ketoconazole is an option in mild-moderate disease.
- Surgery may be indicated for drainage of large abscesses.

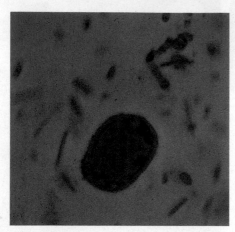

Fig 336-39
Blastocystis hominis. (**A**) Central body form with large "empty" area (appears like a vacuole) with multiple nuclei around the edges (d'Antoni's iodine). (**B**) Three central body forms with the large empty are surrounded by nuclei (trichrome stain).
(From Cohen J, Powderly WG: Infectious Diseases, 2nd ed. St Louis, Mosby, 2004.)

I. SPOROTRICHIOSIS

DEFINITION
Sporotrichosis is a granulomatous disease caused by *Sporothrix schenckii*.

PHYSICAL FINDINGS AND CLINICAL PRESENTATION
- Cutaneous disease
  1. Arises at the site of inoculation
  2. Initial lesion usually located on the distal part of an extremity, although any area may be affected, including the face (Fig. 336–41)
  3. Variable incubation period of approximately 3 weeks once introduced into the skin
  4. Granulomatous reaction provoked
  5. Lesion becomes papulonodular, erythematous, elastic, variable in size
  6. Subsequently, nodule becomes fluctuant, undergoes central necrosis, breaks down, discharges mucoid pus from which fungus may be isolated

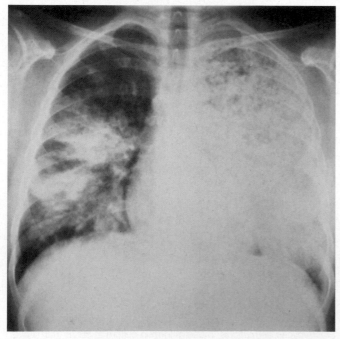

Fig 336-40
Blastomycosis pneumonia showing nonspecific widespread areas of severe consolidation in both lungs.
(From Grainger RG, Allison DJ, Adam A, Dixon AK [eds]: Grainger and Allison's Diagnostic Radiology, 4th ed. Philadelphia, Churchill Livingstone, 2001.)

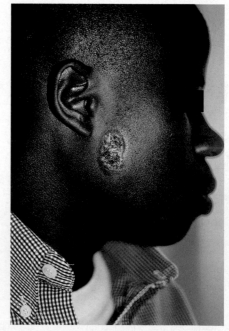

Fig 336-41
Sporotrichosis: localized variant presenting as an ulcerated plaque.
(Courtesy of N. C. Dlova, MD, Nelson R. Mandela School of Medicine, University of Kwa Zulu-Natal, South Africa.)

7. Indolent ulcer with raised erythematous or violaceous borders
8. Secondary lesions:
   a. Develop along superficial lymphatic channels (Fig. 336–42)
   b. Evolve in the same manner as the primary lesion, with subsequent inflammation, induration, and suppuration
- Fixed, or plaque form
  1. Erythematous verrucous, ulcerated, or crusted lesions
  2. Does not spread locally
  3. Does not involve lymphatic vessels
  4. Rarely undergoes spontaneous resolution
  5. More often persists for years without systemic symptoms and within a setting of normal laboratory examinations
- Osteoarticular involvement
  1. Most common extracutaneous form
  2. Usually presents as monoarticular arthritis
  3. Left untreated, may progress to:
     a. Synovitis
     b. Osteitis
     c. Periostitis
     d. All involving elbows, knees, wrists, and ankles
  4. Joint inflamed
     a. Associated with an effusion
     b. Painful on motion
- Early pulmonary disease
  1. Usually associated with a paucity of clinical findings
     a. Low-grade fever
     b. Cough
     c. Fatigue
     d. Malaise
     e. Weight loss
  2. Untreated
     a. Cavitary pulmonary disease
     b. Frank pulmonary dysfunction
  3. Meningitis uncommon
     a. Except perhaps in the immunocompromised patient
     b. Presents with few signs or symptoms of neurologic involvement
  4. Few reported cases
     a. Infection of the ocular adnexa
     b. Endophthalmitis without antecedent trauma
     c. Infections of the testes and epididymis

CAUSE
- *Sporothrix schenckii*
  1. Global in distribution
  2. Often isolated from soil, plants, and plant products
  3. Majority of case reports from tropical and subtropical regions of the Americas
- Occupational or recreational exposure
  1. Hay
  2. Straw
  3. Sphagnum moss
  4. Timber
  5. Thorny plants (e.g., roses and barberry bushes)
- Animal contact
  1. Armadillos
  2. Cats
  3. Squirrels
- Human-to-human transmission
- Tattooing

DIFFERENTIAL DIAGNOSIS
- Fixed, or plaque, sporotrichosis
  1. Bacterial pyoderma
  2. Foreign body granuloma
  3. Tularemia
  4. Anthrax
  5. Other mycoses: blastomycosis, chromoblastomycosis
- Lymphocutaneous sporotrichosis
  1. *Nocardia brasiliensis*
  2. *Leishmania braziliensis*
  3. Atypical mycobacterial disease: *M. marinum, M. kansasii*
- Pulmonary sporotrichosis
  1. Pulmonary TB
  2. Histoplasmosis
  3. Coccidioidomycosis
- Osteoarticular sporotrichosis
  1. Pigmented villonodular synovitis
  2. Gout
  3. Rheumatoid arthritis
  4. Infection with *M. tuberculosis*
  5. Atypical mycobacteria: *M. marinum, M. kansasii, M. avium-intracellulare*
- Meningitis
  1. Histoplasmosis
  2. Cryptococcosis
  3. TB

WORKUP
The diagnosis should be considered in individuals who are occupationally exposed to soil, decaying plant matter, and thorny plants (gardeners, horticulturists, farmers) who present with chronic nonhealing ulcers or lesions with or without associated arthritis or pulmonary symptoms.

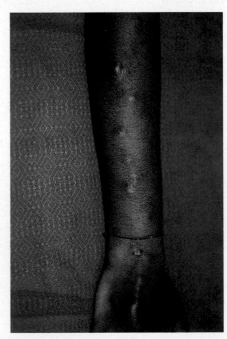

Fig 336–42
Sporotrichosis: multiple nodules are present along the lymphatic channels draining the primary lesion.
(Courtesy of N. C. Dlova, MD, Nelson R. Mandela School of Medicine, University of Kwa Zulu-Natal, South Africa.)

- Diagnosis is made by culture:
  1. Pus
  2. Joint fluid
  3. Sputum
  4. Blood
  5. Skin biopsy
- Isolation of the fungus from any site is considered diagnostic of infection.
- Saprophytic colonization of the respiratory tract has been described.
- A positive blood culture may indicate infection in an immunocompromised host.
- Increasingly sensitive laboratory culturing systems may detect the fungus in the normal host.
- Biopsy specimens are diagnostic if characteristic cigar-shaped, round, oval, or budding yeast forms are seen (Fig. 336–43).
- Despite special staining, the yeast may remain difficult to detect unless multiple sections are examined.
- No standard method of serologic testing is available.
- Previously described techniques have been hampered by the presence of antibody in the absence of infection.

LABORATORY TESTS
- CBCs and serum chemistries are generally normal.
- Elevated ESR is seen with extracutaneous disease.
- CSF analysis in meningeal disease reveals:
  1. Lymphocytic pleocytosis
  2. Elevated protein
  3. Hypoglycorrhachia
- Nested PCR assays represent future clinical modality to rapidly detect *S. schenckii*.

IMAGING STUDIES
- Chest x-ray: unilateral or bilateral upper lobe cavitary or noncavitary lesions
- Radiographic findings of affected joints:
  1. Loss of articular cartilage
  2. Periosteal reaction
  3. Periarticular osteopenia
  4. Cystic changes

TREATMENT
CUTANEOUS AND LYMPHOCUTANEOUS SPOROTRICHOSIS:
- Itraconazole is the drug of choice and should be given for 3 to 6 months.
- Use saturated solution of potassium iodide (SSKI) 5 to 10 drops PO tid or 1.5 mL PO tid, gradually increasing to 40 to 50 drops PO tid or 3 mL PO tid after meals.
- Maximum tolerated dose should be continued until cutaneous lesions have resolved, approximately 6 to 12 weeks.
- Adjunctive therapy with heat is useful and occasionally curative.

DEEP-SEATED MYCOSES (E.G., OSTEOARTICULAR, NONCAVITARY PULMONARY DISEASE)
- Itraconazole
  1. Appropriate initial chemotherapy
  2. Probably as effective as amphotericin B
  3. Less toxic than amphotericin B
  4. Better tolerated than ketoconazole
- Parenteral amphotericin B results in cure in approximately two thirds of cases
  1. Relapses are common.
  2. Amphotericin B–resistant isolates of *S. schenckii* have been reported.
  3. Remains the drug of choice for severely ill patients with disseminated disease
  4. In cavitary pulmonary disease, given perioperatively as an adjunct to surgical resection
  5. In meningitis, amphotericin B may be used alone or in combination with 5-fluorocytosine.
- Fluconazole
  1. Less effective than itraconazole
  2. Requires daily doses of 400 mg/day for lymphocutaneous disease and 800 mg/day for visceral or osteoarticular disease

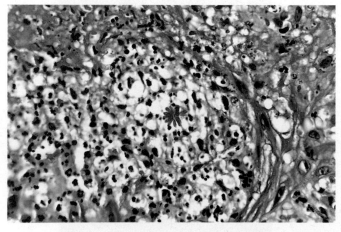

Fig 336–43
Sporotrichosis: the yeast form is characteristically surrounded by radiating eosinophilic spokes (the Splendore-Hoeppli phenomenon). (From McKee PH, Calonje E, Granter SR [eds]: Pathology of the Skin With Clinical Correlations, 3rd ed. St Louis, Mosby, 2005.)

J. MUCORMYCOSIS

DEFINITION

Mucormycosis is a fungal infection by *Zygomycetes* fungi, which include *Mucorales* spp. (*Mucor, Rhizopus, Absidia, Cunninghamella, Mortierella, Saksenaea, Syncephalastrum, Apophysomyces,* and *Thamnidium*) and *Entomophthorales* spp. (*Conidiobolus* and *Basidiobolus*).

PHYSICAL FINDINGS AND CLINICAL PRESENTATION

- Rhinocerebral-rhinoorbital-paranasal syndrome may present with fever, facial and orbital pain, headache, diplopia, loss of vision, facial or orbital cellulitis, facial anesthesia, cranial nerve dysfunction, black nasal discharge, epistaxis, and seizure. Physical findings (Fig. 336–44) in this situation include proptosis, chemosis, nasal, palatal or pharyngeal necrotic ulcerations, and retinal infarction (Fig. 336–45). Thrombosis of the cavernous sinus or internal carotid artery may occur. This form of mucormycosis is found most commonly in diabetics, primarily in the presence of acidosis, and in patients with leukemia and neutropenia.

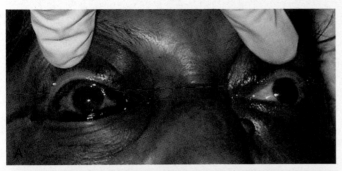

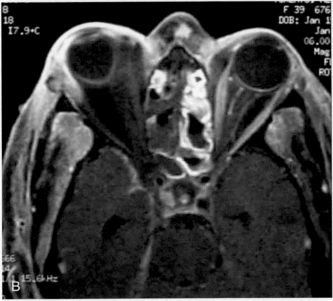

- Pulmonary mucormycosis can present with pneumonia, lung abscess, pulmonary infarction, pleurisy, pleural effusion, hemoptysis, chills, and fever. This form of mucormycosis is found most commonly in immunocompromised neutropenic hosts following chemotherapy for hematologic malignancies.
- Gastrointestinal zygomycosis presents with abdominal pain, diarrhea, GI hemorrhage, ulcers, peritonitis, and bowel infarction. This form of mucormycosis is found most commonly in patients with extreme malnutrition and is believed to arise from ingestion of the fungi.
- Cutaneous zygomycosis presents as nodular lesions (hematogenous seeding) or a wound infection. It involves primarily the epidermis and dermis following use of occlusive dressings that have not been properly sterilized.
- Cardiac mucormycosis is a form of endocarditis.
- Septic arthritis and osteomyelitis
- Brain abscess occurs most often from extension of the fungus from the nose or paranasal sinuses through adjacent bones in severely debilitated patients.
- Disseminated zygomycosis (rare but uniformly fatal)
- Physical findings depend on the location of the infection.

CAUSE AND PATHOGENESIS

The cause of mucormycosis is infection by a fungus of the *Zygomycetes* class (see "Definition"). Normal host defenses include leukocytes and pulmonary macrophages. Quantitative (e.g., neutropenia) or qualitative (e.g., diabetes mellitus or steroid treatment) disruption in the host defenses predisposes the patient to infection.

DIFFERENTIAL DIAGNOSIS

- Infection of the sites described previously by other organisms (bacterial [including TB and leprosy], viral, fungal, or protozoan)
- Noninfectious tissue necrosis (e.g., neoplasia, vasculitis, degenerative) of the sites described previously

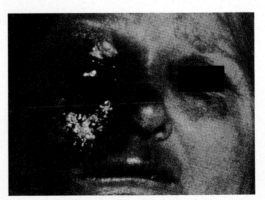

Fig 336–44

A, Patient with mucormycosis of the right orbit, resulting in an orbital apex syndrome. **B,** Axial view from orbital MRI demonstrating mucormycosis of the ethmoid sinuses with extension into orbit.
(From Yanoff M, Duker JS: Ophthalmology, 2nd ed. St Louis, Mosby, 2004.)

Fig 336–45

Patient with mucormycosis. Ocular invasion by mucor in a patient with diabetes mellitus and ketoacidosis.
(From Cohen J, Powderly WG: Infectious Diseases, 2nd ed. St Louis, Mosby, 2004.)

WORKUP

- Biopsy of infected tissue with direct light microscopy examination establishes the diagnosis within minutes of the biopsy in the case of nasopharyngeal infection. Typically the fungi appear as broad (10 to 20 μm in diameter) nonseptate hyphae with branches occurring at right angles (Fig. 336–46).
- Bronchoalveolar lavage or bronchoscopy with biopsy for smear, culture, and histologic examination
- X-rays and other imaging studies of symptomatic sites may be required before infection is suspected and tissue specimens are obtained.

TREATMENT

- Aggressive correction of underlying disease (e.g., hyperglycemia, academia, high steroid doses, use of immunosuppressive drugs) should be undertaken.
- Standard therapy for invasive mucormycosis is treatment with amphotericin B.

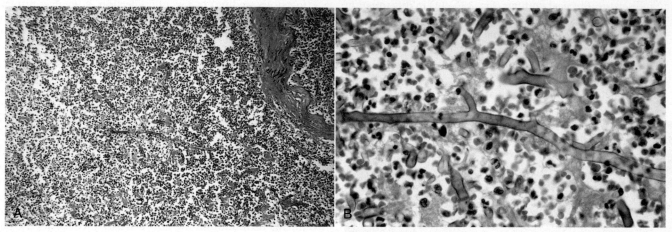

Fig 336–46
Zygomucosis (mucormycosis): (**A**) the fungi are recognizable even at this low-power magnification; (**B**) the hyphae are very broad (much more than *Aspergillus*), are nonseptate, and branch at 90 degrees.
(Courtesy of R. Hay, MD, Institute of Dermatology, London, UK.)

Chapter 337 Rheumatic fever

DEFINITION

- Rheumatic fever is a multisystem inflammatory disease that occurs in the genetically susceptible host after a pharyngeal infection with group A streptococci. It can result in severe damage to the myocardium (Fig. 337–1) and heart valves (Fig. 337–2)
- "Jones Criteria (revised) for Guidance in the Diagnosis of Rheumatic Fever" published by the American Heart Association. One major and two minor criteria if supported by evidence of an antecedent group A streptococcal infection
- Major criteria
  1. Carditis
  2. Migratory arthritis
  3. Chorea
  4. Erythema marginatum
  5. Subcutaneous nodules
- Minor criteria
  1. Previous rheumatic fever or rheumatic heart disease
  2. Fever
  3. Arthralgia
  4. Increased acute-phase reactants
     a. ESR
     b. C-reactive protein
     c. Leukocytosis
  5. Prolonged PR interval

PHYSICAL FINDINGS AND CLINICAL PRESENTATION

- Acute streptococcal pharyngitis, which may be subclinical and not reported by the patient
- After latent period of 1 to 5 weeks (average, 19 days), acute rheumatic attack
- Patient is febrile, with a migratory polyarthritis of knees, ankles, wrists, elbows; typically severe for 1 weeks, remits by 3 to 4 weeks

- Carditis
  1. New heart murmur
     a. Mitral regurgitation
     b. Aortic insufficiency
     c. Diastolic mitral murmur
  2. Cardiomegaly
  3. CHF
  4. Pericardial friction rub or effusion
- Rarely, pancarditis is severe and fatal.
- Subcutaneous nodules can be palpated over extensor tendon surfaces or bony prominences, such as the skull.
- *Chorea (Sydenham's chorea)* is characterized by rapid involuntary movements affecting all muscles.
  1. Muscular weakness
  2. Emotional lability
  3. Rarely seen after adolescence and almost never in adult males
- Erythema marginatum
  1. Evanescent, pink, well-demarcated spreading to trunk and proximal extremities
  2. Not specific
- Arthralgias (joint pain without swelling)
- Abdominal pain

CAUSE

- Group A streptococci not recovered from tissue lesions
- It does not occur in the absence of a streptococcal antibody response.

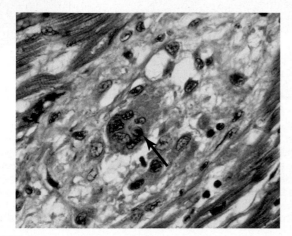

Fig 337–1
Aschoff nodule in the myocardium. The Aschoff nodule is characteristic of rheumatic fever and the nodule consists of multinucleated giant cells (*arrow*) surrounded by macrophages and T lymphocytes. The adjacent myocardial fibers appear intact.
(From Crawford MH, DiMarco JP, Paulus WJ [eds]: Cardiology, 2nd ed. St Louis, Mosby, 2004.)

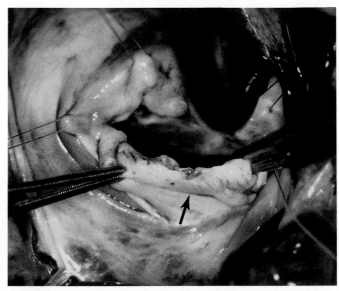

Fig 337–2
View from the left atrium of the mitral valve in a patient with acute rheumatic fever. The leaflets show evidence of rheumatic activity with edematous thickening and verrucous vegetations at the leaflet margins (*arrow*).
(From Crawford MH, DiMarco JP, Paulus WJ [eds]: Cardiology, 2nd ed. St Louis, Mosby, 2004.)

- Immunologic cross-reactivity between certain streptococcal antigens and human tissue antigens suggests an autoimmune etiology.
- Both initial attacks and recurrences can be completely prevented by prompt treatment of streptococcal pharyngitis with penicillin.

DIFFERENTIAL DIAGNOSIS

- Rheumatoid arthritis
- Juvenile rheumatoid arthritis (Still's disease)
- Bacterial endocarditis
- Systemic lupus
- Viral infections
- Serum sickness

LABORATORY TESTS

- Throat cultures are usually negative.
- Streptococcal antibody tests are more useful in establishing the diagnosis.
  1. Peak at the beginning of the attack
  2. Can document a recent streptococcal infection
- ASO (antistreptolysin O) titers peak:
  1. 4 to 5 weeks after a streptococcal throat infection
  2. During the second or third week of illness
- Anti–DNase B (Streptozyme) is also commonly used but is less reliable.
- High-titer streptococcal antibodies:
  1. Are supportive of diagnosis, but not proof
  2. Should be interpreted in the context of clinical criteria

IMAGING STUDIES

- Chest x-ray to assess heart size (Fig. 337–3)
- Echocardiogram (Figs. 337–4 and 337–5):
  1. To evaluate murmurs
  2. To rule out pericardial effusion

TREATMENT

- Course of penicillin to eradicate throat carriage of group A streptococci
- Arthralgia or arthritis without carditis: high dose aspirin or NSAIDs for 6 weeks
- Carditis and heart failure:
  1. Prednisone 40 to 60 mg/day
  2. IV corticosteroids, such as methylprednisolone for severe carditis

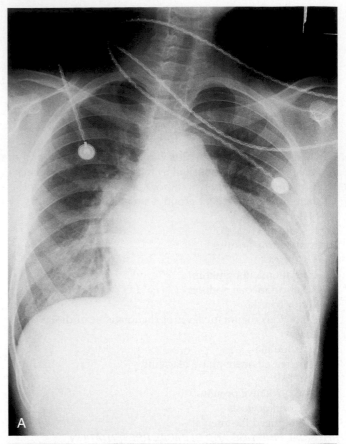

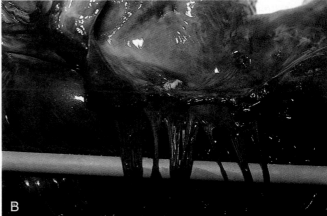

Fig 337–3
(**A**) Chest radiograph of a 15-year-old boy who had multiple recurrences of acute rheumatic fever, showing gross cardiac enlargement and failure. He had mitral regurgitation and stenosis and aortic regurgitation and stenosis. He died 2 days after this radiograph was taken, of intractable cardiac failure. (**B**) Postmortem cardiac examination of the same boy, showing thickened, shortened mitral valve cusps with calcific vegetation and thickened chordae tendinae.
(Photographs kindly provided by Prof. Bard Currie, Darwin, NT, Australia,)

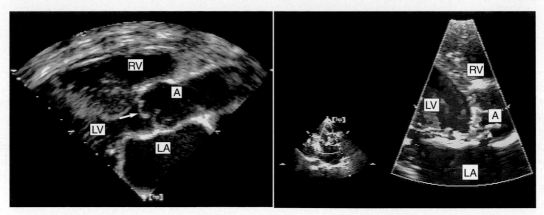

Figs 337–4 and 337–5
Transesophageal long-axis view in a patient with rheumatic fever and severe aortic regurgitation. There is a prolapse of the right coronary cusp. Color Doppler (*right*) confirms a posteriorly directed jet. AO, aorta; LA, left atrium; LV, left ventricle; RV, right ventricle. (From Crawford MH, DiMarco JP, Paulus WJ [eds]: Cardiology, 2nd ed. St Louis, Mosby, 2004.)

Chapter 338 | Infectious mononucleosis

DEFINITION

Mononucleosis is a symptomatic infection caused by Epstein-Barr virus (Fig. 338–1).

PHYSICAL FINDINGS AND CLINICAL PRESENTATION

- Following an incubation period of 1 to 2 months, a prodrome may occur, with fever, chills, malaise, and anorexia for several days. This is followed by the classic triad, which includes pharyngitis, fever, and adenopathy. Although fatigue and malaise may be prominent, pharyngitis is usually the most severe symptom. Exudates (Fig. 338–2) are common.
- Lymphadenopathy (Fig. 338–3) is most prominent in the cervical region but may be diffuse.
- Splenomegaly may occur, most commonly during the second week of illness.
- Rash is uncommon, but will occur in nearly all patients who receive ampicillin.
- At times, infectious mononucleosis (IM) can present as fever and adenopathy without pharyngitis. Although complications may be severe, they are uncommon, and tend to resolve completely. Involvement of the hematologic, pulmonary, cardiac, or nervous system may occur; splenic rupture is rare. IM is usually a self-limited illness, but symptoms of malaise and fatigue may last months before resolving.

CAUSE

The cause of IM is primary infection with Epstein-Barr virus (EBV). Primary infection during childhood causes little or no symptoms. Infection during childhood is more common in lower socioeconomic groups. The frequency of IM in late adolescence is attributed to the onset of social contact between the sexes. Close personal contact is usually necessary for transmission, although EBV has occasionally been transmitted by blood transfusion. Transfer via saliva while kissing may be responsible for many cases.

DIFFERENTIAL DIAGNOSIS

- Heterophile-negative infectious mononucleosis caused by cytomegalovirus (CMV); although clinical presentation may be similar, CMV more frequently follows transfusion
- Bacterial and viral causes of pharyngitis
- Toxoplasmosis
- Acute retroviral syndrome of HIV, lymphoma

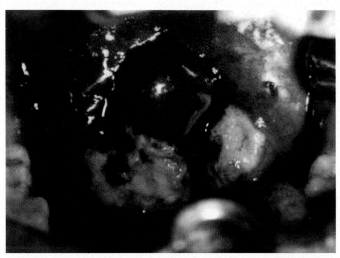

Fig 338–2
Infectious mononucleosis. Note the massive tonsillar enlargement and the cheeselike substance in the crypts.
(From Swartz MH: Textbook of Physical Diagnosis, 5th ed. Philadelphia, WB Saunders, 2006.)

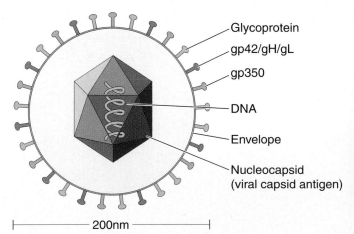

Glycoprotein
gp42/gH/gL
gp350
DNA
Envelope
Nucleocapsid
(viral capsid antigen)

200nm

Fig 338–1
Structure of the Epstein-Barr virus. The virion consists of DNA, the nucleocapsid (which includes the viral capsid antigen), and the envelope (which contains glycoproteins). Glycoprotein 42 (gp42) is part of a trimolecular complex with gH and gL. The virion is approximately 200 nm in diameter.
(From Young NS, Gerson SL, High KA [eds]: Clinical Hematology, St Louis, Mosby, 2006.)

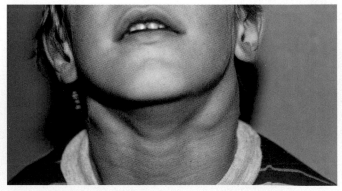

Fig 338–3
Adenopathy associated with Epstein-Barr virus.
(From Cohen J, Powderly WG: Infectious Diseases, 2nd ed. St Louis, Mosby, 2004.)

LABORATORY TESTS

- Increased WBC count is common, with a relative lymphocytosis and neutropenia. Atypical lymphocytes (Fig. 338–4) are the hallmark of IM, but are not pathognomonic. Mild thrombocytopenia is common. A falling hematocrit may signal splenic rupture. Elevated hepatocellular enzymes are often present due to mild hepatitis (Fig. 338–5). Heterophile antibody, as measured by the Monospot test, may be positive at presentation or may appear later in the course of illness. A negative test should be repeated if clinical suspicion is high. If this test remains negative for 8 weeks, other causes of IM are likely. The Monospot usually remains positive for 3 to 6 months but can last for 1 year.
- A positive test has been reported with primary HIV infection.
- In addition to the heterophile antibody, virus-specific antibodies may result in response to IM. Determination of these EBV-specific antibodies is rarely necessary to diagnose IM, although early diagnosis in monospot negative cases may be made by isolating IgM to the viral capsid antigen (VCA), which is usually positive during the acute illness. Figure 338–6 illustrates patterns of EBV serology during acute infection.

IMAGING STUDIES

Chest radiograph may rarely show infiltrates. An elevated left hemidiaphragm may occur in cases of splenic rupture.

TREATMENT

- Supportive rest is advocated by some, but impact on outcome is not clear.
- Splenectomy if rupture occurs. Transfusions for severe anemia or thrombocytopenia.
- Pharmacologic therapy is not indicated in uncomplicated illness.
- The use of steroids is suggested in patients who have severe thrombocytopenia or hemolytic anemia, or impending airway obstruction as a result of enlarged tonsils. There is no role for antiviral agents such as acyclovir in the management of IM.

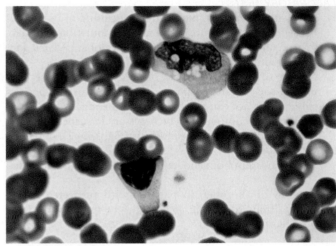

Fig 338–4
Atypical lymphocytes.
(From Young NS, Gerson SL, High KA [eds]: Clinical Hematology, St Louis, Mosby, 2006.)

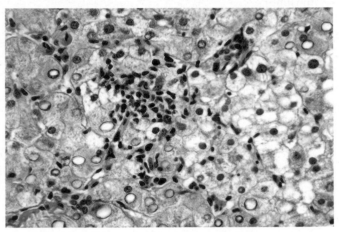

Fig 338–5
Epstein-Barr virus hepatitis. A focus of hepatocellular necrosis and mononuclear infiltrates is seen. Mild hepatitis is common in infectious mononucleosis, but clinical illness that leads to biopsy is unusual (HANDE, ×400).
(From Silverberg SG: Principles and Practice of Surgical Pathology and Cytopathology, 4th ed. Philadelphia, Churchill Livingstone, 2006.)

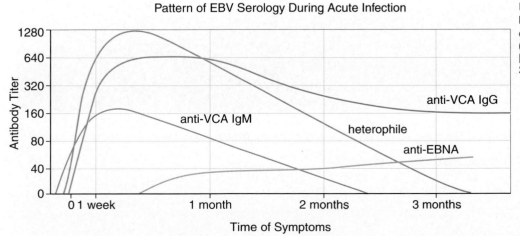

Pattern of EBV Serology During Acute Infection

Fig 338–6
Patterns of Epstein-Barr virus serology during acute infection.
(From Young NS, Gerson SL, High KA [eds]: Clinical Hematology, St Louis, 2006, Mosby.)

Chapter 339 Thrombophlebitis

DEFINITION

Superficial thrombophlebitis is inflammatory thrombosis in subcutaneous veins. **Superficial suppurative thrombophlebitis** is an inflammation of the vein wall due to the presence of microorganisms occurring as a complication of either dermal infection or use of an indwelling intravenous catheter.

PHYSICAL FINDINGS AND CLINICAL PRESENTATION

- Subcutaneous vein is palpable, tender; tender cord is present with erythema and edema of the overlying skin and subcutaneous tissue.
- Induration, redness, and tenderness are localized along the course of the vein. This linear appearance rather than circular appearance is useful to distinguish thrombophlebitis from other conditions (cellulitis, erythema nodosum).
- There is no significant swelling of the limb (superficial thrombophlebitis generally does not produce swelling of the limb).
- Low-grade fever may be present. High fever and chills are suggestive of septic phlebitis.
- Superficial suppurative thrombophlebitis (Fig. 339–1) may be difficult to identify because local findings of inflammation may be absent. Fever is present in 70% of cases but rigors are rare. Local findings (warmth, erythema, tenderness, swelling, lymphangitis) are present in only one third of patients.

CAUSE

- Trauma to preexisting varices.
- Intravenous cannulation of veins (most common cause).
- Abdominal cancer (e.g., carcinoma of the pancreas).
- Infection: *Staphylococcus aureus* was the most common pathogen, found in 65% to 78% of the cases of superficial

suppurative thrombophlebitis before 1970; now most cases are due to Enterobacteriaceae, especially *Klebsiella-Enterobacter* spp. These agents are acquired nosocomially and are often resistant to multiple antibiotics. Infection with fungi or gram-negative aerobic bacilli is often seen in patients who are receiving broad-spectrum antibiotics at the time of the superficial suppurative phlebitis.

- Hypercoagulable state
- Deep venous thrombosis (DVT)

DIFFERENTIAL DIAGNOSIS

- Lymphangitis (see Fig. 28–5)
- Cellulitis (see Fig. 28–4)
- Erythema nodosum (see Fig. 11–2)
- Panniculitis (see Fig. 131–2)
- Kaposi's sarcoma (see Fig. 329–2)

LABORATORY TESTS

- CBC with differential, blood cultures, culture of IV catheter tip (when secondary to intravenous cannulation). Bacteremia occurs in 80% to 90% of the cases of superficial suppurative thrombophlebitis.
- Culture of the catheter may be misleading because even though bacteria are isolated in 60% of the cases, a positive culture does not correlate with inflammation.
- Exploratory venotomy may be necessary in suspected superficial suppurative thrombophlebitis (Fig. 339–2).

IMAGING STUDIES

- Serial ultrasound or venography in patients with suspected DVT
- CT scan of abdomen in patients with suspected malignancy (*Trousseau's syndrome:* recurrent migratory thrombophlebitis)

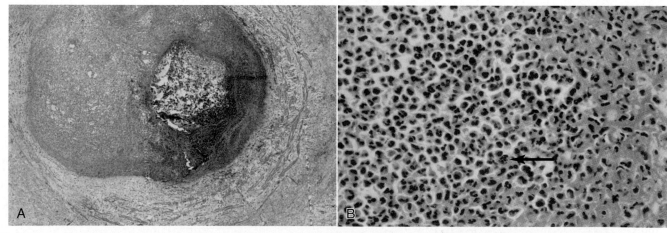

Fig 339–1
Suppurative thrombophlebitis. (**A**) Histologic section of excised vein demonstrating thrombus. (**B**) Microorganisms (Gram-positive cocci) present within the thrombus (*arrow*).
(From Cohen J, Powderly WG: Infectious Diseases, 2nd ed. St Louis, Mosby, 2004.)

TREATMENT

- Warm, moist compresses
- It is not necessary to restrict activity; however, if there is extensive thrombophlebitis, bed rest with the leg elevated will limit the thrombosis and improve symptoms.
- NSAIDs to relieve symptoms
- Treatment of septic thrombophlebitis with antibiotics with adequate coverage of Enterobacteriaceae and *Staphylococcus*. Initial empirical treatment with a semisynthetic penicillin plus either an aminoglycoside or a third-generation cephalosporin or a quinolone
- Ligation and division of the superficial vein at the junction to avoid propagation of the clot in the deep venous system when the thrombophlebitis progresses toward the junction of the involved superficial vein with deep veins
- The role of antifungal therapy for superficial suppurative thrombophlebitis due to *C. albicans* is controversial. Most of these infections can be cured by vein excision. Because of the propensity of these infections for hematogenous spread, a 10- to 14-day course of amphotericin B or fluconazole is advisable.

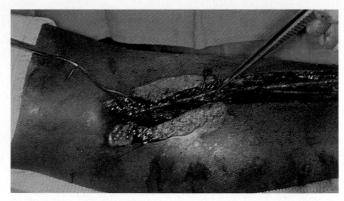

Fig 339–2
Vein resection for suppurative thrombophlebitis.
(From Cohen J, Powderly WG: Infectious Diseases, 2nd ed. St Louis, Mosby, 2004.)

Chapter 340 Leprosy

DEFINITION
Leprosy is a chronic granulomatous infection of humans that primarily affects the skin and peripheral nerves.

PHYSICAL FINDINGS AND CLINICAL PRESENTATION
- Skin lesion: most common initial presentation
- Sensory loss
- Anhidrosis
- Neuritic pain
- Palpable peripheral nerves
- Nerve damage (most commonly affected nerves are ulnar, median, common peroneal, posterior tibial, radial cutaneous nerve of the wrist, facial, and posterior auricular)
- Muscle atrophy and weakness
- Foot drop
- Claw hand and claw toes
- Lagophthalmos, nasal septal perforation, collapse of bridge of nose, loss of eyebrows resulting in **"leonine" facies** (Fig. 340–1)

Leprosy can present along a spectrum from simple cutaneous skin lesions with minimal sensory loss to severe extensive skin involvement (Fig. 340–2), painful neuritis, muscle wasting and contractures, and multiple peripheral nerve damage.

CAUSE
- Leprosy is caused by *Mycobacterium leprae,* an obligate intracellular acid-fast rod.
- The mode of transmission remains elusive. Spread in humans is thought to occur via the respiratory route or entry through broken skin.
- Zoonotic transmission from armadillos has not been proved.
- The majority of people exposed to patients with leprosy do not develop the disease because of their natural immunity.
- Incubation period is 3 to 5 years.

DIAGNOSIS
- The diagnosis of leprosy relies on a detailed history and physical examination and is established by the demonstration of acid-fast bacilli in skin smears or skin biopsies of the affected sites.
- Leprosy has been classified according to the World Health Organization (WHO) system into:
  1. Paucibacillary leprosy defined as fewer than five skin lesions with no bacilli on skin smear
  2. Multibacillary leprosy defined as six or more skin lesions and may be skin-smear positive
- Leprosy has also been classified more specifically according to the type of skin lesions, sensory and motor deficits, and biopsy into:
  1. Indeterminate leprosy
  2. Tuberculoid leprosy (Fig. 340–3) (paucibacillary [few organisms], intense inflammatory reaction; few, well-demarcated skin lesions)
  3. Borderline tuberculoid leprosy (Fig. 340–4)
  4. Borderline lepromatous leprosy
  5. Lepromatous leprosy (Fig. 340–5) (multibacillary [numerous organisms], inadequate host response; diffuse, poorly organized skin lesions)

DIFFERENTIAL DIAGNOSIS
The differential diagnosis of leprosy includes: sarcoidosis, rheumatoid arthritis, systemic lupus erythematosus, lymphomatoid granulomatosis, carpal tunnel syndrome, cutaneous leishmaniasis, fungal infections and other causes of hypopigmented, hyperpigmented, and erythematous skin lesions.

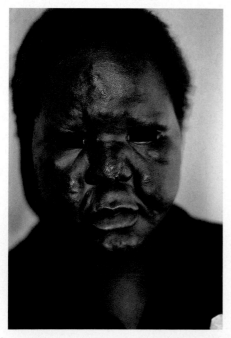

Fig 340–1
Lepromatous leprosy: note the symmetry and characteristic loss of the eyebrows.
(Courtesy of N. C. Dlova, MD, Nelson R. Mandela School of Medicine, University of Kwa Zulu-Natal, South Africa.)

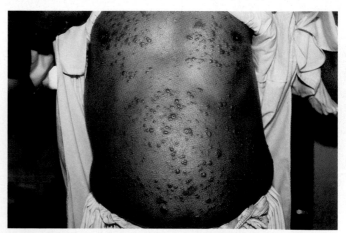

Fig 340–2
Histoid leprosy: these numerous brown papules and nodules may be histologically mistaken for a "fibrohistiocytic" tumor if the clinical information is not available.
(Courtesy of S. Lucas, MD, St Thomas' Hospital, London, UK.)

LABORATORY TESTS

- *Mycobacterium leprae* cannot be cultured on artificial media. The bacteria rapidly proliferate when injected into the footpads of mice or into armadillos and sometimes is used for drug-sensitivity testing.
- Serologic tests, including the antibody to phenolic glyco-lipid 1 (PGL-1), are available and used for diagnostic confirmation and research epidemiologic studies.
- Lepromin intradermal skin test is not diagnostic and not for commercial use.
- Skin smears are taken from active sites or most commonly from the earlobes, elbows, or knees and are stained for acid-fast bacilli.
- Skin biopsies of active sites are stained for acid-fast bacilli (Fig. 340–6).
- Peripheral nerve biopsy can be done in patients with sensory loss and no skin lesions. Common nerves biopsied are the radial cutaneous nerve of the wrist and the sural nerve of the ankle.

TREATMENT

For paucibacillary leprosy:
- Dapsone in an unsupervised setting is the treatment of choice.
- Rifampin in a supervised setting is the recommendation by WHO.
- Ofloxacin or minocycline is another alternative.
  For multibacillary leprosy:
- Rifampin and clofazimine in a supervised setting. Rifampin can be given once monthly without loss of efficacy and at less cost.
- Rifampin and clofazimine in an unsupervised setting.
- Dapsone is sometimes added as triple therapy in this group of patients.
- Clofazimine is usually used in combination with dapsone for better bacteriocidal effect.

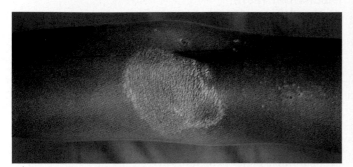

Fig 340–3
Tuberculoid leprosy. Single hypopigmented anesthetic plaque with raised border and dry surface.
(From Cohen J, Powderly WG: Infectious Diseases, 2nd ed. St Louis, Mosby, 2004.)

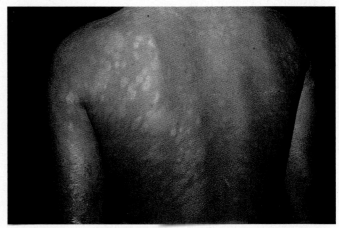

Fig 340–5
Lepromatous leprosy. Multiple, small, slightly erythematous macules with intact sensation and symmetric distribution. The skin smears of both the lesions and intervening skin are positive for acid-fast bacilli.
(From Cohen J, Powderly WG: Infectious Diseases, 2nd ed. St Louis, Mosby, 2004.)

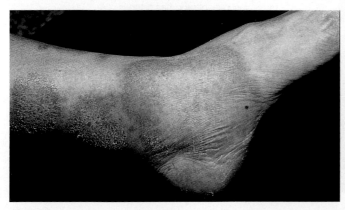

Fig 340–4
Borderline tuberculoid leprosy. Three large well-defined erythematous patches with reduced sensation, spreading borders, and satellite lesion.
(From Cohen J, Powderly WG: Infectious Diseases, 2nd ed. St Louis, Mosby, 2004.)

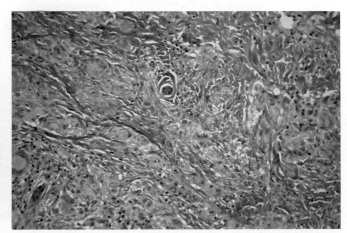

Fig 340–6
Cutaneous leprosy. The dermis is infiltrated with epithelioid macrophages organized into confluent granulomas. Small numbers of acid-fast bacilli are present (HANDE, ×200).
(From Silverberg SG: Principles and Practice of Surgical Pathology and Cytopathology, 4th ed. Philadelphia, Churchill Livingstone, 2006.)

Chapter 341 | **Tetanus**

DEFINITION
Tetanus is a life-threatening illness manifested by muscle rigidity and spasms; it is caused by a neurotoxin (tetanospasmin) produced by *Clostridium tetani*.

PHYSICAL FINDINGS AND CLINICAL PRESENTATION
- Trismus ("lockjaw")
- *Risus sardonicus* ("peculiar grin"), characteristic grimace that results from contraction of the facial muscles (Fig. 341–1)
- Generalized muscle spasms causing severe pain and, at times, respiratory compromise and death
- Rigid abdominal muscles, flexed arms, and extended legs
- Autonomic dysfunction several days after onset of illness
- Leading cause of death: fluctuations in heart rate and blood pressure
- Usually, absence of fever
- Localized tetanus
  1. Rigidity of muscles near the injury
  2. Weakness as a result of lower motor neuron injury
  3. May be self-limited and resolve spontaneously
  4. More often progresses to generalized tetanus
  5. Cephalic tetanus:
     a. May occur with head injuries or chronic otitis with localized ear or mastoid infection with *C. tetani*
     b. Can manifest as cranial nerve dysfunction

CAUSE
- *C. tetani* is a gram-positive, spore-forming bacillus that resides primarily in the soil.
- Majority of cases are caused by punctures and lacerations.
- Toxin is elaborated from organisms in a contaminated wound.

- Local symptoms are caused by inhibition of neurotransmitter at presynaptic sites.
  1. Over the next 2 to 14 days, the toxin travels up the neurons to the CNS, where it acts on inhibitory neurons to prevent neurotransmitter release.
  2. Unopposed motor activity results in tonic contractions of muscles.

DIFFERENTIAL DIAGNOSIS
- Strychnine poisoning
- Dystonic reaction caused by neuroleptic agents
- Local infection (dental or masseter muscle) causing trismus
- Severe hypocalcemia
- Hysteria

WORKUP
- Positive wound culture is not helpful in diagnosis.
- Isolation of organism is possible in patients without the illness.

LABORATORY TESTS
- Usually, normal blood counts and chemistries
- Toxicology of serum and urine to rule out strychnine poisoning

TREATMENT
- Monitoring in a hospital ICU: keep surroundings dark and quiet
- Intubation or tracheostomy for severe laryngospasm
- Débridement of wound
- Human tetanus immunoglobulin (HTIg) via IM injection
- Tetanus toxoid (Td) by IM injection at a different site
- Metronidazole or penicillin G IV
- IV diazepam to control muscle spasms
- Neuromuscular blockade if necessary

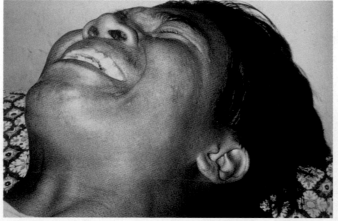

Fig 341–1
Facial spasm and *risus sardonicus* in a Filipino patient who has tetanus. (From Cohen J, Powderly WG: Infectious Diseases, 2nd ed. St Louis, Mosby, 2004.)

Chapter 342 Anaerobic infections

DEFINITION

An anaerobic infection is caused by one of a group of bacteria that require a reduced oxygen tension for growth.

PHYSICAL FINDINGS AND CLINICAL PRESENTATION

- May occur at any site, but most are anatomically related to mucosal surfaces
- Table 342–1 describes clinical signs of anaerobic infection.
- Should be suspected when there is foul-smelling tissue, soft tissue gas, necrotic tissue, or abscesses
- Head and neck
  1. Odontogenic infections from dental or soft tissue possibly progressing to periapical abscesses, at times extending to bone
  2. Both anaerobic and aerobic pathogens in chronic sinusitis, chronic mastoiditis, and chronic otitis media
  3. Peritonsillar abscess possible
  4. Complications: deep neck space infections, brain abscesses, mediastinitis
- Pleuropulmonary
  1. May involve anaerobes present in the oropharynx
  2. Aspiration more common in persons with altered mental status or seizures
  3. Anaerobic bacteria more likely in those with gingivitis or periodontitis
  4. Manifestations: necrotizing pneumonia, empyema, lung abscess
- Intra-abdominal
  1. Disruption of intestinal integrity leading to infection involving anaerobic bacteria
  2. Bacteria from colonic neoplasm, perforated appendicitis, diverticulitis, or bowel surgery, causing bacteremia, peritonitis, at times intra-abdominal abscesses
  3. Resulting infections usually mixed, containing both anaerobes and aerobes

- Female genital tract
  1. Anaerobes in bacterial vaginosis, salpingitis, endometritis, pelvic abscesses, septic abortion; infections tend to be mixed
  2. Possible pelvic thrombophlebitis when resolving pelvic infection is accompanied by new or persistent fever
- Other anaerobic infections
  1. Skin and soft tissue infection at any site (Fig. 342–1)
  2. More commonly associated infections: synergistic gangrene, bite wound infections, infected decubitus ulcers
  3. Clinical significance of anaerobes in diabetic foot infections unclear
  4. Anaerobic bacteremia uncommon with source usually intra-abdominal, followed by female genital tract, pleuropulmonary, and head and neck infections
  5. Osteomyelitis especially when associated with decubitus ulcers or vascular insufficiency
  6. Facial bone osteomyelitis from adjacent infections of the teeth or sinuses

CAUSE

- Most commonly endogenous, arising from bacteria that normally line mucosal surfaces
- Disruption of mucosal barriers resulting from various conditions (trauma, ischemia, surgery, perforation), with infection occurring when organisms gain access to normally sterile sites, causing tissue destruction and abscess formation
- Synergy between different anaerobes or between anaerobes and aerobes important
- Most commonly involved: gram-negative anaerobic bacilli

TABLE 342–1 Clinical signs of anaerobic infection

- Infection adjacent to a mucosal surface
- Foul-smelling discharge
- Necrotic gangrenous tissue and abscess formation
- Free gas in tissue
- Bacteremia or endocarditis with no growth on aerobic blood cultures
- Infection related to the use of antibiotics effective against aerobes only
- Infection related to tumors or other destructive processes
- Infected thrombophlebitis
- Infection after bites
- Black discoloration of exudates containing Batleroides melaninogenicus, which may fluoresce under ultraviolet light
- "Sulfur granules" in discharges caused by actinomycosis
- Clinical presentation of gas gangrene
- Clinical condition predisposing to anaerobic infection (after maternal amnionitis, perforation of bowel, etc.)

From Cohen J, Powderly WG: Infectious Diseases, 2nd ed. St Louis, Mosby, 2004.

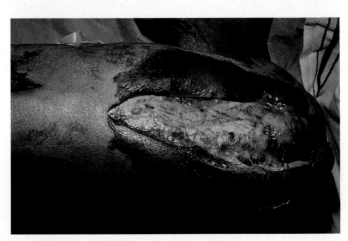

Fig 342–1
Spontaneous necrotizing fasciitis due to *Clostridium septicum*. This patient developed the sudden onset of severe pain in the forearm. Swelling rapidly ensued and he sought medical treatment. Crepitus was present on physical examination, and gas in the soft tissue was verified with routine radiographs. Immediate surgical débridement revealed necrotizing fasciitis but sparing of the muscle. Note the purple-violaceous appearance of the skin.
(From Cohen J, Powderly WG: Infectious Diseases, 2nd ed. St Louis, Mosby, 2004.)

DIFFERENTIAL DIAGNOSIS

- Primary differential possibility is an aerobic bacterial infection without the presence of anaerobic bacteria.
- Ischemic necrosis without accompanying anaerobic infection (or "dry" gangrene [noninfected necrosis] versus "wet" gangrene [infected tissue with anaerobic infection])

WORKUP

- Specimens submitted for culture processed within 30 minutes.
- Large volume of material more likely to have significant growth; swabs less efficient for transporting infected material
- Blood cultures (Fig. 342–2)—preferably before antibiotic administration

LABORATORY TESTS

- Elevated WBC count, with extremely high WBC counts sometimes seen with pseudomembranous colitis
- Positive stool *C. difficile* toxin assay
- Increased lactate levels in ischemia or perforation
- Possible positive blood or wound cultures, but failure to grow anaerobes in culture may be common, attributed to inadequate culturing techniques or fastidious organisms

IMAGING STUDIES

- Plain film of an affected area to show gas in tissues, free air resulting from a perforated viscus, or an air/fluid level inside an abscess
- Ultrasound, CT scan, or MRI to reveal abscesses or tissue destruction

TREATMENT

- Removal of necrotic tissue (Fig. 342–3)
- Drainage of abscesses (accomplished by CT scan–guided percutaneous drainage)

Oral antibiotics with anaerobic activity: clindamycin, metronidazole, and chloramphenicol

- Broader spectrum of activity with amoxicillin/clavulanate
- Penicillin VK in odontogenic infections
- Oral metronidazole for *C. difficile*–associated diarrhea, with oral vancomycin reserved for recurrent or recalcitrant infections

Parenteral antibiotics for more serious illness

- IV clindamycin, metronidazole, and chloramphenicol
- Cephalosporins (anaerobic or mixed infections): cefoxitin and cefotetan
- Extended-spectrum penicillins (e.g., piperacillin) and combination beta-lactamase plus beta-lactamase inhibitor drugs (e.g., clavulanic acid, sulbactam, tazobactam)
  1. Significant anaerobic activity, plus varying degrees of broad-spectrum coverage
  2. Include ampicillin/sulbactam, ticarcillin/clavulanate, and piperacillin/ tazobactam
- Imipenem or other carbapenem such as meropenem or ertapenem: broad-spectrum agents with extensive anaerobic activity

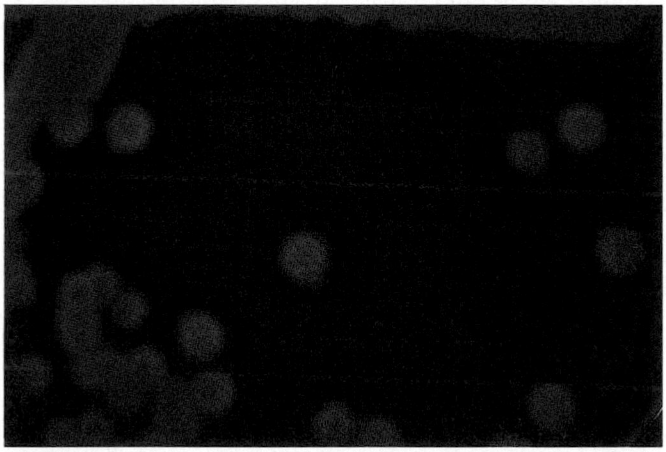

Fig 342–2
Colonies of *Clostridium perfringens* growing on an anaerobic blood agar plate. Theta toxin causes the clear zone of hemolysis closest to the colony. A second area of partial hemolysis is caused by a-toxin, an enzyme with phospholipase C activity.
(From Cohen J, Powderly WG: Infectious Diseases, 2nd ed. St Louis, Mosby, 2004.)

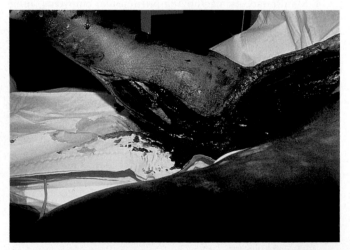

Fig 342–3
Extensive gas gangrene of the arm due to *Clostridium perfringens*. A 35-year-old man sustained a knife wound to the forearm. He did not seek medical care, but 36 hours later experienced severe pain in the upper arm and came to the emergency department. There was extreme tenderness of the arm, and crepitus was easily demonstrated. A radiograph also demonstrated gas in the deep soft tissues. Surgical débridement and antibiotics were instituted, but later amputation at the level of the shoulder was necessary. A pure culture of *C. perfringens* was grown from the deep tissues.
(From Cohen J, Powderly WG: Infectious Diseases, 2nd ed. St Louis, Mosby, 2004.)

Chapter 343 | Diphtheria

DEFINITION
Diphtheria is an infection of the mucous membranes or skin caused by *Coryne bacterium diphtheriae*.

PHYSICAL FINDINGS AND CLINICAL PRESENTATION
RESPIRATORY DIPHTHERIA:
- Commonly presenting as pharyngitis, but any part of the respiratory tract may be involved, including the nasopharynx, larynx, trachea, or bronchi
- Areas of gray or white exudate (Fig. 343–1) coalescing to form a "pseudomembrane" that bleeds when removed
- Possible fever and dysphagia
- Complications: respiratory tract obstruction and pneumonia
- Systemic effects of the toxin: myocarditis and polyneuritis (frequently involving a bulbar distribution)
- Occurs mostly in nonimmune individuals; usually milder and less likely to be complicated in those adequately immunized

CUTANEOUS DIPHTHERIA:
- Usually complicates existing skin lesion (i.e., impetigo or scabies). Typically it has a rolled "crater-like" edge and eschar (Fig. 343–2)

CAUSE
- Caused by *C. diphtheriae*, an aerobic, gram-positive rod
- Transmitted by close contact through droplets of nasopharyngeal secretions
- Symptomatic disease of the respiratory system caused by toxin-producing strains (tox+)
- Systemic effects of toxin: ranging from nausea and vomiting to polyneuropathy, myocarditis, and vascular collapse

- Presence of strains not producing toxin (tox+) in the respiratory tract of asymptomatic carriers and in skin lesions of cutaneous diphtheria

DIFFERENTIAL DIAGNOSIS
- Streptococcus pharyngitis
- Viral pharyngitis
- Mononucleosis

WORKUP
- Presence of a pseudomembrane in the oropharynx suggestive of diagnosis (not always present)
- Gram stains of secretions to show club-shaped organisms, which appear as "Chinese letters" (Fig. 343–3)
- Nasolaryngoscopy to identify lesions in the nares, nasopharynx, larynx, or tracheobronchial tree

LABORATORY TESTS
- Cultures of mucosal lesions or of nasal discharge
  1. Positive culture for *C. diphtheriae* confirms the diagnosis.
  2. Laboratory is notified of the suspected diagnosis so that appropriate culture medium (Tinsdale agar) is used.
- Testing of all isolated organisms for toxin production

IMAGING STUDIES
- Chest x-ray to rule out pneumonia

TREATMENT
- Intubation or tracheostomy if signs of respiratory distress occur
- Nasogastric or parenteral nutrition in those with bulbar signs
- ICU monitoring for patients with signs of systemic toxicity
- Cardiac pacing in patients with heart block
- Respiratory isolation

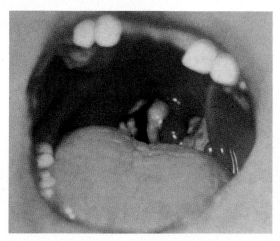

Fig 343–1
Characteristic diphtheria pseudomembrane in a child.
(Courtesy of Dr. Norman Begg.)

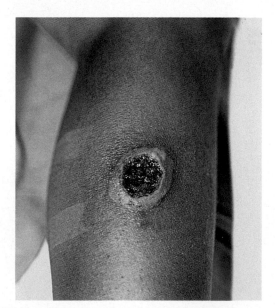

Fig 343–2
Characteristic diphtheria lesion of the lower limb, showing the classic rolled, "crater-like" edge and eschar.
(From Cohen J, Powderly WG: Infectious Diseases, 2nd ed. St Louis, Mosby, 2004.)

- Administration of diphtheria antitoxin once a clinical diagnosis is made
- If tests for hypersensitivity to horse serum are negative: 50,000 U given for mild to moderate disease or 60,000 to 120,000 U for critically ill patients
- IV infusion of antitoxin
- Serum sickness in 10% of treated individuals; those with hypersensitivity to horse serum should be desensitized before administration of antitoxin
- Antibiotics to eradicate the organism in carriers or patients
- For respiratory diphtheria:
  1. Erythromycin PO or IV (clarithromycin and azithromycin are acceptable alternatives) or IM penicillin
  2. Carriers or patients with cutaneous disease: erythromycin or rifampin

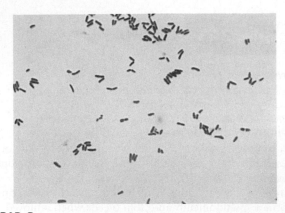

Fig 343-3
Chinese letter and picket-fence appearance of *Corynebacterium* spp. on Gram-stained smears.
(From Cohen J, Powderly WG: Infectious Diseases, 2nd ed. St Louis, Mosby, 2004.)

Chapter 344 Listeriosis

DEFINITION
Listeriosis is a systemic infection caused by the gram-positive aerobic bacterium *Listeria monocytogenes.*

PHYSICAL FINDINGS AND CLINICAL PRESENTATION
- Infections in pregnancy
  1. More common in third trimester
  2. Usually present with fever and chills without localizing symptoms or signs of infection
- Meningoencephalitis
  1. More common in neonates and immunocompromised patients, but up to 30% of adults have no underlying condition
  2. In neonates: poor appetite with or without fever possibly the only presenting signs
  3. In adults: presentation often subacute, with low-grade fever and personality change as only signs
  4. Focal neurologic signs seen without demonstrable brain abscess on CT scan
- Cerebritis/rhombencephalitis:
  1. Headache and fever may be only presenting complaints
  2. Progressive cranial nerve palsies, hemiparesis, seizures, depressed level of consciousness, cerebellar signs, respiratory insufficiency may also be seen
- Focal infections
  1. Ocular infections (purulent conjunctivitis) and skin lesions (granulomatosis infantisepticum) (Fig. 344–1) as a result of inadvertent inoculation by laboratory and veterinary personnel
  2. Others: arthritis, prosthetic joint infections, peritonitis, osteomyelitis, organ abscesses, cholecystitis

CAUSE
- Direct invasion of the skin and eyes has been documented, but mechanism of GI entry is unclear.
- Organism's intracellular life cycle explanatory of:
  1. Importance of cell-mediated immunity in host defense
  2. Increased incidence of infection in neonates, pregnant women, and immunocompromised hosts

DIFFERENTIAL DIAGNOSIS
- Meningitis caused by other bacteria, mycobacteria, or fungi
- CNS sarcoidosis
- Brain neoplasm or abscess
- Tuberculous and fungal (especially cryptococcal) meningitis
- Cerebral toxoplasmosis
- Lyme disease
- Sarcoidosis

LABORATORY TESTS
- Cultures of blood and other appropriate body fluids
- Variable CSF findings, but neutrophils usually predominate
- Organisms uncommonly seen on Gram stain (Fig. 344–2) and may be difficult to identify morphologically
- Monoclonal antibodies, PCR, and DNA probe techniques to detect *Listeria* in foods

IMAGING STUDIES
- If focal cerebral involvement suspected: CT scan or MRI
- MRI most sensitive for evaluation of brainstem and cerebellum

TREATMENT
- Drugs of choice: IV ampicillin
- Alternative: trimethoprim/sulfamethoxazole
- Gentamicin added to provide synergy

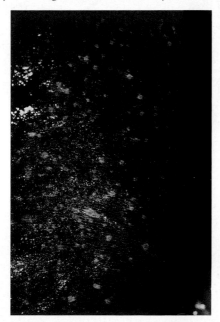

Fig 344–1
Skin rash on premature infant who has sepsis due to *Listeria monocytogenes*. This form of infection, known as granulomatosis infantisepticum, is characterized by disseminated microabscesses on the skin, spleen, and liver. The elevated pale patches (1 to 2 mm in diameter) on the skin are clearly seen in contrast to the bright erythema of surrounding skin.
(From Cohen J, Powderly WG: Infectious Diseases, 2nd ed. St Louis, Mosby, 2004.)

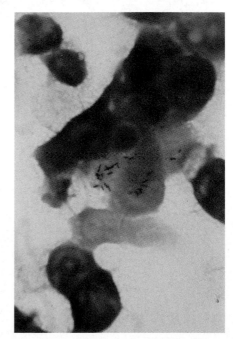

Fig 344–2
Gram stain of clinical specimen showing intra- and extracellular Gram-positive bacilli.
(From Cohen J, Powderly WG: Infectious Diseases, 2nd ed. St Louis, Mosby, 2004.)

Chapter 345   *Yersinia pestis (plague)*

DEFINITION
Zoonosis caused by the Gram-negative bacterium *Yersinia pestis*, which is among the most pathogenic bacteria known. Figure 345–1 describes the transmission cycles of *Y. pestis*.

CLINICAL FEATURES
- Bubonic plague has an incubation period of 2 to 6 days.
- Manifestations include fever, chills, myalgias, arthralgias, headache, and lethargy.
- Within 24 hours, tenderness and pain occur in one or more regional lymph nodes proximal to the site of inoculation of the plague bacillus.
- The femoral and inguinal lymph nodes are most commonly involved.

- The enlarging bubo or buboes become progressively swollen and tender.
- The surrounding tissue becomes erythematous and edematous.
- The bubo of plague differs from lymphadenitis of most other causes by its rapid onset, extreme tenderness, surrounding edema, accompanying signs of toxemia and absence of cellulites or obvious ascending lymphangitis.
- Cough, sputum production, increasing chest pain and dyspnea are suggestive of pneumonic plague. Chest x-ray may reveal extensive infiltrates (Fig. 345–2).
- Septic plague is usually fuminant and fatal.

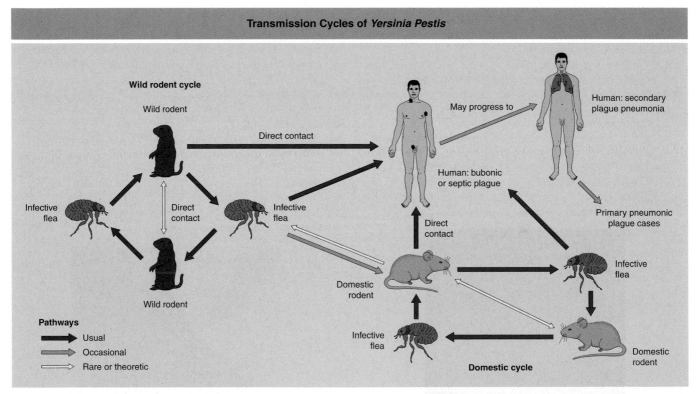

Transmission Cycles of *Yersinia Pestis*

Fig 345–1
Transmission cycles of Yersinia pestis
(From Cohen J, Powderly WG: Infectious Diseases, 2nd ed. St Louis, Mosby, 2004.)

DIAGNOSIS
- Blood and sputum cultures, cultures, and Gram stain from aspirates.
- PCR or ELISA is useful for presumptive identification.
- An immunogold dipstick assay to rapidly detect *Y. pestis* antigens is also available.

TREATMENT
- Antibiotics (streptomycin, gentamicin, tetracycline, doxycycline)

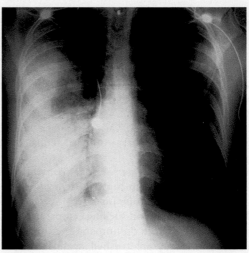

Fig 345-2
Chest radiograph of a patient who has primary plague pneumonia, showing extensive infiltrates in the right middle and lower lung fields. (From Cohen J, Powderly WG: Infectious Diseases, 2nd ed. St Louis, Mosby, 2004.)

Chapter 346 Relapsing fever

DEFINITION
Tick-borne or louse-borne infections manifesting with repeated abrupt episodes of fever, separated by afebrile periods

ETIOLOGY
- Tick-borne relapsing fever: various *Borrelia* species spirochetes transmitted by ticks of the genus *Ornithodoros* (Argasidae)
- Louse-borne relapsing fever: *Borellia recurrentis* spirochete transmitted by the human body louse, *Pediculus humanus*, and the head louse, *Pediculus capitus*.
  - These are obligate blood-sucking ectoparasites that ingest borrelias when they feed on humans and then transmit the organism when they are crushed against broken skin or rubbed on a mucous memberane such as the conjunctiva so that the spirochetes enter the person's blood.
  - Unlike ticks, lice cannot infect their progeny. Humans are the only reservoir.

CLINICAL PRESENTATION
- Tick-borne relapsing fever: fever, headache, muscle and joint pain, profuse sweating occurring after an incubation period of 3 to 18 days following a tick bite.
  - Epistaxis, abdominal pain, neurologic signs (cranial palsies, visual complaints, hemiparesis) may follow.
  - Erythematous rash and petichiae may occur.
  - Symptoms abate after few days and recur 7 to 15 days later but tend to be less severe. As many as eight relapses may occur.
- Louse-borne relapsing fever: fever, chills, headaches, and muscle and body aches occur after an incubation period of 4 to 17 days.
  - Jaundice and subconjunctival hemorrhage may occur (Fig. 346–1).

LABORATORY TESTS
- Leucocytosis, thrombocytopenia, elevated liver transaminases.
- Thin blood smear reveals numerous spirochetes (Fig. 346–2).

TREATMENT
- Louse-borne relapsing fever: tetracycline 500 mg single dose
- Tick-borne relapsing fever: doxycycline 100 mg qd × 10 days

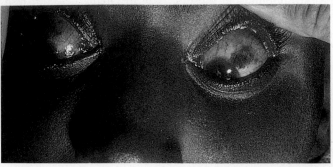

Fig 346–1
Ethiopian patient who has louse-borne relapsing fever 4 days after the start of febrile symptoms, showing subconjunctival hemorrhages and jaundice.
(From Cohen J, Powderly WG: Infectious Diseases, 2nd ed. St Louis, Mosby, 2004.)

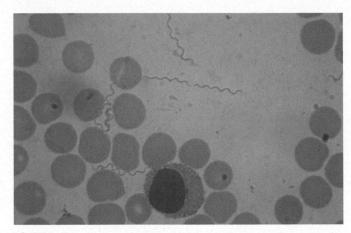

Fig 346–2
Thin blood smear from an Ethiopian patient who has louse-borne relapsing fever (Giemsa stain), showing numerous spirochetes.
(From Cohen J, Powderly WG: Infectious Diseases, 2nd ed. St Louis, Mosby, 2004.)

Chapter 347 Tularemia

DEFINITION

Tularemia is a zoonosis caused by small, facultative gram-negative intracellular coccobacillus *Francisella tularensis*. Clinical manifestations range from asymptomatic illness to septic shock and death. Figure 347–1 describes the clinical types of tularemia.

PHYSICAL FINDINGS AND CLINICAL PRESENTATION

Physical Findings

- Incubation period is 3 to 5 days but may range from 1 to 21 days.
- Most common initial signs and symptoms:
  1. Fever
  2. Chills
  3. Headache
  4. Malaise
  5. Anorexia
  6. Fatigue
  7. Cough
  8. Myalgias
  9. Chest discomfort
  10. Vomiting
  11. Abdominal pain
  12. Diarrhea
  13. Conjunctivitis
  14. Lymphadenitis

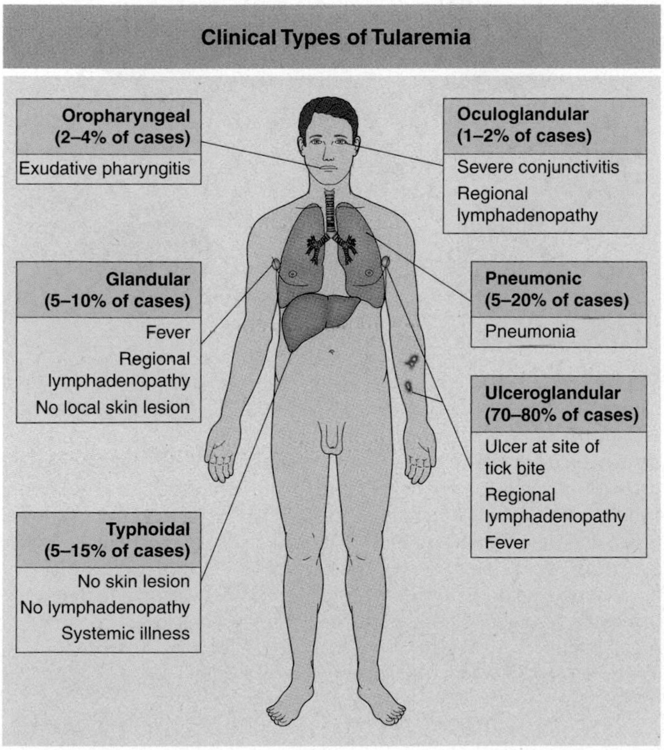

Clinical Presentation

- Ulceroglandular and glandular: account for 75% to 80% of cases. Fever and a single erythematous papuloulcerative lesion with a central eschar (Fig. 347–2) accompanied by tender lymphadenopathy.
- Oculoglandular: accounts for 1% to 2% of cases. Painful inflamed conjunctiva with numerous yellowish nodules and pinpoint ulcers. Purulent conjunctivitis with regional lymphadenopathy (Fig. 347–3). Corneal perforation may occur.
- Oropharyngeal and GI: account for 1% to 4% of cases. Acute exudative membranes pharyngitis associated with cervical lymphadenopathy. Ulcerative intestinal lesion associated with mesenteric lymphadenopathy, diarrhea, abdominal pain, nausea, vomiting, and GI bleeding
- Pulmonary: occurs often in the elderly and has a higher mortality. Symptoms include nonproductive cough, dyspnea, or pleuritic chest pain.
- Typhoidal: 10% of all cases of tularemia. Rare in the United States. Symptoms include high continuous fever, signs of endotoxemia, and severe headache. Mortality can approach 30%.

CAUSE

- Caused by infection with *F. tularensis*.
- Two main biovars of *F. tularensis*: type A and type B. Type A produces severe disease in humans. Type B produces milder subclinical infection.
- Transmitted by ticks, tabanid flies, and mosquitoes. Also acquired by inhalation and ingestion. Figure 347–4 illustrates the life cycles of *Francisella tularensis*.
- Cases also occur after exposure to animals (wild rabbit, squirrels, birds, sheep, beavers, muskrats, and domestic dogs and cats) or animal products.
- Laboratory acquisition is possible.

Clinical Types of Tularemia

Oropharyngeal (2–4% of cases)
Exudative pharyngitis

Oculoglandular (1–2% of cases)
Severe conjunctivitis
Regional lymphadenopathy

Glandular (5–10% of cases)
Fever
Regional lymphadenopathy
No local skin lesion

Pneumonic (5–20% of cases)
Pneumonia

Ulceroglandular (70–80% of cases)
Ulcer at site of tick bite
Regional lymphadenopathy
Fever

Typhoidal (5–15% of cases)
No skin lesion
No lymphadenopathy
Systemic illness

Fig 347–1
Clinical types of tularemia.
(From Cohen J, Powderly WG: Infectious Diseases, 2nd ed. St Louis, Mosby, 2004.)

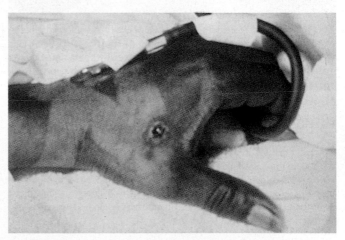

Fig 347–2
Tularemic ulcer with eschar formation after percutaneous inoculation of *Francisella tularensis*.
(From Cohen J, Powderly WG: Infectious Diseases, 2nd ed. St Louis, Mosby, 2004.)

- Pathogenesis: after inoculation into the skin, the organism multiplies locally within 2 to 5 days; then it produces an erythematous tender or pruritic papule. The papule rapidly enlarges and forms an ulcer with a black base. The bacteria spread to the regional lymph nodes producing lymphadenopathy, and with bacteremia may spread to distant organs.

DIFFERENTIAL DIAGNOSIS
- Rickettsial infections
- Meningococcal infections
- Cat scratch disease
- Infectious mononucleosis
- Atypical pneumonia
- Group A streptococcal pharyngitis
- Typhoid fever
- Fungal infection—sporotrichosis
- Anthrax
- Plague
- Bacterial skin infections

LABORATORY TESTS
- WBC count and ESR normal or elevated.
- Rarely seen on Gram-stained smears or tissue biopsy samples.
- Antibodies to *F. tularensis* demonstrated by tube agglutination, microagglutination, heme agglutination, and ELISA; definitive serologic diagnosis requires a fourfold or greater rise in titer between acute and convalescent specimens.
- PCR to facilitate early diagnosis

IMAGING STUDIES
Chest x-ray to show bilateral patchy infiltrate, lobar parenchymal infiltrate, cavitary lesion, pleural effusion, or emphysema

TREATMENT
- Streptomycin or gentamicin
- Tetracycline or doxycycline or chloramphenicol
- Quinolones offer new options for the treatment of tularemia.
- Combination antibiotics required for tularemic meningitis—chloramphenicol plus streptomycin

Surgical therapies are limited to drainage of abscessed lymph nodes and chest tube drainage of empyemas.

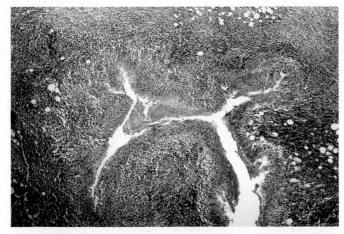

Fig 347–3
Oculoglandular tularemia. A large geographic granuloma with prominent palisading of epithelioid histiocytes and central necrosis occupies a cervical lymph node. The patient had inoculated her eye when she squashed an engorged tick, after which she developed conjunctivitis followed by lymphadenopathy. Tularemia titers were positive and she responded to antibiotic therapy (HANDE, ×15).
(From Silverberg SG: Principles and Practice of Surgical Pathology and Cytopathology, 4th ed. Philadelphia, Churchill Livingstone, 2006.)

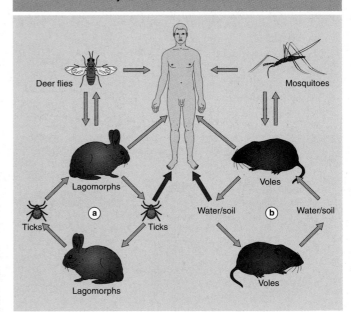

Life Cycles of *Francisella Tularensis*

Fig 347–4
Life cycles of *Francisella tularensis*. The two major life cycles in nature are shown. In cycle (a), which is dominant in North America, *F. tularensis* is maintained predominantly among lagomorphs and hard ticks. In cycle (b), which is dominant in Eurasia, *F. tularensis* is principally maintained among cricetine rodents, especially field voles and mice, water voles, and other aquatic rodents. Humans are incidental hosts that are infected by tick vectors and by the bites of flies or mosquitoes that have contaminated mouthparts, by direct contact with infected animal carcasses or other contaminated materials, by ingestion of contaminated matter, or by inhalation of infectious aerosols or dusts.
(From Cohen J, Powderly WG: Infectious Diseases, 2nd ed. St Louis, Mosby, 2004.)

Chapter 348 | Brucellosis

DEFINITION

Brucellosis is a zoonotic infection caused by one of four species of *Brucella*. It commonly presents as a nondescript febrile illness. Figure 348–1 illustrates clinical manifestations of brucellosis.

PHYSICAL FINDINGS AND CLINICAL PRESENTATION

- Incubation period is 1 weeks to 3 months.
- Patients may be asymptomatic or have nonspecific symptoms such as fever, sweats, malaise, weight loss, depression, arthralgia, and arthritis.
- Fever is the most common finding.
- Hepatomegaly, splenomegaly, or lymphadenopathy is possible.
- Localized disease includes endocarditis, meningitis, spondylitis, sacroiliitis, and osteomyelitis (especially vertebral). Chronic hepatosplenic suppurative brucellosis (CHSB) presents with hepatic or splenic abscesses. This form is thought to be a reactivation and can occur years after the acute infection.

CAUSE

- Caused by infection with *Brucella* species:
  1. Most commonly *B. melitensis*, but also *suis, abortus,* or *canis*
  2. A small, gram-negative coccobacillus

- Acquired through ingestion of organisms (unpasteurized goat or cow's milk), via breaks in the skin, or by inhalation.
- Most cases occur after exposure to animals (sheep, goats, swine, cattle, or dogs) or animal products (i.e., milk, hides, tissue).
- Most cases (in United States) occur in men with occupational exposure to animals (farmers, ranchers, laboratory workers, veterinarians, abattoir workers).

DIFFERENTIAL DIAGNOSIS

Many febrile conditions without localizing manifestations (i.e., TB, endocarditis, typhoid fever, malaria, autoimmune diseases)

WORKUP

- Cultures of blood, bone marrow, or other tissue (lymph node, liver) should be sent and held for 4 weeks, because *Brucella* spp. grow slowly in vitro.
- Granulomas on biopsy (Fig. 348–2) are suggestive of diagnosis.

LABORATORY TESTS

- WBC count: normal or low
- Serology:
  1. Serum agglutination test (SAT) to detect antibodies to *B. abortus, melitensis,* and *suis*
  2. Specific antibody test to identify antibodies to *B. canis*
  3. False-negative SAT possibly resulting from a prozone effect
  4. PCR for *Brucella* spp. specific 16S rRNA or DNA sequences are increasingly used for the diagnosis of brucellosis from blood, tissue samples, and bone marrow.

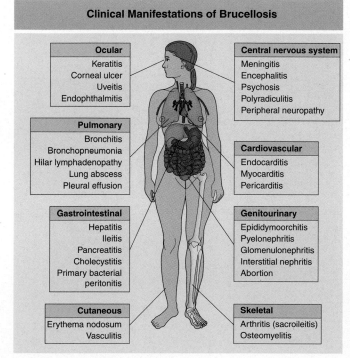

Fig 348–1
Clinical manifestations of brucellosis.
(From Cohen J, Powderly WG: Infectious Diseases, 2nd ed. St Louis, Mosby, 2004.)

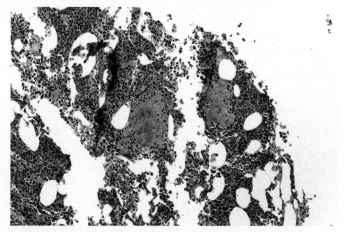

Fig 348–2
Brucellosis. Several small noncaseating granulomas are present in the bone marrow of a patient with an unexplained febrile disease. He was not aware of exposure to *Brucella* in over 30 years (HANDE, ×40, *Brucella suis* isolated from blood cultures).
(From Silverberg SG: Principles and Practice of Surgical Pathology and Cytopathology, 4th ed. Philadelphia, Churchill Livingstone, 2006.)

IMAGING STUDIES

- Radiographs to show splenic or hepatic calcifications in chronic disease
- Bone scan, MRI, and radiographs of the spine (Fig. 348–3) to suggest discitis, spondylitis, or osteomyelitis
- Ultrasound or CT scan of the abdomen to show an enlarged liver or spleen
- Echocardiogram to reveal vegetations in endocarditis

TREATMENT

Combination antibiotics required:

- Doxycycline plus streptomycin
- Drainage of abscesses (Fig. 348–4)
- Valve replacement for endocarditis

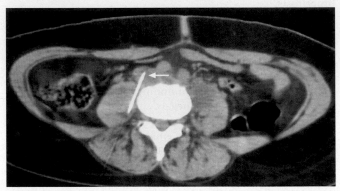

Fig 348–4
CT scan of fine needle aspiration of paraspinal abscess (*arrow*) in a patient with brucellosis.
(From Cohen J, Powderly WG: Infectious Diseases, 2nd ed. St Louis, Mosby, 2004.)

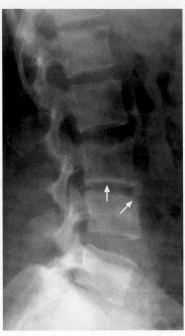

Fig 348–3
Radiograph of the lumbar spine in a patient who has discitis and spondylitis of L3-4 caused by brucellosis. Note the reduced disc space and the destruction of the upper articular margins of L4 (*arrows*).
(From Cohen J, Powderly WG: Infectious Diseases, 2nd ed. St Louis, Mosby, 2004.)

Chapter 349 Cat scratch disease

DEFINITION

Cat scratch disease (CSD) is a syndrome consisting of gradually enlarging regional lymphadenopathy occurring after contact with a feline. Atypical presentations are characterized by a variety of neurologic manifestations as well as granulomatous involvement of the eyes, liver, spleen, and bone. The disease is usually self-limited, and recovery is complete; however, patients with atypical presentations, especially if immunocompromised, may suffer significant morbidity and mortality.

PHYSICAL FINDINGS AND CLINICAL PRESENTATION

- Classic, most common finding: regional lymphadenopathy occurring within 2 weeks of a scratch or contact with felines; usually a new kitten in the household
- Tender, swollen lymph nodes most commonly found in the head and neck, followed by the axillae and the epitrochlear, inguinal, and femoral areas
- Erythematous overlying skin, showing signs of suppuration from involved lymph nodes
- On careful examination; evidence of cutaneous inoculation in the form of a nonpruritic, slightly tender pustule or papule (Fig. 349–1)
- Fever in most patients
- Malaise and headache in fewer than one third of patients
- Atypical presentations in fewer than 15% of cases
  1. Usually in association with lymph-adenopathy and a low-grade or frank fever (>101° F, >38.3° C)
  2. Include granulomatous involvement of the conjunctiva (Parinaud's oculoglandular syndrome) and focal masses in the liver, spleen, and mesenteric nodes
- CNS involvement: neuroretinitis, encephalopathy, encephalitis, transverse myelitis, seizure activity, and coma
- Osteomyelitis in adults and children

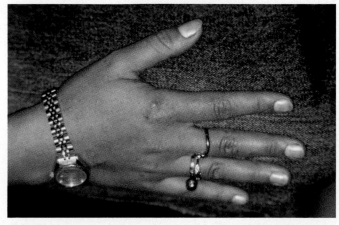

Fig 349–1
Erythematous papule at site of cat scratch. Appearance of erythematous papule at the base of the right index finger after multiple scratches from 1-month-old kitten.
(Courtesy of Ehud Zamir, Hadassah University Hospital, Jerusalem, Israel.)

CAUSE

- Major cause: *Bartonella (Rochalimaea) henselae*
- Mode of transmission: predominantly by direct inoculation through the scratch, bite, or lick of a cat, especially a kitten
- Limited evidence in support of an arthropod (flea) as an alternative vector of infection arising from bacteremic felines
- Rarely, associated with dogs, monkeys, and inanimate objects with which a feline has been in recent contact
- Approximately 2 weeks after introduction of the bacteria into the host, regional lymphatic tissues displaying granulomatous infiltration associated with gradual hypertrophy
- Possible dissemination to distant sites (e.g., liver, spleen, and bone), usually characterized by focal masses or discrete parenchymal lesions

DIFFERENTIAL DIAGNOSIS

Granulomas of this syndrome must be differentiated from those associated with:
- Tularemia
- Tuberculosis or other myobacterial infections
- Brucellosis
- Sarcoidosis
- Sporotrichosis or other fungal diseases
- Toxoplasmosis
- Lymphogranuloma venerum
- Benign and malignant tumors

WORKUP

Diagnosis should be considered in patients who present with a predominant complaint of gradually enlarging regional (focal) lymphadenopathy, often with fever and a recent history of having contact with a cat. A primary ulcer at the site of the cat scratch may or may not be present at the time lymphadenopathy becomes manifest.

LABORATORY TESTS

- Three of four of the following criteria are required:
  1. History of animal contact in the presence of a scratch, dermal, or eye lesion
  2. Culture of lymphatic aspirate that is negative for other causes
  3. Positive CSD skin test
  4. Biopsied lymph node histology consistent with CSD (Fig. 349–2)
- Enhanced culture techniques and serologies will augment establishment of the diagnosis.
- Histopathologically, Warthin-Starry silver stain has been used to identify the bacillus.
- Routine laboratory findings:
  1. Mild leukocytosis or leukopenia
  2. Infrequent eosinophilia
  3. Elevated ESR
- Abnormalities of bilirubin excretion and elevated hepatic transaminases are usually secondary to hepatic obstruction by granuloma, mass, or lymph node.

- In patients with neurologic manifestations, lumbar puncture usually reveals normal CSF, although there may be a mild pleocytosis and modest elevation in protein.
- The diagnosis may be confirmed by specific enzyme immunoassay (EIA) in association with a history of cat contact and a typical clinical presentation.

TREATMENT

- Warm compresses to the affected nodes
- There is no consensus over therapy, especially as the disease is self-limited in a majority of cases.
- It would be prudent to treat severely ill patients, especially if immunocompromised, with antibiotic therapy, because these patients tend to suffer dissemination of infection and increased morbidity.
- *Bartonella* is usually sensitive to aminoglycosides, tetracycline, erythromycin, and the quinolones.
- When the isolate is proved by culture, the patient should receive antibiotic therapy as directed by the obtained sensitivities.
- Antipyretics and NSAIDs may also be used.

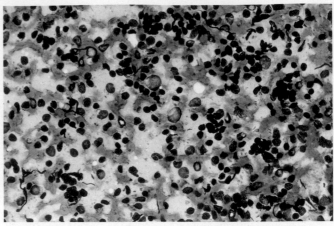

Fig 349–2
Cat scratch disease. Fine needle aspiration of an enlarge lymph node showing evidence of stellate granulomas and abundant acute inflammatory exudates. Clinical correlation along with serologic studies and molecular or immunohistochemical confirmation are required for a definite diagnosis (Diff-Quik, ×600).
(From Silverberg SG: Principles and Practice of Surgical Pathology and Cytopathology, 4th ed. Philadelphia, Churchill Livingstone, 2006.)

Chapter 350 | Leptospirosis

DEFINITION
Leptospirosis (*Weil's disease*) is a zoonosis caused by the spirochete *Leptospira interrogans*.

PHYSICAL FINDINGS AND CLINICAL PRESENTATION
ANICTERIC FORM
- Milder and more common presentation of disease
- A self-limited systemic illness with two stages:
  1. Septicemic stage: presents abruptly with fevers, headache, severe myalgias, rigors, prostration, and sometimes circulatory collapse; conjunctival suffusion is common; skin rash, pharyngitis, lymphadenopathy, hepatomegaly, splenomegaly. Rashes associated with acute spirochetal and rickettsial infections are described in Table 350–1.
  2. Immune stage: occurs a few days after first stage with similar symptoms; hallmark is aseptic meningitis.

ICTERIC LEPTOSPIROSIS (WEIL'S SYNDROME):
  1. Denotes severe cases, with symptoms of hepatic, renal, and vascular dysfunction
  2. Biphasic course: persistence of fever, subconjunctival hemorrhages, jaundice (Fig. 350–1), and azotemia
  3. Complications: oliguria or anuria, hemorrhage, hypotension, vascular collapse

CAUSE
Caused by a spirochete, *L. interrogans*
- Infects a variety of animals, including most mammals
- Specific serotypes associated with different hosts—*pomona* in livestock, *canicola* in dogs, and *icterohaemorrhagiae* in rodents
- Exposure to animal urine or infected water method by which organism penetrates skin or mucous membranes

DIFFERENTIAL DIAGNOSIS
- Bacterial meningitis
- Viral hepatitis
- Influenza
- Legionnaire's disease

WORKUP
Cultures of blood, CSF, and urine:
- Organism can be isolated from blood or CSF during first 10 days of illness.
- Urine should be cultured after first week and for up to 30 days after onset of illness.

LABORATORY TESTS
- Normal or elevated WBCs, at times up to 70,000/mm^3
- Elevated transaminases or bilirubin
- Anemia, azotemia, hypoprothrombinemia in those with icteric illness
- Elevated CK in first phase
- Meningitis in both phases, but aseptic in second phase

IMAGING STUDIES
Chest radiographs to show bilateral nonlobar infiltrates

TREATMENT
- IV penicillin G
- Doxycycline
- Vitamin K administration if hypoprothrombinemia present

TABLE 350–1 Rashes associated with acute spirochetal and rickettsial infections

Agent	Rashes	Comments
Leptospirosis	Hemorrhages Also other rashes	Weil's disease
Borrelia recurrentis (relapsing fever)	Petechiae	Often no rash; sometimes severe hemorrhages
Borrelia burgdorferi (Lyme disease)	Erythema migrans	Sometimes secondary annular or nonspecific rashes
Spirillum minus (rat-bite fever)	Blotchy macular, papular and urticarial rashes, beginning near the bite and spreading	Rashes also in the *Streptobacillus moniliformis* form of rat-bite fever
Rickettsial infections	Macular, papular petechial	Primary eschar (*tache noir*) in some syndromes

From Cohen J, Powderly WG. Infectious Diseases, 2nd ed. St Louis, Mosby, 2004.

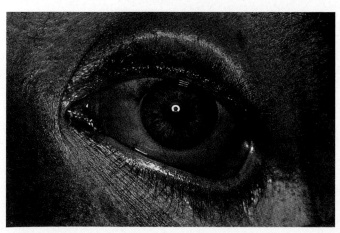

Fig 350–1
Subconjunctival hemorrhages and jaundice in leptospirosis. Asymptomatic or atypical infection probably occurs in 90% of cases and, in some tropical areas, leptospirosis may account for up to 15% of all patients with undiagnosed pyrexia. Although this form can be mild, the infection may develop into a generalized septic form with confusion within 1 to 2 weeks. This is characterized by fever, myalgia, and after subconjunctival hemorrhages. The patient illustrated was in the second week following the onset of symptoms. The most dangerous form (Weil's disease) may be very severe and can involve several organs, with jaundice, renal failure, hemorrhage, vascular collapse, and obtundation.
(From Cohen J, Powderly WG: Infectious Diseases, 2nd ed. St Louis, Mosby, 2004.)

Chapter 351 **Rabies**

DEFINITION

Rabies is a fatal illness caused by the rabies virus and transmitted to humans by the bite of an infected animal.

PHYSICAL FINDINGS AND CLINICAL PRESENTATION

- Incubation period of 10 to 90 days
  1. Shorter with bites of the face
  2. Longer if extremities involved
- Prodrome
  1. Fever
  2. Headache
  3. Malaise
  4. Pain or anesthesia at exposure site
  5. Sore throat
  6. GI symptoms
  7. Psychiatric symptoms
- Acute neurologic period, with objective evidence of CNS involvement
  1. Extreme hyperactivity and bizarre behavior alternating with periods of relative calm
  2. Hallucinations
  3. Disorientation
  4. Seizures
  5. Paralysis may occur
  6. Spasm of the pharynx and larynx, accompanied by severe pain, caused by drinking
  7. Fear elicited by seeing water
  8. Paralysis
  9. Coma
- Possible death from respiratory arrest

CAUSE

- Rabies virus
  - Cases in the United States are associated with bats, raccoons, foxes, and skunks
- In 8 of the 32 cases occurring in the United States since 1980, there was a history of exposure to bats without an actual bite or scratch.
- Imported cases are usually associated with dogs. Figure 351–1 describes the pathogeniesis of rabies.
- Unusual acquisition:
  1. Via organ transplantation
  2. Via aerosol transmission in laboratory workers and spelunkers

DIFFERENTIAL DIAGNOSIS

- Delirium tremens
- Tetanus
- Hysteria
- Psychiatric disorders
- Other viral encephalitides
- Guillain-Barré syndrome
- Poliomyelitis

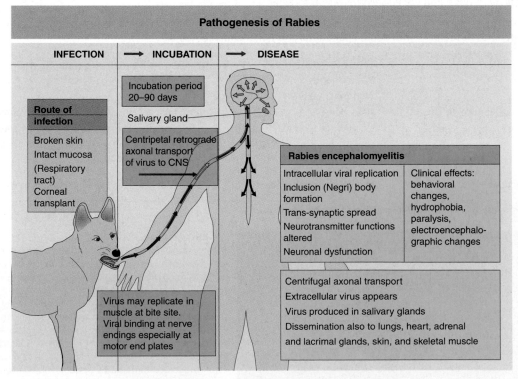

Pathogenesis of Rabies

INFECTION → INCUBATION → DISEASE

Incubation period 20–90 days

Salivary gland

Route of infection

Broken skin

Intact mucosa (Respiratory tract)

Corneal transplant

Centripetal retrograde axonal transport of virus to CNS

Virus may replicate in muscle at bite site. Viral binding at nerve endings especially at motor end plates

Rabies encephalomyelitis

Intracellular viral replication

Inclusion (Negri) body formation

Trans-synaptic spread

Neurotransmitter functions altered

Neuronal dysfunction

Clinical effects: behavioral changes, hydrophobia, paralysis, electroencephalographic changes

Centrifugal axonal transport

Extracellular virus appears

Virus produced in salivary glands

Dissemination also to lungs, heart, adrenal and lacrimal glands, skin, and skeletal muscle

Fig 351–1
Pathogenesis of rabies.
(From Cohen J, Powderly WG: Infectious Diseases, 2nd ed. St Louis, Mosby, 2004.)

WORKUP
- Rabies antibody: serum, CSF
- Viral isolation: saliva, CSF, serum
- Rabies fluorescent antibody: skin biopsy from the hair-covered area of the neck
- Characteristic eosinophilic inclusions (*Negri bodies*) in infected neurons (Fig. 351–2)

TREATMENT
- No known beneficial therapy. A recent report describes a 15-year-old girl who survived rabies and had been treated with a combination of ketamine, midazolam, ribavirin, and amantadine. This therapy seems worth trying despite the fact this is based on a single case report.
- Emphasis placed on prophylaxis of potentially exposed individuals as soon as possible following an exposure:
  1. Thorough wound cleansing
  2. Both active and passive immunization is most effective when used within 72 hours of exposure
- Vaccinations:
  1. Human diploid cell vaccine (HDCV) or rhesus monkey diploid cell vaccine (RVA), 1 mL IM (deltoid) on days 0, 3, 7, 14, and 28
  2. Human rabies hyperimmune globulin (RIG) 20 IU/kg, administered to persons not previously vaccinated. If anatomically feasible, the full dose should be infiltrated around the wounds and any remaining volume should be administered IM at an anatomically distant site from vaccine administration

  Preexposure prophylaxis using HDCV or RVA (1 mL IM days 0, 7, and 21 or 28) in individuals at high risk for acquisition:
  1. Veterinarians
  2. Laboratory workers working with rabies virus
  3. Spelunkers
  4. Visitors to endemic areas

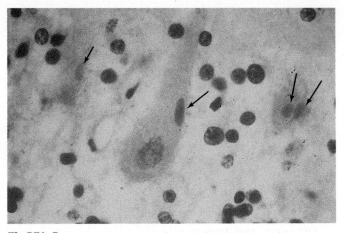

Fig 351–2

Negri bodies in cerebellar Purkinje cells in a human victim of rabies encephalitis. The intracytoplasmic dark-staining Negri bodies are marked with *arrows*.

(Courtesy of the Armed Forces Institute, Bethesda, MD.)

Chapter 352 Toxic shock syndrome

DEFINITION
Toxic shock syndrome (TSS) is an acute febrile illness resulting in multiple organ system dysfunction caused most commonly by a bacterial exotoxin. Disease characteristics also include hypotension, vomiting, myalgia, watery diarrhea, vascular collapse, and an erythematous sunburn-like cutaneous rash that desquamates during recovery.

PHYSICAL FINDINGS AND CLINICAL PRESENTATION
- Fever (≥38.9° C)
- Diffuse macular erythrodermatous rash that desquamates 1 to 2 weeks after disease onset in survivors (Fig. 352–1)
- Orthostatic hypotension
- GI symptoms: vomiting, diarrhea, abdominal tenderness
- Constitutional symptoms: myalgia, headache, photophobia, rigors, altered sensorium, conjunctivitis, arthralgia
- Respiratory symptoms: dysphagia, pharyngeal hyperemia, strawberry tongue
- Genitourinary symptoms: vaginal discharge, vaginal hyperemia, adnexal tenderness
- End-organ failure
- Severe hypotension and acute renal failure
- Hepatic failure
- Cardiovascular symptoms: DIC, pulmonary edema, ARDS, endomyocarditis, heart block

CAUSE
- Menstrually associated TSS: 45% of cases associated with tampons, diaphragm, or vaginal sponge use
- Nonmenstruating associated TSS: 55% of cases associated with puerperal sepsis, post cesarean section endometritis, mastitis, wound or skin infection, insect bite, pelvic inflammatory disease, and postoperative fever

- Causative agent: *S. aureus* infection of a susceptible individual (10% of population lacking sufficient levels of antitoxin antibodies), which liberates the disease mediator TSST-1 (exotoxin)
- Other causative agents: coagulase-negative streptococci producing enterotoxins B or C, and exotoxin A producing group A β-hemolytic streptococci

DIFFERENTIAL DIAGNOSIS
- Staphylococcal food poisoning
- Septic shock
- Scarlet fever
- Rocky Mountain spotted fever
- Meningococcemia
- Toxic epidermal necrolysis
- Kawasaki's syndrome
- Leptospirosis
- Legionnaires' disease
- Hemolytic-uremic syndrome
- Stevens-Johnson syndrome
- Scalded skin syndrome
- Erythema multiforme
- Acute rheumatic fever

WORKUP
Broad-spectrum syndrome with multiorgan system involvement and variable but acute clinical presentation, including the following:
1. Fever ≥38.1° C
2. Classic desquamating (1 to 2 weeks) rash
3. Hypotension/orthostatic SBP 90 or less
4. Syncope
5. Negative throat/CSF cultures

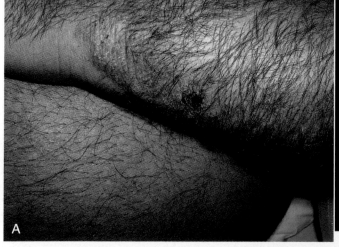
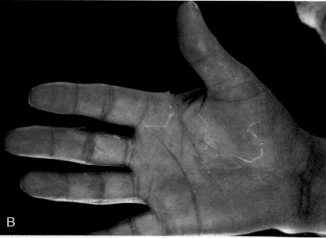

Fig 352–1
Cutaneous changes in toxic shock. (**A**) Localized infection at the edge of a patch of eczema in a patient presenting with staphylococcal toxic shock syndrome. (**B**) Desquamation of the palm following an episode of staphylococcal toxic shock.
(Courtesy of M. Jacobs, London, UK.)

6. Negative serologic test for Rocky Mountain spotted fever, rubeola, and leptospirosis
7. Clinical involvement of three or more of the following:
   a. Cardiopulmonary: ARDS, pulmonary edema, endomyocarditis, second- or third-degree atrioventricular block
   b. CNS: altered sensorium without focal neurologic findings
   c. Hematologic: thrombocytopenia (platelets <100,000)
   d. Liver: elevated LFT results
   e. Renal: >5 WBC/high-power field (HPF), negative urine cultures, azotemia, and increased creatinine double normal
   f. Mucous membrane involvement: vagina, oropharynx, conjunctiva
   g. Musculoskeletal: myalgia, CPK twice normal
   h. GI: vomiting, diarrhea

LABORATORY TESTS
- Pan culture (cervix/vagina, throat, nasal passages, urine, blood, CSF, wound) for *Staphylococcus*, *Streptococcus*, or other pathogenic organisms
- Electrolytes to detect hypokalemia, hyponatremia
- CBC with differential and clotting profile for anemia (normocytic/normochromic), thrombocytopenia, leukocytosis, coagulopathy, and bacteremia
- Chemistry profile to detect decreased protein, increased AST, increased ALT, hypocalcemia, elevated BUN/creatinine, hypophosphatemia, increased LDH, increased CPK
- Urinalysis to detect WBC (>5/HPF), proteinemia, microhematuria
- ABGs to assess respiratory function and acid-base status
- Serologic tests considered for Rocky Mountain spotted fever, rubeola, and leptospirosis

IMAGING STUDIES
- Chest x-ray to evaluate pulmonary edema
- ECG to evaluate arrhythmia
- Sonography/CT scan/MRI considered if pelvic abscess or TOA suspected

TREATMENT
- Aggressive fluid resuscitation (maintenance of circulating volume, CO, systolic blood pressure)
- Thorough search for a localized infection or nidus: incision and drainage, debridement, removal of tampon or vaginal sponge
- Isotonic crystalloid (normal saline solution) for volume replacement
- Electrolyte replacement (K^+, Ca^{2+})
- PRBC/coagulation factor replacement/FFP to treat anemia or D&C
- Vasopressor therapy for hypotension refractory to fluid volume replacement
- Parenteral antibiotic therapy; β-lactamase resistant antibiotic (methicillin, nafcillin, or oxacillin) initiated early

REFERENCES

Bryan CS: Infectious Diseases in Primary Care, Philadelphia, WB Saunders, 2002.

Cohen J, Powderly WG: Infectious Diseases, 2nd ed. St Louis, Mosby, 2004.

Ferri F: Ferri's Clinical Advisor 2007. St Louis, Mosby, 2007.

Ferri F: Practical Guide to the Care of the Medical Patient, 7th ed. St Louis, Mosby, 2007.

Index

Note: Page numbers followed by the letter b refer to boxed material. Those followed by the letter f refer to figures; and those followed by the letter t refer to tables

A

Abdomen, in cirrhosis patients, 616, 617f
Abdominal aortic aneurysm, 470-471, 470f
repair of, 471, 471f
Abdominal distention
assessment of, succussion splash technique in, 620, 620f
mechanical and nonmechanical obstruction in, 578b
Abdominal fat pad biopsy, for amyloidosis, 711, 713f
Abdominal wall veins, dilated, in cirrhosis, 616, 617f
Abdominal-pelvic laparoscopy, 785
ABO-compatible donor blood, selection of, 1060, 1063t
Abortion, 837
recurrent spontaneous, in antiphospholipid antibody syndrome, 965
Abram's needle, for pleural biopsy, 503f
Abrasion, corneal, differential diagnosis of, 263t
Abruptio placentae, 848-849, 848f
Abscess
Bartholin's gland, 776, 779f
brain, 216-219, 216f, 217f, 219f
in endocarditis, 406, 406f
breast, 824, 824f
buccal space, 336, 336f
cranial epidural, 224
liver, 633-635, 633f-635f
amebic, 1165, 1165f
lung, 529-531, 530f, 531f
pancreatic, 610, 611f
perirectal, 606, 606f
renal, 717f
submandibular, 336, 337f
tooth, erythema and edema due to, 337, 337f
vestibular, 336, 336f
Abstinence, as contraceptive method, 789
Acantholytic dermatosis, transient (Grover's disease), 24, 24f
Acantholytic disorder(s), 20f-24f, 21-24. See also specific disorder.
Acanthoma
clear cell, 86, 86f
large cell, 84, 85f, 86
spectacle frame, 84, 85f
Acanthoma fissuratum, 84, 85f
Acanthosis nigricans, 100, 100f
Acarbose, for diabetes mellitus, 920
Accelerated idioventricular rhythm, 434, 434f
Accordion sign, in pseudomembranous colitis, 659, 660f
Acetazolamide, for altitude sickness, 553
Achalasia, 568-569, 568f
Achilles tendon
rupture of, 1024-1025, 1025f
xanthoma of, 923, 925f
Acid-fast bacteria (AFB) stain, 1141, 1141f, 1142f

Acne vulgaris, 72-73, 72f, 73f
classification of, 72
differential diagnosis of, 72
Acoustic neuroma, 311-312, 311f
Acquired ichthyosis, 14, 15f
Acquired immunodeficiency syndrome (AIDS). See Human immunodeficiency virus (HIV) infection.
ACR inhibitors, for chronic renal failure, 699
Acral lentiginous melanoma, 98, 99f
Acral nevus, 93, 94, 94f
Acrochordon, 105, 105f
Acromegaly
clinical presentation of, 859, 861f-863f
differential diagnosis of, 859
medical therapy for, 866
workup for, 861
Acropachy, thyroid, 875, 876f
Actinic (solar) keratosis, 87-88, 88f
Actinic (solar) lentigo, 92, 92f
Actinomycosis, 1203-1204, 1203f
sulfur granules of, 1204, 1204f
Acute bacterial prostatitis, 741, 741t, 742f
treatment of, 742
Acute endocarditis, causes of, 407
Acute febrile neutrophilic dermatosis (Sweet's syndrome), 49-50, 49f, 50f
Acute lymphoblastic leukemia, 1084-1085, 1084f, 1085f
Acute mountain sickness, 552, 552f
Acute myelogenous leukemia, 1085-1087, 1086f, 1087f
Acute renal failure
causes of, 691, 691f, 692t-693t
clinical presentation of, 691, 691f
definition of, 691
imaging studies of, 694, 694f
ischemic
pathologic changes in, 704-705, 704f
phases of, 704
laboratory tests for, 691, 693t, 694
nephrotic, pathologic changes in, 705
treatment of, 694, 695f, 696, 696f
Acute respiratory distress syndrome, 547, 548f
Acute tubular necrosis, 704-705, 704f, 705f
Acyclovir
for chickenpox, 117
for genital herpes, 764
for herpes simplex virus infection, 119
for viral infections, 1157
ADAM 33 gene, in asthma, 485
Adams forward bend test, for scoliosis, 1018, 1018f
Addisonian crisis, 889
Addison's disease, 887, 887f-889f, 889
Adenitis, mesenteric, 658, 658f
Adenocarcinoma
endometrial, 813f
pulmonary, 494
renal cell, 722-723, 723f
Adenoma
parathyroid, 880, 881f
pituitary, 859-866. See also Pituitary adenoma.
Adenoma sebaceum lesions, in tuberous sclerosis, 232, 232f
Adenomatous polyposis, familial, 596, 596f
Adenoviral pharyngitis, 346, 346f
Adenovirus infection, 531
treatment of, 533

Adhesive tape, contact dermatitis due to, 27, 29f
Adjuvant therapy, for colorectal carcinoma, 602
Adrenal hyperplasia, congenital, 903-904, 903f-905f
Adrenocorticotropic hormone (ACTH) syndrome, ectopic, 884, 885f
Adson maneuver, 1014f
Adult renal cystic disease, differential features of, 717t
Age-related cataract, 260
Albendazole
for enterobiasis, 1181
for microsporidiosis, 1158
for trichinosis, 1183
Allergic aspergillosis, 1191
Allergic bronchopulmonary aspergillosis, 1191
Allergic contact dermatitis, 27, 28f
Allergic dermatoconjunctivitis, 267, 267f
Allergic granulomatosis with angiitis (Churg-Strauss syndrome), 56, 58f, 519-520, 520f
Allergic rhinitis, 318-319, 318f, 319f
Allergic vasculitis, 54-55, 54f, 55f
Allopurinol, for uric acid calculi, 736
Alopecia
androgenetic, 67-68, 67f, 68f
syphilitic, 71, 71f
traumatic (trichotillomania), 68, 69f, 70, 70f
Alopecia areata, 68, 68f, 69f
Alpha blockers, for benign prostatic hyperplasia, 740
$Alpha_1$-antitrypsin deficiency, 492, 492f, 493f
5-Alpha-reductase deficiency, in 46,XY males, 772, 773f
5-Alpha-reductase inhibitors, for benign prostatic hyperplasia, 740
Alternating pressure mattress, for decubitus ulcers, 154, 154f
Altitude sickness, 552-553, 552f
Alveolar hemorrhage, in Goodpasture's syndrome, 520, 520f
Alzheimer's disease, 192-193, 193f
diagnosis of, 192
treatment of, 193
Amalgam tattoo, 334-335, 334f
Amaurosis fugax, 290-291, 290f, 291f
Amblyopia, 273, 273f
Amebiasis, 1165-1166, 1165f, 1166f
Amebic liver abscess, 633, 633f, 1165, 1165f
Amiloride, for ascites, 621
Amiodarone, hyperpigmentation due to, 48, 48f
Amniocentesis, 833f
fetal karyotype following, 834f
ultrasound-guided, 834f
Amoxicillin
adverse reactions to, 47, 47f
for Lyme disease, 1045
for typhoid fever, 654
Amoxicillin plus metronidazole, for gastritis, 572
Amsler grid, 252, 256f
Amyloidosis, 711-713, 711f-713f
characteristics of, 711t
Amyotrophic lateral sclerosis, 209-210, 209f, 210f
Anaerobic infections, 1221-1222, 1221f, 1222f
clinical signs of, 1221t
Anal canal, disorders of, 603, 603f, 604f
Anal cancer, HIV-related, 1158
Anal disorders, 603, 603f, 604f
Anal fissure, 605, 605f

Index

Analgesia, for myocardial infarction, 388
Androgen-deprivation therapy, for metastatic
    prostate cancer, 744
Androgenetic alopecia, 67-68, 67f, 68f
Anemia, 1066-1083
    aplastic, 1072-1073, 1073f
    autoimmune hemolytic, 1074f,
        1075-1076, 1075f
        serologic features of, 1134t
    definition of, 1066
    diagnosis of
        algorithm in, 1067f
        history in, 1066
        laboratory results in, 1066, 1068,
            1068f-1070f
        physical examination in, 1066
    iron deficiency, 1070, 1071f
    macrocytic, 1066, 1068, 1069f, 1069t
    microcytic, 1066, 1067t, 1068f
    normocytic, 1066
    pernicious, 1076-1077, 1076f-1078f
    refractory
        with excess blasts in transition,
            1093, 1094f
        with ring sideroblasts, 1093, 1094f
    sickle cell, 1079-1081, 1081f-1083f
    sideroblastic, 1070-1072, 1072f
    thalassemia, 1078-1079, 1079f, 1080f
Aneurysm
    abdominal aortic, 470-471, 470f, 471f
    left ventricular, 394, 394f
    true, in myocardial infarcts, 391, 391f
Angiitis
    allergic granulomatosis with (Churg-Strauss
        syndrome), 56, 58f, 519-520, 520f
    leukocytoclastic, 54-55, 54f, 55f
Angina pectoris
    clinical presentation of, 384
    definition of, 382
    differential diagnosis of, 384
    functional classification of, 383
    microvascular (syndrome X), 383
    Prinzmetal's variant of, 382, 383f
    refractory, 383
    stable (chronic), 382, 382f
    treatment of, 384-385, 385f, 386f
    unstable (rest or crescendo), 382, 382f
Angiography
    coronary, 378, 379f, 380f
    magnetic resonance. See Magnetic resonance
        angiography (MRA).
    of hand, in Buerger's disease, 469f
    of kidney, 686, 686f
        in polyarteritis nodosa, 981f
    of mesenteric ischemia, 661, 661f
    of pulmonary embolism, 555, 557, 557f
    of renal artery stenosis, 720, 721f
    of tetralogy of Fallot, 450f
Angioma
    cherry, 108, 108f
    senile, 108, 108f
    spider, in cirrhosis, 616f
Angiomatosis, bacillary, 140-141, 140f
    in HIV infection, 1157, 1157f
Angioplasty
    balloon, for coarctation of aorta, 455, 456f
    for Budd-Chiari syndrome, 666
Angiotensin receptor blockers, for chronic renal
    failure, 699
Angiotensin-converting enzyme (ACE) inhibitors
    for congestive heart failure, 412
    for myocardial infarction, 389
    for polycystic kidney disease, 715
Ankle fracture, 1023-1024, 1024f

Ankle sprain, 1022-1023, 1023f
Ankylosing spondylitis, 935t, 988, 989f,
    989t, 990f, 991
Ann Arbor staging
    of Hodgkin's lymphoma, 1095
    of non-Hodgkin's lymphoma, 1102
Anomalous pulmonary artery venous
    connection, 444
    imaging of, 444, 445f
    types of, 444, 444f
Anterior drawer test, 936f, 1022-1023, 1023f
Anterior horn cells, in amyotrophic lateral
    sclerosis, 209, 209f
Anterior interosseous nerve syndrome, 1003
Anthrax, 533-534, 534f, 535f
Antiarrhythmic therapy, for congestive heart
    failure, 412
Antibiotics
    for brain abscess, 217, 219
    for cavernous sinus thrombosis, 220-221
    for infective endocarditis, 408
    for otitis externa, 315
    for otitis media, 317
    for sinusitis, 323-324
Anti-CD recombinant immunotoxin, for hairy
    cell leukemia, 1106
Anticonvulsants
    for brain tumors, 185, 188
    for cavernous sinus thrombosis, 221
Antimalarials, for systemic lupus
    erythematosus, 963
Antineutrophil cytoplasmic antibodies
    in ulcerative colitis, 591
    in Wegener's granulomatosis, 518, 518f
    patterns of, 944, 945f
Antinuclear antibodies, patterns of, related to
    diagnosis, 942, 943f, 943t, 944f
Antiphospholipid antibody syndrome, 965-966,
    965f, 1122
Antiplatelet therapy, for myocardial
    infarction, 388
Antithrombin deficiency, 1122
    treatment of, 1125, 1125f
Antithyroid drugs, for hyperthyroidism, 876
Aorta
    abdominal, aneurysm of, 470-471, 470f, 471f
    coarctation of, 455, 456f
    dissection of, 472-473
        classification of, 472, 472f
        imaging studies of, 473, 473f, 474f
        risk factors for, 472
        treatment of, 473, 474f
Aortic valve
    regurgitation of, 401, 401f, 402f
    stenosis of, 399-400, 399f
        imaging of, 400, 400f
Aortic-aortic stent graft, in abdominal aortic
    aneurysm repair, 471, 471f
Aortic-uni-iliac device, with femorofemoral
    crossover graft, in abdominal aortic
    aneurysm repair, 471, 471f
APC gene, in Gardner's syndrome, 598
Aphthous stomatitis, recurrent, 327, 327f
Aplastic anemia, 1072-1073, 1073f
Apocrine hidrocystoma, of eyelid, 280, 280f
Appendicitis, 587, 587f
Arachnid bites, 146-147, 147f
Arcus corneae, 923, 926f
Arcus senilis, 268, 269f
Aromatase inhibitors, for breast cancer, 829
Arrhenoblastoma, associated with polycystic
    ovaries, 910, 911f
Arrhythmias, 427-439. See also specific type of
    arrhythmia.

Arrhythmias (Continued)
    post-infarct, 389, 391
Arterial switch operation, for transposition
    of great arteries, 451, 453f
Arteritis
    giant cell (temporal), 58, 59f, 982-983,
        982f, 983f
    Takayasu's, 59, 59f, 983-984, 983f, 984f
Arthritis
    crystal-related (gout), 933f, 935t, 994-995,
        994f, 995f
    granulomatous, 1040-1041, 1041f
    infectious, 1038, 1038f-1040f, 1039t, 1040
    Lyme, 1044, 1045f
    osteo-. See Osteoarthritis.
    psoriatic, 932f, 935t, 989t, 991-993,
        992f, 993f
    reactive, 935t
    rheumatoid. See Rheumatoid arthritis.
Arthropathy, neuropathic, in diabetes mellitus,
    917, 919f
Arthroscopy, 947, 948f
Asbestos, exposure to, mesothelioma associated
    with, 502. See also Mesothelioma.
Asbestosis, 507, 507f
Ascariasis, 1179, 1181, 1181f
Aschoff nodule, 1211f
Ascites
    clinical presentation of, 620, 620f
    imaging studies of, 620-621, 621f
    in cirrhosis, 616, 617f
    treatment of, 621
Aspergilloma (fungus ball), 1191
    treatment of, 1193
Aspergillosis
    allergic, 1191
    allergic bronchopulmonary, 1191
    extrapulmonary dissemination of, 1191-1192,
        1193f
    invasive, 1191, 1192f
    laboratory tests for, 1193, 1194f
    treatment of, 1193-1194
Aspergillus fumigatus, prick test for, 9f
Aspiration, of joint, 945, 946f
    indications for, 947t
Aspiration pneumonia, 528-529
    community-acquired, 528, 528f
    hospital-acquired, 528, 529f
Aspirin
    for angina pectoris, 385
    for antiphospholipid antibody syndrome,
        during pregnancy, 966
    for headache, in acute mountain
        sickness, 553
    for Kawasaki disease, 129
    for rheumatic fever, 1212
    for secondary Raynaud's phenomenon, 973
Asthma, 485-486, 486f, 487f
Astigmatism, examination of, 252, 256f
Astrocytoma, 186-187
    classification of, 186
Ataxia, Friedreich's, 214, 214f, 215f
Ataxia-telangiectasia, 214-215
Atelectasis, 524, 524f
Atherosclerosis, hypothesis for induction
    of, 923, 923f
Athlete's foot (tinea cruris), 111-112, 112f
ATM gene, in ataxia-telangiectasia, 215
Atopic dermatitis, 25-26, 25f
    differential diagnosis of, 26
    history and location of, 6t
Atrial fibrillation
    causes of, 428
    clinical presentation of, 427-428, 428f

Atrial fibrillation (Continued)
  imaging studies of, 428, 429f
  treatment of, 429-430, 429f
Atrial flutter, 430, 430f
Atrial hypertrophy, left and right, 372
Atrial myxoma, 457-458, 457f, 458f
Atrial septal defect, 442, 442f, 443f, 444
  location of, 442f
Atrial septostomy, for pulmonary
    hypertension, 551
Atrial tachycardia
  multifocal, 427, 428f
  paroxysmal, 427, 427f
Atrioventricular block
  first-degree, 437, 437f
  second-degree (Mobitz types I and II),
    437, 438f
  third-degree (complete), 437, 439, 439f
Atrioventricular conduction defects, 437,
    437f-439f, 439
Atrioventricular pacing, for congestive heart
    failure, 412, 412f
Atrophic glossitis, Candida, 1189f
Atrophic (estrogen-deficient) vulvovaginitis,
    797, 797f
Atrophy, cutaneous, 5b
Auspitz sign, in psoriasis, 33
Autoimmune conditions, oral, 332-333,
    332f, 333f
Autoimmune hemolytic anemia, 1074f,
    1075-1076, 1075f
  serologic features of, 1134t
Autoimmune hepatitis, 643
Avulsion fracture, of long bone, 1052, 1054f
Ayres spatula, Pap smear taken with, 782, 782f
Azacitidine, for myelodysplastic syndrome, 1093
Azidothymidine, nail discoloration due to,
    79, 80f
Azithromycin, for Lyme disease, 1045

B

B cell lymphoma, 1101f
Babesiosis, 1161-1163, 1163f
Babinski's sign, in multiple sclerosis, 207
Bacillary angiomatosis, 140-141, 140f
  in HIV infection, 1157, 1157f
Bacillus anthracis, 534, 534f. See also Anthrax.
Back, rheumatic disorders of, 1014-1019.
    See also specific disorder.
Bacterial arthritis, 1038,
    1038f-1040f, 1040
  agents in, 1039t
Bacterial conjunctivitis, 261, 261f
Bacterial infection(s), 134-142. See also specific
    infection, e.g., Tuberculosis.
Bacterial meningitis, 221-222, 222f
Bacterial pneumonia, 525-528, 525f-527f
Bacterial prostatitis
  acute and chronic, 741, 741t
    treatment of, 742
  Meares and Stamey localization technique
    for, 742f
Bacterial vaginosis, 793, 793f, 794f
Bacteroides fragilis, Gram-stained smear
    of, 1141f
Baker's cyst, 1020-1021, 1021f
Balanitis, 764, 764f
Baldness, common, 67-68, 67f, 68f
Ball-cage prosthesis, for valvular heart disease,
    404, 405f
Balloon dilation angioplasty, for coarctation
    of aorta, 455, 456f
Banal nevus, 93, 93f
Banana fracture, 1051, 1051f

Bandages, compression, for venous ulcers, 461
Barium imaging studies
  of Crohn's disease, 589, 590f
  of diverticular disease, 593, 593f
Barrett's esophagus, 564, 564f
Barrier methods, of contraception, 789,
    789f, 790f
Bartholin's gland, abscess of, 776, 779f
Bartonellosis (Carrión's disease), 141, 141f
Basal cell carcinoma
  definition of, 86
  differential diagnosis of, 86
  of eyelid, 286, 286f
  subtypes of, 86, 86f, 87f
  treatment of, 86-87
Basal layer (stratum basale), of skin, 2
Beau's lines, 77, 78f
Becker nevus, 92, 93f
Becker's muscular dystrophy, 233
Bedbug, 148f
Bedbug bites, 148, 149f
Behçet's syndrome, 50, 50f, 58, 58f,
    984-985, 985f, 986f
Bell's palsy, 238, 238f
Benign prostatic hyperplasia, 739-740,
    739f, 740f
Benztropine, for dystonia, 203
Beta-adrenergic blockers, for myocardial
    infarction, 389
Bicipital tendinitis, clinical tests for, 937f
Bifurcation graft, in abdominal aortic aneurysm
    repair, 471, 471f
Bile duct, common, stones in, 644, 645f
Biliary cirrhosis, primary, 624-625, 624f, 625f
Biliary tract, calculi in, 644-645, 644f, 645f
Bioleaflet prosthesis, for valvular heart disease,
    404, 405f
Bioprosthesis, for valvular heart disease,
    404, 405f
Biopsy
  bone marrow, in myelodysplastic syndrome,
    1093, 1093f
  colposcopic, 784, 785f
  cone, of cervical dysplasia, 803
  CT-guided
    of hepatocellular carcinoma, 631, 632f
    pancreatic, 613, 615f
  duodenal, for Whipple's disease, 657, 657f
  fat pad, for amyloidosis, 711, 713f
  fine-needle aspiration, of cholangiocarcinoma,
    648, 649f
  in lymphomatoid granulomatosis, 522, 523f
  liver, 618
    in alpha₁-antitrypsin deficiency, 492, 493f
    needles for, 619f
    patterns of iron deposition in, 626, 627f
  lung, in Wegener's granulomatosis, 518, 519f
  lymph node, in Hodgkin's lymphoma, 1095,
    1096f
  muscle, 947, 947f
  pleural, 502, 503f
  renal. See Renal biopsy.
  salivary gland, 947, 947f
Bisphosphonates, for osteoporosis, 1032
Bite(s)
  arachnid, 146-147, 147f
    treatment of, 148
  human and animal, 145-146, 146f
  insect, 148-149, 148f, 149f
    treatment of, 149
  snake, 149-151, 151f
    treatment of, 151-152, 152f
Biting injury, chronic, 326, 326f
Biventricular heart failure, 409

Black widow spider, 147f
Blackheads, 72, 73f
Blackwater fever, 1162f
Bladder carcinoma, 737, 737f, 738f
Blastomyces dermatitidis, 1204, 1205f
Blastomycosis, 1204, 1205f, 1206, 1206f
  treatment of, 1206
Blebs, hemorrhagic
  at rattlesnake bite site, 151f
  frostbite with, 157f
Bleeding. See Hemorrhage.
Blepharospasm, 276, 276f
  differential diagnosis of, 277t
Blister(s)
  burn, 156, 156f
  definition of, 16
  oral, 339-340
Blistering disease(s). See also specific disease.
  subepidermal, inherited and autoimmune,
    16-19, 16f-20f
Blood group antigens, 1060
  testing of, 1060, 1062f
Blood group autoantibodies, 1060
  testing of, 1060, 1062f
Blood pressure
  control of, in management of stroke, 178
  high. See Hypertension.
  regulation of
    factors involved in, 478, 479f
    in polycystic kidney disease, 715
Blood smears, peripheral, 1142, 1142f,
    1142t, 1143f
  of babesiosis, 1163f
  of chronic lymphocytic leukemia, 1088, 1089f
  of cold agglutinin syndrome, 1134f
  of hemolytic-uremic syndrome, 1119, 1119f
  of histoplasmosis, 1195, 1196f
  of iron deficiency anemia, 1071f
  of louse-borne relapsing fever, 1228f
  of macrocytic anemia, 1066, 1069f
  of malaria, 1162f
  of microcytic anemia, 1066, 1068f
  of sickle cell anemia, 1083f
  of sideroblastic anemia, 1072f
  of thalassemia, 1080f
  review of erythrocyte morphology in,
    1068, 1070f
Blue bloaters, 488
Blue nevus, common, 96, 97f
Bochdalek hernia, 366, 368f
Body louse (Pediculosis corporis), 144, 144f
Boil (furuncle), 139-140, 139f, 140f
Bone(s), long, fracture of, 1052-1053,
    1053f-1055f
Bone cyst, simple, 1047, 1048f
Bone deformity, in Paget's disease, 1035, 1035f
Bone diseases, 1031-1036. See also specific disease,
    e.g., Osteoporosis.
Bone marrow biopsy, in myelodysplastic
    syndrome, 1093, 1093f
Bone marrow morphology
  in acute myelogenous leukemia, 1085, 1086f
  in aplastic anemia, 1073, 1073f
  in chronic myelogenous leukemia,
    1090, 1091f
Bone marrow transplantation
  and high-dose chemotherapy, for breast
    cancer, 829
  for acute myelogenous leukemia, 1087
  for anaplastic anemia, 1073
  for chronic myelogenous leukemia, 1092
  of acute lymphoblastic leukemia, 1085
Bone mass density, determination of, in
    osteoporosis, 1032, 1032f

Bone tumors, 1047, 1047f-1049f, 1049-1050.
  See also specific tumor.
Borrelia burgdorferi, 1044. *See also* Lyme disease.
Bortezomib, for multiple myeloma, 1109
Botulism, 236t
Botulism toxin injections
  for achalasia, 569
  for blepharospasm, sites of, 276, 276f
Bouchard's nodules, 950f
Boutonniére deformity, 952f
Bow legs, in rickets, 1032, 1032f
Bowen's disease, 88, 89f
  photodynamic therapy for, 12f
Bowman's capsule, 676, 676f
Brain. *See also* Cerebral *entries.*
  abscess of, 216-219, 216f, 217f, 219f
    in endocarditis, 406, 406f
  anatomy of, 162, 162f, 163f
  astrocytoma of, 186-187
  cerebrospinal fluid flow in, 165f
  coverings of, 164f
  craniopharyngioma of, 188-191, 190f
  CT scan of, 168, 168f, 169f
  Cysticercus in, 225, 225f
  developmental disorders of, 206, 206f
  EEG of, 172, 173f, 174f
  glioblastoma multiforme of, 185f
  glioma of, 186f
  infections of, 216-228. *See also specific infection.*
  lymphoma of, 184, 184f, 185f
  meningioma of, 187-188, 188f, 189f
  MRI of, 168, 169f, 170f
  precerebral and cerebral vessels of,
    angiography of, 168, 172,
    172f, 173f
  sections of, 163f
  SPECT scan of, 168, 170f, 171f
  tumors of, 184-191
    histopathology of, 185, 186f
    imaging studies of, 184-185, 184f-186f
    treatment of, 185
Breast
  abscess of, 824, 824f
  changes in, prolactin secretion causing,
    859, 861f
  development of, Tanner stages of, 896, 897f
  female, anatomy of, 821f
  fibrocystic disease of, 821-822, 822f, 823f
  lump in, algorithm for evaluation of, 823f
  Paget's disease of, 830, 831f
  striae gravidarum of, 832, 832f
Breast cancer
  diagnosis of, 826, 827f-829f
  histologic classification of, 826, 827f
  staging of, 826
  treatment of, 826, 828-829
Breast pain, algorithm for evaluation of,
  824, 825f
Breast self-examination, 826, 827f, 828f
Breath odor, in cirrhosis patients, 616
Breech presentation, 841, 841f
Bronchial wall, normal histology of, 488, 488f
Bronchiectasis, 537, 538f
Bronchitis, chronic, 488, 488f
Bronchoalveolar carcinoma, 494. *See also* Lung
  carcinoma.
Bronchogenic cyst, 361, 362f
Bronchopulmonary aspergillosis, allergic, 1191
Bronchoscopic drainage, of lung abscess, 531
Brown casts, muddy, in acute tubular necrosis,
  705, 705f
Brown recluse spider, 147f
Brown recluse spider bite, 147f

Brown tumor, of rib, 880, 880f
Brucellosis, 1231-1232, 1231f, 1232f
  clinical manifestations of, 1231f
Brugada syndrome, 434, 435f
Bubonic plague, 1226
Buccal mucosa
  leukoedema of, 326, 326f
  lipoma of, 328, 329f
  normal histology of, 325, 325f
Buccal space, abscess of, 336, 336f
Budd-Chiari syndrome, 665-666, 666f
Buerger's disease, 58, 58f, 468, 468f, 469f
Bulge sign, 934f
Bulla, 4b
Bullous impetigo, 138
Bullous myringitis, 304, 306f
Bullous pemphigoid, 16-17, 16f
  differential diagnosis of, 6t, 16, 17f
Bunion deformity (hallux abductovalgus),
  1026, 1026f
Burkitt's lymphoma, 1102-1103, 1102f, 1103f
Burning tongue (glossopyrosis), 339
Burns
  classification of, 156
  electrical, 158-159, 159f
  estimating surface area of, rule of nines
    in, 155f
  first-degree, 155, 156f
  marks from, 155f
  second-degree, 156, 156f
  third-degree, 156, 156f
  treatment of, 156-157
Bursitis, 933f
  olecranon, in rheumatoid arthritis, 952, 953f
  septic, 1041-1042, 1042f
  trochanteric, 1019-1020, 1019f
Butterfly erythema, in systemic lupus
  erythematosus, 960, 960f
Buttocks, eruptive xanthoma on, 923, 926f

C

Cachexia, HIV-related, 1158
Café au lait spots, in neurofibromatosis, 96f,
  100, 100f, 229, 230f
Calcification(s)
  eggshell, in sarcoidosis, 515, 515f
  in chronic pancreatitis, 609, 610f, 612
  in chronic renal failure, 697-698, 698f, 699f
Calcinosis, subcutaneous, 975, 975f
Calcium, supplemental, for osteoporosis, 1032
Calcium channel blockers
  for polycystic kidney disease, 715
  for pulmonary hypertension, 551
Calcium fluxes, in normal adult, 880, 881f
Calcium homeostasis, hormonal regulation
  of, 880, 880t
Calcium oxalate stone, 732, 732f
Calcium pyrophosphate dehydrate (CPPD)
  crystal(s)
  in synovial fluid, 996, 997f
  sites of deposition of, 995, 995f
Calcium pyrophosphate dehydrate (CPPD)
  crystal disease, 996, 997f
Calculi
  biliary tract. *See* Cholelithiasis.
  urinary tract. *See* Urolithiasis.
Calve-Legg-Perthes disease, 1020, 1020f
Campbell de Morgan spots, 108, 108f
Candida albicans, culture of, 1143f
Candida liver abscess, 633, 633f
Candidiasis, 1189, 1189f, 1190f
  cutaneous, 113, 114f
  of nails, 79, 80f
  oral (thrush), 339

Candidiasis *(Continued)*
  HIV-related, 1149, 1150f, 1155
  vulvovaginal (moniliasis), 763-764, 763f,
    1189, 1190f
Capillary hemangioma, 108, 108f
  lobular, 108, 109f
  of eyelid, 281, 281f
Caplan's syndrome, 952, 954f
Carbomedic's prosthesis, for valvular heart
    disease, 404, 405f
Carcinoid tumor, 667, 668f-670f
  sites of, 667t
Carcinoma. *See also specific type, e.g.,* Squamous
    cell carcinoma.
  bladder, 737, 737f, 738f
  breast, 826, 827f-829f, 828-829
  cervical, 805-806, 805f, 806f
  colorectal, 600, 600f, 601f, 602
  endometrial, 813, 813f, 814f
  esophageal, 565-566, 565f, 566f
  gastric, 576, 576f, 577f
  hepatocellular, 631-632, 631f, 632f
  lung, 494-499. *See also* Lung carcinoma.
  ovarian, 819, 819f
  pancreatic, 613, 613f-615f
  thyroid, 352-354, 352f-354f
  verrucous, 766, 766f
  vulvar, 798, 798f
Cardiac. *See also* Heart.
Cardiac catheterization, 378, 379f, 380f
  in ventricular septal defect, 446, 447f
Cardiac pacemaker, 440, 441f
  dual chamber, 441f
  features of, definition of, 440t
  for atrial fibrillation, 430
  for congestive heart failure, 412, 412f
  indications for, 440
Cardiac tamponade, in pericarditis, 422, 424
Cardiac thrombus, 428, 429f
Cardiac tumors. *See also specific tumor.*
  common, 457f
Cardiogenic pulmonary edema, 413, 413f
Cardiomyopathy(ies), 414-419
  dilated (congestive), 414, 414f, 415f
    treatment of, 415-416, 416f
  hypertrophic, 417-418, 417f-419f
  restrictive, 416-417, 416f
Cardiovascular system
  cardiac catheterization of, 378, 379f, 380f
  computed tomography of, 380
  diagnostic tests and procedures involving,
    370-381
  echocardiography of, 375, 376f, 377,
    377f, 378t
  electrocardiography of, 370-373, 371f-373f
    exercise, 374-375, 375f
  magnetic resonance angiography of, 381, 381f
  magnetic resonance imaging of, 380, 380f
  nuclear imaging of, 378, 379f
  X-ray of, 373-374, 374f
Carmen ulcer, 577f
Carotid artery, internal, stenosis of, 175, 175f
Carotid artery syndrome, characteristics of,
  175, 175b
Carotid endarterectomy, for stroke, 178
Carpal tunnel
  anatomy of, 1001f
  injection of, 1002, 1002f
Carpal tunnel syndrome, 1001-1002,
  1001f, 1002f
Carrión's disease, 141, 141f
Cat flea, 148f
Cat scratch disease, 1233-1234,
  1233f, 1234f

Cataracts
 treatment of, 259
 types of, 259, 259f, 260f
Catheter(s), peritoneal, 696, 696f
Catheterization, cardiac, 378, 379f, 380f
 in ventricular septal defect, 446, 447f
Cauda equina syndrome, 1014
Cavernous hemangioma, 108, 109f
Cavernous sinus thrombosis, 219-221, 220f
CD4 T cell(s), in HIV infection, 1147
CDKN2 gene, in astrocytomas, 186
Cefotaxime, for meningitis, 222
Ceftriaxone
 for Lyme disease, 1045
 for meningitis, 222
 for typhoid fever, 654
 for Whipple's disease, 657
Celiac disease, 583, 583f, 584f
Celiac plexus block, for pancreatic
  carcinoma, 613
Celiac sprue, 583
Cellulitis, 134-136, 134f, 135f
Central nervous system disorders, in
  antiphospholipid antibody
  syndrome, 965
Cerebral. See also Brain.
Cerebral abscess, 216-219, 216f
 imaging of, 216, 218f, 219f
 in endocarditis, 406, 406f
 sources of, 216, 217f
 treatment of, 217, 219
Cerebral edema, high-altitude, 552
Cerebral malaria, 1161
Cerebral palsy, 239, 239f
Cerebral thrombosis, characteristics of, 177t
Cerebral vessels, angiography of, 168, 172,
  172f, 173f
Cerebritis, 1225
Cerebrospinal fluid, flow of, 165f
Cerebrovascular disease, 175-181, 175b,
  175f-180f, 176t, 177t.
   See also Stroke; Subarachnoid
   hemorrhage; Transient ischemic attack.
Cervical cap, contraceptive, 789, 790f, 791
Cervical lymph nodes, in Hodgkin's lymphoma,
  1095, 1095f
Cervical rib/scalenus syndrome, 1012
Cervical spine, fracture of, 1056, 1056f
Cervicitis, 800, 800f, 801f
Cervicography, 783, 784f
Cerviscope, 783f
Cervix
 cancer of, 805-806, 805f, 806f
  HIV-related, 1158, 1158f
 dysplasia of, 802-803, 803f, 804f
 intraepithelial neoplasia of, 785f
 normal, 776, 781f
 precancerous lesions of, 785f
Cesarean section, 841-842, 843f
 classic, 842
 low cervical, 842
Cestode infestation, 1176, 1176f-1178f
Ceuroxime, for Lyme disease, 1045
Chagas disease, 1170-1172
Chalazion, 284, 284f
Chancroid, 761-762, 761f, 762f
Charcot-Marie-Tooth disease, 212-213, 212f, 213f
Charcot's joints, in diabetes mellitus, 917, 919f
Charcot's triad, in multiple sclerosis, 207
Chemotherapy
 combination
  for esophageal carcinoma, 566
  for Hodgkin's lymphoma, 1098
  for multiple myeloma, 1109

Chemotherapy (Continued)
  for non-small cell lung carcinoma, 499
  for ovarian carcinoma, 819, 819f
 for brain tumors, 185, 187
 for breast cancer
  agents in, 828-829
  high-dose, 829
 for colorectal carcinoma, 600
 for gastric carcinoma, 576
 for hairy cell leukemia, 1106
 for non-small cell lung carcinoma
  postoperative, 499
  preoperative, 498
  with radiation therapy, 499
 for pancreatic carcinoma, 613
Cherry angioma, 108, 108f
Chest radiography. See also Radiography.
 cardiac silhouette on, 373, 374f
 examination of, 373-374
Chest wall, abnormalities of, 358, 358f
Chest wall pain, 1026-1027, 1027f
Chiari malformation, types of, 206, 206f
Chiba needle, for aspiration biopsy, 619f
Chickenpox (varicella), 116-117, 116f, 531
 treatment of, 533
Child, sexual abuse of, signs of, 776, 779f
Chinese letter appearance, of Corynebacterium
  diphtheriae, 1224, 1224f
Chlamydia pneumoniae, 525. See also Pneumonia.
Chlamydia trachomatis, diagnostic tests for, 769t
Chlamydial conjunctivitis, 261, 261f
Chloasma, 64, 64f
 pregnancy, 832f
Chloramphenicol, for actinomycosis, 1204
Cholangiocarcinoma, 648, 648f, 649f
Cholecystectomy, laparoscopic, for gallstones,
  644-645
Cholecystitis, 646-647, 646f, 647f
Cholelithiasis, 644-645, 644f, 645f
Cholera, 655, 655f
Cholesteatoma, of ear, 304, 307f
Cholesterol embolus, in renal artery
  stenosis, 719
Cholesterol stones, 644
Chondrocalcinosis, 995
Chondroma, 1047, 1048f
Chondrosarcoma, 1047
Chordee (penile curvature), 772
Chorioretinitis, HIV-related, 1157
Choroidal vasculitis, in systemic lupus
  erythematosus, 960, 961f
Chromosome abnormality
 in acute myelogenous leukemia,
  1087, 1087f
 in chronic lymphocytic leukemia, 1089, 1089f
Chromosome translocation, in chronic
  myelogenous leukemia, 1090
Chronic bacterial prostatitis, 741, 741t, 742f
 treatment of, 742
Chronic idiopathic myelofibrosis, characteristics
  of, 1113t
Chronic illness, thrombosis risk associated
  with, 1122
Chronic lymphocytic leukemia, 1088-1090,
  1088f, 1089f
 staging of, 1089-1090
Chronic myelogenous (myeloid) leukemia, 1090,
  1091f, 1092, 1092f
 characteristics of, 1113t
 phases of, definition of, 1091t
Chronic obstructive pulmonary disease, 488-491
 clinical presentation of, 488-489, 488f
 definition of, 488
 imaging studies of, 489, 490f-491f

Chronic obstructive pulmonary
  disease (Continued)
 laboratory tests for, 489, 489f
 treatment of, 489, 491
Chronic prostatitis–chronic pelvic pain
  syndrome, 741, 741t
 treatment of, 742
Chronic renal failure
 clinical presentation of, 697-698, 697f-699f
 definition of, 697
 imaging studies of, 699, 700f
 laboratory tests for, 698-699
 treatment of, 699
Churg-Strauss syndrome, 56, 58f, 519-520, 520f
Chvostek's sign
 in acute pancreatitis, 608
 in hypocalcemia, 878, 879f
Chyluria, 1186
Cicatricial pemphigoid, 17-18, 18f
 oral, 332, 332f
Cirrhosis
 causes of, 617
 clinical presentation of, 616-617, 616f, 617f
 imaging studies of, 618, 619f
 laboratory tests for, 617-618, 618f
 primary biliary, 624-625, 624f, 625f
 treatment of, 618
Clarithromycin plus metronidazole, for
  gastritis, 572
Clear cell acanthoma, 86, 86f
Clindamycin
 for bacterial vaginosis, 793
 for lung abscess, 530
Closed fracture, of long bone, 1052
Clostridium difficile, in pseudomembranous
  colitis, 659, 659f
Clostridium perfringens, 1222f
 Gram-stained smear of, 1141f
Clostridium tetani, 1220
Clotrimazole, for oral candidiasis, 1155
Clubbing
 of fingers
  in lung carcinoma, 494, 494f
  in primary biliary cirrhosis, 624, 625f
 of nails, 79, 79f
Coagulation, disseminated intravascular, 60,
  1120-1121, 1120f, 1121f
Coal worker's pneumoconiosis, 509, 509f
Coarctation of aorta, 455, 455f, 456f
Cobalamin
 absorption of, 1076f
 deficiency of
  signs and symptoms of, 1077f
  vitamin B_{12} for, 1077
Cobb angle, measurement of, in scoliosis, 1019f
Coccidioides immitis, 1199, 1200f
Coccidioidomycosis, 1198-1201
 clinical presentation of, 1199, 1199f
 HIV-related, 1155, 1155f
 imaging studies of, 1200, 1201f
 laboratory tests for, 1200, 1200f
 treatment of, 1200-1201
Colchicine, for Peyronie's disease, 774
Cold agglutinin syndrome, 1134, 1134f
Colitis
 amebic, 1165, 1165f
 Crohn's, 589f. See also Crohn's disease.
 HIV-related, 1157
 ischemic, imaging of, 661, 662f
 pseudomembranous, 659, 659f, 660f
 Salmonella, 652, 653f
 ulcerative, 591-592, 591f
Colles fracture, 1053, 1055f
Colonic diverticulum, 593

Index

Colonoscopy
  in colorectal carcinoma, 600, 600f
  in Gardner's syndrome, 599
  in ulcerative colitis, 591, 591f
Colorectal carcinoma, 600, 600f, 601f, 602
  gross appearances of, 601f
Colposcopy, 783, 785f
Comedones
  closed (whiteheads), 72
  open (blackheads), 72, 73f
Comminuted fracture, of long bone, 1052, 1053f
Common blue nevus, 96, 97f
Common wart (verruca vulgaris), 121, 122f
  of eyelid, 285
Community-acquired pneumonia, 528, 528f
Compartment syndrome, 729f
Complex decongestive therapy, for
      lymphedema, 464
Compression bandages, for venous ulcers, 461
Compression fracture, of vertebrae, 1057, 1057f
Compression stockings, for venous ulcers, 461
Computed tomography (CT)
  of abdominal aortic aneurysm, 470, 471f
  of acute lymphoblastic leukemia, 1084,
      1084f, 1085f
  of acute pancreatitis, 609, 610f
  of aortic dissection, 473, 474f
  of appendicitis, 587, 587f
  of ascites, 620, 621f
  of brain, 168, 168f, 169f
  of bronchogenic cyst, 362f
  of brucellosis, 1232, 1232f
  of Budd-Chiari syndrome, 665, 666f
  of carcinoid tumor, 667, 669f
  of cardiovascular system, 380
  of cerebral lymphoma, 184f
  of cervical cancer, 806, 806f
  of cholangiocarcinoma, 648, 648f
  of colorectal carcinoma, 600, 601f
  of congenital adrenal hyperplasia, 904, 905f
  of craniopharyngioma, 190, 191f
  of Crohn's disease, 589, 590f
  of diverticulitis, 593, 594f
  of echinococcosis, 635, 637f
  of gastric carcinoma, 576, 577f
  of glioblastoma multiforme, 185f
  of hepatocellular carcinoma, 631, 631f, 632f
  of Hodgkin's lymphoma, 1095, 1097f
  of hydronephrosis, 728, 728f
  of hypertrophic cardiomyopathy, 418, 419f
  of kidneys, 684, 685f
  of liver abscess, 635, 635f
  of lumbar spine stenosis, 1016, 1016f
  of lung carcinoma, 496, 497f, 498f
  of mediastinal teratoma, 361f
  of meningioma, 188, 189f
  of mesenteric ischemia, 661, 662f
  of mesothelioma, 502, 504f
  of pancreatic carcinoma, 613, 615f
  of paranasal sinuses, 323, 324f
  of pheochromocytoma, 894, 895f
  of polycystic kidney disease, 715, 718f
  of portal vein thrombosis, 663, 664f
  of pseudomembranous colitis, 659, 660f
  of pulmonary embolism, 555, 556f
  of sarcoidosis, 515, 516f
  of stroke, 177, 177f, 178f
  of subarachnoid hemorrhage, 180, 180f
  of ureteric stone, 734, 736f
  of uterine leiomyoma, 810, 810f
  of von Hippel-Lindau disease, 247, 248f
Condoms
  female, 789, 790f, 791
  male, 789, 791

Conductive hearing loss. See also Hearing loss.
  vs. sensorineural hearing loss, 308t
Condyloma acuminatum. See also Wart(s).
  genital, 122, 123f, 758, 758f, 785f
  gingival, 328f
Cone biopsy, of cervical dysplasia, 803
Congenital adrenal hyperplasia, 903-904,
      903f-905f
Congenital cataract, 260
Congenital esotropia, 270, 270f
Congenital granular cell epulis, 325, 326f
Congenital heart disease, 442-456
  anomalous pulmonary artery venous
      connection in, 444, 444f, 445f
  atrial septal defect in, 442, 442f, 443f, 444
  coarctation of aorta in, 455, 455f, 456f
  Ebstein's anomaly in, 453, 453f, 545f
  patent ductus arteriosus in, 453, 455,
      455f, 545f
  tetralogy of Fallot in, 446-448, 448f-450f
  transposition of great arteries in, 450-451,
      451f-453f
  truncus arteriosus in, 450, 450f, 451f
  ventricular septal defect in, 444-446,
      445f-447f
Congenital melanocytic nevus (kissing nevus),
      96, 96f
  of eyelid, 284, 284f
Congestive heart failure, 409-412
  biventricular, 409
  classification of, 409
  clinical presentation of, 409, 411f
  imaging of, 411, 411f
  left ventricular, 409
  right ventricular, 409
  sympathetic activation and parasympathetic
      withdrawal in, mechanism of, 410f
  treatment of, 411-412, 412f
Conjunctiva
  disorders of, 267-268, 267f-269f
  examination of, 252, 254f
Conjunctivitis, 261-262, 261f, 262f
  differential diagnosis of, 263t
  ligneous, 267, 268f
  toxic follicular, 267, 268f
  treatment of, 262
Connective tissue disease
  inherited, 1028-1030, 1028f-1030f
  mixed, 977, 977f
Connective tissue lesions, 104-109.
      See also specific lesion.
Conn's syndrome, 891-892, 891f-893f
Consolidation therapy
  for acute myelogenous leukemia, 1087
  of acute lymphoblastic leukemia, 1085
Contact dermatitis
  allergic, 27, 28f
  clinical presentation of, 27, 27f-29f
  diagnosis of, 28, 29f
  differential diagnosis of, 28
  history and location of, 6t
  irritant, 27, 27f
  treatment of, 28, 30
Contact lens red eye, 261, 262f
Contraception, 789-792
  types of, 789, 789f-791f, 791-792
Contraceptive patch, 792
Coombs' test, 1066
  for autoimmune hemolytic anemia,
      1075, 1075f
Cor pulmonale, 425-426, 425f
Coral snakes, 150, 150f
Corneal abrasion, differential diagnosis of, 263t
Corneal arcus, 268, 269f, 923, 926f

Corneal light reflexes, examination of, 252, 252f
Corneal ulceration (keratitis), 264, 264f, 265f
Coronary angiography, 378, 379f, 380f
Coronary artery, thrombus in, 923, 924f
Coronary artery bypass graft
  for angina pectoris, 385
  for Kawasaki disease, 129-130
Coronary stents, for angina pectoris, 385, 386f
Corrigan's pulse, 401
Cortical cataract, 259f
Corticosteroids
  for cavernous sinus thrombosis, 221
  for idiopathic pulmonary fibrosis, 513
  for sarcoidosis, 516f
  for systemic lupus erythematosus, 963, 964
  for Takayasu's arteritis, 984
  injection of, for epicondylitis, 1008, 1008f
  topical, for Behçet's syndrome, 985
Corticotropin deficiency
  in hypopituitarism, 854
  testing for, 856, 858f
Corynebacterium diphtheriae, 1223.
      See also Diphtheria.
Cosmetic interventions
  for hirsutism, 911
  for skin disorders, 13
Costochondritis, 1026-1027, 1027f
Costoclavicular maneuver, 1013f
Costoclavicular syndrome, 1012
Cover tests, for tropias, 252, 253f
Cowpox, 133, 133f
Crab louse (Phthirus pubis), 144, 144f
Cranial epidural abscess, 224
Craniopharyngioma
  clinical presentation of, 188-189
  histopathology of, 190, 190f
  imaging of, 190, 190f, 191f
  treatment of, 191
C-reactive protein, as inflammatory marker, 944
Creeping eruption (cutaneous larva
      migrans), 145
CREST syndrome, 975, 975f
  digital gangrene in, 976, 976f
Creutzfeldt-Jakob disease, 196-197, 196f, 197f
Crohn's disease
  clinical presentation of, 588, 588f
  endoscopic evaluation of, 589, 589f, 590f
  imaging studies of, 589, 590f
  oral, 331f, 332, 588, 588f
  treatment of, 589-590
Cruciate ligament, tears of, Lachman test
      for, 936f
Crust, cutaneous, 5b
Cryoglobulin(s), classes of, 60-61
Cryoglobulinemia, 60-61, 61f
  hepatitis C–associated
      pulmonary infiltrates in, 640, 641f
      purpura in, 640, 641f
Cryotherapy
  for basal cell carcinoma, 87
  for skin disorders, 10, 11f
  for warts, 123, 124f
Cryptococcosis, 1197-1198, 1197f-1199f
  HIV-related, 1155, 1155f
Cryptococcus neoformans, 1197, 1197f, 1198f
Cryptosporidiosis, 1167-1168, 1168f
Crystal-related arthritis, 933f, 935t, 994-995,
      994f, 995f
Cubital tunnel, anatomy of, 1008f
Cubital tunnel syndrome, 1008-1009, 1008f
Cullen's sign, in acute pancreatitis, 608, 608f
Cultures, 1142, 1143f
Cumulus-oocyte complex, ovulation of,
      776, 777f

Cushing's disease
   clinical presentation of, 859
   differential diagnosis of, 859, 863f
   medical therapy for, 866
   workup for, 861, 864
Cushing's syndrome, 884-885, 884f-886f
   ACTH-dependent vs. ACTH-independent, 884, 886f
Cutaneous. *See also* Skin *entries*.
Cutaneous candidiasis, 113, 114f
Cutaneous cryoglobulinemic vasculitis, 61, 61f
Cutaneous cysts, 102-103, 103f
Cutaneous flushing, carcinoid tumor and, 667, 668f
Cutaneous horn, of eyelid, 278, 278f
Cutaneous larva migrans, 145, 145f
Cutaneous leishmaniasis, 1168, 1169f
Cutaneous lichen planus, 35
Cutaneous neuroendocrine carcinoma, of eyelid, 287, 287f
Cutaneous sensory innervation, of lower extremities, 1014f, 1015f
Cutaneous T-cell lymphoma, 1103, 1103f-1105f
Cutaneous ulcer, in lymphomatoid granulomatosis, 523f
Cutaneous zygomycosis, 1209
Cyclophosphamide
   for Goodpasture's syndrome, 521
   for systemic lupus erythematosus, 964
   intravenous, for glomerulonephritis, 702
Cyclosporine, gingival hyperplasia due to, 329, 330f
Cylindroma
   dermal, 101, 102f
   of eyelid, 281, 281f
Cyst(s), 4b
   Baker's, 1020-1021, 1021f
   bronchogenic, 361, 362f
   dermoid, 103, 103f
      of eyelid, 280, 280f
   epidermal inclusion
      of eyelid, 279, 279f
      vulvar, 798, 799f
   epidermoid, 102, 103f
   epithelial inclusion, conjunctival, 267, 267f
   ganglion, 104, 105f, 1004, 1004f, 1005f
   hepatic
      echinococcal, 635, 636f
      vs. liver abscess, 633, 634f
   lymphoepithelial, oral, 325, 325f
   myxoid, 83, 83f
   ovarian, 815, 816f
   salivary gland, 333
   sebaceous, vulvar, 798, 799f
   simple bone, 1047, 1048f
   thymic, 360, 360f
   thyroglossal duct, 349, 350f
   trichilemmal (pilar), 102, 103f
      surgical excision of, 10f
Cystic fibrosis, 538-540, 539f
Cystic hygroma, mediastinal, 361, 363f
Cysticercosis, 225-226, 225f, 1176, 1178f
Cysticidal therapy, 226
Cystine stone, 732, 732f
Cystocele, 776, 780f
Cytomegalovirus (CMV) pneumonia, 531, 532f, 533f
Cytomegalovirus (CMV) retinitis, HIV-related, 1149, 1151f, 1157

D

Dactylitis, 932f, 988, 988f
Dandy-Walker malformation, 244, 244f

Darier's disease, 23-24, 23f, 24f, 80, 81f
   oral, 339
Dark lesions, oral, 339
De Musset's sign, 401
De Quervain's tenosynovitis, 1005-1006, 1006f
Débridement, of decubitus ulcers, 153, 153f
Decubitus ulcers, 153-154, 153f
Deep vein thrombosis, 465-466, 465f
   clinical algorithm for, 466f
   imaging studies of, 466, 467f
   treatment of, 466, 467f
Deferoxamine
   for hemochromatosis, 627
   for sideroblastic anemia, 1072
Defibrillators, for atrial fibrillation, 430
Dehydration, in cholera, 655, 655f
Dementia, 192-199. *See also specific type.*
   with Lewy bodies, 193-194, 194f
Dental infections, 336-337, 336f, 337f
Depigmentation, 5b
Depo-Provera, contraceptive, 789, 792
Dermal cylindroma, 101, 102f
Dermal melanocytic nevus, 93, 93f
Dermatitis, radiation, 160, 160f
Dermatitis herpetiformis, 18-19, 18f, 19f
   differential diagnosis of, 6t, 18
Dermatoconjunctivitis, allergic, 267, 267f
Dermatographism, 51, 51f
Dermatomyositis, 969-970, 969f
Dermatophyte infection(s), 110-113, 110f-114f.
      See also specific infection.
Dermatophyte test, 9f
Dermatoses. *See also specific type of dermatitis,*
      e.g., Contact dermatitis.
   eczematous
      endogenous, 25-27, 25f-27f
      exogenous, 27-28, 27f-32f, 30-32
      history and location of, 6t
      granulomatous, 41-42, 41f, 42f
      inflammatory, 39-40, 39f, 40f
         of genitalia, 756-757, 756f, 757f
      necrobiotic, 43, 43f
      neutrophilic and eosinophilic, 49-53, 49f-53f
Dermatosis papulosa nigra, 279f
Dermis, structure and function of, 2f, 3
Dermoid
   dumb-bell, 103
   limbal, 267, 267f
Dermoid cyst, 103, 103f
   of eyelid, 280, 280f
Dermolytic pemphigoid, 18, 18f
Desmopressin, for von Willebrand disease, 1130
Dexamethasone
   for altitude sickness, 553
   for meningitis, 1223
   for typhoid fever, 654
Dexamethasone suppression test, for Cushing's syndrome, 884-885
Diabetes insipidus, 867-868, 867f, 868f
Diabetes mellitus, 916-920
   ADA definition of, 916
   clinical presentation of, 916-917, 916f-919f
   laboratory tests for, 917, 919-920
   treatment of, 920
   type 1, 916
   type 2, 916
Diabetic retinopathy, 292, 292f, 916, 916f, 917f
Dialysis. *See also* Hemodialysis; Peritoneal dialysis.
   for chronic renal failure, 699
Diaphragm
   abnormalities of, 366, 366f-368f
   contraceptive, 789, 790f, 791
Diascopy, 8, 8f

Dicloxacillin, for folliculitis, 139
Diet(s)
   for diabetic patient, 920
   gluten-free, for celiac disease, 583, 583f
   low-fat soy protein, for nephrotic syndrome, 708
   nonhydrogenated unsaturated fat, for angina pectoris, 384
   sodium-restricted, for ascites, 621
Diffuse esophageal spasm, 570, 570f
Diffuse idiopathic skeletal hyperostosis (DISH), 1017, 1017f, 1018f
Digit(s). *See* Finger(s); Toe(s).
Dilated cardiomyopathy, 414, 414f, 415f
   treatment of, 415-416, 416f
Diphenhydramine, for dystonia, 203
Diphtheria, 1223-1224, 1223f, 1224f
Diplococcus, Gram-positive, 1140, 1141f
Direct immunofluorescence, of porphyria cutanea tarda, 45, 45f
Discoid eczema, 26, 27f
Discoid lupus erythematosus, 960, 960f
Discoloration, nail, drug-induced, 79, 80f
Disease-modifying drugs, for rheumatoid arthritis, 956
Disseminated intravascular coagulation, 60, 1120-1121, 1120f, 1121f
Distal interphalangeal joint
   osteoarthritis of, 949, 950f
   rheumatic disorders of, 932f
Diuretics
   for ascites, 621
   for chronic renal failure, 699
Diverticular disease
   colonic appearance of, 593, 593f
   imaging studies of, 593, 593f, 594f
   treatment of, 593-594, 594f, 595f
Diverticulitis, 593
   treatment of, 594, 594f, 595f
Diverticulosis, 593
Diverticulum
   colonic, 593
   hemorrhage of, 594, 594f, 595f
   Meckel's, 585, 585f
   Zenker's, 560, 560f
Doll's eye reflex, in progressive supranuclear palsy, 194, 195f
Donovanosis (granuloma inguinale), 760-761, 760f, 761f
Dowager's hump, in osteoporosis, 1031, 1031f
Down syndrome, 240-241, 240f
Doxycycline
   for Lyme disease, 1045
   for syphilis, 760
   for tick-borne relapsing fever, 1228
Drainage
   bronchoscopic, of lung abscess, 531
   surgical
      for cavernous sinus thrombosis, 221
      for sinusitis, 324
Dressler's syndrome, 393-394
Drug(s). *See also named drug or drug group.*
   adverse reactions to, cutaneous, 47-48, 47f, 48f
Drug users, injection in, endocarditis and, 406, 406f
   causes of, 407
Drug-eluting stent, 386f
Drug-induced asthma, 485
Drug-induced nail discoloration, 79, 80f
Duchenne's muscular dystrophy, 233, 234f
Dumb-bell dermoid, 103
Dupuytren's contracture, 1003, 1004f
Dyshidrotic eczema, 27

Index

Dysplasia, cervical, 802-803, 803f, 804f
Dysplastic nevus syndrome, 95, 95f
Dystonia, 202-203, 203f
Dysuria, evaluation of, 794f

E

Ear(s). *See also specific part.*
    anatomy of, 304, 304f
    examination of, 304, 304f-307f
Eaton-Lambert syndrome, in lung
        carcinoma, 494
Ebstein's anomaly, 453, 453f, 545f
Eccrine hidradenoma, 101, 102f
Eccrine hidrocystoma, 100, 101f
    of eyelid, 280, 280f
Eccrine poroma, 100-101, 101f
Echinococcal hepatic cyst, 635, 636f
Echinococcosis, hepatic, 635, 636f,
        637, 637f
Echinococcus granulosus
    life cycle of, 635, 636f
    protoscolex of, 635, 636f
Echocardiography, 375, 376f, 377, 377f
    Doppler, 375, 377f
    of anomalous pulmonary artery venous
            connection, 445f
    of aortic regurgitation, 401, 402f
    of aortic stenosis, 400, 400f
    of atrial myxoma, 458f
    of atrial septal defect, 442, 443f
    of Ebstein's anomaly, 453, 454f
    of hypertrophic cardiomyopathy,
            417-418, 418f
    of left ventricular hypertrophy, 479, 479f
    of mitral regurgitation, 397, 397f
    of mitral valve abnormality, 375, 377f
    of patent ductus arteriosus, 453, 455f
    of pericarditis, 422, 423f
    of restrictive cardiomyopathy, 416, 416f
    of rheumatic fever, 1212, 1213f
    of tetralogy of Fallot, 449f
    of transposition of great arteries, 452f
    of tricuspid regurgitation, 402f
    of ventricular septal defect, 447f
    stress testing in, 377
        high-risk and low-risk, characterization
                of, 378t
        two-dimensional transthoracic imaging
                in, 375, 376f
Ectopic pregnancy, 844-845, 844f, 845f
Ectropion, 275, 275f
Eczema, 25, 25f
    discoid (nummular), 26, 27f
    hand (dyshidrotic), 27
Eczematous dermatoses
    endogenous, 25-27, 25f-27f
    exogenous, 27-28, 27f-32f, 30-32
    history and location of, 6t
Edema, 5b
    cerebral, high-altitude, 552
    facial, tooth abscess causing, 337, 337f
    in nephrotic syndrome, 707, 707f
    joint, testing for, 934, 934f
    pedal, in cirrhosis patients, 617
    pulmonary
        cardiogenic, 413, 413f
        high-altitude, 552
Effusion
    pericardial, 423, 424f
    pleural. *See Pleural effusion.*
Eggshell calcification, in sarcoidosis, 515, 515f
Ehlers-Danlos syndrome, 1028-1029,
        1028f, 1029f
Ehrlichia, genogroups of, 1164t

Ehrlichiosis, human granulocytic, 1163-1165,
        1163f, 1164t
Elbow, rheumatic disorders of, 1007-1009,
        1007f, 1008f
Electrical burns, 158-159, 159f
Electrocardiography
    abnormalities of, 372, 373f
    during pacing, 441f
    exercise, 374-375, 375f
    normal, 370, 370f
    of accelerated idioventricular rhythm, 434f
    of atrial fibrillation, 429f
    of atrial flutter, 430f
    of atrial septal defect, 442f
    of atrioventricular blocks, 437f-439f
    of Brugada syndrome, 435f
    of Ebstein's anomaly, 453, 454f
    of heart failure, in hypothyroid patient,
            871, 873f
    of hypertrophic cardiomyopathy, 418, 419f
    of mitral valve stenosis, 396, 396f
    of multifocal atrial tachycardia, 427f
    of paroxysmal atrial tachycardia, 427f
    of pericarditis, 422-423, 423f
    of pulmonary embolism, 554-555, 554f
    of pulmonary hypertension, 550, 550f
    of sick sinus syndrome, 435, 435f
    of tetralogy of Fallot, 449f
    of torsades de pointes, 433f
    of ventricular fibrillation, 434f
    of ventricular tachycardia, 432f
    of Wolff-Parkinson-White syndrome, 436f
    position of leads and electrodes in, 370, 371f
    systematic approach to, 370-372, 372f
Electrodesiccation/curettage, for basal cell
        carcinoma, 87
Electroencephalography, of brain, 172,
        173f, 174f
    in Creutzfeldt-Jakob disease, 197, 197f
Electron beam therapy, for non-Hodgkin's
        lymphoma, 1105
Elephantiasis, 1186, 1187f
Embolism
    characteristics of, 177t
    pulmonary, 554-555, 554f-557f, 557
    renal artery, causes of, 719
    systemic, 393
Embolization, distal, for aortic dissection,
        473, 474f
Embolus, cholesterol, in renal artery
        stenosis, 719
Embryonal cell carcinoma, 750
Emergency postcoital contraception, 789, 792
Emery-Dreifuss muscular dystrophy, 233
Emmetropia, examination of, 252, 256f
Emphysema, 488
    severe diffuse, 366, 366f, 490f-491f
Empyema, 536-537, 537f
    extradural, 224, 224f
Encephalitis, 222-224
    toxoplasmic, HIV-related, 1149, 1151f
    treatment of, 223-224
    workup for, 223, 223f, 224f
Enchondroma, 1047, 1048f
Endocarditis
    infective
        causes of, 407-408
        clinical presentation of, 406, 406f, 407f
        laboratory tests for, 408, 408f
        types of, 406
    Libman-Sacks, 963, 963f
Endocrine disorder(s). *See also specific disorder,
        e.g., Hypopituitarism.*
    in antiphospholipid antibody syndrome, 965

Endometrial cancer, 813, 813f, 814f
Endometrial polyps, 812, 812f
Endometriosis, 787-788, 787f, 788f
Endoscopic retrograde
        cholangiopancreatography
    of cholecystitis, 647, 647f
    of pancreatic carcinoma, 613, 615f
Engagement, in labor, 837
Entamoeba histolytica, 1166f, 1167f
Entamoeba histolytica liver abscess, 633, 633f
Enterobiasis, 1181, 1181f
Enthesitis, 988, 988f
Entropion, 274, 274f
Environmental trauma, 155-159, 155f-159f
Eosinophilic dermatoses, 49-53, 49f-53f
Ephelides. *See Freckles.*
Epiblepharon, 274, 274f
Epicondylitis, 1007-1008, 1007f, 1008f
Epidermal inclusion cyst
    of eyelid, 279, 279f
    vulvar, 798, 799f
Epidermal nevus, 84, 84f
Epidermis, structure and function of, 2, 2f, 3f
Epidermoid cyst, 102, 103f
Epidermolysis bullosa, differential diagnosis
        of, 6t
Epidermolysis bullosa acquisita, 18, 18f
Epididymitis, 748, 748f, 749f, 749t
Epidural abscess, cranial, 224
Epiglottitis, 348, 348f
Episcleral telangiectasis, in Sturge-Weber
        syndrome, 229, 230f
Episiotomy, 837
    repair of, 840f
Epistaxis (nosebleed), 320
    treatment of, 320f, 321, 321f
Epithelial hyperplasia, focal (Heck's disease),
        331, 331f
Epithelial inclusion cyst, conjunctival, 267, 267f
Epithelial lesions, of genitalia, 765-766,
        765f, 766f
Epstein-Barr virus (EBV)
    Burkitt's lymphoma associated with,
            1102-1103
    in infectious mononucleosis, 1214
    patterns of serology of, in acute infection,
            1215, 1215f
    structure of, 1214f
Erosion, skin, 5b
Erysipelas, 134, 134f
    of outer ear, 314
Erythema, 5b
    butterfly, in systemic lupus erythematosus,
            960, 960f
    of tympanic membrane, 316, 316f
    tooth abscess causing, 337, 337f
Erythema annulare centrifugum, 39, 39f
Erythema infectiosum (fifth disease),
        115-116, 115f
Erythema migrans, of Lyme disease, 1044, 1044f
Erythema multiforme, 36-37, 36f
    differential diagnosis of, 37
Erythema nodosum, 41, 41f
    secondary to sarcoidosis, 514, 514f
Erythematous plaques, sarcoidosis and, 514, 515f
Erythrasma, 137, 137f, 138f, 758, 758f
Erythrocyte morphology, in peripheral blood
        smears, review of, 1068, 1070f
Erythrocyte sedimentation rate, as inflammatory
        marker, 944
Erythroderma, Sézary syndrome causing,
        1103, 1104f
Erythroplakia, oral, 339
Erythropoietin, for chronic renal failure, 699

Erythropoietin therapy, for multiple myeloma, 1110
Esophagitis
  Candida, 1190f
  HIV-related, 1155
Esophagus
  Barrett's, 564, 564f
  carcinoma of, 565-566, 565f, 566f
  motility disorder of, 568-569, 568f
  spasms in, 570, 570f
  varices in, 571, 571f
  webs and rings of, 567, 567f
  Zenker's diverticulum of, 560, 560f
Esotropia
  accommodative, 270
  congenital, 270, 270f
  intermittent, 270, 270f
  paralytic, 270, 271f, 272f
Estrogen receptors, in breast cancer, 826
Estrogen-deficient (atrophic) vulvovaginitis, 797, 797f
Etanercept, for rheumatoid arthritis, 956
Ethambutol, for tuberculosis, 543
Etonogestrel implant, contraceptive, 789, 792
Etretinate, for oral lichen planus, 35
Eventration, diaphragmatic, 366, 368f
Everest nails, 552, 552f
Ewing's sarcoma, 1047, 1048f
Exanthema subitum (roseola), 121, 121f
Exanthematous drug reaction, 47, 47f
Excoriation, 5b
Exenatide, for diabetes mellitus, 920
Exercise electrocardiography, 374-375
  choice of protocols in, 375
  contraindications to, 374
  indications for, 374
  interpretation of, 375, 375f
Exercise-induced asthma, 485
Exostosis, subungual, 82, 82f
External ear canal
  hematoma of, 304, 307f
  wax in, removal of, 304, 305f, 306f
Extradural empyema, 224, 224f
Extrasphincteric fistula, 607
Extremity(ies). *See also specific part.*
  ischemic ulceration of, 459, 459f
  lower, cutaneous sensory innervation of, 1014f, 1015f
Eye(s). *See also specific part.*
  anatomy of, 250, 250f, 251f
  appearance of, in cirrhosis patients, 616
  disorders of. *See specific disorder, e.g.,* Cataracts.
  examination of, 252, 252f-258f, 257
  structure of, 250, 250f
Eyelid(s)
  apocrine hidrocystoma of, 280, 280f
  capillary hemangioma of, 281, 281f
  chalazion of, 284, 284f
  cutaneous horn of, 278, 278f
  cylindroma of, 281, 281f
  dermoid cyst of, 280, 280f
  eccrine hidrocystoma of, 280, 280f
  epidermal inclusion cyst of, 279, 279f
  freckles surrounding, 283, 283f
  hordeolum of, 284-285, 284f, 285f
  keratoacanthoma of, 279, 279f
  malignancies of, 286-287, 286f, 287f
  melanocytic nevi of, 283, 283f
    congenital, 284, 284f
  milia of, 280, 280f
  molluscum contagiosum lesion of, 267, 268f, 285, 285f
  neurofibroma of, 282, 282f
  nevus flammeus surrounding, 281, 281f

Eyelid(s) *(Continued)*
  pyogenic granuloma of, 282, 282f
  seborrheic keratosis of, 278-279, 278f, 279f
  squamous papilloma of, 278, 278f
  verruca vulgaris of, 285
  xanthelasma of, 282, 283f

F

Facial edema, tooth abscess causing, 337, 337f
Facial features
  in acromegaly, 859, 861f
  in postpubertal hypogonadism, 908, 908f
Facial hair, female, 910, 910f
Facial lesions, mimicking lupus, 962t
Facial myokymia, vs. blepharospasm, 277t
Facial seizure, vs. blepharospasm, 277t
Facial spasm, 1220, 1220f
Facial synkinesis, vs. blepharospasm, 277t
Facial telangiectasis, 975, 975f
Facial tic, vs. blepharospasm, 277t
Facioscapulohumeral muscular dystrophy, 233
Factor V Leiden, 1122
Factor VIII concentrates
  for hemophilia A, 1128
  for von Willebrand disease, 1130
Factor IX concentrates, for hemophilia B, 1128
Famiciclovir
  for genital herpes, 764
  for herpes simplex virus infection, 119
Familial atypical multiple mole melanoma syndrome, 95, 95f
Familial polyposis syndrome, 596, 596f
Fasciitis, necrotizing, 136-137, 136f, 137f
Fasciotomy, for rattlesnake bites, 152, 152f
Fasting hypoglycemia, 921
Fat bodies, oval, in nephrotic syndrome, 708, 708f
Fat pad biopsy, for amyloidosis, 711, 713f
Febrile neutrophilic dermatosis, acute (Sweet's syndrome), 49-50, 49f, 50f
Felty's syndrome, 1131, 1131f
Femoral hernia, 586, 586f
Femur, osteomyelitis of, 1042f, 1043f
Ferrous sulfate, for iron deficiency anemia, 1080
Fetal blood sampling, 836f
Fetal descent, during labor, 837
Fetal karyotype, 834f
Fetal monitoring, during labor, 836f
Fetal tachycardia, 836f
Fetal vertex positions, common, 835f
Fetor hepaticus, in cirrhosis, 616
Fetus
  at 12 weeks gestation, 834f
  at 16 weeks gestation, 834f
  at 24 weeks gestation, 835f
  ultrasound growth chart of, 833f
Fever patterns, malarial, 1159, 1159f
Fexofenadine, for Peyronie's disease, 774
Fibrocystic breast disease, 821-822, 822f, 823f
Fibroelastoma, papillary, 457f
Fibroepithelial polyp, 105, 105f
Fibroid(s), uterine, 809-811, 809f-811f
Fibroma
  cardiac, 457f
  oral, 328, 328f
  periungual, 83, 83f
Fibromyalgia, 998-999, 998f, 999f
  tender points in, 998f
Fibrosarcoma, 1047
Fibrosis
  idiopathic pulmonary, 512-513, 512f
  retroperitoneal, causing renal failure, 727, 727f

Fibrous hyperplasia, denture-associated, 328, 329f
Fifth disease (erythema infectiosum), 115-116, 115f
Filariasis, 1186-1188, 1186t, 1187f
Filiform wart, 122, 122f
Fine-needle aspiration biopsy, of cholangiocarcinoma, 648, 649f
Finger(s)
  clubbing of
    in lung carcinoma, 494, 494f
    in primary biliary cirrhosis, 624, 625f
  gangrene of, in CREST syndrome, 976, 976f
  necrosis of, in Raynaud's syndrome, 971, 971f
  osteoarthritis of, 949, 950f
  sausage, 932f, 974f
  trigger, 1004-1005, 1005f
Fire ant lesions, 149, 149f
Fissure, 5b
  anal, 605, 605f
Fistula, 606f, 607
  classification of, 607
Flat wart, 122
Flea bites, 148, 148f
Flexible fiberoptic bronchoscopy, of bronchogenic carcinoma, 495, 496f
Flexor tendons, shrunken, in amyloidosis, 711, 711f
Flow-volume curve
  during expiration, 483f
    with increasing efforts, 484f
  during inspiration, 483f
  in patient with restrictive ventilatory defect, 484f
  in patient with upper airway obstruction, 484f
Flow-volume relationships, definition of, 482
Fluconazole
  for fungal infections, 1155
  for sporotrichosis, 1208
Fluid overload, in acute renal failure, 691, 691f, 694f
Fluorescent in situ hybridization (FISH), 786, 786f
  in breast cancer, 826, 827f
Flushing, cutaneous, carcinoid tumor and, 667, 668f
Focal epithelial hyperplasia (Heck's disease), 331, 331f
Follicular conjunctivitis, toxic, 267, 268f
Folliculitis, 139, 139f
Foot
  ischemic, 459, 459f
  osteoarthritis of, 949, 951f
Foot ulcers, in diabetes mellitus, 917, 919f
Forced expiratory flow
  definition of, 482
  determination of, 483f
Forced expiratory volume, 483f
  definition of, 482
Forced vital capacity, definition of, 482
Forceps delivery, 841, 842f
Forearm entrapment regions, 1003f
Forefoot, rheumatoid, 952f
Forschheimer spots, of rubella, 127, 127f
Foscarnet, for acyclovir-resistant HSV infection, 119
Fourth nerve palsy, strabismus resulting from, 270, 272f
Fracture(s), 1051-1057. *See also specific type of fracture.*
  ankle, 1023-1024, 1024f
  cervical vertebrae, 1056, 1056f
  long bone, 1052-1053, 1053f-1055f

Fracture(s) (Continued)
lumbar vertebrae, 1057, 1057f
assessment of, 1032f
pathologic, 1051, 1051f
pelvic, 1051-1052, 1052f
stress, 1051, 1051f
thoracic vertebrae, 1057, 1057f
Fracture-dislocation
Galeazzi, 1052-1053, 1054f
Monteggia, 1052, 1054f
Framboesia tropica (yaws), 141-142, 141f, 142f
Francisella tularensis. See also Tularemia.
life cycle of, 1230f
Freckles, 91, 91f
around eyelids, 283, 283f
Hutchinson's melanotic, 97, 97f, 98, 99f
of eyelid, 286, 286f
Friedreich's ataxia, 214, 214f, 215f
Frostbite, 157-158, 157f
treatment of, 158, 158f
Fungal infection(s), 1189-1210. See also specific
infection, e.g., Candidiasis.
Fungal vulvovaginitis, 795, 795f
Fungus ball (aspergilloma), 1191
treatment of, 1193
Funnel chest (pectus excavatum), 358, 358f
Furosemide, for ascites, 621
Furuncle (boil), 139-140, 139f, 140f
Furunculosis, of outer ear, 314
Fusobacterium nucleatum, Gram stain of, 146f

G
Gaisböck's syndrome, 1112
Gait disturbance, in Parkinson's disease,
200, 200f
Galeazzi fracture-dislocation, 1052-1053,
1054f
Gallbladder, inflammation of, 646-647,
646f, 647f
Gallstone(s), 644-645, 644f, 645f
pancreatitis due to, 610
Gallstone ileus, 578, 581f
Ganglion cyst, of wrist, 1004, 1004f, 1005f
Gangrene
Clostridium perfringens causing, 1222f
digital, in CREST syndrome, 976, 976f
in systemic lupus erythematosus, 960, 960f
Gardner's syndrome, 598-599, 598f, 599f
colonoscopy in, 599
protein truncation testing for, 599
Gastrectomy, for gastric carcinoma, 576
Gastric carcinoma, 576, 576f, 577f
Gastrinoma (Zollinger-Ellison syndrome),
671, 672f
Gastritis, 572-573
Helicobacter pylori in, 572, 573f
NSAID-induced, 572, 572f
stress, prophylaxis for, 573
Gastroenteritis, viral, 650, 650f, 651f
characteristics of, 650t
treatment of, 654
Gastroesophageal reflux, 561, 561f
Gastrointestinal disorders
arthritis associated with, 989t
endocrine-associated, 667, 667t, 668f-670f
in antiphospholipid antibody syndrome, 965
Gastrointestinal parasite(s), 1166t
Gastrointestinal zygomycosis, 1209
Gaze, diagnostic positions of, 251f
Genetic testing, for hemochromatosis, 627
Genital herpes. See also Herpes simplex virus
(HSV) entries.
HSV-1, 764
HSV-2, 118, 119f, 764, 765f, 1187f

Genital wart (condyloma acuminatum), 122,
123f, 758, 758f, 785f
Genitalia
ambiguous, 903, 904f
cutaneous lesions of
algorithm for evaluation of, 755f
differential diagnosis of, 754t-755t
epithelial lesions of, 765-766, 765f, 766f
infectious diseases of, 758-764. See also specific
infection.
inflammatory dermatoses of, 756-757,
756f, 757f
male, pseudoprecocious puberty and,
903, 903f
Geographic tongue (benign migratory glossitis),
326, 326f, 339
German measles (rubella), 127-128, 127f, 128f
Gianotti-Crosti syndrome, 130, 131f
Giant cell arteritis, 58, 59f, 982-983, 982f, 983f
Giant cell tumor, 1047, 1049f
of tendon sheath, 106, 106f
Giant papillary conjunctivitis, 261, 262f
Giardia lamblia, 1167f
Giardiasis, 1167, 1167f
Gigantism, pituitary, 859, 863f
Gingiva
amalgam tattoo of, 334-335, 334f
condyloma acuminatum of, 328f
hyperplasia of, 329, 330f
nodules of, 329, 329f
Gingivostomatitis, herpetic, 339, 339f
Glaucoma
characteristics of, 297t
closed-angle, 299, 299f, 300f
initial management of, 300f
narrow-angle, differential diagnosis of, 263t
open-angle, 198f, 297-298, 297f
Gleason classification, of prostate cancer,
743, 743f
Glomerulonephritis, 701-702
lupus, 701, 701f
membranoproliferative, 701, 702f
necrotizing, in Wegener's granulomatosis,
517, 517f
poststreptococcal, 702, 703f
Glomerulus, 676, 676f, 677f
Glomus tumor, 108-109, 109f
subungual, 82, 83f
Glossitis
atrophic, Candida, 1189f
benign migratory (geographic tongue), 326,
326f, 339
median rhomboid, 326, 327f
Glossopyrosis (burning tongue), 339
Glucagonoma, 673, 673f
Glucocorticosteroids, for Addison's disease,
889, 889f
Gluten-free diet, for celiac disease, 583, 583f
Glycemic index, 920
Goiter, multinodular, 349, 350f
Goldmann applanation tonometer, 257f
Gonadal abnormalities, 900-901, 900f, 901f
Gonadotropin deficiency
in hypopituitarism, 854
testing for, 856-857
Gonioscopy, 257, 258f
Gonococcal urethritis, 767-768, 767f, 768t
Gonococcemia, 767f
Gonorrhea, Gram-stained smear of, 1141f
Goodpasture's syndrome, 520-521, 520f, 521f
Gorlin's sign, 1028
Gottron's papules, in dermatomyositis, 969, 969f
Gout, 935t, 994-995, 994f, 995f
acute, 933f

Gower's maneuver, 233, 235f
Gram stain, 1140-1141, 1140f, 1141f
Gram-negative rods, 1140-1141
Gram-positive Diplococcus, 1140, 1141f
Gram-positive rods, 1141, 1141f
Gram-positive Staphylococcus, 1140, 1140f
Gram-positive Streptococcus, 1140, 1140f
Granular cell epulis, congenital, 325, 326f
Granular cell layer (stratum granulosum),
of skin, 2
Granulocytic ehrlichiosis, human, 1163-1165,
1163f, 1164t
Granulocytopoiesis, 1060-1061,
1064f, 1065f
Granuloma
in Crohn's disease, 589, 589f
pyogenic, 108, 109f
of eyelid, 282, 282f
oral, 329, 329f
periungual, 82, 82f, 140f
tuberculosis, 545f
ulcerative, traumatic, 327, 327f
Granuloma annulare, 42, 42f
Granuloma gravidarum, mandibular,
329, 329f
Granuloma inguinale (donovanosis),
760-761, 760f, 761f
Granulomatosis
allergic, 56, 58f, 519-520, 520f
lymphomatoid, 522, 522f
Wegener's. See Wegener's granulomatosis.
Granulomatous arthritis, 1040-1041, 1041f
Granulomatous dermatoses, 41-42, 41f, 42f
Graves' disease, 875, 875f, 876f
Graves' ophthalmopathy, 236t
Great arteries, transposition of, 450-451,
451f-453f
Greenstick fracture, 1053, 1055f
Grey Turner's sign, in acute pancreatitis, 608,
608f
Grover's disease, 24, 24f
Growth hormone deficiency
in hypopituitarism, 854, 855f
testing for, 856-857
Guillain-Barré syndrome, 211-212, 211f, 236t
Gut hormone tumor syndromes, 673, 673f
Guttate hypomelanosis, idiopathic, 63, 63f
Guttate psoriasis, 33, 33f
Gynecomastia
diagnosis of, 912, 913f-915f
history and physical examination of, aspects
of, 914b
hormones causing, 912, 912f
pathologic, causes of, 912, 913t
pubertal, bilateral persistent, 915f

H
Hacek organisms, 408
Haemophilus influenzae
cellulitis associated with, 134
epiglottitis associated with, 348, 348f
in meningitis, 222
Hair, diseases of, 67-71, 67f-71f. See also specific
disease.
Hair follicle, normal, 66, 66f, 67f
Hair growth cycle, 66
Hair thinning, hereditary, 67-68, 67f, 68f
Hairy cell leukemia, 1106, 1106f
Hairy leukoplakia, oral, 330-331, 330f, 331f
Hallux abductovalgus (bunion deformity),
1026, 1026f
Halo nevus, 94, 94f
Hamartoma, Peutz-Jeghers, 597, 597f
Hammer toes, 1026, 1026f

Hand(s)
  deformities of, 936f
  osteoarthritis of, 933f, 949, 951f
  rheumatic disorders of, 1001-1007. *See also specific disorder, e.g.,* Dupuytren's contracture.
Hand eczema, 27
Hand-foot-and-mouth disease, 125-126, 125f, 126f
Handwriting sample, of patient with Parkinson's disease, 200, 201f
Hangman's fracture, 1056, 1056f
Hansen's disease, 1218-1219, 1218f, 1219f
Hard palate, verruciform xanthoma of, 328, 328f
Hasimoto's thyroiditis, 355, 356f
Head louse *(Pediculus capitis),* 144, 144f
Hearing loss, 308, 310b
  conductive vs. sensorineural, 308t
  evaluation of, 310f
  Rinne test for, 308, 308f
  Weber test for, 308, 309f
Heart. *See also* Cardiac; Cardio- *entries.*
  chambers of, hypertrophy of, 372
  congenital disease of. *See* Congenital heart disease.
  congestive failure of, 409-412. *See also* Congestive heart failure.
  ischemic disease of, 382-394.
    See also Angina pectoris; Myocardial infarction.
  valvular disease of, 395-405. *See also under specific cardiac valve.*
  surgery for, 404, 405f
Heart rate, determination of, 370
Heart rhythm, determination of, 370
Heart-lung transplantation, for pulmonary hypertension, 551
Heberden's nodules, 950f, 994f
Heck's disease, 331, 331f
Helicobacter pylori
  in gastritis, 572, 573f
  in peptic ulcer disease, 574
HELLP syndrome, 1117-1118, 1118f
Hemangioendothelioma, infantile, 108, 108f
Hemangioma
  capillary, 108, 108f
    lobular, 108, 109f
    of eyelid, 281, 281f
  cavernous, 108, 109f
  juvenile, 108, 108f
Hematoma
  of external ear canal, 304, 307f
  subdural, 183, 183f
Hematopoiesis, 1060, 1060f, 1061f
  definition of, 1060
Hemifacial spasm, vs. blepharospasm, 277t
Hemochromatosis, 626-627, 626f-628f
Hemodialysis system, components of, 695f, 696
Hemoglobinuria
  paroxysmal cold, 1134, 1134f, 1134t
  paroxysmal nocturnal, 1132-1133, 1132f
Hemolysis, immune-related, following transfusion, 1060, 1063f
Hemolytic anemia, autoimmune, 1074f, 1075-1076, 1075f
  serologic features of, 1134t
Hemolytic-uremic syndrome, 1118-1119, 1118f, 1119f
Hemophilia, 1126-1128, 1127f
  differential diagnosis of, 1127t
Hemophilia A, 1127-1128
Hemophilia B, 1128

Hemorrhage
  alveolar, in Goodpasture's syndrome, 520, 520f
  diverticular, 594, 594f, 595f
  postpartum, 837
  splinter, of nails, 79, 79f
  subarachnoid, 180-181, 180f
  subconjunctival, 262f
  variceal, 571
Hemorrhagic blebs
  at rattlesnake bite site, 151f
  frostbite with, 157f
Hemorrhoids, 603, 603f, 604f
Hemostasis, primary, schema for, 1126f
Henoch-Schönlein purpura, 55, 55f, 986-987, 986f
Heparin
  for antiphospholipid antibody syndrome, during pregnancy, 966
  for disseminated intravascular coagulation, 1121
  low-molecular-weight, for thrombosis, 1124
Heparin infusion, for pulmonary embolism, 557
Hepatic. *See also* Liver *entries.*
Hepatic cyst
  echinococcal, 635, 636f
  vs. hepatic abscess, 633, 634f
Hepatic schistosomiasis, 1172, 1175f
Hepatitis
  autoimmune, 643
  Epstein-Barr virus-associated, 1215, 1215f
  viral, 637-642
Hepatitis A, 637-638, 637f
  course of, 638, 638f
Hepatitis B, 638-639, 639f
  chronic, phase of, 639, 640f
Hepatitis B vaccine, for HIV-infected patients, 1152
Hepatitis C, 640-641, 641f, 642f
  cirrhosis due to, 616f
  HIV-related, 1157
Hepatitis D, 642, 642f
Hepatocellular carcinoma, 631-632, 631f, 632f
Hepatomegaly, in cirrhosis, 616
Hepatorenal syndrome, 622-623, 622f
Hepatosplenic candidiasis, 1189f
Herald patch, in pityriasis rosea, 130, 131f
Hereditary hair thinning, 67-68, 67f, 68f
Hernia
  Bochdalek, 366, 368f
  femoral, 586, 586f
  hiatal, 562, 562f
  inguinal, direct and indirect, 586, 586f
  Morgagni, 366, 368f
  umbilical, ascites with, 620, 620f
Herpangina, 338, 338f
Herpes, genital
  HSV-1, 764
  HSV-2, 118, 119f, 764, 765f, 1187f
Herpes simplex virus (HSV), 117-118, 117f
Herpes simplex virus (HSV) encephalitis, 223, 223f, 224f
Herpes simplex virus (HSV) infection, 118-119
  primary and secondary, 118, 118f, 119f
Herpes simplex virus (HSV) stomatitis, 339, 339f
Herpes zoster virus (HZV) infection, 119-120, 120f, 121f
  HIV-related, 1149, 1149f
Hiatal hernia, 562, 562f
Hib vaccine, for HIV-infected patients, 1152
Hidradenitis suppurativa, 52-53, 52f
  differential diagnosis of, 52
Hidradenoma, eccrine, 101, 102f

Hidrocystoma
  apocrine, of eyelid, 280, 280f
  eccrine, 100, 101f
High-altitude cerebral edema, 552
High-altitude pulmonary edema, 552
Highly active antiretroviral therapy (HAART), for HIV infection, 1153, 1153f, 1154f
Hill's sign, 401
Hips, osteoarthritis of, 949, 950f
Hirschberg light reflex method, 252, 252f
Hirsutism, 910-911, 910f, 911f
  in polycystic ovary syndrome, 817, 818f
Histiocytosis X, 1135-1136, 1135f, 1136f
Histoplasmosis, 1194-1197
  clinical presentation of, 1194-1195
  differential diagnosis of, 1195
  endemic distribution of, 1194, 1195f
  HIV-related, 1155-1156, 1156f
  imaging studies of, 1196, 1197f
  laboratory tests for, 1195-1196, 1196f
  treatment of, 1196-1197
HLA-B27-related uveitis, 295f
HLA-DQ8 gene, in celiac sprue, 583
Hodgkin's lymphoma, 1095, 1095f-1097f, 1098
  HIV-related, 1158
Hoffmann's sign, in multiple sclerosis, 207
Homograft valves, for valvular heart disease, 404, 405f
Honeycombing, in idiopathic pulmonary fibrosis, 512, 512f
Hookworm infestation, 1179, 1180f
Hordeolum (stye), 284-285, 284f, 285f
Hormonal events, in ovarian cycle, 776, 777f
Hormonal implants/injectables, as contraceptives, 789, 791-792
Hormonal therapy
  for breast cancer, 829
  for hypospadias, 772
  for renal cell carcinoma, 723
Hormone(s), causing gynecomastia, 912, 912f
Horner's syndrome, 301, 301f, 494
  neuroblastoma and, 245, 245f
Hospital-acquired (nosocomial) pneumonia, 528, 529f
Hot tub folliculitis, 139
Hot water immersion burns, 156f
Human bite, 146f
Human diploid cell vaccine, for rabies, 1237
Human granulocytic ehrlichiosis, 1163-1165, 1163f, 1164t
Human immunodeficiency virus (HIV), replication of, intervention in inhibition of, 1153, 1153f
Human immunodeficiency virus (HIV) infection, 1145-1158
  acute, 1145, 1145f, 1146f
  asymptomatic, 1145-1154
    management strategies for, 1152
  bacterial infections in, management of, 1156-1157, 1157f
  CD4 cells in, 1147
  clinical presentation of, 1148-1149, 1149f-1151f
  differential diagnosis of, 1147
  fungal infections in, management of, 1155-1156, 1155f, 1156f
  highly active antiretroviral therapy for, 1153, 1153f, 1154f
  laboratory tests for, 1148, 1148f, 1149t
  malignancies in, 1158
  opportunistic infections in, prophylaxis for, 1152-1153
  p24 antigen in, 1145, 1146f
  parasitic infections in, 1157-1158

Index

Human immunodeficiency virus (HIV) infection (Continued)
  pathogenesis of, 1147, 1147f, 1148f
  phases of, kinetics of, 1145f
  symptomatic, 1155-1158
  viral infections in, management of, 1157, 1158f
Human immunodeficiency virus-1 (HIV-1), 1145
  life cycle of, 1147f
Human immunodeficiency virus-1 (HIV-1) virion, 1146f
Human papillomavirus (HPV), causing warts, 121, 122, 122f
Human papillomavirus (HPV) infection, HIV-related, 1158, 1158f
Human rabies hyperimmune globulin, 1237
Hungry bones syndrome, 878
Hutchinson's melanotic freckle, 97, 97f, 98, 99f
  of eyelid, 286, 286f
Hutchinson's sign, in herpes zoster, 120, 120f
Hydatid disease
  hepatic, 635, 636f, 637, 637f
  renal, 716f
Hydatidiform mole, 852, 852f
Hydrocele, 745-746, 745f, 746f
  communicating vs. noncommunicating, 745
  transilluminated, 745, 746f
Hydrocephalus, normal-pressure, 242-243, 242f
Hydrochlorothiazide, for hypercalciuria, 736
Hydrocortisone, for Addisonian crisis, 889
Hydronephrosis, 727-728, 727f, 728f
21-Hydroxylase deficiency, in congenital adrenal hyperplasia, 903
Hydroxyzine
  for lichen sclerosis, 757
  for pruritus of chickenpox, 117
Hygroma, cystic, mediastinal, 361, 363f
Hymen
  imperforate, 776, 778f
  septate, 776, 779f
Hyperabduction maneuver, 1013f
Hyperabduction syndrome, 1012
Hyperaldosteronism, 891-892, 891f-893f
Hypercalcemia, 372, 373f
  causes of, 880, 882f
Hypercoagulable states, 1122-1125
  acquired, 1122-1123
  history of, 1122, 1123f
  inherited, 1122, 1124f
  laboratory tests for, 1124, 1125f
  treatment of, 1124-1125, 1125f
  workup for, 1123-1124
Hyperhomocysteinemia, 1122
Hyperkalemia, 372, 373f
Hyperkeratosis, 5b
Hyperlipidemia
  clinical presentation of, 923, 925f-927f
  definition of, 923
  diagnostic approach to, 924
  management of, 924
Hyperopia (farsightedness), examination of, 252, 256f
Hyperparathyroidism
  causes of, 880, 880t, 881f
  clinical presentation of, 880, 880f
  differential diagnosis of, 880, 882f
  imaging studies of, 882, 883f
  laboratory tests for, 882
  treatment of, 882-883
Hyperpigmentation, 5b
  drug-induced, 48, 48f
  in hemochromatosis, 626, 626f

Hyperprolactinemia, 854
  basic mechanisms in, 859, 860f
  testing for, 857
Hypersensitivity syndromes, 36-38, 36f-38f
Hypersensitivity vasculitis, 54-55, 54f, 55f
Hypertension, 478-479, 478f, 479f
  pulmonary, 549-551, 549f-551f
Hypertensive retinopathy, 292, 292f, 478, 478f
Hyperthyroidism
  causes of, 875
  clinical presentation of, 875, 875f, 876f
  imaging studies of, 876, 877f
  treatment of, 876-877
Hypertrophic cardiomyopathy, 417-418, 417f-419f
Hypertrophic osteoarthropathy, 1037, 1037f
Hypoalbuminemia, 878
  treatment of, 879
Hypoaldosteronism, 890
Hypocalcemia, 372, 373f, 878-879, 878f, 879f
Hypoglycemia, 921
Hypogonadism, 908
  laboratory evaluation of, 909f
Hypokalemia, 372, 373f
Hypomagnesemia, 878
  treatment of, 879
Hypomelanosis, guttate, 63, 63f
Hypopigmentation, 5b
Hypopituitarism
  causes of, 854-855, 855f-857f
  clinical presentation of, 854, 854f, 855f
  diagnostic tests of, 856, 858t
  differential diagnosis of, 855-856, 857f
  laboratory tests for, 856-857, 858f
  treatment of, 858
Hypospadias, 771-772
  forms of, 771f
  repair of, 772
Hypothalamo-pituitary-adrenal axis, in adrenocortical insufficiency, 887, 887f
Hypothermia, J or Osborne wave of, 158, 158f
Hypothyroidism
  causes of, 871
  clinical presentation of, 871, 871f-874f
  treatment of, 874
Hypoxemia (secondary polycythemia), 1111
Hysteroscopy, 785

I

Ibuprofen
  for Baker's cyst, 1021
  for exanthema subitum, 121
Ichthyosis, 14, 14f, 15f
Ichthyosis vulgaris, 14, 14f
Ileitis, Crohn's, 590f. See also Crohn's disease.
Ileum
  Meckel's diverticulum of, 585, 585f
  terminal
    cobblestoning of, 589, 590f
    perforating typhoid ulcer of, 652, 652f
Ileus
  gallstone, 578, 581f
  paralytic, 578, 581f
Iliac wing, fracture of, 1051, 1052f
Immune thrombocytopenia, 1114, 1116, 1116f
Immune-related hemolysis, following transfusion, 1060, 1063f
Immunocompromised host, toxoplasmosis in, 226, 227f, 228
Immunoglobulin(s), high-dose, for immune thrombocytopenic purpura, 1116
Immunoglobulin A (IgA) nephropathy, 706, 706f

Immunoglobulin G (IgG), intravenous, for Kawasaki disease, 129
Immunology, diagnostic, 1144, 1144f
Immunosuppressive agents, for autoimmune hemolytic anemia, 1076
Immunotherapy, for renal cell carcinoma, 723
Imperforate hymen, 776, 778f
Impetigo, 138, 138f
  of ear canal, 314
Impingement, of rotator cuff, 1010f
Impingement test, for rotator cuff syndrome, 1009, 1009f
Implantable cardioverter-defibrillator
  electrode configurations of, 433f
  for syncope, 476, 477f
  for torsades de pointes, 433, 434f
Inclusion cysts
  epidermal
    of eyelid, 279, 279f
    vulvar, 798, 799f
  epithelial, conjunctival, 267, 267f
Indomethacin, for Dressler's syndrome, 394
Infantile hemangioendothelioma, 108, 108f
Infantilism, sexual, differential diagnostic features of, 901t
Infarction, myocardial. See Myocardial infarction.
Infection(s). See also specific infection.
  anaerobic, 1221-1222, 1221f, 1221t, 1222f
  bacterial, 134-142, 135t
  dental and periodontal, 336-337, 336f, 337f
  diagnostic tests and procedures for, 1140-1144
  fungal, 1189-1210
  genital, 758-764
  hepatic, 633-642
  oral, 330-331, 330f, 331f
  protozoal, 1159-1175
  respiratory, 525-546
  viral, 115-133, 115t
Infectious mononucleosis, 1214-1215, 1214f, 1215f
Infective dermatitis, 30, 30f
Infective endocarditis
  causes of, 407-408
  clinical presentation of, 406, 406f, 407f
  laboratory tests for, 408, 408f
  types of, 406
Inferior vena cava filter, for deep vein thrombosis, 466, 467f
Infertility, endometriosis-associated, management of, 788
Inflammatory dermatoses, 39-40, 39f, 40f
  of genitalia, 756-757, 756f, 757f
Inflammatory myopathies, idiopathic, 969-970, 969f
Influenza, 531
  treatment of, 532
Inguinal hernia, direct and indirect, 586, 586f
Injection drug users, endocarditis in, 406, 406f
  causes of, 407
Insect stings, 148-149
  treatment of, 149
Insulin, for diabetes mellitus, 920
Insulin tolerance test, 856, 858f
Insulinoma, 921, 922f
Interdigital candidiasis, 1190f
Interphalangeal joint, osteoarthritis of, 949, 951f
Intersphincteric fistula, 607
Interstitial lung disease, 510-511, 510f, 511f
Interstitial nephritis, 709-710, 709f
Intestinal schistosomiasis, 1172
Intestines. See also Large bowel; Small bowel.
  inflammatory disease of. See Crohn's disease.
  normal gas pattern in, 578, 579f

Intestines *(Continued)*
  obstruction of, 578
    abdominal distention in, 578b
    diagnostic imaging of, 578, 579f-582f
    small bowel vs. large bowel, 578t
Intra-aortic balloon pump, principles of, 391-392, 391f
Intraconazole, for histoplasmosis, 1156
Intraepithelial neoplasia, of genitalia, 765, 765f
Intrathoracic herniation, of abdominal content, 366, 368f
Intrauterine devices, contraceptive, 789, 792
Intravenous pyelography, of hydronephrosis, 728
Intravenous urography
  of benign prostatic hyperplasia, 739, 739f
  of kidneys, 682, 682f, 683f
  of urinary stones, 734, 735f
Intumescent cataract, 259f
Iodine, radioactive, for hyperthyroidism, 876
Iontophoresis, for skin disorders, 13
Irinotecan, for colorectal carcinoma, 602
Iritis, differential diagnosis of, 263t
Iron deficiency anemia, 1070, 1071f
Iron index, measurement of, in hemochromatosis, 626, 627f
Irritant contact dermatitis, 27, 27f
Ischemia, mesenteric, 661-662, 661f, 662f
Ischemic foot, 459, 459f
Ischemic heart disease, 382-394. *See also* Angina pectoris; Myocardial infarction.
Isoniazid
  for tuberculosis, 543
  with rifampin, for granulomatous arthritis, 1041
Isopsoriasis, HIV-related, 1158
Isosorbide dinitrate, for achalasia, 569
Itraconazole
  for aspergilloma, 1193
  for aspergillosis, 1193
  for sporotrichosis, 1208
Ivermectin, for cutaneous larva migrans, 145
Ixodes scapularis, life cycle of, 1044, 1044f

J

J wave, of hypothermia, 158, 158f
Jaundice, in cirrhosis patients, 616, 616f
Jock itch (tinea cruris), 111, 111f
Joint(s). *See also specific joint.*
  aspiration or injection of, 945, 946f
    indications for, 947t
  bacterial entry into, 1038, 1038f. *See also* Bacterial arthritis.
  painful, in hemochromatosis, 626, 626f
  pathology of, rheumatic factor in, 942, 942t, 943f
  red-hot, 939t, 1039f
  small, swelling and fluctuation of, 934, 934f
Jones criteria, for diagnosis of rheumatic fever, 1211
Jugular vein, distention of, in congestive heart failure, 409, 411f
Junctional nevus, 93, 93f
Juvenile hemangioma, 108, 108f
Juvenile rheumatoid arthritis
  pauciarticular or oligoarticular form of, 957, 958f
  polyarticular form of, 959, 959f
  systemic or acute febrile, 957, 957f, 958f
Juxtaglomerular apparatus, 676f

K

Kaposi's sarcoma, 1137-1138, 1137f, 1138f
  HIV-related, 1149, 1150f, 1158
  of eyelid, 287, 287f
Kawasaki disease
  clinical manifestations of, 128, 129f
  electrographic abnormalities in, 129, 130f
  treatment of, 129-130
Kawasaki syndrome, 56, 58f
Kayser-Fleischer rings, in Wilson's disease, 202, 202f, 616
Keloid, 104, 105f
Keratin layer (stratum corneum), of skin, 2
Keratinization, disorders of, 14, 14f, 15f
Keratitis (corneal ulceration), 264, 264f, 265f
Keratoacanthoma, 90, 90f
  of eyelid, 279, 279f
  subungual, 82, 82f
Keratoderma, 14, 15f
Keratosis
  actinic (solar), 87-88, 88f
  seborrheic, 84, 84f
    of eyelid, 278-279, 278f, 279f
  smokeless tobacco, 327, 327f
Kidney(s). *See also* Nephr-; Renal *entries.*
  anatomy of, 676, 676f, 677f
  angiography of, 686, 686f
  computed tomography of, 684, 685f
  diabetic changes in, 917, 918f
  diagnostic tests and procedures involving, 678, 678t, 679f-681f, 680
  imaging of, 682
    first-choice techniques in, 682t
    risk of contrast nephrotoxicity in, 682b
  intravenous urography of, 682, 682f, 683f
  magnetic resonance angiography of, 684, 686f
  magnetic resonance imaging of, 684, 685f
  medullary sponge, 716f
  polycystic. *See* Polycystic kidney disease.
  radiography of, 682, 683f
  transplantation of, for chronic renal failure, 699
  tumors of, 722-724, 722f-724f
  ultrasonography of, 682, 684, 684f
Kiesselbach's plexus, epistaxis from, 320, 320f
Kissing nevus, 96, 96f
  of eyelid, 284, 284f
Klatskin tumor, 648, 649f
Klinefelter's syndrome, 900, 900f, 906, 906f
  classic triad in, 906
Knee, rheumatic disorders of, 1020-1022, 1021f, 1022f
Knock knees, in rickets, 1032, 1032f
Knuckle pad, 105, 105f
Koebner's phenomenon, in psoriasis, 33
Koilonychia, 78, 79f
Koplik's spots, in measles, 126, 127f
Krimsky light reflex method, 252, 252f
Kruckenberg tumor, 576, 576f
Kussmaul's sign, 392
Kyphosis, 936f
  scoliosis with, 1018, 1018f

L

Labia majora, sebaceous cysts on, 798, 799f
Labor
  abnormal, 841-842, 841f-843f
    operative delivery in, 841-842, 842f, 843f
    definition of, 841
  fetal monitoring during, 836f
  normal, 837, 838f-839f
  seven cardinal movements of, 837
  stages of, 837

Lachman test, for cruciate ligament tears, 936f
Lactation amenorrhea method, of contraception, 791
Lambert-Eaton myasthenic syndrome, 236t
Laparoscopic cholecystectomy, 644-645
Laparoscopic ovarian diathermy, 818, 818f
Laparoscopy, abdominal-pelvic, 785
Large bowel
  dilatation of, vs. small bowel dilatation, 578t
  obstruction of, 578, 582f
Large cell acanthoma, 84, 85f, 86
Large cell carcinoma, of lungs, 494. *See also* Lung carcinoma.
Larva migrans, cutaneous, 145, 145f
Laser therapy, for skin disorders, 10, 13f
Laser-assisted in situ keratomileusis (LASIK) surgery, technique of, 257, 258f
Latex agglutination, 1144, 1144f
Laurence-Moon-Biedl syndrome, 908
Left atrial hypertrophy, 372
Left bundle-branch block, 371, 372f
Left ventricular aneurysm, 394, 394f
Left ventricular heart failure, 409
Left ventricular hypertrophy, 372, 479, 479f
Leg, rheumatic disorders of, 1020-1022, 1021f, 1022f
Leg ulcers, in rheumatoid arthritis, 952, 954f
Legionella pneumophilia, 525. *See also* Pneumonia.
Leiomyoma
  pilar, 106, 107f
  uterine, 809-811, 809f-811f
Leishman-Donovan bodies, 1170f
Leishmaniasis, 1168-1169, 1169f, 1170f
  geographic distribution of, 1168f
Lenalidomide, for myelodysplastic syndrome, 1093
Lentigo, actinic (solar), 92, 92f
Lentigo maligna, 92, 92f
Lentigo maligna melanoma (Hutchinson freckle), 97, 97f, 98, 99f
  of eyelid, 286, 286f
Lentigo simplex, 91, 91f
LEOPARD syndrome, 65, 65f, 91, 91f
Leprosy (Hansen's disease), 1218-1219, 1218f, 1219f
Leptospirosis, 1235, 1235t
  anicteric form of, 1235
  icteric (Weil's syndrome), 1235, 1235f
Leser-Trélat sign, 84, 85f, 278
Leukemia, 1084-1092
  acute lymphoblastic, 1084-1085, 1084f, 1085f
  acute myelogenous, 1085-1087, 1086f, 1087f
  chronic lymphocytic, 1088-1090, 1088f, 1089f
    staging of, 1089-1090
  chronic myelogenous (myeloid), 1090, 1091f, 1092, 1092f
    characteristics of, 1113t
    phases in, definition of, 1091t
  hairy cell, 1106, 1106f
Leukocytoclastic vasculitis, 54-55, 54f, 55f
Leukoedema, oral, 326, 326f, 339
Leukoencephalopathy, progressive multifocal, 198, 198f
Leukokoria, resulting from retinoblastoma, 289, 289f
Leukoplakia, oral, 334, 334f, 339
  hairy-type, 330-331, 330f, 331f
Levothyroxine
  for hypothyroidism, 874
  for thyroiditis, 355
Lewy bodies, in substantia nigra, 194, 194f
Lhermitte's sign, in multiple sclerosis, 207
Libman-Sacks endocarditis, 963, 963f
Lice infestation, 144, 144f

Lichen planus, 35, 35f
  differential diagnosis of, 6t, 35
  of genitalia, 756, 756f, 757f
  of nails, 80, 80f
  oral, 331f, 332, 339
Lichen planus pemphigoid, 17, 17f
Lichen sclerosus, of genitalia, 756-757, 757f
Lichen simplex chronicus, 30, 30f
Lichenification, 5b
Lichenoid stomatitis, 332
Lidocaine injection
  for epicondylitis, 1008, 1008f
  for trigger finger, 1005, 1005f
LifeSite hemodialysis system, implantation
    of, 695f, 696
Lightning strikes, 158-159, 159f
Ligneous conjunctivitis, 267, 268f
Limbal dermoid, 267, 267f
Limb-girdle muscular dystrophy, 233
Lindsay nails, 78, 78f
Linea nigra, 832f
Linear IgA disease, 19-20, 20f
  oral, 332-333, 333f
Lipemia retinalis, 923, 927f
Lipodystrophy, HIV-related, 1149, 1151f
Lipoma, 104, 104f, 105f
  oral, 328, 329f
Lipoproteins, classes of, composition of,
    923, 925f
Listeria monocytogenes, 1225
  identification of, 1143f
Listeriosis, 1225, 1225f
  HIV-related, 1156
Little's area, epistaxis from, 320
Liver. *See also* Hepatic; Hepato- *entries.*
  cirrhosis of. *See* Cirrhosis.
  infections of, 633-642
  inflammatory disease of. *See* Hepatitis *entries.*
Liver abscess
  amebic, 633, 633f, 1165, 1165f
  causes of, 633, 633f
  differential diagnosis of, 633-634, 634f
  fungal, 633, 633f
  imaging studies of, 634-635, 635f
  pyogenic, 633
  treatment of, 635
Liver biopsy, 618
  in alpha$_1$-antitrypsin deficiency, 492, 493f
  needles for, 619f
  patterns of iron deposition in, 626, 627f
Liver metastasis, from carcinoid tumor,
    667, 669f
Liver palm (palmar erythema), in cirrhosis, 616f
Liver profile, in acute pancreatitis, 609
Liver transplantation
  for Budd-Chiari syndrome, 666
  for cirrhosis, 618
  for hepatorenal syndrome, 623
  for primary biliary cirrhosis, 625
Lobular capillary hemangioma, 108, 109f
Local anesthetic injection, technique of, 7f
Lockjaw (trismus), 1220
Loiasis, 1186, 1186t, 1187f
Long bones, fracture of, 1052-1053,
    1053f-1055f
Long-QT syndrome, 430-431, 431f
Loop recorders, activation of, after syncopal
    episode, 476, 476f
Lordosis, 936f
Louse-borne relapsing fever, 1228, 1228f
Lower extremity(ies). *See also specific part.*
  cutaneous sensory innervation of, 1014f, 1015f
Low-molecular-weight heparin, for
    thrombosis, 1124

Lown-Ganong-Levine syndrome, 436
Lumbar disc syndrome, 1014-1015, 1014f, 1015f
Lumbar spine
  fracture of, 1057, 1057f
    assessment of, 1032f
  stenosis of, 1015-1017, 1016f
Lumpectomy, for stage I and II breast cancer,
    826, 828
Lunelle, contraceptive, 789, 792
Lung(s). *See also* Pulmonary; Respiratory *entries.*
  disease of. *See also specific disease.*
    interstitial, 510-511, 510f, 511f
    occupational, 507-509, 507f-509f
Lung abscess, 529-531, 530f, 531f
Lung biopsy, in Wegener's granulomatosis,
    518, 519f
Lung carcinoma
  characteristics of, 494
  clinical presentation of, 494, 494f, 495f
  differential diagnosis of, 494-495
  imaging studies of, 496, 496f-498f
  laboratory tests for, 495-496, 495f, 496f
  staging of, 496-498
    pretreatment, 498
  survival rates for, 499
  treatment of, 498-499
  types of, 494
Lung transplantation, for pulmonary
    hypertension, 551
Lupus anticoagulant syndrome, 1125f
Lupus glomerulonephritis, 701, 701f
Lupus nephritis, 962, 962f
Lupus pernio, 41, 42f
Lyell's syndrome, 37, 37f
Lyme disease, 1044-1045, 1044f, 1045f
  serologic response in, 1045f
Lymph node(s)
  biopsy, in Hodgkin's lymphoma,
    1095, 1096f
  cervical, in Hodgkin's lymphoma, 1095, 1095f
Lymphadenopathy
  HIV-related, 1148, 1149f
  in infectious mononucleosis, 1214, 1214f
  mediastinal, 360-361, 361f
Lymphangioma, mediastinal, 361, 363f
Lymphedema, 463-464, 463f
Lymphoepithelial cyst, oral, 325, 325f
Lymphogranuloma venereum, 762-763,
    762f, 763f
Lymphoma
  B cell, 1101f
  Burkitt's, 1102-1103, 1102f, 1103f
  CNS, HIV-related, 1158
  cutaneous T-cell, 1103, 1103f-1105f
  Hodgkin's, 1095, 1095f-1097f, 1098
    HIV-related, 1158
  mediastinal, 361, 361f
  non-Hodgkin's, 1099-1105. *See also* Non-
    Hodgkin's lymphoma.
  small bowel, 578, 581f
Lymphomatoid granulomatosis, 522, 522f

M

Macrocytic anemia, 1066, 1068, 1069f, 1069t
Macroglobulinemia, Waldenström's,
    1110, 1110f
Macroglossia
  in acromegaly, 859, 862f
  in amyloidosis, 711, 712f
  in hypothyroidism, 871, 874f
Macular degeneration, 292, 292f
Macule(s), 4b
  in Wegener's granulomatosis, 518, 518f
  melanocytic, oral, 335, 335f

Maculopapular disease(s). *See also specific disease.*
  differential diagnosis of, 6t
Maculopapular rash
  in HIV infection, 1146f
  in interstitial nephritis, 709, 709f
Madura foot (mycetoma), 1201
Magnetic resonance angiography (MRA)
  of cardiovascular system, 381, 381f
  of cerebral arteriovenous malformation,
    177, 179f
  of cerebral vessels, 172, 172f, 173f
  of kidneys, 684, 686f
  of portal vein thrombosis, 663, 664f
  of renal artery stenosis, 720, 721f
Magnetic resonance imaging (MRI)
  of Achilles tendon rupture, 1025, 1025f
  of aortic dissection, 473, 473f
  of benign prostatic hyperplasia, 739, 740f
  of brain, 168, 169f, 170f
  of brain abscess, 216-217, 218f
  of breast, 826, 829f
  of cardiovascular system, 380, 380f
  of cavernous sinus thrombosis, 220, 220f
  of craniopharyngioma, 190, 191f
  of Creutzfeldt-Jakob disease, 197, 197f
  of cysticercosis, 225, 225f
  of Friedreich's ataxia, 214, 215f
  of hemochromatosis, 627, 628f
  of kidneys, 684, 685f
  of lumbar spine stenosis, 1016, 1016f
  of meningioma, 188, 189f
  of Milwaukee shoulder, 1010, 1012f
  of neuroblastoma, 245, 246f
  of normal-pressure hydrocephalus, 242, 242f
  of osteochondritis dissecans, 1022, 1022f
  of progressive multifocal
    leukoencephalopathy, 198, 198f
  of pulmonary hypertension, 550, 551f
  of rotator cuff tear, 1009, 1010f
  of stroke, 177, 179f
  of superior vena cava syndrome, 364, 365f
  of tendinitis, 940f
  of tuberous sclerosis, 232, 232f
  of uterine leiomyoma, 810, 811f
  of Wilms' tumor, 724, 724f
  of wrist ganglion, 1004, 1005f
Malaria
  clinical presentation of, 1159, 1159f,
    1160f, 1161
  laboratory tests for, 1161, 1162f
  treatment of, 1161
Malgaigne complex, fracture of, 1052, 1052f
Malignancy, humoral hypercalcemia of,
    880, 882f
Malignant melanoma. *See* Melanoma.
Malignant mesothelioma. *See* Mesothelioma.
Mallory-Weiss tear, 563, 563f
Malnutrition, in chronic renal failure, 697, 698f
Mammography, 826, 828f
Mandible, granuloma gravidarum of, 329, 329f
Marcus Gunn pupil, in multiple sclerosis, 207
Marfan's syndrome, 1029-1030, 1030f
Mask of pregnancy, 64, 64f
Mastectomy
  bilateral, prophylactic, 829
  radical, for stage III breast cancer, 828
Mastocytosis, maculopapular cutaneous, 53, 53f
Maze procedure, for atrial fibrillation, 430
McBurney's point, 587
Meares and Stamey localization technique, for
    prostatitis, 742f
Measles (rubeola), 126-127, 126f, 127f, 531
  treatment of, 533
Mebendazole, for enterobiasis, 1181

Mechanical ventilation, for Guillain-Barré syndrome, 212
Meckel's diverticulum, 585, 585f
Median nerve, compression of, 1001-1002, 1001f, 1002f
Mediastinal lymphadenopathy, 360-361, 361f, 362f
Mediastinal lymphangioma, 361, 363f
Mediastinal mass(es)
  causes of, 359t
  characteristics of, 359-361, 359f-363f
Mediastinum, anatomic compartments of, 359f
Medullary sponge kidney, 716f
Megacolon
  in trypanosomiasis, 1171, 1171f
  toxic, 578, 582f
Mega-esophagus, in trypanosomiasis, 1171, 1171f
Megakaryocytopoiesis, regulation of, 1061, 1065f
Megaloblastic anemia, hematologic abnormalities in, 1078f
Meige's syndrome, vs. blepharospasm, 277t
Melanocytic macule, oral, 335, 335f
Melanocytic nevus(i), 91-97. See also named nevus.
  of eyelid, 283, 283f
Melanoma
  definition of, 98
  differential diagnosis of, 98
  of eyelid, 286, 286f
  subtypes of, 98, 98f, 99f
  subungual, 81, 81f
  treatment of, 99
Melanonychia, longitudinal, 80, 81f
Melasma, 64, 64f
Meltzer's triad, 61
Membranoproliferative glomerulonephritis, 701, 702f
Meningioma, 187-188
  imaging of, 188, 189f
  whorl formation in, 188, 188f
Meningitis, bacterial, 221-222, 222f
Meningoencephalitis, 1225
Meningomyelocele, 204-205, 205f
Menstrual cycle, hormonal events in, 776, 778f
Mental status testing, in Alzheimer's disease, 192
Merkel cell tumor, of eyelid, 287, 287f
Mesenteric adenitis, 658, 658f
Mesenteric ischemia, 661-662, 661f, 662f
Mesothelioma, 502-503, 503f, 504f
Metacarpophalangeal joint, injection of, 945, 946f
Metastasis
  identification of, whole-body scintigraphy in, 353f, 354
  of carcinoid tumor, 667, 669f, 670f
  of prostate cancer, 743, 743f
Metatarsophalangeal joint, erosive lesions of, in Crohn's disease, 588f
Metformin, for diabetes mellitus, 920
Methylprednisolone
  for giant cell arteritis, 983
  for Reiter's syndrome, 991
  for rheumatic fever, 1212
Metronidazole
  for bacterial vaginosis, 793
  for *Trichomonas* vulvovaginitis, 796
Metronidazole plus penicillin, for lung abscess, 530
Microcytic anemia, 1066, 1067t, 1068f
Microsporidiosis, HIV-related, 1158
Microvascular angina (syndrome X), 383.
  See also Angina pectoris.
Miglitol, for diabetes mellitus, 920

Migratory glossitis, benign (geographic tongue), 326, 326f, 339
Milia, 102, 103f
  of eyelid, 280, 280f
Miliary tuberculosis, 544-546, 544f-546f
Miltefosine, for leishmaniasis, 1169
Milwaukee shoulder, 1009-1010, 1010f, 1012f
Mini pill contraceptive, 789, 791
Minocycline, hyperpigmentation due to, 48, 48f
Mirena Levonorgestrel Intrauterine System (LNGIUS), 792
Mirizzi syndrome, type I, 647, 647f
Mite infestation, 143-144, 143f
Mitral valve
  prolapse of, 398-399, 399f
  regurgitation of, 396-398, 397f
    post-infarct, 391
  repair of, 398, 398f
  stenosis of, 395-396, 395f, 396f
Mitral valvuloplasty, 396, 397f
Mobitz type I (Wenckebach) AV block, 437, 438f
Mobitz type II AV block, 437, 438f
Mohs' surgery
  for basal cell carcinoma, 87
  for skin lesions, 10, 11f
Molecular amplification methods, 1144
Molluscum contagiosum, 124-125, 124f
  of eyelid, 267, 268f, 285, 285f
Molluscum sebaceum (keratoacanthoma), 90, 90f
Monarthritis
  initial approach to, 938f
  selected causes of, 939t
Mongolian blue spot, 96, 97f
Moniliasis (vulvovaginal candidiasis), 763-764, 763f, 1189, 1190f
Monoclonal gammopathy of undetermined significance (MGUS), 1110
Mononucleosis, infectious, 1214-1215, 1214f, 1215f
Monteggia fracture-dislocation, 1052, 1054f
Morgagni hernia, 366, 368f
Morgagnian cataract, 259f
Morpheaform basal cell carcinoma, 86, 87f
Morphine
  for cardiogenic pulmonary edema, 413
  for myocardial infarction, 388
Morton's neuroma, 1025-1026, 1026f
Mosaic wart, 123f
Mosquito bites, 148, 149f
Mouth. *See also* Oral *entries; specific part.*
  autoimmune conditions of, 332-333, 332f, 333f
  infections of, 330-331, 330f, 331f
  leukoplakia of, 334, 334f
  lichenoid and hypersensitivity reactions of, 332, 332f
  normal, 325, 325f
  papillary lesions of, 328, 328f
  pigmented lesions of, 334-335, 334f, 335f
  reactive conditions of, 326-327, 326f, 327f
  tumor-like conditions of, 328-329, 328f-330f
  tumor-like lesions of, 325, 325f, 326f
  ulcerative conditions of, 327, 327f
Mouth ulcers, in systemic lupus erythematosus, 960, 961f
Movement disorders, 200-203. *See also specific disorder.*
Mucocele, oral, 333, 333f
Mucocutaneous lymph node syndrome (Kawasaki syndrome), 56, 58f
Mucosa-associated lymphoid tissue (MALT) lymphoma, 1099, 1099f
Mucosal ulcerations, in HIV infection, 1146f

Muercke's lines, 78, 78f
  in nephrotic syndrome, 707, 707f
Multifocal atrial tachycardia, 427, 428f
Multiple endocrine neoplasia (MEN), 928, 928f
  scintigraphy of, 928, 930f
Multiple myeloma
  clinical presentation of, 1107, 1107f
  laboratory tests for, 1107-1108, 1108f
  prognosis of, 1110
  radiologic evaluation of, 1108, 1109f
  staging of, 1108
  treatment of, 1109-1110
Multiple sclerosis, 207-208, 208f
  differential diagnosis of, 207
Mumps (parotitis), 344-345, 344f, 345f
Murcomycosis, 1209-1210, 1209f, 1210f
Muscle biopsy, 947, 947f
Muscular dystrophy, 233, 234f, 235f
Musculoskeletal pain, in sickle cell disease, 1079-1080
Musculoskeletal system. *See also specific joints, ligaments, and muscles.*
  diagnostic tests and procedures involving, 932-948
  disorders of, 932, 932f, 933f. *See also specific disorder, e.g., Rheumatoid arthritis.*
    clinical signs of, 936, 936f, 936t, 937f
    imaging studies of, 940, 940f-942f
    laboratory tests for, 942, 943f-945f, 943t, 944-945, 952t
    minimally invasive procedures for, 947, 947f, 948f
    pattern recognition in, 938, 938f, 939t
    physical examination of, 932, 932f-934f, 934, 936, 936f, 937f
      characteristic patterns of involvement in, 934, 935t
    specific techniques in, 934, 934t
  skin lesions associated with, 934, 935t
Myasthenia gravis, 233, 235f, 236t, 237, 237f
Mycetoma (Madura foot), 1201
Mycobacterium avium complex, in HIV infection, 1156, 1157f
Mycobacterium avium-intracellulare infection, 142, 142f
Mycobacterium leprae, 1218. *See also* Leprosy (Hansen's disease).
Mycobacterium tuberculosis, 540, 543f. *See also* Tuberculosis.
  in HIV infection, 1156
Mycoplasma pneumoniae, 525. *See also* Pneumonia.
Mycosis fungoides, 1103, 1104f
Myelodysplastic syndrome, 1093, 1093f, 1094f
Myelofibrosis, chronic idiopathic, characteristics of, 1113t
Myeloma, multiple. *See* Multiple myeloma.
Myeloma cast nephropathy, 1107, 1107f
Myelomatosis, 1108, 1109f
Myocardial infarction, 385-394
  cardiac rupture syndromes complicating, 393, 393f
  causes of, 387, 387f, 388f
  characterization of, 385
  clinical presentation of, 386-387
  Dressler's syndrome and, 393-394
  in Kawasaki disease, 129, 130f
  laboratory tests for, 387-388, 388t, 389f
  left ventricular aneurysm in, 394, 394f
  markers for, characteristics of, 388t
  pathologic findings in, 385, 386f
  physical findings in, 387

Myocardial infarction (*Continued*)
post-infarct complications of, 389, 391
treatment of, 391-392
right ventricular, 392-393, 392f
systemic embolism in, 393
treatment of, 388-389
Myocardial infarction with normal coronaries
(MINC) syndrome, 387
Myocardial reperfusion, for myocardial
infarction, 388-389
Myocardial rupture, 393, 393f
Myocarditis, 420-421, 420f, 421f
Myoma, uterine, 809-811, 809f-811f
Myopia (nearsightedness), examination of,
252, 256f
Myotonic dystrophy, 233, 235f
Myringitis, bullous, 304, 306f
Myringotomy, for otitis media, 317
Myxedema, in hypothyroidism, 871, 871f, 872f
Myxoid cyst, 83, 83f
Myxoma, atrial, 457-458, 457f, 458f

N

Nail(s)
anatomy of, 76, 76f
Beau's lines of, 77, 78f
Candida infection of, 79, 80f
clubbing of, 79, 79f
culture specimen of, 7f, 9f
discoloration of, drug-induced, 79, 80f
diseases of, 76-83. *See also specific disorder.*
Everest, 552, 552f
Lindsay, 78, 78f
Muercke's lines of, 78, 78f
pitting of, in psoriatic arthritis, 991, 992f
splinter hemorrhage of, 79, 79f
spoon, 78, 79f
structural relationships of, 76f
Terry, 78, 78f
Naproxen, for Baker's cyst, 1021
Nasal. *See also* Nose.
Nasal oxygen, for myocardial infarction, 388
Nasal pack, insertion of, 320f, 321, 321f
Nasal pinguecula, 268, 268f
Nasal polyps, 318, 319f
National Institutes of Health consensus
classification, of prostatitis syndromes,
741t
Necrobiosis lipoidica, 43, 43f
Necrobiosis lipoidica diabeticorum, in diabetes
mellitus, 917, 919f
Necrobiotic dermatoses, 43, 43f
Necrotizing fasciitis, 136-137, 136f, 137f
Necrotizing glomerulonephritis, in Wegener's
granulomatosis, 517, 517f
Necrotizing (malignant) otitis externa,
314, 315f
Necrotizing scleritis, 266, 266f
Necrotizing vasculitis, in rheumatoid arthritis,
952, 954f
Needle decompression, of tension
pneumothorax, 505, 506f
Negri bodies, 1237, 1237f
Neisseria gonorrhoeae, diagnostic tests for, 768t
Neisseria meningitidis, in meningitis, 222
Nelson's syndrome, 859, 863f
radiation therapy for, 864
Nematode infestations, 1179-1185
Nephrectomy, for renal cell carcinoma, 722, 723f
Nephritis
interstitial, 709-710, 709f
lupus, 962, 962f
Nephroblastoma (Wilms' tumor), 722f,
723-724, 724f

Nephrocalcinosis, hyperparathyroidism causing,
880, 880f
Nephron, 676f
Nephropathy
IgA, 706, 706f
in diabetes mellitus, 917, 918f
myeloma cast, 1107, 1107f
Nephrotic syndrome, 707-708, 707f, 708f
renal vein thrombus in, 719f
Neurilemmoma (schwannoma), 106, 106f
Neuritis, optic, 302-303, 302f
differential diagnosis of, 302b
Neuroblastoma, 245-246, 245f, 246f
Neurocutaneous syndrome(s), 229-232. *See also
specific syndrome.*
Neurodermatitis
circumscribed, 30, 30f
history and location of, 6t
Neuroendocrine carcinoma, of eyelid, 287, 287f
Neurofibroma, 106, 106f
of eyelid, 282, 282f
Neurofibromatosis, 229-231
café au lait spot in, 96f, 100, 100f, 229, 230f
diagnosis of, 230-231
imaging of, 231, 231f
treatment of, 231
type 1, features of, 229-230, 230f
type 2, features of, 230
Neurologic symptoms, in cirrhosis patients, 617
Neuroma
acoustic, 311-312, 311f
Morton's, 1025-1026, 1026f
Neuromuscular junction, disorders of, 233-237.
See also specific disorder.
differential diagnosis of, 236t
Neuropathy(ies), 211-213, 211f-213f. *See also
specific neuropathy.*
in diabetes mellitus, 916-917
Neutrophil(s), differentiation of, 1060, 1064f
Neutrophilic dermatoses, 49-53, 49f-53f
Nevus(i)
acral, 93, 94, 94f
banal, 93, 93f
Becker, 92, 93f
common blue, 96, 97f
congenital melanocytic, 96, 96f
dermal melanocytic, 93, 93f
epidermal, 84, 84f
halo, 94, 94f
junctional, 93, 93f
kissing, 96, 96f
of eyelid, 284, 284f
melanocytic, 91-97
congenital. *See* Nevus(i), kissing.
of eyelid, 283, 283f
spider, 107, 107f
Spitz, 94, 94f
strawberry, 108, 108f
white sponge, 339
Nevus flammeus, around eyelids, 281, 281f
New York criteria, modified, for ankylosing
spondylitis, 988, 989f
Niacin, deficiency of, 46, 46f
Nicotinic stomatitis, 333, 333f
Nifedipine
for achalasia, 569
for high-altitude pulmonary edema, 553
Nitrates, for myocardial infarction, 388
Nocardia asteroides, 1202, 1202f
Nocardiosis, 1201-1203, 1201f, 1202f
Nodular basal cell carcinoma, 86, 86f
Nodular cystic acne, treatment of, 73
Nodular melanoma, 98, 98f
Nodular prurigo, 30-31, 31f

Nodular scleritis, 266, 266f
Nodule(s), 4b
Aschoff, 1211f
gingival, 329, 329f
Mycobacterium avium-intracellulare, 142, 142f
pulmonary, in lymphomatoid granulomatosis,
522, 522f
rheumatoid, 43, 43f, 952, 952f, 953f
Sister Mary Joseph's, 576, 576f
thyroid, 349-351, 349f, 350f
Nonalcoholic steatohepatitis, 629, 629f, 630f
Non-Hodgkin's lymphoma, 1099-1105
cerebral, 1100f
classification of, 1100
clinical presentation of, 1099, 1099f, 1100
diagnosis of, 1103
HIV-related, 1158
patient disposition with, 1102
staging of, 1102
treatment of, 1102, 1105
workup for, 1100, 1101f, 1102f
Non-small cell carcinoma, of lungs. *See also*
Lung carcinoma.
treatment of, 498-499
Nonsteroidal anti-inflammatory drugs
for rheumatoid arthritis, 956
for systemic lupus erythematosus, 963
Noonan's syndrome, 907
Normal-pressure hydrocephalus, 242-243, 242f
Normocytic anemia, 1066
Norplant, contraceptive, 789, 792
Norwegian scabies, 143, 143f
Nose. *See also* Nasal *entries.*
anatomy of, 320f
basal cell carcinoma of, Mohs' surgery for, 11f
examination of, 318, 319f
Nosebleed (epistaxis), 320
treatment of, 320f, 321, 321f
Nosocomial endocarditis, 406
causes of, 408
Nosocomial (hospital-acquired) pneumonia,
528, 529f
Nummular eczema, 26, 27f
Nutritional requirements, in chronic renal
failure, 699
Nutritional support, for acute respiratory distress
syndrome, 547

O

Oblique fracture, of long bone, 1052, 1053f
Occlusal splint, for temporomandibular joint
syndrome, 1001, 1001f
Occupational lung disease, 507-509, 507f-509f.
See also specific disease.
Oculocephalic reflex, in progressive supranuclear
palsy, 194, 195f
Oculopharyngeal muscular dystrophy, 233
Oligodendroglioma, CT scan of, 168, 169f
Olsalazine, for ulcerative colitis, 591
Omega-3 fatty acids, for glomerulonephritis, 702
Onchocerciasis, 1186, 1186f, 1187f
Onychomycosis, 76-77, 76f, 77f
differential diagnosis of, 76-77
Open fracture, of long bone, 1052
Ophthalmoplegia, progressive external, 236t
Opportunistic infections, HIV-related,
prophylaxis for, 1152-1153
Opsoclonus-myoclonus syndrome,
neuroblastoma and, 245
Optic cup asymmetry, in glaucoma,
297, 298f
Optic disc, normal, 251f
Optic neuritis, 302-303, 302f
differential diagnosis of, 302b

Oral candidiasis (thrush), HIV-related, 1149, 1150f, 1155
Oral contraceptives, 789
  combination, 791
Oral hairy leukoplakia, 330-331, 330f, 331f
Oral herpes, HSV-1 in, 118, 118f
Oral lichen planus, 35, 331f, 332
Oral lymphoepithelial cyst, 325, 325f
Oral mucosa, diseases of, 325-335. *See also under* Mouth; *specific disease.*
Oral rehydration, for cholera, 655, 655f
Orbit, sensory nerves of, 251f
Osborne wave, of hypothermia, 158, 158f
Osgood-Schlatter disease, 1021-1022, 1021f, 1022f
Osteoarthritis, 949
  of feet, 949, 951f
  of fingers, 949, 950f
  of hands, 933f, 949, 951f
  of hips, 949, 949f
Osteochondritis dissecans, 1022, 1022f
Osteochondroma, 1047
Osteogenic sarcoma, in Paget's disease, 1036, 1036f
Osteoid osteoma, 1047
  in Gardner's syndrome, 598, 599f
Osteoma, osteoid, 1047
Osteomalacia, 1032-1033, 1033f, 1034f
  hypophosphatemic, 1033f
  serum chemistry in, 1033t
Osteomyelitis, 1042-1044
  chronic, 1043, 1043f
  contiguous, 1043
  hematogenous, 1042, 1042f
  scintigraphy of, 941f
  vertebral, 1042, 1043f
Osteonecrosis, 1034, 1034f, 1035f
Osteoporosis, 1031-1032, 1031f, 1032f
Osteoporosis circumscripta, 1036f. *See also* Paget's disease.
Osteosarcoma, 1047, 1047f
Ostium primum defect, 442
Ostium secundum defect, 442
Otitis externa, 304, 306f, 314-315, 314f, 315f
  diffuse (swimmer's ear), 314
  eczematous, 314
  localized, 314
  necrotizing (malignant), 314, 315f
Otitis media, 316-317, 316f
  treatment of, 317
Otomycosis, 314
Otorhinolaryngeal disease, in relapsing polychondritis, 313, 313f
Ovarian cycle, hormonal events in, 776, 777f
Ovarian diathermy, laparoscopic, 818, 818f
Ovary
  androgen-secreting tumors of, hirsutism associated with, 910, 910f, 911f
  benign lesions of, 815, 816f
  cancer of, 819, 819f
  polycystic, 817-818, 817f, 818f
Ovulation, 776, 777f
Oxaliplatin, for colorectal carcinoma, 602
Oxygen therapy
  for altitude sickness, 553
  for myocardial infarction, 388

P

P24 antigen, in HIV infection, 1145, 1146f
Pacemaker, cardiac. *See* Cardiac pacemaker.
Paget's disease
  of bone, 1035-1036, 1035f, 1036f
  of breast, 830, 831f

Painful subacute thyroiditis, 355
Painless sporadic thyroiditis, 355
Palate
  hard, verruciform xanthoma of, 328, 328f
  normal histology of, 325, 325f
  soft, squamous papilloma of, 328, 328f
Palmar erythema (liver palms), in cirrhosis, 616f
Palmoplantar keratoderma, diffuse, 14, 15f
Pancoast tumor, 494, 495f
Pancreatectomy, for pancreatic carcinoma, 613
Pancreatic abscess, 610, 611f
Pancreatic biopsy, CT-guided, 613, 615f
Pancreatic carcinoma
  clinical presentation of, 613, 613f
  imaging studies of, 613, 614f, 615f
  treatment of, 613
Pancreatic duct, normal, 611f
Pancreatic enzymes, in acute pancreatitis, 609
Pancreatic necrosis, 609, 611f
Pancreatic pseudocyst, 610, 611f
Pancreatitis
  acute, 608-610
    causes of, 608
    clinical presentation of, 608, 608f, 609f
    imaging studies of, 609, 610f, 611f
    treatment of, 609-610, 611f
  chronic, 612, 612f
  gallstone-induced, 610
  necrotizing, 609, 611f
Panhypopituitarism, 854f
Panniculitis, alpha$_1$-antitrypsin deficiency-associated, 492, 492f
Papanicolaou (Pap) smear, 782, 782f, 783f
Papilla, parotid, in mumps, 344, 344f
Papillary fibroelastoma, 457f
Papillary lesions, oral, 328, 328f
Papillary muscle rupture, in myocardial infarcts, 390f, 391
Papilloma, squamous
  of eyelid, 278, 278f
  of soft palate, 328, 328f
Pappenheimer bodies, 1072, 1072f
Papule(s), 4b
  in Wegener's granulomatosis, 518, 518f
Para-aminobenzoic acid, for Peyronie's disease, 774
Paralytic ileus, 578, 581f
Parameningeal pyogenic infections, 224, 224f
Parasite(s), gastrointestinal, 1166t
Parasitic infection(s), HIV-related, 1157-1158
Parathyroid adenoma, 880, 881f
Parkinsonism, 193
Parkinson's disease, 200-201, 200f, 201f
  treatment of, 201
  with dementia, 193
Paronychia, 77, 77f
Parotitis (mumps), 344-345, 344f, 345f
Paroxysmal atrial tachycardia, 427, 427f
Paroxysmal cold hemoglobinuria, 1134, 1134f, 1134t
Paroxysmal nocturnal hemoglobinuria, 1132-1133, 1132f
Parturition, 837
Parvovirus B19, in fifth disease, 115
Patch, for amblyopia, 273, 273f
Patch testing, 8, 9f
  for contact dermatitis, 28, 29f
Patent ductus arteriosus, 453, 455, 455f
  types of, 453, 454f
Peak flowmeter, asthma patient using, 486f
Pectus carinatum (pigeon chest), 358, 358f
Pectus excavatum (funnel chest), 358, 358f
Pedal edema, in cirrhosis patients, 617
Pediculosis, 144, 144f

Pediculosis corporis (body louse), 144, 144f
Pediculus capitis (head louse), 144, 144f
Pellagra, 46, 46f
Pelvic inflammatory disease, 820, 820f
Pelvis
  female
    anatomy of, 776, 776f
    bimanual examination of, 776, 780f
    diagnostic tests and procedures involving, 782-786. *See also specific test.*
  fracture of, 1051-1052, 1052f
Pemberton's sign, in hypothyroidism, 871, 872f
Pemphigoid
  bullous, 6t, 16-17, 16f
  cicatricial, 17-18, 18f
  oral, 332, 332f
  dermolytic, 18, 18f
  lichen planus, 17, 17f
Pemphigoid gestations, 17, 17f
Pemphigus, 21-23
  oral, 332, 332f
Pemphigus erythematosus, 23, 23f
Pemphigus foliaceus, 22, 22f
Pemphigus vegetans, 22, 23f
Pemphigus vulgaris, 21-22, 21f, 22f
  differential diagnosis of, 6t, 22
  oral, 332, 332f
Penicillin, for lung abscess, 530
Penicillin G, for syphilis, 760
Penicillin V, for sickle cell anemia, 1081
Penile curvature (chordee), 772
Penile ulcer, in HIV infection, 1146f
Penis, verrucous carcinoma of, 766, 766f
Pentooxifylline, for venous ulcers, 462
Peptic ulcer, 574, 574f, 575f
Percutaneous coronary intervention, for angina pectoris, 385, 385f
Perianal region, disorders of, 603, 603f, 604f
Pericardial Carpentier Perimount bioprosthesis, for valvular heart disease, 404, 405f
Pericardial effusion, 423, 424f
  in systemic lupus erythematosus, 960, 961f
Pericardial friction rub, 422
Pericarditis
  causes of, 422
  chronic constrictive, 424
  clinical presentation of, 422
  complications of, 423-424
  effusive-constrictive, 424
  imaging studies of, 422-423, 423f, 424f
  in rheumatoid arthritis, 952, 954f
  treatment of, 423
Periodontal infections, 336-337, 336f, 337f
Periorbital edema, in nephrotic syndrome, 707, 707f
Periorbital purpura, in amyloidosis, 711, 712f
Peripheral arterial disease, 459-460, 459f, 460f
Peripheral blood smears. *See* Blood smears, peripheral.
Perirectal abscess, 606, 606f
Peritoneal dialysis, 696, 696f
Periungual fibroma, 83, 83f
Periungual pyogenic granuloma, 82, 82f, 140f
Pernicious anemia, 1076-1077, 1076f-1078f
Peruvian wart, 141, 141f
Peutz-Jeghers syndrome, 64, 64f, 91, 92f, 597, 597f
Peyer's patches, ulceration of, 652, 652f
Peyronie's disease, 774, 774f
Phalen's test, for carpal tunnel syndrome, 1001, 1002f
Pharyngitis, 346-347, 346f, 347f

Index

Pheochromocytoma, 894, 894f, 895f
Philadelphia chromosome, in chronic myelogenous leukemia, 1090, 1092f
Phlebotomy
    for sideroblastic anemia, 1072
    weekly, for hemochromatosis, 627
Photoallergic drug reaction, 47-48, 48f
Photodermatitis, 39, 39f
Photodynamic therapy, for skin disorders, 10, 12f
Phototherapy, for skin disorder, 13, 13f
Phototoxic drug reaction, 47-48, 47f
Phthirus pubis (crab louse, pubic louse), 144, 144f
Pick bodies, 198, 199f
Pick cells, 198, 199f
Pick's disease, 198, 199f
Pigeon chest (pectus carinatum), 358, 358f
Pigment stones, 644
Pigmentation disorder(s), cutaneous, 62-66. *See also specific disorder.*
Pigmented lesions, oral, benign, 334-335, 334f, 335f
Pigmented spindle cell tumor of Reed, 95, 95f
Pilar cyst, 102, 103f
    surgical excision of, 10f
Pilar leiomyoma, 106, 107f
Pili incarnati (shaving bumps), 139-140
Pinguecula, nasal, 268, 268f
Pink puffers, 488
Pinta, 142, 142f
Pinworms, 1181, 1181f
Pioglitazone, for diabetes mellitus, 920
Pit viper bites, 150, 151f
Pituitary adenoma
    clinical presentation of, 859, 861f-863f
    corticotropin-secreting. *See* Cushing's disease.
    differential diagnosis of, 859-860, 863f
    growth hormone-secreting. *See* Acromegaly.
    nonsecretory, 859, 860, 864, 866
    radiologic classification of, 864, 864f
    thyrotropin-secreting, 859, 860, 864, 866
    treatment of, 864, 865f, 866
    workup for, 860-861, 861f
Pityriasis alba, 32, 32f, 63, 63f
Pityriasis rosea, 130, 131f, 132
    differential diagnosis of, 6t, 132
Pivot shift test, 937f
Placenta, delivery of, 837
Placental abruption, 848-849, 848f
Placenta previa, 850-851, 850f
Plague, 1226-1227, 1227f
Plane wart (verruca plana), 122, 122f
Plantar calcaneal spur, imaging of, 940f
Plantar wart, 122, 123f
Plaque, 4b
    senile scleral, 268, 269f
Plaque psoriasis, 33, 33f
Plaques
    erythematous, sarcoidosis and, 514, 515f
    pleural, in asbestosis, 507, 507f
Plasma, milky appearance of, hyperlipidemia and, 923, 927f
Plasma cell dyscrasias, 1107-1110. *See also specific type.*
Plasma exchange therapy, for glomerulonephritis, 702
Plasmapheresis, for systemic lupus erythematosus, 964
Plasmodium falciparum malaria, 1159, 1159f, 1160f
Plasmodium malariae malaria, 1161
Plasmodium ovale malaria, 1161
Plasmodium vivax, life cycle of, 1160f

Plasmodium vivax malaria, 1159
Pleura, diseases of, 500-506. *See also specific disease.*
Pleural biopsy, 502, 503f
Pleural effusion
    diagnostic thoracentesis for, 500-501, 501f
    examination of fluid in, 502t
    localization of, 500, 500f
    subpulmonary, tension, 366, 367f
Pleural plaques, in asbestosis, 507, 507f
Pleurisy, systemic lupus erythematosus causing, 960, 961f
Pleurodesis, for mesothelioma, 503
Plummer-Vinson syndrome, 567
Pneumococcal vaccine, for HIV-infected patients, 1152
Pneumoconiosis, 509, 509f
Pneumocystis jiroveci (carinii) infection, 535, 535f, 536f
    HIV-related, 1149, 1150f, 1156
Pneumonia
    Aspergillus, 1191, 1192f
    aspiration, 528-529
    community-acquired, 528, 528f
    hospital-acquired, 528, 529f
    bacterial, 525-528
    causes of, 525, 525f-527f
    imaging studies of, 527-528, 527f
    treatment of, 528
    cytomegalovirus, 531, 532f, 533f
    interstitial, 523, 523f
    Pneumocystis jiroveci (carinii), 535, 535f, 536f
    HIV-related, 1149, 1150f, 1156
    viral, 531-533, 532f, 533f
Pneumothorax
    clinical presentation of, 503
    imaging studies of, 504, 505f
    tension, 366, 367f, 505f
    treatment of, 505, 506f
    treatment of, 505
Poison ivy dermatitis, 27, 28f, 29f
Poison oak dermatitis, 27, 28f
Poloxamer, for sickle cell anemia, 1081
Polyarteritis, cutaneous, Crohn's disease and, 588f
Polyarteritis nodosa, 56, 57f, 980-981, 981f
Polyarthritis, classification of, 939t
Polychondritis, relapsing, 313, 313f
Polycystic kidney disease, 714-718
    autosomal dominant
        extrarenal manifestations of, 715f
        vascular manifestations of, 714f
    clinical presentation of, 714, 714f, 715f
    differential diagnosis of, 715, 715f-717f
    differential features of, 717t
    imaging studies of, 715, 718f
    treatment of, 715
Polycystic liver disease, vs. hepatic abscess, 633, 634f
Polycystic ovary syndrome, 817-818, 817f, 818f
Polycythemia
    secondary (hypoxemia), 1111
    stress (Gaisböck's syndrome), 1112
Polycythemia vera, 1111-1112, 1111f, 1112f
    characteristics of, 1113t
Polydipsia, causes of, 867, 867f
    differentiating, 868, 868f
Polymorphous light eruption (photodermatitis), 39, 39f
Polymyalgia rheumatica, 981-982
Polymyositis, 969-970

Polyp(s)
    fibroepithelial, 105, 105f
    inflammatory, ulcerative colitis with, 591, 591f
    nasal, 318, 319f
    uterine, 812, 812f
Polyposis, familial adenomatous, 596, 596f
Polyuria, causes of, 867, 867f
Pompholyx, 27, 27f
Poroma, eccrine, 100-101, 101f
Porphyria cutanea tarda, 44-45, 44f
    laboratory tests for, 45, 45f
Portal vein thrombosis, 663, 663f, 664f
Port-wine stain, 106-107, 107f
    laser therapy for, 13f
Positron emission tomography
    of frontal glioma, 185, 186f
    of lung carcinoma, 496, 498f
    of pheochromocytoma, 894
    of thyroid carcinoma, 354, 354f
Postcoital contraception, emergency, 789, 792
Postpartum hemorrhage, 837
Poststreptococcal glomerulonephritis, 702, 703f
Posture instability, in Parkinson's disease, 200
Potassium hydroxide preparation, of skin swabs, 8, 9f
Potassium iodide solution, for sporotrichosis, 1208
Pott's disease, 1041f
PR interval, 370
Prader's orchiodometer, 896f
Prader-Willi syndrome, 908
    obesity in, 900, 900f
Pramlintide, for diabetes mellitus, 920
Precocious puberty, 898-899, 898f
    protocol for investigation of, 899t
Prednisone
    for Addisonian crisis, 889
    for aspergillosis, 1193
    for autoimmune hemolytic anemia, 1076
    for celiac disease, 583
    for cirrhosis, 618
    for cutaneous lichen planus, 35
    for Dressler's syndrome, 394
    for erythema multiforme, 37
    for giant cell arteritis, 982-983
    for Goodpasture's syndrome, 521
    for Henoch-Schönlein purpura, 987
    for histoplasmosis, 1197
    for immune thrombocytopenic purpura, 1116
    for nephrotic syndrome, 708
    for *Pneumocystis carinii* infection, 1156
    for polyarteritis nodosa, 981
    for polymyalgia rheumatica, 982
    for rheumatic fever, 1212
    for thyroiditis, 355
Prednisone plus cyclophosphamide, for Wegener's granulomatosis, 519
Preeclampsia, 846-847, 846f, 847f
    definitions of, 846
Preexcitation, in Wolff-Parkinson-White syndrome, 436f
Pregnancy
    antiphospholipid antibody syndrome and, management of, 966
    ectopic, 844-845, 844f, 845f
    physiologic changes and prenatal monitoring during, 832, 832f-836f
    toxoplasmosis in, 228
    thrombosis risk associated with, 1122-1123
Premature labor, 837
Prick test, for *Aspergillus fumigatus*, 9f
Prickle cell layer (stratum spinosum), of skin, 2
Primary biliary cirrhosis, 624-625, 624f, 625f

Prinzmetal's angina, 382, 383f. *See also* Angina pectoris.
Prion disease, neuropathology of, 196, 196f
Procaine penicillin plus probenecid, for syphilis, 760
Prognathism, in acromegaly, 859, 862f
Progressive multifocal leukoencephalopathy, 198, 198f
  HIV-related, 1157
Progressive supranuclear palsy, 194-195, 195f
Prolactinoma
  clinical presentation of, 859, 861f
  differential diagnosis of, 859
  medical therapy for, 864
  workup for, 860
Pronator syndrome, 1003, 1003f
Propionibacterium acnes, 72.
    See also Acne vulgaris.
Propranolol, for thyroiditis, 355
Prostate, benign hyperplasia of, 739-740, 739f, 740f
Prostate cancer
  Gleason classification of, 743, 743f
  imaging studies of, 743, 743f, 744f
  staging of, 743
  treatment of, 744
Prostatectomy, radical, for prostate cancer, 744
Prostatitis, 741-742
  Meares and Stamey localization technique for, 742f
  NIH consensus classification of, 741t
Prosthetic valve endocarditis, causes of, 408
Protein C, 1122
  deficiency of, 1122, 1124f
    treatment of, 1124
Protein electrophoretic patterns, in multiple myeloma, 1108, 1108f
Protein S, 1122
  deficiency of, 1122
Protein truncation testing, for Gardner's syndrome, 599
Proteinuria, definition of, 846
Prothrombin G20210A mutation, 1122
Protozoal infection(s), 1159-1175.
    See also specific infection.
Prurigo nodularis, 30-31, 31f
  in chronic renal failure, 697, 697f
Pruritus, in primary biliary cirrhosis, 624
Pseudoaneurysm, in myocardial infarcts, 391, 391f
Pseudocyst, pancreatic, 610, 611f
Pseudofolliculitis (shaving bumps), 139-140
Pseudogout, 995-997, 996f, 997f
Pseudohypoparathyroidism, 878, 878f, 879f
Pseudomembrane, diphtheria, 1223, 1223f
Pseudomembranous colitis, 659, 659f, 660f
Pseudoporphyria, in chronic renal failure, 697, 697f
Pseudoprecocious puberty, 903, 903f
Psoralen plus ultraviolet A (PUVA) therapy, for non-Hodgkin's lymphoma, 1105
Psoriasis, 33-34, 33f
  definition of, 33
  differential diagnosis of, 6t, 33
  nail, 77, 77f
  of genitalia, 756, 756f
Psoriatic arthritis, 932f, 935t, 989t, 991-993, 992f, 993f
Pterygium, double, 268, 269f
Puberty
  delayed, 900-901, 900f
    differential diagnostic features of, 901t
    evaluation of, 902f

Puberty *(Continued)*
  normal, 896, 896f, 897f
  precocious, 898-899, 898f
    protocol for investigation of, 899t
  pseudoprecocious, 903, 903f
Pubic hair, development of, Tanner stages of, 896, 897f
Pubic louse *(Phthirus pubis)*, 144, 144f
Pulmonary. *See also* Lung *entries.*
Pulmonary disorders, in antiphospholipid antibody syndrome, 965
Pulmonary edema
  cardiogenic, 413, 413f
  high-altitude, 552
Pulmonary embolism
  clinical algorithm for, 555f
  clinical presentation and causes of, 554
  imaging studies of, 555, 556f, 557f
  laboratory tests for, 554-555, 554f
  treatment of, 557
Pulmonary fibrosis, idiopathic, 512-513, 512f
Pulmonary hypertension
  causes of, 549, 549f
  imaging studies of, 550, 551f
  laboratory tests for, 550, 550f
  primary, 549
  secondary, 549
  treatment of, 550-551
  workup for, 549-550
Pulmonary infiltrations, 514-523. *See also specific disorder.*
  in hepatitis C–associated cryoglobulinemia, 640, 641f
Pulmonary nodules, in lymphomatoid granulomatosis, 522, 522f
Purpura
  Henoch-Schönlein, 55, 55f
  immune thrombocytopenic, 1114-1116, 1116f
  in hepatitis C–associated cryoglobulinemia, 640, 641f
  in Sjögren's syndrome, 967, 967f
  periorbital, in amyloidosis, 711, 712f
  thrombotic thrombocytopenic, 1116-1117, 1117f
Purpura fulminans, 60, 61f
Pustular acne, treatment of, 72-73
Pyelography
  intravenous, of hydronephrosis, 728
  retrograde, of urinary stones, 734, 735f
Pyelonephritis, 725, 725f, 726f
Pyoderma gangrenosum, 49, 49f
Pyogenic granuloma, 108, 109f
  of eyelid, 282, 282f
  oral, 329, 329f
  periungual, 82, 82f, 140f
Pyogenic liver abscess, 633
Pyrazinamide, for tuberculosis, 543
Pyrimethamine plus leucovorin, for toxoplasmosis, 228

Q

QRS interval, 370
QT interval, 371
  prolongation of, 372, 373f
QuantiFERON TB gold test, 542
Quincke's pulse, 401

R

Rabies, 1236-1237, 1237f
  pathogenesis of, 1236f
Radiation dermatitis, 160, 160f
Radiation therapy
  for basal cell carcinoma, 87

Radiation therapy *(Continued)*
  for brain tumors, 185, 187, 188
  for colorectal carcinoma, 600
  for esophageal carcinoma, 566
  for Hodgkin's lymphoma, 1098
  for Nelson's syndrome, 864
  for pancreatic carcinoma, 613
  for pituitary adenoma, 864, 865f
  for prostate cancer, 744
  with chemotherapy, for non-small cell lung carcinoma, 499
Radioactive iodine, for hyperthyroidism, 876
Radiofrequency ablation, catheter-based, for atrial fibrillation, 429-430, 429f
Radiography
  chest
    cardiac silhouette on, 373, 374f
    examination of, 373-374
  of acute lymphoblastic leukemia, 1084, 1085f
  of acute respiratory distress syndrome, 547, 548f
  of ankylosing spondylitis, 988, 990f
  of anomalous pulmonary artery venous connection, 445f
  of aortic dissection, 473, 473f
  of aortic regurgitation, 401, 401f
  of aortic stenosis, 400, 400f
  of ascites, 620, 621f
  of atrial septal defect, 442, 443f
  of bacterial pneumonia, 525f-527f, 527
  of bronchial carcinoma, 496, 496f
  of brucellosis, 1232, 1232f
  of carcinoid tumor, 667, 668f
  of cardiogenic pulmonary edema, 413, 413f
  of chronic pancreatitis, 609, 610f
  of coarctation of aorta, 455f, 456f
  of coccidioidomycosis, 1200, 1201f
  of cryptococcosis, 1198, 1199f
  of diaphragm abnormalities, 366, 366f-368f
  of dilated cardiomyopathy, treatment of, 415, 415f, 416f
  of heart failure, in hypothyroid patient, 871, 873f
  of histoplasmosis, 1196, 1197f
  of Hodgkin's lymphoma, 1095, 1097f
  of hypertrophic cardiomyopathy, 417, 418f
  of hypertrophic osteoarthropathy, 1037, 1037f
  of kidneys, 682, 683f
  of maxillary sinus opacification, 323, 323f
  of mediastinal masses, 359f-363f
  of mesothelioma, 502, 504f
  of Milwaukee shoulder, 1010, 1012f
  of mitral valve disease, 395, 396f
  of pericarditis, 423, 424f
  of plantar calcaneal spur, 940f
  of pleural effusion, 500, 500f
  of pneumothorax, 504, 505f
  of pulmonary embolism, 555, 556f
  of pulmonary hypertension, 550, 551f
  of rheumatic fever, 1212, 1212f
  of sarcoidosis, 515, 515f
  of transposition of great arteries, 451f
  of tricuspid stenosis, 402, 403f
  of truncus arteriosus, 451f
  of ventricular septal defect, 446f
  of Wegener's granulomatosis, 518, 518f
Radiology, of tetralogy of Fallot, 448f
Raised lesions, oral, 339
Ramsay-Hunt syndrome, 238
Ranula, oral, 333, 333f
Rash(es)
  associated with bacterial infections, 135t
  associated with inflammatory myopathies, 969, 969f

Rash(es) (Continued)
  associated with spirochetal and rickettsial
    infections, 1235t
  associated with viral infections, 115t
    non-specific, 130, 131f
  classic distribution of, 4, 5f
  maculopapular
    in HIV infection, 1146f
    in interstitial nephritis, 709, 709f
Rattlesnake, 150f
Rattlesnake bites, 150, 151f
  fasciotomy for, 152, 152f
Raynaud's phenomenon
  differential diagnosis of, 972t
  in connective tissue disease, 977, 977f
  in systemic sclerosis, 975, 975f
Raynaud's syndrome, 971-973, 971f
Reactive arthritis, 935t
Rectal biopsy, in amyloidosis, 712, 712f
Rectal examination, in cirrhosis patients, 617
Rectocele, 776, 780f
Red eye
  contact lens, 261, 262f
  differential diagnosis of, 263t
Red lesions, oral, 339
Reed-Sternberg cells, in Hodgkin's lymphoma,
    1095, 1096f
Reflex sympathetic dystrophy, 1006-1007,
    1007f
Reflux, gastroesophageal, 561, 561f
Refractory anemia
  with excess blasts in transition, 1093, 1094f
  with ring sideroblasts, 1093, 1094f
Refractory angina, 383. See also Angina pectoris.
Reiter's syndrome, 756, 756f, 989t, 991, 992f
Relapsing fever, 1228, 1228f
Relapsing polychondritis, 313, 313f
Renal. See also Kidney(s).
Renal abscess, 717f
Renal artery, stenosis/thrombosis of, 719-720,
    719f-721f
Renal biopsy, 686-687
  contraindications to, 687t
  evaluation of specimen from, 688,
    689f, 690f
  in Goodpasture's syndrome, 521, 521f
  ultrasound-guided, 687, 687f, 688f
  workup for, 687, 687f
Renal biopsy gun, 687, 687f
Renal cell carcinoma, 722-723, 723f
Renal corpuscle, 676f
Renal cystic disease, adult, differential features
    of, 717t
Renal failure
  acute, 691-696. See also Acute renal failure.
  chronic, 697-699, 697f-700f
  retroperitoneal fibrosis causing, 727, 727f
Renal insufficiency, 878
Renal stones. See also Urolithiasis.
  laboratory tests for, 734t
Renal vein, thrombus in, 719f
Renography, captopril-enhanced, of renal artery
    stenosis, 720, 720f
Resisted wrist extension test, 1007, 1007f, 1008f
Respiratory distress syndrome, acute, 547, 548f
Respiratory function, measurement of, 482,
    482f-484f
Respiratory infections, 525-546. See also specific
    infection.
Respiratory syncytial virus (RSV)
    infection, 531
  treatment of, 532
Restrictive cardiomyopathy, 416-417, 416f
Reticulocyte count, in anemia, 1066, 1067f

Retina, 250f
  detachment of, 293, 293f, 294f
  pigmented epithelium of, congenital
    hypertrophy of, 599
Retinal artery, occlusion of, 290, 290f
Retinitis
  cytomegalovirus, HIV-related, 1149,
    1151f, 1157
  toxoplasmic, 226, 226f
Retinitis pigmentosa, 288, 288f
Retinoblastoma, 289, 289f
Retinopathy
  diabetic, 292, 292f, 916, 916f, 917f
  hypertensive, 292, 292f, 478, 478f
  proliferative, 916, 917f
Retrograde pyelography, of urinary stones, 734,
    735f
Rhabdomyolysis, 729-730
  alcohol-related, 729f
  pathophysiology of, 730f
Rhabdomyoma, 457f
Rheumatic disorders, regional, 1000-1027. See
    also at specific anatomic site.
Rheumatic factor
  in joint pathology, 942, 943f
  sensitivity and specificity of, 942t
Rheumatic fever, 1211-1212, 1211f-1213f
Rheumatoid arthritis, 935t, 952-956
  causes of, 953
  clinical presentation of, 952-953,
    952f-954f, 955t
  differential diagnosis of, 954
  imaging studies of, 940f, 956, 956f
  juvenile, 957, 957f-959f, 959
  laboratory tests for, 954
  treatment of, 956
Rheumatoid nodules, 43, 43f, 952,
    952f, 953f
Rhinitis, allergic, 318-319, 318f, 319f
Rhinocerebral-rhinoorbital-paranasal syndrome,
    1208
Rhinophyma, 74, 75f
Rhombencephalitis, 1225
Rhomboid glossitis, median, 326, 327f
Rhythm method, of contraception,
    789, 791
Rib, brown tumor of, 880, 880f
Rickets
  childhood, 1032-1033, 1032f
  hypophosphatemic, 1033f
Riedel's thyroiditis, 355
Rifampin
  for folliculitis, 139
  for tuberculosis, 543
Rifapentine, for tuberculosis, 543
Right atrial hypertrophy, 372
Right bundle-branch block, 371, 372f
Right ventricular heart failure, 409
Right ventricular hypertrophy, 372
Right ventricular infarct, 392-393, 392f
Rigidity, in Parkinson's disease, 200
Ring pessary therapy, for uterine prolapse,
    808, 808f
Ringworm
  body (tinea corporis), 110, 110f
  scalp (tinea capitis), 110-111, 110f
Rinne test, for hearing loss, 308, 308f
Rituximab, for immune thrombocytopenic
    purpura, 1116
Rocky Mountain spotted fever, 1045-1046,
    1046f
Rods
  Gram-negative, 1140-1141
  Gram-positive, 1141, 1141f

Romaña's sign, 1170, 1170f
Rosacea, 74-75, 74f, 75f
  differential diagnosis of, 74
  subtypes of, 74
Rose spots, in salmonellosis, 652, 652f
Roseola (exanthema subitum), 121, 121f
Rosiglitazone, for diabetes mellitus, 920
Rotator cuff syndrome, 1009, 1009f, 1010f
Rotator cuff tear, 1010, 1010f
Roundworms, 1182, 1182f
  life cycle of, 1180f
Rovsing's sign, 587
Rubella (German measles), 127-128, 127f, 128f
Rubeola (measles), 126-127, 126f, 127f, 531
  treatment of, 533
Rule of nines, in estimating surface area of
    burns, 155f

S

Sacroiliitis, in inflammatory bowel disease,
    591, 591f
Saddle-nose deformity, in Wegener's
    granulomatosis, 517, 517f
Saint Anne-Mayo grading system, of
    astrocytomas, 186
Salivary gland(s)
  biopsy of, 947, 947f
  cysts of, 333
  enlargement of, in Sjögren's syndrome,
    967, 967f
  malignant, 342
  tumors of, benign, 342, 343f
Salmonella infection, HIV-related, 1156
Salmonellosis, 652-654, 652f, 653f
Salpingectomy, for ectopic pregnancy, 845
Salpingitis, acute, 820f
Sarcoid uveitis, 295f
Sarcoidosis, 41, 41f, 42f, 514-516, 514f-516f
  hilar lymph node enlargement due to, 361, 362f
Sarcoma. See specific type, e.g., Kaposi's sarcoma.
Scabies, 143-144, 143f
Scale, cutaneous, 5b
Scalp, ringworm of (tinea capitis), 110-111, 110f
Scaphoid, osteonecrosis of, 1035f
Scar, 5b
Scarlet fever, 341, 341f
Schatzki's ring, 567, 567f
Schirmer's test, for Sjögren's syndrome, 967, 968f
Schistosomes
  geographic distribution of, 1173t
  life cycle of, 1173f
Schistosomiasis, 1172-1173, 1173f-1175f, 1175
Schmorl's nodes, 1057, 1057f
Schrober's test, modified, for ankylosing
    spondylitis, 988, 989f
Schwannoma (neurilemmoma), 106, 106f
Scintigraphy
  of avascular necrosis, 1034, 1034f
  of carcinoid tumor, 667, 670f
  of cardiovascular system, 378, 379f
  of cholecystitis, 646f, 647
  of Conn's syndrome, 892, 893f
  of gastrinoma, 671, 672f
  of Graves' disease, 355, 356f
  of hyperthyroidism, 876, 877f
  of hypertrophic osteoarthropathy, 1037, 1037f
  of Meckel's diverticulum, 585, 585f
  of multiple endocrine neoplasia (MEN) type
    IIB, 928, 930f
  of neuroblastoma, 245, 246f
  of normal thyroid, 355, 356f
  of osteomyelitis, 941f
  of pheochromocytoma, 894, 895f
  of prostate cancer, 743, 743f

Scintigraphy *(Continued)*
  of pulmonary embolism, 555, 556f
  of sarcoidosis, 515, 516f
  of stress fracture, 942f
  of thyroid nodule, 349, 349f, 350f, 351
  whole-body, metastasis identification with, 353f, 354
Scleral plaque, senile, 268, 269f
Scleritis, 266, 266f
  in rheumatoid arthritis, 952, 953f
Scleroderma, 974-976, 974f-976f
Scoliosis, 936f, 1017-1019, 1018f
  Cobb angle in, measurement of, 1019f
  kyphosis with, 1018, 1018f
Scorpion stings, 147
  treatment of, 148
Scrofuloderma, in tuberculosis, 545, 546f
Scrotum
  acute, differential diagnosis of, 753t
  contents of, anatomy of, 745f
Sebaceous cysts, vulvar, 798, 799f
Sebaceous gland carcinoma, of eyelid, 286, 286f
Seborrheic dermatitis, 26, 26f
  differential diagnosis of, 6t
Seborrheic keratosis, 84, 84f
  of eyelid, 278-279, 278f, 279f
Seminoma, 750, 750f, 751f
Senile angioma, 108, 108f
Senile scleral plaque, 268, 269f
Sensorineural hearing loss. *See also* Hearing loss.
  vs. conductive hearing loss, 308t
Sensory nerves, of orbit, 251f
Septal defect(s)
  atrial, 442, 442f, 443f, 444
  ventricular, 444-446, 445f-447f
Septate hymen, 776, 779f
Septic arthritis, 1039f, 1040f. *See also* Bacterial arthritis.
Septic bursitis, 1041-1042, 1042f
Septic plague, 1226
Sex-linked ichthyosis, 14, 15f
Sexual abuse, signs of, in child, 776, 779f
Sexual infantilism, differential diagnostic features of, 901t
Sexually transmitted diseases (STDs). *See specific disease, e.g.,* Syphilis.
Sézary cells, in lymphoma, 1103, 1105f
Sézary syndrome, 1103, 1104f
Shark bite, 146f
Shawl sign, 969
Sheehan's syndrome, vs. hypopituitarism, 855-856, 857f
Shingles (herpes zoster), 119-120, 120f, 121f
Shoulder, rheumatic disorders of, 1009-1014. *See also specific disorder.*
Shoulder pain, differential diagnosis of, 1011t
Sick sinus syndrome, 435, 435f
Sickle cell anemia, 1079-1081, 1081f-1083f
Sickle cell disease, 1079
  chronic nonhematologic complications of, 1082f, 1083
  pathophysiology of, 1081f
Sideroblastic anemia, 1070-1072, 1072f
Silicosis, 508, 508f
Single-photon emission computed tomography (SPECT), of brain, 168, 170f, 171f
Sinus venous defect, 442
Sinusitis, 322-324, 322f
  Aspergillus, 1191, 1193f
  treatment of, 323-324
  workup for, 323, 323f, 324f
Sister Mary Joseph's nodule, 576, 576f
Sixth nerve palsy, strabismus resulting from, 270, 273f

Sjögren's syndrome, 967-968, 967f, 968f
Skin. *See also* Cutaneous *entries.*
  appearance of, in cirrhosis patients, 616, 616f, 617f
  properties of, 2b
  structure and function of, 2-3, 2f
Skin disorder(s). *See also specific disorder.*
  acantholytic, 21-24
  classic distribution of rashes in, 4, 5f
  diagnostic tests and procedures involving, 6-9
  diascopy for, 8, 8f
  drug-induced, 47-48, 47f, 48f
  eczematous, 6t, 25-32
  evaluation of, 4-13
  granulomatous and necrobiotic, 41-43
  history and physical examination of, 4-6
    questions in, 4b
  hypersensitivity in, 36-38
  in antiphospholipid antibody syndrome, 965, 965f
  inflammatory, 39-40, 39f, 40f
  keratinization in, 14-20
  laboratory tests for, 8, 8f-10f
  maculopapular, 6t
  neutrophilic and eosinophilic, 49-53
  pigmentation, 62-66
  specimen collection in, 6, 7f
  therapeutic interventions for, 10, 10f-13f, 13
  vascular, 54-61
  vesiculobulbous, 6t
  Wood's light examination of, 8, 8f
Skin lesions. *See also named lesion.*
  disseminated, in chronic lymphocytic leukemia, 1088, 1088f
  genital
    algorithm for evaluation of, 755f
    differential diagnosis of, 754t-755t
    primary, 4b
    secondary, 5b
    specimen collection from, techniques of, 6, 7f
Skin tag, 105, 105f
Skin ulcer, ischemic, trauma-induced, 459, 459f
Slit lamp, 252, 257f
Small bowel
  dilatation of, vs. large bowel dilatation, 578t
  fluid levels in, causes of, 578t
  lymphoma in, 578, 581f
  obstruction of, 578, 580f
Small cell carcinoma, of lungs. *See also* Lung carcinoma.
  treatment of, 499
Smallpox (variola), 132-133, 132f
Smokeless tobacco keratosis, 327, 327f
Snake bites, 149-151, 151f
  treatment of, 151-152, 152f
Snellen eye chart, 252, 255f
Soft palate, squamous papilloma of, 328, 328f
Solar (actinic) keratosis, 87-88, 88f
Solar (actinic) lentigo, 92, 92f
Spasms, esophageal, 570, 570f
Spastic quadriplegia, in cerebral palsy, 239, 239f
Spectacle frame acanthoma, 84, 85f
Speculae, used in gynecologic examination, 776, 781f
Spermatic cord, twisting of. *See* Testicular torsion.
Spermicides, contraceptive, 791
Spider angioma, in cirrhosis, 616f
Spider bites, 146-147, 147f
  treatment of, 148
Spider nevus, 107, 107f
Spina bifida, 204, 205f
Spinal canal, lumbar, healthy and diseased, 1015, 1016f

Spinal cord, developmental disorders of, 204-205, 204f, 205f
Spinal nerve(s), 166f
  dermatome distribution of, 167f
Spinal stenosis, lumbar, 1015-1017, 1016f
Spindle cell tumor of Reed, pigmented, 95, 95f
Spine
  curvature of. *See* Kyphosis; Lordosis; Scoliosis.
  deformation of, 936f, 936f
  fracture of
    cervical, 1056, 1056f
    lumbar, 1057, 1057f
      assessment of, 1032f
    thoracic, 1057, 1057f
  tuberculosis of (Pott's disease), 1041f
Spiral fracture, of long bone, 1052, 1053f
Spirography, 482, 482f
Spironolactone, for ascites, 621
Spitz nevus, 94, 94f
Splenectomy
  for autoimmune hemolytic anemia, 1076
  for immune thrombocytopenic purpura, 1116
Splint
  occlusal, 1001, 1001f
  wrist and hand, 956, 956f
Splinter hemorrhage, of nails, 79, 79f
Spondyloarthtopathy(ies), 988-993.
  See also specific type.
  seronegative, 989t
Spoon nail (koilonychia), 78, 79f
Sporothrix schenckii, 1206, 1207
Sporotrichosis, 1206-1208, 1206f-1208f
Sprain, ankle, 1022-1023, 1023f
Sprue, celiac, 583
Spurious thrombocytopenia, 1114
Squamous cell carcinoma, 88-89, 88f, 89f
  definition of, 88
  differential diagnosis of, 89
  of eyelid, 286
  of oral cavity, 334, 334f
  pulmonary, 494, 495f. *See also* Lung carcinoma.
  subungual, 81, 81f
  treatment of, 89
  vulvar, 765-766, 766f
Squamous cell carcinoma in situ (Bowen's disease), 88, 89f
Squamous intraepithelial lesion
  high-grade, 783f, 804f
  low-grade, 783f, 803f
Squamous papilloma
  of eyelid, 278, 278f
  of soft palate, 328, 328f
Stable angina, 382. *See also* Angina pectoris.
Staphylococcal scalded skin syndrome, 136, 136f
Staphylococcus
  Gram-positive, 1140, 1140f
  in cellulitis, 134, 134f
Stasis dermatitis, 31, 31f
  chronic, 461-462, 461f
  history and location of, 6t
Steatohepatitis, nonalcoholic, 629, 629f, 630f
Stem cell transplantation
  for anaplastic anemia, 1073
  for chronic myelogenous leukemia, 1092
  for multiple myeloma, 1109
  for myelodysplastic syndrome, 1093
  for sickle cell anemia, 1081
Stenosis. *See at anatomic site.*
Stents
  coronary, for angina pectoris, 385
  drug-eluting, 386f

Sterilization
female (tubal ligation), 789, 790f, 791
male (vasectomy), 789, 791, 791f
Steroids. *See* Corticosteroids; *specific steroid.*
Stevens-Johnson syndrome, 37-38, 37f, 38f
differential diagnosis of, 38
Still's disease, 957, 957f-959f, 959
Sting(s)
insect, 148-149
treatment of, 149
scorpion, 147
treatment of, 148
Stockings, compression, for venous ulcers, 461
Stomatitis, 339-340, 339f
aphthous, recurrent, 327, 327f
lichenoid, 332
nicotinic, 333, 333f
Stomatocytes, in cirrhosis patients, 617, 618f
Strabismus
common forms of, 270, 270f-272f
cover test detection of, 252, 253f
definition of, 270
treatment of, 272, 272f
Strawberry nevus, 108, 108f
Streptococcus
culture of, 1143f
Gram-positive, 1140, 1140f
pharyngitis associated with, 346, 347f
Stress fracture, 1051, 1051f
scintigraphy of, 942f
Stress gastritis, prophylaxis for, 573
Stress polycythemia (Gaisböck's syndrome), 1112
String sign, in terminal ileum, 589
Stroke, 176-178, 180
causes of, 176
characteristics of, 177t
imaging studies of, 177, 177f-179f
selected syndromes of, 176t
treatment of, 177-178, 180
Strongyloides stercoralis, life cycle of, 1184f
Strongyloidiasis, 1183, 1184f, 1185f
Sturge-Weber syndrome, 229, 230f
Stye (hordeolum), 284-285, 284f, 285f
Subacute endocarditis, 406
causes of, 407
Subarachnoid hemorrhage, 180-181, 180f
Subclavian steal syndrome, 182, 182f
Subconjunctival hemorrhage, 262f
Subcutaneous tissue, structure and function
of, 2, 2f
Subdural empyema, 224
Subdural hematoma, 183, 183f
Subepidermal blistering disease(s). *See also*
specific disease.
inherited and autoimmune, 16-19, 16f-20f
Submandibular abscess, 336, 337f
Substantia nigra, Lewy bodies in, 194, 194f
Subungual exostosis, 82, 82f
Subungual glomus tumor, 82, 83f
Subungual keratoacanthoma, 82, 82f
Subungual melanoma, 81, 81f
Subungual squamous cell carcinoma, 81, 81f
Succussion splash technique, in assessment of
abdominal distention, 620, 620f
Sulfadiazine, for nocardiosis, 1203
Sulfonylureas, for diabetes mellitus, 920
Sulfur granules, of actinomycosis, 1204, 1204f
Superficial basal cell carcinoma, 86, 87f
Superficial spreading melanoma, 98, 98f
Superior vena cava syndrome, 364-365,
364f, 365f
in lung carcinoma, 494
Suppurative thyroiditis, 355
Suprasphincteric fistula, 607

Surgical drainage
for cavernous sinus thrombosis, 221
for sinusitis, 324
Surgical excision
of clot, from thrombosed hemorrhoid,
603, 604f
of skin lesions, 10, 10f
Surgical resection. *See also named procedure.*
of carcinoid tumor, 667, 670f
of colorectal carcinoma, 600, 601f
of esophageal carcinoma, 566
of hepatocellular carcinoma, 631
of non-small cell lung carcinoma, 498
trans-sphenoidal, of pituitary adenoma, 864,
865f
Swan-neck deformity, 933f, 952f
Sweat gland(s), tumors of, 100-101, 101f, 102f
Sweet's syndrome, 49-50, 49f, 50f
Swelling. *See* Edema.
Swimmer's ear (diffuse otitis externa), 314
Sycosis barbae, follicular papules/pustules in, 139
Syncope
causes of, 475
imaging studies of, 476, 476f, 477f
prognosis of, 477
tilt-table testing in, 476, 477f
treatment of, 476
workup for, 475-476
Syndrome of inappropriate ADH secretion
(SIADH), 869-870, 869f
Synovial fluid
analysis of, 945, 945f, 945t, 946f
calcium pyrophosphate dehydrate crystals in,
996, 997f
Syphilis, 758-760
differential diagnosis of, 760, 760f
latent, 760
primary, 759, 759f
secondary, 759-760, 759f
treatment of, 760
Syphilitic alopecia, 71, 71f
Syringoma, 101, 101f
Syringomyelia, 204, 204f
Systemic lupus erythematosus
clinical presentation of, 960, 960f-961f
differential diagnosis of, 960, 962t
imaging studies of, 963, 963f
treatment of, 963-964
workup for, 962-963, 962f, 963f
Systemic sclerosis (scleroderma), 974

T

Tachycardia
atrial
multifocal, 427, 428f
paroxysmal, 427, 427f
fetal, 836f
ventricular, 431, 432f
Tachycardia-bradycardia syndrome, 435, 435f
Taenia saginata, 1176, 1176f, 1178f
Takayasu's arteritis, 59, 59f, 983-984,
983f, 984f
Tamoxifen, prophylactic, for breast cancer, 829
Tapeworms
infestation with, 1176, 1176f-1178f
life cycle of, 1176, 1177f
Tarsal tunnel, anatomy of, 1025f
Tarsal tunnel syndrome, 1025
T-cell lymphoma, cutaneous, 1103, 1103f-1105f
Telangiectasis, facial, 975, 975f
Telogen effluvium, 70, 70f, 71f
Temno biopsy needle, 619f
Temporal arteritis, 58, 59f, 982-983,
982f, 983f

Temporomandibular joint syndrome,
1000-1001, 1000f
occlusal splint for, 1001, 1001f
Tendinitis
bicipital, clinical tests for, 937f
magnetic resonance imaging of, 940f
Tendon sheath, giant cell tumor of, 106, 106f
Tenosynovitis, de Quervain's, 1005-1006, 1006f
Tension pneumothorax, 366, 367f, 505f
treatment of, 505, 506f
Teratocarcinoma, 750
Teratoma, 750, 750f, 751f
mediastinal, 360, 361f
Terry nails, 78, 78f
Testicular atrophy, in cirrhosis patients, 617
Testicular torsion, 749f, 749t, 752, 752f, 753f
Testicular tumor, 749f-751f, 749t, 750
Tetanus, 1220, 1220f
Tetanus toxoid, 1220
Tetanus-diphtheria vaccine, for HIV-infected
patients, 1152
Tetracycline
adverse reactions to, 48f
for Behçet's syndrome, 985
for louse-borne relapsing fever, 1228
Tetralogy of Fallot
clinical presentation of, 446-447
imaging studies of, 448, 448f-450f
treatment of, 448
variants of, 446, 448f
Texas coral snake, 150f
Thalassemia, 1078-1079, 1079f, 1080f
α, 1078, 1079
β, 1078, 1079
Thalidomide, for multiple myeloma, 1109
Thenar muscle atrophy, 1001, 1002f
Thiabendazole, for strongyloidiasis, 1183
Thionamides, for hyperthyroidism, 876
Third nerve palsy
in herpes zoster, 120, 121f
strabismus resulting from, 270, 272f
Thoracentesis, diagnostic, 500-501, 501f
Thoracic outlet, anatomy of, 1013f
Thoracic outlet syndrome, 1012-1014,
1013f, 1014f
types of, 1012
Thoracic spine, fracture of, 1057, 1057f
Three-part modular device, in abdominal aortic
aneurysm repair, 471, 471f
Thromboangiitis obliterans (Buerger's disease),
58, 58f, 468, 468f, 469f
Thrombocythemia, essential, 1111, 1112f
characteristics of, 1113t
Thrombocytopenia
causes of, 1114
clinical presentation of, 1114, 1114f
diagnostic approach to, 1114, 1115f
immune, 1114, 1116, 1116f
spurious, 1114
Thrombolytic agents, for pulmonary
embolism, 557
Thrombophlebitis, 1216-1217, 1216f, 1217f
Thrombosis
cavernous sinus, 219-221, 220f
cerebral, characteristics of, 177t
deep vein, 465-466, 465f-467f
in antiphospholipid antibody syndrome, 965
increased risk of, medical conditions
associated with, 1122-1125
portal vein, 663, 663f, 664f
renal artery, 719-720, 719f-721f
causes of, 719
spontaneous, in thrombophilia, 1122, 1123f
treatment of, 1124

Thrombotic thrombocytopenic purpura, 1116-1117, 1117f
Thrombus
 cardiac, 428, 429f
 coronary artery, 923, 924f
 electron micrograph of, 465f
 renal vein, 719f
Thrush (oral candidiasis), 339
 HIV-related, 1149, 1150f, 1155
Thymic cyst, 360, 360f
Thymoma, 360, 360f
Thyroglossal duct cyst, 349, 350f
Thyroid acropachy, 875, 876f
Thyroid carcinoma, 352-354, 352f-354f
 anaplastic, 353
 follicular, 352f, 353
 medullary, 353
 papillary, 352-353, 352f
 treatment of, 354
Thyroid dermopathy, 875, 876f
Thyroid disorders, endocrine-associated. See Hyperthyroidism; Hypothyroidism.
Thyroid mass, intrathoracic, 359, 359f
Thyroid nodule, 349-351, 349f, 350f
Thyroidectomy, subtotal, for hyperthyroidism, 877
Thyroiditis, 355, 356f
Thyrotropin deficiency
 in hypopituitarism, 854
 testing for, 856
Tick bites, 147
 treatment of, 148
Tick-borne relapsing fever, 1228
Tilting disk prosthesis, for valvular heart disease, 404, 405f
Tilt-table testing, in syncope, 476, 477f
Timber rattlesnake, 150f
Tinea capitis, 110-111, 110f
Tinea corporis, 110, 110f
Tinea cruris, 111-112, 111f, 112f
Tinea versicolor, 112-113, 113f
 differential diagnosis of, 6t
Tinel's sign, in carpal tunnel syndrome, 1001, 1002f
Tinidazole, for Trichomonas vulvovaginitis, 796
Tissue plasminogen activator (tPA), in management of stroke, 178, 180
TMP/SMX therapy
 for salmonellosis, 654
 for Wegener's granulomatosis, 519
 for Whipple's disease, 657
Toe(s)
 gout of, 994f, 995f. See also Gout.
 hammer, 1026, 1026f
 sausage, 932f, 988f
Tongue
 burning (glossopyrosis), 339
 fibroma of, 328, 328f
 geographic (benign migratory glossitis), 326, 326f, 339
 traumatic ulcerative granuloma of, 327, 327f
Tongue wasting, in amyotrophic lateral sclerosis, 209, 210f
Tonometry, 252, 257f
Tonsillitis, 346-347
Tooth abscess, erythema and edema due to, 337, 337f
Torsades de pointes, 432-433, 433f, 434f
Torsion, testicular, 749f, 749t, 752, 752f, 753f
Torus fracture, 1053, 1055f
Toxic epidermal necrolysis (Lyell's syndrome), 37, 37f
Toxic follicular conjunctivitis, 267, 268f
Toxic megacolon, 578, 582f

Toxic shock syndrome, 1238-1239, 1238f
Toxocara canis, life cycle, 1182f
Toxocariasis, 1182, 1182f
Toxoplasmosis
 clinical presentation of, 226, 226f
 congenital, 228
 HIV-related, 1149, 1151f, 1157
 in immunocompromised host, 226, 227f, 228
 in pregnancy, 228
 treatment of, 228
Transfusion
 ABO-compatible donor for, 1060, 1063t
 immune-related hemolysis following, 1060, 1063f
Transient ischemic attack, 175-176, 175b, 175f
Transillumination, sinus, 323, 324f
Transitional cell carcinoma, of bladder, 737f, 738f
Transjugular intrahepatic portosystemic shunt
 for ascites, 621, 621f
 for Budd-Chiari syndrome, 666
Transplantation. See specific type, e.g., Liver transplantation.
Transposition of great arteries, 450-451, 451f-453f
Trans-sphenoidal surgical resection, of pituitary adenoma, 864, 865f
Transsphincteric fistula, 607
Trastuzumab (Herceptin), for breast cancer, 829
Trauma. See also specific type of injury.
 environmental, 155-159, 155f-159f
Traumatic cataract, 260
Traumatic ulcerative granuloma, 327, 327f
Traverse fracture, of long bone, 1052
Treadmill exercise tolerance test, 374
Tremor, in Parkinson's disease, 200
Triamcinolone
 for Baker's cyst, 1021
 injection of, for trigger finger, 1005, 1005f
Trichilemmal (pilar) cyst, 102, 103f
 surgical excision of, 10f
Trichinella spiralis, 1183f
Trichinosis, 1182-1183, 1183f
Trichomonas vulvovaginitis, 796, 796f
Trichotillomania, 68, 69f, 70, 70f
Tricuspid valve
 Ebstein's anomaly of, 453, 453f
 endocarditis of, 406, 406f
 prolapse of, 404f
 regurgitation of, 402f, 403-404
 stenosis of, 402-403, 402f, 403f
Trigger finger, 1004-1005, 1005f
Trismus (lockjaw), 1220
Trochanteric bursitis, 1019-1020, 1019f
Tropheryma whippelii, in Whipple's disease, 656
Tropias, cover tests for, 252, 253f
Trousseau's sign
 in acute pancreatitis, 608
 in hypocalcemia, 878
Truncus arteriosus
 clinical presentation of, 450, 451f
 types of, 450, 450f
Trypanosoma cruzi, 1170, 1172f
 life cycle of, 1170f
Trypanosomiasis, 1170-1172, 1170f-1172f
Tubal ligation, 789, 790f, 791
Tuberculoid leprosy, 1218, 1219f
Tuberculosis
 drug-resistant, 543
 genitourinary, 544f
 HIV-related, 1149, 1149f, 1156
 imaging studies of, 542, 543f
 laboratory tests for, 542, 542f, 543f

Tuberculosis (Continued)
 miliary, 544-546, 544f-546f
 of spine (Pott's disease), 1041f
 pathogenesis of, 540-541
 primary, 361, 362f
 sputum culturing and staining in, 540, 540f, 541f
 treatment of, 543
 workup for, 541-542
Tuberous sclerosis, 231-232, 231f, 232f, 716f
Tularemia, 1229-1230, 1229f, 1230f
 clinical types of, 1229, 1229f
Tumor(s), 4b. See also specific tumor.
 bone, 1047, 1047f-1049f, 1049-1050
 brain, 184-191, 184f-186f
 epithelial, 84-90
 kidney, 722-724, 722f-724f
 salivary gland, 342, 343f
 sweat gland, 100-101, 101f, 102f
 testicular, 749f-751f, 749t, 750
Turner's syndrome, 900, 901f, 907
Tympanic membrane
 erythema of, 316, 316f
 normal landmarks of, 304, 305f
 perforation of, 304, 307f
Tympanostomy, for otitis media, 317
Typhoid fever, 653, 653f
 treatment of, 654
Typhoid ulcer, perforating, of terminal ileum, 652, 652f
Tzanck smear, of herpes simplex virus infection, 118, 119f

U
Ulcer (ulceration), 5b
 Carmen, 577f
 corneal, 264, 264f, 265f
 cutaneous, in lymphomatoid granulomatosis, 523f
 decubitus, 153-154, 153f
 foot, in diabetes mellitus, 917, 919f
 ischemic, of extremities, 459, 459f
 leg, in rheumatoid arthritis, 952, 954f
 mouth, 327, 327f
  in systemic lupus erythematosus, 960, 961f
 mucosal, in HIV infection, 1146f
 penile, in HIV infection, 1146f
 peptic, 574, 574f, 575f
 tularemic, 1229, 1229f
 typhoid, perforating, of terminal ileum, 652, 652f
 venous, 461-462
Ulcerative basal cell carcinoma, 86, 87f
Ulcerative colitis, 591-592, 591f
Ulcerative granuloma, traumatic, 327, 327f
Ulcerocavernous lesions, in tuberculosis, 545f
Ulnar nerve, compression of, 1008-1009, 1008f
Ultrasonography
 compression, of deep vein thrombosis, 466, 467f
 obstetric, 833f
 of abdominal aortic aneurysm, 470, 471f
 of appendicitis, 587, 587f
 of benign prostatic hyperplasia, 739, 739f
 of cerebral vessels, 168, 172, 172f
 of cholangiocarcinoma, 648, 648f
 of cholecystitis, 646f, 647
 of ectopic pregnancy, 845, 845f
 of hydatidiform mole, 852, 852f
 of hydrocele, 746f
 of hydronephrosis, 728, 728f
 of kidneys, 682, 684, 684f
 of liver abscess, 634, 635f

Ultrasonography (Continued)
of ovarian carcinoma, 819, 819f
of ovarian cyst, 815, 816f
of polycystic kidney disease, 715, 718f
of polycystic ovary syndrome, 817, 818f
of portal vein thrombosis, 663, 663f
of prostate cancer, 743, 744f
of renal cell carcinoma, 722, 723f
of thyroid, 350, 350f
of uterine leiomyoma, 810, 810f
of varicocele, 747, 747f
Ultrasound growth chart, of normal fetus, 833f
Umbilical hernia, ascites with, 620, 620f
Unstable angina, 382. See also Angina pectoris.
Urethritis
gonococcal, 767-768, 767f, 768t
nongonococcal, 769-770, 769f
Urinalysis, 678, 678t, 679f-681f, 680
Urinary casts, 678, 680f
clinical significance of, 678t
Urinary crystals, 678, 680, 681f
Urinary schistosomiasis, 1173
Urinary sediment cells, 678, 679f
Urinary tract, calculi in, 732-736. See also
Urolithiasis.
Urine, chemistry, in acute renal failure, 693t
Urine crystals, 733, 733f
Urine dipstick testing, 678t
Urography, intravenous
of benign prostatic hyperplasia, 739, 739f
of kidneys, 682, 682f, 683f
of urinary stones, 734, 735f
Urolithiasis
causes of, 732
clinical presentation of, 732, 733f
imaging studies of, 734, 734f-736f
laboratory tests for, 733, 733f, 734t
treatment of, 734, 736
types of stones in, 732, 732f
Ursodiol therapy, long-term, for cirrhosis, 618
Urticaria, 51-52, 51f
definition of, 50
differential diagnosis of, 51
Urticaria pigmentosa, 53, 53f
Urticarial vasculitis, 40, 40f, 55-56, 56f
Uterine cervix. See Cervix.
Uterus
leiomyomas (fibroids) of, 809-811, 809f-811f
polyps of, 812, 812f
pregnant, 832, 832f
prolapse of, 807-808, 807f, 808f
Uveitis, 295-296, 295f
history taking in, 296b
treatment of, 296

V

Vaccinations
for HIV-infected patients, 1152
rabies, 1237
Vaccinia, 133, 133f
Vaginal contraceptive ring, 792
Vaginal discharge
characteristics of, 794t
evaluation of, 794f
Vaginosis, bacterial, 793, 793f, 794f
Valacyclovir
for genital herpes, 764
for herpes simplex virus infection, 119
Valvular heart disease, 395-405. See also under
specific cardiac valve.
surgery for, 404, 405f

Vancomycin, for meningitis, 222
Vancomycin plus rifampin, for infective
endocarditis, 408
Varicella (chickenpox), 116-117, 116f, 531
treatment of, 533
Varicocele, 747, 747f
Variola (smallpox), 132-133, 132f
Varix (varices)
esophageal, 571, 571f
hemorrhoidal, 603, 603f
of popliteal fossa, 460f
Vascular disease(s), of skin, 54-61.
See also specific disease.
Vasculitis
choroidal, in systemic lupus erythematosus,
960, 961f
cutaneous cryoglobulinemic, 61, 61f
leukocytoclastic, 54-55, 54f, 55f
necrotizing, 980, 981f
in rheumatoid arthritis, 952, 954f
noninfectious, categories of, 979f
pathogenesis of, 980f
secondary to sarcoidosis, 514, 514f
systemic, 978-987. See also specific types.
classification of, 978t
investigative approach to, 979t
mimics of, 978t
urticarial, 40, 40f, 55-56, 56f
Vasectomy, 789, 791, 791f
Vasopressin deficiency
in hypopituitarism, 854
testing for, 857
Vein(s), varicose. See Varix (varices).
Venography
of deep vein thrombosis, 466, 467f
of superior vena cava syndrome, 364, 365f
Venous lake, 107, 107f
Venous stasis, 461-462, 461f
Venous ulcers, 461-462
Ventilatory support, for acute respiratory distress
syndrome, 547
Ventricular aneurysm, left, 394, 394f
Ventricular fibrillation, 433, 434f
Ventricular heart failure, 409
Ventricular hypertrophy
left, 372, 479, 479f
right, 372
Ventricular infarct, right, 392-393, 392f
Ventricular septal defect
anatomic varieties of, 445, 445f
clinical presentation of, 445-446
imaging studies of, 446, 446f, 447f
treatment of, 446
Ventricular tachycardia, 431, 432f
Vernal conjunctivitis, 261, 262f
Verniar acuity test, 273f
Vernier spatial localization test, for
amblyopia, 273f
Verruca. See also Wart(s).
Verruca peruana, in bartonellosis, 141, 141f
Verruca vulgaris, 121, 122f
of eyelid, 285
Verruciform xanthoma, of hard palate, 328, 328f
Verrucous carcinoma
of genitalia, 766, 766f
vulvar, 798, 798f
Vertebrae, fracture of
assessment of, 1032f
cervical, 1056, 1056f
lumbar, 1057, 1057f
assessment of, 1032f
thoracic, 1057, 1057f

Vertebrobasilar artery syndrome, characteristics
of, 175, 175b
Vesicle, 4b
Vesiculobullous disease(s). See also specific
disease.
differential diagnosis of, 6t
Vestibular abscess, 336, 336f
Vibrio cholere, in cholera, 655
Vibrio vulnificus cellulitis, 134
Viral conjunctivitis, 261, 261f
Viral encephalitis, 223, 223f, 224f
Viral gastroenteritis, 650, 650f, 651f
characteristics of, 650t
treatment of, 654
Viral hepatitis, 637-642. See also Hepatitis entries.
Viral infection(s), 115-133. See also specific
infection, e.g., Human immunodeficiency
virus (HIV) infection.
HIV-related, management of, 1157, 1158f
rashes associated with, 115t
Viral markers, in HIV infection, kinetics of, 1146f
Viral pneumonia, 531-533, 532f, 533f
Virion, HIV-1, 1146f
Virtual colonoscopy, in colorectal
carcinoma, 600
Viscerotrophic leishmaniasis, 1168, 1169f
Vision, temporary loss of, 290-291, 290f, 291f
Visual acuity chart, 252, 255f
Visual field
defects of, 190f
examination of, 252, 253f
Vitamin B_6, for sideroblastic anemia, 1072
Vitamin B_{12}, for cobalamin deficiency, 1077
Vitamin D
deficiency of, 878
supplemental, for osteoporosis, 1032
Vitamin E, for Peyronie's disease, 774
Vitiligo, 62-63, 62f
differential diagnosis of, 62
Von Hippel-Lindau disease, 247, 248f
Von Willebrand disease, 1129-1130, 1130f
classification of, 1129t
Vulva
atrophic, 797f
cancer of, 798-799, 798f, 799f
normal, 776, 778f
squamous cell carcinoma of, 765-766, 766f
verrucous carcinoma of, 766, 766f
Vulvar intraepithelial neoplasia, 798, 798f
Vulvovaginal candidiasis (moniliasis), 763-764,
763f, 1189, 1190f
Vulvovaginitis
atrophic (estrogen-deficient), 797, 797f
fungal, 795, 795f
Trichomonas, 796, 796f

W

Waldenström's macroglobulinemia, 1110, 1110f
Warfarin
for antiphospholipid antibody syndrome, 966
for protein C deficiency, 1124
for pulmonary embolism, 557
Wart(s), 121-124
common, 121, 122f
differential diagnosis of, 123
filiform, 122, 122f
flat or plane, 122, 122f
genital, 122, 123f, 758, 758f, 785f
human papillomavirus causing, 121,
122, 122f

Wart(s) *(Continued)*
Peruvian, 141, 141f
plantar, 122, 123f
removal of, cryotherapy for, 11f
treatment of, 123, 124f
Watchful waiting, for prostate cancer, 744
Weber test, for hearing loss, 308, 309f
Webs, esophageal, 567, 567f
Wegener's granulomatosis, 56, 57f
antineutrophil cytoplasmic antibodies in, 518, 518f
classic triad of, 516
clinical presentation of, 517-518, 517f, 518f
imaging studies of, 518, 518f, 519f
oral, 332, 332f
treatment of, 519
Weil's syndrome (icteric leptospirosis), 1235, 1235f
Western blot assay, 1144, 1144f
for HIV infection, 1148, 1148f
Wheal, 4b
Whipple's disease, 656-657, 656f, 657f
Whipple's procedure, for pancreatic carcinoma, 613
White lesions, oral, 339
White sponge nevus, 339
Whiteheads, 72

Wilms' tumor (nephroblastoma), 722f, 723-724, 724f
Wilson's disease, 201-202
Kayser-Fleischer rings in, 202, 202f, 616
Withdrawal method, of contraception, 789, 791
Wolff-Parkinson-White syndrome, 436-437, 436f
variants of, 436
Wood's light, skin examination by, 8, 8f
World Health Organization (WHO) classification, of astrocytomas, 186
World Health Organization (WHO) criteria, for chronic myelogenous (myeloid) leukemia, 1091t
Wound(s), bite, 145-146, 146f
Wrist
ganglion of, 1004, 1004f, 1005f
rheumatic disorders of, 1001-1007. *See also specific disorder.*
Wrist and hand splint, 956, 956f
Wrist extension test, resisted, 1007, 1007f, 1008f

X

Xanthelasma, 923, 925f
in nephrotic syndrome, 707, 707f
of eyelid, 282, 283f

Xanthoma
Achilles tendon, 923, 925f
eruptive
in primary biliary cirrhosis, 624, 624f
on buttocks, 923, 926f
verruciform, of hard palate, 328, 328f
X-rays. *See* Radiography.
46,XY males, 5-alpha-reductase deficiency in, 772, 773f

Y

Yaws (framboesia tropica), 141-142, 141f, 142f
Yellow nail syndrome, 79-80, 80f
Yersinia, in mesenteric lymphadenitis, 658, 658f
Yersinia pestis
infection with (plague), 1226-1227, 1227f
transmission cycle of, 1226f

Z

Zenker's diverticulum, 560, 560f
Zollinger-Ellison syndrome, 671, 672f
Zygomycosis, 1209, 1210f

Diseases/Disorders	ICD-9 CM
Hypospadias	752.61
Hypothyroidism	244
Ichthosis	701.1
Ichtyosis vulgaris	757.1
Idiopathic guttate hypomelanosis	709.09
Idiopathic inflammatory myopathies (dermatomyositis, polymyositis)	710.3
Idiopathic pulmonary fibrosis	516.3
IgA nephropathy	583.81
Immune thrombocytopenia (ITP)	287.3
Impetigo	684
Inappropriate secretion of antidiuretic hormone	253.6
Infectious arthritis	711.9
Infectious mononucleosis	075
Infective dermatitis	686.9
Infective endocarditis	421.0
Inguinal hernia	550.9
Insulinoma	M8151/0
Interstitial cystitis	595.1
Interstitial lung disease	136.3
Interstitial nephritis	583
Interstitial pneumonia	516.8
Intestinal obstruction	560.9
Intraepithelial neoplasia	173.9
Iron deficiency anemia	280.9
Juvenile rheumatoid arthritis	714.3
Kaposi's sarcoma	173.9
Kawasaki syndrome (mucocutaneous lymph node syndrome)	446.1
Keloid	701.4
Keratoacanthoma	238.2
Keratoderma	701.1
Klinefelter's syndrome	578.7
Knuckle pad	728.79
Koilonychia	703.8
Large cell acanthoma	M8070/0
Leishmaniasis	085.9
Lentigo maligna (Hutchinson's melanotic freckle)	M8742/2
Lentigo simplex (lentigines)	709.09
Leprosy	030.9
Leptospirosis	100.9
Leukocytoclastic vasculitis	446.29
Leukoedema	528.79
Leukoplakia	528.6
Lichen planus	697.0
Lichen planus pemphigoid	697.0
Lichen sclerosus	701.0
Lichen simplex chronicus (circumscribed neurodermatitis)	693.3
Ligneous Conjunctivitis	372.00
Limbal Dermoid	M9084/0
Lipoma	214.9
Listeriosis	027.0
Long QT syndrome	427.9
Lumbar disc syndrome	724.4
Lung abscess	513.0
Lung neoplasm	162.9
Lyme disease	088.8
Lymphedema	457.1

Diseases/Disorders	ICD-9 CM
Lymphogranuloma venereum	099.1
Lymphomatoid granulomatosis	686.1
Macular degeneration	362.50
Malaria	084.6
Malignant melanoma	172.9
Mallory-Weiss tear	530.7
Marfan's syndrome	759.82
Meckel's diverticulum	751.0
Median rhomboid glossitis	529.2
Melanocytic nevi	M8720/0
Melanoma	172.9
Melasma (Chloasma, mask of pregnancy)	709.09
Meningiomas	225.2
Meningomyelocele	741.9
Merkel cell tumor (Cutaneous neuroendocrine carcinoma)	173.9
Mesenteric adenitis	289.2
Mesenteric ischemia	557.1
Mesothelioma	199.1
Milia	706.2
Mitral regurgitation	424.0
Mitral stenosis	394.0
Mitral valve prolapse	424.0
Mixed connective tissue disease	710.9
Molluscum contagiosum	078.0
Monoclonal gammopathy of undetermined significance (MGUS)	273.1
Mongolian blue spot	757.33
Morton's neuroma	355.6
Mucormycosis	117.7
Multiple myeloma	203.0
Multiple sclerosis	340
Muscular dystrophy	359
Myasthenia gravis	358.0
Myelodysplastic syndrome	238.7
Mycobacterium avium intracellulare (MAI)	031.2
Myocardial infarction	410.9
Mucocele (ranula, salivary gland cyst)	528.9
Multifocal atrial tachycardia	427.89
Mumps	072.9
Myocarditis	429.0
Myxoid cyst	M8840/0
Necrotizing fasciitis	728.86
Nephrotic syndrome	581.9
Neurilemmoma (schwannomas)	M9560/0
Neuroblastoma	194.0
Neurofibroma	M9540/0
Neurofibromatosis	237.71
Nevus flammeus	757.32
Nicotinic stomatitis	528.0
Nocardiosis	039.9
Nodular prurigo (prurigo nodularis)	698.3
Non-alcoholic steatohepatitis	571.8
Non-Hodgkin's lymphoma	201.9
Non-specific viral rash, Gianotti-Crosti syndrome (GCS)	782.1
Normal pressure hydrocephalus	331.3

Diseases/Disorders	ICD-9 CM
Onychomycosis	110.1
Optic neuritis	377.3
Oral lymphoepithelial cyst	528.4
Oral melanocytic macule	709.8
Orchitis	098.13
Osgood-Schlatter disease	732.4
Osteoarthritis	715.0
Osteochondritis dissecans	732.7
Osteoporosis	733.0
Osteomyelitis	730.2
Osteonecrosis	733.40
Otitis externa	38.10
Otitis media	382.9
Ovarian cancer	183.0
Paget's disease of bone	731.0
Parkinson's disease	332.0
Paronychia	681.9
Paroxysmal atrial tachycardia	427.0
Paroxysmal cold hemoglobinuria	283.2
Patent ductus arteriosus	747.0
Pediculosis (lice)	132.9
Pellagra	265.2
Pelvic inflammatory disease	614.9
Pemphigoid gestionalis	694.5
Pemphigus erythematosus	694.4
Pemphigus vegetans	694.4
Pemphigus vulgaris	694.4
Peptic ulcer	536.8
Pericarditis	420.91
Peripheral arterial disease	443.9
Perirectal abscess	566
Periungal fibroma	M8810/0
Pernicious anemia	281.0
Peyronie's disease	607.89
Peutz-Jeghers syndrome	759.6
Pharyngitis/Tonsillitis	462
Pheochromocytoma	194.0
Phototoxic and photoallergic reactions	692.72
Pilar leiomyoma	M8890/0
Pinguecula	372.51
Pinta	103.9
Pituitary adenoma	253
Pityarisis alba	696.5
Pityarisis rosea	696.3
Placenta previa	641.1
Pleural effusion	511.9
Pneumoconiosis	505
Pneumocystis pneumonia	136.3
Pneumothorax	512.0
Polyarteritis nodosa	446.0
Polycystic kidney disease	753.13
Polycystic ovary syndrome	256.4
Polycythemia vera	238.4
Polymorphous light eruption (photodermatitis)	692.72
Polymyalgia rheumatica	725.0
Porphiria cutanea tarda (PCT)	277.1
Port wine stain	757.32
Portal vein thrombosis	452
Precocious puberty	259.1
Preeclampsia	642.6
Primary biliary cirrhosis	571.6
Progressive supranuclear palsy	333.0
Progressive multifocal leucoencephalopathy (PML)	046.3

Continued on the next page